ENDURANCE IN SPORT

IOC MEDICAL COMMISSION

SUB-COMMISSION ON PUBLICATIONS IN THE SPORT SCIENCES

Howard G. Knuttgen PhD (Co-ordinator)
Boston, Massachusetts, USA

Francesco Conconi MD
Ferrara, Italy

Harm Kuipers MD, PhD
Maastricht, The Netherlands

Per A.F.H. Renström MD, PhD
Stockholm, Sweden

Richard H. Strauss MD
Los Angeles, California, USA

ENDURANCE IN SPORT

VOLUME II OF THE ENCYCLOPAEDIA OF SPORTS MEDICINE

AN IOC MEDICAL COMMISSION PUBLICATION

IN COLLABORATION WITH THE

INTERNATIONAL FEDERATION OF SPORTS MEDICINE

EDITED BY

R.J. SHEPHARD AND P.-O. ÅSTRAND

SECOND EDITION

**Blackwell
Science**

© 1992, 2000 International Olympic
Committee

Published by
Blackwell Science Ltd
Editorial Offices:
Osney Mead, Oxford OX2 0EL
25 John Street, London WC1N 2BL
23 Ainslie Place, Edinburgh EH3 6AJ
350 Main Street, Malden
   MA 02148 5018, USA
54 University Street, Carlton
   Victoria 3053, Australia
10, rue Casimir Delavigne
   75006 Paris, France

Other Editorial Offices:
Blackwell Wissenschafts-Verlag GmbH
Kurfürstendamm 57
10707 Berlin, Germany

Blackwell Science KK
MG Kodenmacho Building
7–10 Kodenmacho Nihombashi
Chuo-ku, Tokyo 104, Japan

First published 1992
Reprinted 1993, 1995
Second edition 2000

Part title illustration by Grahame Baker

A catalogue record for this title
is available from the British Library

ISBN   978-0-632-05348-3

Library of Congress
Cataloging-in-publication Data

Endurance in sport / edited by R.J.
   Shephard & P.-O. Astrand. — 2nd ed.
      p.   cm. (Volume II of the
Encyclopaedia of sports medicine)
   "An IOC Medical Commission
publication, in collaboration with the
International Federation of Sports
Medicine."
   Includes bibliographical references
and index.
   ISBN 978-0-632-05348-3
   1. Endurance sports.   2. Exercise—
Physiological aspects.   3. Physical
fitness.   I. Shephard, Roy J.
II. Åstrand, Per-Olof.   III. IOC
Medical Commission.
IV. International Federation of Sports
Medicine.   V. Series: Encyclopaedia of
sports medicine; v. 2.
RC1220.E53E53   2000
613.7′1—dc21
                                    99-38456
                                    CIP

DISTRIBUTORS

Marston Book Services Ltd
PO Box 269
Abingdon, Oxon OX14 4YN
(*Orders*: Tel: 01235 465500
            Fax: 01235 465555)

USA
   Blackwell Science, Inc.
   Commerce Place
   350 Main Street
   Malden, MA 02148 5018
   (*Orders*: Tel: 800 759 6102
                    781 388 8250
              Fax: 781 388 8255)

Canada
   Login Brothers Book Company
   324 Saulteaux Crescent
   Winnipeg, Manitoba R3J 3T2
   (*Orders*: Tel: 204 837 2987)

Australia
   Blackwell Science Pty Ltd
   54 University Street
   Carlton, Victoria 3053
   (*Orders*: Tel: 3 9347 0300
              Fax: 3 9347 5001)

For further information on
Blackwell Science, visit our website:
www.blackwell-science.com

Contents

List of Contributors, ix

Forewords, xiii

Preface to the First Edition, xiv

Preface to the Second Edition, xvi

Part 1: Definitions

1 Semantic and Physiological Definitions, 3
R.J. SHEPHARD

2 Endurance Sports, 9
P.-O. ÅSTRAND

Part 2: Basic Scientific Considerations

Part 2a: Biological Bases of Endurance Performance and the Associated Functional Capacities

3 Determinants of Endurance Performance, 21
R.J. SHEPHARD

4 Body Size and Endurance Performance, 37
J.C. EISENMANN & R.M. MALINA

5 Pulmonary System and Endurance Exercise, 52
T.J. WETTER & J.A. DEMPSEY

6 The Athlete's Heart, 68
J. GOODMAN

7 Skeletal Muscle Blood Flow and Endurance Exercise: Limiting Factors and Dynamic Responses, 84
J.W.E. RUSH, C.R. WOODMAN, A.P. AAKER, W.G. SCHRAGE & M.H. LAUGHLIN

8 Endurance Exercise and the Regulation of Visceral and Cutaneous Blood Flow, 103
J.M. JOHNSON

9 Cellular Metabolism and Endurance, 118
J. HENRIKSSON

10 Influence of Endurance Training and Detraining on Motoneurone and Sensory Neurone Morphology and Metabolism, 136
R.R. ROY, V.R. EDGERTON & A. ISHIHARA

11 Muscular Factors in Endurance, 158
H.J. GREEN

12 Endocrine Factors in Endurance, 184
M.S. TREMBLAY & J.L. COPELAND

13 The Importance of Carbohydrate, Fat and Protein for the Endurance Athlete, 197
T.E. GRAHAM

Part 2b: Psychological Aspects of Endurance Performance

14 Psychology in Endurance Performance, 212
J.S. RAGLIN & G.S. WILSON

Part 2c: Genetic Determinants of Endurance Performance

15   Genetic Determinants of
     Endurance Performance, 223
     C. BOUCHARD, B. WOLFARTH, M.A.
     RIVERA, J. GAGNON & J.-A. SIMONEAU

Part 2d: Physical Limitations of Endurance Performance

16   Biomechanical Constraints and Economy of
     Movement in Endurance Performance, 245
     K.R. WILLIAMS

17   Endurance in Hot and Cold Environments, 259
     G.W. MACK & E.R. NADEL

Part 3: Measurements in Endurance Sport

18   Factors to be Measured, 271
     P.-O. ÅSTRAND

19   Sport-Specific Testing in Laboratory and
     Field, 273
     A. DAL MONTE, M. FAINA & G. MIRRI

20   Assessment of Environmental Extremes and
     Competitive Strategies, 287
     K.B. PANDOLF & A.J. YOUNG

21   Maximal Oxygen Intake, 301
     R.J. SHEPHARD

22   Anaerobic Metabolism and
     Endurance Performance, 311
     R.J. SHEPHARD

23   Metabolism in the Contracting
     Skeletal Muscle, 328
     J. HENRIKSSON

24   Body Composition of
     the Endurance Performer, 346
     S. GOING & V. MULLINS

25   Personality Structure of the
     Endurance Performer, 366
     L.M. LEITH

26   Perception of Effort During Endurance
     Training and Performance, 374
     B.J. NOBLE & J.M. NOBLE

Part 4: Principles of Endurance Preparation

27   Influences of Biological Age and Selection, 397
     P.-O. ÅSTRAND

28   Endurance Conditioning, 402
     J. SVEDENHAG

29   Food and Fluids Before, During and After
     Prolonged Exercise, 409
     R.J. MAUGHAN

30   Haemoglobin, Blood Volume
     and Endurance, 423
     N. GLEDHILL & D. WARBURTON

31   Smoking, Alcohol, Ergogenic Aids, Doping
     and the Endurance Performer, 438
     M.H. WILLIAMS

32   Psychological Preparation of
     Endurance Performers, 451
     S. TUFFEY

33   Prevention of Injuries in Endurance
     Athletes, 458
     P.A.F.H. RENSTRÖM & P. KANNUS

34   Monitoring for Overtraining in the
     Endurance Performer, 486
     D.G. ROWBOTTOM, A.R. MORTON &
     D. KEAST

Part 5: Specific Population Groups and Endurance Training

35   Endurance Training and Children, 507
     T.W. ROWLAND

36 Endurance Training for Women, 517
M.L. O'TOOLE

37 Pregnant Women and Endurance Exercise, 531
L.A. WOLFE

38 The Elderly and Endurance Training, 547
M.L. POLLOCK, D.T. LOWENTHAL,
J.F. CARROLL & J.E. GRAVES

39 Endurance Training for Persons
with Disabilities, 565
K.H. PITETTI & J.L. DURSTINE

**Part 6: Environmental Aspects of
Endurance Training**

40 Hyperthermia, Hypothermia and
Problems of Hydration, 591
T.D. NOAKES

41 Problems of High Altitude, 614
R.J. SHEPHARD

42 Air Pollutants and Endurance Performance,
628
L.J. FOLINSBEE & E.S. SCHELEGLE

43 Endurance Performers and
Time-Zone Shifts, 639
T. REILLY, G. ATKINSON & J. WATERHOUSE

**Part 7: Clinical Aspects of
Endurance Training**

44 Medical Surveillance of Endurance Sport, 653
R.J. SHEPHARD

45 Considerations for Preparticipation
Cardiovascular Screening in Young
Competitive Athletes, 667
B.J. MARON

46 Lung Fluid Movements in Endurance Sport,
682
N.H. SECHER

47 Cardiovascular Benefits of
Endurance Exercise, 688
A.R. FOLSOM & M.A. PEREIRA

48 Cardiovascular Risks of Endurance Sport, 708
R.J. SHEPHARD

49 Reproductive Changes and the
Endurance Athlete, 718
A.B. LOUCKS

50 Endurance Exercise and the
Immune Response, 731
D.C. NIEMAN

51 Other Health Benefits of Physical Activity, 747
R.J. SHEPHARD

52 Overuse Syndromes, 766
A.J. MALLOCH & J.E. TAUNTON

53 Countering Inflammation, 800
H. NORTHOFF & A. BERG

**Part 8: Specific Issues in
Individual and Team Sports**

54 Energetics of Running, 813
P.E. DI PRAMPERO

55 Swimming as an Endurance Sport, 824
L. GULLSTRAND

56 Rowing, 836
N.H. SECHER

57 Cross-Country Ski Racing, 844
U. BERGH & A. FORSBERG

58 Cycling, 857
G. NEUMANN

59 The Triathlon, 872
G.G. SLEIVERT

60   Canoeing, 888
     A. DAL MONTE, P. FACCINI & G. MIRRI

61   Endurance Aspects of Soccer and
     Other Field Games, 900
     T. REILLY

62   Mountaineering, 931
     R.B. SCHOENE & T.F. HORNBEIN

63   The Physiology of Human-Powered Flight,
     942
     E.R. NADEL & S.R. BUSSOLARI

64   Endurance in Other Sports, 945
     P.-O. ÅSTRAND

     Index, 947

List of Contributors

AARON P. AAKER MS, *Department of Medical Physiology, University of Missouri-Colombia, Colombia, MO, USA*

PER-OLOF ÅSTRAND MD PhD, *Department of Physiology & Pharmacology, Karolinska Institute, Stockholm, Sweden*

GREG ATKINSON PhD, *Reasearch Institute for Sport and Exercise Sciences, Liverpool John Moores' University, Liverpool, UK*

ALOIS BERG MD, *Department of Prevention, Rehabilitation and Sports Medicine, University of Freiburg, Freiburg, Germany*

ULF BERGH PhD, *Defence Research Institute, S-17290, Stockholm, Sweden*

CLAUDE BOUCHARD PhD, *Pennington Biomedical Reasearch Center, Louisiana State University, Baton Rouge, LA, USA*

STEVEN R. BUSSOLARI PhD, *Department of Aeronautics and Astronautics, Massachusetts Institute of Technology, Cambridge, MA, USA*

JOAN F. CARROLL PhD, *Department of Integrative Physiology, University of North Texas Health Science Center, Fort Worth, TX, USA*

JENNIFER L. COPELAND MSc, *Faculty of Kinesiology, University of New Brunswick, Fredericton, New Brunswick, Canada*

JEROME A. DEMPSEY PhD, *Department of Preventive Medicine, University of Wisconsin at Madison, 504 N Walnut, Madison, WI, USA*

J.LARRY DURSTINE PhD, *Department of Exercise Science, University of South Carolina, Columbia, SC, USA*

V. REGINALD EDGERTON PhD, *Life Science Center, University of California, Los Angeles, CA, USA*

JOEY C. EISENMANN MA, *Institute for the Study of Youth Sports, 213 IM Sports Circle, Michigan State University, East Lansing, MI, USA*

PIERRO FACCINI PhD, *Institute of Sports Science, Italian National Olympic Committee, Rome, Italy*

MARCELLO FAINA PhD, *Institute of Sports Science, Italian National Olympic Committee, Rome, Italy*

LAWRENCE J. FOLINSBEE PhD, *National Center for Environmental Assessment, U.S. Environmental Protection Agency, Research Triangle Park, NC, USA*

AARON R. FOLSOM MD MPH, *Division of Epidemiology, School of Public Health, University of Minnesota, Minneapolis, MN, USA*

ARTUR FORSBERG DPE, *Swedish National Center for Research in Sports, Stockholm, Sweden*

JACQUES GAGNON PhD, *Physical Activity Sciences Laboratory, Division of Kinesiology, Faculty of Medicine, Université Laval, Ste-Foy, Quebec, Canada*

NORMAN GLEDHILL PhD, *Department of Kinesiology and Health Science, Bethune College, York University, Toronto, Ontario, Canada*

SCOTT GOING PhD, *Department of Physiology, University of Arizona, Tucson, AZ, USA*

JACK GOODMAN PhD, *Faculty of Physical Education & Health, University of Toronto, Toronto, Ontario, Canada*

TERRY E. GRAHAM PhD, *Human Biology and Nutritional Sciences, University of Guelph, Guelph, Ontario, Canada*

JAMES E. GRAVES PhD, *Department of Exercise Science, Syracuse University, New York, USA*

HOWARD J. GREEN PhD, *Department of Kinesiology, University of Waterloo, Waterloo, Ontario, Canada*

LENNART GULLSTRAND PhD, *Bosön Institute of Sport, S-181 47, Lidingö, Sweden*

JAN HENRIKSSON MD PhD, *Department of Physiology & Pharmacology, Karolinska Institute, Stockholm, Sweden*

TOM F. HORNBEIN PhD, *Department of Medicine, University of Washington, Harborview Medical Center, Seattle, WA, USA*

AKIHIKO ISHIHARA PhD, *Laboratory of Neurochemistry, Faculty of Integrated Human Studies, Kyoto University, Kyoto, Japan*

JOHN M. JOHNSON PhD, *Department of Physiology, University of Texas Health Science Center, San Antonio, TX, USA*

PEKKA KANNUS MD PhD, *Tampere Research Station of Sports Medicine, Tampere, Finland*

DAVID KEAST PhD, *Department of Microbiology, The University of Western Australia, Queen Elizabeth II Medical Centre, Nedlands, WA, Australia*

M.H. LAUGHLIN PhD, *Department of Veterinary Biomedical Sciences & Medical Physiology, and Dalton Cardiovascular Research Center, University of Missouri-Colombia, MO, USA*

LARRY M. LEITH MA PhD, *Faculty of Physical Education & Health, University of Toronto, Toronto, Ontario, Canada*

ANNE B. LOUCKS PhD, *Department of Biological Sciences, Ohio University, Athens, OH, USA*

DAVID T. LOWENTHAL MD PhD, *Department of Medicine, Pharmacology, Exercise and Sport Sciences, University of Florida and Gregg VA Medical Center, Gainsville, FL, USA*

GARY W. MACK PhD, *John B. Pierce Laboratory, and Department of Epidemiology and Public Health, Yale University School of Medicine, 290 Congress Avenue, New Haven, CT, USA*

ROBERT M. MALINA PhD, *Institute for the Study of Youth Sports, 213 IM Sports Circle, Michigan State University, East Lansing, MI, USA*

ANDREW J. MALLOCH MB ChB, *Sports Medicine Center, University of British Columbia, BC, Columbia*

BARRY J. MARON MD, *Minneapolis Heart Institute Foundation, 920 East 28th Street, Minneapolis, MN, USA*

RONALD J. MAUGHAN PhD, *Department of Biomedical Sciences, University Medical School, Aberdeen, UK*

GIOVANNI MIRRI PhD, *Institute of Sports Science, Italian National Olympic Committee, Rome, Italy*

ANTONIO DAL MONTE PhD, *Italian National Olympic Committee, Institute of Sports Science, Via dei Campi Sportivi, Rome, Italy*

ALAN R. MORTON EdD FACSM, *Department of Human Movement & Exercise Science, The University of Western Australia, Nedlands, WA, Australia*

VERONICA MULLINS MS RD, *Department of Nutritional Sciences, University of Arizona, Tucson, AZ, USA*

ETHAN R. NADEL PhD, *John B. Pierce Laboratory and Departments of Cellular and Molecular Physiology, and Epidemiology and Public Health, Yale University School of Medicine, New Haven, CT, USA (Dr E.R. Nadel unfortunately passed away during production of this volume.)*

GEORG NEUMANN MD, *Department of Sports Medicine, Institute for Applied Training Science, Leipzig, Germany*

DAVID C. NIEMAN PhD, *Department of Health, Leisure and Exercise Science, Appalachian State University, Boone, NC, USA*

TIMOTHY D. NOAKES MD, *Department of Exercise and Sports Science, University of Cape Town, and Sports Science Institute of South Africa, Newlands, South Africa*

BRUCE J. NOBLE PhD, *Purdue University, Madison, WI, USA*

JOHN M. NOBLE PhD, *HPER Building, University of Nebraska at Omaha, Omaha, NE, USA*

HINNAK NORTHOFF MD, *Department of Transfusion Medicine, University of Tübingen, Abteilung Transfusionsmedizin, Tübingen, Germany*

MARY L. O'TOOLE PhD, *Department of Obstetrics and Gynaecology and Women's Health, Saint Louis University, St Louis, MO, USA*

KENT B. PANDOLF PhD, *U.S. Army Research Institute of Environmental Medicine, Natick, MA, USA*

MARK A. PEREIRA PhD, *Division of Epidemiology, School of Public Health, University of Minnesota, Minneapolis, MN, USA*

KENNETH H. PITETTI PhD, *Department of Public Health Sciences, College of Health Professions, Witchita State University, Witchita, KS, USA*

MICHAEL L. POLLOCK PhD, *Center for Exercise Science, College of Medicine, University of Florida, Gainsville, FL, USA*
(Dr M.L. Pollock unfortunately passed away during the production of this volume.)

PIETRO E. DI PRAMPERO MD PhD, *Department of Biomedical Sciences, University of Udine, Udine, Italy*

JOHN S. RAGLIN PhD, *Department of Kinesiology, Indiana University, Bloomington, IN, USA*

THOMAS REILLY PhD DSc, *Research Institute for Sport & Exercise Sciences, Liverpool John Moores' University, Liverpool, UK*

PER A.F.H. RENSTRÖM MD PhD, *Department of Orthopaedic Sports Medicine, Karolinska Hospital, Stockholm, Sweden*

MIGUEL A. RIVERA PhD, *Departments of Physiology and Physical Medicine and Sports Medicine, University of Puerto Rico Medical School, San Juan, Puerto Rico*

DAVID G. ROWBOTTOM PhD, *School of Human Movement Studies, Queensland University of Technology, Kelvin Grove, QLD, Australia*

THOMAS W. ROWLAND MD, *Department of Pediatric Cardiology, Baystate Medical Center, Springfield, MA, USA*

ROLAND R. ROY PhD, *Brain Research Institute, University of California, Los Angeles, CA, USA*

JAMES W.E. RUSH PhD, *Department of Veterinary Biomedical Sciences and Dalton Cardiovascular Research Center, University of Missouri-Columbia, MO, USA*

EDWARD S. SCHELEGLE PhD, *School of Veterinary Medicine, Department of Anatomy, Physiology and Cell Biology, University of California, CA, USA*

ROBERT B. SCHOENE MD, *Department of Medicine, University of Washington, Harborview Medical Center, Seattle, WA, USA*

WILLIAM G. SCHRAGE MS, *Department of Medical Physiology, University of Missouri-Columbia, Colombia, MO, USA*

NIELS H. SECHER MD PhD, *Department of Anaesthesia, Rigshospitalet, Blegdamsveg 9, Copenhagen, Denmark*

ROY J. SHEPHARD MD PhD DPE, *Professor Emeritus of Applied Physiology, PO Box 521, Brackendale, British Colombia, Canada*

JEAN-AIMÉ SIMONEAU PhD, *Physical Activity Sciences Laboratory, Division of Kinesiology, Faculty of Medicne, Université Laval Ste-Foy, Quebec, Canada*
(*Dr J.A. Simoneau unfortunately passed away during the production of this volume.*)

GORDON G. SLEIVERT PhD, *Human Performance Centre, School of Physical Education, University of Otago, Dunedin, New Zealand*

JAN SVEDENHAG MD PhD, *Department of Clinical Physiology, St Göran's Hospital, Stockholm, Sweden*

JACK E. TAUNTON MD PhD, *Sports Medicine Center, University of British Colombia, Vancouver, BC, Canada*

MARK S. TREMBLAY PhD, *Faculty of Kinesiology, University of New Brunswick, Fredericton, New Brunswick, Canada*

SUZANNE TUFFEY PhD, *Sport Psychology Director, USA Swimming, Colorado Springs, CO, USA*

DARREN WARBURTON MSc, *Faculty of Physical Education and Recreation, University of Alberta, Edmonton, Alberta, Canada*

JIM WATERHOUSE DPhil, *Research Institute for Sport and Exercie Sciences, Liverpool John Moores' University, Liverpool, UK*

THOMAS J. WETTER MS, *Department of Preventive Medicine, University of Wisconsin at Madison, Madison, WI, USA*

MELVIN H. WILLIAMS PhD, *Department of Exercise Science, Old Dominion University, Norfolk, VA, USA*

KEITH R. WILLIAMS PhD, *Department of Exercise Science, University of California at Davis, Davis, CA, USA*

GREGORY S. WILSON PED, *Department of Human Kinetics and Sports Medicine, University of Evansville, Evansville, IL, USA*

BERN WOLFARTH PhD, *Department of Rehabilitation and Preventive Sports Medicine, Freiburg University, Freiburg, Germany*

LARRY A. WOLFE PhD, *School of Physical & Health Education, Department of Physiology, Queen's University, Kingston, Ontario, Canada*

CHRISTOPHER R. WOODMAN PhD, *Department of Veterinary Biomedical Sciences, and Dalton Cardiovascular Research Center, University of Missouri-Colombia, Colombia, MO, USA*

ANDREW J. YOUNG PhD, *Thermal and Mountain Medicine Division, U.S. Army Research Institute of Environmental Medicine, Natick, MA, USA*

Forewords

Nine years have passed since the publication of Volume II *Endurance in Sport* for the IOC Medical Commission Encyclopaedia of Sports Medicine Series. Reflecting the tremendous research activity that has taken place relative to the topic of endurance, Professors Shephard and Åstrand have succeeded in collecting the input of 85 authors of international renown to produce a completely revised second edition of this publication.

Endurance in Sport includes basic and applied scientific information on cellular metabolism, genetics, physiological function, environment, laboratory testing, and conditioning programs as related to endurance performance. Special attention is given to children, women, the elderly, and the disabled. Special attention is also given to a variety of Olympic sports in separate chapters dealing with such activities as running, swimming, rowing, skiing, cycling, and team sports.

This publication in its new and expanded edition will prove to be of great value as an authoritative reference to scientists, clinicians, and graduate students around the world for many years to come.

Prince Alexandre de Merode
Chairman IOC Medical Commission

This new edition will offer all those involved in the field of sport sciences updated information indispensable to an improved perception of sport in general, just as the first edition did nine years ago.

This new volume will enhance the intrinsic value of the IOC Medical Commission's collection of Sports Medicine Encyclopaedias.

I hope it will be just as successful as the first edition.

Juan Antonio Samaranch
Marqués de Samaranch

Preface to the First Edition

Relatively brief physical activities such as a 1500-m race have sometimes been characterized as 'endurance sport'. However, in this book we have deliberately focussed our attention upon events where the competition itself and/or the required training lasts for 1 hour or longer. There were several reasons for this decision. Certainly, we were instructed to do this by the series editors, since they are currently planning other volumes that will cover shorter periods of activity. However, we are not exactly famous for following arbitrary directives from editors, and our eventual compliance with the 1-hour criterion was assured by more persuasive arguments.

Firstly, we both view international competition as the ultimate challenge to the various regulatory systems of the body, physiological, biochemical, biomechanical and psychological. If the body finds difficulty in regulating the constancy of the *milieu intérieur* over a 4-min mile, how much greater is the challenge to accommodate the metabolic, thermal and other demands of a marathon race run in the heat of summer, or the Vasa Loppet in the depths of winter, and how much more exciting it is to unravel details of the adaptive mechanisms that allow such feats to be accomplished!

We recognize that there have been a number of previous monographs looking at various physiological aspects of prolonged exercise, but much of the work described in such texts has been conducted in the laboratory. There remains a dearth of scientific information on the stresses encountered and the adaptive responses demanded by actual participa-

tion in the various potential forms of prolonged athletic competition. The present volume was thus conceived to fill this void in a comprehensive fashion.

In completing such a major undertaking, we have been fortunate to draw upon more than 60 of the world's authorities in all areas of the sport sciences. The volume thus offers a broad international perspective upon the challenge of human participation in endurance events. The material is divided into seven sections: (1) a brief definition of fundamental terms and concepts, (2) a full review of basic scientific considerations that ranges over anatomy, biomechanics, physiology, biochemistry, nutrition, humoral and immune function, psychological factors, genetics and environmental constraints, (3) methods of measuring the various determinants of endurance performance in the field and in the laboratory, (4) optimal principles of preparation for various types of endurance competition, (5) endurance training in special population groups, (6) prevention of medical and surgical problems during endurance training and competition, with a discussion of the potential health benefits of such activities, and (7) an exploration of issues specific to individual types of endurance performance ranging from cross-country skiing to human-powered flight.

The material is presented in a format that will be accessible to all with some background in the sport sciences. It is anticipated that the volume will appeal particularly to sport scientists and physicians involved in the preparation of endurance competitors, but the broad picture of human regulatory mechanisms during extended exercise will also attract the interest of a much wider audience in physiology, biochemistry and psychology, and this volume will undoubtedly become required reading for many graduate programmes in medicine and the science of sport.

Roy J. Shephard, *Toronto*
Per-Olof Åstrand, *Stockholm*
1991

Preface to the Second Edition

The first edition of *Endurance in Sport* was designed to offer state-of-the-art information on current topics of clinical and scientific importance for endurance sport, provided by a panel of international experts in a form that would be appropriate for professional personnel working with athletes and sports teams. For our purpose, endurance sport was arbitrarily defined as an event where the competition itself or the associated training lasted for 1 hour or longer.

We recognized that relatively brief physical activities such as a 1500-m race were sometimes characterized as 'endurance sport'. The 60-minute criterion was established in discussion with the IOC Publications Advisory Committee, who were planning other volumes covering competitions of shorter duration. Nevertheless, the editors of the present volume were also intrigued by the ultimate challenge that prolonged international competition presented to the body systems regulating physiological, biochemical, biomechanical and psychological variables. If the body found difficulty in regulating the constancy of the *milieu intérieur* over a 4-minute mile, how much greater was the challenge to accommodate the metabolic, thermal and other demands of a marathon race run in the heat of summer, or the Vasa Loppet in the depths of winter.

We immediately recognized that a number of monographs and specialist symposia had looked at various physiological aspects of prolonged exercise, but we also noted that much of the work described had been conducted in the laboratory. There remained a dearth of authoritative scientific information on the stresses encountered and the adaptive responses demanded by actual participation in the various potential forms of prolonged athletic competition. The book *Endurance in Sport* was thus conceived to fill this void.

The information was directed to individuals and groups representing a wide range of disciplines, particularly sports scientists, sports physicians, medical doctors in family practice, physical therapists and athletic trainers, and the growing number of graduate students in the sports sciences and other health-related professions. The first edition was generously received by critics, and achieved a very large world-wide distribution relative to its size and cost. However, almost 8 years have elapsed since the appearance of the first edition, and in order that potential readers might still have access to state-of-the-art information, it was thought important to embark upon a second edition. This has followed the same general plan as the first edition, although the volume has necessarily undergone considerable expansion. Many new international experts have been recruited, and all of the remaining chapters have been thoroughly revised and updated. The volume thus offers a broad and current perspective on the challenges associated with human participation in endurance events.

The material is now divided into eight main sections: (i) a brief description of fundamental terms and concepts; (ii) a full review of the basic scientific principles underlying the optimization of endurance performance, including anthropometry, biomechanics, physiology, biochemistry, nutrition, humoral and immune function, psychological factors, and genetic and environmental constraints;

(iii) methods of measuring the various determinants of endurance performance in the field and in the laboratory; (iv) principles of preparation for various types of endurance competition; (v) the response to endurance training in various special population groups; (vi) environmental aspects of endurance training; (vii) the prevention of medical and surgical problems during endurance training and competition, with a discussion of the potential health benefits of such activities; and (viii) an exploration of issues specific to various types of individual and team endurance performance, ranging from cross-country skiing, mountaineering and human-powered flight to soccer and other team games.

The material is once again presented in a format that will be accessible to all with some background in the sports sciences. Although the volume will continue to appeal particularly to sport scientists and physicians involved in the preparation of endurance competitors, the broad analysis of human regulatory mechanisms during prolonged exercise will attract the interest of a much wider audience in physiology, biochemistry and psychology. It will continue to be required reading for many graduate programmes in medicine and the science of sport.

Roy J. Shephard, *Toronto*
Per-Olof Åstrand, *Stockholm*
1999

PART 1

DEFINITIONS

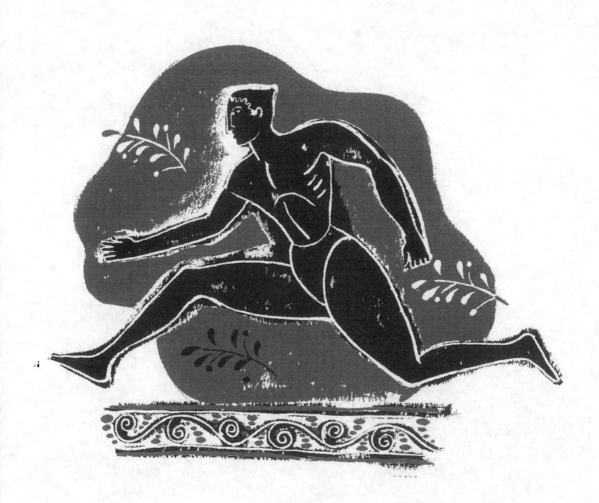

Chapter 1

Semantic and Physiological Definitions

ROY J. SHEPHARD

Physical activity, exercise and physical fitness

The distinction between such terms as physical activity, exercise and physical fitness has been sharpened through the contributions of Caspersen *et al.* (1985) and Bouchard and Shephard (1994), as discussed below.

Physical activity

Physical activity may be considered as any form of body movement that makes a significant metabolic demand. Thus defined, it encompasses not only preparation for, and participation in, competitive sports, but also other aspects of an athlete's life, such as the pursuit of a strenuous physical occupation, the undertaking of household chores (including the care of children and ageing relatives, and in some countries the production of food), certain methods of transportation (walking, cycling, the operation of hand-propelled watercraft) and engaging in voluntary leisure activities that are unrelated to the individual's primary sport interests.

Exercise

Physical exercise is usually considered as the voluntary component of a person's physical activity inventory, although in the case of professional athletes it may be a form of employment. It is occasionally spontaneous and playful, but more usually it is performed with a specific objective in view (such as preparation for competition, rehabilitation

following injury or the maintenance of personal fitness). Some forms of play and recreational exercise contribute to the primary performance of a major athlete, either by developing biological function (for example, the adoption of a land-based training programme when a rower cannot exercise on water, Wright *et al.* 1976) or by offering relaxation and psychological *détente* between competitive seasons. However, other physically active pursuits are disadvantageous to the performance of an athlete, encouraging an inappropriate development of physique, occupying time that should have been allocated to more specific forms of training and sometimes (through a process of 'negative transfer') degrading established psychomotor skills.

Physical fitness

The concept of physical fitness has been discussed in detail elsewhere (Shephard 1977, 1994). Its definition remains controversial, but in the context of high-performance sport, it implies an optimal combination of those physical, physiological, biochemical, biomechanical and psychological characteristics that contribute to competitive success. The physical fitness of an athlete is usually highly specific to a given class of competition, although in the pentathlon and decathlon the successful contestant requires a more broadly based type of fitness. Further, an optimal combination of biological characteristics does not guarantee success in any given event; for example, psychological hardiness has sometimes allowed a very successful competitive

3

performance by a person with a body form that is very unfavourable from a biomechanical or a physiological standpoint.

Repeated bouts of vigorous physical activity normally enhance fitness. But this is not inevitably the case. An inappropriate type of conditioning can induce disadvantageous changes. For example, an overemphasis upon strength training can handicap a distance runner by causing an excessive increase in body mass. Moreover, if the intensity and/or duration of training are excessive, a combination of physiological and psychological reactions leads to a deterioration of fitness (the situation of 'staleness' or 'overtraining'), with microinjuries of muscle, suppression of immune function and an increased vulnerability to infections (Shephard 1997).

Argument continues as to how far physical fitness is inherited, how far it is determined by a person's family environment, and how far it can be acquired through an appropriate conditioning programme (Bouchard & Malina 1983; Bouchard & Pérusse 1994). Plainly, body build makes a major contribution to success in many events; body fat content can increase with overeating and severe malnutrition can stunt growth, but in general the shape of the human body is an immutable inherited characteristic. With respect to physiological characteristics such as peak oxygen transport, an attempt can be made to partition observed interindividual differences into components of variance attributable to constitution, a constitutional susceptibility to training, domestic environment (for example, a household where high-level competition is the expected norm) and a residual response to training that could have been elicited through adequate motivation of any growing child or young adult (Bouchard & Pérusse 1994).

A clarification of the relative contributions of genes and environment to competitive success is important for the coach, who must decide whether to allocate resources to talent scouting or to improvement of training methods (Fig. 1.1). Unfortunately, results obtained through comparisons between twins and other closely related family members have to date proved rather unstable. Some authors have inferred that physical fitness has a large genetic component, but others have found that constitution has only a minor influence on the determinants of endurance performance. It is possible that completion of the human genome project will resolve this issue. But given current uncertainty in the partition of variance for easily quantified biological data such as maximal oxygen intake, it is hardly surprising that little is known about the contribution of inheritance to other more subjective determinants of endurance fitness.

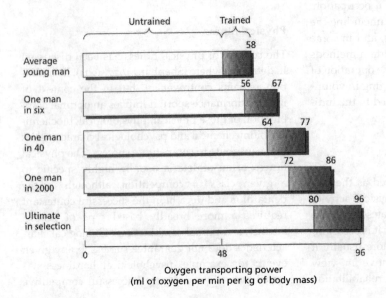

Fig. 1.1 Diagram illustrating the relative importance of athletic selection and rigorous training to the development of a competitor with a large maximal oxygen intake. Assumptions are made that: (i) the peak effect of training is a 20% increase in oxygen transport; and (ii) the constitutional variance in maximal oxygen intake is normally distributed, with a standard deviation of 8 ml·[kg·min]$^{-1}$. From Shephard (1978), with permission.

Force, work and power: the choice of units

The terms force, work and power have a long-standing mechanical significance; they have been defined in a biological context by Ellis (1971), Knuttgen (1984) and Knuttgen & Komi (1992).

Force

Early reports expressed peak muscle force in pounds weight or kilograms force. Force is more properly expressed in newtons (N), the SI unit of force (Ellis 1971; Table 1.1). For example, a mass of 1 kg exerts a force of 9.81 N when in unit gravitational field. Gravitational acceleration (and thus the weight of an object) varies with changes in its latitude or altitude, reflecting corresponding differences in the object's distance from the centre of the Earth. The effects (up to 3%) are large enough to have an appreciable influence on sport performance.

Work

Work is the product of force and distance. If a force of 1 N is sustained over a distance of 1 m, 1 newton-metre, or 1 joule (J) of work is performed. Older texts on nutrition express work and stored food energy in calories; under standard conditions, 1 calorie is equal to 4.186 J.

The body must perform work whenever physical activity is undertaken. Stores of potential energy are modified, viscous work is performed against internal or external resistance, and the kinetic energy of the body and associated equipment is altered. Body stores of chemical energy are used to effect these changes, and reserves are later replenished through the consumption of food.

Metabolic energy expenditure is still commonly expressed in $kcal \cdot min^{-1}$ or $kJ \cdot min^{-1}$, although in the future these may be replaced by the SI unit (Watts). Likewise, the SI unit of heat accumulation or dissipation in unit time is the Watt.

The athlete may increase the *potential energy* stores of the body and/or sports equipment by performing sustained work against gravity, for example when propelling a bicycle up a steep hill. The accumulated potential energy may be calculated as the product of the vertical ascent (in metres) and the mass of the rider plus machine (in newtons). The potential energy of individual body segments may also change in the course of a bout of physical activity, for example when an arm and racquet are raised in a tennis serve.

A good example of external *viscous work* is encountered when cross-country skis glide over a snow-covered surface. The external viscous work

Table 1.1 Recommended standard international (SI, Système International (d'Unités)) units of force, work and power (based on recommendations of The International Bureau of Weights and Measures 1970, Ellis 1971 and Knuttgen & Komi 1992).

Mass	= kilogram (kg)
Force	= newton (N) ($1 \, kg \cdot m \cdot s^{-2}$; a mass of 1 kg exerts a force of 9.81 N in a standard gravitational field)
Distance	= metre (m)
Time	= second (s)
Velocity	= metres per second ($m \cdot s^{-1}$)
Acceleration	= metres per second^2 ($m \cdot s^{-2}$)
Torque	= newton-metre (N·m)
Angle	= radian (rad)
Angular velocity	= radians per second ($rads \cdot s^{-1}$)
Work	= force × distance = N·m = joule (J)
Power	= work/time = $J \cdot s^{-1}$ = watt (W)
Pressure	= force/area = $N \cdot m^{-2}$ = pascal (Pa)
Volume	= litre (l)
Amount of substance	= mole (mol)

performed by the ski competitor may be calculated as the distance travelled times the resisting force (the product of gravitational acceleration, the mass of the competitor plus skis and the coefficient of sliding friction for a given wax, temperature and snow condition).

The body accumulates *kinetic energy* when its speed of movement is increased, as when a runner accelerates from the blocks. A single limb and associated equipment may also gain kinetic energy (for example, as the arm and racquet accelerate during a tennis serve). The developed force is proportional to the product of the mass of the moving part plus equipment and its acceleration; the work performed is again the product of this force and the distance over which it has operated. Work may be performed not only in accelerating the body or its parts, but also in deceleration (for instance, the eccentric muscle contractions that control the descent of the body when running downhill).

Power

The quantity of work performed in unit time has the dimensions of power. It is best expressed in watts ($1\,W = 1\,N{\cdot}s^{-1}$, or $1\,J{\cdot}s^{-1}$). A distinction must be drawn between the external power output, readily measured on a device such as a cycle ergometer, and the internal energy consumption. The latter is usually at least four times as great, reflecting not only energy consumed by the muscles engaged in the primary task, but also the resting energy consumption, unavoidable ancillary costs of the activity (such as increases of energy expenditure in the heart and the respiratory muscles) and (particularly if the regimen includes resistance exercise) the energy costs of synthesizing additional lean tissue.

Other units

In general, the SI system of units (Ellis 1971) is now well accepted by exercise physiologists. However, two exceptions are the systemic blood pressure (still commonly expressed in mmHg rather than in kPa; $100\,mmHg = 13.3\,kPa$), and oxygen transport (still expressed in $l{\cdot}min^{-1}$ STPD rather than as $mmol{\cdot}s^{-1}$; $1\,l = 44.6\,mmol$).

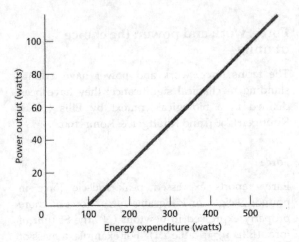

Fig. 1.2 Relationship between rate of energy expenditure and power available for performance of sport. The intercept on the abcissa reflects the resulting rate of energy expenditure, and the slope of the line indicates net efficiency (20% in the example illustrated). Adapted from Shephard (1982), with permission.

Mechanical efficiency

Like most human-designed machines, the body is an imperfect device for converting stored food energy into external work. The gross mechanical efficiency expresses the ratio of the external work performed to the food energy that has been consumed. Commonly, resting energy expenditure is deducted from the gross energy cost to yield a *net efficiency value*. The net efficiency varies from around 25%* when operating a machine such as a bicycle or a cycle ergometer (Fig. 1.2) to a figure as low as 1% in a novice swimmer. In activities such as swimming, the difference in mechanical efficiency (and thus the energy cost of a given performance) between a novice and a highly skilled international competitor is at least four-fold, and a novice can make very substantial gains of performance from an upgrading of technique, even if the individual shows no increase of maximal oxygen intake.

The difference between the external work performed and the food energy that is consumed nor-

---

*The mechanical efficiency can sometimes rise above the theoretical ceiling of 25% suggested by biochemical analyses (Shephard 1982), for instance if stored energy is recouped from sources such as the stretched tendons of a runner during a stride rebound.

mally appears as heat. In many circumstances, the endurance athlete has problems in dissipating the waste heat, but in some types of event (such as distance swimming in very cold water), heat production helps to conserve body core temperature.

Strength and endurance

Physically demanding sports may be broadly classified into events that demand great strength (well typified by competitive weightlifting) and events that demand tremendous endurance (for example, participation in an ultramarathon run). The first type of competition requires an unusual development of the skeletal muscles (particularly fast-twitch, type II muscle fibres), but performance in the second category of event is favoured by the predominance of slow-twitch, type I fibres (Fig. 1.3). Endurance performance depends on an ability to supply the active muscle fibres with adequate amounts of oxygen and essential nutrients, to eliminate metabolic heat, carbon dioxide and other waste products and to sustain homeostasis in the body as a whole.

Strength events are examined in a companion volume in this series (Komi 1992). The present book is thus limited almost exclusively to a discussion of endurance activities, typically events that require an hour or more of physical activity.

In many classes of prolonged athletic competition, central factors (particularly the pumping ability of the heart) appear important to success, but in some events (for example, the dinghy sailor who must make repeated 'hiking' movements to counterbalance a small boat), an ability to sustain load-bearing muscle contractions (isometric muscle endurance) is a critical factor. In other instances (such as a prolonged tennis tournament) repeated powerful arm movements (isotonic muscular endurance) are needed for success.

The distance runner requires, above all, cardiovascular endurance. A large blood flow to the working muscles must be sustained as preloading of the heart is reduced by sweating and an extravasation of fluid into the active tissues, and peripheral resistance is diminished by a rising core temperature (Saltin *et al.* 1972).

In ultra-long distance events, performance is threatened by other factors—a depletion of intramuscular and hepatic glycogen reserves, a dispersal of the sarcoplasmic calcium ion reserves needed to initiate muscle contraction and an escape of intracellular potassium ions that threatens the electrical function of the muscle membranes.

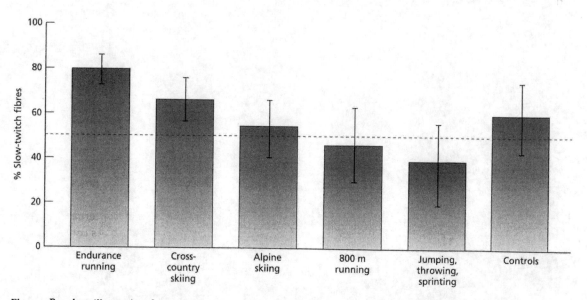

Fig. 1.3 Bar chart illustrating the preponderance of slow-twitch (type I) muscle fibres among successful endurance competitors. From Dirix *et al.* (1988), with permission.

Finally, irrespective of the type of event, there is a need for psychological toughness—a motivation to endure and to excel in the face of pain and discouragement. Individual competitors may have an advantage in any of these domains, giving them an unusual endurance relative to their rivals.

Acknowledgement

Dr Shephard's studies are funded in part by research grants from the Defence and Civil Institute of Environmental Medicine, Toronto, ON.

References

Bouchard, C. & Malina, R. (1983) Genetics of physiological fitness and motor performance. *Exercise and Sports Sciences Reviews* 11, 306–339.

Bouchard, C. & Pérusse, L. (1994) Heredity, activity level, fitness and health. In: Bouchard, C., Shephard, R.J. & Stephens, T. (eds) *Physical Activity, Fitness and Health*, pp. 106–118. Human Kinetics, Champaign, IL.

Bouchard, C. & Shephard, R.J. (1994) Physical activity, fitness and health: The model and key concepts. In: Bouchard, C., Shephard, R.J. & Stephens, T. (eds) *Physical Activity, Fitness and Health*, pp. 77–88. Human Kinetics, Champaign, IL.

Caspersen, C.J., Powell, K.E. & Christensen, G.M. (1985) Physical activity, exercise and physical fitness: definitions and distinctions for health related research. *Public Health Reports* 100, 126–131.

Dirix, A., Knuttgen, H.G. & Tittel, K. (eds)

(1988) *The Olympic Book of Sports Medicine*. Blackwell Scientific Publications, Oxford.

Ellis, G. (1971) *Units, Symbols and Abbreviations. A Guide for Biological and Medical Editors and Authors*. Royal Society of Medicine, London.

International Bureau of Weights and Measures (1970) *SI. The International Systems of Units* (Approved translation). Her Majesty's Stationery Office, London.

Knuttgen, H. (1984) Instructions to authors. *Medicine and Science in Sports and Exercise* 16, xviii–xix.

Knuttgen H.G. & Komi, P.V. (1992) Basic definitions for exercise. In Komi, P.V. (ed.) *Strength and Power in Sport*, pp. 3–6. Blackwell Scientific Publications, Oxford.

Komi, P.V. (1992) *Strength and Power in Sport*. Blackwell Scientific Publications, Oxford.

Saltin, B., Gagge, A.P., Bergh, V. & Stilwijk, J.A.J. (1972) Body temperature and sweating during exhausting exercise. *Journal of Applied Physiology* 32, 635–643.

Shephard, R.J. (1977) *Endurance Fitness*, 2nd edn. University of Toronto Press, Toronto.

Shephard, R.J. (1978) *The Fit Athlete*. Oxford University Press, Oxford.

Shephard, R.J. (1982) *Physiology and Biochemistry of Exercise*. Praeger Publications, New York, NY.

Shephard, R.J. (1994) *Aerobic Fitness and Health*. Human Kinetics, Champaign, IL.

Shephard, R.J. (1997) *Physical Activity, Training and the Immune Response*. Cooper Publications, Carmel, IN.

Wright, G.R., Bompa, T. & Shephard, R.J. (1976) Physiological evaluation of a winter training programme for oarsmen. *Journal of Sports Medicine and Physical Fitness* 16, 22–37.

Chapter 2

Endurance Sports

PER-OLOF ÅSTRAND

Introduction

Which sport events call for endurance? Certainly running a marathon, cycling 180 km and, still more so, participating in the triathlon. What about running 10 000 m? Rather arbitrarily, physical activity that lasted for 1 h or longer was taken as a guide in this volume. However, each training session for a 10 000-m race usually lasts for many hours. A tennis match can last for 4 h or more. Team sports are activities with intermittent exercise: the regulation time in team handball is two periods of 30 min, in basketball 2 × 20 min, in American football 4 × 15 min, and in Australian football 4 × 25 min; volleyball consists of three sets and the time for a set is from 15 to 30 min, field hockey is 2 × 35 min, water polo is 4 × 5 min and netball is 4 × 15 min; in ice hockey, where the effective time is 3 × 20 min, individual players except for the goalkeeper participate for only part of this time.

The total time taken for a game is often much longer than the 'regulation time'. In a world cup soccer championship held in Italy, many matches were not settled after two 45-min periods; two 15-min periods were added, with short breaks in between.

The physiological response to continuous exercise can be very different when compared with the response to intermittent exercise, i.e. short bursts of intensive exercise. This chapter describes the physiology of intermittent exercise (bouts of less than 1 min), interval exercise (2–6-min bouts) and continuous exercise (over longer periods of time).

Intermittent exercise

A man was able to exercise at a high work rate, 412 W, but after 3 min of continuous cycling he was exhausted (Åstrand et al. 1960). When exercising intermittently for 1 min and resting for 2 min, etc., the same man was able to continue for 24 min before being totally exhausted, with a blood lactate concentration of 15.7 mM. On another day, the periods of exercise were reduced to 10 s and the rest periods to 20 s. He could then complete the intended work production of 247 kJ within 30 min with no severe feeling of strain. On this occasion, his blood lactate concentration did not exceed 2 mM, indicating an almost balanced oxygen supply to his heavily stressed muscles (Fig. 2.1a). With periods of exercise and rest of 30 s and 60 s, respectively, intermediate results were obtained. Thus, if 10-s exercise bouts were interrupted by 20-s rest periods, the engaged muscles and their metabolic processes could be subjected to great demands without undue fatigue. How can we explain the fact that a power which demands an oxygen consumption exceeding the subject's maximal oxygen intake, measured at the 'lung level', can be performed without noticeable support from anaerobic processes? Figure 2.1(b) attempts to give an answer.

When a person exercises intermittently in 10-s periods there is a vasodilatation of the vessels supplying active muscles; this will secure a good blood supply, and therefore a good oxygen supply, during exercise as well as during rest intervals. In addition, there is an oxygen store in the myoglobin which can be consumed during the bout of exercise. During the

9

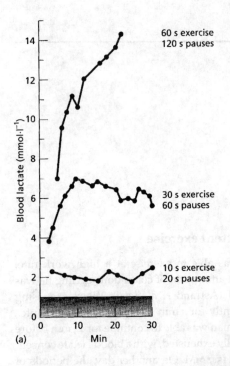

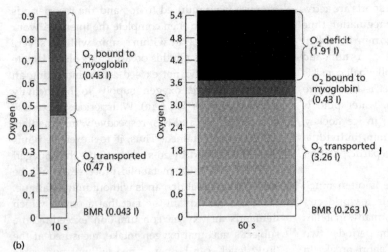

Fig. 2.1 (a) Blood lactate concentration in a total work production of 247 kJ in 30 min. The exercise was accomplished with a power of 412 W, the exercise periods being 10, 30 and 60 s, and the rest periods 20, 60 and 120 s, respectively. The lower shaded area shows lactate concentration at rest. (b) Oxygen requirement for 10 s and 60 s power of 412 W. The schematic drawing indicates the basal metabolic rate (BMR), the calculated fractions of oxygen bound to myoglobin and transported by the blood, and the oxygen deficit. From Åstrand *et al.* (1960).

following rest interval, this depot is quickly refilled with oxygen. The calculated oxygen store in this experiment was approximately 0.4 l. With the period of exercise prolonged to 60 s, it was calculated that 1.9 l of oxygen were 'missing' (Fig. 2.1b) and therefore anaerobic processes must have been contributing to exercise metabolism.

In another experiment, by running for 10 s and resting for 5 s, a subject was able to prolong the total exercise plus rest period to 30 min at a speed that would normally have exhausted him after about 4 min of continuous running. During exercise, there is a reduction in adenosine triphosphate (ATP) and phosphocreatine concentrations; however, this can be restored during the period of rest, evidently by aerobic processes. If intermittent exercise is performed at the same work rate as continuous exercise, less glycogen is utilized and the lactate concentration in the muscles is much lower. Thirteen times more ATP can be replenished when glycogen is metabolized aerobically, compared with the efficiency of anaerobic breakdown of glycogen to lactate (for references to these studies, see Åstrand & Rodahl 1986, pp. 304–307).

If maximal effort is extended to 1 min, followed by rest for 4 min, and the sequence is repeated four or five times, very high lactate concentrations can be attained both in the active muscles ($>25\,mM\cdot kg^{-1}$ wet muscle) and in the blood ($>20\,mM\cdot l^{-1}$); indeed the pH in arterial blood can drop to 7.0. It is very fatiguing to train using this protocol, and such a regimen is usually not introduced until a month or two before the competitive season.

Interval exercise

Figure 2.2 illustrates interval exercise, performed with the intent of bringing oxygen intake, heart rate and cardiac output up to maximal values. After warming up, maximal rates can be reached within 1 min. When running, well-trained and highly motivated athletes can maintain maximal oxygen intake for some 20 min, but a more 'normal' time is well below 10 min. One hundred per cent of maximal oxygen intake can be attained even if speed and perceived exertion are submaximal. If oxygen demand exceeds the individual's maximal oxygen intake, the deficit must be covered by anaerobic processes, with the consequence that muscle and blood proton (and lactate) concentrations increase. We cannot explain the mechanisms, but marked proton accumulations interfere negatively with performance and are correlated with fatigue. Training at maximal oxygen intake is an effective way of improving maximal aerobic power (see Wenger & Bell 1986). The balancing act is to find a work rate just high enough to tax this maximum without requiring too much anaerobic support. On a cycle ergometer, a power demand of 300W may cause exhaustion after 5 min, but 250W is enough to

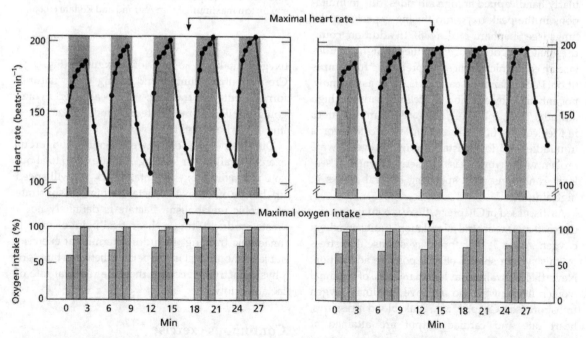

Fig. 2.2 Heart rate and oxygen uptake recorded in two subjects during training with alternating 3-min periods of running (shaded areas) and rest (unshaded areas). The efforts were not maximal, but the oxygen uptake reached maximal values, as did the heart rate. From Saltin *et al.* (1968).

engage the oxygen transport system at maximal power (Åstrand & Rodahl 1986, p. 300). When running on a treadmill at a speed of 13 km·min^{-1}, the maximal time for one subject was 4 min. His speed could be reduced by several km·min^{-1} without reducing maximal oxygen intake (see Åstrand & Rodahl 1986, p. 443). These examples illustrate how maximal aerobic power can be attained at submaximal work rates.

There are no studies indicating that an aerobic training regimen is more effective if combined with hypoxia and anaerobic conditions. There is an ongoing discussion about training at high altitude (see Chapters 30 and 41). In endurance events, a period of several weeks of acclimatization is an essential part of the preparation for competition at an altitude of 2000 m or higher (see Jackson & Sharkey 1988). It is unfortunate that organizers of world cups, world championships and the Olympic games give in to pressure groups for economic reasons and select high-altitude locations for competition. Data indicate that athletes with a very high oxygen intake per kilogram of body mass are particularly handicapped at high altitudes, due to limitations in the peak oxygen diffusing capacity of the lungs (see Shephard *et al.* 1988). In addition, countries that lack good sports facilities at high altitudes face an economic handicap in preparing for competition. Performance at sea-level is, as far as we know, not enhanced by a period of acclimatization at high altitude. Thus, following the 1968 Olympic Games in Mexico City (altitude 2300 m), no world records in middle- and long-distance running events were broken when world-class runners returned to sea-level conditions after spending several weeks at high altitude.

As discussed in Chapter 3, there is convincing evidence that the central circulation limits maximal oxygen intake. It therefore makes sense that stress on this system should elicit a positive adaptation. Nevertheless, training at less than 100% of maximal oxygen intake will also improve maximal oxygen transport (see Chapter 28). Peak blood pressures, heart rate and cardiac output are attained at approximately the same work rate as when oxygen intake reaches its maximum. However, stroke volume has already reached a maximum when

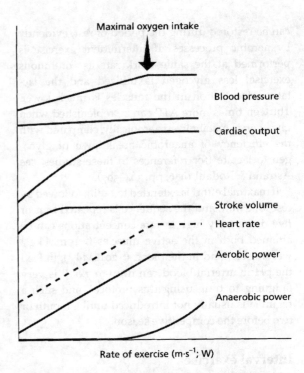

Fig. 2.3 Schematic diagram showing some of the major cardiovascular responses to exercise of increasing intensity up to a maximum. From Åstrand and Rodahl (1986).

oxygen intake is 40–50% of maximum (Fig. 2.3). Cross-country running and skiing offer 'natural' forms of interval training, with peak efforts when going uphill and moderate demands when travelling on the horizontal or downhill.

During the periods between bouts of vigorous exercise, walking or jogging at a rate of up to about 50% of maximal oxygen intake ($\dot{V}o_{2max}$) will speed up the rate of removal of lactate, which is a substrate in aerobic metabolism. Lactate is definitely not a waste product! From a theoretical point of view if 'anaerobic training' includes intermittent exercise, subjects should rest in the periods between bursts of physical activity, because then the removal rate of lactate is slow.

Continuous exercise

The endurance time is limited in types of exercises that demand maximal oxygen intake. Therefore, if continuous exercise is performed for 10–20 min or longer, as in running, cycling, skiing, swimming or canoeing, the intensity must be submaximal. The skeletal muscle cells of endurance-trained individuals are characterized by a high density of mitochondria and therefore a high concentration of the enzymes involved in aerobic metabolism. In fact, fast-twitch (type II) and slow-twitch (type I) muscle fibres have similar metabolic profiles in such subjects. Capillary density is also high and, at any given time, more blood is available for the exchange of gases, nutrients and waste products with the tissues. Promotion of the oxidation of free fatty acids has a glycogen-saving effect (see Chapter 13). It was mentioned above that the central circulation seems to be the limiting factor for maximal aerobic power. In endurance events, peripheral factors are quite decisive. An élite marathon runner has a high maximal oxygen intake per kilogram of body mass and a good running economy, and she or he can run at a high percentage of maximal aerobic power without accumulation of protons and lactate (see Sjödin & Svedenhag 1985). As indicated in Fig. 2.4, marathon runners are not necessarily champions in terms of their maximal oxygen intake. Other qualities, just mentioned, are very important for success. Élite marathon runners and cross-country skiers have a high percentage of slow-twitch fibres, about 80%, compared with about 50% in unselected subject groups. It is still an open question whether the high percentage of slow-twitch fibres is a consequence of adaptation to endurance training or is an innate, inherited characteristic (see Chapters 9, 11 and 15). Coggan *et al.* (1990) found that master athletes in endurance events, with a mean age of 63 years, had a similar distribution of fibre types to younger runners with a mean age of 26 years (60% type I and very few type IIb fibres in the gastrocnemius muscle). One interpretation of their finding could be that years of endurance training do not modify fibre distribution (from type II to I).

The literature related to exercise physiology reveals a great interest in the anaerobic threshold concept, i.e. the work rate or percentage of maximal oxygen intake that can be attained at a given blood lactate concentration (Chapter 22). Alternative methods of establishing the threshold are non-

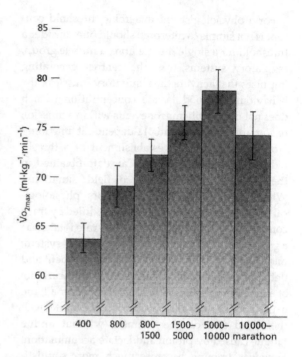

Fig. 2.4 Maximal oxygen intake in track athletes who represented the Swedish national team. From Svedenhag and Sjödin (1984).

invasive. With increasing work rate, pulmonary ventilation increases linearly with oxygen intake to a point where ventilation increases non-linearly (the ventilation per litre of oxygen intake increases). There are data indicating that this 'ventilatory threshold' occurs at a work rate associated with an increase in blood lactate concentration. However, other reports do not support the idea of similar ventilatory and lactate thresholds (Loat & Rhodes 1993). There are also large individual variations in the responses (for discussion, see Åstrand & Rodahl 1986, pp. 327–330; Orok *et al.* 1989; Chapter 22). Droghetti *et al.* (1985) found a linear relationship between power output and heart rate up to a certain submaximal rate, beyond which the increase in heart rate slowed down. This deflection point where non-linearity in the heart rate response was found correlated significantly with the anaerobic threshold ('Conconi test'). Other researchers have been unable to confirm this finding (see Francis *et al.* 1989).

For a physiologist, the anaerobic threshold concept is not simple to interpret: should one consider a threshold for a single muscle fibre, a muscle group, regulatory systems (e.g. the centres generating impulses that activate the respiratory muscles), the behaviour of blood lactate concentration (which does not necessarily mirror events within a muscle), or some other lactate- and pH-dependent functions? How important is the establishment of a threshold as a guide in coaching? Can data obtained in the laboratory be applied to field situations? When running is performed outdoors, physiological responses at a given speed are modified by track conditions, terrain and wind. If heart rate is taken as a guide to demands on the oxygen transport system, one must keep in mind that a hot environment and dehydration can dramatically increase the heart rate at a given oxygen intake (Chapter 40). After all, the experienced endurance athlete knows quite well the speed that can be tolerated without undue fatigue caused by proton and lactate accumulation. However, training becomes much more sophisticated when the coach can give instructions based on blood lactate data.

Recommendations about the intensity of endurance training are often based on a percentage of maximal oxygen intake or heart rate. Perceived exertion is also used as a guide (see Purvis & Cureton 1981; Chapter 26).

From a practical viewpoint, few coaches have access to laboratories that can measure pulmonary ventilation, oxygen intake or lactate concentration, particularly in developing countries. Therefore heart rate recordings or, if equipment is not available, just recording the time taken for a fixed number of heart beats, are often the only objective measurements available. Taking group mean values, 50% of $\dot{V}_{O_{2max}}$ corresponds to about 65% of maximal heart rate; 80% of $\dot{V}_{O_{2max}}$ corresponds to about 87% of maximal heart rate. If heart rate is calculated as a percentage of 'heart rate reserve', the value comes, on average, very close to the corresponding percentage of $\dot{V}_{O_{2max}}$. One can generalize and take 60 beats·min^{-1} as the resting heart rate. If the maximal heart rate is 190 beats·min^{-1}, then the 'reserve' is $190 - 60 = 130$ beats·min^{-1}. If the purpose is to train at 80% of 'heart rate reserve', the required

value is 104 beats·min^{-1}. Adding the resting heart rate of 60 beats·min^{-1}, we end up with a heart rate of $104 + 60 = 164$ beats·min^{-1}. In the example given above, 80% of $\dot{V}_{O_{2max}}$ should correspond to 87% of the maximal heart rate: 87% of $190 = 165$ beats·min^{-1}. If the individual's maximal heart rate is not known, an age group mean value is often used. However, because this mean value has a standard deviation of ± 10 beats·min^{-1} it is quite useless as a guide. In healthy, trained people, the individual's maximal heart rate can easily be established with a stopwatch. After warming up, the subject runs at a speed close to maximum for a couple of minutes and then makes a 1-min spurt, preferably uphill. Immediately afterwards the subject sits down and a stopwatch is used to record the time taken for exactly 10 beats, with palpation over the carotid artery or the radial artery, or on the chest over the heart. Because the heart rate drops rapidly, it is important that counting of the heart rate should start immediately after exercise (make a countdown of '5–4–3–2–1–0', and on '0', start the stopwatch). A table can be constructed to convert the 10-beat time to heart rate in beats·min^{-1}.

A similar protocol can be applied when the exercise is skiing, cycling, swimming or rowing; the peak heart rate in these activities is similar to that of running. Again it should be emphasized that exercise in a hot environment and resulting dehydration will gradually increase the heart rate at a given submaximal oxygen intake.

Conclusion

This volume concentrates on a scientific analysis of endurance sports, focusing particularly on events with continuous activation of large muscle groups for 1 h or more. However, it is important to include also a basic discussion of training for many sports events of short duration because they may demand hours of daily exercise. In this chapter, the physiological responses involved in three different types of training have been discussed.

1 Intermittent exercise with repeated bursts of vigorous activity of short duration (less than 1 min, followed by rest). Intermittent exercise in periods of 10 s or less can be performed almost exclusively

aerobically, thanks to unloading and recharging of myoglobin oxygen stores.

2 Interval exercise, where repeated 3–6-min periods of vigorous activity are interspersed with periods of walking or jogging. Such exercise can effectively load the oxygen transport system up to maximum. A balancing act is needed to find a power level that is high enough to tax this maximum while requiring only a modest contribution from the anaerobic breakdown of glycogen.

3 Continuous, relatively long duration exercise at submaximal oxygen intake. This type of training seems effective as a stimulus to increase the mass

and density of mitochondria in skeletal muscle. The oxidation of free fatty acids is thus enhanced, with a glycogen-saving effect.

A simple method of establishing an individual's maximal heart rate is described, and a formula is given by which the percentage of maximal oxygen intake can be converted to the percentage of maximal heart rate. Other chapters give more detailed discussion of muscular endurance, including the 'anaerobic threshold' (Chapter 22), endurance conditioning (Chapter 28) and training for specific sport events (Chapters 54–64).

References

Åstrand, P.-O. & Rodahl, K. (1986) *Textbook of Work Physiology*. McGraw-Hill, New York.

Åstrand, I., Åstrand, P.-O., Christensen, E.H. & Hedman, R. (1960) Myoglobin as an oxygen-store in man. *Acta Physiologica Scandinavica* **48**, 454–460.

Coggan, A.R., Spina, R.J., Rogers, M.A. *et al.* (1990) Histochemical and enzymatic characteristics of skeletal muscle in master athletes. *Journal of Applied Physiology* **68**, 1896–1901.

Droghetti, P., Borsetto, C. & Casoni, I. (1985) Noninvasive determination of the anaerobic threshold in canoeing, cross-country skiing, rolling and ice skating, rowing and walking. *European Journal of Applied Physiology* **53**, 299–303.

Francis, K.T., McClatchey, P.R., Sumsion, J.R. & Hansen, D.E. (1989) The relationship between an aerobic threshold and

heart rate linearity during cycling ergometry. *European Journal of Applied Physiology* **59**, 273–277.

Jackson, C.G.R. & Sharkey, B.J. (1988) Altitude, training and human performance. *Sports Medicine* **6**, 279–284.

Loat, C.E. & Rhodes, E.C. (1993) Relationship between the lactate and ventilatory thresholds during prolonged exercise. *Sports Medicine* **15**, 104–115.

Orok, C.J., Hughson, R.L., Green, H.J. & Thomson, J.A. (1989) Blood lactate responses in incremental exercise as predictors of constant load performance. *European Journal of Applied Physiology* **59**, 262–267.

Purvis, J.W. & Cureton, K.J. (1981) Ratings of perceived exertion at the anaerobic threshold. *Ergonomics* **16**, 595–600.

Saltin, B., Blomqvist, G., Mitchell, J.H., Johnson, R.L. Jr, Wildenthal, K. & Chapman, C.B. (1968) Response to sub-

maximal and maximal exercise after bed rest and training. *Circulation* **38** (Suppl. 7), 1–78.

Shephard, R.F., Bouhlel, E., Vanderwalle, H. & Monod, H. (1988) Peak oxygen intake and hypoxia: influence of physical fitness. *International Journal of Sports Medicine* **9**, 279–283.

Sjödin, B. & Svedenhag, J. (1985) Applied physiology of marathon running. *Sports Medicine* **2**, 83–99.

Svedenhag, J. & Sjödin, B. (1984) Maximal and submaximal oxygen uptakes and blood lactate levels in élite male middle- and long-distance runners. *International Journal of Sports Medicine* **5**, 255–261.

Wenger, H.A. & Bell, G.J. (1986) The interactions of intensity, frequency and duration of exercise training in altering cardiorespiratory fitness. *Sports Medicine* **3**, 346–356.

PART 2

BASIC SCIENTIFIC CONSIDERATIONS

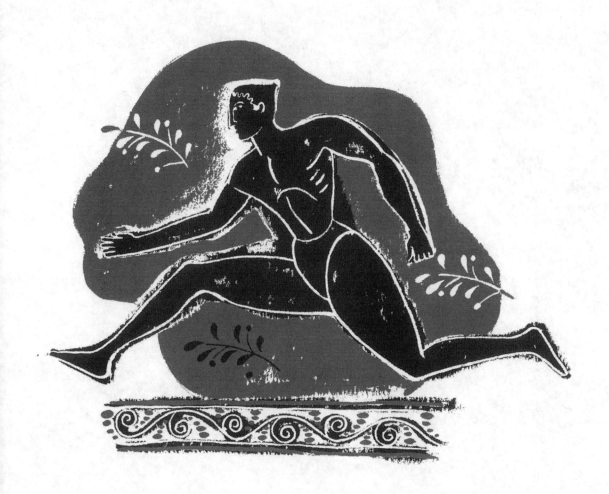

Part 2a

Biological Bases of Endurance Performance and the Associated Functional Capacities

Chapter 3

Determinants of Endurance Performance

ROY J. SHEPHARD

General considerations

This section of the monograph examines the basic determinants of endurance performance: physical, biological, psychological and genetic. In essence, competitive success depends on the individual's ability to maximize biological function, technical skills and psychological preparedness, thus optimizing his or her potential to perform athletically useful work against the inevitable constraints imposed by body form and environment.

Much of the focus of this section is upon biological factors. Nevertheless, the psychological make-up of the individual is a major determinant of the athlete's willingness to maximize biological function by continuing rigorous training over many months. Psychological hardiness also allows a person to sustain an all-out competitive effort in the face of physical pain and discouragement. Genetic factors contribute to the individual's initial physical and physiological status, as well as modulating a competitor's responsiveness to training; constitution seems a significant determinant of the susceptibility of both whole organs and specific enzyme systems to conditioning programmes. Finally, the immediate physical circumstances (for example, a change in the type of equipment that is permitted, or the choice of a high-altitude location for training or competition) can substantially influence the physical performance that is achieved for a given expenditure of metabolic energy.

Because the human body obeys the basic laws of thermodynamics, the energy that is needed to perform external work must be derived from the physical or chemical stores of the body. Individuals differ greatly in the mechanical efficiency with which they can convert the chemical energy of foods into athletically useful work. Such discrepancies reflect inherent differences in body build, the progressive acquisition of technical skills and the learning of competitive tactics such as the choice of a moderate aerobic pace rather than a faster speed that demands costly and inefficient anaerobic effort. Realization of the individual's potential in terms of technical skills and the learning of optimal tactics are important goals of prolonged, sport-specific training.

Discounting special cases such as an athlete who is reducing reserves of potential energy by releasing a stretched tendon or descending a hill, the active muscle fibres meet their immediate energy needs through the breakdown of a small local reserve of high-energy phosphate compounds (the phosphagens adenosine triphosphate (ATP) and creatine phosphate (CP)). During a bout of physical activity, the ATP is usually degraded to adenosine diphosphate (ADP) and occasionally to adenosine monophosphate (AMP), whereas CP is converted to creatine. Each gram molecule of phosphate that is liberated by the breakdown of these several phosphagens yields a 'free' energy of about $46\,kJ\cdot mol^{-1}$. This can be applied to the actin–myosin interaction that is needed to initiate a muscle contraction. Unfortunately, the total usable store of high-energy phosphagens is only about $30\,mmol\cdot kg^{-1}$ muscle (wet weight), a reserve that can be exhausted by 2 s or less of all-out effort. The endurance competitor must therefore resynthesize ATP and CP repeatedly, using energy derived from the metabolic break-down of other food reserves (Newsholme 1983; Shephard 1984).

Prolonged athletic performance depends not only on the extent of local food stores within the active muscles, but also on the ability to mobilize reserves held elsewhere in the body and to transport them to the working tissues. Furthermore, the cardiorespiratory system must be equal to the task of transporting the oxygen needed for aerobic metabolism, and of removing the waste products of metabolism (carbon dioxide, heat and such substances as lactate). Moreover, function must be sustained in regions of the body other than muscle as exercise proceeds. For instance, an inadequate blood flow to the brain may lead to a poor competitive performance because of mental confusion or impaired muscular coordination. Likewise, in sports that demand forward planning or teamwork, either an excessive rise in core body temperature or a drop in blood sugar concentration may lead to impaired thinking, irritability and a lack of cooperation between team members. The next section of this chapter discusses factors influencing the transport of oxygen, carbon dioxide, lactate, heat and metabolic fuels in terms of a generalized conductance equation.

Ultimately, fatigue develops as various homeostatic mechanisms fail. A final section of the chapter thus looks at physiological, psychological and medical aspects of fatigue, discussing whether the primary site of fatigue is central or peripheral.

Conductance theory

The physiological and biochemical systems involved in metabolism are arranged as a tightly interlinked sequence of transport mechanisms extending from the environment to the enzymes of the mitochondrial cristae within the active muscle cells (Shephard 1977, 1994).

The various links in the transport chain can be conceptualized as a series of conductances. A conductance ($\dot{g}$) is the reciprocal of the corresponding resistance (r): $\dot{g} = 1/r$, or $r = 1/\dot{g}$. Thus, it is conventional to think of the gas transporting function of the chest bellows as the respiratory minute volume that can be sustained during vigorous exercise (a maximum of perhaps $100\,l\cdot min^{-1}$). It is possible to think of an electrical or mechanical analogue for any conductance. The electrical analogue is governed by Ohm's law, with the electrical driving pressure or voltage (e) across an individual link in the system being proportional to the product of flux (I) and resistance ($e = Ir$, or $e = I/\dot{g}$). The overall resistance of the system is then given by reciprocal summation of the individual conductances:

$$R = 1/\dot{G} = 1/\dot{g}_1 + 1/\dot{g}_2 + 1/\dot{g}_3 \ldots + 1/\dot{g}_n$$

One purpose of such a conductance analysis is to identify potential bottlenecks in the processes of transport and metabolism. Performance can then be bettered as these bottlenecks are eliminated through an appropriate combination of initial selection and extensive conditioning of the competitor. We shall look first at the conductance chain for the transport of oxygen, and will then examine more briefly analogous systems for the transport of carbon dioxide, lactate heat and metabolic fuels between the working muscles and the external environment (Shephard 1976, 1982).

Oxygen conductance

When analysing any of the conductances in the human model, the driving pressure must be expressed in dimensionless units. For example, ambient air normally contains about 20.9% oxygen, and the partial pressure of oxygen in the active muscle fibres is close to zero. Thus, the total driving pressure (E) from ambient air to the muscle mitochondria may be expressed as $209\,ml\cdot l^{-1}$, or the corresponding fraction of an atmosphere (0.209). To apply this concept in a practical sense, let us assume that an endurance competitor can develop a maximal oxygen flux of $6\,l\cdot min^{-1}$. The overall conductance for oxygen ($\dot{G} = I/E$) is then 6/0.209, or $28.7\,l\cdot min^{-1}$. If the driving pressure from the atmosphere to alveolar gas is 0.06 of an atmosphere, and the maximal alveolar ventilation during exercise is $100\,l\cdot min^{-1}$, then the overall oxygen flux can be derived from the product of the regional pressure gradient and the corresponding conductance ($I = e\dot{g}$, 100×0.06, or again $6\,l\cdot min^{-1}$).

It is more difficult to analyse data describing the

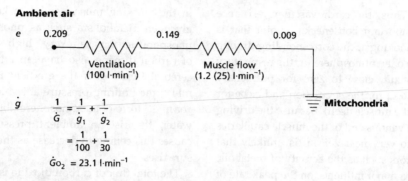

Fig. 3.1 Diagram illustrating in terms of electrical conductances the main barriers to the transport of oxygen from ambient air to the working muscles. The total pressure gradient (E) from ambient air to the muscle mitochondria (0.209 atm) is distributed between ventilation ($e = 0.06$), muscle blood flow ($e = 0.149$) and the residual intramuscular gradient ($e = 0.009$), the distribution being determined by the reciprocal of the individual conductances (for ventilation, $\dot{g}_1 = 100\,l\cdot min^{-1}$, and for muscle blood flow, $\dot{g}_2$ becomes $30\,l\cdot min^{-1}$ after allowing for an average solubility coefficient of 1.2; see Fig. 3.2).

transfer of oxygen from the alveolar spaces of the lungs to the pulmonary capillaries, and from the muscle capillaries to the muscle sarcoplasm, because the driving pressure changes continually, over the respiratory cycle in the case of the lungs, and at both sites the pressure gradient decreases progressively along the length of the capillaries. In both the lungs and the skeletal muscles, equilibration is almost complete on reaching the venous end of the capillaries. An accurate modelling of gas exchange in either capillary bed would require an integration of pressure gradients along individual capillary pathways, and an averaging of integrals across parallel pathways. But because equilibration is almost complete at the venous end of the capillaries, both in the lungs and in muscle, to a first approximation the overall process conducting oxygen from ambient air to the muscle sarcoplasm can be simplified to a series arrangement of respiratory and cardiovascular conductances (Fig. 3.1).

There is a change of phase on passing from alveolar gas into the bloodstream. Thus, it is necessary to introduce an appropriate solubility factor (technically, an air–liquid partition coefficient) in order to describe the cardiovascular conductance relative to the chosen measure of driving pressure. This solubility factor corresponds to the average slope of the oxygen dissociation curve between arterial and muscle venous blood. During vigorous endurance

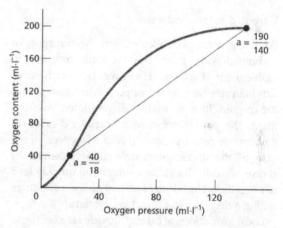

Fig. 3.2 Graph illustrating the calculation of an average blood solubility factor (air–liquid partition coefficient) for oxygen during a bout of maximal aerobic exercise. At the arterial point on the oxygen dissociation curve, an oxygen pressure of $140\,ml\cdot l^{-1}$ is associated with a blood oxygen content of $190\,ml\cdot l^{-1}$, while at the venous point the corresponding figures are 18 and $40\,ml\cdot l^{-1}$. The slope between the arterial and venous points during maximal aerobic activity thus averages $150/122$, or 1.2.

exercise, a linear average value of 1.2 may be assumed (Fig. 3.2). A peak muscle blood flow of $25\,l\cdot min^{-1}$ thus yields a bloodstream conductance of $30\,l\cdot min^{-1}$.

Plainly, when considering oxygen transport, the cardiovascular conductance is the smallest element in the chain. Thus, the cardiovascular resistance is the most important bottleneck, a point that is confirmed by looking at the corresponding driving pressures (0.06 of an atmosphere for the respiratory part of the circuit, close to zero for pulmonary gas exchange, 0.14 for the circulation and 0.009 for events within the muscle itself). Because the driving pressure at the venous end of the muscle capillaries has dropped to very near zero, it is unlikely that peripheral factors such as the activity of metabolic enzymes have a major influence on the peak rate of oxygen consumption during sustained endurance effort.

The overall oxygen conductance can be approximated by reciprocal summation of the respiratory and cardiovascular components. In our example, it amounts to $23.1 \, l \cdot min^{-1}$ (see Fig. 3.1).

Carbon dioxide conductance

Similar general principles govern the transport of carbon dioxide from the working muscles to ambient air (Fig. 3.3). However, the gradient of driving pressure is in the opposite direction to that for oxygen. In a normal, well-ventilated environment, the partial pressure of carbon dioxide in ambient air remains close to zero. However, in the case of the underwater athlete, inefficiencies of carbon dioxide absorbing systems can quickly lead to a significant build-up of carbon dioxide pressures within a closed-circuit breathing system.

Local toxic effects of carbon dioxide set a ceiling to driving pressures at the muscular end of the system. Specifically, a rising hydrogen ion concentration in the working muscles inhibits key enzymes of glycogen metabolism such as phosphorylase and phosphofructokinase. Very high concentrations of carbon dioxide also have an adverse effect on cerebral function. If the gradient is expressed in $ml \cdot l^{-1}$, the limiting pressure at sea-level is perhaps $100 \, ml \cdot l^{-1}$ (0.10 of an atmosphere), but when underwater, the rise in ambient pressure necessarily causes this ceiling to decrease as the ambient pressure rises.

The total flux of carbon dioxide is usually a little less than that for oxygen. At the beginning of an endurance event, the respiratory quotient (the ratio of carbon dioxide output to oxygen intake) is likely to exceed 0.9, signifying that carbohydrate metabolism is providing most of the food the body requires. Thus, if the maximal oxygen transport is $6 \, l \cdot min^{-1}$, the initial maximal flux of carbon dioxide is 6.0×0.9, or $5.4 \, l \cdot min^{-1}$. However, the body reserves of glycogen become exhausted if an event continues for longer than about 100 min. The main source of energy then becomes fat. At this stage, the respiratory quotient may drop to 0.8 or lower, corresponding to a maximal carbon dioxide flux of $4.8 \, l \cdot min^{-1}$. Note also that as the respiratory quotient falls, there is a progressive decrease in the quantity of energy transformed for each litre of oxygen that has been transported; the yield is 10% poorer for fat than for carbohydrate metabolism.

The blood solubility factor is larger for carbon dioxide than for oxygen. As with oxygen, we are in essence dealing with the corresponding blood dissociation curve. Over the normal operating range from the venous end of the muscle capillaries to

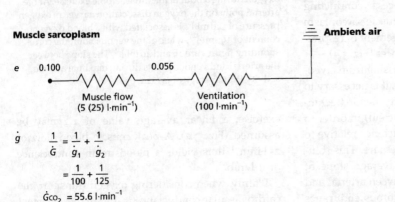

Muscle sarcoplasm　　　　　　　　　　　　　**Ambient air**

e　0.100　　　　　　0.056

Muscle flow
$(5 \, (25) \, l \cdot min^{-1})$

Ventilation
$(100 \, l \cdot min^{-1})$

$\dot{g}$

$$\frac{1}{\dot{G}} = \frac{1}{\dot{g}_1} + \frac{1}{\dot{g}_2}$$

$$= \frac{1}{100} + \frac{1}{125}$$

$$\dot{G}_{CO_2} = 55.6 \, l \cdot min^{-1}$$

Fig. 3.3 Diagram illustrating the conductance of carbon dioxide from the exercising muscles to the atmosphere. The total pressure gradient from the working muscles to ambient air (E, 0.100 atm) is distributed between ventilation ($e = 0.056$) and muscle blood flow ($e = 0.044$) according to the reciprocal of the individual conductances (for ventilation, $\dot{g}_1 = 100 \, l \cdot min^{-1}$, and for muscle blood flow, $\dot{g}_2 = 125 \, l \cdot min^{-1}$ after allowing for a solubility coefficient of 5.0).

arterialized blood, the curve for carbon dioxide may be approximated by a linear solubility coefficient of 5.0. Thus, in our hypothetical example, the overall conductance for carbon dioxide becomes $1/100 + 1/5(25)$, or $55.5\,l\cdot min^{-1}$. Given also that the peak flux is smaller for carbon dioxide than for oxygen, it is unlikely that carbon dioxide transport will limit most types of competition, despite the fact that the overall pressure gradient is smaller for carbon dioxide than for oxygen. Exceptions are found in the underwater environment and in patients with chest disease (situations where the alveolar ventilatory conductance may be reduced by an increase in gas density, and spasm of the airways or a poor distribution of inspired gas, respectively).

Lactate conductance

Lactate is normally converted to pyruvate, and is then broken down to carbon dioxide and water via the Krebs cycle. However, it tends to accumulate in the active muscles whenever the local oxygen supply is inadequate to support aerobic metabolism (Shephard 1982). Lactate that cannot be metabolized locally either passes from the active muscles into the bloodstream (Fig. 3.4) and thence to the liver (where glucose and glycogen can be synthesized from the lactate residues), or it diffuses locally to other better oxygenated tissues (where it can be converted back to pyruvate and then metabolized through the Krebs cycle) (Gladden 1989).

The pressure driving lactate from the muscle sarcoplasm into the bloodstream is the local concentra-

tion within the active tissues, acting on a 30–40 kD lactate transporting protein (McCullagh & Bonen 1995). The rate of transport is also influenced by the local tissue pH (Bonen & McCullagh 1994). The maximal intramuscular lactate concentration $(30–40\,mmol\cdot l^{-1})$ is set by the rising local hydrogen ion concentration and the resultant inhibition of glycolytic enzymes (Shephard 1984). The peak arterial concentration in young adults is typically $10–15\,mmol\cdot l^{-1}$, although lower values are seen in young adolescents and in elderly individuals. Arterial concentrations as high as $30\,mmol\cdot l^{-1}$ have been reached when conditions have allowed equilibration between muscle and blood (for instance, when several brief bouts of exhausting large muscle work have been repeated over the space of 20 min). Peak lactate values are usually larger in athletes than in sedentary individuals, and at any given level of training they are also greater in individuals who have a high proportion of Type I muscle fibres (Pilegaard et al. 1994). Bangsbo et al. (1994) further noted that during 'active' recovery (a period of light exercise following endurance exercise), lactate concentrations decreased more rapidly than with passive recovery. The main basis for this was an increase of metabolism within the muscle rather than a speeding of bloodstream transport to other parts of the body.

The flux of lactate from the active muscle to the bloodstream and other, better oxygenated muscles typically reaches a rate of about $10\,mmol\cdot min^{-1}$ during maximal effort, although some authors have suggested figures as low as $2\,mmol\cdot min^{-1}$

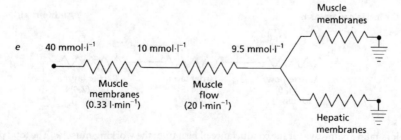

Fig. 3.4 Diagram illustrating possible pathways for the conductance of lactate from the working muscles. The pressure gradient E is a lactate concentration of $40\,mmol\cdot l^{-1}$, extending from the muscle sarcoplasm to the sites of lactate metabolism in resting muscle and liver. The main gradient (and thus the smallest conductance) is from muscle sarcoplasm into the bloodstream.

(Shephard 1976). Taking the 10 mmol·min^{-1} figure, and assuming a muscle blood flow of 20 l·min^{-1}, the arteriovenous concentration gradient would reach the typically observed experimental value of 0.5 mmol·l^{-1}, compared with a gradient of 30 mmol·l^{-1} from muscle sarcoplasm to the capillary bed.

Based on these driving pressures, we may conclude that the conductance term describing the outward transport of lactate from muscle into the bloodstream and other muscle fibres is only about one-sixtieth of that describing bloodstream transport, the equivalent of a local blood flow of 0.33 l·min^{-1}. The reverse conductance of lactate, from the bloodstream into resting or moderately active muscle, proceeds more rapidly than the efflux, probably reaching a peak rate of about 40 mmol·min^{-1}.

These figures still remain relatively imprecise, and there have been suggestions that the bottleneck in lactate transport across the muscle cell membrane can be reduced substantially if the local hydrogen ion gradient is manipulated by the administration of bicarbonate solutions. There is thus a temptation to enhance athletic performance by 'bicarbonate doping' (Gledhill 1984). Over medium distances, this may confer an advantage of about 3%, but such a practice may not confer any advantage in long-distance events, since an increase of blood bicarbonate slows the transfer of lactate from the blood into resting muscle (Grainer et al. 1996). Bicarbonate is a normal body constituent, so there is little possibility of regulating this practice by blood or urine testing.

Heat conductance

During vigorous exercise, metabolic heat follows a pathway from muscle to skin (Fig. 3.5). It is then normally dissipated by a combination of sweating and convection (Nadel 1977, 1987). The driving pressure is a temperature difference, measured between the active deep tissues and either the skin surface (in a partial analysis) or the ambient air (in a total analysis).

There is competition between muscle and skin blood flow when vigorous exercise is being performed in a hot environment. Skin blood flow usually peaks at 5 l·min^{-1} or less. When the data are analysed in terms of a conductance analogue, it is necessary to apply a solubility factor describing the heat-carrying capacity of the blood (its specific heat, about 3.4 kJ·l^{-1} per degree centigrade). The total heat conductance of the body is then approximated by reciprocal summation as $(1/20 + 1/5)\ 1/3.4$, or 14 kJ·l^{-1}·min^{-1} per degree centigrade.

Assuming a net mechanical efficiency of 25%, 75% of body metabolism appears as heat. Further, each litre of oxygen that is consumed generates some 21 kJ of heat. If the oxygen flux is 6 l·min^{-1}, the total heat flux is then 0.75 (6.0) 21 kJ·min^{-1}, or about 95 kJ·min^{-1}. Given also a total conductance of 14 kJ·min^{-1} per degree centigrade, a thermal gradient of about 7°C is necessary for circulatory transfer to the skin surface of all the heat that is produced by the working muscles. A core temperature in excess of 41°C is regarded as a dangerous level of hyperthermia. The implication is that the skin temperature should not exceed 34°C if a prolonged bout of

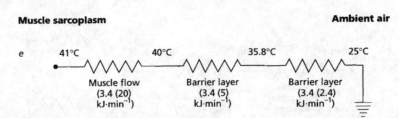

Fig. 3.5 Diagram illustrating pathways for the conductance of heat from the working muscles. The total pressure gradient (measured in degrees centigrade) depends on the ambient air temperature (25°C in the example). The bloodstream conductance of heat is given by the product of blood flow and a 'heat solubility factor' of 3.4 kJ·l^{-1}·°C^{-1}. If transfer of heat across the barrier layer of still air around the body is expressed in the same units, it can be seen that normally this is the smallest of the three conductances, and thus it has the largest influence on heat loss from the body.

strenuous physical activity is to be performed under warm conditions.

The peak oxygen intake is more commonly $4 \, l \cdot min^{-1}$ rather than $6 \, l \cdot min^{-1}$ during prolonged endurance events; this reduces the total heat flux from 95 to about $65 \, kJ \cdot min^{-1}$. Moreover, some heat is conducted directly from muscle through the overlying tissues, without transfer to the bloodstream. The required skin temperature can thus rise to around 35.8°C rather than 34°C. Nevertheless, it may remain difficult for an athlete to achieve thermal homeostasis if an event is performed under hot and humid conditions. A rising core temperature commonly becomes an important factor limiting sustained physical activity in a warm environment.

Finally, it is worth noticing that under temperate environmental conditions, a major portion of the overall thermal gradient is from the skin surface to ambient air. A thin film of stationary air (the 'boundary layer') offers a major barrier to heat dissipation. Assuming an air temperature of 25°C, the thermal gradient from skin to air (10.8°C in our example) is more than twice that from core to skin (5.2°C), implying that the barrier to heat exchange is at least twice as great for the boundary layer as for the maximal circulatory conductance.

Heat transfer across the boundary layer changes dramatically from the laboratory treadmill (where there is normally little air movement or displacement of the body) to the athletic field (where body movement greatly reduces the effectiveness of the barrier layer, particularly for competitors such as cyclists, skiers and speed skaters. The conductance of heat across the barrier layer depends on the density and thermal conductivity of gases in the body's immediate microenvironment. Conductance falls with the decrease of gas density which occurs at high altitudes, but it is greatly increased in the diver who is using not only a high-pressure breathing system, but also a gas mixture that contains a substantial fraction of helium (a gas with a high thermal conductivity).

The thermal conductivity of water is much larger than that of air, and boundary layer effects are also much less important when a person is immersed in water. The outward heat flux is thus much greater when swimming than when on land, and a distance swimmer may encounter physiological problems due to a fall in core body temperature over the course of competition.

Conductance of metabolites

Depending somewhat upon the state of training of the individual, carbohydrate provides about two-thirds of the energy needed by an endurance athlete at the beginning of an endurance event. Intramuscular reserves of glycogen are used at a rate of about $2–4 \, g \cdot min^{-1}$ (about $16 \, mmol \cdot min^{-1}$ of the equivalent glucosyl units), while a further $1 \, g \cdot min^{-1}$ ($5.3 \, mmol \cdot min^{-1}$ of glucosyl units) is transported from the liver to the active tissues. There is no evidence that performance is limited by the transport of metabolites to the working muscle, at least until the local reserves of glycogen have dropped to quite low levels (Hultman 1971; Karlsson 1979; Conlee 1986; Greenhaff et al. 1993; see Chapter 13). At this stage, corresponding to the running of a distance of perhaps 30–35 km, the speed of a distance competitor shows an appreciable decline, and contestants speak of 'hitting the wall'.

The rate of muscle glycogen depletion depends on the tactics that are adopted by the competitor. Fat metabolism is oxygen dependent, so that the choice of an over-rapid pace increases the likelihood of local oxygen lack, boosting the proportion of energy that must be obtained from carbohydrate rather than fat in the early part of a race. The ideal plan is for the competitor to operate just below his or her anaerobic threshold. The experienced participant in endurance events adopts this pattern of exercise, reserving a burst of anaerobic activity for the final sprint to the finishing line. Endurance training also influences the situation; as conditioning increases the activity of the aerobic enzymes, the contestant is able to obtain a larger fraction of the needed energy by metabolism of fat (Greenhaff et al. 1993).

On occasion, an attempt is made to eke out the carbohydrate reserves of the athlete by the drinking of a glucose or glucose/polymer solution during competition (Murray 1987; Shephard & Leatt 1987). The maximum rate of ingestion and absorption of sweetened fluid seems to be achieved when drinking a 5% solution of glucose. The peak intake is then about $600\,ml\cdot h^{-1}$ ($0.5\,g\cdot min^{-1}$ glucosyl units, or $92.6\,mmol\cdot min^{-1}$). This makes some contribution to metabolic demand, although it represents only a small fraction of total carbohydrate metabolism, at least until muscle glycogen reserves have been depleted.

In very prolonged effort, performance may be limited by the ability to mobilize fat from the adipose tissue and/or the ability to transport fatty acids to the working muscles (Bülow 1987). In view of the limited blood supply of adipose tissue and the variations in the rates of triglyceride metabolism with changes in blood levels of fatty acids, one might suspect the problem is in part a local limitation of vascular conductance within the fat depots. On the other hand, training increases the ability to mobilize triglyceride metabolites, in addition to its effect in increasing the activity of fat-metabolizing enzymes within the working muscle. Presumably, these changes contribute to a sparing of glycogen in the early stages of an endurance competition.

Nature and location of fatigue

Acute and chronic forms of fatigue (Simonson 1971; Green 1987; MacLaren *et al.* 1989) are common complaints of the endurance competitor. The problem may be physiological, psychological or occasionally medical in nature, and it can be local (confined to a particular group of muscles) or general (affecting the body as a whole).

Physiological fatigue

Physiological fatigue is seen as a deterioration of performance, either over the course of a specific competition, or as a task is repeated from one day to another. For example, the pace of a runner may become slow, or the force of repeated maximal isotonic muscular contractions may diminish. There are usually associated signs of failing homeostasis; for example, the cardiorespiratory system is marked by a rising heart rate, respiratory rate, respiratory minute volume or respiratory gas exchange ratio at any given intensity of effort, and there are parallel increments in blood lactate and core temperature. However, there remain substantial interindividual

differences in the limiting values for each of these variables, and often there is only a limited relationship between subjective reports of tiredness and changes in objective measures of fatigue. For many people, there is a substantial gap between the physiologically possible and the psychologically acceptable, a gap that can be narrowed by either hypnosis or the roar of a cheering crowd.

The proximal cause of fatigue may be central (a lack of appropriate signals to drive the active muscle fibres, resulting in a decrease of motor unit discharge, fibre recruitment and tension development), or peripheral (a failure of force generation due to problems in replenishing the high-energy phosphate molecules needed to power muscle contractions). There may also be more general problems of homeostasis associated with the accumulation of the waste products of metabolism (lactate, hydrions, phosphate and ammonia), disturbances of the ionic balance across membranes (Simonson 1971; Dawson *et al.* 1986), progressive fluid depletion, or an excessive accumulation of heat and resulting circulatory collapse (see Chapters 17 and 40).

FAILURE OF DRIVE MECHANISMS

Muscle contractions are normally initiated by a coordinated volley of impulses originating in the motor cortex and/or the cerebellum. The electrical signal passes through several synapses in the brain and spinal cord, traverses the neuromuscular junction and penetrates the transverse tubules, finally activating the muscle fibre by liberating calcium ions from the sarcoplasmic reticulum. The calcium ions in turn are one key component in a triggering mechanism that initiates the formation of crossbridges between actin and myosin molecules, using energy stored in ATP.

In theory, fatigue could originate at any point in the chain of command. The brain has little capacity for vasodilatation, and is thus dependent on the ability of the heart to maintain an adequate perfusion pressure. Moreover, cerebral tissue can only metabolize carbohydrate, so that the progressive decrease in blood sugar which develops after several hours of large muscle activity and/or severe shivering may cause errors of judgement, loss of teamwork, failure of coordination and a cerebral form of fatigue. In some instances (for example, soccer matches), team performance has improved when players have been given small doses of glucose or sugar at half-time (Shephard & Leatt 1987). A poor coordination of movement is one expression of cerebral fatigue, although it may reflect either a poor circulation to the brain or a low blood sugar level. Clumsiness is exacerbated by changes in the sensitivity of the spindle organs that detect muscle tension, and by attempts to sustain a given level of performance using muscle groups other than those which have been trained to undertake a given task.

Evidence for a neural component to fatigue can be seen in both a decrease of discharge frequency in fast-twitch motor units and an altered pattern of movement as a person becomes tired (Green 1987; Bigland-Ritchie 1990; Figs 3.6 & 3.7). Recordings of action potentials from the working muscles show that the slow frequency component of the electromyogram increases as fatigue develops. This could represent an attempt to recruit fibres that are not yet exhausted from some alternative muscle group. Among many suggested causes of the slower average rate of firing we may note: (i) a voluntary inhibition of effort (the peak muscle force of an 'exhausted' competitor can often be increased by techniques such as hypnosis or cheering); (ii) a lessening of synchronization of firing between individual motor units; (iii) the recruitment of slowly firing, high-threshold motor fibres; (iv) alterations in the electrophysiological characteristics of the conducting membranes; and (v) an inhibitory feedback from muscular afferents designed to maintain optimal muscle function in the face of a prolonged force transient and a slow relaxation of the contracting muscle (Fitts & Metzger 1993; Nicol & Komi 1996). There is little evidence that the carriage of impulses along the nerve fibres or neuromuscular transmission itself is adversely affected by the fatigue of endurance competition. Fatigued muscles generate the same tension whether they are stimulated directly or via the motor nerve (Fitts & Metzger 1993).

Within the muscle, there is sometimes evidence of a slowing of calcium pumping; this process is essential to a recovery of function both at the neuromuscular junction and in the sarcoplasmic reticulum of the active muscle fibres. Hydrogen ion accumulation may competitively inhibit the binding of calcium ions to troponin, thus preventing activation of the muscle cross-bridges; it may also inhibit the shift of the cross-bridges from a low to a high

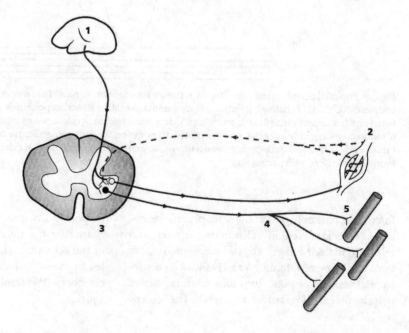

Fig. 3.6 Potential sites of central fatigue: 1, supraspinal failure; 2, segmental afferent inhibition; 3, depression of motoneurone excitability; 4, loss of excitation at branch points; 5, presynaptic failure. From Green (1987), with permission.

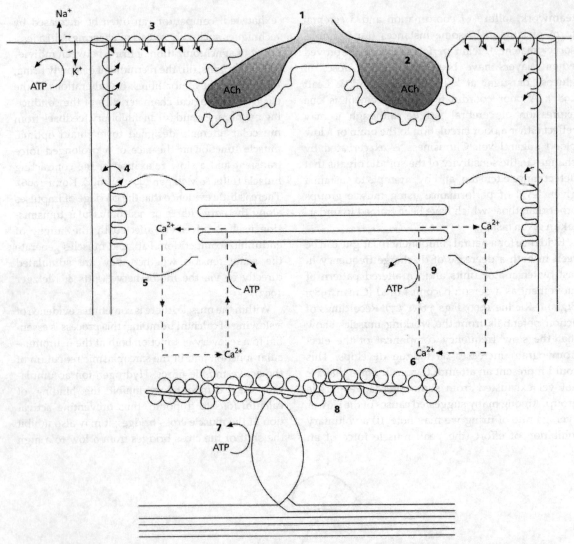

Fig. 3.7 Potential peripheral sites of fatigue: 1, presynaptic failure; 2, inability to develop an action potential at the motor endplate (ACh, acetyl choline); 3, failure of sarcolemma to sustain an action potential; 4, loss of coupling of excitation between t-tubule and sarcoplasmic reticulum; 5, depressed release of calcium ions from the sarcoplasmic reticulum; 6, reduced binding affinity of the receptor protein troponin on the actin molecule; 7, a failure in the actin–myosin cross-bridge cycle; 8, delayed cross-bridge dissociation; 9, depressed reaccumulation of calcium ions by sarcoplasmic reticulum. From Green (1987), with permission.

force state, or it may inhibit the sarcoplasmic reticular ATPase involved in calcium ion uptake and release (Fitts & Metzger 1993). Furthermore, both local and general fatiguing exercise lead to a substantial leakage of potassium ions from the active muscle fibres (Sjögaard *et al.* 1985). The escape of potassium ions adversely affects the electrical charge on the muscle membrane and conduction of the activating signal along the transverse tubules to the site of calcium release within the muscle fibres (Westerblad *et al.* 1990; Fitts & Metzger 1993).

FAILURE OF POWER SUPPLY

We have noted that the release of energy needed for the resynthesis of ATP can be threatened by an inadequate supply of oxygen, an inhibition of the enzymes involved in glycogen breakdown due to an accumulation of carbon dioxide, hydrogen ions or lactate, a product inhibition from the accumulation of phosphate radicals (Dawson *et al.* 1986), or a depletion of food reserves locally within the active muscle fibres. However, there is surprisingly little correlation between the onset of fatigue and the exhaustion of local reserves of CP and ATP (Thompson & Fitts 1992).

A competitor can use 100% of maximal oxygen transport for a few minutes of large muscle effort, but during an extended competition such as a marathon run, fatigue generally develops if the intensity of effort averages more than 75% of maximal oxygen intake (Costill 1972). The probable explanation of this ceiling is that the blood supply to the muscle fibres is non-uniform. Thus, if the intensity of effort exceeds 75% of the overall oxygen-transporting capacity, the capillary supply to some parts of the working muscle is no longer sufficient to avert anaerobic metabolism (Antonutto & DiPrampero 1995). One factor that profoundly influences the local blood supply in heavy rhythmic and isotonic activity is the development of a high intramuscular pressure as the muscles contract; this occludes the arterial supply. The problem can be countered by a reduction of intramuscular pressure (for instance, by using a lower gear ratio on a bicycle, or strengthening the active muscles through appropriate training). Such tactics enable a distance competitor to exercise at more than 75% of maximal oxygen intake for long periods without becoming fatigued (Chapter 7). Likewise, in a sport that requires repeated vigorous isotonic efforts, the decrease in peak force over 50 such contractions may be much less marked after suitable training.

Carbon dioxide accumulation does not contribute significantly either to local or to general fatigue, except in special circumstances such as prolonged underwater exploration. At depth underwater, the ventilatory component of overall conductance (more important for carbon dioxide output than for the intake of oxygen) is limited both by the increase in gas density and by the added dead space and external resistance of breathing equipment.

Glycogen reserves are almost completely depleted after 100 min of endurance work (Hultman 1971; Conlee 1986; Chapter 13). Stores can also be exhausted by the frequent accelerations and decelerations needed in team sports such as soccer and ice hockey. A third possible scenario is a sequence of 10–12 near-maximal contractions of a given muscle group, particularly if individual efforts have been sustained to the point of fatigue. The transport of fatty acids from depot fat to the working muscles can subsequently sustain an intensity of aerobic activity equivalent to about 50% of the competitor's maximal oxygen intake, but unfortunately, fat metabolism cannot provide fuel for anaerobic activity. The potential to synthesize glucose in the liver (the process of hepatic gluconeogenesis; Wahren & Björkman 1981; Winder 1985) draws on such precursor resources as hepatic glycogen, amino acids, glycerol and lactate. Nevertheless, the peak rate of gluconeogenesis is quite limited; the blood glucose may thus drop as low as $3 \, mmol \cdot l^{-1}$ in some very prolonged events such as ultramarathon running. Once muscle glycogen stores have been depleted, a sensation of intense weakness and fatigue develops whenever postural, isometric or heavy isotonic muscle activity must be performed.

FAILURE OF HOMEOSTASIS

With very prolonged activity, a general failure of homeostasis may develop. This can involve the circulation, the kidneys and/or the endocrine glands. Sometimes, there is also an excessive rise or fall of body temperature. A local failure of homeostasis is a further possibility, particularly if one specific group of muscles is engaged in repeated and intensive isotonic or isometric effort.

General circulatory problems arise from a decrease in the fraction of the total blood volume stored in the central part of the circulation (Saltin 1964; Senay & Pivarnik 1985; Convertino 1987). Many factors contribute to the depletion of central blood volume, including: (i) a dilatation of the peripheral capacitance vessels (the major veins); (ii) sweating (which may cause a fluid loss of as much as $2 l \cdot h^{-1}$); (3) exudation of fluid into the active tissues (a loss of fluid which has the potential to decrease total blood volume by up to 20% over 30 min of vigorous physical activity); and (iv) possible exhaustion of the neural and hormonal regulatory systems. Dominant features of central circulatory failure include a decline in blood pressure and cardiac stroke volume with an increase in heart rate for any given intensity of effort.

Local circulatory problems arise when blood flow is restricted by a forceful muscle contraction. Perfusion of a given muscle decreases when contractions exceed 15% of the maximal voluntary force for a given muscle group. Occlusion of the local blood supply becomes complete at 70% of maximal voluntary force (Shephard 1982). Because of the effective decrease in local systolic pressure, the situation is worsened if the arm is held above the head (as in rock-climbing or a tennis serve). The perfusion pressure in the upper limb is then decreased because the heart must pump blood to a greater height, but the force of muscle contraction and thus of vascular compression is unchanged by limb position.

If subjects compete repeatedly in a very hot environment, a progressive failure of circulatory homeostasis may develop over several weeks (Wyndham & Strydom 1972). The problem seems to involve a chronic depletion of sodium and other mineral ions, with an associated loss of water and thus blood volume.

There have been occasional reports of renal failure following prolonged events such as marathon and ultramarathon races. Generally, there is evidence of an associated hyperthermia. The primary cause of the problem seems to be a restriction of visceral blood flow, in an attempt to maintain blood flow to other 'more vital' parts of the circulation. However, such a shift in blood flow distribution is not always advantageous; late-stage renal failure has possible links to tissue injury, a generalized septic response, excessive inflammation and the multiple organ dysfunction syndrome (Shephard & Shek 1998).

Restriction of visceral flow may allow a penetration of the gut wall by intestinal bacteria, or cause a failure of the adrenal cortex (the final stage of Selye's stress reaction). Damage to the adrenal cortex limits the production of the hormones regulating potassium and sodium ions (aldosterone) and water and carbohydrate stores (cortisol). If competition is perceived as unusually stressful from a psychological perspective, there can be an interaction between physiological and psychological stress, exacerbating hormonal fatigue. There may be an associated deterioration in immune function (Keast *et al.* 1988; Shephard 1997). This leaves the athlete temporarily more vulnerable to viral infection. Moreover, any infection can further exacerbate both physical and psychological fatigue.

A failure of circulatory homeostasis may be linked with an excessive rise in core body temperature (Nadel 1987). Because the rising core temperature diverts blood flow from the brain and the working muscles to the skin, it exacerbates feelings of fatigue, and precipitates a failure of circulatory homeostasis (Rowell 1986).

Repeated bouts of prolonged exercise in a hot climate can produce cumulative chronic fatigue; this condition can be associated with mineral ion and water depletion, unless care has been taken to replenish mineral stores between bouts of physical activity.

Too low a core body temperature can also induce fatigue. In a cold environment, the local blood flow to the limbs is reduced, an increase of muscle viscosity augments the internal work that must be performed during physical activity, and a cooling of peripheral neural receptors leads to a more clumsy performance of many tasks.

Psychological fatigue

Although psychological fatigue is hard to pinpoint, it is a very real phenomenon, particularly in athletes who have pursued heavy training to the point of 'staleness'.

The tiredness can arise acutely, but more often its onset is gradual and chronic. Typically, symptoms have a situational or even an emotional rather than a firm physiological basis. Factor analyses of subjective reports from athletes (Kinsman *et al.* 1973) distinguish three elements: *projected fatigue* (noted in such sensations as leg weakness, shaking or aching muscles, a pounding heart, shortness of breath and a dry mouth—many of the somatic manifestations of an anxiety state); *task aversion* (perceived as sweating, discomfort and a wish to do something other than train or compete); and *poor motivation*, encompassing feelings of reduced drive, lack of vigour and a want of determination.

The athlete becomes bored with the routine of seemingly endless and unchanging training sessions, and there is an adverse reaction to the restrictions imposed by the coach, with the associated loss of social life. Discouragement develops as the rewards of a progressive improvement in performance disappear, despite the ever-increasing demands of training. The affected individual is typically underaroused, and fails to achieve his or her physiological potential. An associated loss of vigilance may increase the risk of accidents. In contrast with physical exhaustion, the psychologically fatigued athlete demands a change rather than a rest. An unpleasant or unfamiliar environment (for example, competition in a foreign country, sleeping in an uncomfortable hotel room at an unaccustomed altitude or temperature, conflict with the coach or a series of defeats) can exacerbate the problem, not by any direct physiological mechanism, but rather by increasing task aversion.

Short-term training programmes apparently do little to change the perception of a given intensity of physical effort (Pandolf 1983). However, highly trained athletes undoubtedly habituate themselves to situations that lesser competitors would find psychologically fatiguing.

Medical aspects of fatigue

Fatiguing effort may induce disturbances of tissue function that are only slowly reversed. Lesions range from a slight muscular stiffness and/or pain, reported for a few days following intensive competition, to chronic tendon injuries, fatigue fractures of bones and disturbances of immune function. The immunosuppression increases susceptibility to intercurrent infections (Chapter 50) and, at least theoretically, augments the risk of various types of tumour.

The minor muscle lesions are subcellular in type. It is unclear how far they arise simply from mechanical overload, how far they are attributable to local hypoxia, and how far they are a consequence of increased local concentrations of reactive species of oxygen (Hellsten 1996; Jackson 1996). Evidence of increased membrane permeability can be found in: (i) modifications of ionic balance (a shift of potassium ions from within the active muscles to extracellular fluid, plasma and inactive tissues); (ii) the liberation of various intracellular enzymes such as lactate dehydrogenase and creatine kinase into the bloodstream; and (iii) the appearance of low molecular weight proteins in the urine (Poortmans 1985; Rogers *et al.* 1985; Armstrong 1986).

The majority of observers have detected evidence of mitochondrial damage and other ultrastructural changes in fatigued muscle, heart and nerve at electron microscopy (Banister 1971; Oscai & Palmer 1988; McCutcheon *et al.* 1992). It seems likely that these ultrastructural changes contribute to perceptions of chronic fatigue—particularly in terms of such feelings as stiffness and muscle pain. Some authors have suggested that the subcellular changes are a necessary concomitant of an adaptive response to heavy training, including the increased synthesis of muscle protein. However, the dividing line that separates such phenomena from irreversible tissue injury is fine.

Immune disturbances may reflect a decrease in plasma levels of glutamine and other amino acids needed for cell proliferation (Newsholme *et al.* 1991), inhibitory effects of prostaglandins on natural killer (NK) cell function (Pedersen 1997), and direct influences of mood state upon the immune system (LaPerrière *et al.* 1994).

In some instances, reports of fatigue may be an indication that an athlete is developing an anxiety state, as a reaction to the stresses of competition or other adverse personal circumstances.

Interindividual differences

Susceptibility to central fatigue depends largely on the psychological hardiness of the individual and his or her willingness to continue exercise in the face of weakness, pain and other symptoms.

The speed of onset of peripheral fatigue is influenced markedly by the relative proportion of type I and type II fibres in the individual's musculature. Subjects with a high proportion of type I fibres are less susceptible to fatigue (Komi & Tesch 1979).

Central versus peripheral limitations of endurance effort

There has been much debate as to whether a typical endurance performance such as distance running is limited by central or peripheral factors (Shephard 1982). The issue is important for both the physiologist and the coach who seek to augment human performance, since it indicates whether investigative effort and conditioning programmes should focus on methods of boosting cardiorespiratory function, or whether attention should be directed towards enhancing the cellular and subcellular processes of metabolism.

In forms of exercise that involve activation of a large proportion of the total musculature, the conductance theorem (this chapter) offers persuasive arguments favouring a central limitation of effort. Arguments for a peripheral limitation of function have been considered and rejected (Shephard 1982). Given 20 kg of active muscle and a peak muscle blood flow of $25\,l\cdot min^{-1}$, the regional blood flow to the legs of a distance runner averages about $800\,ml\cdot min^{-1}$ per litre of tissue. There are good reasons to believe that the blood vessels in a large muscle could accept three to four times this flow if the heart were able to sustain a greater rate of tissue perfusion (Savard et al. 1987; Reading et al. 1993).

In forms of exercise where the volume of active muscle is more limited, the likelihood of a peripheral limitation of effort is correspondingly increased (Shephard et al. 1988). During cycling, a surprisingly large proportion of the total effort is sustained by the quadriceps muscle. Poorly trained individuals thus complain that their maximal effort on a bicycle or cycle ergometer is limited by muscular fatigue, rather than by indications of impending cardiovascular collapse such as incoordination, mental confusion or loss of consciousness (Shephard 1977). Because of local hypertrophy of the limb muscles, muscle fatigue is less likely in those who are well trained. Wheelchair athletes, for example, can use the greatly hypertrophied muscles of their arms and shoulder girdles to develop as large a maximal oxygen intake as an average person can produce when running on the treadmill. Acquired skill is a further important consideration. Thus, the experienced cyclist uses toe clips and oscillatory movements of the body mass against the handlebars to distribute effort over a large fraction of the total muscle mass, avoiding local problems of quadriceps fatigue.

During some types of heavy dynamic work, the volume of active muscle is very small. The intensity of effort that is demanded then approaches maximal voluntary force very quickly. Local blood flow becomes entirely occluded, and a peripheral limitation of exercise is the norm (Shephard et al. 1988).

Even if a sport does involve use of a large fraction of the total muscle mass, the distinction between a central and a peripheral limitation of endurance performance becomes less clear cut as the determinants of cardiac output are considered. Determinants include preloading of the ventricles, myocardial contractility, the chronotropic response of the heart and the afterloading of the ventricles. Preloading reflects the rate of venous return to the heart. Thus, in wheelchair athletes with muscular paralysis, a loss of the muscle pump may cause blood to accumulate in the paralysed limbs, reducing preloading and restricting cardiac output (Shephard 1990; Glaser 1992). The sympathetically controlled increase of myocardial contractility quickly augments the stroke volume during exercise, and the chronotropic increase in heart rate is also mediated largely via sympathetic β-receptors. However, some authors have argued that local, limb-specific peripheral responses to training can play an important role in modulating the extent of these responses. Perhaps there is less peripheral stimulation of ergoreceptors as the active muscles become stronger, or perhaps there is a reduction of central command to the working muscles and thus a lesser irradiation of impulses to the cardiovascular control centres in the brain. Finally, the extent of afterloading, the force opposing ventricular emptying, is strongly influenced by the exercise-induced rise in systemic blood pressure; this depends in turn on the fraction of the maximal voluntary force which is exerted by the working muscles, and thus on the local muscular strength (Shephard 1982). From many points of view, the distinction between central and peripheral limitation is thus somewhat arbitrary, and tends to be a matter of semantics.

Acknowledgement

The studies of Dr Shephard are supported in part by research grants from the Defence and Civil Institute of Environmental Medicine, Toronto, ON.

References

Antonutto, G. & DiPrampero, P.E. (1995) The concept of lactate threshold. A short review. *Journal of Sports Medicine and Physical Fitness* **35**, 6–12.

Armstrong, R.B. (1986) Muscle damage and endurance events. *Sports Medicine* **3**, 370–381.

Bangsbo, J., Graham, T., Johansen, L. & Saltin, B. (1994) Muscle lactate metabolism in recovery from intense exhaustive exercise: impact of light exercise. *Journal of Applied Physiology* **77**, 1890–1895.

Banister, E. (1971) Energetics of muscular contraction. In: Shephard, R.J. (ed.) *Frontiers of Fitness*, pp. 5–36. C.C. Thomas, Springfield, IL.

Bigland-Ritchie, B. (1990) Discussion: nervous system and sensory adaptation. In: Bouchard C., Shephard, R.J., Stephens, T., Sutton, J. & McPherson, B. (eds) *Exercise, Fitness and Health*, pp. 377–384. Human Kinetics, Champaign, IL.

Bonen, A. & McCullagh, K.J.A. (1994) Effects of exercise on lactate transport into mouse skeletal muscles. *Canadian Journal of Applied Physiology* **19**, 275–285.

Bülow, J. (1987) Regulation of lipid mobilization in exercise. *Canadian Journal of Sport Sciences* **12** (Suppl. 1), 117S–119S.

Conlee, R.K. (1986) Muscle glycogen and exercise endurance. *Exercise and Sport Sciences Reviews* **15**, 1–28.

Convertino, V.A. (1987) Fluid shifts and hydration state: effects of long-term exercise. *Canadian Journal of Sport Sciences* **12** (Suppl. 1), 136S–139S.

Costill, D.L. (1972) Physiology of marathon running. *Journal of the American Medical Association* **221**, 1024–1029.

Dawson, M.J., Smith, S. & Wilkie, D.R. (1986) The [$H_2PO_4^{-1}$] may determine cross-bridge cycling rate and force production in living fatiguing muscle. *Biophysics Journal* **49**, 268a.

Fitts, R.H. & Metzger, J.M. (1993) Mechanisms of muscular fatigue. In: Poortmans, J.R. (ed.) *Principles of Exercise Biochemistry*, 2nd edn, pp. 248–268. Karger, Basel.

Gladden, L.B. (1989) Lactate uptake by skeletal muscle. *Exercise and Sport Sciences Reviews* **17**, 115–156.

Glaser, R.M. (1992) Cardiovascular problems of the wheelchair disabled. In: Shephard, R.J. & Miller, H.S. (eds) *Exercise and the Heart in Health and Disease*, pp. 467–500. Marcel Dekker, New York.

Gledhill, N. (1984) Bicarbonate ingestion and anaerobic performance. *Sports Medicine* **1**, 177–180.

Granier, P.L., Dubouchard, H., Mercier, B.M., Mercier, J.G., Ahmaidi, S. & Préfaut, C. (1996) Effect of $NaHCO_3$ on lactate kinetics in forearm muscles during leg exercise in man. *Medicine and Science in Sports and Exercise* **28**, 692–697.

Green, H.J. (1987) Neuromuscular aspects of fatigue. *Canadian Journal of Sport Sciences* **12** (Suppl. 1), 7S–19S.

Greenhaff, P.L., Hultman, E. & Harris, R.C. (1993) Carbohydrate metabolism. In: Poortmans, J.R. (ed.) *Principles of Exercise Biochemistry*, 2nd edn, pp. 89–136. Karger, Basel.

Hellsten, Y. (1996) Adenine nucleotide metabolism—a role for free radical generation and protection? In: Marconnet, P., Saltin, B., Komi, P.V. & Poortmans, J.R. (eds) *Human Muscular Function During Dynamic Exercise*, pp. 102–120. Karger, Basel.

Hultman, E. (1971) Muscle glycogen stores and prolonged exercise. In: Shephard, R.J. (ed.) *Frontiers of Fitness*, pp. 37–60. C.C. Thomas, Springfield, IL.

Hultman, E. (1978) Regulation of carbohydrate metabolism in the liver during rest and exercise, with special reference to diet. In: Landry, F. & Orban, W.A.R. (eds) *Third International Symposium on the Biochemistry of Exercise*, pp. 99–126. Symposia Specialists, Miami, FL.

Jackson, M.J. (1996) Oxygen radical production and muscle damage during running exercise. In: Marconnet, P., Saltin, B., Komi, P.V. & Poortmans, J. (eds) *Human Muscular Function During Dynamic Exercise*, pp. 121–133. Karger, Basel.

Karlsson, J. (1979) Localized muscular

fatigue: role of muscle metabolism and substrate depletion. *Exercise and Sport Sciences Reviews* **7**, 1–42.

Keast, D., Cameron, K. & Morton, A.R. (1988) Exercise and the immune response. *Sports Medicine* **5**, 248–267.

Kinsman, R.A., Weiser, P.C. & Stamper, D.A. (1973) Multidimensional analysis of subjective symptomatology during prolonged strenuous exercise. *Ergonomics* **16**, 211–226.

Komi, P.V. & Tesch, P. (1979) EMG frequency spectrum, muscle structure, and fatigue during dynamic contractions in man. *European Journal of Applied Physiology* **42**, 41–50.

LaPerrière, A., Ironson, G., Antoni, M.T., Schneiderman, N., Klimas, N. & Fletcher, M.A. (1994) Exercise and psychoneuroimmunology. *Medicine and Science in Sports and Exercise* **26**, 182–190.

McCullagh, K.J.A. & Bonen, A. (1995) L (+)-lactate binding to a protein in rat skeletal muscle plasma membranes. *Canadian Journal of Applied Physiology* **20**, 112–124.

McCutcheon, L.J., Byrd, S.K. & Hodgson, D.R. (1992) Ultrastructural changes in skeletal muscle after fatiguing exercise. *Journal of Applied Physiology* **72**, 1111–1117.

MacLaren, D.P., Gibson, H., Parry-Billings, M. & Edwards, R.H.T. (1989) A review of metabolic and physiological factors in fatigue. *Exercise and Sport Sciences Reviews* **17**, 29–66.

Murray, R. (1987) The effects of consuming carbohydrate–electrolyte beverages on gastric emptying and fluid absorption during and following exercise. *Sports Medicine* **4**, 322–351.

Nadel, E.R. (1977) *Problems with Temperature Regulation During Exercise*. Academic Press, New York.

Nadel, E.R. (1987) Prolonged exercise at high and low ambient temperatures. *Canadian Journal of Sport Sciences* **12** (Suppl. 1), 140S–142S.

Newsholme, E.A. (1983) Control of metabolism and the integration of fuel supply for the marathon runner. In: Knuttgen, H.G., Vogel, J.A. & Poortmans, J. (eds)

Biochemistry of Exercise, pp. 144–150.
Human Kinetics, Champaign, IL.

Newsholme, E., Parry-Billings, M.,
McAndrew, N. & Budgett, R. (1991) A
biochemical mechanism to explain some
characteristics of overtraining. *Medicine
and Science in Sports and Exercise* 32,
79–93.

Nicol, C. & Komi, P.V. (1996) Neuromuscu-
lar fatigue in stretch-shortening cycle
exercises. In: Marconnet, P., Saltin, B.,
Komi, P.V. & Poortmans, J.R. (eds)
*Human Muscular Function During
Dynamic Exercise*, pp. 134–148. Karger,
Basel.

Oscai, L.B. & Palmer, W.K. (1988) Muscle
lipolysis during exercise: an up-date.
Sports Medicine 6, 23–28.

Pandolf, K.B. (1983) Advances in the study
and application of perceived exertion.
Exercise and Sport Sciences Reviews 11,
118–158.

Pedersen, B.K. (1997) *Exercise Immunology*.
Chapman & Hall, London.

Pilegaard, H., Bangsbo, J., Richter, E.A. &
Juel, C. (1994) Lactate transport studied
in sarcolemmal giant vesicles from
human muscle biopsies: relation to training status. *Journal of Applied Physiology*
77, 1858–1862.

Poortmans, J.R. (1985) Effects of long-
lasting exercise and training on protein
metabolism. In: Howald, H. & Poortmans, J.R. (eds) *Metabolic Adaptations to
Prolonged Physical Exercise*, pp. 212–228.
Birkhäuser Verlag, Basel.

Reading, J., Goodman, J., Plyley, M. *et al.*
(1993) Relationship of skeletal muscle
vascular conductance to aerobic power
and left ventricular function. Data for
sedentary patients, endurance athletes
and patients with congestive failure.
Journal of Applied Physiology 74, 567–573.

Rogers, M.A., Stull, G.A. & Apple, F.S.
(1985) Creatine kinase isoenzyme activities in men and women following a
marathon race. *Medicine and Science in
Sports and Exercise* 17, 679–682.

Rowell, L.B. (1986) *Human Circulation:
Regulation During Physical Stress*. Oxford
University Press, New York.

Saltin, L.B. (1964) Aerobic work capacity
and circulation at exercise in man. *Acta
Physiologica Scandinavica* 62 (Suppl.), 230.

Savard, G., Kiens, B. & Saltin, B. (1987)
Limb blood flow in prolonged exercise:
magnitude and implications for cardiovascular control during muscular work
in man. *Canadian Journal of Sport Sciences*
12 (Suppl. 1), 89S–101S.

Senay, L.C. & Pivarnik, J.M. (1985) Fluid
shifts during exercise. *Exercise and Sport
Sciences Reviews* 13, 335–387.

Shephard, R.J. (1976) A new look at aerobic
power. In: Jokl, E., Anand, R.L. & Stoboy,
H. (eds) *Medicine and Sport*, Vol. 9, pp.
61–84. Karger Publishing, Basel.

Shephard, R.J. (1977) *Endurance Fitness*,
2nd edn. University of Toronto Press,
Toronto.

Shephard, R.J. (1982) *Physiology and Biochemistry of Exercise*. Praeger Publications, New York.

Shephard, R.J. (1984) *Biochemistry of Physical Activity*. C.C. Thomas, Springfield, IL.

Shephard, R.J. (1990) *Fitness in Special
Populations*. Human Kinetics, Champaign, IL.

Shephard, R.J. (1994) *Aerobic Fitness and
Health*. Human Kinetics, Champaign, IL.

Shephard, R.J. (1997) *Physical Activity,
Training and the Immune Response*.
Cooper Publications, Carmel, IN.

Shephard, R.J. & Leatt, P. (1987) Carbohydrate and fluid needs of the soccer
player. *Sports Medicine* 4, 164–176.

Shephard, R.J. & Shek, P.N. (1998) Immune
responses to inflammation and trauma: a
physical training model. *Canadian
Journal of Physiology and Pharmacology* 76
469–472.

Shephard, R.J., Bouhlel, E., Vandewalle,
H. & Monod, H. (1988) Muscle mass
as a factor limiting physical work.
Journal of Applied Physiology 64, 1472–
1479.

Simonson, E. (1971) *Physiology of Work
Capacity and Fatigue*. C.C. Thomas,
Springfield, IL.

Sjögaard, G., Adams, R.B. & Saltin, B.
(1985) Water and ion shifts in skeletal
muscle of humans with intense dynamic
knee extension. *American Journal of
Physiology* 248, R190–R196.

Thompson, L.V. & Fitts, R.V. (1992) Muscle
fatigue in the frog semi-tendinosus;
role of high energy phosphate and P_i.
American Journal of Physiology 263, C803–
C809.

Wahren, J. & Björkman, O. (1981) Hormones, exercise and regulation of
splanchnic glucose output in normal
man. In: Poortmans, J. & Nisset, G. (eds)
Biochemistry of Exercise, IVa. University
Park Press, Baltimore.

Westerblad, H., Lee, J.A., Lännergren, J. &
Allen, D.G. (1990) Spatial gradients of
intracellular calcium in skeletal muscle
during fatigue. *Pflügers Archives* 415,
734–740.

Winder, W. (1985) Regulation of hepatic
glucose production during exercise.
Exercise and Sport Sciences Reviews 13,
1–32.

Wyndham, C. & Strydom, N.B. (1972) Kör-
perliche Arbeit bei höher Temperatur. In:
Hollmann, W. (ed.) *Zentrale Themen der
Sport Medizin*, pp. 131–149. Springer-
Verlag, Berlin.

Chapter 4

Body Size and Endurance Performance

JOEY C. EISENMANN AND ROBERT M. MALINA

Introduction

Many of the same questions that we ask today about body size and sports performance were addressed a century ago by one of the first 'exercise scientists', Harvard professor of physical training, Dudley A. Sargent (Carter & Heath 1990). The main question was, 'Are there certain structural (anthropometric) requirements for various sports?' The general hypothesis is that body size and physique are important selective factors necessary for élite performance in a particular sport (Tanner 1964; Carter 1970).

Successful athletes in many sports or in specific events within a sport often have many morphological characteristics in common. Further, 'ideal' values for a given sport are based upon reported values for élite performers and are often used to predict success in a given sport. Although the ideal values appear to cluster around the mean of a given morphological parameter, interindividual variability is considerable. Given such variability, what are the consequences of body size for endurance performance? This chapter provides an overview of the anthropometric characteristics of endurance athletes in several sports and then discusses the issue of scaling body size for differences in endurance performance. The adult and child endurance athletes are considered. 'Endurance' refers to the ability of the organism to maintain muscular activity for a period of time that depends upon aerobic metabolism as the predominant energy system.

Assessment of body size and physique

The size and shape of the body can be measured with a series of systematized techniques that comprise anthropometry (Malina 1995). The number of measurements that can be taken on an individual is almost limitless. However, the selection of measurements should depend on the purpose of the study and the specific questions under consideration. In this chapter, we focus on overall body size and physique, although many other measures such as segment lengths, skeletal breadths, circumferences and skinfold thicknesses, and various ratios and proportions have been described for athletes in a variety of sports.

Several methodological issues must be considered in reviewing studies of the anthropometric characteristics of athletes. Some include self-report of body size, equipment, inter- and intraobserver measurement reliability, and diurnal variation. These issues may be especially relevant when considering the stature and body mass of Olympic athletes as reported in the descriptive summaries for each sport at specific Olympic competitions. Although anthropometry is quite easy, it is often taken for granted and used without considering its limitations.

Physique is an individual's body form, the configuration of the entire body. The assessment of physique is most often expressed as the somatotype, which consists of three components: endomorphy (predominance of roundness of contours throughout the body); mesomorphy (predominance of muscularity); and ectomorphy (predominance of linearity). It should be emphasized that the somatotype should be treated as a unit, i.e. the contributions of endomorphy, mesomorphy and ectomorphy should be considered together and not in isolation. Most of the somatotype data used in this chapter are from Carter and Heath (1990). The Heath–Carter anthropometric protocol is the method of estimating somatotype most commonly used in studying athletes.

Anthropometric characteristics of adult endurance athletes

Mean stature and body mass vary among endurance athletes in different endurance sports (Tables 4.1 & 4.2; Fig. 4.1a,b). Although certain events in swimming constitute endurance activity, studies often fail to stratify by distance. Body size and physique differ among élite short-, middle- and long-distance swimmers (Table 4.3). Therefore, only a limited number of studies of swimmers are reported here.

Among endurance athletes in a particular sport, mean values are similar. The stature and body mass of rowers and swimmers are the greatest, while body size is smallest in distance runners. Based on a model of the effects of gravity on endurance performance, Tittel and Wutscherk (1992) suggested that

Table 4.1 Age, body size and physique of adult male endurance athletes.

Sample	Number	Age (years)	Stature (m)	Mass (kg)	Somatotype
Cyclists					
Mexico City Olympics, 1968	67	24.0 (3.4)	1.75 (0.07)	68.7 (6.9)	1.8–4.9–2.7 0.5–0.8–0.7
British Olympic Squad, 1982	14	22.4	1.76 (0.07)	68.4 (5.8)	1.6–4.2–2.8 0.3–1.1–0.8
Cuba, 1976–80	16	21.5 (3.9)	1.72 (0.04)	65.8 (4.8)	2.0–4.8–2.5 0.4–0.7–0.6
Rowing					
Mexico City Olympics, 1968	85	24.3 (3.3)	1.85 (0.06)	82.6 (7.4)	2.1–5.3–2.4 0.6–0.9–0.8
Montreal Olympics, 1976	65	24.2 (3.3)	1.91 (0.06)	90.0 (5.6)	2.3–5.0–2.7 0.6–0.9–0.8
Cuba, 1976–80	24	22.2 (2.3)	1.87 (0.04)	86.3 (4.0)	2.3–5.3–2.5 0.6–0.8–0.6
South Australia					
Heavyweight	7	24.7 (1.9)	1.92 (0.04)	88.7 (4.7)	2.0–5.2–3.0 0.5–0.7–0.5
Lightweight	5	21.3 (2.4)	1.82 (0.03)	72.0 (4.1)	2.1–4.3–3.4 0.2–0.4–0.7
World Championships, 1985 (lightweight)	144	24.3 (3.3)	1.81 (0.04)	70.3 (1.9)	1.6–4.0–3.4 0.3–0.8–0.7
San Diego State University, 1967	21	20.2	1.84	79.8	2.7–5.1–2.6
USA Olympic Trials, 1968					
Singles	11	25.0 (4.0)	1.86 (0.08)	84.9 (6.7)	2.3–5.9–2.5 0.7–0.8–0.7
Eights	32	21.6 (1.4)	1.91 (0.03)	88.6 (4.7)	2.1–5.3–2.7 0.4–0.5–0.6

Continued

Table 4.1 *(Continued)*

Sample	Number	Age (years)	Stature (m)	Mass (kg)	Somatotype
New Zealand National Team, 1967–68	16	24.8 (2.3)	1.87 (0.05)	85.6 (5.1)	2.5–5.2–2.5
Distance running					
Mexico City Olympics, 1968*					
800–1500 m	41	22.9 (3.0)	1.77 (0.06)	65.0 (5.6)	1.5–4.2–3.6
					0.2–0.6–0.7
3000–10 000 m	34	25.3 (4.5)	1.72 (0.05)	59.8 (5.4)	1.4–4.1–3.6
					0.5–0.7–0.9
Marathon	20	26.4 (4.8)	1.69 (0.06)	56.6 (3.7)	1.4–4.3–3.5
					0.5–0.8–0.9
US, 1977†					
Distance	11		1.76 (0.05)	63.1 (5.3)	
Marathon	8		1.77 (0.06)	62.1 (3.7)	
Bulgaria (élite)‡					
Marathon	53		1.73 (0.06)	64.3 (6.4)	2.0–4.7–3.0
					0.5–0.9–1.0
Cross-country skiing					
Czechoslovakia, 1968	46	25.2	1.75 (0.04)	70.6 (5.1)	1.7–6.3–2.0
					0.6–0.7–0.7
European, 1976	26	22.1	1.76 (0.05)	69.3 (6.3)	1.9–5.3–2.8
US National Team, 1975	11	22.8 (1.9)	1.79 (0.05)	71.8 (5.4)	2.0–4.5–3.0
					0.5–0.4–0.3
Bulgaria (élite), 1984	30	21.7	1.77	70.0	2.1–5.4–2.7
Triathlon					
USA National Team, 1984	7	28.9 (3.2)	1.83 (0.03)	75.6 (4.3)	1.7–4.3–3.1
					0.6–0.3–0.6
US, 1989§	9	28.7	1.82	73.8	
	25	27.2	1.76	69.4	
	9	27.6	1.79	72.8	
	8	30.5	1.79	74.7	
	10	30.5	1.82	76.6	
Swimming					
World Championships, 1991¶					
1500 m	10	19.5	1.83	74.3	1.5–4.8–3.4
25 km	13	22.0	1.80	78.1	2.5–5.3–2.3
Bulgaria (élite)‡	16		1.75 (0.06)	65.0 (9.3)	2.1–4.0–3.2
					0.6–1.1–1.1

All values are adapted from Carter and Heath (1990) except as indicated.

Mean (SD) except for somatotype where SD is indicated below the mean.

* Data from de Garay *et al.* (1974).

† Data from Pollock *et al.* (1977).

‡ Data from Toteva (1992).

§ As reported in Roalstad (1989).

¶ Data from Carter and Ackland (1994).

Table 4.2 Age, body size and physique of adult female endurance athletes.

Sample	Number	Age (years)	Stature (m)	Mass (kg)	Somatotype
Rowing					
Montreal Olympics, 1976	51	23.8 (2.7)	1.74 (0.05)	67.4 (5.3)	3.1–3.9–2.8 0.8–0.9–0.8
World Championships, 1985	50	24.1 (3.7)	1.67	57.1 (2.0)	2.4–3.0–3.5 0.8–1.1–1.0
Distance running					
England, 1983 'élite' marathon	11	29.4 (7.6)	1.66 (0.04)	54.7 (5.6)	2.8–3.6–4.6 0.5–0.8–0.6
Brighton Polytechnic, 1986	5		1.67 (0.03)	55.0 (5.8)	2.7–3.6–4.1 1.0–0.9–1.0
San Diego, 1981					
Eumenorrhoeic	23	29.4 (6.6)	1.66 (0.06)	54.2 (5.9)	3.0–3.2–3.5 1.0–0.9–0.8
Oligoamenorrhoeic	16	25.1 (6.3)	1.65 (0.07)	50.4 (6.2)	2.6–2.8–4.1 0.8–1.1–1.0
University of Texas, 1985–95*	30	19.3 (1.2)	1.65 (0.05)	52.2 (3.7)	2.4–2.8–3.7 0.6–0.8–1.0
Cross-country skiing					
USA, 1976	5	23.5 (4.7)	1.64 (0.03)	53.9 (1.1)	3.5–4.3–2.3 0.7–0.5–0.8
Triathlon					
Southern California, 1987	16	24.2 (4.3)	1.62 (0.06)	55.2 (4.6)	3.1–4.3–2.6 1.0–0.8–0.9
US, 1989†	6	31.3	1.63	56.4	
	8	31.3	1.68	58.9	
Swimming					
University of Texas, 1985–95*	14	18.7 (0.8)	1.70 (0.05)	61.4 (5.0)	3.4–3.8–3.0 0.6–0.7–0.8
World Championships, 1991‡					
800 m	6	19.3	1.72	63.5	2.4–3.8–3.0
25 km	10	22.8	1.63	62.2	4.4–4.7–1.7
Bulgaria (élite)§	16		1.65 (0.04)	52.9 (6.6)	2.7–3.3–3.6 0.8–0.6–0.9

All values are adapted from Carter and Heath (1990) except as indicated.
Mean (SD) except for somatotype where SD is indicated below the mean.
*Unpublished data, Malina.
† As reported by Roalstad (1989).
‡ Data from Carter and Ackland (1994).
§ Data from Toteva (1992).

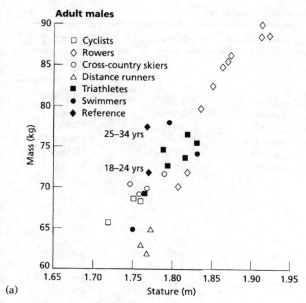

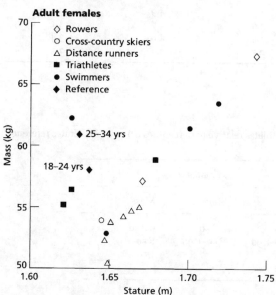

Fig. 4.1 (a,b) Distribution of male and female endurance athletes based on mean mass and stature.

endurance athletes are low in endomorphy, ranging from 1.4 in distance runners to 2.5 in rowers for males and from 2.4 in distance runners and rowers (lightweight) to 3.5 in cross-country skiers in females. Mesomorphy is lowest in distance runners and highest in cross-country skiers in both sexes. Ectomorphy is relatively similar in all groups of endurance athletes, but distance runners generally have the highest ratings.

Anthropometric characteristics of child and adolescent endurance athletes

Two other questions proposed by Sargent that are still of interest today include, 'Are body size parameters of child and adolescent endurance athletes comparable to adult endurance athletes?' and 'Can athletic success in adulthood be predicted during childhood or adolescence?' In general, studies of child and adolescent endurance athletes indicate that body size (Table 4.4) and physique (Malina 1994) resemble those of adult endurance athletes in the corresponding sports. However, the ability to predict future athletic ability assumes that growth in body size and physique is stable throughout childhood and adolescence. The stability of stature ($r = 0.8$) and mass ($r = 0.6$–0.8) tends to be moderately high to high and stable from the age of 2–3 years until early adulthood (Malina & Bouchard 1991), whereas the stability of somatotype during growth is only moderate ($r = 0.4$–0.6). Therefore, those interested in identifying young athletes on the basis of body size and physique alone need to be aware of the growth- and especially maturity-associated variation related to the timing and tempo of the adolescent growth spurt. Selection at an early age implies the exclusion of other potentially talented youth and, given the limited precision of talent identification and selection programmes, the exclusion factor needs to be considered carefully.

Another issue in the area of body size and endurance performance of child and adolescent athletes is whether intensive training during childhood and adolescence perturbs the processes of linear growth and biological maturation. Presently the available data for young athletes, including distance

the lowest values are seen in sports where the body mass acts in an unrestricted manner against gravity, whereas the highest values are in endurance sports that require a greater level of strength.

Mean somatotypes for endurance athletes also vary among sports (Tables 4.1 & 4.2). In general,

Table 4.3 Differences in body size and physique of swimmers stratified by distance.

Distance	Stature (m)	Mass (kg)	Endomorphy	Mesomorphy	Ectomorphy
*University**					
Females					
Sprint (*n* = 39)	1.74 (0.05)	64.2 (5.1)	2.8 (0.6)	3.7 (0.6)	3.2 (0.7)
	1.62–1.85	55.1–74.8	1.7–4.1	2.5–5.0	1.7–4.7
Middle (*n* = 34)	1.70 (0.06)	62.2 (5.1)	3.1 (0.6)	3.9 (0.7)	2.9 (0.7)
	1.56–1.84	50.3–72.6	1.9–4.4	2.7–5.7	1.0–4.4
Long (*n* = 14)	1.70 (0.05)	61.4 (5.0)	3.4 (0.6)	3.9 (0.7)	3.0 (0.8)
	1.61–1.78	53.3–70.8	2.3–4.8	2.7–5.1	1.5–4.5
World Championships, 1991†					
Females					
Sprint (*n* = 31)	1.74	65.0	2.8	3.7	3.2
Middle (*n* = 27)	1.74	64.6	2.9	3.7	3.2
Long (*n* = 6)	1.72	63.5	2.4	3.8	3.0
Ultra (*n* = 10)	1.63	62.2	4.4	4.7	1.7
Males					
Sprint (*n* = 47)	1.86	79.8	1.7	4.9	3.2
Middle (*n* = 34)	1.85	79.1	1.9	4.7	3.1
Long (*n* = 10)	1.83	74.3	1.5	4.8	3.4
Ultra (*n* = 13)	1.80	78.1	2.5	5.3	2.3

*Unpublished data, Malina. Mean (SD) and range provided.
†Means from Carter and Ackland (1994).

Table 4.4 Stature and mass of child and adolescent endurance athletes relative to percentiles (P) of United States reference data. Based on data reported in Malina (1994, 1998).

Sport	Males		Females	
	Stature	Mass	Stature	Mass
Distance running	P 50±	≤ P 50	≥ P 50	< P 50
Swimming	P 50–P 90	> P 50–P 90	P 50–P 90	P 50–P 90
Cycling	> P 50	± P 50		
Rowing/canoeing	> P 50	> P 50		

runners, do not meet epidemiological criteria allowing us to assert that any relationship between training and growth and maturation has a causal basis (Malina 1998).

Individual variability

Although typical values for body size and physique may assist in identifying and developing athletes, one must also recognize the variability in body size and physique among élite performers. For example, the range of body size of long-distance (3000–10 000 m) runners in the 1968 Mexico City Olympics was considerable (Table 4.5). Researchers in the sport sciences, as a rule, have tended to emphasize analysis of central tendencies in studies of élite athletes. In this context, the mean values quite often become the main focus of analysis and comparison,

Table 4.5 Range of body size and somatotype variables for male long-distance (3000–10 000 m) runners from the 1968 Mexico City Olympics. Data from de Garay *et al.* (1974).

Variable	Minimum	Maximum
Stature (m)	1.56	1.86
Mass (kg)	48.7	71.7
Endomorphy	1.0	3.0
Mesomorphy	2.5	5.5
Ectomorphy	1.5	5.0

and variation surrounding the means is overlooked. This is especially apparent when considering the body size and shape of athletes. By focusing on 'the tyranny of the Golden Mean', interesting biological problems and questions may be overlooked (Bennett 1987).

Some physiological and biomechanical considerations of body size and endurance performance

In the two-compartment model of body composition, body mass is divided into estimated fat-free mass (FFM) and fat mass. The various methods and limitations of body composition assessment are beyond the scope of this discussion (see Roche *et al.* 1996 and Chapter 24). Values for the absolute and relative fat mass of endurance athletes are rather low compared to other athletes (Houtkooper & Going 1994). It is reasonable to assume that excess body fatness has a negative influence on locomotion, since it increases the 'non-functional' load (i.e. the increased mass does not contribute to the ability to generate neuromuscular force). Cureton *et al.* (1978) examined the effects of an increased load (i.e. weight belt) on the physiological response to exercise and performance. Treadmill time to exhaustion, $\dot{V}O_{2max}$ and 12-min run performance decreased linearly when increasing loads (5, 10 and 15% additional external weight) were worn. By inference, excess body mass has a negative influence on running performance.

The thermoregulatory properties of an individual exercising in a hot environment are also modified adversely by an increase in fat mass. The thermal conductivity and rate of heat flow are lower in fat tissue than in other tissues, including skin (see Chapter 17). From a thermoregulatory perspective, the surface area of the body may also be an important consideration, since an increased surface area allows for greater heat transfer to the external environment.

Among the groups examined in this chapter, rowers are the largest. In this sport, the ability to generate force against an external resistance (i.e. water) is necessary. Therefore, the higher body masses of these athletes probably reflect an increased FFM. On the other hand, athletes in other sports require the translocation of the body, where higher values of body mass (and FFM) may affect endurance performance adversely (Cureton *et al.* 1978).

Implications

The implications of body size for endurance performance highlight the limitations of human performance and sport selection. Given the general characteristics of body size among and between endurance athletes, and the results of experimental studies that have manipulated body mass, 'ideal' values are only suggestive of the requirements for optimal performance in a given endurance sport.

Does scaling for body size affect endurance performance or the interpretation of endurance performance?

The size and shape of the body influence several physiological variables that are important for performance (Schmidt-Nielsen 1984). A relevant question is, 'How should performance be compared among animals (humans) of various sizes?' In this context, the biological principle of scaling is central. Scaling can be defined as the structural and functional consequences of changes in size or scale among otherwise similar organisms (Schmidt-Nielsen 1984). The historical background and basic principles of scaling, and the scaling of submaximal and maximal oxygen consumption ($\dot{V}O_{2submax}$ and $\dot{V}O_{2max}$, respectively) and endurance performance are briefly reviewed. $\dot{V}_{O_{2submax}}$ and $\dot{V}_{O_{2max}}$ were chosen since they are two main determinants of endurance performance (Coyle 1995 and Chapter 3).

Basic principles and historical background of scaling

The concept of scaling is a fundamental principle of engineering and a basic concept in the zoological sciences, particularly among comparative mammalian physiologists. Such investigators regard it as a cornerstone in the search for unifying principles among animals of differing body mass (M_b) and shape (White 1987). Engineers have long recognized that when the size of a structure is increased, three parameters could possibly change—the dimensions, the materials or the design of the structure. In animals, linear dimensions and body mass can easily be measured.

The principles of scaling are based on dimensionality theory, where surface area is proportional to the volume raised to the 2/3 power. Thus, as the volume of a body increases, its surface area does not increase in the same proportion, but rather as the 2/3 power of the volume. However, this argument holds only for an isometric body; animals are not isometric, since certain proportions change in a regular fashion. Non-isometric scaling is referred to as allometric scaling (Schmidt-Nielsen 1984).

A fundamental question related to scaling is, 'How should differences in body size be partitioned mathematically or statistically?' Several authors have addressed this question (Smith 1984; Winter 1992, 1996; Nevill 1997). Traditionally, exercise physiologists have expressed physiological measurements as a ratio standard (i.e. $\dot{V}_{O_2}$ as $ml \cdot kg^{-1} \cdot min^{-1}$). About 50 years ago, Tanner (1949) addressed the theoretically fallacious and misleading practice of expressing physiological measurements per unit of body mass or per unit of surface area. Although acknowledged periodically thereafter, the issue of scaling of $\dot{V}_{O_2}$ has not been systematically addressed in humans until recently (Winter 1992, 1996; Nevill 1997). Nevertheless, the use of ratio standards remains common in exercise science.

Perhaps, this question can best be answered by the following three points made by Packard and Boardman (1987) in a critical review of the use and misuse of ratios in ecological physiology:

1 biologists were influenced by competent biometricians to use ratio standards to scale physiological data;

2 ratios are easy to compute; and

3 it is hard to imagine that ratios can be misleading, because they are so easy to compute and comprehend.

Due to the theoretical and statistical limitations of the ratio standard, other statistical methods including linear regression, analysis of covariance (ANCOVA), allometric models, power functions and multilevel modelling have recently gained attention in the exercise sciences (Winter 1992, 1996; Baxter-Jones et al. 1993; Armstrong & Welsman 1994). The most widely used of these models is allometry. The allometric equation has the general form $y = ax^b$. In biological problems related to body size, the independent variable (x) is M_b so that the allometric equation is expressed as, $y = aM_b{}^b$. In the present context, aerobic energy metabolism or endurance performance represent y, or the dependent variable.

Early studies on a wide range of animals from rodent to elephant indicated that a scaling factor b of approximately 0.74 best describes the relationship between body size and resting metabolic rate (Kleiber 1932; Brody 1945). Taylor and Weibel (1981) (see also Taylor et al. 1981) used allometric scaling to compare the size of various structures in the oxygen transport system with $\dot{V}_{O_{2max}}$ in wild African and domestic mammals ranging from 0.5 kg (dwarf mongoose) to 263 kg (Zebu cattle). These authors found that $\dot{V}_{O_{2max}}$ scaled approximately to $M_b{}^{0.75}$.

An additional question is, 'When should allometry be used?' Calder (1987, p. 112) suggests that 'as useful as allometry may be, we lack general consensus on principles of its application'. To clarify the application of allometry, the following points have been emphasized by Schmidt-Nielsen (1984, p. 32).

1 Allometric equations are descriptive; they are not biological laws.

2 Allometric equations are useful for showing how a variable quantity is related to body size, all other things being equal.

3 Allometric equations are valuable tools because

they may reveal principles and connections that otherwise remain obscure.

4 Allometric equations are useful as a basis for comparisons and can reveal deviations from a general pattern.

5 Allometric equations are useful in estimating the expected magnitude of some variable for a given body size.

6 Allometric equations cannot be used to extrapolate beyond the range of the data on which they are based.

Body size and $\dot{V}O_{2max}$

$\dot{V}O_{2max}$ increases as a function of body size throughout the animal kingdom (Schmidt-Nielsen 1984). As noted above, $\dot{V}O_{2max}$ in wild and domestic mammals scales approximately proportionally to the theoretical value of $M_b^{0.75}$ (Taylor *et al.* 1981). In humans, the $\dot{V}O_{2max}$–body mass relationship also exists, particularly during growth and maturation (Fig. 4.2). Much of the attention on scaling $\dot{V}O_{2max}$ for body size has been directed at children and adolescents, given variation and change in body size associated

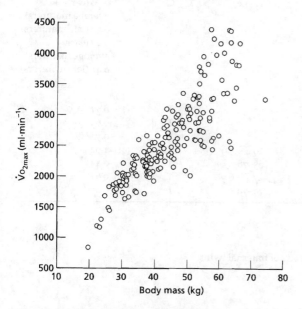

Fig. 4.2 The body size–$\dot{V}O_{2max}$ relationship in competitive young distance runners aged 8–18 years. Unpublished data from the Michigan State University Young Runners Study (1982–86), Institute for the Study of Youth Sports.

with growth and maturation. Table 4.6 provides a summary of reported scaling factors for $\dot{V}O_{2max}$ in children, adolescents and adults. Mean scaling factors for $\dot{V}O_{2max}$ range from 0.27 to 1.09. Fewer studies have examined the scaling of $\dot{V}O_{2max}$ in adults, but the results also show wide variability in the scaling exponent, ranging from 0.43 in older men to 1.02 in young adults.

An argument can be made that just as many scaling factors approximate $M_b^{1.0}$ as those that approximate the theoretical values of 0.67 and 0.75. This observation has led to the recommendation that $\dot{V}O_{2max}$ be expressed as a simple ratio standard in children and adolescents (Bar-Or 1983); indeed, the same recommendations could perhaps be extended to adults, based on the observations shown here. However, Armstrong and Welsman (1994) argue against the expression of $\dot{V}O_{2max}$ as a ratio standard for growth-related comparisons, stating that it clouds the understanding of growth and maturational changes in the oxygen transport system. The general understanding is that $\dot{V}O_{2max}$ expressed per unit body mass remains relatively stable during childhood and adolescence in boys and decreases with age in girls, particularly during adolescence (Fig. 4.3). To explore the growth-related changes in $\dot{V}O_{2max}$, Armstrong and colleagues (1994, 1998; Welsman *et al.* 1996, 1997) have used allometric scaling. Adjusted means (ANCOVA controlling for body mass) for $\dot{V}O_{2max}$ were similar between 10- and 15-year-old boys (2.21 and 2.30 l·min⁻¹, respectively). In a subsequent paper, a significant increase in $\dot{V}O_{2max}$ across prepubertal, circumpubertal and adult males, and between prepubertal and circumpubertal girls was noted when data were fitted by linear and log-linear allometric models adjusted for body mass (Welsman *et al.* 1996). Adjusted means were similar between circumpubertal and adult females, suggesting that $\dot{V}O_{2max}$ remains constant during this period. These results are intriguing, given past assumptions about growth-related changes in $\dot{V}O_{2max}$. Recently, Armstrong *et al.* (1998) also demonstrated a maturity-associated increase in $\dot{V}O_{2max}$ in 12-year-old boys and girls. Log-linear adjusted means increased from 2.01 to 2.30 l·min⁻¹ in boys and from 1.78 to 1.99 l·min⁻¹ in girls grouped by stage of pubic hair development.

Table 4.6 Summary of scaling factors for maximal oxygen intake ($\dot{V}_{O_2 max}$) in children and adolescents and in adults.

Study	Number	Sex	Age (years)	Mode	M_b exponent
Children and adolescents					
Cross-sectional					
Åstrand (1952)	68	M, F	6–17	T	0.95*
Cooper et al. (1984)	58	M	6–17	C	1.09
	51	F			0.83
	109	M, F			1.01
Rogers et al. (1995)	25	M, F	6.6–9.5		0.47
	27	M, F	11.1–14.2		0.62
Welsman et al. (1997)	32	M, F	9–10	T	0.52
Armstrong et al. (1998)	212	M, F	12	T	0.65
Mixed-longitudinal					
Eisenmann (unpublished data)	27	M	8–18	T	0.94
	27	F	8–18	T	0.83
Longitudinal					
Åstrand et al. (1963)	30	F	12–16		0.97‡
Daniels & Oldridge (1971)	14	M	10–15	T	1.07‡
Klissouras (1971)	50†		7–13		0.88‡
Bailey et al. (1978)	51	M	8–15	T	0.82*
Paterson et al. (1987)	18	M	11–15	T	1.02
Sjödin & Svedenhag (1992)	8 (trained)	M	11–15	T	1.01
	4 (untrained)	M			0.78
Beunen et al. (1997)	47	M	11–14	C	0.80 (early + average maturers) 0.57 (late maturers)
	31	F			0.27 (early + average maturers) 0.42 (late maturers)
Adults					
Bergh et al. (1991)	114	M, F	17–44	T	0.71
Nevill et al. (1992)	179	M	?	T	0.63
	129	F			0.72
Rogers et al. (1995)	29	M, F	20.4–25.9	T	1.02
Davies et al. (1995)	73	M	65–78	T	0.43
Vanderburgh et al. (1996)	94	F	27.4 + 6.7	T	0.61
Heil (1997)	440	M, F	20–79	T	0.65

M_b, body mass; C, cycle ergometer; T, treadmill.
Table adapted from Rowland (1996).
* As reported by Rowland (1996).
† 25 sets of twins including 15 pairs of identical twins and 10 pairs of fraternal twins.
‡ As estimated by McMiken (1976).

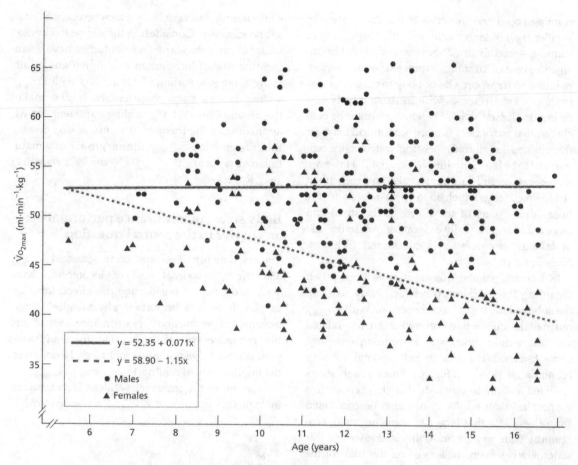

Fig. 4.3 Age-related changes in $\dot{V}O_{2max}$, expressed per unit of body mass, during childhood and adolescence. Data points represent mean values from published studies. Reproduced with permission from Krahenbuhl *et al.* (1985).

The preceding results are based on cross-sectional analyses. Thus, although the findings provide insight into the growth and maturation of the oxygen transport system, their implications for our understanding of growth- and maturity-related changes in endurance performance remain unknown. Evidence from a short-term longitudinal study on an 11–14-year age group suggests that among boys who are active in sport (track, wrestling, basketball), scaling $\dot{V}O_2$ for body mass and stature varies with the maturity status of the individual, and that there is considerable interindividual variation in scaling coefficients during early and mid-adolescence. In early and average maturing boys, $\dot{V}O_{2max}$ increases at a slightly higher rate

than expected from the increase in body mass, whereas in later maturing boys the increase is smaller than expected. In contrast, over this same age range, the increase of $\dot{V}O_{2max}$ in girls active in sport (track, rowing) is generally unrelated to the increase in body mass or stature (Beunen *et al.* 1997). These results, although limited to early and mid-adolescence, suggest maturity-associated variation in growth of the oxygen transport system.

Body size and submaximal energy cost of locomotion

Animal studies have indicated that $\dot{V}O_2$ per unit body mass per unit time is greater at a given running speed and increases to a greater extent in smaller than in larger animals with an increase of running speed (Schmidt-Nielsen 1984). Additionally, the cost of running, expressed as the oxygen required to transport 1 kg of body mass over a distance of 1 km, decreases with increasing body size (Schmidt-Nielsen 1984). Therefore, it might be concluded that movement is more economical in larger than in smaller animals, or simply, it is more economical to be big (Schmidt-Nielsen 1984). However, the energy cost of locomotion also depends upon stride frequency, which in turn is related to the linear dimensions of the limbs. Thus, small and large animals are equally economical, when the cost of taking a single step is considered (Schmidt-Nielsen 1984).

In humans, similar questions have been raised regarding the relationship between body size and the submaximal cost of locomotion. As with $\dot{V}O_{2max}$, much of the attention has centred on growth-related and adult–child differences in running economy. Growth-related changes in submaximal running economy are shown in Fig. 4.4. These observations have led authors to conclude that children are less economical than adults. It can also be concluded from these data that larger humans are more economical than smaller individuals. However, this statement has been challenged on the basis of the confounding effects of body size when expressed as a ratio standard. Considering the suggested limited utility of ratio standards, a few studies have examined the cost of locomotion in children and adults using allometric scaling (Table 4.7). As with $\dot{V}O_{2max}$, scaling factors vary considerably. If one makes the assumption that the scaling exponent for M_b approximates the theoretical values of 0.67 or 0.75, the difference in $\dot{V}O_{2submax}$ during growth and maturation disappears (Fig. 4.5) (Sjodin & Svedenhag 1992; Rogers et al. 1995).

Body size and endurance performance: an answer to the central question?

The relationships between body size and $\dot{V}O_{2max}$ and the submaximal cost of locomotion have been addressed. Considering the effects of scaling on these two important physiological determinants of endurance performance, what are the consequences of body size for endurance performance? Svedenhag (1995) recently reviewed the implications of scaling $\dot{V}O_{2max}$ and $\dot{V}O_{2submax}$ for evaluations of the endurance athlete. He suggested that whether $\dot{V}O_{2max}$ and $\dot{V}O_{2submax}$ are scaled to $M_b^{1.0}$

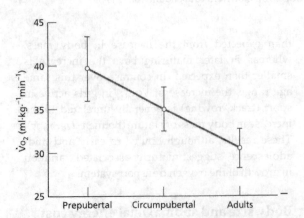

Fig. 4.4 Submaximal oxygen cost of running, expressed as ml·kg^{-1}·min^{-1}, at 8.0 km·h^{-1} in prepubertal and circumpubertal children, and adults. Data from Rogers et al. (1995).

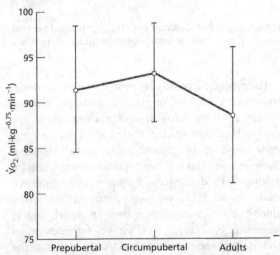

Fig. 4.5 Submaximal oxygen cost of running, expressed as ml·kg$^{-0.75}$·min^{-1}, at 8.0 km·h^{-1} in prepubertal and circumpubertal children, and adults. Data from Rogers et al. (1995).

Table 4.7 Summary of scaling factors for submaximal $\dot{V}_{O_2}$, or anaerobic/ventilatory threshold in children and adolescents and adults.

Study	Number	Sex	Age (years)	Mode	Intensity	M_b exponent
Children and adolescents						
Cross-sectional						
Cooper *et al.* (1984)	51	M	6–17	C	AT	0.99
	58	F				0.77
	109	M, F				0.92
Rogers *et al.* (1995)	25	M, F	6.6–9.5	T	8.0 km·h⁻¹*	0.74
	27	M, F	11.1–14.2			0.81
Longitudinal						
Paterson *et al.* (1987)	18	M	11–15	T	VT	1.13
Sjödin & Svedenhag (1992)	12	M	11–15	T	15 km·h⁻¹	0.75
Adults						
Bergh *et al.* (1991)	114	M, F	17–44	T	14 km·h⁻¹	0.76
Rogers *et al.* (1995)	29	M, F	20.4–25.9	T	8.0 km·h⁻¹*	0.96
Davies *et al.* (1997)	12	M	18–34	T	12.9 km·h⁻¹*	1.07
	12	F				0.86
	24	M, F				1.01

AT, anaerobic threshold; M_b, body mass; C, cycle ergometer; T, treadmill; VT, ventilatory threshold.
*Converted from mph, or m·min⁻¹ to km·h⁻¹.

Table 4.8 A comparison of two élite distance runners of differing body mass and the interpretation of submaximal and maximal $\dot{V}_{O_2}$ based on simple ratio standard and allometric scaling. See text for explanation. Adapted from Svedenhag (1995).

	Mass (kg)	FU (%)	$\dot{V}_{O_{2submax}}$		$\dot{V}_{O_{2max}}$	
			ml·kg⁻¹·min⁻¹	ml·kg⁻⁰·⁷⁵·min⁻¹	ml·kg⁻¹·min⁻¹	ml·kg⁻⁰·⁷⁵·min⁻¹
Runner A	80	75	55.5	166	74.0	221
Runner B	50	75	61.5	164	82.0	218

FU, fractional utilization ($\dot{V}_{O_{2submax}}/\dot{V}_{O_{2max}}$).

or $M_b^{0.75}$ may influence the evaluation of and the selection of a training programme for an endurance athlete (Table 4.8). In this example, Runners A and B have an equivalent fractional utilization of $\dot{V}_{O_2}$ (%$\dot{V}_{O_2}$) and similar performance levels. Based on the traditional ratio standard for $\dot{V}_{O_{2submax}}$ and $\dot{V}_{O_{2max}}$ (ml·kg⁻¹·min⁻¹), Runner A has a better running economy but a lower $\dot{V}_{O_{2max}}$, whereas Runner B has a poorer running economy and a higher $\dot{V}_{O_{2max}}$. This may lead a coach or athlete to manipulate training in

an attempt to improve upon the poorer functional capacity. In contrast, if values are expressed per unit $kg^{0.75}$, the runners have similar values, or perhaps results contrary to the initial analysis. Thus, scaling $\dot{V}_{O_{2submax}}$ and $\dot{V}_{O_{2max}}$ may influence the findings at evaluation and the resultant training programmes for endurance athletes.

However, the argument advanced by Svedenhag (1995) still does not answer the central question, 'How does scaling for body size affect endurance performance?' Vanderburgh *et al.* (1996) (see also Vanderburgh & Mahar 1995) have examined the application of allometric scaling to assessments of endurance performance in the 3.2-km (2-mile) run and indoor rowing. In a study of 59 male, college-age military cadets, a body mass coefficient of 0.40 was determined for the 3.2-km run. The authors suggest the use of allometric scaling as a tool for 'handicapping' in certain competitive events where age and body size may 'bias' results. In this regard, appropriate allowance would be made for differences in body size before evaluation of performance (Vanderburgh *et al.* 1996). If this principle was applied in competitive athletics, the athlete who crossed the finishing line first would not always be the winner, unless of course his/her time remained first after adjusting for body size! Such statistical manipulation of performance would detract from the selective pressures of athletics.

Conclusions

The general statement, 'he/she looks like an (endurance) athlete' has some basis. However, body size and physique are only two determinants of performance. Although available data suggest central tendencies for the size and physique of endurance athletes, variability also needs to be taken into consideration.

With regard to allometric scaling, body size is a confounder in understanding the structural and functional aspects of an organism. However, endurance performance *per se* should not be governed by the statistical adjustments of allometry. Absolute speed is the standard that is applied when evaluating locomotor performance for an individual who is competing in real time (Jones & Lindstedt 1993). Exercise scientists have been criticized for not recognizing the imperfections of ratio standards and being unaware of alternative methods for partitioning the effects of body size in human studies (Winter 1996), but it remains to be demonstrated that allometric scaling among a small magnitude of difference in body sizes warrants such statistical manipulation. According to Calder (1987, p. 116), 'small size ranges within species obscure overall trends, patterns, and constraints of size.' Thus, scaling differences in body size among a small range in body size to understand variation in biological function may be of limited value. In contrast, others argue that scaling body size helps us to understand the growth and maturation of the oxygen transport system, its response to submaximal and maximal exercise (Armstrong & Welsman 1994), and evaluations of endurance athletes (Svedenhag 1995). In turn, scaling may contribute to a better understanding of endurance performance as a whole.

References

Armstrong, N. & Welsman, J.R. (1994) Assessment and interpretation of aerobic fitness in children and adolescents. *Exercise and Sports Sciences Reviews* 22, 435–476.

Armstrong, N., Welsman, J. & Kirby, B. (1998) Peak oxygen uptake and maturation in 12-year olds. *Medicine and Science in Sports and Exercise* 30, 165–169.

Åstrand, P.O. (1952) *Experimental Studies of Physical Work Capacity in Relation to Sex and Age.* Ejnar Munksgaard, Copenhagen.

Åstrand, P.O., Engstrom, L., Eriksson, B.O., Karlberg, P., Nylander, I., Saltin, B. & Thoren, C. (1963) *Girl Swimmers.* Acta Paediatrica Scandinavica (Suppl. 147).

Bailey, D.A., Ross, W.D., Mirwald, R.L. & Weese, C. (1978) Size dissociation of maximal aerobic power during growth in boys. In: Borms, J. & Hebbelinck, M.

(eds.) *Medicine and Sport* (Vol. 11), pp. 140–151. S. Karger, Basel.

Bar-Or, O. (1983) *Pediatric Sports Medicine for the Practitioner.* Springer-Verlag, New York.

Baxter-Jones, A., Goldstein, H. & Helms, P. (1993) The development of aerobic power in young athletes. *Journal of Applied Physiology* 75, 1160–1167.

Bennett, A. (1987) Interindividual variability: an underutilized resource. In: Feder, M., Bennett, A., Burggren W. & Huey, R. (eds) *New Directions in Ecological Physiology,* pp. 147–166. Cambridge University Press, Cambridge.

Bergh, U., Sjödin, B., Forsberg, A. & Svedenhag, J. (1991) The relationship between body mass and oxygen uptake during running in humans. *Medicine and Science in Sports and Exercise* 23, 205–211.

Beunen, G.P., Rogers, D.M., Woynarowska,

B. & Malina, R.M. (1997) Longitudinal study of ontogenetic allometry of oxygen uptake in boys and girls grouped by maturity status. *Annals of Human Biology* 24, 33–43.

Brody, S. (1945) *Bioenergetics and Growth, with Special Reference to the Efficiency Complex in Domestic Animals.* Reinhold, New York.

Calder, W.A. (1987) Scaling energetics of homeothermic vertebrates: an operational allometry. *Annual Review of Physiology* 49, 107–120.

Carter, J.E.L. (1970) The somatotypes of athletes: a review. *Human Biology* 42, 535–569.

Carter, J.E.L. & Ackland, T.R. (1994) *Kinanthropometry in Aquatic Sports.* Human Kinetics, Champaign, IL.

Carter, J.E.L. & Heath, B.H. (1990) *Somatotyping—Development and Applications.*

Cambridge University Press, Cambridge.

Cooper, D.M., Weiler-Ravell, D., Whipp, B.J. & Wasserman, K. (1984) Aerobic parameters of exercise as a function of body size during growth in children. *Journal of Applied Physiology* 56, 628–634.

Coyle, E. (1995) Integration of the physiological factors determining endurance performance ability. *Exercise and Sport Sciences Reviews* 23, 25–63.

Cureton, K.J., Sparling, P.B., Evans, B.W., Johnson, S.M., Kong, U.D. & Purvis, J.W. (1978) Effect of experimental alterations in excess weight on aerobic capacity and distance running performance. *Medicine and Science in Sports* 10, 194–199.

Daniels, J.T. & Oldridge, N. (1971) Oxygen consumption and growth of young boys during running training. *Medicine and Science in Sports* 3, 161–165.

Davies, M.J., Dalsky, G.P. & Vanderburgh, P. (1995) Allometric scaling of $\dot{V}_{O_{2max}}$ by body mass and lean body mass in older men. *Journal of Aging and Physical Activity* 3, 324–331.

Davies, M.J., Maher, M.T. & Cunningham, L.N. (1997) Running economy: comparison of body mass adjustment methods. *Research Quarterly for Exercise and Sport* 68, 177–181.

de Garay, A.L., Levine, L. & Carter, J.E.L. (1974) *Genetic and Anthropological Studies of Olympic Athletes*. Academic Press, New York.

Heil, D.P. (1997) Body mass scaling of peak oxygen uptake in 20- to 79-yr-old adults. *Medicine and Science in Sports and Exercise* 29, 1602–1608.

Houtkooper, L.B. & Going, S.B. (1994) Body composition: how should it be measured? Does it affect sport performance? *Sport Sciences Exchange* 7, 33–42.

Jones, J. & Lindstedt, S. (1993) Limits to maximal performance. *Annual Review of Physiology* 55, 547–569.

Kleiber, M. (1932) Body size and metabolism. *Hilgardia* 6, 315–353.

Klissouras, V. (1971) Heritability of adaptive variation. *Journal of Applied Physiology* 31, 338–344.

Krahenbuhl, G.S., Skinner, J.S. & Kohrt, W.M. (1985) Developmental aspects of maximal aerobic power in children. *Exercise and Sport Sciences Reviews* 13, 503–538.

Malina, R.M. (1994) Physical growth and biological maturation of young athletes. *Exercise and Sport Sciences Reviews* 22, 389–433.

Malina, R.M. (1995) Anthropometry. In: Maud, P.J. & Foster, C. (eds) *Physiological Assessment of Human Fitness*, pp. 205–219. Human Kinetics, Champaign, IL.

Malina, R.M. (1998) Growth and maturation of young athletes— is training for sport a factor? In: Chan, K.M. & Micheli, L.J. (eds) *Sports and Children*, pp. 133–161. Williams & Wilkins, Hong Kong.

Malina, R.M. & Bouchard, C. (1991) *Growth, Maturation, and Physical Activity*. Human Kinetics, Champaign, IL.

McMiken, D.F. (1976) Maximum aerobic power and physical dimensions of children. *Annals of Human Biology* 3, 141–147.

Nevill, A. (1997) The appropriate use of scaling techniques in exercise physiology. *Pediatric Exercise Science* 9, 295–298.

Nevill, A.M., Ramsbottom, R. & Williams, C. (1992) Scaling physiological measurements for individuals of different body size. *European Journal of Applied Physiology* 65, 110–117.

Packard, G. & Boardman, T. (1987) The misuse of ratios to scale physiological data that vary allometrically with body size. In: Feder, M., Bennet, A., Burggren W. & Huey, R. (eds) *New Directions in Ecological Physiology*, pp. 216–236. Cambridge University Press, Cambridge.

Paterson, D., McLellan, T., Stella, R. & Cunningham, D. (1987) Longitudinal study of ventilation threshold and maximal O_2 uptake in athletic boys. *Journal of Applied Physiology* 62, 2051–2057.

Pollock, M.L., Gettman, L.R., Jackson, A., Ayres, J., Ward, A. & Linnerud, A.C. (1977) Body composition of élite class distance runners. *Annals of the New York Academy of Science* 301, 361–370.

Roalstad, M. (1989) Physiologic testing of the ultraendurance triathlete. *Medicine and Science in Sports and Exercise* 21, S200–S204.

Roche, A.F., Heysmfield, S.B. & Lohman, T.G. (eds) (1996) *Human Body Composition*. Human Kinetics, Champaign, IL.

Rogers, D.M., Olson, B.L. & Wilmore, J.H. (1995) Scaling for the $\dot{V}_{O_2}$-to-body size relationship among children and adults. *Journal of Applied Physiology* 79, 958–967.

Rowland, T.W. (1996) *Developmental Exercise Physiology*. Human Kinetics, Champaign, IL.

Schmidt-Nielsen, K. (1984) *Scaling: Why Is Animal Size So Important?* Cambridge University Press, Cambridge.

Sjödin, B. & Svedenhag, J. (1992) Oxygen uptake during running as related to body mass in circumpubertal boys: a longitudinal study. *European Journal of Applied Physiology* 65, 150–157.

Smith, R. (1984) Allometric scaling in comparative biology: problems of concept

and method. *American Journal of Physiology* 246, R152–R160.

Svedenhag, J. (1995) Maximal and submaximal oxygen uptake during running: how should body mass be accounted for? *Scandinavian Journal of Medicine and Science in Sports* 5, 175–180.

Tanner, J.M. (1949) Fallacy of per-weight and per-surface area standards, and their relation to spurious correlation. *Journal of Applied Physiology* 2, 1–15.

Tanner, J.M. (1964) *The Physique of the Olympic Athlete*. George Allen and Unwin, London.

Taylor, C.R. & Weibel, E.R. (1981) Design of the mammalian respiratory system. *Respiration Physiology* 44, 1–164.

Taylor, C.R., Maloiy, G.M.O., Weibel, E.W. et al. (1981) Scaling maximum aerobic capacity to body mass: wild and domestic mammals. *Respiration Physiology* 44, 3–37.

Tittel, K. & Wutscherk, H. (1992) Anatomical and anthropometric fundamentals of endurance. In: Shephard, R.J. & Åstrand, P.-O. (eds) *Endurance in Sport*, pp. 35–45. Blackwell Scientific Publications, Oxford.

Toteva, M. (1992) *Somatotyping in Sports*. National Sports Academy, Sofia (in Bulgarian).

Vanderburgh, P. & Mahar, M. (1995) Scaling of 2-mile run times by body weight and fat-free weight in college-age men. *Journal of Strength and Conditioning Research* 9, 67–70.

Vanderburgh, P., Katch, F., Schoenleber, J., Balabinis, C. & Elliott, R. (1996) Multivariate allometric scaling of men's world indoor rowing championship performance. *Medicine and Science in Sports and Exercise* 28, 626–630.

Welsman, J.R., Armstrong, N., Nevill, A.M., Winter, E.M. & Kirby, B.J. (1996) Scaling peak $\dot{V}_{O_2}$ for differences in body size. *Medicine and Science in Sports and Exercise* 28, 259–265.

Welsman, J.R., Armstrong, N., Kirby, B.J., Winsley, R.J., Parsons, G. & Sharpe, P. (1997) Exercise performance and magnetic resonance imaging-determined thigh muscle, in children. *European Journal of Applied Physiology* 76, 92–97.

White, F. (1987) Scaling and structure–function relationships. *Annual Review of Physiology* 49, 105–106.

Winter, E.M. (1992) Scaling: partitioning out differences in size. *Pediatric Exercise Science* 4, 296–301.

Winter, E.M. (1996) Importance and principles of scaling for size differences. In: Bar-Or, O. (ed.) *The Child and Adolescent Athlete*, pp. 673–679. Blackwell Science, Oxford.

Chapter 5

Pulmonary System and Endurance Exercise

THOMAS J. WETTER AND JEROME A. DEMPSEY

The main function of the pulmonary system is to ensure an adequate supply of oxygen and facilitate the removal of carbon dioxide from the body, thus maintaining homeostasis of arterial blood gases. During endurance exercise the pulmonary system fulfils this function even though carbon dioxide production may increase dramatically and oxygen saturation in mixed venous blood may fall to very low levels. Furthermore, it accomplishes the exchange of gases over a time that becomes increasingly short as total cardiac output and pulmonary blood flow increase with exercise intensity. The work required by the respiratory muscles to ensure adequate ventilation requires a substantial local oxygen delivery, blood supply and pressure-generating capacity that must be maintained throughout exercise. Failure in either the gas exchange or muscular component of the pulmonary system during exercise would reduce oxygen supply to and lead to acidification of the working muscles. We present an overview of basic responses of the pulmonary system to endurance exercise in terms of gas exchange, mechanics and ventilatory regulation. These topics have been covered in greater detail previously (Dempsey *et al.* 1988). The present review emphasizes two additional themes, namely: (i) limitations to effort and exercise performance that may occur as a result of inputs from the pulmonary system; and (ii) adaptations of the respiratory system to endurance exercise training and to specific training of the respiratory muscles.

Basic responses to exercise

Gas exchange

As exercise intensity increases from mild to moderate effort, alveolar ventilation ($\dot{V}_A$) must increase proportionally to prevent a build-up of carbon dioxide which would soon acidify the arterial blood; furthermore, the oxygen removed by working muscle must be replenished. Pulmonary capillary blood flow and blood volume increase and the alveolar to arterial oxygen difference widens. This widening with an increase in exercise intensity, however, has little effect on arterial blood gases; partial pressures of oxygen and carbon dioxide (Po_2 and Pco_2) stay fairly constant. The rise in $\dot{V}_A$ parallels the increase in carbon dioxide production until very strenuous exercise is reached, when alveolar hyperventilation develops and arterial Pco_2 falls. The effects of this last response are to buffer the decrease in pH as lactic acid production increases, and to prevent arterial hypoxaemia (this is essentially a respiratory compensation for metabolic acidosis). During prolonged exercise, gas exchange is well maintained in most cases; only occasionally does arterial Po_2 remain low throughout prolonged exercise requiring 70–85% of maximal oxygen intake ($\dot{V}o_{2max}$) (Dempsey *et al.* 1988). Blood pH generally remains near resting levels or can even become slightly alkaline with exercise of a long duration. This reflects a relatively steady circulating lactate level combined with increases in $\dot{V}_A$. Pulmonary arterial pressure increases at a slightly slower rate than pulmonary blood flow as exercise intensity is increased, and it may actually fall with prolonged exercise. The diffusing capacity of the lungs increases with exercise intensity, due to the recruitment of previously closed pulmonary capillaries and the dilatation of existing ones. Increases in pulmonary blood flow and alveolar–capillary surface area increase leakage of plasma into the interstitial fluid space during exercise, but increases in lymphatic drainage, the dilatation of the pulmonary vasculature and a fall in pressure over time, along with decreases in osmotic and hydrostatic pressure gradients, prevent fluid accumulation (O'Brodovich & Coates 1991). Even so, evidence for the accumulation of extravascular water or the narrowing of small airways has been found by some investigators after long-distance events such as a marathon and this has been proposed as evidence for a degree of pulmonary oedema; however, pulmonary oedema is likely only under extreme situations (McKechnie *et al.* 1979; Young *et al.* 1987) (see further, Chapter 46). Impairment of the pulmonary blood–gas barrier in élite athletes has recently been studied (Hopkins *et al.* 1997, 1998a); compared to non-exercising control subjects, higher concentrations of red blood cells and protein have been found in the bronchoalveolar lavage fluid of athletes after an acute bout of high-intensity effort but not after prolonged submaximal exercise. This suggests that the mechanical stress of high capillary pressures may alter the structure and function of the blood–gas interface, but only during intense exercise. However, because the athletes did not serve as their own control (i.e. there was no pre-exercise bronchoalveolar lavage done in the athletes) and the absolute value for red blood cell concentration was much higher (8×) in the athletes after the prolonged exercise bout compared to the athletes after high-intensity exercise, scepticism is warranted. Asthma precipitated by exposure to environmental pollutants can also affect pulmonary function. One example is the response to high levels of ozone which can increase airway resistance, stimulate airway (C-fibre) receptors and provoke rapid and shallow breathing (Lauritzen & Adams 1985) (Chapter 42). It is not known whether endurance exercise, where prolonged exposure to irritants is possible, has potentially negative effects on gas exchange.

Mechanics of breathing during exercise

The increase in minute ventilation ($\dot{V}_E$) that accompanies exercise is brought about by increasing both the frequency of breathing (f_B) and tidal volume (V_T). The latter expands into both inspiratory and expiratory reserve volumes, and is the dominant response during mild to moderate exercise. During heavy exercise, once V_T reaches ~60% of vital capacity, V_T plateaus and further increases in ventilation are brought about by an increase of f_B alone. This pattern of response is effective in that it limits the amount of dead space ventilation. The dead space to tidal volume ratio ($V_D : V_T$) falls with increases in V_T, up to the point where further increases in V_T must overcome the increasing elastic forces of an expanding lung. The resistance of the airway remains constant during exercise even though flow rates may increase five-fold, because of a stiffening of the upper airway, a shift from primarily nasal to oral ventilation, and dilatation of the intrathoracic airways. During heavy-intensity exercise, f_B may increase greatly, leading to increases in the proportion of turbulent air flow and thus flow-resistive work. As expiratory time is shortened, expiratory flow rates may increase to the point where they approach the limits of the flow–volume loop. The peak pressures exerted by the inspiratory muscles may increase from ~50% of maximum to close to their maximal dynamic capacity. The mechanical action of the respiratory muscles results in changing intrathoracic pressures which aid venous return (the respiratory pump). Severe inspiratory efforts may collapse the inferior vena cava and potentially reduce venous return, but this is unlikely to occur with the efforts made during exercise (Cummin *et al.* 1986; Harms *et al.* 1998a).

During prolonged exercise, the respiratory muscles must sustain an adequate alveolar ventilation. To accomplish this, the respiratory muscles require a substantial blood flow and oxygen supply. The oxygen cost of ventilation has been estimated at ~2 ml O_2 per l·min^{-1} of $\dot{V}_E$ at moderate ventilatory rates (3–5% of total oxygen consumption). Values increase to $3\,ml\,O_2$ per $l\cdot min^{-1}$ of $\dot{V}_E$ (8–10% of total oxygen consumption) during work above the ventilatory threshold, as accessory respiratory muscles must be called into action for both inspiration and expiration (Aaron *et al.* 1992). The estimates of oxygen cost during heavy exercise probably depend on the amount of expiratory flow limitation present, as the total cost of ventilation at $\dot{V}_E$ rates above $120\,l\cdot min^{-1}$ can reach 13–15% of total oxygen consumption.

Regulation of exercise hyperpnoea

It is generally thought that both neural and chemical factors are responsible for controlling the rate of ventilation during exercise of any intensity or duration. Feed-forward mechanisms activating both medullary respiratory neurones and the motor pathways to limb locomotor muscles and feedback afferents in working limb muscles may serve to match locomotor power output with $\dot{V}_E$, although little is known about the processing and integration of these inputs. Chemoreceptor feedback is sensitive to changes in acid–base status and arterial oxygenation; it keeps arterial Pco_2 and pH near resting levels during mild and moderate exercise. The idea that carbon dioxide flow is sensed and controls $\dot{V}_E$ is appealing because carbon dioxide production is closely matched with $\dot{V}_E$. However, no receptors in the lungs or venous circuit have yet been identified to account for this matching.

As the exercise intensity increases to ~65–75% of maximal aerobic power, hyperventilation usually develops and chemical stimuli become increasingly important in regulating ventilation. Hydrogen ion (H^+), potassium and norepinephrine have all been implicated. The close matching of the ventilatory threshold with the lactate threshold (under most conditions) has led to speculation that increased H^+, resulting from lactic acidosis, may be the signal for this ventilatory response. However, hyperventilation still occurs despite unchanged pH levels in patients with McArdle's disease (Hagberg *et al.* 1982) and in glycogen-depleted subjects (Hughes *et al.* 1982), thus providing strong evidence that H^+ accumulation is not necessary to increase $\dot{V}_E$. The accumulation of potassium in working muscles may activate local receptors and rising concentrations of potassium in arterial blood may stimulate the carotid bodies, both of which could contribute to increases in $\dot{V}_E$. Nevertheless, the increase in $\dot{V}_E$ obtained by artificially increasing circulating potassium is relatively small, indicating that a build-up of potassium is not the only stimulus to exercise-induced hyperventilation (Eldridge & Waldrop 1991). An alternative explanation for the hyperventilatory response is an increased central command. This is directed in parallel to fatiguing locomotor muscles (as more motor units must be recruited) and to the respiratory muscles. Diaphragmatic fatigue or mechanical constraints to ventilation can become important factors controlling $\dot{V}_E$ and may constrain ventilation as evidenced by smaller than normal declines in arterial Pco_2 during maximal exercise in some athletes (see excessive work of breathing during prolonged exercise, below).

With prolonged exercise, there is a tachypnoeic drift, similar to and coincident with the cardiovascular drift. This can increase $\dot{V}_E$ by 15–35% and may be more pronounced under hot and humid conditions (Hanson *et al.* 1982). The main reason for this drift is unknown, but increases in body temperature (Hagberg *et al.* 1978), accumulation of humoral factors such as norepinephrine (Martin *et al.* 1981), increased lung extravascular water (Paintal 1973) and respiratory muscle fatigue (Roussos & Moxham 1986) have all been implicated. The ventilatory drift is adaptive, in that arterial Po_2 and pH are maintained constant (indeed pH may even show a slight alkalosis). However, the process is highly inefficient, as V_D/V_T increases, and the normal entrainment of breathing rhythm with limb contraction may be lost. If this leads to respiratory muscle fatigue, $\dot{V}_E$ can still continue unabated; the diaphragm may be recruited less, but other, albeit less efficient, accessory muscles take over (Johnson *et al.* 1993; Sliwinski *et al.* 1996).

Does the pulmonary system fail and, if so, do failures contribute to limitations of endurance performance?

First, we summarize ways in which the pulmonary system might limit endurance performance.

1 Exercise-induced arterial hypoxaemia (EIAH) limits systemic oxygen transport to muscle. Systemic oxygen transport is also reduced to the heart, brain and respiratory muscles—all of which may have indirect influences on skeletal muscle performance.

2 Excessive work of breathing may have four types of influences, all of which could potentially affect performance:

   (i) alveolar ventilation may be limited, causing arterial hypoxaemia;

   (ii) respiratory muscle fatigue may develop;

   (iii) high levels of respiratory work demand high levels of metabolism, and therefore substantial levels of blood flow. These demands may limit the blood flow available to the working locomotor muscles;

   (iv) any one of the above may induce severe and progressive dyspnoea, causing a cessation of exercise.

Exercise-induced arterial hypoxaemia

The lung is not always a near perfect gas exchanger, and many highly trained athletes develop significant EIAH during peak short-term exercise (Dempsey *et al.* 1984; Powers *et al.* 1988). In the lung of the untrained individual, the alveolar to arterial partial pressure gradient (A–aDO_2) at $\dot{V}O_{2max}$ is some two- to three-fold greater than at rest (0.7–1.3 to 2.7–3.3 kPa); this is mainly because of a falling mixed venous oxygen content in combination with a small anatomical right-to-left shunt, and an imperfect, slightly non-uniform ventilation to perfusion ($\dot{V}_A:\dot{Q}$) distribution. The widened A–aDO_2 is compensated by alveolar hyperventilation, which lowers arterial PCO_2 and raises alveolar PO_2 sufficiently to maintain arterial PO_2 near resting levels. However, in many highly trained young male, female and elderly athletes (Dempsey *et al.* 1984; McClaran *et al.* 1995; Harms *et al.* 1998a; McClaran *et al.* 1998), the maximum metabolic demand increases although the lung structure remains virtually unchanged relative to their untrained counterparts (see effects of endurance training on the pulmonary system, below). Thus, A–aDO_2 widens further, probably because of alveolar to capillary

diffusion limitations. At the same time, compensatory hyperventilation is less effective in these subjects, because their ventilation is mechanically constrained by flow limitation (see below). Hence, arterial hypoxaemia develops. This reduces systemic oxygen transport and also $\dot{V}O_{2max}$, as shown by experiments where prevention of the fall in oxygen saturation (via small increases in inspired oxygen concentration) increased $\dot{V}O_{2max}$ by an increase in oxygen intake at the same heavy work rate, an increase in exercise duration at this work rate, and an increase in peak work rate in a minority of subjects (Powers *et al.* 1989; Harms *et al.* 1997b). Systemic oxygen transport is probably important to both endurance and short-term maximum performance, as shown by the longer endurance times achieved by use of a hyperoxic inspirate (Welch 1987). Conversely, the hypoxia of high altitude severely limits both $\dot{V}O_{2max}$ and endurance performance (Chapter 41), although this effect may reflect not only a reduced oxygen transport to the working skeletal muscle, but also a hypoxia of the central nervous system (Sutton *et al.* 1988) or the myocardium (Noakes 1998).

It is not clear if EIAH is an important factor during long-term endurance exercise at sea-level. Theoretically, EIAH is highly possible because the uniformity of $\dot{V}_A:\dot{Q}$ distribution worsens as moderate-intensity exercise continues (Hopkins *et al.* 1998b). Alveolar to end-capillary diffusion disequilibrium does not occur during moderate-intensity exercise. The maldistribution of $\dot{V}_A:\dot{Q}$ is attributable to a 'cuffing' of oedema fluid around medium-sized vessels and/or airways. It is associated with a falling pulmonary arterial pressure, a decreasing pulmonary vascular resistance and a modest widening of A–aDO_2. The lung gas exchange capability is jeopardized, presumably because of sustained high levels of pulmonary vascular perfusion—but there is little evidence of EIAH in sustained submaximal exercise. We have previously reported that 1 h of submaximal exercise, including competitive road racing (Hanson *et al.* 1982), resulted in very little or no EIAH in the highly trained athlete (Dempsey 1987). In fact, only three of 10 subjects who had previously shown severe EIAH in maximum short-term exercise showed sustained modest EIAH during long-term exercise at 65–75% of $\dot{V}_{O_{2max}}$. The time-dependent hyperventilation that develops during prolonged exercise appears to compensate for modest increases in A–aD_{O_2}.

So, available findings would not implicate EIAH as an important determinant of oxygen transport, and, therefore, performance in prolonged submaximal exercise. None the less, at least two types of descriptive studies need to be carried out.

First, higher intensities of exercise (in the 80–90% of $\dot{V}_{O_{2max}}$ range) must be examined, because at least in young fit males, the prevalence of EIAH is greatest at high intensities; this may be because a high blood flow increases the likelihood of diffusion limitation, secondary to a reduction of red cell transit time through the pulmonary capillaries when pulmonary capillary blood volume plateaus. Secondly, the effects of various intensities of long-term exercise need to be tested in susceptible subjects—such as the elderly, and especially fit young women. The latter group are of special interest, because many show EIAH even during short-term submaximal exercise (Harms et al. 1998a).

Excessive work of breathing during prolonged exercise

The work of the respiratory muscles increases with time during prolonged heavy exercise, because of two major factors. Firstly, the upward drift in f_B and therefore $\dot{V}_E$, demands an increased velocity of shortening of respiratory muscles to overcome flow resistance. Secondly, if flow rate increases sufficiently, expiratory flow limitation (EFL) occurs; this increases both end-expiratory and end-inspiratory lung volumes, thereby increasing the amount of elastic work performed during inspiration. The work rate of the expiratory muscles is high, but it rarely increases further, once EFL has developed. In fact, the increase in end-expiratory lung volume begins even when EFL is only being 'approached', i.e. when the tidal flow–volume loop intersects small portions of the maximal flow–volume loop. The probable mechanism is that expiratory effort is sharply inhibited and inspiration abruptly initiated by an inhibitory feedback from airway pressure receptors (Pelligrino et al. 1993).

EFFECTS ON HYPERPNOEA

Mechanical constraints on hyperventilation develop in heavy exercise, especially through EFL. This has been shown by the use of a helium–oxygen gas mixture, with added resistances in the measurement system apparatus so that the special gas mixture only reduced the *internal* component of airway resistance (Krishnan et al. 1997; McClaran et al. 1999). Helium–oxygen increased the maximum flow–volume envelope and thus allowed an increase in the ventilatory response to heavy exercise, but only under conditions where EFL or 'impending' EFL had been attained. However, the mechanical constraint on ventilation is never sufficient to cause a retention of carbon dioxide in healthy exercising subjects, regardless of the degree of EFL (Johnson et al. 1992). Rather, it may limit the hyperventilatory response to long-term heavy exercise, keeping arterial P_{CO_2} at near normal levels and lowering alveolar, and therefore, arterial P_{O_2}. Such an effect would contribute to EIAH only in cases where the A–aD_{O_2} widened excessively (see above).

EXERCISE-INDUCED RESPIRATORY MUSCLE FATIGUE

Studies using supramaximal phrenic nerve stimulation show that the diaphragm fatigues during heavy endurance exercise in healthy subjects (see Fig. 5.1) (Johnson et al. 1993; Mador et al. 1993; Babcock et al. 1995b; Mador & Dahuja 1996). Thus, the increase in transdiaphragmatic pressure induced by phrenic nerve stimulation at 1–100 Hz is reduced 15–45% immediately following endurance exercise, and it takes more than 1 h to recover a normal capacity for force development. Diaphragmatic fatigue is seen only if the exercise intensity exceeds 85% of $\dot{V}_{O_{2max}}$ and exercise is sustained to exhaustion. Hypoxia potentiates this fatigue and increases recovery times (Babcock et al. 1995a). The fatigue is attributable to a combination of high levels of respiratory muscle work and blood flow limitations imposed by the high demand for blood flow to the active limb muscles. Volitional tests of maximal expiratory pressure also suggest that heavy endurance exercise

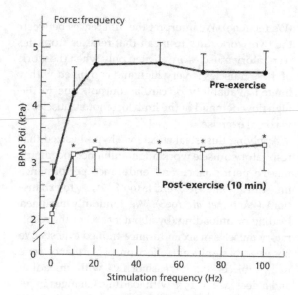

Fig. 5.1 The transdiaphragmatic pressure (Pdi) response to supramaximal twitch and paired stimuli using bilateral phrenic nerve stimulation (BPNS) at frequencies of 10, 20, 50, 70 and 100 Hz before and after exercise at 93% $\dot{V}_{O_{2max}}$ (time to exhaustion = 10 min). The BPNS Pdi response was substantially reduced at all frequencies after intense whole-body exercise. *The postexercise value was significantly different from the pre-exercise value at the same frequency of stimulation, $P < 0.05$. From Babcock *et al.* (1998).

may cause expiratory muscle 'fatigue' (Fuller *et al.* 1996).

If respiratory muscle fatigue is produced through voluntary hyperpnoea to the point of task failure in resting subjects, this reduces subsequent exercise performance times in some subjects (Mador & Acevedo 1991; Sliwinski *et al.* 1996). So, there is potential for respiratory muscle fatigue to influence exercise performance. Nevertheless, the relevance of these findings to physiological, exercise-induced diaphragm fatigue is questionable, because a much greater reduction in maximal respiratory muscle force is produced by the sustained voluntary efforts than by exercise. Fatigue of a muscle (defined as significant reduction in force output for a given motor drive) and 'task failure' are not necessarily synonymous events. In fact, if a high force production and velocity of shortening of the diaphragm are maintained long enough to cause diaphragm fatigue in

resting subjects (as documented by supramaximal phrenic nerve stimulation), subjects can still maintain a substantial submaximal level of transdiaphragmatic pressure almost indefinitely (Aaron *et al.* 1992; Babcock *et al.* 1995b).

There is now ample evidence to show that heavy endurance exercise will cause diaphragmatic fatigue. However, multiple 'respiratory' muscles can be recruited to meet even very high ventilatory demands, so hypoventilation does not occur in prolonged heavy exercise, even in the face of substantial reductions in diaphragmatic force output (Johnson *et al.* 1993; Babcock *et al.* 1995a). In fact, extreme respiratory muscle fatigue (again produced by voluntary effort) may elicit a subsequent tachypnoea and hyperventilatory response (Sliwinski *et al.* 1996). In summary, it is not clear at this time whether exercise-induced diaphragmatic fatigue has any serious consequences for endurance exercise performance.

STEAL OF LOCOMOTOR MUSCLE PERFUSION BY THE RESPIRATORY MUSCLES

This seems the most likely aspect of respiratory muscle work limiting endurance performance. The oxygen cost of breathing increases progressively to about 10% of $\dot{V}_{O_{2max}}$ (at $\dot{V}_E < 120 l \cdot min^{-1}$) and reaches as much as 15% of $\dot{V}_{O_{2max}}$ in the highly trained ($\dot{V}_E > 150 l \cdot min^{-1}$ + EFL). Harms *et al.* (1998b) used respiratory muscle loading and unloading to show that with brief maximum exercise, the work of the human expiratory muscles has two significant cardiovascular consequences: (i) it demands as much as 14–16% of the total cardiac output—a value comparable to that shown by microsphere measurements in exercising ponies (Manohar 1986a) and deduced from the oxygen cost of hyperpnoea in resting subjects (Aaron *et al.* 1992); and (ii) it causes a reflex vasoconstriction, reducing blood flow to the limb locomotor muscles, as evidenced by changes in limb vascular resistance and norepinephrine spillover across the limb during respiratory muscle unloading and loading (see Fig. 5.2). We think the reflex is initiated in type III/IV receptors of the diaphragm, which when stimulated increase efferent sympathetic vasoconstrictor activity. During

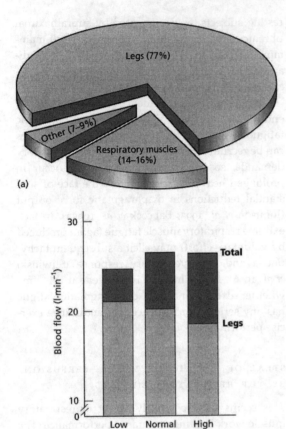

(a)

(b)

Fig. 5.2 (a) Distribution of total cardiac output among legs, respiratory muscles and other metabolically active tissues (skin, heart, brain, kidneys and liver) at $\dot{V}_{O_{2max}}$. (b) Total cardiac output and leg blood flow were measured under control conditions (normal work of breathing), with respiratory muscle unloading (low work of breathing) and with respiratory muscle loading (high work of breathing). Respiratory muscle blood flow at $\dot{V}_{O_{2max}}$ was assumed to be equal to the fall in CO_2 obtained with respiratory muscle unloading and extrapolated to zero work of breathing. Based on data from Harms *et al.* (1998b) and Harms *et al.* (1997a).

Note. The term 'work of breathing' is common in respiratory physiology. Technically, it means the energy used per unit of time (power) in order to sustain a given level of pulmonary ventilation (volume per unit of time).

submaximal exercise (up to 75% $\dot{V}_{O_{2max}}$), respiratory muscle loading and unloading affect total oxygen intake and probably cardiac output, but do not change limb vascular resistance or limb blood flow

(Wetter 1999). We interpret the differences between the two work rates to mean that reflexes from the respiratory muscles are elicited only when the work of these muscles is very high and combined with a limited availability of cardiac output, due to the high flow demand of the limb locomotor muscles at maximal exercise.

Applying this 'steal effect', we hypothesized that respiratory muscle work might influence locomotor muscle performance and endurance performance time during intense exercise (90% $\dot{V}_{O_{2max}}$ to exhaustion) (Wetter *et al.* 1998). We randomly assigned loading or unloading (by about ±50%) of the respiratory muscles in six endurance-trained cyclists. We observed a significant effect on performance time in all subjects—an increase of 14% with unloading and a decrease of 15% with loading. Changes in respiratory muscle loading also altered whole-body oxygen consumption as well as the perceived efforts of both the limbs and ventilation throughout exercise. We do not know precisely why performance was modified. Gallagher and colleagues did not observe this effect of unloading (Gallagher & Younes 1989; Marciniuk *et al.* 1994; Krishnan *et al.* 1996); but, unlike us, they found no change in oxygen consumption. Perhaps the studies differed in the magnitude of respiratory unloading that was achieved.

The effects of loading and unloading on dyspnoeic sensations might explain some of the increase in performance during unloading. We found that unloading also prevented exercise-induced diaphragm fatigue in prolonged heavy exercise. The decreased perception of limb effort with unloading might be related to reflex vasodilatation and increased blood flow to the limbs; nevertheless, we emphasize that these effects on limb flow represent a change of only 5–10% relative to control (Harms *et al.* 1997a) and they only occur during maximal or near-maximal exercise.

The effects of respiratory muscle work on limb blood flow and exercise performance might be more sensitive and widespread in patients with heart failure (Clark *et al.* 1995) and in healthy subjects when facing the chronic hypoxia of high altitudes. Both heart failure and chronic hypoxia reduce cardiac output at any given work rate, as well as augmenting the hyperventilatory response and increasing the work of breathing. This combination of changes greatly increases the probability of producing reflex effects on the limb vasculature that originate from the respiratory muscles.

SUMMARY

In summary, respiratory muscle unloading sufficient to reduce oxygen consumption shows that respiratory muscle work normally has a negative influence on endurance exercise performance. The development of diaphragmatic fatigue during prolonged heavy exercise indicates that 'failure' can occur within the pulmonary system. On the other hand, the redundancy made available by recruitment of accessory respiratory muscles normally prevents ventilatory failure. Furthermore, even though the force output of the diaphragm decreases in response to supramaximal stimulation after exhaustive exercise, this magnificent muscle still has a substantial reserve and does not undergo substantial glycogen depletion or task failure. Accordingly, we do not believe that exercise-induced diaphragm fatigue, *per se*, limits exercise performance. The high levels of work performed and the energy and blood flow required by the respiratory muscles during heavy endurance exercise have two major effects, namely, an increase in the severity of dyspnoea and a reduction in limb blood flow because of a sympathoexcitatory reflex from the working/fatiguing diaphragm. We believe these are the important contributions of the respiratory system to a limitation of exercise performance.

Effects of endurance training on the pulmonary system

An untrained person running next to a well-trained athlete would hardly question that the pulmonary system *responds* to exercise differently after endurance training. As the untrained person gasps for air, the well-trained athlete engages in a lengthy discourse of future racing plans. But does endurance training induce specific *adaptations* that improve pulmonary system function in a manner analogous to the responses of the cardiovascular and muscular systems? Comparative anatomical data from athletic versus non-athletic animals show a relative absence of adaptation in the lungs when compared with the adaptations seen in the heart and muscles (Weibel *et al*. 1992). Is this also true in humans?

An increase in pulmonary diffusing capacity would be an appropriate response to endurance training, since both maximal cardiac output and pulmonary blood flow increase with training. Reported differences in this variable for highly fit athletes may be biased by preselection, as a greater diffusing capacity would be an obvious benefit at high work intensities. There are no studies indicating structural changes (such as a decreased diffusion distance, an increased diffusion area, an increased diffusion time or an increased pulmonary capillary volume) as a result of endurance training in either humans or animals (Babcock & Dempsey 1994). Instead, the transit time of red blood cells through the pulmonary capillaries is decreased and diffusion limitation becomes possible at the high cardiac outputs seen in élite athletes. Therefore, it appears that the structural elements involved in lung–blood gas exchange do not change appreciably with training, despite their increased importance for function during exercise. Is it possible that the exercise training is not an intense enough stimulus to cause adaptation? The answer appears to be yes, as changes in diffusing capacity are seen both with long-term exposure to hypoxia and in the genetic adaptation of high-altitude natives (Cerny *et al*. 1973).

In terms of static lung volumes, maximal inspiratory and expiratory flow rates, and maximal voluntary ventilation, the competitive or élite athlete does not differ significantly from an untrained person (Martin & Stager 1981; Mahler *et al*. 1982). The exceptional case may be in competitive swimmers, especially long-distance swimmers, who sometimes have a larger than average vital capacity and total lung capacity (Shephard *et al*. 1974; Clanton *et al*. 1987). Whether endurance exercise in young athletes whose pulmonary system may still be developing results in lasting pulmonary function changes is unknown. With endurance exercise training in the already fit adult, static lung volumes may be altered, but only very slightly, as demonstrated by increases in vital capacity, functional residual capacity and total lung capacity in collegiate swimmers after a period of heavy swim training (Clanton *et al.* 1987). After endurance training, sedentary subjects show little change in static lung volumes, but there may be changes in volitional pulmonary function tests such as increases in peak pressures and maximal voluntary ventilation (Robinson & Kjeldgaard 1982). Loss of pulmonary function (decreased lung elastic recoil) with ageing is not prevented by endurance training (McClaran *et al.* 1995).

Changes in the endurance capacity of the respiratory muscles would be a likely consequence of exercise training and this appears to be the case as indicated by increases in maximal sustainable ventilatory capacity (Robinson & Kjeldgaard 1982). It is logical that respiratory muscles adapt to training overload much as any other skeletal muscle, and changes in contractile and biochemical properties of the muscle would be expected. Unfortunately, it is not easy to test this in humans, as respiratory muscle biopsies are uncommon. Data from exercise-trained animals show 10–30% increases in oxidative enzyme capacities (Powers *et al.* 1992), increases in the proportion of slow-twitch fibres (Lieberman *et al.* 1972) and decreased rates of fatigue (Farkas & Roussos 1982). The changes in enzyme content are approximately one-half of that which occurs in locomotor muscles of similar fibre type, suggesting that during exercise training the respiratory muscles either do not respond as much, or are not recruited to the same degree as working limb muscles. More severe and chronic stresses such as tracheal banding can produce larger changes in the oxidative capacity of the respiratory muscles (Keens *et al.* 1978). The slightly lower oxygen extraction of the diaphragm, relative to the working limbs, suggests that the respiratory muscles are always adequately supplied with oxygen and that they are working submaximally during exercise (Poole *et al.* 1997). On the other hand, the limb muscle vasculature vasodilates further when adenosine is administered during heavy exercise, whereas the respiratory muscle vasculature does not, and this may indicate that exercise stresses the respiratory muscles to the point of eliciting the highest attainable blood flow (Manohar 1986b).

After endurance training, $\dot{V}_E$ is commonly lower at the same work rate, although the mechanical work of breathing is the same in a trained versus an untrained person ventilating at the same rate (Milic-Emili *et al.* 1962). At a given power output or oxygen uptake however, the work of breathing is lower in the trained versus the untrained, because there is a ~20% decrease in $\dot{V}_E$ at a given work rate in the trained subject. The decrease varies with work rate. No change in $\dot{V}_E$ is seen at light work rates. The greatest change occurs at or near the anaerobic threshold, and it is apparent throughout exercise (Coggan *et al.* 1993). Because fewer chemical stimuli are produced by the working limbs at the same absolute intensity of effort after training, the decrease in $\dot{V}_E$ is often attributed to a decrease in lactate production (Casaburi *et al.* 1987). There is a tight correlation between these two variables. However, there is not necessarily a cause–effect relationship, as the exact stimulus to the increase of $\dot{V}_E$ is not known. A decrease in central command may recruit fewer lower efficiency fast-twitch fibres in working muscles after endurance training, and theoretically this could be coupled with a decreased drive to the respiratory motor output. Thus, the lactate–ventilation relationship may be coincidental (Mateika & Duffin 1994). An increased fat utilization (at the same absolute work rate) after training would produce less carbon dioxide per litre of oxygen consumed and would perhaps result in a smaller ventilatory stimulus. A decrease in $\dot{V}_E$ would be likely to decrease the oxygen cost of breathing at a given work rate and it would possibly lower total oxygen consumption, although on the other hand, increases in $\dot{V}_E$ do not always increase total oxygen consumption (Boutellier 1998). We do know that increasing or decreasing the work of the respiratory muscles, without altering $\dot{V}_E$, will raise or lower total body oxygen consumption, respectively (Harms *et al.* 1997a). Although the ventilation rate at a given power output is lower after exercise training, the absolute ventilation rates at $\dot{V}_{O_{2max}}$ are higher in trained athletes than in sedentary people because the athletes achieve much higher power outputs. After training, an athlete is able to exercise at intensities which require ventilation rates and pressure-generating capabilities that are closer to the maximal capacity of the respiratory system. At prolonged high work rates, there is ample evidence that the respiratory muscles fatigue (see previous section on exercise-induced respiratory muscle fatigue), although whether whole-body endurance training protects against (Anholm *et al.* 1989) or increases the chance of (Ker & Schultz 1996) diaphragm fatigue is debatable. Both highly fit and normally fit people show a similar amount of diaphragmatic fatigue at the end of exercise (Babcock *et al.* 1996). However, in highly fit, endurance-trained individuals, this fatigue is observed after exercising at a much higher absolute work rate, $\dot{V}_E$ and diaphragm force output than in their less fit peers.

Does specific respiratory muscle training improve endurance performance?

Recent research has brought renewed interest to the question of whether the respiratory muscles can themselves be trained (independently of whole-body exercise), and whether specific respiratory muscle training (RMT) can enhance performance. Leith and Bradley (1976) documented the effects of specific training of the respiratory muscles for strength and endurance. Although there were only minor changes in vital capacity and total lung capacity, respiratory muscle endurance (measured by maximal sustainable ventilatory capacity) and strength (measured by maximal inspiratory and expiratory pressures) improved and were specific to the strength or endurance type of training. Since then, many others have shown changes in volitional respiratory muscle function tests (maximal voluntary ventilation, maximal sustainable ventilatory capacity and maximal inspiratory and expiratory pressure generation) in a wide variety of subjects (untrained, trained, elderly, chronic obstructive lung disease and cystic fibrosis patients) in response to several weeks of specific RMT (Keens *et al.* 1977; Levine *et al.* 1986; Clanton *et al.* 1987; Morgan *et al.* 1987; Belman & Gaesser 1988; Fairbarn *et al.* 1991). In cystic fibrosis patients, respiratory muscle endurance was improved equally after specific RMT or upper body endurance exercise (Keens *et al.* 1977). In swim-trained females, slightly greater improvements in some aspects of respiratory muscle function were seen when specific RMT was combined with endurance training when compared

with endurance training alone (Clanton *et al.* 1987). Apparently, no one has compared the effects of specific RMT and endurance training on outcomes of respiratory muscle endurance in normal subjects; thus, the relative benefits of general endurance exercise versus specific RMT are unknown, but perhaps depend on the outcome measure.

The outcome of most concern to a competitive endurance athlete is whether RMT can improve track performance, that is, 'Will I be able to go faster?'. In laboratory trials, this outcome is usually not examined; measures such as $\dot{V}_{O_2\,max}$ or time to exhaustion are more common. A universal finding is that $\dot{V}_{O_2max}$ does not change with specific RMT. Time to exhaustion during very high intensity cycle ergometry (90–95% $\dot{V}_{O_2max}$) is also unaffected (Morgan *et al.* 1987; Fairbarn *et al.* 1991). However, dramatic increases in endurance performance have been found in both untrained (Boutellier & Piwko 1992) and trained (Boutellier *et al.* 1992) cyclists after 4 weeks of isocapnic hyperpnoea (30 min·day^{-1}). Time to exhaustion during cycle ergometry at 64% (untrained) or 77% (trained) of peak oxygen consumption increased by 50% in untrained and 38% in trained cyclists.

These effects are surprisingly large, and the results demand excessive proof. As many of the outcome measures require maximal volitional efforts, a placebo group is needed to control for systematic effects of learning upon retesting, the attention given to subjects, and any purely psychological benefits (i.e. increased motivation) which might be perceived as due to the intervention *per se*. This form of RMT has not always produced global gains in exercise performance at these submaximal intensities (Kohl *et al.* 1997). Kohl *et al.* (1997) postulated that perhaps too short a recovery time (5–7 days) after the last RMT session led to a lack of performance gains. It seems unlikely that the respiratory muscles would require this amount of time to recover from any type of fatigue. While low-frequency diaphragmatic fatigue persists for at least 24 h, based on the rate of recovery from fatigue, decrements in peak diaphragmatic tension should be very small 3 days after a fatiguing protocol (Laghi *et al.* 1995). Furthermore, in subjects faced with daily exposure to RMT, recovery from any fatigue due to the training would be expected to be enhanced. More recent data from the same laboratory (presented in abstract form) showed a 28% increase in time to exhaustion post-RMT in 20 endurance athletes; moreover, improvements were seen immediately after training, as well as 1 week later (Spengler *et al.* 1994). In addition, increases in mean time to exhaustion for subjects engaged in RMT only (29% increase over control) were only slightly lower than for subjects who engaged in whole-body endurance training (39% increase over control) (Spengler *et al.* 1998).

Mechanisms for improvement in endurance performance

Because of the small muscle mass involved, it is unlikely that RMT would result in any central circulatory adaptations such as increases in stroke volume or maximal cardiac output. Therefore changes with RMT are likely to be confined to the respiratory muscle, although they may ultimately involve interactions with the brain or working locomotor muscles (see Fig. 5.3). We define some of the possible adaptations to RMT and detail how these changes could specifically enhance endurance performance.

A strengthening of the respiratory muscles, possibly the result of fibre hypertrophy (Rollier *et al.* 1998), may allow higher ventilation rates to be achieved during heavy exercise, at least in athletes whose ventilatory requirements are so high that tidal inspiratory pressures reach ~90% of capacity (Johnson *et al.* 1992). If individuals in this group develop EIAH, and if the cause of the EIAH is at least in part a relative lack of hyperventilation, they may benefit from increases in inspiratory muscle

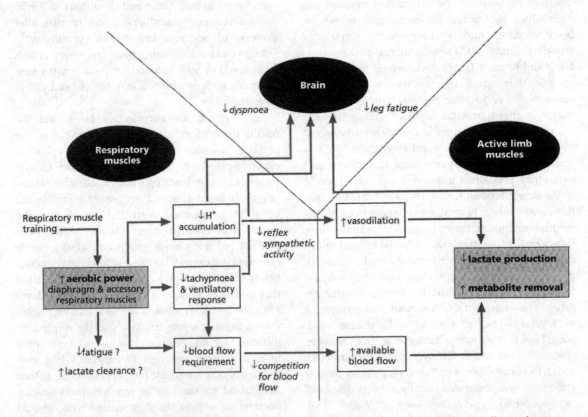

Fig. 5.3 Simplified scheme of possible effects of respiratory muscle training on parameters which may affect endurance performance. It is likely that time to exhaustion tests are terminated by the overall sensation of discomfort (both dyspnoea and leg fatigue). Metabolic adaptations in the respiratory muscles could potentially modify either of these effects.

strength, provided that a lack of strength was the cause of underventilation. In this group, increased ventilation might allow maintenance of higher arterial P_{O_2} levels. In addition, if RMT increased the velocity of diaphragm shortening, this would lead to a faster inspiratory time (and allow the expiratory time to be extended); this in turn would keep end-expiratory lung volume from climbing, thus allowing the diaphragm to contract nearer to its optimal length and reducing the elastic recoil forces to be overcome because of inspiration to large lung volumes. No benefits would be expected from increased expiratory muscle strength since, at high ventilation rates, people already approach the effort-independent part of the flow–volume loop where further increases in expiratory effort do not augment flow rate. That respiratory muscle strength is *not* a likely limitation of endurance performance is confirmed by the lack of significant changes in $\dot{V}_E$ during incremental maximal tests or in endurance tests >90% of $\dot{V}_{O_{2max}}$, and most importantly by the lack of significant performance gains in tests conducted at these high intensities after RMT. Increased respiratory muscle strength alone is of minimal benefit for performance at either maximal or submaximal intensities, except in rare cases.

Increases in respiratory muscle endurance are a more likely explanation of performance enhancement following RMT. An increase in aerobic efficiency of the (already efficient) diaphragm and (less efficient) accessory respiratory muscles could allow ventilation rates that were similar to pretraining to be sustained for a longer time after RMT. It could also potentially reduce or delay the upward time-related drift in f_B and $\dot{V}_E$ during heavy endurance exercise. The greater maximal sustainable ventilation after RMT provides evidence that respiratory muscle endurance capacity is increased. The basis for the increased endurance capacity seems similar to that for the metabolic changes seen in any muscle with endurance training: increased capillary and mitochondrial density and increased aerobic enzyme activities, with a decreased reliance on glycolysis, less lactate production, less decrease in intracellular pH and an overall improvement in cellular homeostasis. The ability to take up and use lactate as a fuel may also be enhanced. These mecha-

nisms could reduce the fatiguability of the respiratory muscles, but would also alter the inhibitory feedback from fatiguing respiratory muscles to the working limbs and higher brain centres.

How would these changes, specific to respiratory muscles, lead to increased endurance performance? After training, the respiratory muscles would be working at a lower relative intensity and therefore they would produce fewer metabolic stimuli. This could signal a decreased need for vasodilatation in the respiratory muscles, and allow a greater blood supply to be directed to the working legs. Alternatively, a reduction in chemical stimuli could reduce the output from respiratory muscles to the working limbs via reflex pathways (type III/IV afferents) reducing vasoconstriction in the limbs. In either case, increased leg blood flow may result in greater oxygen delivery to the limbs and reduced limb fatigue. Data indicating that changes in the amount of respiratory muscle work affect locomotor blood flow support this idea. However, benefit is only likely in near-maximal exercise conditions (see Steal of locomotor perfusion by the respiratory muscles). As mentioned previously, the amount of work performed by the respiratory muscles during exercise determines exercise performance to some extent. Reducing the work of breathing increases the time to exhaustion and increasing the work of breathing has the opposite effect. Thus, it is possible that a delay in fatigue of the respiratory muscles after RMT would have a direct impact on the working limbs.

Does RMT lead to decreased lactate accumulation? A correlation between decreased levels of lactate during exercise and improved endurance time after RMT has been reported (Spengler *et al.* 1994); further, it has been suggested that these decreases are the *result* of RMT, but are not responsible for the increased whole-body performance (Boutellier 1998). This viewpoint is based on a study where RMT reduced lactate accumulation, yet endurance time was not increased (Kohl *et al.* 1997). Unloading or loading the respiratory muscles by 40–60% during exercise intensities of 50–100% of $\dot{V}_{O_{2max}}$ did not change arterial or femoral venous lactate concentrations in our studies. This suggests that reducing the work of breathing has a minimal impact on either lactate production by the working legs or lactate production or clearance by the respiratory muscles. Because RMT probably alters the oxidative capacity of the respiratory muscles, while unloading does not, it is possible that the effects on lactate accumulation differ between the two protocols. Highly oxidative muscle like the diaphragm can and does utilize lactate as a fuel source. It seems unlikely, however, that improvements in the endurance capacity of this small muscle (0.5% of body mass) could alter circulating lactate accumulation significantly by a lesser production or a greater removal of lactate.

Are the ventilation rate and breathing pattern during endurance exercise altered after RMT? Lower $\dot{V}_E$ and less tachypnoea have been reported (Boutellier 1998); these changes would be consistent with a reduction in respiratory muscle fatigue as a bout of endurance exercise is continued over time. Would these changes enhance performance? Lower $\dot{V}_E$ would certainly reduce the oxygen cost of breathing, and reductions in f_B could reduce the dead space ventilation, thus allowing an increased $\dot{V}_A$ at a similar $\dot{V}_E$. These effects may be important during maximal exercise, where cardiac output and the oxygen supply to the working muscle are usually limiting. However, such changes would be less important in submaximal work.

Is it possible that RMT leads to a reduction in the relative levels of sensory stimuli to higher brain centres and that this enhances performance? A decrease in the accumulation of end-products (H^+) in the respiratory muscles during exercise could cause less sensory input to the central nervous system and thus reduce the stimulus to dyspnoea. It is also possible that after repeated bouts of high rates of ventilation or generation of large pressures, as with RMT, the level of sensory input from the respiratory muscles to the brain during exercise is processed as being less severe than initially and that this reduces dyspnoea. This would only help perfor-

mance if dyspnoeic sensations contributed to limitation of exercise. However, both before and after RMT, fit and sedentary subjects usually report that they stop an endurance test due to leg fatigue rather than dyspnoea. Since we know very little of the causes of dyspnoea and how central feedback alters exercise performance, it is possible that reducing dyspnoea could enhance performance, even if it is not sensed as the limiting factor at the end of exercise.

Additional well-controlled studies need to be conducted to confirm that RMT benefits endurance exercise. If results are confirmed, the mechanism(s) responsible need to be investigated. There are several unknowns.

• Whether there are exercise intensities or modes of exercise where RMT is of particular benefit (for example, rowing, where entrainment is especially important).
• Whether the mechanics of breathing are modified; does mechanical efficiency change so that less pleural pressure is developed at a given $\dot{V}_E$; are there changes in end-expiratory lung volume or breathing pattern?
• Whether arterial lactate levels change after RMT; is leg lactate production decreased; does respiratory muscle clearance or production of lactate change?
• Whether RMT increases performance not only in terms of time to exhaustion, but also in measures more applicable to race situations, such as a time trial over a fixed distance.

Conclusions

Once commonly held as 'overbuilt', the pulmonary system faces extreme challenges during endurance exercise. These challenges are accentuated in the élite or highly trained athlete who engages in endurance exercise which requires a substantial percentage of $\dot{V}_{O_{2max}}$.

References

Aaron, E.A., Seow, K.C. & Johnson, B.D. (1992) Oxygen cost of exercise hyperpnea: implications for performance. *Journal of Applied Physiology* 72, 1818–1825.

Anholm, J.D., Stray-Gundersen, J., Ramanathan, M. & Johnson, R.L. (1989) Sustained maximal ventilation after endurance exercise in athletes. *Journal of Applied Physiology* 67, 1759–1763.

Babcock, M.A. & Dempsey, J.A. (1994) Pulmonary system adaptations: limitations to exercise. In: Bouchard, C., Shepard, R.J. & Stephens, T. (eds) *Physical Activity, Fitness, and Health*, pp.

320–330. Human Kinetics, Champaign, IL.

Babcock, M.A., Johnson, B.D., Pegelow, D.F., Suman, O.E., Griffin, D. & Dempsey, J.A. (1995a) Hypoxic effects on exercise-induced diaphragmatic fatigue in normal healthy humans. *Journal of Applied Physiology* **78**, 82–92.

Babcock, M.A., Pegelow, D.F., McClaran, S.R., Suman, O.E. & Dempsey, J.A. (1995b) Contribution of diaphragmatic power output to exercise-induced diaphragm fatigue. *Journal of Applied Physiology* **78**, 1710–1719.

Babcock, M.A., Pegelow, D.F., Johnson, B.D. & Dempsey, J.A. (1996) Aerobic fitness effects on exercise-induced low-frequency diaphragm fatigue. *Journal of Applied Physiology* **81**, 2156–2164.

Babcock, M.A., Pegelow, D.F., Taha, B.H. & Dempsey, J.A. (1998) High frequency diaphragmatic fatigue detected with paired stimuli in humans. *Medicine and Science in Sports and Exercise* **30**, 506–511.

Belman, M.J. & Gaesser, G.A. (1988) Ventilatory muscle training in the elderly. *Journal of Applied Physiology* **64**, 899–905.

Boutellier, U. (1998) Respiratory muscle fitness and exercise endurance in healthy humans. *Medicine and Science in Sports and Exercise* **30**, 1169–1172.

Boutellier, U. & Piwko, P. (1992) The respiratory system as an exercise limiting factor in normal sedentary subjects. *European Journal of Applied Physiology* **64**, 145–152.

Boutellier, U., Buchel, R., Kundert, A. & Spengler, C. (1992) The respiratory system as an exercise limiting factor in normal trained subjects. *European Journal of Applied Physiology* **65**, 347–353.

Casaburi, R., Storer, T.W. & Wasserman, K. (1987) Mediation of reduced ventilatory response to exercise after endurance training. *Journal of Applied Physiology* **63**, 1533–1538.

Cerny, F.C., Dempsey, J.A. & Reddan, W.G. (1973) Pulmonary gas exchange in non-native residents of high altitude. *Journal of Clinical Investigation* **52**, 2993–2999.

Clanton, T.L., Dixon, G.F., Drake, J. & Gadek, J.E. (1987) Effects of swim training on lung volumes and inspiratory muscle conditioning. *Journal of Applied Physiology* **62**, 39–46.

Clark, A.L., Sparrow, J.L. & Coats, A.J. (1995) Muscle fatigue and dyspnoea in chronic heart failure: two sides of the same coin? *European Heart Journal* **16**, 49–52.

Coggan, A.R., Habash, D.L., Mendenhall, L.A., Swanson, S.C. & Kien, C.L. (1993) Isotopic estimation of CO_2 production during exercise before and after endurance training. *Journal of Applied Physiology* **75**, 70–75.

Cummin, A.R.C., Iyawe, V.I., Jacobi, M.S., Mehta, N., Patil, C.P. & Saunders, K.B. (1986) Immediate ventilation response to sudden changes in venous return in humans. *Journal of Physiology (London)* **380**, 45–49.

Dempsey, J.A. (1987) Exercise-induced imperfections in pulmonary gas exchange. *Canadian Journal of Sport Sciences* **12** (Suppl.), 66–71.

Dempsey, J.A., Hanson, P.G. & Henderson, K.S. (1984) Exercise-induced arterial hypoxemia in healthy human subjects at sea level. *Journal of Physiology (London)* **355**, 161–175.

Dempsey, J.A., Aaron, E. & Martin, B.J. (1988) Pulmonary function and prolonged exercise. In: Lamb, D.R. & Murray, R. (eds) *Perspectives in Exercise Science and Sports Medicine*, Vol. 1. *Prolonged Exercise*, pp. 75–119. Benchmark Press, Indianapolis.

Eldridge, F.L. & Waldrop, T.G. (1991) Neural control of breathing during exercise. In: Whipp, B.J. & Wasserman, K. (eds) *Exercise: Pulmonary Physiology and Pathophysiology*, pp. 309–370. Marcel Dekker, New York.

Fairbarn, M.S., Coutts, K.C., Pardy, R.L. & McKenzie, D.C. (1991) Improved respiratory muscle endurance of highly trained cyclists and the effects on maximal exercise performance. *International Journal of Sports Medicine* **12**, 66–70.

Farkas, G.A. & Roussos, C. (1982) Adaptability of the hamster diaphragm to exercise and/or emphysema. *Journal of Applied Physiology* **53**, 1263–1272.

Fuller, D., Sullivan, J. & Fregosi, R.F. (1996) Expiratory muscle endurance performance after exhaustive submaximal exercise. *Journal of Applied Physiology* **80**, 1495–1502.

Gallagher, C.G. & Younes, M. (1989) Effect of pressure assist on ventilation and respiratory mechanics in heavy exercise. *Journal of Applied Physiology* **66**, 1824–1837.

Hagberg, J.M., Mullin, J.P. & Nagle, F.J. (1978) Oxygen consumption during constant-load exercise. *Journal of Applied Physiology* **45**, 381–384.

Hagberg, J.M., Coyle, E.F., Carroll, J.E., Miller, J.M., Martin, W.H. & Brooke, M.H. (1982) Exercise hyperventilation in patients with McArdle's disease. *Journal of Applied Physiology* **52**, 991–994.

Hanson, P., Claremont, A., Dempsey, J.A. & Reddan, W. (1982) Determinants and consequences of ventilatory responses to competitive endurance running. *Journal of Applied Physiology* **52**, 615–623.

Harms, C.A., Babcock, M.A., McClaran, S.R. *et al.* (1997a) Respiratory muscle work compromises leg blood flow during maximal exercise. *Journal of Applied Physiology* **82**, 1573–1583.

Harms, C.A., McClaran, S.R., Nickele, G., Pegelow, D. & Dempsey, J.A. (1997b) High prevalence of exercise-induced arterial hypoxemia and expiratory flow limitation in healthy young women. *American Journal of Respiratory and Critical Care Medicine* **155**, A910.

Harms, C.A., McClaran, S.R., Nickele, G.A., Pegelow, D.F., Nelson, W.B. & Dempsey, J.A. (1998a) Exercise-induced arterial hypoxaemia in healthy young women. *Journal of Physiology (London)* **507**, 619–628.

Harms, C.A., Wetter, T.J., McClaran, S.R. *et al.* (1998b) Effects of respiratory muscle work on cardiac output and its distribution during maximal exercise. *Journal of Applied Physiology* **85**, 609–618.

Hopkins, S.R., Schoene, R.B., Henderson, W.R., Spragg, R.G., Martin, T.R. & West, J.B. (1997) Intense exercise impairs the integrity of the pulmonary blood–gas barrier in élite athletes. *American Journal of Respiratory and Critical Care Medicine* **155**, 1090–1094.

Hopkins, S.R., Schoene, R.B., Henderson, W.R., Spragg, R.G. & West, J.B. (1998a) Sustained submaximal exercise does not alter the integrity of the lung blood–gas barrier in élite athletes. *Journal of Applied Physiology* **84**, 1185–1189.

Hopkins, S.R., Gavin, T.P., Siafakas, N.M. *et al.* (1998b) Effect of prolonged, heavy exercise on pulmonary gas exchange in athletes. *Journal of Applied Physiology* **85**, 1523–1532.

Hughes, E.F., Turner, S.C. & Brooks, G.A. (1982) Effects of glycogen depletion and pedaling speed on 'anaerobic threshold'. *Journal of Applied Physiology* **52**, 1598–1607.

Johnson, B.D., Saupe, K.W. & Dempsey, J.A. (1992) Mechanical constraints on exercise hyperpnea in endurance athletes. *Journal of Applied Physiology* **73**, 874–886.

Johnson, B.D., Babcock, M.A., Suman, O.E. & Dempsey, J.A. (1993) Exercise-induced diaphragmatic fatigue in healthy humans. *Journal of Physiology (London)* **460**, 385–405.

Keens, T.G., Krastins, I.R., Wannamaker, E.M., Levison, H., Crozier, D.N. & Bryan, A.C. (1977) Ventilatory muscle endurance training in normal subjects and patients with cystic fibrosis. *American Review of Respiratory Disease* **116**, 853–860.

Keens, T.G., Chen, V., Patel, P.O., Brien, P.,

Levison, H. & Ianuzzo, C.D. (1978) Cellular adaptations of the ventilatory muscles to a chronic increased respiratory load. *Journal of Applied Physiology* **44**, 905–908.

Ker, J.A. & Schultz, C.M. (1996) Respiratory muscle fatigue after an ultramarathon measured as inspiratory task failure. *International Journal of Sports Medicine* **17**, 493–496.

Kohl, J., Koller, E.A., Brandenberger, M., Cardenas, M. & Boutellier, U. (1997) Effect of exercise-induced hyperventilation on airway resistance and cycling endurance. *European Journal of Applied Physiology* **75**, 305–311.

Krishnan, B., Zintel, T., McParland, C. & Gallagher, C.G. (1996) Lack of importance of respiratory muscle load in ventilatory regulation during heavy exercise in humans. *Journal of Physiology (London)* **490**, 537–550.

Krishnan, B.S., Clemens, R.E., Zintel, T.A., Stockwell, M.J. & Gallagher, C.G. (1997) Ventilatory response to helium–oxygen breathing during exercise: effect of airway anesthesia. *Journal of Applied Physiology* **83**, 82–88.

Laghi, F.D., Alfonso, N. & Tobin, M.J. (1995) Pattern of recovery from diaphragmatic fatigue over 24 hours. *Journal of Applied Physiology* **79**, 539–546.

Lauritzen, S.K. & Adams, W.C. (1985) Ozone inhalation effects consequent to continuous exercise in females; comparison to males. *Journal of Applied Physiology* **59**, 1601–1606.

Leith, D.E. & Bradley, M. (1976) Ventilatory muscle strength and endurance training. *Journal of Applied Physiology* **41**, 508–516.

Levine, S., Weiser, P. & Gillen, J. (1986) Evaluation of a ventilatory muscle endurance training program in the rehabilitation of patients with chronic obstructive pulmonary disease. *American Review of Respiratory Disease* **133**, 400–406.

Lieberman, D.A., Maxwell, L.C. & Faulkner, J.A. (1972) Adaptations of guinea pig diaphragm muscle to aging and endurance training. *American Journal of Physiology* **222**, 556–560.

McClaran, S.R., Babcock, M.A., Pegelow, D.F., Reddan, W.G. & Dempsey, J.A. (1995) Longitudinal effects of aging on lung function at rest and exercise in healthy active fit elderly adults. *Journal of Applied Physiology* **78**, 1957–1968.

McClaran, S.R., Harms, C.A., Pegelow, D.F. & Dempsey, J.A. (1998) Smaller lungs in women affect exercise hyperpnea. *Journal of Applied Physiology* **84**, 1872–1881.

McClaran, S.R., Wetter, T.J., Pegelow, D.F. & Dempsey, J.A. (1999) Role of expiratory flow limitation in determining lung volumes and ventilation during exercise. *Journal of Applied Physiology* **86**, 1357–1366.

McKechnie, J.K., Leary, W.P., Noakes, T.D., Kallmeyer, J.C., MacSearraigh, E.T. & Olivier, L.R. (1979) Acute pulmonary edema in two athletes during a 90-km running race. *South African Medical Journal* **56**, 261–265.

Mador, M.J. & Acevedo, F.A. (1991) Effect of respiratory muscle fatigue on subsequent exercise performance. *Journal of Applied Physiology* **70**, 2059–2065.

Mador, M.J. & Dahuja, M. (1996) Mechanisms for diaphragmatic fatigue following high-intensity leg exercise. *American Journal of Respiratory and Critical Care Medicine* **154**, 1484–1489.

Mador, M.J., Magalang, U.J., Rodis, A. & Kufel, T.J. (1993) Diaphragmatic fatigue after exercise in healthy human subjects. *American Review of Respiratory Disease* **148**, 1571–1575.

Mahler, D.A., Moritz, E.D. & Loke, J. (1982) Ventilatory responses at rest and during exercise in marathon runners. *Journal of Applied Physiology* **52**, 388–392.

Manohar, M. (1986a) Blood flow to the respiratory and limb muscles and to abdominal organs during maximal exertion in ponies. *Journal of Physiology (London)* **377**, 25–35.

Manohar, M. (1986b) Vasodilator reserve in respiratory muscles during maximal exertion in ponies. *Journal of Applied Physiology* **60**, 1571–1577.

Marciniuk, D., McKim, D., Sanii, R. & Younes, M. (1994) Role of central respiratory muscle fatigue in endurance exercise in normal subjects. *Journal of Applied Physiology* **76**, 236–241.

Martin, B.J. & Stager, J.M. (1981) Ventilatory endurance in athletes and nonathletes. *Medicine and Science in Sports and Exercise* **13**, 21–26.

Martin, B.J., Morgan, E.J., Zwillich, C.W. & Weil, J.V. (1981) Control of breathing during prolonged exercise. *Journal of Applied Physiology* **50**, 27–31.

Mateika, J.A. & Duffin, J. (1994) Coincidental changes in ventilation and electromyographic activity during consecutive incremental exercise tests. *European Journal of Applied Physiology* **68**, 54–61.

Milic-Emili, G., Petit, J.M. & Deroanne, R. (1962) Mechanical work of breathing during exercise in trained and untrained subjects. *Journal of Applied Physiology* **17**, 43–46.

Morgan, D.W., Kohrt, W.M., Bates, B.J. & Skinner, J.S. (1987) Effects of respiratory muscle endurance training on ventilatory and endurance performance of moderately trained cyclists. *International Journal of Sports Medicine* **8**, 88–93.

Noakes, T.D. (1998) Maximal oxygen uptake: 'classical' versus 'contemporary' viewpoints: a rebuttal. *Medicine and Science in Sports and Exercise* **30**, 1381–1398.

O'Brodovich, H. & Coates, G. (1991) Lung water and solute movement during exercise. In: Whipp, B.J. & Wasserman, K. (eds) *Exercise. Pulmonary Physiology and Pathophysiology*, pp. 253–270. Marcel Dekker, New York.

Paintal, A.S. (1973) Vagal sensory receptors and their reflex effects. *Physiological Reviews* **53**, 159–227.

Pelligrino, R., Brusasco, V., Rodarte, J.R. & Babb, T.G. (1993) Expiratory flow limitation and regulation of end-expiratory lung volume during exercise. *Journal of Applied Physiology* **74**, 2552–2558.

Poole, D.C., Sexton, W.L., Farkas, G.A., Powers, S.K. & Reid, M.B. (1997) Diaphragm structure and function in health and disease. *Medicine and Science in Sports and Exercise* **29**, 738–754.

Powers, S.K., Dodd, S., Lawler, J. *et al.* (1988) Incidence of exercise induced hypoxemia in élite endurance athletes at sea level. *European Journal of Applied Physiology* **58**, 298–302.

Powers, S.K., Lawler, J., Dempsey, J.A., Dodd, S. & Landry, G. (1989) Effects of incomplete pulmonary gas exchange on $\dot{V}O_{2max}$. *Journal of Applied Physiology* **66**, 2491–2495.

Powers, S.K., Grinton, S., Lawler, J., Criswell, D. & Dodd, S. (1992) High intensity exercise training-induced metabolic alterations in respiratory muscles. *Respiration Physiology* **89**, 169–177.

Robinson, E.P. & Kjeldgaard, J.M. (1982) Improvement in ventilatory muscle function with running. *Journal of Applied Physiology* **52**, 1400–1406.

Rollier, H., Bisschop, A., Gayan-Ramirez, G., Gosselink, R. & Decramer, M. (1998) Low load inspiratory muscle training increases diaphragmatic fiber dimensions in rats. *American Journal of Respiratory and Critical Care Medicine* **157**, 833–839.

Roussos, C.H. & Moxham, J. (1986) Respiratory muscle fatigue. In: Roussos, C.H. & Macklem, P. (eds) *The Thorax*, pp. 829–870. Marcel Dekker, New York.

Shephard, R.J., Godin, G. & Campbell, R. (1974) Characteristics of sprint, medium and long-distance swimmers. *European Journal of Applied Physiology* **32**, 99–116.

Sliwinski, P., Yan, S., Gauthier, A.P. & Macklem, P. (1996) Influence of global inspiratory muscle fatigue on breathing during exercise. *Journal of Applied Physiology* **80**, 1270–1278.

Spengler, C.M., Roos, M., Laube, S. & Boutellier, U. (1994) Respiratory endurance training increases exercise endurance and reduces blood lactate accumulation in healthy subjects. *European Journal of Applied Physiology* **69**, S13.

Spengler, C.M., Lenzin, C., Markov, G., Stussi, C. & Boutellier, U. (1998)

Improved cycling endurance after respiratory endurance training without cardiovascular improvement. *FASEB Journal* **12**, A1117.

Sutton, J.R., Reeves, J.T., Wagner, P.D. *et al.* (1988) Operation Everest II: oxygen transport during exercise at extreme simulated altitude. *Journal of Applied Physiology* **64**, 1309–1321.

Weibel, E.R., Taylor, C.R. & Hoppeler, H. (1992) Variations in function and design: testing symmorphosis in the respiratory system. *Respiration Physiology* **87**, 325–348.

Welch, H.G. (1987) Effects of hyperoxia on human performance. *Exercise and Sport Sciences Reviews* **15**, 191–221.

Wetter, T.J., Harms, C.A., Nelson, W.B., Pegelow, D.F. & Dempsey, J.A. (1999) Influence of respiratory work on Vo_2 and leg blood flow during submaximal exercise. *Journal of Applied Physiology* **87**, 643–651.

Wetter, T.J., Harms, C.A., St. Croix, C., Pegelow, D.F. & Dempsey, J.A. (1998) Effects of respiratory muscle loading and unloading on time to exhaustion during cycle ergometry. *Medicine and Science in Sports and Exercise* **30**, S190.

Young, M., Sciurba, F. & Rinaldo, J. (1987) Delirium and pulmonary edema after completing a marathon. *American Review of Respiratory Disease* **136**, 737–739.

Chapter 6

The Athlete's Heart

JACK GOODMAN

Historical perspectives

Early developments

The historical debate surrounding the effects of exercise on the heart extends well back into history. In 492 BC, the ancient Greek Philipides ran over 100 miles to pronounce victory for the Athenians over the Persians, and then promptly died of what might be the first reported case of exercise-induced cardiac sudden death. Today, the distinction of physiological cardiac adaptation associated with exercise training from pathological changes remains a diagnostic dilemma. In addition, there is a persistent debate about the safety of exercise, particularly in athletes with enlarged hearts.

Initially, cardiac enlargement was observed in wild animals compared to their domesticated counterparts in the late 1800s (Rost 1997) and, in 1892, Osler suggested that a large heart was necessary for success in sport (Osler 1892). Eight years later, Henschen (1899), performing percussion of the chest to estimate heart size in cross-country skiers, first used the term 'athlete's heart': '...skiing causes an enlargement of the heart, and that this enlarged heart can perform more work than the normal heart. There is therefore a physiologic enlargement of the heart, due to athletic activity: the athlete's heart.' (From Rost 1997, p. 493.)

Henschen's work was remarkably comprehensive for its time. He proposed that enlargement was secondary to both hypertrophy and dilatation of the chambers, and that the dilatation was symmetrical (left and right sided); this remains a distinguishing feature between physiological and pathological enlargement today. However, the view that participation in athletics contributed to benign cardiac enlargement was not uniformly held during that time. There were some who believed that exercise-induced cardiac enlargement would inevitably lead to cardiovascular collapse (Deutsch & Kauf 1924), or that it was secondary to a pre-existing weakness (Deutsch & Moritz 1908). As Rost (1997) summarizes, the commonly held view in the late 1800s and early 1900s was that an athlete had a shortened lifespan compared to the general population! This belief continued well into the 20th century and in fact, identification of heart murmurs of any kind could lead to disqualification from athletic competition, as was the case for the legendary marathon runner Clarence DeMar in the 1910s and Wally Hayward in the 1930s (Noakes 1991). In the case of DeMar, an autopsy performed after his death (from bowel cancer) revealed a normal cardiac anatomy, and earlier diagnoses of heart murmurs were attributed to the athletic heart syndrome. Some 70 years after DeMar's incorrect diagnosis, it was reported that the majority of long-distance runners present with benign heart murmurs and additional (third and fourth) heart sounds (Parker *et al.* 1978). Current epidemiological evidence suggests that the lifespan for individuals with athlete's heart is at least equal to those with normal-sized hearts (Rost 1997), and there is some evidence that world-class athletes outlive the general population (Sarna *et al.* 1993).

68

Technical advances in diagnosis

Technical advances in cardiac assessment have certainly contributed to greater precision in distinguishing pathological and physiological cardiac enlargement. Radiological techniques have improved considerably since their introduction and by the early 1960s, the oxygen pulse was used in conjunction with radiological examination to differentiate physiological from pathological hypertrophy (Rost 1997). Cardiothoracic ratios exceeding the normal ceiling of 0.50 were observed in athletes as early as the 1960s using radiographs (Shephard 1996).

Electrocardiographic (ECG) voltages were later used in detection of left ventricular hypertrophy (LVH) and right ventricular hypertrophy (RVH); LVH was considered if the sum of the ECG waves SV1 + RV5 exceeded 35 mm and RVH was diagnosed if the sum of RV1 + SV5 exceeded 10.5 mm. Using this technology, a high percentage of athletes could be classified as having LVH (Shephard 1996) and incomplete right bundle branch block (Rost 1997). However, the use of ECG alone to predict LVH is of dubious value in this population because of the increased thoracic skeletal muscle mass (Park & Crawford 1985), and the wide range of abnormal ECG patterns that are associated with endurance training (Holly et al. 1998).

The widespread use of echocardiography in the early 1970s greatly accelerated research on the athlete's heart. Although Morganroth and colleagues (Morganroth et al. 1975) are frequently cited in the North American literature as the first to describe echocardiographic data on the athlete's heart, Rost and colleagues (cited in Rost 1997) reported LVH in athletes using M-mode echocardiography at the Munich Olympics in 1972. It appears that two-dimensional echocardiography has more precision than M-mode techniques, when magnetic resonance imaging (MRI) is used as the gold-standard comparison (Pluim et al. 1997). Texture analysis to quantify the collagen content in hypertensive and athletic hearts has recently been used in conjunction with two-dimensional echocardiography (Di Bello et al. 1997). MRI has further refined imaging of the athletic heart (Milliken et al. 1988),

and now MRI techniques can be supplemented with functional and metabolic measures of the athletic heart (Pluim et al. 1998). Despite the application of modern-day cardiac imaging technologies, the task of distinguishing pathological from physiological hypertrophy remains elusive because of the overlap in morphological findings between the athletic heart and diseased states such as dilated and hypertrophic cardiomyopathy.

Aside from morphological evidence of the athlete's heart, reports of acute 'cardiac fatigue' during prolonged endurance events (Niemela et al. 1984, 1987; Douglas et al. 1987, 1990a,b; Vanoverschelde et al. 1991; Ketelhut et al. 1992) and exercise-induced sudden cardiac death in athletes (Van Camp & Choi 1988; Thompson 1993; Goodman 1995) have helped to maintain interest in this topic.

Ventricular performance and the athletic heart: effects of training

The human left ventricle is capable of profound changes in size and shape in response to a broad range of stimuli. Now commonly referred to as ventricular remodelling, these changes relate to global changes in size, shape and wall thickness, in addition to alterations at the cellular and molecular levels (Sabbah & Goldstein 1993).

Left ventricular chamber size

Training-induced changes in LV volume can occur with less than 3 months of endurance training (Ehsani et al. 1978), and LV diastolic chamber size may increase within 1 week of endurance training (Rubal et al. 1987). The hallmark feature of training-induced increases in $\dot{V}_{O_{2max}}$ is an increase in stroke volume (Clausen 1977). The mechanisms responsible for the increase in stroke volume include: (i) proportional increases in LV chamber diameter and wall thickness (Ehsani et al. 1978; Ehsani & Spina 1997; Fagard 1997); (ii) enhanced LV contractility due to enhanced β-adrenergic sensitivity (Spina et al. 1992, 1998; Seals et al. 1994; Stratton et al. 1994); and (iii) enhanced diastolic filling (Forman et al. 1992; Takemoto et al. 1992; Brandao et al. 1993; Levy et al. 1993).

Systolic and diastolic function

Despite the training-induced increased LV wall thickness, it remains unclear if systolic performance is actually enhanced in trained athletes. An increased contractile reserve has been reported in older male adults following training (Ehsani *et al.* 1991; Seals *et al.* 1994; Spina *et al.* 1994, 1997, 1998; Schulman *et al.* 1996), but a number of investigators have failed to demonstrate similar findings in younger athletes (Brandao *et al.* 1993) participating in a wide range of endurance sports (Fagard 1997). Determination of contractile function remains problematic in the intact heart, given that indirect measures of contractility are influenced by heart rate, preload and afterload. If the various determinants of systolic shortening are considered, it becomes questionable whether contractility is enhanced. But in contrast with the reduced contractility seen in enlarged and diseased hearts, contractility appears to be normal in the athletic heart (Colan 1997). There is more evidence to support a training-induced enhancement in diastolic function in both young and older individuals (Levy *et al.* 1993; Stratton *et al.* 1994).

Physiological basis of cardiac enlargement in the athlete's heart

Haemodynamic basis of hypertrophy in the athlete's heart

The ventricular remodelling that is brought about by long-term adherence to endurance training reflects chronic haemodynamic overloading (Pelliccia & Maron 1997; Richey & Brown 1998). In general, the nature of the hypertrophy reflects the nature of the stimulus and the function of the hypertrophied heart reflects its biochemistry (Scheuer & Buttrick 1987). The precise stimulus inducing hypertrophy in the athletic heart is unknown, but it is probable that the total work load 'seen' by the heart acts as a primary stimulus (pressure and volume overload). Prolonged exposure to catecholamines may act in an independent fashion (Scheuer & Buttrick 1987). In both physiological and pathological hypertrophy, the increased wall thickness is a compensatory

response that reduces LV wall stress (Grossman 1980; Scheuer & Buttrick. 1987; Maron *et al.* 1995; Opie 1998; Richey & Brown 1998). However, in pathological hypertrophy, remodelling fails to meet myocardial demands, and the result is a decline in function due to ischaemia or 'slippage' of the contractile apparatus, producing heart failure.

In endurance athletes, the chronic exposure to volume overload is secondary to an increased cardiac output and venous return. The prolonged bradycardia, reduced afterload and enhanced preload contribute to a volume overload stimulus, leading to ventricular remodelling (Opie 1998; Fig. 6.1). Volume overloading produced by endurance training increases the LV end-diastolic volume during exercise (enhanced use of the Frank–Starling

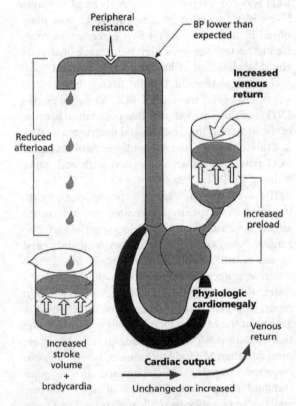

Fig. 6.1 The athlete's heart. As a simplification, the adaptations involved in dynamic exercise training may be regarded as compensatory responses to a chronic volume load, including physiological cardiomegaly. BP, blood pressure. From Opie (1998, p. 465), with permission.

mechanism). It is likely to be secondary to an exercise-induced hypervolaemia (Convertino *et al.* 1980; Blomqvist & Saltin 1983; Convertino 1991; Green *et al.* 1991; Schwartz *et al.* 1992; Levine 1993). The eccentric LV adaptation, aided by a training-induced bradycardia, contributes to a prolonged ventricular filling time and a more efficient filling pattern (Colan *et al.* 1987; Levine 1993; Levy *et al.* 1993).

Balanced enlargement and normalizing wall stress

The law of Laplace dictates that LV wall tension (T) is a function of both the intraventricular pressure (P) and radius (r), and LV wall thickness (H), where:

$$T = Pr/2H$$

Implicit in this relationship is the fact that a dilated heart is at a mechanical disadvantage. In fact, if the diameter of the heart were to be doubled, the radius of curvature would also be doubled, resulting in a doubling of the tension per unit length of ventricular wall in order to produce the same systolic blood pressure. If linear dimensions of the heart are doubled (to account for the longitudinal axis), the total tension of the ventricle is actually quadrupled (Burton 1965). The normalizing of ventricular wall tension (or 'wall stress') and thus myocardial oxygen demand can be achieved rather simply by modest hypertrophy of the ventricular wall.

In the context of endurance training, LV chamber dilatation is indeed accompanied by modest hypertrophy, whereas in pathological states (see also Chapter 48), dilatation is associated with thin-walled ventricles and poor function. The actual measurement of LV wall stress is complex, in part because wall stress in the LV acts in three directions—circumferential, meridional and radial. The actual measurement requires simultaneous measures of intraventricular pressure and LV wall diameter by echocardiography across the minor axis (Little & Braunwald 1997). Although the basic equation for calculating wall stress (above) is an oversimplification, it emphasizes the interaction between ventricular volume and wall thickness. Figure 6.2 provides hypothetical examples of how endurance training elicits remodelling in a manner that normalizes wall stress, and thereby enhances ventricular output without increasing myocardial O_2 demands significantly, compared to a non-physiological strategy.

Molecular triggers for hypertrophy

Three main triggers for hypertrophy link haemodynamic loading and cardiac growth. These triggers include: (i) *stretching* of muscle cells, brought about by augmented preload and afterload; (ii) *agonists*, including angiotensin II, catecholamines and endothelin (which act on protein kinase C (PKC)); and (iii) *growth factors*, such as insulin-like growth factor (IGF) and transforming growth factor (TGF), which act through phosphorylation (Opie 1998). Although myocyte stretch is the most widely accepted signal to hypertrophy (Opie 1998), exposure to different types of overload (i.e. pressure versus volume) is known to influence gene expression (Schwartz *et al.* 1992). Given the wide variation in loading conditions produced by different types of exercise (e.g. static versus dynamic exercise, intensity of training, etc.), it is not surprising to see different types (and extents) of hypertrophy in the broad athletic population.

Characterizing the athletic heart

Distinguishing pathological and physiological hypertrophy

Hypertrophic patterns in the athletic heart often resemble those typically seen in pathological states, yet the mechanisms, haemodynamic responses and functional characteristics differ considerably in the two types of cardiac enlargement (Table 6.1).

Differentiating the athletic and diseased ventricle has posed a challenge to the clinician. A number of criteria can be considered, including the upper limits for various LV wall thicknesses and wall thickness ratios, cavity dimensions, and systolic and diastolic function. Nevertheless, there is still no single reliable criterion to distinguish hypertrophic cardiomyopathy (HCM) from the physiological hypertrophy associated with the athletic heart.

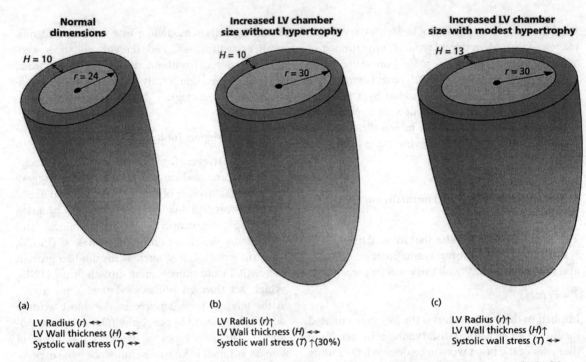

Normal dimensions	**Increased LV chamber size without hypertrophy**	**Increased LV chamber size with modest hypertrophy**
(a)	(b)	(c)
LV Radius (*r*) ↔	LV Radius (*r*)↑	LV Radius (*r*)↑
LV Wall thickness (*H*) ↔	LV Wall thickness (*H*) ↔	LV Wall thickness (*H*)↑
Systolic wall stress (*T*) ↔	Systolic wall stress (*T*) ↑(30%)	Systolic wall stress (*T*) ↔

Fig. 6.2 Interaction between left ventricular dimensions and wall stress (a) in a normal left ventricle (untrained), (b) following chamber enlargement without left ventricular hypertrophy (i.e. cardiomyopathy) and (c) following endurance training (increased ventricular chamber volume and modest hypertrophy).

Many athletes can demonstrate hypertrophic changes that fall between pathological and physiological limits. Nevertheless, various clinical and morphological criteria have been suggested (Maron *et al.* 1995) and can be used jointly when ruling out pathology in athletes (Fig. 6.3).

When an athlete presents with LV morphology that exceeds the generally accepted upper limits of normality, a period of deconditioning will usually produce regression of the LVH, establishing the physiological nature of the hypertrophy (Fig. 6.4). A number of studies have shown rapid reversal of LV dimensions (Ehsani *et al.* 1978; Maron *et al.* 1993; Ehsani & Spina 1997) upon cessation of endurance training, a trend not seen in athletes with diagnosed HCM (Maron *et al.* 1993). The cause of this reversal is unknown; however, it seems logical that a loss in plasma volume and the chronic exposure to a volume load (e.g. stretch stimulus) produced by an elevated cardiac output are contributing factors.

WALL THICKNESS AND CAVITY DIMENSIONS

Echocardiographically determined criteria specify a wide range of normal cardiac dimensions. These include an arbitrary ceiling for LV wall thickness of 12 mm, a septal/free wall thickness ratio of 1.3 and a septal/posterior wall thickness ratio of 1.2:1. The upper normal limit for the LV mass index (LVMI) is 130 g per square of body surface area, and the normal LV chamber cross-sectional diameter is said to range between 45 mm and 55 mm. However, the 'upper limits' of normal are frequently exceeded in the athlete's heart. LV wall thickness is typically 15% greater than normal, and cavity dimensions are often 10% beyond the normal range (Pelliccia *et al.* 1996). The latter figure represents a 33% increase in end-diastolic volume, owing to the cubic relationship of dimension to volume (Maron 1986; Shapiro 1997).

Table 6.1 Left ventricular hypertrophic patterns and related haemodynamic mechanisms in physiological and pathological hypertrophy. Adapted from Richey and Brown (1998).

	Physiological LVH (athlete's heart)		Pathological LVH	
	Concentric	Eccentric	Concentric	Eccentric
Possible haemodynamic triggers	Increased afterload and wall stress	Increased preload (volume/stretch)	Increased afterload and wall stress	Increased preload (volume/stretch)
Aetiology	*Dominant:* strength/static exercise *Secondary:* endurance (dynamic) exercise	*Dominant:* endurance (dynamic) exercise *Secondary:* static exercise	Hypertension, aortic stenosis	Valvular disease, idiopathic dilated cardiomyopathy
Myofibular characteristics	New myofibrils in parallel (individual thickening)	New sarcomeres added in series	New myofibrils in parallel (individual thickening), necrosis and fibrosis and inflammation	New sarcomeres added in series; wall thinning; necrosis and fibrosis
Ventricular dimensions	Modest increases in LV wall thickness and small changes in chamber size	Increase in chamber volume and increases in wall thickness	Pronounced wall thickness with relatively small chamber size	Pronounced increase in chamber volume without compensatory wall thickening
Cellular characteristics	Increased capillarity and mitochondrial volume	Increased capillarity and mitochondrial volume	Inadequate capillary growth to match myofibular hypertrophy	Inadequate capillary growth to match increased wall stress
Functional characteristics	Normal or augmented systolic function; normal diastolic function	Normal systolic function; normal or enhanced diastolic function	Diastolic dysfunction and depressed contractility	Impaired contractility ('slippage') and sometimes diastolic dysfunction
Regression possible	Yes	Yes	No	No

LVH, left ventricular hypertrophy.

Few studies have examined the shape of the athletic heart in comparison to untrained subjects. It appears that the athlete's heart reflects a pattern of remodelling that promotes dilatation along the longitudinal axis (measured from the mitral valve to the apex) (Turpeinen *et al.* 1996; Pelliccia & Maron 1997). This is in contrast to cardiomyopathies, which normally see remodelling towards a spherical or horizontally elongated shape (Pelliccia & Maron 1997). Both pathological and physiological adaptations show interindividual differences in hypertrophic patterns; certainly, the pattern of hypertrophy is not uniform from one athlete to another.

Most echocardiographic data used to establish normal limits for the athletic population have been

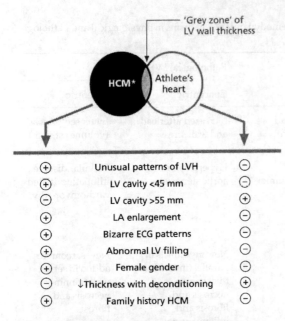

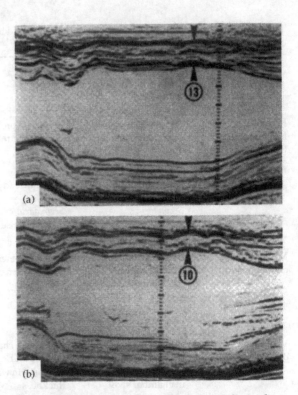

Fig. 6.3 Criteria used to distinguish hypertrophic cardiomyopathy from athlete's heart. The shaded area (grey zone) indicates overlap between the two diagnoses, and the criteria listed below indicate which diagnosis would be favoured (+) or less likely (–) for each criterion. ↓, decreased; ECG, electrocardiograph; HCM, hypertrophic cardiomyopathy; LA, left atrial; LV, left ventricular; LVH, left ventricular hypertrophy. *Assumes that systolic anterior motion of the mitral valve is absent because its presence would indicate the presence of hypertrophic cardiomyopathy even in an athlete. From Maron *et al.* (1995, p. 1596), with permission.

Fig. 6.4 M-mode echocardiographic tracings obtained from an élite male rower at the peak of athletic conditioning (a) and after an 8-week deconditioning period (b). The ventricular septum shows a reduction in thickness from 13 mm (a) to 10 mm (b). From Pelliccia & Maron (1997, p. 390), with permission.

cross-sectional, based on athletes who have participated in their respective sports for some time. Most, but not all, longitudinal training studies have demonstrated modest increases in the wall thickness and LV internal diameter of healthy non-athletic volunteers relative to a control group (Fagard 1996, 1997). The limit of resolution for the M-mode echocardiography (2 mm) that was used in earlier studies is similar to the typical differences between trained and untrained individuals (Perreault & Turcotte 1994; Shephard 1996). When endurance training is intense, as in élite athletes, the accepted normal ranges are easily exceeded, and in some cases values approach the range seen in advanced pathology. Some 2% of athletes from a variety of disciplines demonstrate LV wall thicken-

ing greater than 13 mm, and 15% of athletes present with an end-diastolic cross-sectional diameter greater than 60 mm (Pelliccia *et al.* 1991; Pelliccia & Maron 1997). At the international level of competition, it is common for these athletes to present with cardiac dimensions that are well beyond the normal range; however, pronounced LV dilatation is typically balanced by increases in LV wall thickness in order to normalize wall stress (Fig. 6.5).

In most endurance athletes, LVH is dominant in the anterior septum. However, the pattern of hypertrophy is far more uniform than that seen in HCM, where the average LV wall thickness is 20 mm, but can exceed 60 mm in some cases (Maron *et al.* 1995). Both pathological and physiological adaptations show differing patterns of hypertrophy (eccentric or

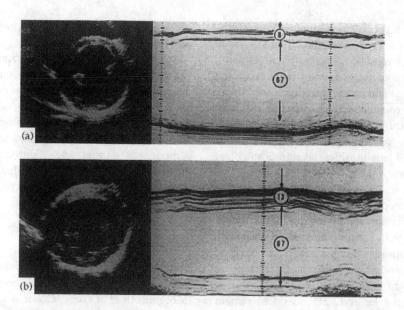

Fig. 6.5 Comparative echocardiographic images of left ventricular dilatation in a 20-year-old asymptomatic patient with idiopathic dilated cardiomyopathy (a) and extreme expression of athlete's heart in a 26-year-old highly trained élite rower, who was a participant in the 1992 Olympic Games (b). Parasternal long-axis and M-mode recordings, at the same calibration in the cardiomyopathy patient and in the élite athlete, showing a markedly enlarged left ventricular cavity (end-diastolic diameter 67 mm in both instances); the ventricular septum is relatively thin (8 mm) in the patient with dilated cardiomyopathy, but is mildly increased (13 mm) in the highly trained rower. Septal and free wall excursion are mildly reduced in the patient (suggesting decreased contractility), but are normal in the rower. From Pelliccia A. & Maron, B.J. (1986) Differentiation of cardiovascular disease from the physiological changes of the highly trained athlete. *Sport, Exercise and Injury* **2**, 64–71, cited in Pelliccia & Maron (1997), p. 393, with permission.

concentric), depending on the type and extent of haemodynamic loading.

BIOCHEMICAL AND CELLULAR CHANGES

The changes in biochemical and cellular characteristics of the athletic heart reflect the nature of the stimulus. A key adaptive feature of the athletic heart is the proportional increase in cellular content and enhanced vascular function. The increase in LV muscle mass is matched by a maintenance of a normal mitochondrial/myofibril volume ratio (Crisman & Tomanek 1985; Richey & Brown 1998), and in particular, by an enhanced coronary vascular reserve and capillarity (Hudlicka *et al.* 1995; Laughlin 1995; Laughlin *et al.* 1996, 1998; Zhao *et al.* 1997). These physiological adaptations are the complete opposite of what is observed in HCM and other cardiomyopathies (Richey & Brown 1998).

VENTRICULAR FUNCTION

A key feature of physiological adaptation in endurance athletes is normal (and sometimes supranormal) diastolic filling (Forman *et al.* 1992; Takemoto *et al.* 1992; Brandao *et al.* 1993; Levy *et al.* 1993). In contrast, filling is commonly impaired in HCM (Spirito *et al.* 1985; Maron *et al.* 1987; Spirito & Maron 1988). As mentioned above, systolic function is typically normal in the athletic heart (Colan 1997), whereas in HCM indices of LV systolic function are profoundly impaired (Pelliccia & Maron 1997; Wynne & Braunwald 1997).

Gender issues

Women athletes appear to develop mild but significant increases in LV cavity size, wall thickness and mass, and like their male counterparts, these changes are most pronounced among those participating in endurance competition (Pelliccia *et al.* 1996). From a review of 600 élite female athletes, Pelliccia *et al.* (1996) showed a mean increase of 6% for LV cavity size and a 14% increase in wall thickness compared to age- and sex-matched sedentary controls. These differences persist even when values are normalized for body surface area (BSA), but the advantage of female athletes is significantly less than that of their male counterparts. Only 1% of female athletes had figures in the 'upper limit' of 'normal' hypertrophy (i.e. Maron's 'grey zone', an LV thickness of 11 mm), and none had LV wall thicknesses of more than 13 mm. This is in contrast with male athletes, some of whom have had values of 16 mm or more, and 2% of whom had LV thicknesses in excess of 12 mm.

Reasons for the lesser LVH in women remain unclear. A smaller body size is only a partial explanation, since normalizing values with BSA still yields values that are less than in men. Differences in the cardiovascular response to exercise (Spina *et al.* 1993), a lower absolute training intensity (which may reduce the cardiac loading) and possible androgenic influences on myocardial protein synthesis (Koenig *et al.* 1982; Marsh *et al.* 1998) may offer some explanation.

Influence of type of sport on physiological hypertrophy

The type and intensity of training have considerable influence on LV dimensions (Morganroth *et al.* 1975; Keul *et al.* 1981; Longhurst *et al.* 1981; Fisher *et al.* 1989; Pelliccia *et al.* 1991, 1993; Spirito *et al.* 1994) (Table 6.2). Factors including the length of training, haemodynamic loads and phase of training all influence the adaptive response. In addition, overall body size strongly influences findings (Pelliccia *et al.* 1991; Urhausen *et al.* 1996b, 1997), making absolute comparisons unreliable. Unfortunately, these factors are often described sparsely in the literature, particularly when large samples of athletes from a variety of disciplines are reported.

Endurance sports

The pattern of hypertrophy is generally eccentric in athletes engaged in dynamic endurance activity (Morganroth *et al.* 1975; Colan *et al.* 1987; Fagard 1997; Richey & Brown 1998). However, some reports have demonstrated a high occurrence of concentric hypertrophy (Rodriguez Reguero *et al.* 1995). In distance runners, the ventricular mass at rest and during exercise is related largely to an increased ventricular chamber volume (compared to controls). However, increased LV septal and posterior wall thicknesses have also been reported in endurance athletes (Morganroth *et al.* 1975; Ehsani *et al.* 1978; Colan *et al.* 1987; Maron *et al.* 1995; Fagard 1996; Pluim *et al.* 1996; Pelliccia & Maron 1997).

In a comprehensive meta-analysis, Fagard (1996) combined studies in which competitive long-distance runners had been compared to matched

Table 6.2 Typical cardiac dimensions in a range of sports.

	Normal range	Runners‡	Cyclists‡	Strength athletes	Basketball players
$LVID_d$ (mm)	37–55	53.2±0.68*	55.1±0.33*	53.2±0.99*	59†
$IVST_d$ (mm)	6–14	10.8±0.27*	11.7±0.6*	10.3±0.48*	11.4†
PWT_d (mm)	6–11	10.5±0.29*	11.6±0.75*	9.5±0.55*	11.4†
LVM (g)	200–300	200–215	240–270	190–200	284†
LVMI (g·m⁻²)	65–90	100–130	110–138	85–90	118.3†
BSA (m²)	1.45–2.22	1.81	1.89	1.98	2.4†

$LVID_d$, left ventricular internal diameter; $IVST_d$, interventricular septal thickness;
PWT_d, posterior wall thickness; LVM, left ventricular mass; LVMI, left ventricular mass index;
BSA, body surface area.
*Data cited in Fagard (1997).
†Data from Van Decker *et al.* (1989).
‡Endurance events; no specific distance provided.

non-athletic controls. In runners, the LV internal diameter was 10% higher, and the LV wall thickness was 18% greater. LV mass was 48% greater in runners, whereas cyclists showed a 64% larger mass than the controls. In another large study of élite endurance cyclists, only a small proportion of the sample demonstrated an LV wall thickness in excess of 12 mm (Pelliccia *et al.* 1991). The most pronounced dimensional changes are seen in élite athletes who combine upper- and lower-body work during endurance events, including cycling, rowing and cross-country skiing. The static nature of the arm work may stimulate more pronounced changes in LV wall thickness, whereas 'pure' endurance sports such as running are dominated by changes in cavity dimension and modest changes in wall thickness (Pelliccia & Maron 1997). There are few data on swimmers, and few details are offered regarding the training regimen and type of swimmer studied. Morganroth *et al.* (1975) found modest dimensional changes in male collegiate swimmers who had been swimming for at least 3 years. In general, swimmers demonstrate only modest eccentric hypertrophy with significantly larger LV internal diameters (Fagard 1997). In sports which combine several types of training regimens, such as the triathlon, increases in LV mass have been observed (Fagard 1997), but only one study showed changes in wall thickness (Douglas *et al.* 1986).

The literature describing the 'endurance athlete' remains limited, primarily because of the broad scope of sports studied, often without mention of specific events in which athlete groups competed. For example, in one of the largest studies involving 25 sports, only 'vigorous training' was provided as a description of training status (Pelliccia *et al.* 1991). In most reports, as in that of Pelliccia *et al.* (1991), the majority of athletes studied have been of an international calibre.

Strength training

Strength training regimens may be considered 'static exercise' (Longhurst & Stebbens 1997). Weightlifting produces transient increases in systolic pressure in excess of 300–350 mmHg (Mac-Dougall *et al.* 1985), due to increases in intrathoracic and intra-abdominal pressures (Palatini *et al.* 1989)

and a significant pressor reflex originating from the active muscle mass. This extreme haemodynamic load is not accompanied by any significant change in cardiac output or ventricular filling during activity.

The lack of a significant preload may explain why these athletes fail to show the same degree of ventricular remodelling that is seen in endurance exercise (Longhurst & Stebbens 1997). Notwithstanding, when allowance is made for body mass, the LV mass and wall thickness of strength training athletes are increased on average by 25% and 12%, respectively (Fagard 1996, 1997). The pattern of hypertrophy is predominantly concentric, but can also involve eccentric hypertrophy. In athletes who use weightlifting to supplement endurance training (for example, rowers), the pattern of LV enlargement is dominated by increases in cavity size, with less change in wall thickness (Urhausen *et al.* 1996a). Changes in wall thickness do not appear to be augmented by use of anabolic steroids (Urhausen *et al.* 1989; Palatini *et al.* 1996), but steroid use may contribute to an increased LV stiffness (Wight & Salem 1995). The influence of steroid use on ventricular hypertrophy requires further research.

Exercise and sudden death

Some 2000 years after Philipides' pronouncement of victory of the Athenians, Bassler (1977) suggested that marathon running provided immunity against coronary heart disease. The so-called 'Bassler hypothesis' has since been dismissed; it is widely accepted that atherosclerosis can develop in distance runners, and indeed is a major culprit in exercise-related sudden death, even amongst veteran marathon runners and those with a long history of physical activity. Contrary to the assertions of Bassler, there are now a number of reports of advanced coronary disease in marathon runners (Noakes 1987), proving that sudden cardiac death (SCD) can occur as a result of occlusive atherosclerotic disease despite a high commitment to endurance training. In addition, a number of reports have described exercise-induced SCD in young athletes (less than 35 years of age), who upon autopsy had mild to extreme LVH. The question remains:

given the widespread prevalence of LVH in endurance athletes, are they at greater risk?

To date, there have been over 600 reported cases of exercise-related sudden deaths occurring either during or immediately after participation in a wide range of sports. These reports have raised questions about the athlete's heart. Careful inspection of autopsy data has established that the vast majority of SCD cases in those above an age of 30–35 years are secondary to acute complications of atherosclerosis (Waller 1985). However, SCD in those less than 30–35 years of age is commonly ascribed to disorders of myocardial structure and/or conduction (Waller 1985; Maron *et al.* 1986), secondary to various congenital conditions, the most common being HCM. Irrespective of aetiology, the immediate mechanism of death is probably fatal LV dysrhythmia. Females represent only a small fraction of SCD cases (approximately 10% of reported incidents).

The incidence of SCD in endurance athletes is extremely low—0.002% or 1 in 50 000 race finishers ranging in age from 19 to 58 years (average age = 37) (Maron *et al.* 1996). Fissuring of a previously fragile but non-occlusive plaque with thrombus formation and total occlusion is thought to account for most deaths with postmortem evidence of acute myocardial infarction. However, a fresh occlusive thrombus is found in only a small percentage of cases (Northcote *et al.* 1986). In the absence of myocardial damage, transient myocardial ischaemia is another possible mechanism of death; fissuring of a plaque may partially occlude a major coronary vessel, the lesion being sufficient to induce ischaemia and/or vasospasm which evolves to a malignant dysrhythmia.

In non-exercise cases of SCD, acute rupture or partial thrombosis evolving from a plaque is responsible for over 90% of cases, occlusions often occurring at what had previously been thought to be non-critical lesions (Davies & Thomas 1985; Thompson 1993). This may explain why some individuals have previously been symptom free, and/or have failed to demonstrate ECG changes during a stress test; there is an acute progression of the disease in the moments immediately preceding death (Kohl *et al.* 1992). Associated pathologies that increase the risk of sudden death include LV outflow tract obstruction, endocardial mural plaques, mitral valve disease, atrial dilatation, abnormal intramural coronary arteries, and a disorganization of myocardial fibres in the septum.

Hypertrophic cardiomyopathy

Hypertrophic cardiomyopathy is widely held to be the most common cause of exercise-related sudden death in sedentary and athletic individuals under the age of 35 years (Maron *et al.* 1980, 1986) (Fig. 6.6) (see also Chapter 48). Although HCM is rare in the general population (0.1% in young adults), 40% of HCM-related sudden deaths are associated with exertion of some type (Maron & Fananapazir 1992; Maron 1993). The primary morphological abnormality lies in the septum, which exceeds the diameter of the free ventricular wall by a factor of 1.4 or more (Goodwin *et al.* 1982; Maron *et al.* 1986, 1995), but the abnormal histology involves more than 5% of the total cardiac muscle mass (Burke *et al.* 1992).

As described above, most endurance athletes have only modest wall thickening (12–14 mm), but demonstrate proportionally enlarged ventricular cavities with uniform hypertrophy (Fig. 6.4). The most striking feature of the pathological hypertrophy seen in HCM is a focal disarray of the myocardial fibres down to the level of the myofilament. This feature is seen in 90% of those with HCM (Maron *et al.* 1981). The morphological characteristics produce LV systolic dysfunction, including a reduction in diastolic filling characteristics, whereas they are often enhanced in the athletic heart. Outflow tract obstruction is often associated with sudden death in HCM, but it occurs in only 25% of reported cases (Maron 1993).

The mechanism of exercise-related SCD in athletes with HCM is most likely arrhythmogenic (Maron & Fananapazir 1992; Maron *et al.* 1986, 1993). The action potential is lengthened in hypertrophied myocytes, and some experimental data suggest an ionic basis for this abnormality (Pye & Cobbe 1992). Accessory conduction pathways and a mechanical stretching of myocytes (which can increase ectopic beat frequency) are other possible bases for the dysrhythmias.

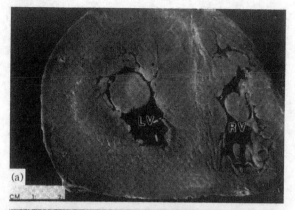

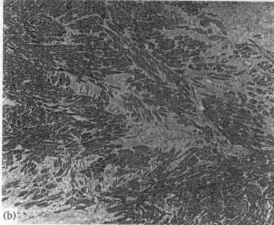

Fig. 6.6 Hypertrophic cardiomyopathy. A 20-year-old man died suddenly during a basketball game. The heart weighed 690 g with asymmetric septal hypertrophy (anterior septum 3 cm and left ventricular free wall 2.1 cm) with microscopic, focal areas of fibrosis within the area of the greatest hypertrophy. There was a discrete outflow tract plaque noted on gross examination. Sections of the ventricular septum showed marked fibromuscular disarray (b) with intramyocardial coronary artery thickening. LV, left ventricle; RV, right ventricle. From Virmani *et al.* (1997, p. 447).

Conduction abnormalities

A number of ECG syndromes are associated with the sudden death of athletes, including the Wolff–Parkinson–White syndrome and Lown–Ganong–Levine syndrome (Sadaniantz & Thompson 1990; Holly *et al.* 1998). Isolated conduction abnormalities may be a 'concealed' cause of death in young athletes with normal histology, because the conduction systems are rarely examined thoroughly (Corrado

et al. 1990; Sadaniantz & Thompson 1990; Holly *et al.* 1998). Atrioventricular (AV) and nodoventricular accessory pathways have been suggested as culprits in some cases of exercise-related SCD (Corrado *et al.* 1990; Holly *et al.* 1998). However, the lack of prior ECG evidence of such disorders in many of the athletes who die makes such speculations difficult to prove or disprove. In addition, various dysrhythmias (e.g. paroxysmal supraventricular tachycardia, non-sustained ventricular tachycardia) are frequently reported in athletes, but are rarely lethal.

The distribution of sudden deaths in various sports shows a predominance of squash relative to other types of active leisure pursuits. This may simply reflect the popularity of the sport (Northcote & Ballantyne 1985; Corrado *et al.* 1990; Sadaniantz & Thompson 1990; Holly *et al.* 1998). The sudden bursts of isometric activity seen with squash may provoke SCD if the individual has a severe cardiac pathology, yet the pressor response to this sport is similar to cycle ergometry (Brigdgen *et al.* 1992). In addition, recreational players, if older, are more likely to have advanced coronary artery disease (Northcote *et al.* 1986).

Potential triggers of sudden death

In establishing a *de facto* cause of exercise-induced SCD, a '*trigger*' must act as a substrate within a *pathophysiologic milieu*, typically multifactorial in nature (Kohl *et al.* 1992).

Humoral and other blood-borne triggers act to precipitate SCD in individuals who are free of coronary heart disease. The abnormalities identified include magnesium ion (Mg) deficiency (Eisenberg 1992; Rowe 1993), hyperlipidaemia and hyperglycaemia (Stendig-Lindberg 1992). Mg deficiency often develops after prolonged effort, and can persist more than 12 weeks following competition. Because Mg deficiency usually elicits vasoconstriction (Stendig-Lindberg 1992), it has been proposed as a trigger of vasospasm-induced SCD (Rowe 1993), and even pronounced silent ischaemia in a world-class marathon runner (Rowe 1991). In addition, Mg deficiency may precipitate complex dysrhythmias (Eisenberg 1992) which may progress to ventricular fibrillation in HCM. Plasma catecholamines may invoke electrical instability, producing abnormal electrical conduction and depolarization.

Sudden exercise and/or abrupt cessation of exercise may also precipitate SCD in vulnerable individuals, including those with abnormal ECG and ventricular function (Foster *et al.* 1991). Prolonged endurance running in itself is an unlikely, but possible long-term trigger for SCD (Rowe 1993). Prolonged effort may increase the risk of SCD via increases in core temperature, dehydration and Mg depletion (Eisenberg 1992). Impaired diastolic and systolic performance (referred to as 'cardiac fatigue') has been reported following prolonged effort (Niemela *et al.* 1984, 1987; Douglas *et al.* 1987, 1990a,b; Vanoverschelde *et al.* 1991; Ketelhut *et al.* 1992). However, a recent report suggests this activity is not associated with myocardial tissue damage (Laslett & Eisenbud 1997).

Conclusions

The athlete's heart is the product of physiological hypertrophy secondary to extensive participation in physical activity, usually performed at an international competitive level. The nature and extent of LV remodelling are dependent on the amount of exercise performed and, to some extent, the type of activity. The most profound morphological changes are seen in élite endurance athletes. More modest changes are seen in the general population who are involved in less intensive, fitness-related activity. In extreme cases of conditioning, LV dimensions can approach those seen in pathological states. The majority of endurance athletes have cardiac dimensions that fall within the normal range, but often dimensions are classified as 'high-normal'. However, the evidence strongly supports the physiological nature of this adaptation, which includes increases in LV chamber size and modest wall thickening, concomitant with normal or enhanced systolic and diastolic function. Consequently, the athlete's heart reflects appropriate physiological remodelling that maintains or enhances performance.

References

Bassler, T.J. (1977) Marathon running and immunity to atherosclerosis. *Annals of the New York Academy of Sciences* **301**, 579–592.

Blomqvist, C.G. & Saltin, B. (1983) Cardiovascular adaptations to physical training. *Annual Review of Physiology* **45**, 169–189.

Brandao, M.U., Wajngarten, M., Rondon, E., Giorgi, M.C., Hironaka, F. & Negrao, C.E. (1993) Left ventricular function during dynamic exercise in untrained and moderately trained subjects. *Journal of Applied Physiology* **75** (5), 1989–1995.

Brigdgen, G.S., Hughes, L.O., Broadhurst, P. & Raftery, E.B. (1992) Blood pressure changes during the game of squash. *European Heart Journal* **13**, 1084–1087.

Burke, A.P., Farb, A. & Virmani, R. (1992) Causes of sudden death in athletes. *Cardiology Clinics* (B. J. Maron, ed.) **10**, 303–317.

Burton, A.C. (1965) Hemodynamics and the physics of the circulation. In: Ruch, T.C. & Patton, H.D. (eds) *Physiology and Biophysics*, pp. 523–542. W.B. Saunders, Philadelphia.

Clausen, J.P. (1977) Effect of physical training on cardiovascular adjustments to exercise in man. *Physiological Reviews* **57**, 779–815.

Colan, S.D. (1997) Mechanics of left ventricular systolic and diastolic function in physiologic hypertrophy of the athlete's heart. *Cardiology Clinics* **15** (3), 355–372.

Colan, S.D., Sanders, S.P. & Borow, K.M. (1987) Physiologic hypertrophy: effects on left ventricular systolic mechanics in athletes. *Journal of the American College of Cardiology* **9**, 776–783.

Convertino, V.F. (1991) Blood, its adaptation to endurance training. *Medicine and Science in Sports and Exercise* **23**, 1338–1348.

Convertino, V.F., Brock, P.J., Keil, L.C., Bernauer, E.M. & Greenleaf, J.E. (1980) Exercise training-induced hypervolemia: role of plasma albumin, renin, and vasopressin. *Journal of Applied Physiology* **48**, 665–669.

Corrado, D., Thiene, G., Nava, A., Rossi, L. & Penelli, N. (1990) Sudden death in young competitive athletes: clinicopathologic correlations in 22 cases. *American Journal of Medicine* **89**, 588–595.

Crisman, R.P. & Tomanek, R.J. (1985) Exercise training modifies myocardial mitochondria and myofibril growth in spontaneously hypertensive rats. *American Journal of Physiology* **248**, H8–H14.

Davies, M.J. & Thomas, A.C. (1985) Plaque fissuring—the cause of acute myocardial infarction, sudden ischaemic death, and crescendo angina. *British Heart Journal* **53**, 363–373.

Deutsch, F. & Kauf, E. (1924) *Herz und Sport*. Bern, Wein.

Deutsch, F. & Moritz, F. (1908) Über das Verhalten des Herzens nach langendauerndem und anstrengendem Radfahren (translation). *Münchener Medizinische Wochenschrift* **55**, 489.

Di Bello, V., Pedrinelli, R., Giorgi, D. *et al.* (1997) Ultrasonic videodensitometric analysis of two different models of left ventricular hypertrophy. Athlete's heart and hypertension. *Hypertension* **29** (4), 937–944.

Douglas, P.S., O'Toole, M.L. & Hiller, W.D.B. (1986) Left ventricular structure and function by echocardiography in ultraendurance athletes. *American Journal of Cardiology* **58**, 505–511.

Douglas, P.S., O'Toole, M.L., Hiller, D.B., Hackney, K. & Reichek, N. (1987) Cardiac fatigue after prolonged exercise. *Circulation* **76**, 1206–1213.

Douglas, P.S., O'Toole, M.L., Hiller, W.D. & Reichek, N. (1990a) Different effects of prolonged exercise on the right and left ventricles. *Journal of the American College of Cardiology* **15**, 64–69.

Douglas, P.S., O'Toole, M.L. & Woolard, J. (1990b) Regional wall motion abnormalities after prolonged exercise in the normal left ventricle. *Circulation* **82**, 2108–2114.

Ehsani, A.A. & Spina, R.J. (1997) Loss of cardiovascular adaptations after physical inactivity. *Cardiology Clinics* **15**, 431–437.

Ehsani, A.A., Hagberg, J.M. & Hickson, R.C. (1978) Rapid changes in left ventricular dimensions and mass in response to physical conditioning and deconditioning. *American Journal of Cardiology* **42**, 52–56.

Ehsani, A.A., Ogawa, T., Miller, T.R., Spina, R.J. & Jilka, S.M. (1991) Exercise training improves left ventricular systolic function in older men. *Circulation* **83**, 96–103.

Eisenberg, M.J. (1992) Magnesium deficiency and sudden death. *American Heart Journal* **124**, 544–548.

Fagard, R.H. (1996) Athlete's heart: a meta-analysis of the echocardiographic experience. *International Journal of Sports Medicine* **17** (Suppl. 3), S140–S144.

Fagard, R.H. (1997) Impact of different sports and training on cardiac structure and function. *Cardiology Clinics* **15** (3), 397–412.

Fisher, A.G., Adams, T.D., Yanowitz, F.G., Ridges, J.D., Orsmond, G. & Nelson, A.G. (1989) Noninvasive evaluation of world class athletes engaged in different modes of training. *American Journal of Cardiology* **63**, 337–341.

Forman, D.E., Manning, W.J., Hauser, R., Gervino, E.V., Evans, W.J. & Wei, J.Y. (1992) Enhanced left ventricular diastolic filling associated with long-term endurance training. *Journals of Gerontology* **47** (2), M56–M58.

Foster, C., Anholm, J.D., Hellman, C.K., Carpenter, J., Pollock, M.L. & Schmidt, D.H. (1991) Left ventricular function during sudden strenuous exercise. *Circulation* **63**, 592–596.

Goodman, J. (1995) Exercise and cardiac sudden death: etiology in apparently healthy individuals. *Sport Science Reviews* **4** (2), 14–30.

Goodwin, J.F., Roberts, W.C. & Wenger, N.K. (1982) Cardiomyopathy. In: Hurst, J.W. (ed.) *The Heart Arteries and Veins*, pp. 1299–1362. McGraw-Hill, New York.

Green, H.J., Coates, G., Sutton, J.R. & Jones, S. (1991) Early adaptations in gas exchange, cardiac function and haematology to prolonged exercise training in man. *European Journal of Applied Physiology* **63**, 17–23.

Grossman, W. (1980) Cardiac hypertrophy: useful adaptation or pathological process? *American Journal of Medicine* **69**, 576–583.

Henschen, S. (1899) *Skilanglauf und Skiwettlauf. Eine Medizinische Sportstudie*. Jena, Mitt med Klin Uppsala (cited by Rost 1997).

Holly, R.G., Shaffrath, J.D. & Amsterdam, E.A. (1998) Electrocardiographic alterations associated with the hearts of athletes. *Sports Medicine* **25** (3), 139–148.

Hudlicka, O., Brown, M.D., Walter, H., Weiss, J.B. & Bate, A. (1995) Factors involved in capillary growth in the heart. *Molecular and Cellular Biochemistry* **147** (1–2), 57–68.

Ketelhut, R., Losem, C.J. & Messerli, F.H. (1992) Depressed systolic and diastolic function after prolonged aerobic exercise in healthy subjects. *International Journal of Sports Medicine* **13**, 293–297.

Keul, J., Dickhuth, H.-H., Simon, G. & Lehmann, M. (1981) Effect of static and dynamic exercise on heart, contractility, and left ventricular dimensions. *Circulation Research* **48** (Suppl. 1), I-162–I-170.

Koenig, H., Goldstone, A. & Lu, C.Y. (1982) Testosterone-mediated sexual dimorphism of the rodent heart. *Circulation Research* **50**, 782–787.

Kohl, H.W., Powell, K.E., Gordon, N.F., Blair, S.N. & Paffenbarger, R.S. (1992) Physical activity, physical fitness and sudden cardiac death. *Epidemiological Reviews* **14**, 37–58.

Laslett, L. & Eisenbud, E. (1997) Lack of detection of myocardial injury during competitive races of 100 miles lasting 18–30 hours. *American Journal of Cardiology* **80**, 379–380.

Laughlin, M.H. (1995) Endothelium-mediated control of coronary vascular tone after chronic exercise training. *Medicine and Science in Sports and Exercise* **27**, 1135–1144.

Laughlin, M.H., McAllister, R.M., Jasperse, J.L., Crader, S.E., Williams, D.A. & Huxley, V.H. (1996) Endothelium-mediated control of the coronary circulation. Exercise training-induced vascular adaptations. *Sports Medicine* **22**, 228–250.

Laughlin, M.H., Oltman, C.L. & Bowles, D.K. (1998) Exercise training-induced adaptations in the coronary circulation. *Medicine and Science in Sports and Exercise* **30**, 352–360.

Levine, B.D. (1993) Regulation of central blood and cardiac filling in endurance athletes: the Frank–Starling mechanism as a determinant of orthostatic tolerance. *Medicine and Science in Sports and Exercise* **25**, 727–732.

Levy, W.C., Cerqueira, M.D., Abrass, I.B., Schwartz, R.S. & Stratton, J.R. (1993) Endurance exercise training augments diastolic filling at rest and during exercise in healthy young and older men. *Circulation* **88**, 116–126.

Little, W.C. & Braunwald, E. (1997) Assessment of Cardiac Function. In: Braunwald, E. (ed.) *Heart Disease: A Textbook of Cardiovascular Medicine*, pp. 421–444. W.B. Saunders, Philadelphia.

Longhurst, J.C. & Stebbens, C.L. (1997) The power athlete. *Cardiology Clinics* **15**, 413–429.

Longhurst, J.C., Kelly, A.R., Gonyea, W.J. & Mitchell, J.H. (1981) Chronic training with static and dynamic exercise: cardiovascular adaptation and response to exercise. *Circulation Research* **48** (Suppl. 1), I-171–I-178.

MacDougall, J.D., Tuxen, D., Sale, D.G., Moroz, J.R. & Sutton, J.R. (1985) Arterial blood pressure response to heavy resistance exercise. *Journal of Applied Physiology* **58** (3), 785–790.

Maron, B.J. (1986) Structural features of the athletic heart as defined by echocardiography. *Journal of the American College of Cardiology* **7**, 190–203.

Maron, B.J. (1993) Hypertrophic cardiomyopathy in athletes: catching a killer. *Physician and Sportsmedicine* **21** (9), 83–91.

Maron, B.J. & Fananapazir, L. (1992) Sudden cardiac death in hypertrophic cardiomyopathy. *Circulation* **85** (Suppl. 1), I-57–I-63.

Maron, B.J., Roberts, W.C., McAllister, H.A., Rosing, D.R. & Epstein, S.E. (1980) Sudden death in young athletes. *Circulation* **62**, 218–229.

Maron, B.J., Anan, T.J. & Roberts, W.C. (1981) Quantitative analysis of the distribution of cardiac muscle cell disorganization in the left ventricular wall of patients with hypertrophic cardiomyopathy. *Circulation* **63**, 882–894.

Maron, B.J., Epstein, S.E. & Roberts, W.C. (1986) Causes of sudden death in competitive athletes. *Journal of the American College of Cardiology* **7**, 204–214.

Maron, B.J., Spirito, P., Green, K.J., Wesley, Y.E., Bonow, R.O. & Arce, J. (1987) Noninvasive assessment of left ventricular diastolic function by pulsed Doppler echocardiography in patients with hypertrophic cardiomyopathy. *Journal of* the American College of Cardiology 10, 733–742.

Maron, B.J., Pelliccia, A., Spataro, A. & Granata, M. (1993) Reduction in left ventricular wall thickness after deconditioning in highly trained Olympic athletes. *British Heart Journal* 69, 125–128.

Maron, B.J., Pelliccia, A. & Spirito, P. (1995) Cardiac disease in young trained athletes. Insights into methods for distinguishing athlete's heart from structural heart disease, with particular emphasis on hypertrophic cardiomyopathy. *Circulation* 91, 1596–1601.

Maron, B.J., Poliac, L.C. & Roberts, W.O. (1996) Risk for sudden cardiac death associated with marathon running. *Journal of the American College of Cardiology* 28, 428–431.

Marsh, J.D., Lehmann, M.H., Ritchie, R.H., Gwathmey, J.K., Green, G.E. & Schiebinger, R.J. (1998) Androgen receptors mediate hypertrophy in cardiac myocytes. *Circulation* 98, 256–261.

Milliken, M.C., Stray-Gunersen, J., Pesjock, R.M., Katz, J. & Mitchell, J.H. (1988) Left ventricular mass as determined by magnetic resonance imaging in male endurance athletes. *American Journal of Cardiology* 62, 301–305.

Morganroth, J., Maron, B.J., Henry, W.L. & Epstein, S.E. (1975) Comparative left ventricular dimensions in athletes. *Annals of Internal Medicine* 82, 521–524.

Niemela, K.O., Palatsi, I.J., Ikaheimo, M.J., Takkunen, J.T. & Vuori, J.J. (1984) Evidence of impaired left ventricular performance after an uninterrupted competitive 24 hour run. *Circulation* 70, 350–356.

Niemela, K., Palatsi, I., Ikaheimo, M., Airaksinen, J. & Takkunen, J. (1987) Impaired left ventricular diastolic function in athletes after utterly strenuous prolonged exercise. *International Journal of Sports Medicine* 8, 61–65.

Noakes, T. (1987) Heart disease in marathon runners: a review. *Medicine and Science in Sports and Exercise* 19, 187–194.

Noakes, T. (1991) *Lore of Running*. Leisure Press, Champaign, IL.

Northcote, R.J. & Ballantyne, D. (1985) Cardiovascular implications of strenuous exercise. *International Journal of Cardiology* 8, 3–12.

Northcote, R.J., Flannigan, C. & Ballantyne, D. (1986) Sudden death and vigorous exercise—a study of 60 deaths associated with squash. *British Heart Journal* 55, 198–203.

Opie, L.H. (1998) *The Heart: Physiology, From Cell to Circulation*. Lippincott-Raven, Philadelphia.

Osler, W. (1892) *The Principles and Practice of Medicine*. Appleton, New York.

Palatini, P., Mos, L., Munari, L. *et al.* (1989) Blood pressure changes during heavy-resistance exercise. *Journal of Hypertension* Suppl. 7 (6), S72–S73.

Palatini, P., Giada, F., Garavelli, G. *et al.* (1996) Cardiovascular effects of anabolic steroids in weight-trained subjects. *Journal of Clinical Pharmacology* 12, 1132–1140.

Park, R.C. & Crawford, M.H. (1985) Heart of the athlete. *Current Problems in Cardiology* 10, 1–73.

Parker, B.M., Londeree, B.R., Cupp, G.V. & Dubiel, J.P. (1978) The non-invasive cardiac evaluation of long-distance runners. *Chest* 73, 376–381.

Pelliccia, A. & Maron, B.J. (1997) Outer limits of the athlete's heart, the effect of gender, and relevance to the differential diagnosis with primary cardiac diseases. *Cardiology Clinics* 15, 381–396.

Pelliccia, A., Maron, B.J., Spataro, A., Proschan, M.A. & Spirito, P. (1991) The upper limit of physiologic cardiac hypertrophy in highly trained endurance athletes. *New England Journal of Medicine* 324, 295–301.

Pelliccia, A., Maron, B.J., Spataro, A. & Caselli, G. (1993) Absence of left ventricular hypertrophy in athletes engaged in intense power training. *American Journal of Cardiology* 72, 1048–1054.

Pelliccia, A., Maron, B.J., Culasso, F., Spataro, A. & Caselli, G. (1996) Athlete's heart in women. Echocardiographic characterization of highly trained élite female athletes. *Journal of the American Medical Association* 276, 211–215.

Perreault, H. & Turcotte, R.A. (1994) Exercise-induced cardiac hypertrophy. Fact or fallacy? *Sports Medicine* 17, 283–288.

Pluim, B.M., Chin, J.C., De Roos, A. *et al.* (1996) Cardiac anatomy, function and metabolism in élite cyclists assessed by magnetic resonance imaging and spectroscopy [see comments]. *European Heart Journal* 17, 1271–1278.

Pluim, B.M., Beyerbacht, H.P., Chin, J.C. *et al.* (1997) Comparison of echocardiography with magnetic resonance imaging in the assessment of the athlete's heart. *European Heart Journal* 18, 1505–1513.

Pluim, B.M., Lamb, H.J., Kayser, H.W. *et al.* (1998) Functional and metabolic evaluation of the athlete's heart by magnetic resonance imaging and dobutamine stress magnetic resonance spectroscopy. *Circulation* 97, 666–672.

Pye, M.P. & Cobbe, S.M. (1992) Mechanisms of ventricular arrhythmias in cardiac failure and hypertrophy. *Cardiovascular Research* 26, 740–750.

Richey, P.A. & Brown, S.P. (1998) Pathological versus physiological left ventricular hypertrophy: a review. *Journal of Sports Sciences* 16, 129–141.

Rodriguez Reguero, J.J., Iglesias Cubero, G., Lopez de la Iglesia, J. *et al.* (1995) Prevalence and upper limit of cardiac hypertrophy in professional cyclists. *European Journal of Applied Physiology and Occupational Physiology* 70, 375–378.

Rost, R. (1997) The athlete's heart. Historical perspectives—solved and unsolved problems. *Cardiology Clinics* 15, 493–512.

Rowe, W.J. (1991) A world record marathon runner with silent ischemia without coronary atherosclerosis. *Chest* 99, 1306–1308.

Rowe, W.J. (1993) Endurance exercise and injury to the heart. *Sports Medicine* 16, 73–79.

Rubal, B.J., Al-Muhailani, R.R. & Rosentswieg, J. (1987) Effects of physical conditioning on the heart size and wall thickness of college women. *Medicine and Science in Sports and Exercise* 19, 423–429.

Sabbah, H.N. & Goldstein, S. (1993) Ventricular remodelling: consequences and therapy. *European Heart Journal* 14, 24–29.

Sadaniantz, A. & Thompson, P.D. (1990) The problem of sudden death in athletes as illustrated by case studies. *Sports Medicine* 9, 199–204.

Sarna, S., Sahi, T., Koskwenvuo, M. & Kaprio, J. (1993) Increased life expectancy of world class male athletes. *Medicine and Science in Sports and Exercise* 25, 237–244.

Scheuer, J. & Buttrick, P. (1987) The cardiac hypertrophic responses to pathologic and physiologic loads. *Circulation* 75 (Suppl. 1, Part 2), I-63–I-68.

Schulman, S.P., Fleg, J.L., Goldberg, A.P. *et al.* (1996) Continuum of cardiovascular performance across a broad range of fitness levels in healthy older men. *Circulation* 94, 359–367.

Schwartz, K., Boheler, K.R., De La Bastie, D., Lompre, A.-M. & Mercadier, J.-J. (1992) Switches in cardiac muscle gene expression as a result of pressure and volume overload. *American Journal of Physiology* 31, R364–R369.

Seals, D.R., Hagberg, J.M., Spina, R.J., Rogers, M.A., Schechtman, K.B. & Ehsani, A.A. (1994) Enhanced left ventricular performance in endurance trained older men. *Circulation* **89**, 198–205.

Shapiro, L.M. (1997) The morphologic consequences of systemic training. *Cardiology Clinics* **15**, 373–379.

Shephard, R.J. (1996) The athlete's heart: is big beautiful? *British Journal of Sports Medicine* **30**, 5–10.

Spina, R.J., Ogawa, T., Coggan, A.R., Holloszy, J.O. & Ehsani, A.A. (1992) Exercise training improves left ventricular contractile response to beta-adrenergic agonist. *Journal of Applied Physiology* **72**, 307–311.

Spina, R.J., Ogawa, T., Kohrt, W.M., Martin, W.H.D., Holloszy, J.O. & Ehsani, A.A. (1993) Differences in cardiovascular adaptations to endurance exercise training between older men and women. *Journal of Applied Physiology* **75**, 849–855.

Spina, R.J., Bourey, R.E., Ogawa, T. & Ehsani, A.A. (1994) Effects of exercise training on alpha-adrenergic mediated pressor responses and baroreflex function in older subjects. *Journal of Gerontology* **49**, B277–B281.

Spina, R.J., Turner, M.J. & Ehsani, A.A. (1997) Exercise training enhances cardiac function in response to an afterload stress in older men. *American Journal of Physiology* **272**, H995–H1000.

Spina, R.J., Turner, M.J. & Ehsani, A.A. (1998) Beta-adrenergic-mediated improvement in left ventricular function by exercise training in older men. *American Journal of Physiology* **274**, H397–H404.

Spirito, P. & Maron, B.J. (1988) Doppler echocardiography for assessing left ventricular diastolic function. *Annals of Internal Medicine* **109**, 122–126.

Spirito, P., Maron, B.J., Chiarella, F. *et al.* (1985) Diastolic abnormalities in patients with hypertrophic cardiomyopathy: relation to magnitude of left ventricular hypertrophy. *Circulation* **72**, 310–316.

Spirito, P., Pelliccia, A., Proschan, M.A. *et al.* (1994) Morphology of the 'athlete's

heart' assessed by echocardiography in 947 élite athletes representing 27 sports. *American Journal of Cardiology* **74**, 802–806.

Stendig-Lindberg, G. (1992) Sudden death of athletes: is it due to long-term changes in serum magnesium, lipids and blood sugar? *Journal of Basic and Clinical Physiology and Pharmacology* **3**, 153–164.

Stratton, J.R., Levy, W.C., Schwartz, R.S., Abrass, I.B. & Cerqueira, M.D. (1994) Beta-adrenergic effects on left ventricular filling: influence of aging and exercise training. *Journal of Applied Physiology* **77**, 2522–2529.

Takemoto, K.A., Bernstein, L., Lopez, J.F., Marshak, D., Rahimtoola, S.H. & Chandraratna, P.A. (1992) Abnormalities of diastolic filling of the left ventricle associated with aging are less pronounced in exercise-trained individuals. *American Heart Journal* **124**, 143–148.

Thompson, P.D. (1993) Athletes, athletics and sudden cardiac death. *Medicine and Science in Sports and Exercise* **25**, 981–984.

Turpeinen, A.K., Kuikka, J.T., Vanninen, E. *et al.* (1996) Athletic heart: a metabolic, anatomical, and functional study. *Medicine and Science in Sports and Exercise* **28**, 33–40.

Urhausen, A., Holpes, R. & Kindermann, W. (1989) One- and two-dimensional echocardiography in bodybuilders using anabolic steroids. *European Journal of Applied Physiology* **58**, 633–640.

Urhausen, A., Monz, T. & Kindermann, W. (1996a) Sports-specific adaptation of left ventricular muscle mass in athlete's heart. I. An echocardiographic study with combined isometric and dynamic exercise trained athletes (male and female rowers). *International Journal of Sports Medicine* **17** (Suppl. 3), S145–S151.

Urhausen, A., Monz, T. & Kindermann, W. (1996b) Sports-specific adaptation of left ventricular muscle mass in athlete's heart. II. An echocardiographic study

with 400-m runners and soccer players. *International Journal of Sports Medicine* **17** (Suppl. 3), S152–S156.

Urhausen, A., Monz, T. & Kindermann, W. (1997) Echocardiographic criteria of physiological left ventricular hypertrophy in combined strength- and endurance-trained athletes. *International Journal of Cardiac Imaging* **13**, 43–52.

Van Camp, S.P. & Choi, J.H. (1988) Exercise and sudden death. *Physician and Sportsmedicine* **16** (3), 49–52.

Van Decker, W., Panidis, I.P., Boyle, K., Gonzales, R. & Bove, A.A. (1989) Left ventricular structure and function in professional basketball players. *American Journal of Cardiology* **64**, 1072–1074.

Vanoverschelde, J.-L.J., Younis, L.T., Melin, J.A. *et al.* (1991) Prolonged exercise induces left ventricular dysfunction in healthy subjects. *Journal of Applied Physiology* **70**, 1356–1363.

Virmani, R., Burke, A.P., Farb, A. & Kark, J.A. (1997) Causes of sudden death in young and middle-aged competitive athletes. *Cardiology Clinics* **15**, 439–466.

Waller, B.F. (1985) Exercise-related sudden death in young (age < 30 years) and old (age > 30 years) conditioned subjects. *Cardiology Clinics* **15**(2), 9–73.

Wight, J.N. Jr & Salem, D. (1995) Sudden cardiac death and the 'athlete's heart'. *Archives of Internal Medicine* **155** (14), 1473–1480.

Wynne, J. & Braunwald, E. (1997) The cardiomyopathies and myocarditis. In: Braunwald, E. (ed.) *Heart Disease: A Textbook of Cardiovascular Medicine*, pp. 1404–1463. W.B. Saunders, Philadelphia.

Zhao, G., Zhang, X., Xu, X., Ochoa, M. & Hintze, T.H. (1997) Short-term exercise training enhances reflex cholinergic nitric oxide-dependent coronary vasodilation in conscious dogs. *Circulation Research* **80**, 868–876.

Chapter 7

Skeletal Muscle Blood Flow and Endurance Exercise: Limiting Factors and Dynamic Responses

JAMES W. E. RUSH, CHRISTOPHER R. WOODMAN, AARON P. AAKER, WILLIAM G. SCHRAGE AND M. HAROLD LAUGHLIN

Introduction

Endurance exercise performance is absolutely dependent upon adequate blood flow to deliver sufficient oxygen to active skeletal muscle. Both local and central mechanisms control the blood flow response to exercise, which is dictated by the type and intensity of muscle contractions. The purpose of this chapter is to discuss several important basic features of skeletal muscle blood flow and its relationship to endurance exercise.

The profound impact of the inherent energy supply and demand characteristics of different muscle fibres on the capacity for blood flow and oxygen exchange is described, to establish the axiom that different fibre types have different functional properties. The balance between energy supply and demand is so delicate, in fact, that when energy supply is limited, endurance is severely impaired. This is illustrated by discussing cardiovascular disease states which limit skeletal muscle blood flow as a paradigm for limited energy supply. The nature of the blood flow response during the transition from rest to exercise and during steady-state exercise is described, as are some local regulatory mechanisms believed to be important in realizing the appropriate amount of skeletal muscle blood flow. Throughout the chapter, an attempt has been made to demonstrate that skeletal muscle blood flow and related responses to exercise are dependent upon the type of muscle fibres involved in the exercise, and that under normal circumstances there is an impressive matching of blood flow to muscle energy demand. Relevant effects of endurance exercise training on these responses have also been indicated.

Skeletal muscle design, blood flow and oxygen exchange capacity

The ability to maintain exercise at a given intensity requires that the rate of energy utilization in the active muscle (i.e. the rate of adenosine triphosphate (ATP) hydrolysis) be precisely matched by the rate of energy supply (i.e. the rate of ATP resynthesis). The energy supply during sustainable exercise of more than a few minutes' duration depends almost entirely on aerobic metabolism. If the rate of energy utilization exceeds the rate of aerobic energy supply, exercise cannot be maintained. Under these circumstances either frank fatigue rapidly develops, coincident with a net degradation of muscle high-energy phosphates if an effort is made to maintain energy utilization and force production, or force production is reduced to a level at which aerobic metabolism can meet the energy demand (Terjung et al. 1985; Whitlock & Terjung 1987; Meyer & Foley 1996). The ability to meet the energy demand of muscle during endurance exercise depends on the inherent aerobic capacity of the muscle, and on the ability to deliver sufficient oxygen through adequate convective blood flow, and diffusive blood–muscle oxygen exchange. In this section the relationship of blood flow and diffusional exchange capacities to the aerobic capacity of different muscle fibre types is examined.

Heterogeneity of skeletal muscle energy supply and demand

Adult mammalian skeletal muscle is not a homogeneous tissue; rather, it is composed of a continuum of skeletal muscle fibre types which result from the expression of unique complements of contractile and metabolic protein isoforms (Table 7.1; Saltin & Gollnick 1983; Booth & Baldwin 1996; Chapter 11). It is useful to classify skeletal muscle fibres into one of three groups, based on their functional and metabolic properties: slow-twitch oxidative (SO), fast-twitch oxidative glycolytic (FOG) and fast-twitch glycolytic (FG) (Table 7.1; Peter *et al.* 1972). An alternative classification system defines these fibre types as types I, IIa and IIb, respectively (Spurway 1981).

Energy utilization characteristics of the fibre types set limits on the peak rates of tension development and relaxation (Booth & Baldwin 1996; Meyer & Foley 1996). Thus, fast-twitch fibres express myosin- and Ca^{2+}-ATPase isoforms with high inherent ATPase rates, allowing for rapid shortening and relaxation velocities, respectively (Table 7.1). Fast-twitch fibres are therefore capable of relatively high rates of energy utilization. In contrast slow-twitch fibres express myosin- and Ca^{2+}-ATPase isoforms with relatively lower inherent rates, and thus have slower maximal shortening and relaxation velocities (Table 7.1). The rates of energy utilization in slow-twitch fibres are correspondingly lower.

The ability to meet the ATPase energy utilization rate by aerobic energy supply determines the fatigue resistance of fibres. Aerobic energy supply depends on muscle oxidative enzyme capacity, muscle blood flow capacity and blood–muscle oxygen exchange capacity. Muscle oxidative enzyme capacity (the ability of the muscle to consume oxygen) is set by the inherent mitochondrial endowment, estimated as the maximal *in vitro* activity of mitochondrial enzymes (Holloszy 1967; McAllister & Terjung 1990). Highly oxidative fibres by definition have a greater mitochondrial content and therefore higher mitochondrial enzyme activities (FOG > SO > FG, see Table 7.1; Baldwin *et al.* 1972; Maxwell *et al.* 1977; Saltin & Gollnick 1983). Maximal oxygen delivery and uptake depend on the blood flow and oxygen exchange capacities, respectively. Both of these parameters are greater in more oxidative muscle fibres (Maxwell *et al.* 1977; Mackie & Terjung 1983; Saltin & Gollnick 1983; Armstrong & Laughlin 1984, 1985; Armstrong *et al.* 1992). Together, high oxidative enzyme capacity, high blood flow capacity and high oxygen exchange capacity confer resistance to fatigue, the efficacy of which is inversely related to the maximal rate of ATP utilization that can be generated in a given fibre type (Table 7.1).

These considerations make it clear that skeletal muscle cannot be regarded as a homogeneous tissue if the bases for its functional properties are to be understood in any detail. The particular endowment of contractile and metabolic proteins that are

Table 7.1 Relative biochemical and functional properties of different skeletal muscle fibre types.

Property	Fibre type		
	SO	FOG	FG
Myosin-ATPase activity	Low	High	Very high
SR Ca^{2+}-ATPase activity	Low	High	Very high
Contractile speed	Slow	Fast	Fast
Glycolytic enzyme activity	Low	High	Very high
Mitochondrial (oxidative) enzyme activity	High	Very high	Low
Blood flow	High	Very high	Low
Fatiguability	Low	Moderate	High

Values are indicated in arbitrary relative terms to give a general sense of fibre type-specific properties.
FG, fast-twitch glycolytic; FOG, fast-twitch oxidative glycolytic; SO, slow-twitch oxidative; SR, sarcoplasmic reticulum.

expressed defines the unique phenotype of different fibres; the fibre type composition of a given muscle in turn determines its physiological characteristics. The balance between ATPase activity and oxidative energy provision influences the functional characteristics of different fibre types. The phenotype of different fibres is important for the function of exercising muscle only when the fibres are recruited during exercise. Muscle recruitment patterns during exercise are not random. Rather, recruitment is dictated by the central nervous system to meet the demands of a given activity.

Fibre distribution, recruitment and fatigue

The degree to which energy supply and utilization mechanisms are matched in different fibre types is consistent with their functions and recruitment patterns during locomotory exercise. The combination of high mitochondrial capacity, high blood flow capacity and low ATPase activity of SO fibres furnishes these fibres with the ability to maintain relatively low levels of force production for prolonged periods without fatigue, as long as blood flow is adequate (Table 7.1; Dudley *et al.* 1982; Terjung *et al.* 1985; Whitlock & Terjung 1987; Meyer & Foley 1996). This is the precise role that these fibres play *in vivo*. The limb antigravity extensor muscles of quadrupedal mammals such as the rat tend to be predominantly SO with some FOG fibres (Baldwin *et al.* 1972; Ariano *et al.* 1973; Armstrong & Phelps 1984). These muscles are recruited at relatively low work intensities to maintain posture and to power slow walking movements (Sullivan & Armstrong 1978; Walmsley *et al.* 1978). The high mitochondrial content, high blood flow capacity and high ATPase rates in FOG fibres endow these fibres both with relatively high rates of force production and with fatigue resistance (Table 7.1). These fibres, typically concentrated in deeper portions of the extensor muscles of quadrupedal mammals, but distributed throughout (Baldwin *et al.* 1972; Armstrong & Phelps 1984), are progressively recruited as exercise intensity is increased (Armstrong *et al.* 1977; Sullivan & Armstrong 1978; Saltin & Gollnick 1983). A large fraction of the force production during

endurance exercise is thus provided by FOG fibres. The high ATPase rate of FG fibres ideally suits them for high rates of force production. However, the combination of high ATPase rate with a low aerobic capacity and low blood flow capacity in these fibres results in a relative ease of fatiguability (Table 7.1). These fibres are typically concentrated in superficial regions of the limb extensor muscles of quadrupedal mammals (Baldwin *et al.* 1972; Armstrong & Phelps 1984). Their utility is limited to short periods of intense force production and energy turnover; they are recruited last during exercise of progressively increasing intensity (Armstrong *et al.* 1977; Sullivan & Armstrong 1978; Walmsley *et al.* 1978). Fatigue is imminent when FG fibres are recruited (Sullivan & Armstrong 1978; Dudley *et al.* 1982).

The localization of like fibres into discrete muscle sections in some quadrupedal mammals facilitates the study of muscle recruitment, regional-specific blood flow and fibre-specific metabolism. In human muscles, however, there appears to be less stratification of muscle into distinct sections of like fibres (Edgerton *et al.* 1975; Saltin & Gollnick 1983). Instead, there appears to be a more homogeneous dispersion of the different fibre types, and rarely is a fibre of a given type surrounded by like fibres (Saltin & Gollnick 1983). In human quadriceps muscle for instance, the fibre type distribution is approximately 50% slow twitch:50% fast twitch, with little regional specificity in fibre type distribution (Saltin & Gollnick 1983). Although it is likely that muscle fibre recruitment patterns during locomotory exercise in humans are similar to those described above for quadrupedal mammals (Burke 1981; Saltin & Gollnick 1983), the lack of fibre stratification hinders the study of fibre-specific blood flow and metabolic responses in humans.

In summary, a heterogeneity in muscle is established by the expression of differences in energy supply and utilization characteristics, which in turn determine the functional properties of different fibre types. The capacities for convective blood flow and oxygen exchange are two functional properties of muscle that are related to the oxidative capacity of different fibre types. The balance between these aerobic energy supply mechanisms and the energy utilization properties of different fibres determines their endurance capacities (their fatigue resistance; Table 7.1).

Skeletal muscle blood flow capacity is related to its oxidative enzymatic capacity

In both whole-body exercise and isolated working muscle preparations, maximal muscle oxygen consumption scales linearly with the mitochondrial enzymatic capacity of the working muscle, and with its blood flow capacity (Maxwell *et al.* 1977; Saltin & Gollnick 1983). This results from an exquisite matching between regional blood flow capacity ($\dot{Q}_{cap}$) and mitochondrial enzymatic capacity across muscles of differing fibre type composition, both within and between species (Fig. 7.1; Maxwell *et al.* 1977; Mackie & Terjung 1983; Saltin & Gollnick 1983; Armstrong & Laughlin 1984, 1985). For instance, the deep lateral portion of the rat gastrocnemius muscle (the red gastrocnemius, G_r) is composed predominantly of FOG fibres (60% FOG, 35% SO) and is therefore endowed with a high inherent oxidative enzyme capacity; it also has a high blood flow capacity (Table 7.1; Fig. 7.1). In contrast, the superficial medial rat gastrocnemius (the white gastrocnemius, G_w) is predominantly composed of FG fibres (90% FG, 10% FOG), and thus has a relatively low oxidative enzyme capacity; it also has a low blood flow capacity (Table 7.1; Fig. 7.1). The rat soleus (Sol) is predominantly composed of SO fibres (90% SO, 10% FOG) and has oxidative enzyme and blood flow capacities intermediate between the G_r and G_w muscles (Table 7.1; Fig. 7.1; Armstrong & Laughlin 1985). Data for various dog muscles (Maxwell *et al.* 1977; Musch *et al.* 1987b) and for human mixed quadriceps muscle (Andersen & Saltin 1985; Rowell *et al.* 1986) fit the relationship between $\dot{Q}_{cap}$ and mitochondrial enzymatic capacity established across different rat muscles (Fig. 7.1).

It is important to be specific in the definition of $\dot{Q}_{cap}$ at this juncture; it is the maximal flow possible to a defined region of tissue at a given physiological pressure gradient (arterial pressure ~100–140

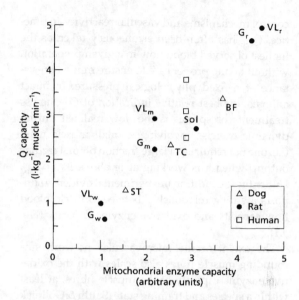

Fig. 7.1 Blood flow capacity ($\dot{Q}_{cap}$) graphed as a function of muscle mitochondrial enzymatic capacity (expressed relative to the value for rat white vastus lateralis) in limb muscles of variable fibre type composition from various mammals. Rat data are from Armstrong and Laughlin (1984, 1985); dog data are from Musch *et al.* (1987a) and Maxwell *et al.* (1977); human data are from Saltin and Gollnick (1983), Andersen and Saltin (1985), Rowell *et al.* (1986) and Richardson *et al.* (1993). Arterial pressure varied from 128 to 142 mmHg across the various studies. VL_r, VL_m and VL_w refer to the red, mixed and white portions of the vastus lateralis muscle, respectively; G_r, G_m and G_w refer to the red, mixed and white portions of the gastrocnemius muscle, respectively; BF, biceps femoris; Sol, soleus; ST, semitendinosus; TC, tibialis cranialis. Human data are from mixed quadriceps muscle. In all cases blood flow measurements were made at or above $\dot{V}_{O_{2max}}$ in rhythmically contracting muscle.

mmHg, depending on species) under conditions of minimal vascular resistance. Minimal resistance may be induced either by the administration of potent vasodilatory agents or by the vasodilatory effect of intense muscle contractions. $\dot{Q}_{cap}$ cannot be used to predict the relative blood flow between different muscle regions at any submaximal exercise intensity, since muscle recruitment, microvascular recruitment and blood flow redistribution also affect regional blood flow during exercise. Ideally, determinations of $\dot{Q}_{cap}$ are independent of vascular control mechanisms and vascular reactivity. In practice, $\dot{Q}_{cap}$ has often been erroneously taken as the highest observed blood flow in a given preparation without taking proper care to ensure minimal resistance at a fixed physiological pressure. In intact animals, the best relative indication of $\dot{Q}_{cap}$ across treatments or species is the flow realized during dynamic exercise involving a small muscle mass (i.e. one not requiring a large fraction of total cardiac output) when it is working at or above its $\dot{V}_{O_{2max}}$. Under these conditions, experimental evidence supports a strong relationship between muscle blood flow capacity and oxidative enzyme capacity (Fig. 7.1).

The extent of the microvascular network surrounding muscle fibres also scales with the oxidative enzyme capacity of the muscle fibres, at least within a species and training state (Saltin & Gollnick 1983; Gute *et al.* 1994, 1996). The microvascular network includes the arterioles, the capillaries and the venules. Arterioles are precapillary and are the main site of vascular resistance; capillaries are the primary exchange vessels, which form the interface between blood and muscle; and venules are the postcapillary collecting vessels which unite to form veins. In general, the three vessel types composing the microvascular network scale with each other, so that changes in the number of one usually indicate the degree of change in the others. Thus, although muscle capillarity (the number of capillaries per fibre or per mm^2 of muscle cross-sectional area) is often the variable that is quantified and used to describe the extent of the microvascular network, the role of the arterioles and venules must be kept in mind. Since the microvascular network generally scales with the oxidative enzyme capacity of the fibres that it surrounds, the rank order for capillarity in the sedentary rat hindlimb muscle sections is $G_r >$ Sol $> G_m > G_w$ (Fig. 7.2; Gute *et al.* 1994, 1996; G_m is fast-twitch, mixed gastrocnemius).

The rank order for $\dot{Q}_{cap}$ is exactly the same as for capillarity (Fig. 7.1; Table 7.1). The relationship between muscle fibre type-specific $\dot{Q}_{cap}$ and the extent of the microvascular network results from the simple fact that the inverses of parallel resistances, R, are additive (parallel conductances, g, are additive; Equation 1; see Chapter 3).

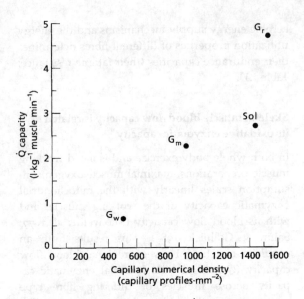

Fig. 7.2 Muscle blood flow capacity ($\dot{Q}_{cap}$) graphed as a function of capillarity in limb muscles of variable fibre type composition from sedentary rats. Abbreviations are defined in the legend to Fig. 7.1. Arterial pressure was 129 mmHg in the $\dot{Q}_{cap}$ studies. $\dot{Q}_{cap}$ data are from Armstrong and Laughlin (1985); capillarity data are from Gute *et al.* (1994, 1996). The relationship is similar if capillarity is expressed as either the number of capillaries per fibre, or the capillary surface area density instead of capillary profiles/mm^2 (see Gute *et al.* 1994, 1996). Capillarity is used as an indication of the extent of the entire microvascular network.

$$1/R_{total} = 1/R_1 + 1/R_2 \ldots 1/R_n \text{ or}$$

$$\dot{g}_{total} = \dot{g}_1 + \dot{g}_2 + \ldots \dot{g}_n \tag{1}$$

Ohm's law adapted for haemodynamics (Equation 2) states that

$$\dot{Q} = \Delta P / R_{total} \tag{2}$$

where $\dot{Q}$ is blood flow through a defined circuit, ΔP is the pressure gradient across the circuit and R_{total} is the total resistance across the circuit. At any given arterial-to-venous ΔP across a maximally dilated muscle vascular circuit, a greater number of microvessels (greater number of parallel conductances) results in lower total resistance and greater maximal convective blood flow (Fig. 7.2). Although this point is illustrated in Fig. 7.2 using capillarity as an index of the extent of the microvascular network, the reduction of resistance that results in greater $\dot{Q}_{cap}$ is primarily a function of a greater number of arterioles, since these vessels are the principal site of resistance. Thus, skeletal muscle is remarkably well adapted to provide a higher $\dot{Q}_{cap}$ to muscle fibres of higher oxidative capacity, primarily by utilizing a greater vascular network to bathe the muscle fibres in blood more effectively. This adaptation contributes to the greater maximal oxygen consumption and fatigue resistance of these fibres.

The greater convective blood flow capacity of the more aerobic fibres is important in delivering oxygen in an amount appropriate to support the muscle oxidative capacity. As will be outlined below, features of the more aerobic muscle fibres themselves and of the surrounding vasculature also favour a greater oxygen diffusion capacity; the maximal ability to exchange oxygen between blood and muscle.

Oxygen exchange capacity is coupled to capillarity and muscle oxidative capacity

For the more aerobic fibres to benefit from their greater $\dot{Q}_{cap}$, the blood–muscle oxygen exchange capacity must also be greater. Fick's first law (Equation 3) states

$$\dot{J} = (dc/dx) \cdot DA \qquad (3)$$

where $\dot{J}$ is the instantaneous diffusive flux of oxygen; dc is the difference in concentration between two points (e.g. a red blood cell in a capillary and a skeletal muscle fibre mitochondrion) separated by dx, the distance over which flux occurs; D is a proportionality constant which reflects the permeability of the diffusional barrier; and A is the surface area over which exchange can occur. The blood–muscle oxygen exchange capacity of a given fibre is a function of the variables of Fick's first law; more oxidative fibres are predicted to have a greater $\dot{J}$. It is generally believed that blood of the same composition perfuses all fibre types. Thus, the dc term, which depends mostly upon the oxygen content of arterial blood, does not influence possible differences in $\dot{J}$ across fibre types. Assuming again the case of maximal dilatation across a muscle vascular circuit, a higher capillarity is expected to

increase diffusion capacity for oxygen and substrate by increasing the surface area for diffusion (A; Gute et al. 1994, 1996). For an individual capillary, A is the product of the circumference multiplied by its length. Thus, total A in a defined volume of muscle is the sum of the A values for each of the individual capillaries therein. The surface area available for blood–muscle oxygen exchange is greater in more oxidative fibres, which are surrounded by a greater number of capillaries (Gute et al. 1994, 1996), and this favours increased diffusive flux. Shortening the diffusional path length between capillary and mitochondrion is also expected to increase $\dot{J}$. The dx is decreased in two ways in more oxidative fibres: increased capillary density (Fig. 7.2; Saltin & Gollnick 1983; Gute et al. 1994, 1996) and increased mitochondrial density (Table 7.1; Fig. 7.1; Baldwin et al. 1972; Dudley et al. 1982; Armstrong & Laughlin 1984). Differences in the permeability (D) of capillaries supplying different muscle fibre types would also affect the diffusive flux of oxygen and substrate. The relative impact of this parameter is not known, however, since the inherent permeability characteristics of capillaries supplying different skeletal muscle fibre types have not been determined experimentally.

$\dot{J}$ is the diffusive oxygen flux; integrated over time, the oxygen exchange capacity also depends on how long an oxygen-carrying red blood cell is in an exchange vessel (the transit time). Reported values for transit time vary, but there is general agreement that the transit time is in excess of the minimal value required for haemoglobin oxygen unloading (Hudlicka et al. 1982; Sarelius 1986; Yamaguchi et al. 1987), even at $\dot{V}O_{2max}$ (Kayar et al. 1992). This suggests that transit time does not normally present a limitation for oxygen unloading. Greater capillary density and branching in more oxidative muscle fibres (Fig. 7.2; Hudlicka 1977; Saltin & Gollnick 1983; Gute et al. 1994, 1996) increase the total capillary volume and therefore increase the transit time at a given total capillary flow rate. Increased time available for exchange facilitates greater total oxygen flux as blood passes through the muscle vascular circuit.

In summary, the combination of greater mitochondrial content and capillarity provides a greater blood–muscle oxygen exchange capacity to more oxidative muscle fibres by decreasing the diffusive path length for oxygen and increasing the surface area available for exchange. Improved oxygen exchange capacity complements enhanced convective blood delivery in the fine matching of oxygen delivery to oxidative capacity of muscle. This matching is essential in order to maintain aerobic energy production and resistance to fatigue during dynamic exercise.

Effects of training on $\dot{Q}_{cap}$ and $\dot{J}$

Muscle $\dot{V}_{O_{2max}}$ is absolutely dependent upon the mitochondrial electron flux capacity; if any fraction of this is inhibited, muscle $\dot{V}_{O_{2max}}$ and performance decrease (McAllister & Terjung 1990). A hallmark of the muscle adaptation to exercise training is an increase in mitochondrial enzyme activities. This adaptation is specific to the fibres recruited during an exercise training programme (Holloszy 1967; Dudley *et al.* 1982; Holloszy & Coyle 1984). The increased $\dot{V}_{O_{2max}}$ of trained muscle is also absolutely dependent upon expansion of the mitochondrial electron flux capacity that occurs with training. If pharmacological agents are used to inhibit the electron flux capacity of trained muscle such that it remains at pretraining levels, the increases in $\dot{V}_{O_{2max}}$ and performance that normally occur as a result of exercise training are lost (Robinson *et al.* 1994). Whether the increased oxidative enzyme capacity of trained muscle necessarily depends on an increase in $\dot{Q}_{cap}$ in order to realize a greater $\dot{V}_{O_{2max}}$ is unclear, however, because the $\dot{Q}_{cap}$ of normal untrained skeletal muscle is already very high. It is so high, in fact, that cardiac output could not increase sufficiently to perfuse the entire vasculature of human skeletal muscle if it were to dilate maximally (Andersen & Saltin 1985). In addition, oxygen extraction can increase to meet the oxygen demand of trained muscle (Saltin *et al.* 1976; McAllister & Terjung 1991). Greater mitochondrial and capillary densities, which are important determinants of oxygen diffusion capacity, facilitate greater oxygen extraction in trained muscle. In light of the already high $\dot{Q}_{cap}$ and increased oxygen extraction, it does not seem necessary to increase $\dot{Q}_{cap}$ in trained

muscle. Nevertheless, $\dot{Q}_{cap}$ can in fact increase to various extents as a result of training (usually < 20% increase: Mackie & Terjung 1983; Musch *et al.* 1987b; Sexton & Laughlin 1994).

Increases in muscle $\dot{V}_{O_{2max}}$, mitochondrial enzyme activity and muscle oxygen extraction established by exercise training are often accompanied by increases in capillarity in human muscle (Saltin & Gollnick 1983). Whether increases in regional $\dot{Q}_{cap}$ also occur with training remains unknown. When the relationships between changes in regional specific $\dot{Q}_{cap}$, capillarity and mitochondrial capacity due to exercise training are examined in other animals in which muscle fibre recruitment during exercise can be better controlled, it is found that these parameters can change independently. For instance, high-intensity aerobic training in rats resulted in significant increases in oxidative capacity and capillarity in gastrocnemius and soleus muscles (Dudley *et al.* 1982; Gute *et al.* 1996), but it had a minimal effect on $\dot{Q}_{cap}$ in any region of these muscles (Sexton & Laughlin 1994). Conversely, low-intensity training produced significant increases in oxidative capacity and $\dot{Q}_{cap}$ in all regions (Dudley *et al.* 1982; Laughlin & Ripperger 1987), but it resulted in either no or minimal increases in capillarity (Gute *et al.* 1994). Thus, the evidence does not support a necessary coincidence of increased capillarity and $\dot{Q}_{cap}$ with increased muscle oxidative capacity due to exercise training. It must be emphasized that although capillarity reflects the extent of the other components of the microvascular network, there are exceptional cases in which arterioles (most important in determining $\dot{Q}_{cap}$) and capillaries (most important in determining $\dot{J}$) may not adapt in a coordinated manner.

It is abundantly clear that all skeletal muscle fibres are not created equally. Differences in the matching of inherent energy demand and supply rates determine the fatiguability of fibres, which in turn is related to their recruitment pattern during exercise, and their contribution to the work output of the intact muscle and organism. Convective blood flow and oxygen exchange capacities are two important determinants of the ability to supply aerobic energy; they usually scale with the extent of the microvascular network and with the inherent muscle oxidative capacity established by the mitochondrial content. Aerobic exercise training can increase each of these variables, but the changes in one do not necessarily predict the changes (or lack of changes) in another. It is important to emphasize that the discussion thus far has focused on the *capacities* of various parameters. These quantities set limits on the range of dynamic responses to exercise stresses, but they may not always be predictive of the relative response of each during submaximal exercise. It is strikingly evident, however, that the blood flow capacity is a strong determinant of the endurance performance of skeletal muscle. In disease states which disrupt the skeletal muscle blood flow capacity, endurance is compromised.

Cardiovascular disease states emphasize the importance of skeletal muscle blood flow for endurance

The importance of skeletal muscle blood flow to endurance performance is evident in the dramatic decrease in endurance and exercise tolerance associated with conditions that limit blood flow. The two most common causes of limited skeletal muscle blood flow are peripheral arterial occlusive diseases and congestive heart failure (CHF). Patients with either condition have very limited abilities to perform endurance exercise.

Acute ligation of the arterial supply to an active limb results in rapid loss of locomotory function in the affected limb of walking rats (Armstrong & Peterson 1981). In humans, acute arterial occlusion can occur due to thrombosis, embolism, dissection or trauma, and this results in a sudden onset of severe limb ischaemia, preventing any sustained motor function (Halperin & Creager 1996). Exercise simply cannot be maintained in the absence of blood flow to the active skeletal muscle. Intermittent claudication is a common symptom of obstructive arterial disease in the lower extremities. Intermittent claudication is a complex of symptoms including pain and weakness which are only present or prominent during walking. These symptoms intensify progressively during acute exercise, until further physical activity becomes impossible. Symptoms diminish with time if the patient stops exercise.

Exercise training can increase exercise tolerance and endurance, both in humans with peripheral vascular disease (Zetterquist 1970; Strandness & Sumner 1975) and in experimental models of arterial occlusive disease (Terjung et al. 1988; Mathien & Terjung 1990). In humans, these improvements in exercise endurance appear to result from enhanced collateral vessel development and increased blood flow (Strandness & Sumner 1975; Terjung et al. 1988). Zetterquist (1970) proposed that the beneficial effects of training on exercise performance in humans with peripheral vascular disease were related more to altered distribution of blood flow in the limb than to increases in total limb blood flow. More detailed experiments in animal models of peripheral vascular disease support the hypothesis that exercise training has a greater effect on the distribution of blood flow within the affected limb than on total blood flow (Terjung et al. 1988; Mathien & Terjung 1990).

The most common complaints of patients with CHF are dyspnoea, exercise intolerance and decreased endurance. Decreased exercise tolerance appears to be primarily the result of an insufficient skeletal muscle blood flow during exercise (Wiener et al. 1986; Massie et al. 1988; Wilson et al. 1994). Consistent with the view that limited skeletal muscle blood flow is the cause of exercise intolerance in CHF are reports of the early onset of anaerobic metabolism in CHF patients during exercise (Weber & Janicki 1985; Sullivan et al. 1989). The metabolic disturbance appears to result in part from reduced skeletal muscle blood flow and in part from abnormalities of skeletal muscle metabolism which occur because of chronic limitation of blood flow (Wiener et al. 1986; Massie et al. 1988; Sullivan et al. 1989; Wilson et al. 1994). The limitation in muscle blood flow during exercise is not simply the result of limited cardiac output. The vascular beds of skeletal muscle in CHF patients appear to have an impaired ability to vasodilate (Zelis et al. 1969; Wiener et al. 1986; Wilson et al. 1994). Isnard et al. (1996) found that CHF patients exhibited normal exercise-induced vasodilatation during submaximal exercise. In contrast, it appears that maximal exercise capacity is limited in CHF patients in part due to impaired ability of skeletal muscle vascular beds to vasodilate (LeJemtel *et al.* 1986; Wiener *et al.* 1986; Massie *et al.* 1988; Jondeau *et al.* 1992; Wilson *et al.* 1994) and that skeletal muscle vascular beds show other signs of altered vasoregulation (Zelis *et al.* 1969). However, there remains controversy about whether vasoregulation is abnormal in the skeletal muscle of CHF patients during submaximal exercise (Isnard *et al.* 1996).

The blunted ability to vasodilate in the arteries of CHF patients appears to be due at least in part to a decreased endothelium-dependent vasodilatation (Kubo *et al.* 1991; Drexler *et al.* 1992). Katz *et al.* (1997) reported that exercise training increased exercise tolerance in CHF patients, and they suggested that these changes might be the result of enhanced endothelium-dependent vasodilatation in skeletal muscle. Thus, both common causes of exercise intolerance emanating from inadequate skeletal muscle blood flow are ameliorated by exercise training. The improved exercise endurance in these patients is partially the result of improved blood flow and its distribution in skeletal muscle. This is further evidence that adequate skeletal muscle blood flow is required for endurance exercise.

The discussion of disease states which limit skeletal muscle blood flow serves to emphasize that when the normal delicate matching of blood flow to metabolism is disrupted, exercise endurance is profoundly impaired. In healthy skeletal muscle, the blood flow during steady-state dynamic exercise is dictated by the metabolic needs of the tissue. The actual nature of the blood flow response in the transition from rest to steady-state exercise, however, is dependent upon the intensity and frequency of the contractions.

Nature of the blood flow response to exercise

During graded-intensity dynamic exercise, blood flow to contracting skeletal muscle increases in direct proportion to the increase in exercise intensity, matching the increase in metabolic demand (Saltin *et al.* 1998). At an exercise intensity that elicits $\dot{V}_{O_{2max}}$, blood flow to human mixed fibre type limb muscle can be up to 100-fold greater than resting

values (Saltin *et al.* 1998). Indeed, blood flow values of $> 2 l \cdot kg^{-1} \cdot min^{-1}$ have been reported in fit human subjects (Andersen & Saltin 1985; Kim *et al.* 1995), and values approaching $4 l \cdot kg^{-1} \cdot min^{-1}$ have been reported in highly trained subjects (Fig. 7.1; Richardson *et al.* 1993; Blomstrand *et al.* 1997).

Blood flow increases rapidly at the onset of exercise (Shoemaker *et al.* 1994; Tschakovsky *et al.* 1995; Radegran 1997). An increase in blood flow is observed immediately following the first contraction of exercise. Its extent depends on the rate of contraction (i.e. the running speed), but in some animal models can be independent of the metabolic requirements of the contraction (Fig. 7.3; Pollack & Wood 1949; Sheriff *et al.* 1993a; Sheriff & Van Bibber 1998). A steady-state blood flow is achieved within ~30–120 s, depending on the intensity of the exercise and the fitness level of the subjects (Fig. 7.3; Sheriff *et al.* 1993a; Radegran 1997; Saltin *et al.* 1998). During normal steady-state exercise both rats and humans match convective

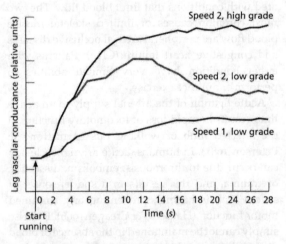

Fig. 7.3 Skeletal muscle vascular conductance at the onset of dynamic exercise. Arbitrary curves have been depicted based on the data of Sheriff *et al.* (1993a). Calculated conductance (*C*) is blood flow normalized for perfusion pressure (*C = Q/P*). Note that there are two general phases: initial hyperaemia (~0–5 s) and steady state (after ~20 s). Speed 2 is greater than speed 1. Speed depends on frequency of contractions, grade determines intensity of contractions.

blood flow exquisitely to the energy demand (oxygen demand) of the muscle, and exercise can be sustained for a prolonged period of time without large variations in muscle blood flow or oxygen uptake (Laughlin & Armstrong 1983; Armstrong *et al.* 1987; Savard *et al.* 1987). In contrast, steady-state conditions may not be achieved during brief, heavy-intensity exercise, and skeletal muscle blood flow may increase gradually over the time course of such an exercise bout (Armstrong & Laughlin 1983).

Dynamic muscle contractions can generate intramuscular pressures of 100–300 mmHg (Gaffney *et al.* 1990). Because mean intravascular pressure is only ~100–130 mmHg during exercise, muscle contraction at forces equal to 10–15% of maximum voluntary contraction (MVC) significantly impede blood flow (Shepherd 1983). This impedance is removed, however, during relaxation of the skeletal muscle, allowing flow to increase in proportion to the strength of the preceding contraction (Corcondilas *et al.* 1964; Folkow *et al.* 1970; Bystrom & Kilbom 1990). Sustained isometric contractions at >25% MVC for instance, markedly inhibit blood flow during the contraction, but the postcontraction blood flow is much higher than occurs after 15% MVC contractions. Thus, blood flow to contracting muscle does not occur at a steady rate independently of the muscle activity. Rather, blood flow is phasic and depends on the skeletal muscle contraction–relaxation cycle during exercise (see 'Muscle pump control of skeletal muscle blood flow', below). Therefore, even though each contraction impedes arterial blood flow, the net effect of dynamic exercise is to increase muscle blood flow.

Data collected from exercising animals indicate that the increase in blood flow during exercise does not occur uniformly throughout skeletal muscle (Laughlin & Armstrong 1982; Armstrong & Laughlin 1984). Rather, the increase in blood flow is distributed preferentially to the muscle fibres that are recruited to perform the exercise. Whether this pattern of response occurs in human skeletal muscle during exercise is not known. The lack of both fibre type stratification and regional-specific recruitment makes it difficult to assess the matching of regional-specific blood flow and recruitment responses in human muscle. It is clear from animal studies, however, that the matching of regional-specific blood flow to active muscle contributes to the observed tight coupling between limb blood flow and oxygen uptake.

Following a programme of endurance exercise training, blood flow to contracting skeletal muscle at any given submaximal exercise intensity is lower than in the untrained state (Clausen 1977). In contrast, blood flow during exercise is the same before and after training when exercise is performed at the same *relative* exercise intensity (i.e. a fixed percentage of $\dot{V}_{O_{2max}}$, Clausen 1977). The lower blood flow during submaximal exercise (despite similar levels of oxygen consumption) is attributed to the improved ability of skeletal muscle to extract and utilize oxygen (see 'Effects of training on $\dot{Q}_{cap}$ and $\dot{J}$).

It is apparent that oxygen delivery is the controlled variable and that blood flow is adjusted to deliver oxygen according to the tissue needs; during arterial hyperoxia, blood flow is decreased at a given work rate (Welch 1982), and during hypoxia or anaemia in which arterial oxygen content is decreased, blood flow is increased at a given work rate (Koskolou *et al.* 1997; Richardson *et al.* 1998). We next examine some of the potential blood flow regulatory mechanisms which result in this tight coupling between oxygen delivery and oxygen consumption.

Regulation of skeletal muscle blood flow during exercise

During exercise, the increase in blood flow to active skeletal muscle is mediated by a reduced vascular resistance in the skeletal muscle and an increased perfusion pressure (i.e. mean arterial pressure). Resistance to flow through cylindrical vessels can be defined as

$$R = 8l \cdot \eta / \pi \cdot r^4 \tag{4}$$

where R is the resistance to flow through the vessel, l is the length of the vessel, η is the viscosity of the blood flowing through the vessel and r is the inner radius of the vessel (Equation 4). Substituting Equation 4 into Equation 2

$$\dot{Q} = \pi \, \Delta P \cdot r^4 / 8\eta \cdot l \qquad (5)$$

results in Poiseuille's law of flow through cylindrical vessels (Equation 5). Since flow is directly proportional to the fourth power of the vessel radius, even small changes in radius can have substantial effects on flow. The reduction in vascular resistance mediated by an increased vessel radius (vasodilatation) is so powerful, in fact, that it is the primary mechanism by which skeletal muscle blood flow increases during exercise (Hermansen *et al.* 1970; Poliner *et al.* 1980). In contrast, when humans perform dynamic exercise, the increase in mean arterial pressure is modest, and the vessel length and blood viscosity do not change appreciably.

Systemic vascular resistance decreases rapidly during large muscle dynamic exercise; the magnitude of the reduction is dependent on the exercise intensity (Hermansen *et al.* 1970). Several mechanisms of local blood flow control (i.e. signals produced at or around the vascular bed being affected) have been proposed as contributing to the reduction in vascular resistance and increased perfusion during exercise. These include metabolic control, myogenic control, endothelium-mediated control

and the muscle pump (Fig. 7.4; Laughlin *et al.* 1996; Delp & Laughlin 1998). These factors are independent of central and neural control of skeletal muscle blood flow, topics that will not be covered in this chapter.

Metabolic control of skeletal muscle blood flow

According to the metabolic control hypothesis, products of cellular activity in the active skeletal muscle contribute to the dilatation of arterioles via direct effects on vascular smooth muscle and endothelium, or indirectly by interrupting the vasoconstrictor impulses of the sympathetic neurones (Fig. 7.4; Shepherd 1983). As exercise intensity increases, metabolism increases, and more metabolites diffuse to the interstitial space to elicit greater vasorelaxation. Many candidates for eliciting relaxation of vascular smooth muscle have been identified. These include, but are not limited to, K^+, H^+, hypoxia and adenosine (Fig. 7.4; Laughlin *et al.* 1996; Delp & Laughlin 1998). To date, however, no single metabolite has been demonstrated as exclusively essential for eliciting the increase in skeletal muscle blood flow during exercise. Some of the factors associated with metabolic control of skeletal muscle blood flow have also been identified as potential

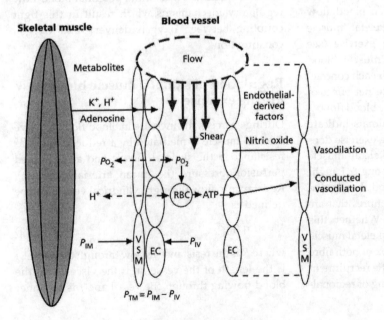

Fig. 7.4 Some of the local factors that may contribute to the control of skeletal muscle blood flow by affecting vascular tone. Not drawn to scale. EC, endothelial cell; P_{IM}, intramuscular pressure; P_{IV}, intravascular pressure; P_{TM}, transmural pressure; RBC, red blood cell; VSM, vascular smooth muscle cell. The VSM has been schematically pulled away from the EC on the right side of the figure (dashed lines) to depict the interaction of endothelial-derived factors with VSM.

factors contributing to skeletal muscle fatigue. Thus, the direct effects of a metabolic by-product on muscle fatigue could be balanced by its vasodilatory effects, which would tend to combat fatigue by increasing local blood flow. Examples of metabolic products that are implicated both in muscle fatigue and in regulation of skeletal muscle blood flow include K^+ and H^+. Evidence of the possible involvement of these factors in skeletal muscle fatigue and vasodilatation is briefly reviewed.

During high-intensity exercise, K^+ is released from active skeletal muscle, and interstitial $[K^+]$ can approach 10mM (Hirsch et al. 1980; Vyskocil et al. 1983). Such concentrations can reduce force production in isolated muscle preparations (Clausen & Everts 1991; Renaud & Light 1992). It appears that interstitial K^+ is associated with fatigue during high-, but not low-intensity exercise (Sjogaard 1996); this is probably because less K^+ accumulates in the interstitium during low-intensity exercise. Although the mechanism of K^+-induced reduction in force is not understood (Fitts & Balog 1996), K^+-induced depolarization may reduce the size of the skeletal muscle action potential, and thus result in a decreased Ca^{2+} release from the sarcoplasmic reticulum (Renaud & Light 1992). In addition to its effects on skeletal muscle, K^+ at low concentrations has been reported to have vasodilatory effects (Fig. 7.4; Duling 1975), but the mechanism remains unclear. It is likely to be a complicated process, since higher concentrations of K^+ result in vascular smooth muscle contraction, and vasoconstriction. Exercise training appears to result in better regulation of K^+. Thus, exercise induces a lesser increase in plasma K^+ after training (Kjeldsen et al. 1986; McKenna et al. 1993), presumably reflecting decreased interstitial K^+. Increased Na^+/K^+ pump density in trained skeletal muscle (Kjeldsen et al. 1986; McKenna et al. 1993) may contribute to the better regulation of K^+. The impact of this training effect on possible K^+-induced vasodilatation will not be clear until the mechanism and relative importance of K^+-induced vasodilatation are better understood.

Production of H^+ and the associated reduction in pH may be related to fatigue during high-intensity exercise. Intracellular pH may drop as low as 6.2 during high-intensity exercise (Wilson et al. 1988),

and acidosis reduces the developed tension in skinned muscle fibres (Fabiato & Fabiato 1978; Metzger & Moss 1987). Acidosis appears to produce fatigue by several mechanisms, including direct inhibition of the contractile apparatus and alteration of sarcoplasmic reticular function (Fitts 1996). During low-intensity exercise, however, pH probably does not become acidic enough to inhibit skeletal muscle contractile function (Fitts 1996). Vascular smooth muscle, in several vascular beds including skeletal muscle, relaxes in response to decreased pH, with resulting vasodilatation (Fig. 7.4; Deal & Green 1954). Elevations in H^+ may cause vasodilatation in direct and indirect ways. Directly, vasodilatation results from the activation of ATP-sensitive K^+ channels in vascular smooth muscle cells by H^+ (Ishizaka & Kuo 1996). Indirectly, a reduced pH results in the release of small amounts of ATP from red blood cells (Ellsworth et al. 1995). Since micromolar concentrations of ATP result in arteriolar vasodilatation that can be conducted to larger upstream arterial vessels (Collins et al. 1998), this could potentially contribute to increased flow during exercise.

Muscle fibre type influences the potential signalling by H^+, insomuch as the H^+ production and release are expected to be much greater from low oxidative, high glycolytic fibres (FG) than from more oxidative fibre types. Thus, the muscle recruitment pattern influences the response of H^+, and in turn its potential influence on fatigue and vasodilatation.

Large increases in blood flow can occur under conditions that do not result in significant accumulation of K^+ or H^+ (i.e. at low and moderate exercise intensities). Whether K^+- or H^+-dependent vasodilatation becomes relatively more important in increasing blood flow at a very high intensity of exercise is not known. Thus, although K^+ and H^+ have been associated with both muscle fatigue and vasodilatation, their contributions to the vasodilatory effect of low- and moderate-intensity exercise remain uncertain. Other local factors, not necessarily associated with muscle fatigue, may contribute to vasodilatation. Two examples of these are the blood Po_2 and the concentration of the adenine nucleotide degradation product, adenosine.

Measures of intracellular oxygen tension (Po_2) suggest that oxygen availability to active skeletal muscle is sufficient for mitochondrial respiration during exercise (> 0.5 torr; Chance & Quistorff 1978). Recently, Richardson *et al.* (1998) utilized magnetic resonance spectroscopy to assess myoglobin saturation in exercising humans. They observed that intramuscular Po_2 remained above 2 torr during maximal exercise, whether the subjects breathed normoxic or hypoxic gas mixtures resulting in respective capillary Po_2 values of 42 and 30 mmHg. Leg blood flow increased in the subjects breathing hypoxic gas, such that the oxygen delivery was similar to that in subjects breathing normoxic gas. Oxygen extraction was also elevated in the hypoxic subjects. The local blood flow regulatory mechanisms that participate in the response to hypoxia are not entirely clear. Recently, however, it has been reported that low Po_2 results in the release of micromolar amounts of ATP from red blood cells (Bergfeld & Forrester 1992; Ellsworth *et al.* 1995). As mentioned above, micromolar amounts of ATP result in significant conducted vasodilatation, even from venules across the capillary bed to arterioles (Fig. 7.4; Collins *et al.* 1998). This mechanism could play a role in distributing flow to regions experiencing high energy demands relative to supply, manifest as a decreased venous Po_2. The exact mechanism of ATP-induced conducted vasodilatation is not known, but it may involve nitric oxide signalling (Collins *et al.* 1998).

Adenosine in the interstitial space can result in vasodilatation via an intracellular signalling pathway that is stimulated by the interaction of adenosine with adenosine receptors on vascular smooth muscle cells (Fig. 7.4). Interstitial adenosine concentration has recently been reported to increase several-fold in human muscle during exercise (Hellsten *et al.* 1998). Adenosine can be released from skeletal muscle as such, or can be formed extracellularly by dephosphorylation of adenosine monophosphate (AMP) catalysed by an ecto-5′-nucleotidase. Although the interstitial concentrations of adenosine surrounding different skeletal muscle fibre types during exercise are not known, it is known that greater adenosine formation occurs in more oxidative fibres at a given high energy utiliza-

tion rate (Whitlock & Terjung 1987). In such fibres, adenosine formation occurs due to ATP breakdown when aerobic energy supply processes are inadequate to meet the energy utilization rate, as established by inadequacy of blood flow.

Myogenic control of skeletal muscle blood flow

The myogenic model of vascular control suggests that vessels can constrict in response to increased transmural pressure (the difference between the intravascular and intramuscular pressures; Fig. 7.4), and the same vessels can dilate in response to decreased transmural pressure. Myogenic control is thought to aid in maintaining relatively constant capillary hydrostatic pressures. According to Meininger and Davis (1992), increased vessel wall stress results in stretch, which activates stretch-activated cation channels and phospholipid signalling pathways, both of which ultimately result in increased cytosolic Ca^{2+}. Thus, activation of these signalling pathways during increased stretch of the vessel wall is expected to result in vascular smooth muscle contraction, and vasoconstriction. In contrast, decreased transmural pressure, as can occur via arteriolar compression during skeletal muscle contraction, results in decreased stretch of the vessel wall, and therefore a decreased stretch-dependent Ca^{2+} signalling. Vascular smooth muscle therefore relaxes when transmural pressure decreases, causing vasodilatation. Although the myogenic response is clearly important in determining vasomotor tone in resting skeletal muscle, this mechanism is likely to be of only minor importance in initiating the blood flow response to exercise (Sheriff *et al.* 1993a) or in matching blood flow to muscle energy demand during prolonged exercise (Bacchus *et al.* 1981).

Endothelium-dependent control of skeletal muscle blood flow

The endothelium-dependent, flow-induced dilatation model of vascular control predicts that vasodilatory factors are released from endothelial cells in response to elevations in blood flow and vessel wall shear stress during exercise (Fig. 7.4).

Nitric oxide is one such factor. It can be released from the endothelium in response to increased flow, and can activate a cascade in vascular smooth muscle that ultimately results in decreased cytosolic Ca^{2+} and vasodilatation. Although there are several published studies that have attempted to assess the role of nitric oxide in the hyperaemic response to exercise, the role nitric oxide plays in regulating blood flow during exercise in humans is unclear. Some studies using handgrip exercise indicate that if nitric oxide synthesis is inhibited, this attenuates the rise in blood flow at the onset of exercise (Gilligan et al. 1994) and reduces forearm blood flow during steady-state exercise (Dyke et al. 1995). In contrast, other studies suggest that nitric oxide is not essential to the increase in blood flow during handgrip exercise (Wilson & Kapoor 1993; Endo et al. 1994). Data collected from exercising animals have yielded conflicting results. When nitric oxide synthesis is inhibited with arginine analogues, blood flow to the hindlimbs of rats is significantly reduced during submaximal treadmill exercise (Hirai et al. 1994). In contrast, skeletal muscle blood flow in dogs exercising on a motorized treadmill is not altered by the inhibition of nitric oxide synthesis (O'Leary et al. 1994). Collectively, these data indicate that nitric oxide may play a modest role in the skeletal muscle blood flow response to light- and moderate-intensity exercise, but it is not essential for exercise hyperaemia. The role nitric oxide plays in the blood flow response of human subjects to high-intensity exercise as well as exercise performed using a larger muscle mass (i.e. running or cycling) is not known. In addition, the contribution of nitric oxide to blood flow regulation during prolonged exercise remains to be determined.

Muscle pump control of skeletal muscle blood flow

The muscle pump model predicts that during large muscle dynamic exercise, perfusion is enhanced by the rhythmic contraction of skeletal muscle (Pollack & Wood 1949; Folkow et al. 1970; Laughlin 1987). During skeletal muscle contraction, the venous vasculature is compressed, the kinetic energy of the venous blood increases, and blood is forced towards

the heart; one-way venous valves prevent retrograde flow. This aids venous return to the heart (and augments right atrial pressure), a response which is essential for maintaining the high cardiac output required during endurance exercise (Sheriff et al. 1993b). During relaxation of the skeletal muscle, venous pressure drops, and ΔP across the vascular circuit increases. The kinetic energy of the venous blood is essentially zero at this time, because venous outflow is zero, whereas the kinetic energy of the arterial blood increases (due to cardiac systole). Refilling of the veins with blood facilitates perfusion of the muscle during relaxation (Folkow et al. 1970; Laughlin 1987; Tschakovsky et al. 1996).

The upright posture creates a hydrostatic column of blood in the veins at all points below the heart, reducing ΔP across the affected circuit. Since back pressure created by the hydrostatic column is greatest at the feet, this could limit blood flow to the calf and thigh muscles. A classic study of humans with venous valve incompetence provided strong support for the role of venous valves and the muscle pump mechanism in maintaining adequate leg blood flow during exercise (Pollack et al. 1949). Humans walking at 2.7 km per hour had a reduced ankle venous pressure, which remained depressed while they were in motion, but increased as walking slowed or stopped (Pollack & Wood 1949). In contrast, patients with incompetent leg vein valves did not exhibit a reduced ankle venous pressure during walking, and they often experienced muscle pain and fatigue, possibly due to inadequate muscle blood flow (Pollack et al. 1949). Critical to the efficacy of the muscle pump is the contraction frequency; in this study, if the walking speed was reduced below 2.7 km per hour, there was sufficient time for the venous vasculature to fill with blood from the capillaries, and the venous pressure at the ankle was not reduced. Additional studies in humans have confirmed the potential role of the muscle pump in other muscle groups. For instance, Tschakovsky et al. (1996) found that the forearm muscle blood flow was enhanced when forearm exercise was performed below the level of the heart. Recently, Sheriff and Van Bibber (1998) have demonstrated the flow-generating capability of the isolated skeletal muscle pump. They utilized an abdominal aortic shunt in pigs to eliminate cardiac pump-derived perfusion pressure. In this model, the pumping action caused by electrically induced skeletal muscle contractions was the only potential generator of perfusion pressure. The rhythmically contracting hindlimb muscles of the pig maintained perfusion for at least 10s, indicating that the muscle pump acts on the muscle vasculature in a manner which enhances perfusion during exercise.

Thus, the muscle pump may function by decreasing venous pressure during skeletal muscle relaxation, and by increasing the kinetic energy of venous blood during skeletal muscle contraction to promote venous return. The muscle pump probably contributes to the increased blood flow at the onset of exercise, and during prolonged endurance exercise in humans (Laughlin *et al.* 1996; Tschakovsky *et al.* 1996; Sheriff & Van Bibber 1998).

Reduced vascular resistance, mediated by relaxation of vascular smooth muscle and subsequent vasodilatation, is the major mechanism by which skeletal muscle blood flow is elevated during exercise. In addition to central and neural effects, local regulation plays a major role in controlling skeletal muscle vascular resistance. This type of control is linked to the metabolic and contractile characteristics of the skeletal muscle, and is therefore affected by the type and number of muscle fibres recruited to perform the exercise. The pumping action of skeletal muscle contraction aids the mechanisms of reduced vascular resistance in enhancing skeletal muscle blood flow during exercise. These local control mechanisms are an important component of the matching of oxygen delivery to oxygen utilization in skeletal muscle during exercise.

Implications for the endurance competitor

Adaptations to endurance exercise training are complex and the coordinated changes of muscle cell phenotype and the vasculature supplying the muscle are likely to be of great importance in supporting the enhanced endurance performance after training. These adaptations ultimately improve the balance of aerobic energy supply to demand. Thus, training is one important factor determining perfor-

mance of both the endurance competitor and the recreational athlete. Detraining induced by inactivity can rapidly eliminate the beneficial adaptations induced by endurance exercise training; thus, maintenance of the endurance-trained state requires a certain minimum level of maintained activity. The exact amount of activity required to maintain the trained state is probably specific to the adaptation under consideration. Genetic predisposition sets the baseline upon which training can cause muscle and vascular adaptations. For example, although endurance training does not produce major shifts in the contractile properties of muscle fibre populations from fast-twitch to slow-twitch fibres, competitive endurance athletes generally have a predominance of slow-twitch fibres with high aerobic capacity and capillarity. This genetic endowment may be important in cultivating the dedication to training required for the endurance competitor to excel.

Conclusions

Energy utilization and supply processes must be balanced for exercise to be maintained at a given intensity. Skeletal muscle energy utilization is ultimately determined by ATPase rate, whereas energy supply depends on muscle oxidative enzyme capacity, and the blood flow and oxygen exchange capacities. These determinants of energy utilization and supply differ in different skeletal muscle fibre types, and the balance achieved between the two in a given fibre type determines its utility in a given type of exercise. Endurance performance and resistance to fatigue are greatest in fibres which have relatively high oxidative enzyme, blood flow and oxygen exchange capacities compared to their inherent ATPase rates. Exercise training can result in increases in all of the determinants of aerobic energy supply, but the changes do not always occur in concert. Disruption of the energy supply processes by diseases which limit skeletal muscle blood flow severely impairs exercise endurance. This attests to the powerful influence of blood flow on muscle performance.

During dynamic exercise, increased skeletal muscle blood flow occurs primarily as a result of decreased vascular resistance. This is mediated primarily by increasing the radius of blood vessels supplying the active skeletal muscle (vasodilatation). Many local mechanisms contribute to the steady-state blood flow response to exercise, including metabolic factors, myogenic control, endothelium-dependent control and the action of the muscle pump. The function of these control mechanisms is determined by the metabolic and contractile demands of the exercise being performed. They are therefore ultimately dependent upon the specific muscle fibre types recruited during exercise. The local mechanisms of blood flow control and the blood flow response itself both adapt to exercise training. In the trained state blood flow at any absolute, submaximal intensity is less than in the untrained state, primarily due to enhanced oxygen extraction. Central and neural mechanisms also contribute to the regulation of skeletal muscle blood flow during exercise, but have not been discussed in this chapter.

Acknowledgements

Work in the authors' laboratory is supported by grants HL-36088 and HL-52490 from the National Institutes of Health, United States of America.

References

Andersen, P. & Saltin, B. (1985) Maximal perfusion of skeletal muscle in man. *Journal of Physiology (London)* **366**, 233–249.

Ariano, M.A., Armstrong, R.B. & Edgerton, V.R. (1973) Hindlimb muscle fiber populations of five mammals. *Journal of Histochemistry and Cytochemistry* **21**, 51–55.

Armstrong, R.B. & Laughlin, M.H. (1983) Blood flows within and among rat muscles as a function of time during high speed treadmill exercise. *Journal of Physiology (London)* **344**, 189–208.

Armstrong, R.B. & Laughlin, M.H. (1984) Exercise blood flow patterns within and among rat muscles after training. *American Journal of Physiology* **246**, H59–H68.

Armstrong, R.B. & Laughlin, M.H. (1985) Rat muscle blood flows during high-speed locomotion. *Journal of Applied Physiology* **59**, 1322–1328.

Armstrong, R.B. & Peterson, D.F. (1981) Patterns of glycogen loss in muscle fibers: response to arterial occlusion during exercise. *Journal of Applied Physiology* **51**, 552–556.

Armstrong, R.B. & Phelps, R.O. (1984) Muscle fiber composition of the rat hindlimb. *American Journal of Anatomy* **171**, 259–272.

Armstrong, R.B., Marum, P., Saubert, C.W., Seeherman, H.W. & Taylor, C.R. (1977) Muscle fiber activity as a function of speed and gait. *Journal of Applied Physiology* **43**, 672–677.

Armstrong, R.B., Delp, M.D., Goljan, E.F. & Laughlin, M.H. (1987) Progressive elevations in muscle blood flow during prolonged exercise in swine. *Journal of Applied Physiology* **63**, 285–291.

Armstrong, R.B., Essen-Gustavsson, B., Hoppeler, H. *et al.* (1992) O_2 delivery at $\dot{V}O_{2max}$ and oxidative capacity of Standardbred horses. *Journal of Applied Physiology* **73**, 2274–2282.

Bacchus, A., Gamble, G., Anderson, D. & Scott, J. (1981) Role of the myogenic response in exercise hyperemia. *Microvascular Research* **21**, 92–102.

Baldwin, K.M., Klinkerfuss, G.H., Terjung, R.L., Mole, P.A. & Holloszy, J.O. (1972) Respiratory capacity of white, red, and intermediate muscle: adaptive response to exercise. *American Journal of Physiology* **222**, 373–378.

Bergfeld, G.R. & Forrester, T. (1992) Release of ATP from human erythrocytes in response to a brief period of hypoxia and hypercapnia. *Cardiovascular Research* **26**, 440–447.

Blomstrand, E., Radegran, G. & Saltin, B. (1997) Maximum rate of oxygen uptake by human skeletal muscle in relation to maximal activities of enzymes in the Krebs cycle. *Journal of Physiology (London)* **501**, 455–460.

Booth, F.W. & Baldwin, K.M. (1996) Muscle plasticity: energy demand supply processes. In: Rowell, L.B. & Shepherd, J.T. (eds) *Handbook of Physiology*, Section 12, *Exercise: Regulation and Integration of Multiple Systems* (Brooks, V.M., Brodhart, J.M. & Mountcastle, V.B., eds), pp. 1075–1123. Oxford University Press, New York.

Burke, R.E. (1981) Motor units: anatomy, physiology, and functional organization. In: *Handbook of Physiology*, Section 1, *The Nervous System*, pp. 345–422. American Physiological Society, Bethesda, MD.

Bystrom, S.E.G. & Kilbom, A. (1990) Physiological response in the forearm during and after isometric intermittent handgrip. *European Journal of Applied Physiology* **60**, 457–466.

Chance, B. & Quistorff, B. (1978) Study of tissue oxygen gradients by single and multiple indicators. *Advances in Experimental Medicine and Biology* **94**, 331–338.

Clausen, J.P. (1977) Effect of physical training on cardiovascular adjustments to exercise in man. *Physiological Reviews* **57**, 799–815.

Clausen, T. & Everts, M.E. (1991) K^+-induced inhibition of contractile force in rat skeletal muscle: role of active Na^+-K^+ transport. *American Journal of Physiology* **261**, C799–C807.

Collins, D.M., McCullough, W.T. & Ellsworth, M.L. (1998) Conducted vascular responses: communication across the capillary bed. *Microvascular Research* **56**, 43–53.

Corcondilas, A., Koroxenidis, G.T. & Shepherd, J.T. (1964) Effect of a brief contraction of forearm muscles on forearm blood flow. *Journal of Applied Physiology* **19** (1), 142–146.

Deal, C.P. Jr & Green, H.D. (1954) Effects of pH on blood flow and peripheral resistance in muscular and cutaneous vascular beds in the hind limb of the pentobarbitalized dog. *Circulation Research* **2**, 148–154.

Delp, M.D. & Laughlin, M.H. (1998) Regulation of skeletal muscle perfusion during exercise. *Acta Physiologica Scandinavica* **162**, 411–419.

Drexler, H., Banhardt, U., Meinertz, T., Wollschlager, H., Lehmann, M. & Just,

H. (1992) Endothelial function in congestive heart failure. *American Journal of Cardiology* **69**, 1596–1601.

Dudley, G.A., Abraham, W.M. & Terjung, R.L. (1982) Influence of exercise intensity and duration on biochemical adaptations in skeletal muscle. *Journal of Applied Physiology* **53**, 844–850.

Duling, B.R. (1975) Effects of potassium on the microcirculation of the hamster. *Circulation Research* **37**, 325–332.

Dyke, C.K., Proctor, D.N., Dietz, N.M. & Joyner, M.J. (1995) Role of nitric oxide in exercise hyperaemia during prolonged rhythmic handgripping in humans. *Journal of Physiology (London)* **488**, 259–265.

Edgerton, V.R., Smith, J.L. & Simpson, D.R. (1975) Muscle fibre type populations of human leg muscles. *Histochemical Journal* **7**, 259–266.

Ellsworth, M.L., Forrester, T., Ellis, C.G. & Dietrich, H.H. (1995) The erythrocyte as a regulator of vascular tone. *American Journal of Physiology* **272**, H1364–H1371.

Endo, T., Imaizumi, T., Tagawa, T., Shiramoto, M., Ando, S. & Takeshita, A. (1994) Role of nitric oxide in exercise-induced vasodilation of the forearm. *Circulation* **90**, 2886–2890.

Fabiato, A. & Fabiato, F. (1978) Effects of pH on the myofilaments and the sarcoplasmic reticulum of skinned cells from cardiac and skeletal muscles. *Journal of Physiology (London)* **276**, 233–255.

Fitts, R.H. (1996) Cellular, molecular, and metabolic basis of muscle fatigue. In: Rowell, L.B. & Shepherd, J.T. (eds) *Handbook of Physiology*, Section 12, *Exercise: Regulation and Integration of Multiple Systems*, pp. 1151–1183. Oxford University Press, New York.

Fitts, R.H. & Balog, E.M. (1996) Effect of intracellular and extracellular ion changes on E–C coupling and skeletal muscle fatigue. *Acta Physiologica Scandinavica* **156**, 169–181.

Folkow, B., Gaskell, P. & Waaler, B.A. (1970) Blood flow through limb muscles during heavy rhythmic exercise. *Acta Physiologica Scandinavica* **80**, 61–72.

Gaffney, F.A., Sjogaard, G. & Saltin, B. (1990) Cardiovascular and metabolic responses to static contraction in man. *Acta Physiologica Scandinavica* **138**, 249–258.

Gilligan, D.M., Panza, J.A., Kilcoyne, C.M., Waclawiw, M.A., Casino, P.R. & Quyyumi, A.A. (1994) Contribution of endothelium-derived nitric oxide to exercise-induced vasodilation. *Circulation* **90**, 2853–2858.

Gute, D., Laughlin, M.H. & Amann, J.F. (1994) Regional changes in capillary supply in skeletal muscle of interval-sprint and low-intensity, endurance-trained rats. *Microcirculation* **1**, 183–193.

Gute, D., Fraga, C., Laughlin, M.H. & Amann, J.F. (1996) Regional changes in capillary supply in skeletal muscle of high-intensity endurance-trained rats. *Journal of Applied Physiology* **81**, 619–626.

Halperin, J.L. & Creager, M.A. (1996) Arterial obstructive diseases of the extremities. In Loscalzo, J., Creager, M.A. & Dzau, V.J. (eds) *Vascular Medicine*, pp. 825–852. Little, Brown, New York.

Hellsten, Y., Maclean, D., Radegran, G., Saltin, B. & Bangsbo, J. (1998) Adenosine concentrations in the interstitium of resting and contracting human skeletal muscle. *Circulation* **98**, 6–8.

Hermansen, L., Ekblom, B. & Saltin, B. (1970) Cardiac output during submaximal and maximal treadmill and bicycle exercise. *Journal of Applied Physiology* **29**, 82–86.

Hirai, T., Visneski, M.D., Kearns, K.J., Zelis, R. & Musch, T.I. (1994) Effects of NO synthase inhibition on the muscular blood flow response to treadmill exercise in rats. *Journal of Applied Physiology* **77**, 1288–1293.

Hirsch, H., Schumacher, E. & Hageman, H. (1980) Extracellular K^+ concentration and K^+ balance of the gastrocnemius muscle of the dog during exercise. *Pflügers Archives* **387**, 231–237.

Holloszy, J.O. (1967) Biochemical adaptations in muscle. Effects of exercise on mitochondrial oxygen uptake and respiratory enzyme activity in skeletal muscle. *Journal of Biological Chemistry* **242**, 2278–2282.

Holloszy, J.O. & Coyle, E.F. (1984) Adaptations of skeletal muscle to endurance exercise and their metabolic consequences. *Journal of Applied Physiology* **56**, 831–838.

Hudlicka, O. (1977) Effect of training on the macro- and microcirculatory changes in exercise. *Exercise and Sport Sciences Reviews* **5**, 181–230.

Hudlicka, O., Zweifach, B.W. & Tyler, K.R. (1982) Capillary recruitment and flow velocity in skeletal muscle after contractions. *Microvascular Research* **23**, 201–213.

Ishizaka, H. & Kuo, L. (1996) Acidosis-induced coronary arteriolar dilation is mediated by ATP-sensitive potassium channels in vascular smooth muscle. *Circulation Research* **78**, 50–57.

Isnard, R., Lechat, P., Kalotka, H. *et al.* (1996) Muscular blood flow response to submaximal leg exercise in normal subjects and in patients with heart failure. *Journal of Applied Physiology* **81**, 2571–2579.

Jondeau, G., Katz, S.D., Zohman, L.R. *et al.* (1992) Active skeletal muscle mass and cardiopulmonary reserve: failure to attain peak aerobic capacity during maximal exercise in patients with congestive heart failure. *Circulation* **86**, 1351–1356.

Katz, S.D., Yuen, J., Bijou, R. & Lejemtel, T.H. (1997) Training improves endothelium-dependent vasodilation in resistance vessels of patients with heart failure. *Journal of Applied Physiology* **82**, 1488–1492.

Kayar, S.R., Hoppeler, H., Armstrong, R.B. *et al.* (1992) Estimating transit time for capillary blood in selected muscles of exercising animals. *Pflügers Archives— European Journal of Physiology* **421**, 578–584.

Kim, C.K., Strange, S., Bangsbo, J. & Saltin, B. (1995) Skeletal muscle perfusion in electrically induced dynamic exercise in humans. *Acta Physiologica Scandinavica* **153**, 279–287.

Kjeldsen, K., Richter, E.A., Galbo, H., Lortie, G. & Clausen, T. (1986) Training increases the concentration of [^{3}H] ouabain-binding sites in rat skeletal muscle. *Biochimica et Biophysica Acta* **860**, 708–712.

Koskolou, M.D., Calbet, J.A.L., Radegran, G. & Roach, R.C. (1997) Hypoxia and the cardiovascular response to dynamic knee extensor exercise. *American Journal of Physiology* **272**, H2655–H2663.

Kubo, S.H., Rector, T.S., Bank, A.J., Williams, R.E. & Heifetz, S.M. (1991) Endothelium-dependent vasodilation is attenuated in patients with heart failure. *Circulation* **84**, 1589–1596.

Laughlin, M.H. (1987) Skeletal muscle blood flow capacity: role of muscle pump in exercise hyperemia. *American Journal of Physiology* **253**, H993–H1004.

Laughlin, M.H. & Armstrong, R.B. (1982) Muscular blood flow distribution patterns as a function of running speed in rats. *American Journal of Physiology* **243**, H296–H306.

Laughlin, M.H. & Armstrong, R.B. (1983) Rat muscle blood flow as a function of time during prolonged slow treadmill exercise. *American Journal of Physiology* **244**, H814–H824.

Laughlin, M.H. & Ripperger, J. (1987) Vascular transport capacity of hindlimb muscles of exercise-trained rats. *Journal of Applied Physiology* **62**, 438–443.

Laughlin, M.H., Korthuis, R.J., Dunker, D.J. & Bache, R.J. (1996) Control of blood flow to cardiac and skeletal muscle during exercise. In: Rowell, L.B. & Shepherd, J.T. (eds) *Handbook of Physiology*, Section 12, *Exercise: Regulation and Integration of Multiple Systems*, pp. 705–769. Oxford University Press, New York.

LeJemtel, T.H., Maskin, C.S., Lucido, D. & Chadwick, B.J. (1986) Failure to augment maximal blood flow in response to lone-leg versus two-leg exercise in patients with congestive heart failure. *Circulation* 74, 245–251.

Mackie, B. & Terjung, R. (1983) Influence of training on blood flow to different skeletal muscle fiber types. *Journal of Applied Physiology* 55, 1072–1078.

Massie, B., Conway, M., Rajagopalan, B. *et al.* (1988) Skeletal muscle metabolism during exercise under ischemic conditions in congestive heart failure. *Circulation* 78, 320–326.

Mathien, G.M. & Terjung, R.L. (1990) Muscle blood flow in trained rats with peripheral arterial insufficiency. *American Journal of Physiology* 258, H759–H765.

Maxwell, L.C., Barclay, J.K., Mohrman, D.E. & Faulkner, J.A. (1977) Physiological characteristics of skeletal muscles of dogs and cats. *American Journal of Physiology* 233, C14–C18.

McAllister, R.M. & Terjung, R.L. (1990) Acute inhibition of respiratory capacity of muscle reduces peak oxygen consumption. *American Journal of Physiology* 259, C889–C896.

McAllister, R.M. & Terjung, R.L. (1991) Training-induced muscle adaptations: increased performance and oxygen consumption. *Journal of Applied Physiology* 70, 1569–1574.

McKenna, M.J., Schmidt, T.A., Hargreaves, M., Cameron, L., Skinner, S.L. & Kjeldsen, K. (1993) Sprint training increases human skeletal muscle Na$^+$-K$^+$-ATPase concentration and improves K$^+$ regulation. *Journal of Applied Physiology* 75, 173–180.

Meininger, G.A. & Davis, M.J. (1992) Cellular mechanisms involved in the vascular myogenic response. *American Journal of Physiology* 63, H647–H659.

Metzger, J.M. & Moss, R.L. (1987) Greater hydrogen ion-induced depression of tension and velocity in skinned single fibres of rat fast than slow muscles. *Journal of Physiology (London)* 393, 727–742.

Meyer, R.A. & Foley, J.M. (1996) Cellular processes integrating the metabolic response to exercise. In: Rowell, L.B. &

Shepherd, J.T. (eds) *Handbook of Physiology*, Section 12, *Exercise: Regulation and Integration of Multiple Systems*, pp. 841–869. Oxford University Press, New York.

Musch, T.I., Friedman, D.B., Pitetti, K.H. *et al.* (1987a) Regional distribution of blood flow of dogs during graded dynamic exercise. *Journal of Applied Physiology* 63, 2269–2277.

Musch, T.I., Haidet, G.C., Ordway, G.A., Longhurst, J.C. & Mitchell, J.H. (1987b) Training effects on regional blood flow response to maximal exercise in foxhounds. *Journal of Applied Physiology* 62, 1724–1732.

O'Leary, D.S., Dunlap, R.C. & Glover, K.W. (1994) Role of endothelium-derived relaxing factor in hindlimb reactive and active hyperemia in conscious dogs. *American Journal of Physiology* 266, R1213–R1219.

Peter, J.B., Barnard, R.J., Edgerton, V.R., Gillespie, C.A. & Stemel, K.E. (1972) Metabolic profiles of three types of skeletal muscle in guinea pigs and rabbits. *Biochemistry* 11, 2627–2633.

Poliner, L.R., Dehmer, G.J., Lewis, S.E., Parkey, R.W., Blomqvist, C.G. & Willerson, J.T. (1980) Left ventricular performance in normal subjects: a comparison of the responses to exercise in the upright and supine positions. *Circulation* 62, 528–534.

Pollack, A.A. & Wood, E.H. (1949) Venous pressure in the saphenous vein at the ankle in man during exercise and changes in posture. *Journal of Applied Physiology* 1, 649–662.

Pollack, A.A., Taylor, B.E., Myers, T.T. & Wood, E.H. (1949) The effect of exercise and body position in patients having valvular defects. *Journal of Clinical Investigation* 23, 559–563.

Radegran, G. (1997) Ultrasound Doppler estimates of femoral artery blood flow during dynamic knee extensor exercise in man. *Journal of Applied Physiology* 83, 1383–1388.

Renaud, J.M. & Light, P. (1992) Effects of K$^+$ on the twitch and tetanic contraction of the sartorius muscle of the frog, *Rana pipiens*. Implication for fatigue *in vivo*. *Canadian Journal of Physiology and Pharmacology* 70, 1236–1246.

Richardson, R.S., Poole, D.C., Knight, D.R. *et al.* (1993) High muscle blood flow in man, is maximal O$_2$ extraction compromised? *Journal of Applied Physiology* 75, 1911–1916.

Richardson, R.S., Noyszewski, E.A., Leigh, J.S. & Wagner, P.W. (1998) Lactate efflux

from exercising human skeletal muscle: role in intracellular P$_{O_2}$. *Journal of Applied Physiology* 85, 627–634.

Robinson, D.M., Ogilvie, R.W., Tullson, P.C. & Terjung, R.L. (1994) Increased peak oxygen consumption of trained muscle requires increased electron flux capacity. *Journal of Applied Physiology* 77, 1941–1952.

Rowell, L.B., Saltin, B., Kiens, B. & Christensen, N.J. (1986) Is peak quadriceps blood flow in humans even higher during exercise with hypoxemia? *American Journal of Physiology* 251, H1038–H1044.

Saltin, B. & Gollnick, P.D. (1983) Skeletal muscle adaptability: significance for metabolism and performance. In: Peachey, L.D. (ed) *Handbook of Physiology*, Section 10, *Skeletal Muscle*, pp. 555–631. Williams & Wilkins, Baltimore, MD.

Saltin, B., Nazar, K., Costill, D.L. *et al.* (1976) The nature of the training response: peripheral and central adaptations to one-legged exercise. *Acta Physiologica Scandinavica* 96, 289–305.

Saltin, B., Radegran, G., Koskolou, M.D. & Roach, R.C. (1998) Skeletal muscle blood flow in humans and its regulation during exercise. *Acta Physiologica Scandinavica* 162, 421–436.

Sarelius, I.H. (1986) Cell flow path influences transit time through striated muscle capillaries. *American Journal of Physiology* 250, H899–H907.

Savard, G.K., Kiens, B. & Saltin, B. (1987) Limb blood flow in prolonged exercise; magnitude and implication for cardiovascular control during muscular work in man. *Canadian Journal of Sport Sciences* 12, S89–S101.

Sexton, W.L. & Laughlin, M.H. (1994) Influence of endurance exercise training on distribution of vascular adaptations in rat skeletal muscle. *American Journal of Physiology* 266, H483–H490.

Shepherd, J.T. (1983) Circulation to skeletal muscle. In: Shepherd, J.T. (ed.) *Handbook of Physiology*, Section 2, *The Cardiovascular System: Peripheral Circulation and Organ Blood Flow*, pp. 319–370. American Physiological Society, Bethesda, MD.

Sheriff, D.D. & Van Bibber, R.V. (1998) Flow-generating capability of the isolated skeletal muscle pump. *American Journal of Physiology* 274, H1502–H1508.

Sheriff, D.D., Rowell, L.B. & Scher, A.M. (1993a) Is rapid rise in vascular conductance at onset of dynamic exercise due to muscle pump? *American Journal of Physiology* 265, H1227–H1234.

Sheriff, D.D., Zhou, X.P., Scher, A.M. & Rowell, L.B. (1993b) Dependence of cardiac filling pressure on cardiac output during rest and dynamic exercise in dogs. *American Journal of Physiology* **265**, H316–H322.

Shoemaker, J.K., Hodge, L. & Hughson, R.L. (1994) Cardiorespiratory kinetics and femoral artery blood velocity during dynamic knee extension exercise. *Journal of Applied Physiology* **77**, 2625–2632.

Sjogaard, G. (1996) Potassium and fatigue: the pros and cons. *Acta Physiologica Scandinavica* **156**, 257–264.

Spurway, N.C. (1981) Interrelationship between myosin-based and metabolism-based classifications of skeletal muscle fibers. *Journal of Histochemistry and Cytochemistry* **29**, 87–88.

Strandness, D.E. & Sumner, D.S. (1975) *Hemodynamics for Surgeons.* Grune and Stratton, New York.

Sullivan, T.E. & Armstrong, R.B. (1978) Rat locomotory muscle fiber activity during trotting and galloping. *Journal of Applied Physiology* **44**, 358–363.

Sullivan, M.J., Knithe, D., Higginbotham, M.B. & Cobb, F.R. (1989) Relation between central and peripheral hemodynamics during exercise in patients with chronic heart failure. Muscle blood flow is reduced with maintenance of arterial perfusion pressure. *Circulation* **80**, 769–781.

Terjung, R.L., Dudley, G.A. & Meyer, R.A. (1985) Metabolic and circulatory limitations to muscular performance at the organ level. *Journal of Experimental Biology* **115**, 307–318.

Terjung, R.L., Mathien, G.M., Erney, T.P. & Ogilvie, R.W. (1988) Peripheral adaptations to low blood flow in muscle during exercise. *American Journal of Cardiology* **62**, 15E–19E.

Tschakovsky, M.E., Shoemaker, J.K. & Hughson, R.L. (1995) Beat-by-beat forearm blood flow with Doppler ultrasound and strain-gauge plethysmography. *Journal of Applied Physiology* **79**, 713–719.

Tschakovsky, M.E., Shoemaker, J.K. & Hughson, R.L. (1996) Vasodilation and muscle pump contribution to immediate exercise hyperemia. *American Journal of Physiology* **271**, H169–H1701.

Vyskocil, F., Hnik, P., Rehfeldt, H., Vejsada, R. & Ujec, E. (1983) The measurement of K_e^+ concentration changes in human muscles during volitional contractions. *Pflügers Archives* **399**, 235–238.

Walmsley, B., Hodgson, J.A. & Burke, R.E. (1978) Forces produced by medial gastrocnemius and soleus muscles during locomotion in freely moving cats. *Journal of Neurophysiology* **41**, 1203–1216.

Weber, K.T. & Janicki, J.S. (1985) Lactate production during maximal and submaximal exercise in patients with chronic heart failure. *Journal of the American College of Cardiology* **6**, 717–724.

Welch, H.G. (1982) Hyperoxia and human performance: a brief review. *Medicine and Science in Sports and Exercise* **14**, 253–262.

Whitlock, D.M. & Terjung, R.L. (1987) ATP depletion in slow-twitch red muscle of rat. *American Journal of Physiology* **253**, C426–C432.

Wiener, D.H., Fink, L.I., Maris, J., Jones, R.A., Chance, B. & Wilson, J.R. (1986) Abnormal skeletal muscle bioenergetics during exercise in patients with heart failure: role of reduced muscle blood flow. *Circulation* **73**, 1127–1136.

Wilson, J.R. & Kapoor, S. (1993) Contribution of endothelium-derived relaxing factor to exercise-induced vasodilation in humans. *Journal of Applied Physiology* **75**, 2740–2744.

Wilson, J.R., McCully, K.K., Mancini, D.M., Boden, B. & Chance, B. (1988) Relationship of muscular fatigue to pH and diprotonated P_i in humans: a ^{31}P-NMR study. *Journal of Applied Physiology* **64**, 2333–2339.

Wilson, J.R., Martin, J.L., Schwartz, D. & Ferraro, N. (1994) Exercise intolerance in patients with chronic heart failure: role of impaired nutritive flow to skeletal muscle. *Circulation* **69**, 1079–1087.

Yamaguchi, K., Glahn, J., Scheid, P. & Piiper, J. (1987) Oxygen transfer conductance of human red blood cells at varied pH and temperature. *Respiration Physiology* **67**, 209–223.

Zelis, R., Mason, D.T. & Brunwald, E. (1969) A comparison of the effects of vasodilator stimuli on peripheral resistance vessels in normal subjects and in patients with congestive heart failure. *Journal of Clinical Investigation* **47**, 960–969.

Zetterquist, S. (1970) The effect of active training on the nutritive blood flow in exercising ischemic legs. *Scandinavian Journal of Clinical and Laboratory Investigation* **25**, 101–111.

Chapter 8

Endurance Exercise and the Regulation of Visceral and Cutaneous Blood Flow

JOHN M. JOHNSON

A primary function of the autonomic nervous system and of reflex control of the circulation during endurance exercise is to provide for an efficient distribution of blood flow. This efficiency requires a redistribution of blood flow from inactive regions to active tissues (muscle, heart), reducing the demand to increase cardiac output to meet the metabolic needs of active skeletal muscle. In this chapter, several important elements in the control of the distribution of the cardiac output are examined. These elements include the quantitative importance of regional circulatory responses during endurance exercise to oxygen delivery and to blood pressure. The circulation to the skin is treated as a special case because, as endurance exercise progresses, competing thermoregulatory demands for higher skin blood flow succeed an initial cutaneous vasoconstriction. Finally, modifications of control—specifically of body temperature and of blood pressure—that accompany endurance exercise are examined.

Oxygen delivery and extraction

As illustrated by the Fick principle, there is a fixed relationship among blood flow, oxygen consumption and oxygen extraction. Applied either to an organ or to the entire systemic circulation, the oxygen consumption is equal to the product of the blood flow through the region in question and the arteriovenous difference in oxygen content across that region. Table 8.1 indicates that relationship for the entire body, for muscle and for the splanchnic circulation, both at rest and during heavy exercise.

For the entire circulation, this represents the relationship among whole-body oxygen consumption, cardiac output and the difference in oxygen content between the systemic arterial blood and that of mixed systemic venous blood as sampled in the pulmonary artery. As an aside, although right atrial blood also represents whole-body venous blood, it is not always so well mixed as to provide a sample that is faithfully representative of the entire venous system. The increased oxygen consumption of the muscle is seen to arise both from increased muscle blood flow and from an increased arteriovenous oxygen difference (see Chapter 7). The increased extraction is also applicable to non-active regions. Several characteristics give regional circulations of inactive tissues importance as targets for redistribution. Firstly, they claim a significant blood flow in resting conditions. Together, the kidney and the splanchnic circulations comprise 45–50% of the cardiac output in a supine, resting human, or about $2.5–3 \, l \cdot min^{-1}$ (Bradley 1963; Chapman & Mitchell 1965; Rowell 1974, 1986; Valtin 1983). Secondly, this blood flow greatly exceeds that required to meet the metabolic needs of those organs. The arteriovenous oxygen difference across the gastrointestinal–hepatic organs, i.e. the splanchnic circulation, shows that only about 25% of the available oxygen is removed from the arterial blood (Bradley 1963; Clausen & Trap-Jensen 1974; Rowell 1974, 1986). An even lower oxygen extraction is found for the renal circulation in resting conditions (Valtin 1983; Haywood et al. 1993). It is clear that splanchnic tissue oxygen consumption can be sustained in the face of a major reduction in blood flow if reductions

Table 8.1 Relationship among oxygen consumption ($\dot{V}o_2$), blood flow ($\dot{Q}$) and arteriovenous oxygen difference ($C_ao_2 - C_\bar{v}o_2$) as applied to the whole body, to skeletal muscle and to the splanchnic circulation at rest and during exercise. In each case, the oxygen consumption is equal to the flow through that region and the arteriovenous oxygen difference across it. Note that the increased oxygen consumption of muscle is met by both increased blood flow and increased arteriovenous oxygen difference and that splanchnic oxygen consumption is preserved during exercise by an increased extraction balancing the reduced blood flow.

$$\dot{V}o_2\,(\text{ml·min}^{-1}) = \dot{Q}\,(\text{l·min}^{-1}) \times (C_ao_2 - C_\bar{v}o_2)\,(\text{ml·l}^{-1})$$

Body	$\dot{V}o_2 = \dot{Q} \times (C_ao_2 - C_\bar{v}o_2)$
Rest	$300 = 6 \times (200 - 150)$
Exercise	$3000 = 22 \times (200 - 64)$
Muscle	$\dot{V}o_2 = \dot{Q}_m \times (C_ao_2 - C_\overline{mv}o_2)$
Rest	$50 = 1 \times (200 - 150)$
Exercise	$2700 = 18 \times (200 - 50)$
Splanchnic	$\dot{V}o_2 = \dot{Q}_s \times (C_ao_2 - C_\overline{hv}o_2)$
Rest	$60 = 1.5 \times (200 - 160)$
Exercise	$60 = 0.5 \times (200 - 80)$

$\dot{Q}_m$, muscle blood flow; $\dot{Q}_s$, splanchnic blood flow; $\dot{Q}$, cardiac output; C_ao_2, systemic arterial oxygen content; $C_\bar{v}o_2$, systemic venous oxygen content; $C_\overline{mv}o_2$, oxygen content in venous blood from muscle; $C_\overline{hv}o_2$, hepatic venous oxygen content.

in perfusion are matched by increases in oxygen extraction as reflected by an expanded arteriovenous difference in oxygen content (Clausen & Trap-Jensen 1974). The redistribution from the splanchnic circulation in the example of Table 8.1 would provide $1\,\text{l·min}^{-1}$ of blood flow to muscle. Similar reductions in renal blood flow (Radigan & Robinson 1949; Grimby 1965; Castenfors & Piscator 1967; Haywood *et al.* 1993) and in other inactive regions might provide another $1-1.5\,\text{l·min}^{-1}$ for muscle, or a total redistribution to active muscle (and the coronary circulation) of over $2\,\text{l·min}^{-1}$. This represents blood flow that the heart does not have to furnish in the form of further increases in cardiac output, and provides $300-600\,\text{ml}\,O_2\cdot\text{min}^{-1}$ of the increased oxygen consumption of active muscle (Chapman & Mitchell 1965; Rowell 1986). Hence, the ability of visceral organs, like active muscle, to increase their oxygen extraction aids in meeting the metabolic demands of exercise.

Blood pressure maintenance and peripheral vasoconstriction

The reflex reductions in blood flow to visceral organs also help to maintain arterial blood pressure.

Metabolic vasodilatation in active skeletal muscle challenges blood pressure because total peripheral resistance falls markedly and rapidly. Table 8.2 shows examples of the relationships among blood pressure, blood flow and vascular resistance for the whole body, the muscle circulation and the splanchnic circulation. These are shown for rest and the same level of heavy exercise as assumed in Table 8.1. The arterial blood pressure is the same for all regions. The venous pressure is not, but for the convenience of this example it is low enough to be ignored. The reduction in muscle vascular resistance to 5–6% of its value at rest has a large effect on total peripheral resistance. This, however, is moderated to some degree by simultaneous increases in vascular resistance in the splanchnic region (Table 8.2), the kidneys and other inactive regions (Chapman & Mitchell 1965; Grimby 1965; Bevegård & Shepherd 1966b; Castenfors & Piscator 1967; Rowell 1974, 1986; Clausen 1977; Haywood *et al.* 1993; Kenney & Ho 1995; Ho *et al.* 1997). Note in this example that splanchnic vascular resistance rose to over 350% of its resting value. Similar responses in renal blood flow and in other non-active regions contribute further to preventing total peripheral resistance from falling more than it does. If, for

Table 8.2 Relationship among blood pressure (BP), blood flow and vascular resistance (R) for the whole body, skeletal muscle and the splanchnic circulation at rest and during exercise. The level of exercise is the same as in the example in Table 8.1. In all cases the blood pressure is equal to the product of the blood flow through that region and the vascular resistance of that region.

$$BP\,(mmHg) = \dot{Q}\,(l\cdot min^{-1}) \times R\,(mmHg\cdot min\cdot l^{-1})$$

Body	$BP = \dot{Q} \times TPR$
Rest	$90 = 6 \times 15$
Exercise	$110 = 22 \times 5$
Muscle	$BP = \dot{Q}_m \times MVR$
Rest	$90 = 1 \times 90$
Exercise	$110 = 18 \times 6$
Splanchnic	$BP = \dot{Q}_s \times SVR$
Rest	$90 = 1.5 \times 60$
Exercise	$110 = 0.5 \times 220$

TPR, total peripheral resistance; MVR, muscle vascular resistance; SVR, splanchnic vascular resistance; other abbreviations as in Table 8.1. BP is arterial pressure (venous pressure has been assumed to be low and negligible). Note the marked increase in SVR accompanying the fall in MVR.

example, visceral vasoconstriction during exercise were to revert suddenly to resting levels without simultaneous changes in either cardiac output or muscle vascular resistance, blood pressure would fall by about 15 mmHg in this example. The quantitative effect of such vasoconstriction on blood pressure depends on the level of exercise, the degree of vasoconstriction and the cardiac output (Rowell 1974). A similar contribution to blood pressure maintenance from renal vasoconstriction adds to the importance of the visceral circulations with respect to blood pressure control, as well as to the delivery of oxygen.

The gastrointestinal circulation is a target for vasodilatation during digestion. In humans, this vasodilatation can be significantly reversed by exercise (Eriksen & Waaler 1994; Puvi-Rajasingham et al. 1997b), although such a response is not consistently observed in exercising dogs (Fronek & Fronek 1970). In humans, Doppler ultrasound measurements of superior mesenteric arterial blood flow revealed a more marked exercise-induced vasoconstriction in the fed state, as compared to the response when fasted (Eriksen & Waaler 1994; Puvi-Rajasingham et al. 1997b).

The consequences of a loss of vasoconstrictor response to exercise are illustrated by patients with autonomic failure. Such patients have a marked reduction in blood pressure with exercise (Puvi-Rajasingham et al. 1997a). Ironically, they also have about the same reduction in blood flow in the superior mesenteric artery as do healthy controls. The difference is that in the case of the patients with autonomic failure, a passive reduction in blood flow accompanies the fall in blood pressure, whereas in the controls the reduction is due to sympathetically mediated vasoconstriction and an increased vascular resistance.

Graded vasoconstrictor responses to endurance exercise

The examples developed in Tables 8.1 and 8.2 focus on rest and a single level of fairly heavy exercise. For intermediate levels of exercise, intermediate degrees of vasoconstriction are seen (Grimby 1965; Castenfors & Piscator 1967; Rowell 1974, 1986; Clausen 1977; Rowell et al. 1996). Figure 8.1 summarizes data for splanchnic blood flow from a number of studies in exercising humans (Rowell et al. 1964, 1965; Blackmon et al. 1967; Clausen et al. 1973). Observations include athletes, sedentary subjects and patients with mitral stenosis, i.e. subjects with very different endurance capacities. Figure 8.1a shows that each group responds to exercise by a vasoconstriction and, as the intensity of exercise

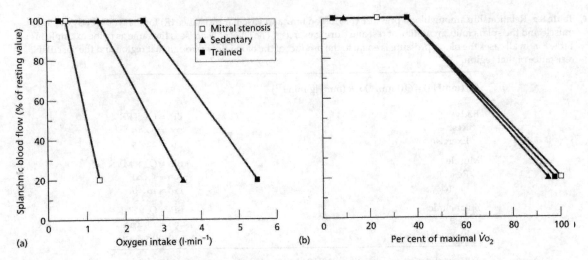

Fig. 8.1 Relationship of splanchnic blood flow (percentage of resting value) to the level of exercise for three groups: patients with mitral stenosis, sedentary healthy subjects and trained athletes. Splanchnic blood flow is related to oxygen consumption on an absolute scale (a), and to the percentage of each individual's maximal oxygen intake (b). On the relative scale, response patterns among these groups with very different exercise capacities are similar. After Rowell (1973).

increases (shown by increasing oxygen consumption on the abscissae), splanchnic blood flow is proportionally reduced (Rowell 1973; Rowell 1974). The same is true for renal blood flow (Grimby 1965; Castenfors & Piscator 1967; Kenney & Zappe 1994). However, for a given increase in absolute work rate, the groups show differing reductions in splanchnic blood flow. The degree of vasoconstriction is in inverse relation to the pumping capacity of the heart: greatest in mitral stenosis and least in athletes. When cardiac output is limited, the need to redistribute blood flow becomes greater (Blackmon et al. 1967; Rowell 1973, 1974; Clausen 1977; Ho et al. 1997). Indeed, Rowell (1974) estimates that as much as 40% of the oxygen delivered to active muscle at maximal exercise in patients limited by mitral stenosis is met by the redistribution from the splanchnic region, whereas the corresponding values are only 9% in the athletes and 15% in the sedentary group. An interesting corollary to this is seen in patients following cardiac transplantation (Haywood et al. 1993). Such patients have a limited ability to increase heart rate and cardiac output and consequently show a more marked renal vasoconstriction than their healthy counterparts, despite a lower level of exercise.

Although the absolute reduction in splanchnic blood flow for a given increase in work rate differs among these groups, similar patterns of response emerge. This is illustrated in Fig. 8.1b, in which data for splanchnic blood flow are plotted relative to the percentage of maximal oxygen intake (Rowell 1973). When individuals with very different exercise capacities exercise at the same fraction of their individual maximal oxygen intake, they experience similar reductions in splanchnic blood flow, although the absolute work rates are quite different. Thus reflex responses relate more closely to the difficulty of work for the individual, and not so much to the absolute work rate or oxygen requirement. The inverse relationship between visceral vasoconstriction and the pumping capacity of the heart among cardiac patients, healthy humans and athletes transcends species. The Alaskan sled dog has essentially no visceral vasoconstriction (Van Citters & Franklin 1969). Dogs generally show little exercise-induced visceral vasoconstriction (Van Citters & Franklin 1969; Vatner et al. 1971, 1972; Delgado et al. 1975; Musch et al. 1987) unless challenged by limitations to oxygen delivery such as heart block or anaemia (Vatner et al. 1971, 1972). Baboons and swine, presumably less fit, have marked vasoconstrictor responses to exercise (Sanders *et al.* 1976; Hohimer & Smith 1979).

The relationship between the reflex vasoconstrictor response to exercise and the percentage of the maximal oxygen intake is very similar to previous analyses of the heart rate response to exercise. In particular, different populations show similar heart rate responses to endurance exercise when the level of work is expressed relative to the individual maximal oxygen intake (Åstrand & Rodahl 1970). Thus, there is a parallel behaviour between splanchnic vasoconstriction and increased heart rate (Rowell 1974; Clausen 1977). During endurance exercise requiring heart rates above 100 beats·min^{-1}, the degree of reduction in splanchnic or renal blood flow is proportional to the increase in heart rate (Grimby 1965; Rowell 1974; Clausen 1977; Kenney & Zappe 1994). A reasonable interpretation of this relationship is that parasympathetic withdrawal accounts for most of the heart rate increase up to 100 beats·min^{-1} (with no change in splanchnic vascular resistance); with heavier exercise, sympathetic activity is increased both to the sinoatrial node (raising heart rate further) and to the visceral circulations (raising vascular resistance and reducing blood flow) (Rowell 1974). The sensitivity of the relationship is remarkably consistent among athletes, healthy subjects, patients with mitral stenosis, patients with coronary artery disease and subjects before and following training (Blackmon *et al.* 1967; Clausen *et al.* 1973; Rowell 1974, 1986; Clausen 1977).

Influence of ageing

Ageing is associated with some modifications in the peripheral vascular responses to endurance exercise. At mild levels of exercise, changes in splanchnic and renal blood flow are similar among different age groups (Kenney & Zappe 1994; Kenney & Ho 1995), although there is an apparent interaction between age and fitness in the visceral vascular response to endurance exercise (Kenney & Ho 1995; Ho *et al.* 1997). At levels of exercise requiring 60% of maximal oxygen intake or more, healthy older individuals show somewhat reduced splanchnic and renal vasoconstrictor responses (Kenney & Ho 1995;

Ho *et al.* 1997). Responses in heart rate and in plasma norepinephrine are also reduced (Ho *et al.* 1997), indicating that reduced sympathetic activation is at least part of the cause. The relationship between visceral vasoconstriction and plasma norepinephrine or heart rate appears to be the same as in younger subjects.

Other regions

The focus on the splanchnic and renal circulations derives from the large number of studies, in humans, of these regions as targets for the reflexes associated with exercise, their high blood flows and the consequent potential for significant redistribution of blood flow from them. The patterns of response seen in the renal and gastrointestinal circulations do not uniformly anticipate those that occur in other regions, however. Blood flow to resting skeletal muscle is predictably reduced by endurance exercise (e.g. Bevegård & Shepherd 1966b; Zelis *et al.* 1969). On the other hand, blood flow to adipose tissue and bone usually increases during endurance exercise (Bülow & Madsen 1978, 1986; Tondevold & Bülow 1983). Although changes in total cerebral blood flow are often unremarkable (Foreman *et al.* 1976; Gross *et al.* 1980), some authors report generalized increases in cerebral blood flow (Herholz *et al.* 1987; Jorgensen *et al.* 1992). One consistent feature of exercise is an increased blood flow in cerebellar areas (Gross *et al.* 1980; Manohar 1986). Finally, significant reductions in uterine blood flow have been noted in pregnant females (Bell *et al.* 1983; Lotgering *et al.* 1983) Fortunately, the reduction in placental blood flow is small (Hohimer *et al.* 1984; Rauramo & Forss 1988), and unlikely to have negative consequences for pregnancy (Jones *et al.* 1990).

Skin: a special case

The distribution of blood flow to and away from skin follows a more complicated pattern than that for the viscera because the metabolic heat production by the active muscle increases body temperature and ultimately engages heat loss mechanisms. These include sweating and, importantly, increased skin blood flow. Thus, there is an inherent competition between the necessity for increased blood flow to active muscle to meet its metabolic needs and the thermoregulatory drive to increase blood flow to skin (Johnson 1986, 1992; Kenney & Johnson 1992).

The heat production associated with metabolic activity is approximately 4.8 kcal or 20 kJ per litre of oxygen (Brengelmann 1989). In a resting human weighing 75 kg and consuming $250 \, ml O_2 \cdot min^{-1}$, body temperature would rise by about $1°C \cdot h^{-1}$ if all of the heat produced were stored, with no caloric loss to the environment (Nadel 1977). With the same constraint on heat loss, the rise in body temperature would be about $10°C \cdot h^{-1}$ during moderate exercise requiring an oxygen consumption of $2.5 \, l \cdot min^{-1}$. Such a rate of increase in body temperature cannot be tolerated more than briefly and heat loss mechanisms must be engaged such exercise is to continue.

In the first 5–10 min of exercise, most of the increased heat generation is actually stored, leading to a brisk rise in body temperature. Some increase in heat loss does occur via ventilation and via convection from the motion of the athlete's body through the air, but this loss is small relative to heat production (Saltin & Hermansen 1966; Nadel 1977). Thus, the maximal rates of heat gain and body temperature increase suggested above are nearly achieved in the very early stages of endurance exercise.

As exercise continues, however, body temperature reaches a level at which heat loss mechanisms are activated, in particular cutaneous vasodilatation and sweating. The threshold internal temperature at which vasodilatation or sweating begins is not a fixed temperature; it changes during the day (Stephenson & Kolka 1985), as a function of acclimatization (Fox *et al.* 1958; Roberts *et al.* 1977; Johnson 1998) and in women during the phases of the menstrual cycle (Stephenson & Kolka 1985, 1993; Charkoudian & Johnson 1997). Exercising individuals with hypertension also demonstrate a delayed cutaneous vasodilator response to dynamic exercise (Kenney 1985).

Dynamic exercise influences the threshold for vasodilatation, so that the increase in blood flow begins at a higher internal temperature during exercise than under resting conditions (Johnson & Park 1981; Taylor *et al.* 1988; Kellogg *et al.* 1991; Smolan-

der *et al.* 1991; Mack *et al.* 1994) (see Fig. 8.2.) It does not appear, however, that exercise has the same influence on the internal temperature threshold for the onset of sweating (Johnson & Park 1981). This observation speaks against the hypothesis of a mechanistic role for sweat gland activation in the control of skin blood flow (see Johnson & Proppe 1996). The difference between the control of sweating and of blood flow reflects an efficiency of modified thermoregulatory control by exercise, because it allows evaporative heat loss to continue unaffected while permitting a distribution of the cardiac output which reflects the various demands for blood flow. Thermoregulatory demands are not as completely met as at rest, thereby contributing to the higher body temperatures of exercise.

The influence of exercise on the threshold for cutaneous vasodilatation is one expression of the competition between the drives to increase blood flow to skin and to muscle during dynamic exercise. This competition also reveals itself in other ways. For example, the initiation of dynamic exercise is associated with a cutaneous vasoconstriction (Zelis *et al.* 1969; Johnson & Park 1982; Taylor *et al.* 1988, 1990), which persists in the face of elevated skin and

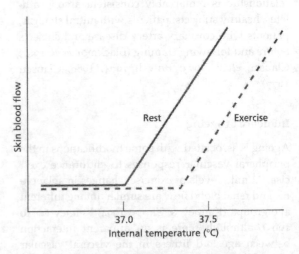

Fig. 8.2 Relationship of skin blood flow to internal temperature in resting conditions and during moderate dynamic exercise. Blood flow rises in response to increased body temperature in both cases, but during exercise the increase of flow begins at a higher internal temperature. After Johnson and Park (1981).

internal temperatures (Johnson & Park 1982). The degree of vasoconstriction is such that the competition between the drive from exercise to reduce skin blood flow and the drive from elevated internal temperature to increase it is seen: the level to which skin blood flow falls is low relative to thermoregulatory demands, but is still relatively high considering the competing demands by active muscle (Johnson & Park 1982). The cutaneous vasoconstrictor response at the onset of exercise is most pronounced in the hands, perhaps reflecting an important contribution of arteriovenous anastomoses in this region (Midttun & Sejrsen 1998), but it is seen in non-glabrous skin as well (Zelis *et al.* 1969; Johnson & Park 1982; Taylor *et al.* 1988, 1990). The vasoconstriction is reversed in relatively short order to a net vasodilatation. Although this may appear to refute a persistent vasoconstrictor role for exercise, *per se*, closer analysis reveals that the levels of skin blood flow reached during exercise are lower than they are in resting conditions for the same combination of skin and internal temperatures (Johnson & Park 1981, 1982).

With longer periods of exercise, the cutaneous vasodilatation reaches an apparent upper limit as body temperature exceeds about 38°C (Brengelmann *et al.* 1977; Nadel *et al.* 1979; Kenney & Johnson 1992; Kellogg *et al.* 1993). As illustrated by Fig. 8.3, significant increases in internal temperature beyond 38°C are accompanied by little or no further increase in blood flow to the skin. This upper limit is characteristic of dynamic exercise; it is not seen with body heating at rest. The apparent upper limit during endurance exercise is at about 60% of maximal skin blood flow, implying that exercise constrains further vasodilatation (Brengelmann *et al.* 1977; Kellogg *et al.* 1993).

Cardiovascular drift

The elevation in skin blood flow during exercise is thought by some to be the origin of the steady increase in heart rate during prolonged endurance exercise, which has been termed 'cardiovascular drift' (Ekelund 1967). The steady rise in heart rate is associated with declines in stroke volume, pulmonary vascular pressures and arterial pulse

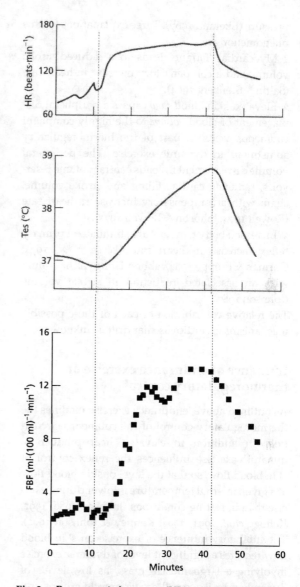

Fig. 8.3 Responses in heart rate (HR), internal temperature (measured in the oesophagus) (Tes) and skin blood flow (measured as increases in forearm blood flow) (FBF) during 30 min of moderate dynamic exercise (indicated by the vertical lines) at a warm (38°C) skin temperature. Skin blood flow rises with internal temperature only to a point, after which further vasodilatation is limited despite a further 1°C increase in internal temperature. After Brengelmann *et al.* (1977).

pressure (Ekelund 1967). Three explanations for this phenomenon are:

1 Myocardial 'fatigue' leads to a reduced stroke volume and a compensatory increase in heart rate (Saltin & Stenberg 1964).

2 Elevated skin blood *flow* causes a peripheral displacement of blood *volume* to the highly compliant cutaneous veins as part of the thermoregulatory adjustment to dynamic exercise. The peripheral volume displacement unloads central volume reservoirs, reducing cardiac filling and stroke volume, again with a compensatory increase in heart rate (Rowell 1974; Johnson & Rowell 1975).

3 Increased body temperature stimulates a primary reflex increase in heart rate (Wyss *et al.* 1974; Gorman & Proppe 1984), abbreviating cardiac filling with an associated reduction in stroke volume (Johnson 1987).

The relative contribution of each of these possible mechanisms to cardiovascular drift is unknown.

Influence of endurance exercise on thermoregulatory control

As outlined above, endurance exercise modifies the thermoregulatory control of the cutaneous circulation. In addition to elevated heat production, dynamic exercise influences the reflex control of skin blood flow, so that the level of skin blood flow at a given internal temperature is lower during exercise than in resting conditions (Johnson 1986, 1992; Kellogg *et al.* 1991, 1993; Kenney & Johnson 1992). The inhibitory influence of exercise on skin blood flow requires a significant level of dynamic exercise involving a large muscle mass, as low levels of dynamic exercise, small active muscle groups and static exercise do not cause an important redistribution of blood flow from the skin (Kilbom & Brundin 1976; Taylor *et al.* 1988, 1989, 1990; Crandall *et al.* 1995). Ironically, the endurance exercise with the greatest vasoconstrictor influence on skin also has the greatest heat production.

The combination of limited heat loss and elevated heat production dictates that the body temperature will rise during endurance exercise. Whether the increased body temperature reflects an increase in the thermoregulatory 'set point' or is a consequence of the competition between thermoregulatory and non-thermoregulatory reflex control of skin blood flow is not resolved (see Johnson 1986, 1992). Arguments can be made for dynamic exercise causing an increased thermoregulatory set point, a reduced set point, or no change. The delayed onset of vasodilatation, plus the other effects inhibitory to the increase in skin blood flow, suggest a regulated increase in body temperature. However, the lack of similar effects of endurance exercise on the control of sweating argue for an alternative in which competition for the control of skin blood flow occurs at some central site different from the primary thermoregulatory centres (Johnson & Proppe 1996).

Influence of temperature regulation on endurance exercise

It is clear that demands for blood flow from skeletal muscle are met in part by redistribution of blood flow from inactive regions and by limits on the increases in blood flow to skin. It is also clear that a hot environment is associated with reduced capacity to perform prolonged activity. Endurance time is reduced in warm conditions (Nielsen *et al.* 1993; Febbraio *et al.* 1994; Galloway & Maughan 1997). In particular, the time to exhaustion is abbreviated for endurance activity in a hot environment and it can be extended when the activity follows a precooling period (Schmidt & Brück 1981; Olschewski & Brück 1988; Kruk *et al.* 1990; Nielsen *et al.* 1993; Lee & Haymes 1995; Booth *et al.* 1997).

Does the demand for blood flow by skin limit the delivery of blood flow to active muscle? Active muscle will vasoconstrict when sympathetic nerve activity increases (Donald *et al.* 1970; Laughlin *et al.* 1996; Rowell *et al.* 1996; Saltin *et al.* 1998) and hyperthermia has vasoconstrictor effects on non-cutaneous regions (Radigan & Robinson 1949; Rowell 1973, 1974; Kenney & Johnson 1992; Johnson & Proppe 1996; Ho *et al.* 1997). The possibility of a thermoregulatory-induced vasoconstriction in active muscle was raised to explain the source of the increased skin blood flow during prolonged exercise (Johnson & Rowell 1975) in the face of a presumed constant cardiac output (Ekelund 1967). Small reductions in blood flow to active muscle (relative to the total) could account for significantly increased skin blood flow (again, relative to the total).

Demonstration of a thermoregulatory influence on skeletal muscle blood flow has not been forthcoming. The observation of increased blood lactate during hyperthermic exercise (Fink *et al.* 1980) is indirect evidence for a compromised skeletal muscle blood flow, i.e. a lower blood flow and earlier or more pronounced anaerobic metabolism. However, this observation is not universal. Other studies find no evidence for enhanced glycogenolysis or lactic acidosis during exercise in the heat (Savard *et al.* 1988; Nielsen *et al.* 1990). Also, elevated plasma lactate concentrations could reflect limited removal due to reduced liver blood flow rather than an enhanced production caused by a reduced blood flow to active muscle. Indeed, direct measurements during exercise in the heat indicate such a vasoconstrictor effect of heat stress is absent in humans (Nielsen *et al.* 1990, 1993; Savard *et al.* 1988), although it has been demonstrated in sheep (Bell *et al.* 1986).

In humans, the evidence against a reduction in blood flow to active skeletal muscle in a hot environment is very strong, but fails to explain why fatigue becomes so prominent in that environment. The best available evidence currently indicates temperature, *per se*, to be the source of the problem (Nielsen *et al.* 1993). Nielsen *et al.* (1993) studied the time to fatigue during uncompensable hyperthermia: exercise under conditions in which body temperature continues to rise rather than reaching a steady-state level. Daily exercise to fatigue in a hot (41°C) environment led to acclimatization and an increased time to fatigue. Two related observations from that study stand out. As acclimatization proceeded, the internal temperature at the beginning of exercise was lower than in the unacclimatized state and it remained lower after any given duration of exercise. Secondly, the internal temperature at fatigue did not change from the beginning to the end of acclimatization. These findings strongly indicate that it is the internal temperature which limits endurance time

during exercise in the heat. The authors detected no signs of circulatory collapse in the form of falling blood pressure or reduced muscle blood flow. The exact site at which the high body temperature exerts its limiting effects is unknown, but possibilities are motor control areas of the central nervous system (see Nielsen *et al.* 1993) and skeletal muscle contractile function (Brooks *et al.* 1971; Febbraio *et al.* 1994, 1996).

An important practical implication for endurance exercise and for competition is that fatigue depends on reaching this apparently critical internal temperature. In the study by Nielsen *et al.* (1993), the average endurance time increased from 48 min before acclimatization to 80 min after 9–12 days of acclimatization. Tolerance depends not on the ability to cope voluntarily with a higher body temperature, but on how long it takes to reach the critical temperature. Acclimatization increases this time, both by reducing the initial body temperature and by engaging heat loss mechanisms at lower temperatures. The increase in endurance time varies both with the extent of acclimatization and with the test procedures. For example, in a follow-up study with lower levels of exercise and less extreme environmental heating, acclimatization increased the exercise time to fatigue by only 7 min (Nielsen *et al.* 1997). Although protocol dependent, the clear message is that procedures which provide lower initial body temperatures (body cooling, acclimatization) also increase the time to fatigue for those performing endurance exercise in a hot environment.

Visceral vasoconstriction during hyperthermic exercise

Although blood flow to active muscle is apparently not reduced by hyperthermia, blood flow to the gastrointestinal organs and to the kidneys is reduced by exercise and is further reduced by hyperthermic exercise (Radigan & Robinson 1949; Rowell *et al.* 1965; Rowell 1974). Hyperthermia, alone, causes a splanchnic vasoconstriction (Rowell 1974, 1986; Johnson & Proppe 1996). It is therefore not surprising that exercise-induced splanchnic vasoconstriction becomes more intense in a hot environment (Rowell *et al.* 1965). Figure 8.4 shows this result for exercise in neutral and hot environments. Radigan and Robinson (1949) made similar observations for renal blood flow.

Ageing modifies the extent, although not the pattern, of visceral vasoconstriction during endurance exercise in warm conditions. In particular, Ho *et al.* (1997) found that healthy 65-year-old subjects exercising in the heat had smaller reductions in splanchnic and renal blood flows than did their 25-year-old counterparts. The smaller reduction in the older group was due in part to a lower visceral blood flow at rest, as the levels reached during exercise did not differ between age groups. Importantly, the increase in skin blood flow with body heating or during exercise is also reduced by ageing (Rooke *et al.* 1994; Kenney & Ho 1995; Ho *et al.* 1997; Minson & Kenney 1997), so that the requirement for blood flow redistribution is less.

Thus, exercise in a hot environment has two associated challenges to the distribution of the cardiac output: to muscle (to support its metabolic activity), and to skin (to protect body temperature). Targets for each of these demands include the gastrointestinal and renal circulations and the sinoatrial node of the heart. The controls of these elements of the cardiovascular system operate very much in parallel. By combining findings from a large number of studies of splanchnic vasoconstrictor responses to exercise, heat stress and their combination, Rowell (1974) found that the increase in heart rate and the reduction in splanchnic blood flow were highly correlated. As maximal heart rate is approached, so is maximal vasoconstriction in the organs making up the splanchnic circulation. Because of additional demands for heat elimination, however, high heart rates and low splanchnic blood flows are reached at lower power outputs in the heat than in cool or thermoneutral conditions. Demands for more blood flow from further increases in exercise level and/or thermal stress cannot be met adequately, leading to compromises in temperature regulation and to early fatigue (Nielsen *et al.* 1993, 1997; Galloway & Maughan 1997). It is also at this point that intense visceral vasoconstriction leads to a situation wherein the reduction in oxygen delivery to the gastrointestinal system and kidneys can no longer be balanced by further increases in oxygen extraction. The risk is then of an ischaemic liver, intestines and/or kidneys. Indeed, the oxygen content of blood draining the liver falls as low as $0.5\,ml\,O_2\cdot dl^{-1}$. Repeated, prolonged exposures to intense work in hot environments could lead to tissue damage from multiple ischaemic episodes.

Baroreflex control modifications

It is clear that endurance exercise can significantly modify how body temperature is regulated (see above). Whether and how the reflex control of blood pressure is modified by endurance exercise and how the baroreflex affects circulatory control during exercise have only recently gained some clarity. Indeed, it was believed for some time that the baroreflex was 'switched off' by dynamic exercise. When blood pressure is forced to rise by an exogenous means such as the infusion of norepinephrine, heart rate falls in a classical baroreflex fashion. However, when blood pressure increases at the start of exercise, heart rate does not fall. It has been argued from these observations that the baroreflex is reduced in sensitivity or even becomes nonfunctional during exercise (Bristow *et al.* 1971).

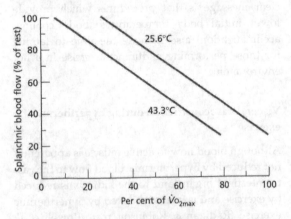

Fig. 8.4 Relationship of splanchnic blood flow to the level of exercise, expressed as the percentage of maximal oxygen intake, at neutral (25.6°C) and hot (43.3°C) ambient temperatures. For any given level of exercise, blood flow is lower in the hot environment. After Rowell (1973).

The above conclusion has come into question and more recent syntheses now accord the baroreflex a central position with respect to the reflex adjustments to endurance exercise (Rowell *et al.* 1996). In dogs without baroreceptor connections to the central nervous system, blood pressure falls precipitously at the onset of exercise, whereas in intact animals blood pressure is maintained or rises (Walgenbach & Donald 1983). This observation indicates that the baroreflex has a functional significance in the control of blood pressure during exercise and is certainly not 'switched off'. The same series of experiments provided further evidence for a functional baroreflex by selectively controlling blood pressure in the carotid sinus, a major sensory area for blood pressure regulation. When blood pressure in the area was caused to rise or fall, reflex changes in heart rate and peripheral resistance resulted. Indeed, baroreflex sensitivity was not much different from that seen in resting conditions (Walgenbach & Donald 1983). Results similar to these have been seen in humans in whom the carotid sinus distension was controlled by an external device generating positive or negative pressure around the neck (Bevegård & Shepherd 1966a; Strange *et al.* 1990; Potts *et al.* 1993; Papelier *et al.* 1997). These studies and others in which blood pressure regulation was challenged during exercise (Mack *et al.* 1988) clearly show that reflex responses to acute stimulation or unloading of baroreceptors are not eliminated by exercise.

What role does the baroreflex play during exercise? It appears that the reflex not only acts to prevent a fall in blood pressure, but also assists in causing an increase. One current postulate is that during endurance exercise central command and/or muscle metaboreceptor pathways (Mitchell 1990; Williamson *et al.* 1995, 1996) act centrally, 'resetting' the baroreceptor reflex, and thereby shifting the relationship between blood pressure and sympathetic activity (Fig. 8.5) (DiCarlo & Bishop 1992; Rowell *et al.* 1996; Raven *et al.* 1997). Indeed, the entire feedback reflex is modified to raise blood pressure, rather than to return it to pre-exercise levels. This conclusion has considerable irony when it is recalled that the baroreflex was once thought to be suppressed or even 'switched off' during exer-

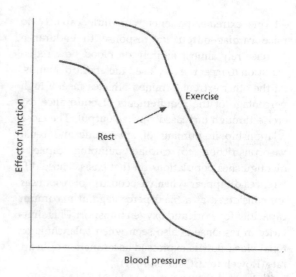

Fig. 8.5 Effect of endurance exercise on the reflex control of blood pressure. Increases or decreases in blood pressure (abscissa) lead to reflex changes in sympathetic nerve activity and heart rate (indicated collectively as 'effector function' on the ordinate). During exercise the relationship is shifted to the right and upward, indicating a 'resetting' of the reflex to higher blood pressures by endurance exercise. After Rowell *et al.* (1996) and Raven *et al.* (1997).

cise. Because the targets for the increased sympathetic activity are the heart and the resistance vessels, the redistribution of blood flow that accompanies endurance exercise is, by this hypothesis, partially due to a modification of the baroreflex.

Conclusions

The redistribution of blood flow from inactive to active regions during endurance exercise is an important component of the overall strategy of the cardiovascular system and its control elements to maximize the delivery of oxygen to active muscle and to maintain arterial blood pressure. Major targets for the redistribution of blood flow are the splanchnic and renal circulations, which have high levels of blood flow at rest but remove only 20–25% of the available oxygen. These characteristics permit major reductions in blood flow, with maintenance of tissue oxygen delivery through concomitantly increased extraction. The importance of this redistribution is inversely tied to cardiac pumping capacity.

At one extreme, patients with little capacity to raise cardiac output in response to endurance exercise rely almost entirely on blood flow redistribution to meet the increased metabolic demands. At the other extreme, trained athletes meet a high percentage of the requirements of endurance exercise through increased cardiac output. The close relationship in humans of splanchnic and renal vasoconstriction to cardiac pumping capacity distinguishes populations on that basis. Those differences disappear when vasoconstrictor responses are considered at a fixed percentage of maximum capacities for work and oxygen transport. This similarity in response is also seen when splanchnic or renal blood flow is expressed as a function of heart rate (Rowell 1974; Clausen 1977).

Such response patterns also obtain for some other regions (e.g. resting skeletal muscle), but not for others (cerebral, coronary). The cutaneous circulation presents a unique pattern of response because of competition between different reflexes. Initial responses include cutaneous vasoconstriction (which furnishes more blood flow to active muscle). As exercise continues and body temperature rises, skin blood flow increases to levels well above those seen at rest. The competing demands from skeletal muscle persist, however, and are expressed as an upward movement in the threshold internal temperature for vasodilatation, and as an upper limit to the increase in skin blood flow. Cutaneous vasoconstriction no longer provides more blood flow for muscle. Instead, cutaneous vasodilatation now competes with active muscle for blood flow. Available data indicate that the increase in skin blood flow is not supplied by a reduction in blood flow to active muscle (Savard *et al.* 1988; Nielsen *et al.* 1993). It is likely that the demands for blood flow to skin are met by a combination of greater reductions in blood flow to the splanchnic and renal regions and a modest increase in cardiac output. The earlier onset of fatigue with endurance exercise in the heat occurs because a critical internal temperature is reached sooner, suggesting a central nervous system failure rather than reduced muscle blood flow or sudden fall in blood pressure (Nielsen *et al.* 1993).

The competing control for the cutaneous circulation between thermoregulatory reflexes and the reflexes associated with exercise causes a modification in temperature regulation. Blood pressure control is also modified by exercise. Although at one time it was argued that the baroreceptor reflex was inhibited by exercise, recent analyses indicate that the baroreflex is 'reset' to higher levels by exercise. Further, this resetting is probably the major mechanism responsible for the reflex vasoconstriction and tachycardia of exercise.

Acknowledgements

The author acknowledges the many contributions by colleagues to our understanding of the circulatory adjustments to endurance exercise. Much of this chapter reflects synthesis by those fellow investigators. In particular, the outstanding contributions of Loring B. Rowell and Jere H. Mitchell are recognized. Colleagues in the author's laboratory who made invaluable contributions to the work reported here include Myung Park, W. Fred Taylor, Donal O'Leary, Dean L. Kellogg Jr, Pablo Pérgola, Craig Crandall and Nisha Charkoudian. Support for this research by the National Institutes of Health (HL20663, HL36080, HL08861 and HL59166) is also gratefully acknowledged.

References

Åstrand, P.O. & Rodahl, K. (1970) *Textbook of Work Physiology*. McGraw-Hill, New York.

Bell, A.W., Hales, J.R.S., King, R.B. & Fawcett, A.A. (1983) Influence of heat stress on exercise-induced changes in regional blood flow in sheep. *Journal of Applied Physiology* 55, 1916–1923.

Bell, A.W., Hales, J.R.S., Fawcett, A.A. & King, R.B. (1986) Effects of exercise and heat stress on regional blood flow in pregnant sheep. *Journal of Applied Physiology* 60, 1759–1764.

Bevegård, B.S. & Shepherd, J.T. (1966a) Circulatory effects of stimulating the carotid arterial stretch receptors in man at rest and during exercise. *Journal of Clinical Investigation* 45, 132–142.

Bevegård, B.S. & Shepherd, J.T. (1966b) Reaction in man of resistance and capacity vessels in forearm and hand to leg exercise. *Journal of Applied Physiology* 21, 123–132.

Blackmon, J.R., Rowell, L.B., Kennedy, J.W., Twiss, R.D. & Conn, R.D. (1967)

Physiological significance of maximal oxygen intake in pure mitral stenosis. *Circulation* **36**, 497–510.

Booth, J., Marino, F. & Ward, J.J. (1997) Improved running performance in hot humid conditions following whole body precooling. *Medicine and Science in Sports and Exercise* **29**, 943–949.

Bradley, S.E. (1963) The hepatic circulation. In: Hamilton, W.F. & Dow, P. (eds) *Handbook of Physiology*, Section 2, Vol. II, *Circulation*, pp. 1387–1438. American Physiological Society, Washington, DC.

Brengelmann, G.L. (1989) Body temperature regulation. In: Patton, H.D., Fuchs, A.F., Hille, B., Scher, A.M. & Steiner R. (eds) *Textbook of Physiology*, Vol. 2, pp. 1584–1596. W.B. Saunders, Philadelphia.

Brengelmann, G.L., Johnson, J.M., Hermansen, L. & Rowell, L.B. (1977) Altered control of skin blood flow during exercise at high internal temperatures. *Journal of Applied Physiology* **43**, 790–794.

Bristow, J.D., Brown, E.B. Jr, Cunningham, D.J.C. *et al.* (1971) Effect of bicycling on the baroreflex regulation of pulse interval. *Circulation Research* **28**, 582–592.

Brooks, G.A., Hittleman, K.J., Faulkner, J.A. & Beyer, R.A. (1971) Temperature, skeletal muscle mitochondrial functions and oxygen debt. *American Journal of Physiology* **220**, 1053–1059.

Bülow, J. & Madsen, J. (1978) Human adipose tissue blood flow during prolonged exercise II. *Pflügers Archives* **376**, 41–45.

Bülow, J. & Madsen, J. (1986) Exercise-induced increase in dog adipose tissue blood flow before and after denervation. *Acta Physiologica Scandinavica* **128**, 471–474.

Castenfors, J. & Piscator, M. (1967) Renal haemodynamics, urine flow and urinary protein excretion during exercise in supine position at different loads. *Acta Medica Scandinavica* **472** (Suppl.), 231–244.

Chapman, C.B. & Mitchell, J.H. (1965) The physiology of exercise. *Scientific American* **212**, 88–96.

Charkoudian, N. & Johnson, J.M. (1997) Modification of active cutaneous vasodilatation by oral contraceptive hormones. *Journal of Applied Physiology* **83**, 2012–2018.

Clausen, J.P. (1977) Circulatory adjustments to dynamic exercise and effect of physical training in normal subjects and in patients with coronary artery disease. In: Sonnenblick, E.H. & Lesch, M. (eds) *Exercise and Heart Disease*, pp. 39–75. Grune & Stratton, New York.

Clausen, J.P. & Trap-Jensen, J. (1974) Arteriohepatic venous oxygen difference and heart rate during initial phases of exercise. *Journal of Applied Physiology* **37**, 716–719.

Clausen, J.P., Klausen, K., Rasmussen, B. & Trap-Jensen, J. (1973) Central and peripheral circulatory changes after training of the arms or legs. *American Journal of Physiology* **225**, 675–682.

Crandall, C.G., Musick, J., Hatch, J.P., Kellogg, D.L. Jr & Johnson, J.M. (1995) Cutaneous vascular and sudomotor responses to isometric exercise in humans. *Journal of Applied Physiology* **79**, 1946–1950.

Delgado, R., Sanders, T.M. & Bloor, C.M. (1975) Renal blood flow distribution during steady-state exercise and exhaustion in conscious dogs. *Journal of Applied Physiology* **39**, 475–478.

DiCarlo, S.E. & Bishop, V.S. (1992) Onset of exercise shifts operating point of arterial baroreflex to higher pressures. *American Journal of Physiology* **262**, H303–H307.

Donald, D.E., Rowlands, D.J. & Ferguson, D.A. (1970) Similarity of blood flow in the normal and the sympathectomized dog hind limb during graded exercise. *Circulation Research* **26**, 185–199.

Ekelund, L.-G. (1967) Circulatory and respiratory adaptations during prolonged exercise. *Acta Physiologica Scandinavica* **70** (Suppl. 292).

Eriksen, M. & Waaler, B.A. (1994) Priority of blood flow to splanchnic organs in humans during pre- and post-meal exercise. *Acta Physiologica Scandinavica* **150**, 363–372.

Febbraio, M.A., Snow, R.J., Stathis, C.G., Hargreaves, M. & Carey, M.F. (1994) Effect of heat stress on muscle energy metabolism during exercise. *Journal of Applied Physiology* **77**, 2827–2831.

Febbraio, M.A., Carey, M.F., Snow, R.J., Stathis, C.G. & Hargreaves, M. (1996) Influence of elevated muscle temperature on metabolism during intense, dynamic exercise. *American Journal of Physiology* **271**, R1251–R1255.

Fink, W.J., Costill, D.L. & VanHandel, P.J. (1980) Leg muscle metabolism during exercise in heat and cold. *European Journal of Applied and Occupational Physiology* **34**, 183–190.

Foreman, D.L., Sanders, M. & Bloor, C.M. (1976) Total and regional cerebral blood flow during moderate and severe exercise in miniature swine. *Journal of Applied Physiology* **40**, 191–195.

Fox, R.H., Goldsmith, R., Kidd, D.J. & Lewis, H.E. (1958) Acclimatization to the heat in man by controlled elevation of body temperature. *Journal of Physiology (London)* **142**, 219–232.

Fronek, K. & Fronek, A. (1970) Combined effect of exercise and digestion on hemodynamics in conscious dogs. *American Journal of Physiology* **218**, 555–559.

Galloway, S.D.R. & Maughan, R.J. (1997) Effects of ambient temperature on the capacity to perform prolonged exercise in man. *Medicine and Science in Sports and Exercise* **29**, 1240–1249.

Gorman, A.J. & Proppe, D.W. (1984) Mechanisms producing tachycardia in conscious baboons during environmental heat stress. *Journal of Applied Physiology* **56**, 441–446.

Grimby, G. (1965) Renal clearances during prolonged supine exercise at different loads. *Journal of Applied Physiology* **20**, 1294–1298.

Gross, P.M., Marcus, M.L. & Heistad, D.D. (1980) Regional distribution of cerebral blood flow during exercise in dogs. *Journal of Applied Physiology* **48**, 213–217.

Haywood, G.A., Counihan, P.J., Sneddon, J.F., Jennison, S.H., Bashir, Y. & McKenna, W.J. (1993) Increased renal and forearm vasoconstriction in response to exercise after heart transplantation. *British Heart Journal* **70**, 247–251.

Herholz, K., Buskies, W., Rist, M., Pawlik, G., Hollman, W. & Heiss, W.D. (1987) Regional cerebral blood flow in man at rest and during exercise. *Journal of Neurology* **234**, 9–13.

Ho, C.W., Beard, J.L., Farrell, P.A., Minson, C.T. & Kenney, W.L. (1997) Age, fitness, and regional blood flow during exercise in the heat. *Journal of Applied Physiology* **82**, 1126–1135.

Hohimer, A.R. & Smith, O.A. (1979) Decreased renal blood flow in the baboon during mild dynamic leg exercise. *American Journal of Physiology* **236**, H141–H150.

Hohimer, A.R., Bissonette, J.M., Metcalfe, J. & McKean, T.A. (1984) Effect of exercise on uterine blood flow in the pregnant pygmy goat. *American Journal of Physiology* **246**, H207–H212.

Johnson, J.M. (1986) Nonthermoregulatory control of human skin blood flow. *Journal of Applied Physiology* **61**, 1613–1622.

Johnson, J.M. (1987) Central and peripheral adjustments to long-term exercise in humans. *Canadian Journal of Sport Sciences* **12** (Suppl. 1), 84S–88S.

Johnson, J.M. (1992) Exercise and the cutaneous circulation. *Exercise and Sport Sciences Reviews* **20**, 59–97.

Johnson, J.M. (1998) Physical training and the control of skin blood flow. *Medicine and Science in Sports and Exercise* **30**, 382–386.

Johnson, J.M. & Park, M.K. (1981) Effect of upright exercise on threshold for cutaneous vasodilatation and sweating. *Journal of Applied Physiology* **50**, 814–818.

Johnson, J.M. & Park, M.K. (1982) Effect of heat stress on cutaneous vascular responses to the initiation of exercise. *Journal of Applied Physiology* **53**, 744–749.

Johnson, J.M. & Proppe, D.W. (1996) Cardiovascular adjustments to heat stress. In: Fregley, M.L. & Blatteis, C.M. (eds) *Handbook of Physiology*, Section 4, Vol. 1, *Environmental Physiology*, pp. 215–244. Oxford University Press, New York, NY.

Johnson, J.M. & Rowell, L.B. (1975) Forearm skin and muscle vascular responses to prolonged leg exercise in man. *Journal of Applied Physiology* **39**, 920–924.

Jones, M.T., Norton, K.I., Dengel, D.R. & Armstrong, R.B. (1990) Effects of training on reproductive tissue blood flow in exercising pregnant rats. *Journal of Applied Physiology* **69**, 2097–2103.

Jorgensen, L.G., Perko, M., Hanel, B., Schroeder, T.V. & Secher, N.H. (1992) Middle cerebral artery flow velocity and blood flow during exercise and muscle ischemia in humans. *Journal of Applied Physiology* **72**, 1123–1132.

Kellogg, D.L. Jr, Johnson, J.M. & Kosiba, W.A. (1991) Control of internal temperature threshold for active cutaneous vasodilatation by dynamic exercise. *Journal of Applied Physiology* **71**, 2476–2482.

Kellogg, D.L. Jr, Johnson, J.M., Kenney, W.L., Pérgola, P.E. & Kosiba, W.A. (1993) Mechanisms of control of skin blood flow during prolonged exercise in humans. *American Journal of Physiology* **265**, H562–H568.

Kenney, W.L. (1985) Decreased core-to-skin heat transfer in mild essential hypertensives exercising in the heat. *Clinical and Experimental Hypertension. Part A Theory and Practice* **7**, 1165–1172.

Kenney, W.L. & Ho, C.W. (1995) Age alters regional distribution of blood flow during moderate intensity exercise. *Journal of Applied Physiology* **79**, 1112–1119.

Kenney, W.L. & Johnson, J.M. (1992) Control of skin blood flow during exercise. *Medicine and Science in Sports and Exercise* **24**, 303–312.

Kenney, W.L. & Zappe, D.H. (1994) Effect of age on renal blood flow during exercise. *Aging Clinical and Experimental Research* **6**, 293–302.

Kilbom, Å. & Brundin, T. (1976) Circulatory effects of isometric muscle contractions, performed separately and in combination with dynamic exercise. *European Journal of Applied and Occupational Physiology* **36**, 7–17.

Kruk, B., Pekkarinen, H., Harri, M. & Hänninen, O. (1990) Thermoregulatory responses to exercise at low ambient temperature performed after precooling or preheating. *European Journal of Applied and Occupational Physiology* **59**, 416–420.

Laughlin, M.H., Korthuis, R.J., Duncker, D.J. & Bache, R.J. (1996) Control of blood flow to cardiac and skeletal muscle during exercise. In: Rowell, L.B. & Shepherd, J.T. (eds) *Handbook of Physiology*, Section 12, *Exercise: Regulation and Integration of Multiple Systems*, pp. 705–769. Oxford University Press, New York.

Lee, D.T. & Haymes, M.N. (1995) Exercise duration and thermoregulatory responses after whole body cooling. *Journal of Applied Physiology* **79**, 1971–1976.

Lotgering, F.K., Gilbert, R.D. & Longo, L.D. (1983) Exercise responses in pregnant sheep: oxygen consumption, uterine blood flow and blood volume. *Journal of Applied Physiology* **55**, 834–841.

Mack, G., Nose, H. & Nadel, E.R. (1988) Role of cardiopulmonary baroreflexes during dynamic exercise. *Journal of Applied Physiology* **65**, 1827–1832.

Mack, G.W., Nose, H., Takamata, A., Okuno, T. & Morimoto, T. (1994) Influence of exercise intensity and plasma, on active cutaneous vasodilatation in humans. *Medicine and Science in Sports and Exercise* **26**, 209–216.

Manohar, M. (1986) Regional brain blood flow and O_2 delivery during severe exertion in the pony. *Respiration Physiology* **64**, 339–349.

Midttun, M. & Sejrsen, P. (1998) Cutaneous blood flow rate in areas with and without arteriovenous anastomoses during exercise. *Scandinavian Journal of Medicine and Science in Sports* **8**, 84–90.

Minson, C.T. & Kenney, W.L. (1997) Age and cardiac output during cycle exercise in thermoneutral and warm environments. *Medicine and Science in Sports and Exercise* **29**, 75–81.

Mitchell, J.H. (1990) Neural control of the circulation during exercise. *Medicine and Science in Sports and Exercise* **22**, 141–154.

Musch, T.I., Friedman, D.B., Pitetti, K.H. *et al.* (1987) Regional distribution of blood flow of dogs during graded dynamic exercise. *Journal of Applied Physiology* **63**, 2269–2277.

Nadel, E.R. (1977) A brief overview. In: Nadel, E.R. (ed.) *Problems with Temperature During Exercise*, pp. 1–10. Academic Press, New York.

Nadel, E.R., Cafarelli, E., Roberts, M.F. & Wenger, C.B. (1979) Circulatory regulation during exercise in different ambient temperatures. *Journal of Applied Physiology* **46**, 430–437.

Nielsen, B., Savard, G., Richter, E.A., Hargreaves, M. & Saltin, B. (1990) Muscle blood flow and metabolism during exercise and heat stress. *Journal of Applied Physiology* **69**, 1040–1046.

Nielsen, B., Hales, J.R.S., Strange, S., Christensen, N.J., Warberg, J. & Saltin, B. (1993) Human circulatory and thermoregulatory adaptations with heat acclimation and exercise in a hot, dry environment. *Journal of Physiology (London)* **460**, 467–485.

Nielsen, B., Strange, S., Christensen, N.J., Warberg, J. & Saltin, B. (1997) Acute and adaptative responses to exercise in a warm, humid environment. *Pflügers Archives* **434**, 49–56.

Olschewski, H. & Brück, K. (1988) Thermoregulatory, cardiovascular and muscular factors related to exercise after precooling. *Journal of Applied Physiology* **64**, 803–811.

Papelier, Y., Escourrou, P., Helloco, F. & Rowell, L.B. (1997) Muscle chemoreflex alters carotid sinus baroreflex response in humans. *Journal of Applied Physiology* **82**, 577–583.

Potts, J.T., Shi, X. & Raven, P.B. (1993) Carotid baroreflex responsiveness during dynamic exercise in humans. *American Journal of Physiology* **265**, H1928–H1938.

Puvi-Rajasingham, S., Smith, G.D., Akinola, A. & Mathias, C.J. (1997a) Abnormal regional blood flow responses during and after exercise in human sympathetic denervation. *Journal of Physiology (London)* **505**, 841–849.

Puvi-Rajasingham, S., Wijeyekoon, B., Natarajan, P. & Mathias, C.J. (1997b) Systemic and regional (including superior mesenteric) haemodynamic responses during supine exercise while fasted and fed in normal men. *Clinical Autonomic Research* **7**, 149–154.

Radigan, L.R. & Robinson, S. (1949) Effects of environmental heat stress and exercise on renal blood flow and filtration rate. *Journal of Applied Physiology* **2**, 185–191.

Rauramo, I. & Forss, M. (1988) Effect of exercise on maternal hemodynamics and placental blood flow in healthy women. *Acta Obstetrica et Gynecologica Scandinavica* **67**, 21–25.

Raven, P.B., Potts, J.T. & Shi, X. (1997) Baroreflex regulation of blood pressure during dynamic exercise. *Exercise and Sport Sciences Reviews* **25**, 365–389.

Roberts, M.F., Wenger, C.B., Stolwijk, J.A.J. & Nadel, E.R. (1977) Skin blood flow and sweating changes following exercise training and heat acclimation. *Journal of Applied Physiology* **43**, 133–137.

Rooke, G.A., Savage, M.V. & Brengelmann, G.L. (1994) Maximal skin blood flow is decreased in elderly men. *Journal of Applied Physiology* **77**, 11–14.

Rowell, L.B. (1973) Regulation of splanchnic blood flow in man. *Physiologist* **16**, 127–142.

Rowell, L.B. (1974) Human cardiovascular adjustments to exercise and thermal stress. *Physiological Reviews* **54**, 75–159.

Rowell, L.B. (1986) *Human Circulation: Regulation During Physical Stress.* Oxford University Press, New York.

Rowell, L.B. & O'Leary, D.S. (1990) Reflex control of the circulation during exercise: chemoreflexes and mechanoreflexes. *Journal of Applied Physiology* **69**, 407–418.

Rowell, L.B., Blackmon, J.R. & Bruce, R.A. (1964) Indocyanine green clearance and estimated hepatic blood flow during mild to maximal exercise in upright man. *Journal of Clinical Investigation* **43**, 1677–1690.

Rowell, L.B., Blackmon, J.R., Martin, R.H., Mazzarella, J.A. & Bruce, R.A. (1965) Hepatic clearance of indocyanine green in man under thermal and exercise stresses. *Journal of Applied Physiology* **20**, 384–394.

Rowell, L.B., Wyss, C.R. & Brengelmann, G.L. (1973) Sustained human skin and muscle vasoconstriction with reduced baroreceptor activity. *Journal of Applied Physiology* **34**, 639–643.

Rowell, L.B., O'Leary, D.S. & Kellogg, D.L. Jr (1996) Integration of cardiovascular control systems in dynamic exercise. In: Rowell, L.B. & Shepherd, J.T. (eds) *Handbook of Physiology, Section 12, Exercise: Regulation and Integration of Multiple Systems,* pp. 770–838. Oxford University Press, New York.

Saltin, B. & Hermansen, L. (1966) Esophageal, rectal and muscle temperature during exercise. *Journal of Applied Physiology* **21**, 1757–1762.

Saltin, B. & Stenberg, J. (1964) Circulatory response to prolonged severe exercise. *Journal of Applied Physiology* **19**, 833–838.

Saltin, B., Rådegren, G., Koskolou, M.D. & Roach, R.C. (1998) Skeletal muscle blood flow in humans and its regulation during exercise. *Acta Physiologica Scandinavica* **162**, 421–436.

Sanders, M., Rasmussen, S., Cooper, D. & Bloor, C. (1976) Renal and intrarenal blood flow distribution in swine during severe exercise. *Journal of Applied Physiology* **40**, 932–935.

Savard, G.K., Nielsen, B., Laszczynska, I., Larsen, B.E. & Saltin, B. (1988) Muscle blood flow is not reduced in humans during moderate exercise and heat stress. *Journal of Applied Physiology* **64**, 649–657.

Schmidt, V. & Brück, K. (1981) Effect of a precooling maneuver on body temperature and exercise performance. *Journal of Applied Physiology* **50**, 772–778.

Smolander, J., Saalo, J. & Korhonen, O. (1991) Effect of work load on cutaneous vascular response to exercise. *Journal of Applied Physiology* **71**, 1614–1619.

Stephenson, L.A. & Kolka, M.A. (1985) Menstrual phase and time of day alter reference signal controlling arm blood flow and sweating. *American Journal of Physiology* **249**, R186–R191.

Stephenson, L.A. & Kolka, M.A. (1993) Thermoregulation in women. *Exercise and Sport Sciences Reviews* **21**, 231–262.

Strange, S., Secher, N.H., Christensen, N.J. & Saltin, B. (1990) Cardiovascular responses to carotid sinus baroreceptor stimulation during moderate to severe exercise in man. *Acta Physiologica Scandinavica* **138**, 145–153.

Taylor, W.F., Johnson, J.M., Kosiba, W.A. & Kwan, C.M. (1988) Graded cutaneous vascular responses to dynamic leg exercise. *Journal of Applied Physiology* **64**, 1803–1809.

Taylor, W.F., Johnson, J.M., Kosiba, W.A. & Kwan, C.M. (1989) Cutaneous vascular responses to isometric handgrip exercise. *Journal of Applied Physiology* **66**, 1586–1592.

Taylor, W.F., Johnson, J.M. & Kosiba, W.A. (1990) Roles of absolute and relative load in skin vasoconstrictor responses to exercise. *Journal of Applied Physiology* **69**, 1131–1136.

Tondevold, E. & Bülow, J. (1983) Bone blood flow in conscious dogs at rest and during exercise. *Acta Orthopedica Scandinavica* **54**, 53–57.

Valtin, H. (1983) *Renal Function.* Little, Brown, Boston.

Van Citters, R.L. & Franklin, D.L. (1969) Cardiovascular performance of Alaska sled dogs during exercise. *Circulation Research* **24**, 33–42.

Vatner, S.F., Higgins, C.B., White, S., Patrick, T. & Franklin, D. (1971) The peripheral vascular response to severe exercise in untethered dogs before and after complete heart block. *Journal of Clinical Investigation* **50**, 1950–1960.

Vatner, S.F., Higgins, C.B. & Franklin, D. (1972) Regional circulatory adjustments to moderate and severe chronic anemia in conscious dogs at rest and during exercise. *Circulation Research* **30**, 731–740.

Walgenbach, S.C. & Donald, D.E. (1983) Inhibition by carotid baroreflex of exercise-induced increases in arterial pressure. *Circulation Research* **52**, 253–262.

Williamson, J.W., Nobrega, A.C., Winchester, P.K., Zim, S. & Mitchell, J.H. (1995) Instantaneous heart rate increase with dynamic exercise: central command and muscle–heart reflex contributions. *Journal of Applied Physiology* **78**, 1273–1279.

Williamson, J.W., Olesen, H.L., Pott, F., Mitchell, J.H. & Secher, N.H. (1996) Central command increases cardiac output during static exercise in humans. *Acta Physiologica Scandinavica* **156**, 429–434.

Wyss, C.R., Brengelmann, G.L., Johnson, J.M., Rowell, L.B. & Niederberger, M. (1974) Control of skin blood flow, sweating and heart rate: role of skin vs. core temperature. *Journal of Applied Physiology* **36**, 726–733.

Zelis, R., Mason, D.T. & Braunwald, E. (1969) Partition of blood flow to the cutaneous and muscular beds of the forearm at rest and during leg exercise in normal subjects and in patients with heart failure. *Circulation Research* **24**, 799–806.

Chapter 9

Cellular Metabolism and Endurance

JAN HENRIKSSON

The capacity of skeletal muscle cells for adaptation to changes in metabolic demand is quite remarkable. Endurance training induces marked adaptive changes in several structural components and metabolic variables in the engaged skeletal muscles. Among the changes observed with different training regimens are those involving the muscle's content of metabolic enzymes, the sensitivity to hormones and the composition of the contracting filaments. Other adaptations affect membrane transport processes and the muscular capillary network. Since these adaptive changes occur regularly in response to endurance training, they are likely to be important determinants of an individual's physical working capacity. The adaptive changes in metabolic enzymes and capillaries are well-described consequences of endurance training and are probably also important adaptations enhancing the muscle's capacity to perform prolonged work. This chapter takes a closer look at the cellular adaptation to endurance training, with particular regard to changes in these two variables.

How to determine the metabolic capacity of skeletal muscle

The introduction of the muscle biopsy procedure (Bergström 1962), whereby small (10–100 mg) muscle pieces can be sampled, and the development of sensitive biochemical techniques have made it possible to estimate the capacity of different metabolic pathways in human muscle. Using micromethods, this can be done even at the single fibre level (Lowry & Passonneau 1973). The most important

metabolic pathways for energy delivery in exercising muscle are glycolysis/glycogenolysis, fatty acid oxidation, the citric acid cycle and the respiratory chain (for a detailed discussion, see Chapter 23, 'Metabolism in the Contracting Skeletal Muscle'). The capacity of a metabolic pathway is limited mainly by the amount of pathway enzymes contained in the cell. In this context, some enzymes (the rate-limiting or flux-generating ones) are more important than others. Such an enzyme has low activity and constitutes a bottleneck in a pathway. Theoretically, an increased concentration of the rate-limiting enzyme with unchanged concentrations of the other pathway enzymes would be sufficient to increase the capacity of the entire metabolic pathway (see Newsholme & Leech 1983). In practice, with a change in the capacity of a metabolic pathway, e.g. due to training or inactivity, the content of all enzymes, whether rate limiting or not, changes in the same direction. This can be illustrated by the response of the anterior tibial muscle of the rabbit to chronic electrical stimulation. In this situation, there is an almost identical decrease in all glycolytic and glycogenolytic enzymes, although only one, phosphofructokinase, is considered to be rate limiting (see Figs 9.1 & 9.2). The reason for this is not entirely clear, but it may be that relatively constant proportions of the different enzymes in a given metabolic pathway are necessary in order to maintain metabolic equilibrium within a cell. It is therefore possible to make a good estimate of the cellular capacity of a specific metabolic pathway by measuring the content (maximal activity) of any one of its enzymes. The choice of

Fig. 9.1 Enzyme changes induced by chronic electrical muscle stimulation. The rabbit anterior tibial muscle was stimulated at 10 impulses per second, 24 hours a day, for differing periods (3 days–10 weeks). The figure depicts changes in the muscle content of three oxidative and two glycolytic enzymes. SDH (succinate dehydrogenase), CS (citrate synthase) and MDH (malate dehydrogenase) are enzymes in the citric acid cycle; LDH (lactate dehydrogenase) and PFK (6-phosphofructokinase) are involved in glycolysis. The value for unstimulated control muscles has been set at 100%. From Henriksson *et al.* (1986); modified with the permission of the *American Journal of Physiology*.

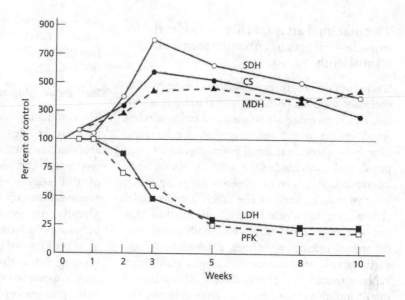

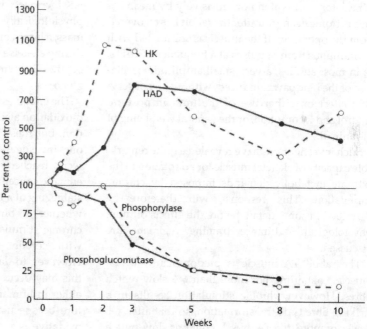

Fig. 9.2 Enzyme changes induced by chronic electrical muscle stimulation. HAD (3-hydroxyacyl CoA dehydrogenase) represents the fat degradation (fatty acid oxidation) system, and phosphorylase and phosphoglucomutase glycolysis. The main function of the enzyme HK (hexokinase) is to make glucose—taken up from the blood—available to the muscle cell by channelling it into the glycolytic pathway. For further explanation, see the legend to Fig. 9.1. From Henriksson *et al.* (1986); modified with the permission of the *American Journal of Physiology*.

enzymes for analysis depends largely on the simplicity and speed of available analytical methods. Levels of the following enzymes are commonly used to measure the capacity of their respective metabolic pathways.

(a) *Glycolysis*: phosphofructokinase (PFK), lactate dehydrogenase (LDH).

(b) *Fatty acid oxidation*: 3-hydroxyacyl CoA dehydrogenase (HAD).

(c) *Citric acid cycle*: citrate synthase (CS), succinate dehydrogenase (SDH).

(d) *Respiratory chain*: cytochrome c oxidase.

The location of these enzymes in the pathways is shown in Fig. 23.5.

The maximal adaptability of skeletal muscle — effects of chronic electrical stimulation

It is of considerable theoretical interest to know how skeletal muscle adapts to a maximal training stimulus. This knowledge can be used as a frame of reference, against which the effects of, for instance, different endurance training regimens can be compared and evaluated. One way to obtain such information has been to subject a normally rather inactive muscle, such as the rabbit anterior tibial (TA) muscle, to chronic electrical stimulation. This can be done in a way that is essentially painless to the animal. During anaesthesia, a stimulator (of fingertip size) is implanted under aseptic conditions. When activated, this allows chronic stimulation of the TA muscle via the common peroneal nerve. The stimulator is activated non-invasively by means of an electronic flash-gun after the rabbit has recovered from the operation. If the muscle is stimulated with a continuous train of pulses at a frequency of 10 Hz, as in most studies, a very small amplitude oscillation of the hindpaw is induced, without any observable effect on either use of the limb in postural control and locomotion, or the general well-being of the animal.

Such investigations have revealed a quite remarkable capacity of skeletal muscle for adaptation to the extreme metabolic demands imposed by chronic stimulation. This response will therefore be described in some detail, before the effects of more physiological endurance training regimens are discussed.

The rabbit TA muscle is predominantly a fast muscle, containing not more than 6% slow-twitch fibres. However, chronic stimulation results in a striking fibre type transformation, so that after 5–6 weeks or more, the TA muscle contains slow-twitch fibres only. Simultaneously, the normally very fatiguable TA muscle becomes highly fatigue resistant. The increased endurance is most likely mainly a result of the pronounced enzyme and microcirculatory adaptations induced by chronic stimulation, but the fibre type transformation may also have major importance in this respect. For a more detailed description of the effects of chronic stimula-

tion on muscles, see reviews by Salmons and Henriksson (1981), Jolesz and Sreter (1981) and Pette (1984).

Enzyme adaptation

The stimulation-induced enzyme changes are summarized in Figs 9.1 and 9.2. Of all enzymes analysed, hexokinase (HK) shows the most rapid response to chronic stimulation. The main function of this enzyme is to channel (phosphorylate) glucose, taken up by muscle, into the muscle cell's glycolytic or glycogen synthetic pathway. An HK increase (which on chronic stimulation was 11-fold at its peak) is not normally seen during endurance training, but it illustrates the capacity of skeletal muscle to adapt rapidly to the use of blood glucose as the preferred energy substrate. The absence of an HK increase with endurance training makes sense physiologically since, with a large trained muscle mass, a large consumption of blood-derived glucose during exercise would rapidly override the capacity of the liver to replenish the consumed blood glucose.

The enzymes of the citric acid cycle and fatty acid β-oxidation also display large increases on stimulation, but these increases occur somewhat later. In our investigations, maximal changes (6–12-fold) were reached after 2–5 weeks. Thereafter, the enzyme concentrations decreased somewhat before stabilizing at a lower level (Fig. 9.1). It is not known whether this biphasic pattern of change is specific to chronic stimulation or whether it may also occur with certain endurance training programmes. However, to date there have been no reports that this may occur in response to endurance training, either in humans or in other species. It may therefore be speculated that the secondary decline in oxidative enzymes is related to the fast- to slow-twitch fibre type transformation; this occurs with prolonged chronic stimulation, but not with short-term exercise training programmes. It is believed that slow-twitch fibres are more energy efficient than fast-twitch fibres at slow contraction speeds; thus, it is possible that, everything else remaining equal, the level of oxidative enzymes could be kept lower in a slow-twitch than in a fast-twitch muscle fibre. Contrary to the oxidative enzymes, the gly-colytic enzymes, as well as creatine kinase (i.e. the enzymes supplying energy to the muscle during short-term, intense exercise), decreased drastically with chronic stimulation. After 2 months of continu-ous stimulation only one-fifth of the initial gly-colytic enzyme content remained in the TA muscle. On discontinuing stimulation, the enzymes whose activity had increased again declined towards the initial level, at first rapidly and later more slowly, and had returned to their normal values after 5–6 weeks. The opposite was also true of the glycolytic enzymes, which increased when stimulation was stopped, although with these enzymes normaliza-tion of activity occurred more rectilinearly (Brown *et al.* 1989).

Figure 9.3 shows that the normally large variation in enzyme content among different fibres in the same muscle, and even between fibres of the same

type, is reduced with chronic stimulation. No corre-sponding information is available with regard to the effect of endurance training, although some infor-mation can be found in Chi *et al.* (1983).

Other stimulation-induced changes

There is a doubling of the number of blood capillar-ies per unit of muscle cross-sectional area with stim-ulation, thus greatly improving the muscle's blood supply (Brown *et al.* 1976). The time course of this change has not been studied in detail, but prelimi-nary data indicate that it is roughly similar to that of the oxidative enzymes. Concomitant with these changes there is, as mentioned above, a dramatic improvement in the muscle's endurance. In our investigations, this variable has been measured as an index: the muscle force remaining after a 5-min protocol of intense muscle stimulation divided by

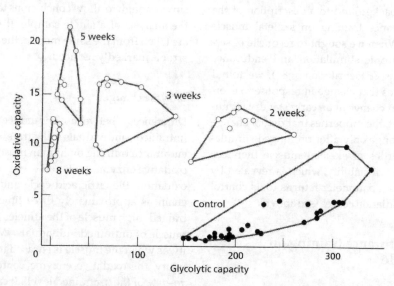

Fig. 9.3 Enzyme changes in single skeletal muscle fibres induced by chronic electrical muscle stimulation. The anterior tibial muscle of the rabbit was stimulated as described in the legend to Fig. 9.1. Single fibres were isolated by microdissec-tion from muscles stimulated for differing periods (2, 3, 5 and 8 weeks, respectively) and from unstimulated control muscles. The fibres were subsequently analysed for two enzymes, citrate synthase, as a measure of the fibre's oxidative capacity, and fructose bisphosphatase, as a measure of its glycolytic capacity. Citrate synthase is a member of the citric acid cycle and fructose bisphosphatase catalyses reversal of the 6-phosphofructokinase reaction in glycolysis. All fibres in a normal unstimulated (control) muscle have a high content of glycolytic enzymes, whereas the content of oxidative enzymes varies 10-fold. Chronic stimulation induces a high oxidative capacity in all fibres, whereas the glycolytic capacity decreases to low levels. Figures are moles (citrate synthase) or millimoles (fructose bisphosphatase) per kilogram dry weight per hour at 20°C. From Chi *et al.* (1986), with the permission of the *American Journal of Physiology*.

the muscle force exerted during the first few contractions. This index increases from a normal value
of 0.5 to 1.0 in muscle that has been stimulated continuously for 6 weeks. Following discontinuation of
chronic stimulation, fatiguability again increases,
the time needed for a normalization of responses
(5–6 weeks) being similar to that of the metabolic
enzymes and the capillary supply. The different biochemical and morphological adaptations to chronic
stimulation fit into a 'first in, last out' pattern for the
response to stimulation and recovery. The earlier the
stage at which a parameter changes during stimulation, the later the stage at which it returns to control
levels during recovery. For further information on
this point, see Brown et al. (1989); it may be a general
rule governing training adaptations, and it implies
that a threshold level of muscle activity must be
exceeded in order to induce and maintain a specific
adaptation.

This summary of what is likely to be the maximal
activity-induced adaptability of skeletal muscle
may serve as a background to a description of the
effects of endurance training on skeletal muscle
characteristics. When we sought to reconcile observations from chronic stimulation and endurance
training (Salmons & Henriksson 1981), we found
that the properties that change in response to exercise are those that change at an early stage of stimulation; in contrast, the properties that do not change
with exercise change only after prolonged stimulation. The properties of skeletal muscle therefore
show a hierarchy of stability, which is revealed by
the rate at which a parameter returns to its control
value when stimulation ceases (see above).

Effects of endurance training on human muscle

Background

Russian investigators studied the effects of
endurance training on metabolic enzymes in skeletal muscle of the rat during the 1950s, but the first
detailed investigation was completed by Holloszy et
al. (see Holloszy & Booth 1976). Petrén et al. had
shown the influence of training on the capillary
network of rat skeletal muscle as early as 1937. The
first human studies on muscle metabolic enzymes
were published around 1970 (Varnauskas et al. 1970;
Morgan et al. 1971). During the 1970s and 1980s,
improved methodology allowed more detailed
studies on both humans and other species. For the
human studies, small muscle biopsy specimens
(20–100 mg) were obtained, usually from the thigh
muscle, but also from other muscles like the gastrocnemius, deltoid and triceps. Different groups of
individuals were compared, e.g. untrained persons
versus athletes participating in various sports or,
alternatively, previously untrained individuals
were studied repeatedly during a training period.
Different parts of a given muscle often differ in fibre
type composition, capillary density and enzyme
content, but nevertheless the muscle biopsy technique has proven surprisingly useful. A change in
enzyme content or capillary density of 15–20% can
be detected when a group of five or six subjects is
studied by single biopsies before and after training.
However, the biopsy technique is generally not sensitive enough to allow conclusions to be drawn from
the analysis of a single sample. If several samples
are taken from the same muscle, the methodological
error is markedly reduced.

Enzyme changes

Differences between endurance athletes and
untrained individuals illustrate the effects of
endurance training on human muscle (Fig. 9.4). The
oxidative enzyme content (i.e. enzymes of fatty acid
oxidation, the citric acid cycle and the respiratory
chain) is approximately three times greater in the
trained thigh muscle of the athletes than in the thigh
muscle of untrained individuals. With total inactivity, as when the muscle is encased in plaster after an
injury, the oxidative enzyme content decreases to
70–75% of the 'untrained level'. It can be speculated
that levels lower than this would not be compatible
with survival of the muscle cell. The maximal range
of change of oxidative enzyme content in human
thigh muscle is therefore approximately four-fold,
although it can be assumed that a very long training
time would be required for an individual to cover
this entire range. A comparison with chronically
stimulated rabbit muscle (Fig. 9.4) reveals that the

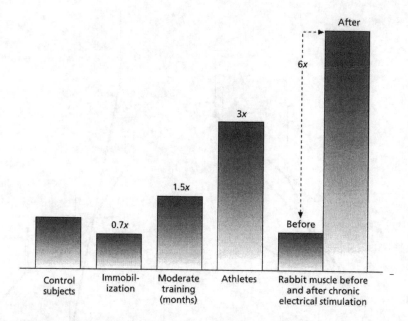

Fig. 9.4 The influence of physical fitness on skeletal muscle oxidative capacity, measured as the content of citrate synthase. Muscle tissue from normal sedentary individuals is compared to muscle subjected to encasement in plaster after injury or to 2–3 months of moderate endurance training. Values are also shown for top-class cyclists and long-distance runners. As a further comparison, the corresponding values from the rabbit anterior tibial muscle before and after 3–5 weeks of chronic electrical stimulation are indicated on the right. (The human data have generously been placed at my disposal by Dr Eva Jansson, Department of Clinical Physiology, Karolinska Hospital, Stockholm; the results regarding chronic stimulation are from Henriksson *et al.* 1986.)

muscles of endurance athletes have approximately 40% lower levels of oxidative enzymes than those found in chronically stimulated muscles. The difference with respect to fat oxidation enzymes is somewhat larger. Ignoring the issue of possible differences in response between rabbits and humans, this result may be taken to indicate that the trained muscles of the best endurance athletes have an oxidative capacity that is half to two-thirds of the theoretically attainable maximal level.

Another important question concerns the magnitude of the enzyme changes that can be attained with a few weeks or months of more moderate endurance training. Here, information is available from a large number of investigations, in which different research groups have studied the effects of 2–3 months of training on the oxidative enzyme content of leg or arm muscles. Such studies have usually involved bouts of 30–60 min of exercise at intensities corresponding to 70–80% of maximal

oxgen intake ($\dot{V}O_{2max}$), three to five times per week. With a group of previously untrained individuals, the general finding is an increase in the content of oxidative enzymes of approximately 40–50% in the trained muscles (Fig. 9.5). This increase occurs gradually over 6–8 weeks, with the most rapid change taking place during the first 3 weeks of training (see Saltin & Gollnick 1983). Recent work has shown that the metabolic changes associated with exercise training may occur faster than was previously thought. Seven to 10 days of training (2 h per day) is sufficient to induce a marked reduction in both lactate production and glycogen utilization during an acute bout of exercise, as well as a lowering of the respiratory quotient (RQ). Spina *et al.* (1996) and Chesley *et al.* (1996), but not Green *et al.* (1992), found a mitochondrial adaptation on the same timescale; this could explain the glycogen-sparing effect that develops early during exercise training.

The number of nuclei in skeletal muscle cells may

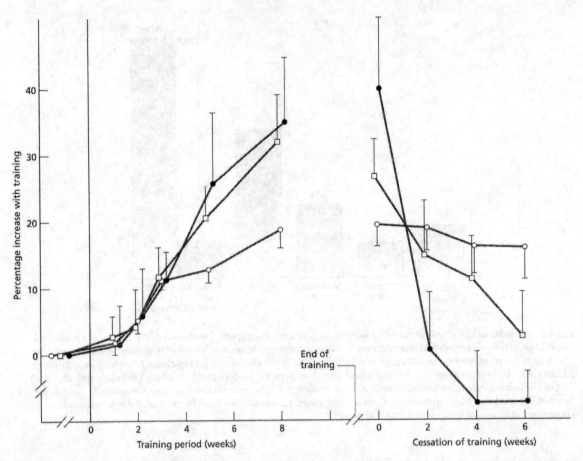

Fig. 9.5 The effect of endurance training on the oxidative enzyme content of human skeletal muscle. A group of previously untrained subjects trained on cycle ergometers (40 min per day, 4 days per week for 10–14 weeks). The work rate corresponded to 80% of the individual's maximal oxygen intake. Biopsy samples were obtained from the thigh muscle at different intervals during training, as well as 2, 4 and 6 weeks after cessation of training. The muscle samples were analysed for the oxidative enzymes succinate dehydrogenase (of the citric acid cycle) (□) and cytochrome c oxidase (the last enzyme in the respiratory chain) (●). In addition, the subjects' maximal oxygen intakes were determined using the Douglas bag technique (O). In the post-training period, the whole-body $\dot{V}_{O_{2max}}$ was maintained significantly longer than the muscle oxidative enzyme content. From Henriksson and Reitman (1977); modified with the permission of *Acta Physiologica Scandinavica*.

change with training. It is therefore possible that variations in the amount of available nuclear DNA may be one factor of importance for adaptability in muscle size and enzyme content (Allen *et al.* 1995). There are two separate pools of mitochondria in skeletal muscle, the subsarcolemmal pool immediately below the cellular membrane and the intermyofibrillar pool that is interspersed among the myofibrils. In trained subjects the subsarcolemmal

mitochondria account for 30% of total mitochondria, as compared to only 14% in untrained subjects (Puntschart *et al.* 1995). It is believed that this mitochondrial pool is involved in supplying energy to different membrane transport processes, so this finding may indicate that the relative increase in energy demand of the membrane transport processes with exercise training may be even greater than that of the contracting filaments.

The importance of exercise intensity and duration of training

Data from experimental animals

A question of practical importance is the intensity and duration of training needed to obtain optimal results with respect to enzyme adaptation. A person who is untrained but not inactive can obtain some increase in the muscle content of oxidative enzymes by fairly light running (jogging), but the enzyme adaptation becomes much more marked if training is increased to work rates demanding 70–80% of the individual's $\dot{V}_{O_{2max}}$. In theory, even higher training intensities would further enhance the muscle's oxidative capacity, but in practical terms this may not be so, because the duration of training bouts is another important factor. There are no conclusive human data illustrating the interdependency between exercise intensity and duration, but infor-

mation can be deduced from a detailed study on the rat (Dudley *et al.* 1982); rats were subjected to 2 months of treadmill running, 5 days per week, at varying speeds and for varying daily training periods (Fig. 9.6). The running speeds demanded approximately 60%, 70%, 80%, 95%, 105% and 115% of their $\dot{V}_{O_{2max}}$, the two highest speeds being performed intermittently. The muscle enzyme adaptation increased with the duration of daily exercise at any given speed, but no additional training effect was noted when the daily duration of exercise exceeded 45–60 min. At the two highest speeds, the rats could only tolerate exercise for 15 and 30 min, respectively, but this was sufficient to induce marked training effects; responses were similar (red vastus, fast-twitch oxidative glycolytic fibres) or much greater (white vastus, fast-twitch glycolytic fibres) than those observed at the highest exercise intensity that could be tolerated for 60 min (95% of $\dot{V}_{O_{2max}}$). However, in the slow-twitch soleus muscle,

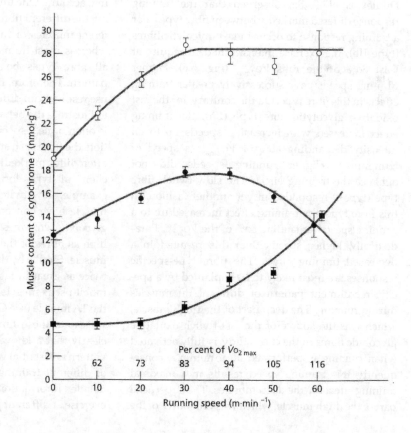

Fig. 9.6 The effects of endurance training on the oxidative enzyme content of different muscles in the rat. The rats were trained on a treadmill for 2 months, 5 days per week (usually for 45–60 min daily, at varying running speeds). The muscle content of cytochrome c, a respiratory chain component, was used as an indicator of muscle oxidative capacity. Three muscles were chosen to represent different fibre types: fast-twitch oxidative glycolytic (○) (type IIa), slow-twitch (●) (type I) and fast-twitch glycolytic (■) (type IIb) fibres. The approximate percentage of the rat's maximal oxygen intake demanded at each speed is indicated. From Dudley *et al.* (1982); modified with the permission of the *Journal of Applied Physiology*.

the enzyme changes at the two highest speeds were less than at slower speeds. This could indicate that 15–30 min of daily exercise was insufficient to result in maximal enzyme adaptation in the soleus muscle. As might be expected, the initial portion of the daily exercise bout gave the largest training effect per unit of training time, with progressively smaller effects in subsequent periods. In a previous study, Fitts *et al.* (1975) trained rats on a motor-driven treadmill for 10, 30, 60 or 120 min·day^{-1}; animals displayed progressively larger increases in the gastrocnemius muscle oxidative capacity with increasing exercise duration, but beyond 120 min of exercise there were no further increases. The available data thus indicate that beyond a certain time, a law of diminishing returns applies, i.e. less adaptation occurs per unit increase in training duration.

Effect of the fibre type-specific recruitment pattern

Dudley *et al.* (1982) observed that the training response differed markedly between fibre types. For a training response to occur in fast glycolytic fibres (type IIb), the exercise intensity had to require at least 80% of the rat's $\dot{V}_{O_{2max}}$ (Fig. 9.6). Higher running speeds gave successively greater training effects in this fibre type. On the contrary, for the fast oxidative glycolytic fibre type (IIa), the training effect increased with increasing speeds up to an intensity demanding 80% of $\dot{V}_{O_{2max}}$ (a speed of 30 m·min^{-1}). Higher running speeds did not enhance the training effect. The slow-twitch fibre type (type I) responded in yet another fashion. In this fibre type, the training effect increased up to a running speed demanding 80% of the $\dot{V}_{O_{2max}}$. Paradoxically, higher speeds than this resulted in a decreased training effect. The fibre type-specific responses are most likely to be explained by a specific recruitment pattern of different rat muscles during running. The deep part of the thigh muscle, which was the source of the fast-twitch oxidative glycolytic fibres in the cited study, is fully activated when running is performed at 30 m·min^{-1}; consequently, this training speed results in a maximal training effect for the deep muscles. The superficial part of the thigh muscle, which was the source of the

fast-twitch glycolytic fibres, has a higher activation threshold. No training effect is therefore seen in this region at low running speeds, but above the activation threshold there is a linear relationship between running speed and training effect. The soleus muscle, which contains almost exclusively slow-twitch (type I) fibres, is fully activated at 30 m·min^{-1}. Therefore, we would not expect higher running speeds than this to increase the training effect. However, there is no obvious explanation for the finding (Dudley *et al.* 1982) that running speeds higher than 30 m·min^{-1} resulted in a progressive diminution of training effect in this muscle, but not in the fast-twitch oxidative glycolytic deep vastus muscle.

Effects of fibre type recruitment in humans

Can these findings in the rat predict the effects of endurance training in humans? The answer is likely to be yes, provided that species differences are taken into account. One important difference is that, in the rat, the different fibre types are largely located in different muscles or in different parts of one muscle, whereas most human muscles are mixed muscles, all fibre types being intermingled in a mosaic pattern. Therefore, it may not be entirely correct to use results from different muscles or muscle groups to illustrate the behaviour of a specific fibre type, as is often done, especially in rodent studies. In addition, the fibres of a specific type found in one muscle often differ markedly from fibres of the same histochemical type located in another muscle. For example, slow-twitch (type I) fibres in the rabbit TA muscle have concentrations of both oxidative and glycolytic enzymes approximately three times as high as fibres of the same type in the rabbit soleus muscle. Similarly, the glycolytic enzyme content is twice as great in fast-twitch glycolytic fibres of the rabbit psoas muscle as in fibres of the same type in the TA muscle (see Chi *et al.* 1986).

Despite these limitations, the rat data illustrate clearly that a knowledge of fibre type recruitment pattern is essential when trying to predict the effects of different training regimens. For humans, quite detailed information is available on cycle ergometer exercise at different power outputs. As in the rat, the slow-twitch (type I) muscle fibres are the first to be activated and are kept activated even at higher exercise intensities. With increasing rates of work, there is a recruitment of fast-twitch motor units, type IIa followed by type IIb. It is believed that fibres (motor units) of all types are recruited at exercise intensities demanding more than 80–85% of the $\dot{V}_{O_{2max}}$. However, very strenuous exercise is probably required to activate maximally all type IIb motor units in a given muscle (for references, see Saltin & Gollnick 1983).

This fibre type recruitment pattern probably applies to other activities, such as running. However, the recruitment of high-threshold IIb units may be less marked in running than in cycling, especially at high exercise intensities, when cycling may involve quite forceful pedalling. Training at an exercise intensity slightly above that resulting in a marked increase in blood lactate concentration is generally sufficient to ensure maximal recruitment of the muscle's slow-twitch (type I) fibres. However, there is no evidence that more intense exercise would decrease the training effect in this fibre type as it did in the rat studies discussed above. Maximal training of the muscle's IIa and IIb fibres demands higher rates of work—how high may depend on the percentage fibre type composition of a particular muscle. Available evidence indicates that with prolonged exercise, and the resulting glycogen depletion, there is a time-dependent increase in the recruitment of higher threshold motor units; therefore long-duration exercise would be expected to result in an increased training effect (Saltin & Gollnick 1983; Vollestad et al. 1984; Ball-Burnett et al. 1991).

It may be concluded that it is advisable to use high training intensities to obtain a large training effect per unit of training time. However, with very heavy exercise, the duration of the exercise bouts may be insufficient to achieve an optimal training effect. The rat study by Dudley et al. (1982) gives some hints about the optimal balance between the intensity and duration of training, but there are still insufficient human data. The importance of this balance at the cellular level may be illustrated by a study from our laboratory that compared two different training protocols: (i) 72–79% of $\dot{V}_{O_{2max}}$, 30 min

daily; and (ii) 100% of $\dot{V}_{O_{2max}}$ performed as interval training with 4 min of exercise and 2 min of rest, five times daily. The training was performed on cycle ergometers, three times weekly for a period of 2 months. The oxidative enzyme content of the thigh muscle (measured as the maximal activity of the enzyme SDH) increased by approximately 25% with both training protocols. On the other hand, if a microscale SDH analysis was performed on the different fibre types, clear differences between the two training groups were apparent. In those training at the lower exercise intensity, SDH increased only in the slow-twitch type I fibres, whereas interval training at high exercise intensities resulted in an SDH increase mainly in the fast-twitch type II fibres (Henriksson & Reitman 1976). These results stress the importance of training at the exercise intensity at which an improvement is most desirable.

Effect of endurance training on glycolytic enzymes, capillarization and fibre types

The muscle cell's content of glycolytic enzymes is not, or is only marginally, affected by endurance training programmes of 2–6 months' duration. The content of glycolytic enzymes in the skeletal muscles of endurance athletes is normally low, but this finding is explained entirely by the large percentage of slow-twitch fibres in their muscles. The glycolytic enzyme content of this fibre type is normally only half that of the fast-twitch fibres. The mean glycolytic enzyme level in the slow-twitch and fast-twitch muscle fibres of athletes is thus normal, or even slightly enhanced (Chi et al. 1983; Essén-Gustavsson & Henriksson 1984). This finding is in accord with what has been observed during chronic stimulation in the rabbit (see above), when there is a complete fibre type transformation from fast-twitch glycolytic (type IIb) to slow-twitch (type I) fibres. In this situation, the glycolytic enzyme content of the muscle is decreased to 20% of its initial level (Figs 9.1–9.3), a decrease which reflects the large difference in glycolytic potential between fast-twitch glycolytic and slow-twitch fibres in the rabbit (Chi et al. 1986). It can therefore be concluded that the type of muscle fibre, based on its myofibrillar protein composition, is a strong determinant of its glycolytic enzyme content. The same is not true of most oxidative enzymes; their levels change with training and physical inactivity, completely independently of the specific myofibrillar protein isoforms of the fibre.

Human skeletal muscle capillarization is enhanced rapidly with endurance training; 2 months of training at high submaximal exercise intensities is sufficient to increase the total number of muscle capillaries by 50% (Andersen & Henriksson 1977a; Brodal et al. 1977; Ingjer 1979; Fig. 9.7). The capillary count per muscle fibre (leg muscles) differs two- to three-fold between endurance athletes and untrained individuals (Saltin & Gollnick 1983). Information is lacking on the extent to which formation of new capillaries depends on training intensity and duration. It is known, however, that less intense training often results in oxidative enzyme increases without any change in capillarization.

When stains for myofibrillar adenosine triphosphatase (ATPase) have been used to classify fibre type, most longitudinal studies in humans have failed to demonstrate any interconversion of fibre types (i.e. fast twitch to slow twitch) in response to endurance training. The stable nature of a muscle's fibre type composition is further illustrated by the consequences of chronic stimulation in rabbits. In this situation, there is a gradual and complete replacement of fast-twitch by slow-twitch fibres, but quite long periods of chronic stimulation are required. Fibre type changes are also the first factor to revert to normal when stimulation is discontinued (Brown et al. 1989). On the basis of these findings, the high percentage of slow-twitch (type I) fibres in endurance athletes and the opposite finding in sprinters have been ascribed to genetic factors (Komi et al. 1976). Endurance training is known, however, to lead to a complete type transformation within fast-twitch (type II) fibres, from type IIb to type IIa (Andersen & Henriksson 1977b; Jansson & Kaijser 1977).

The concept that endurance training does not change the relative occurrence of fast- and slow-

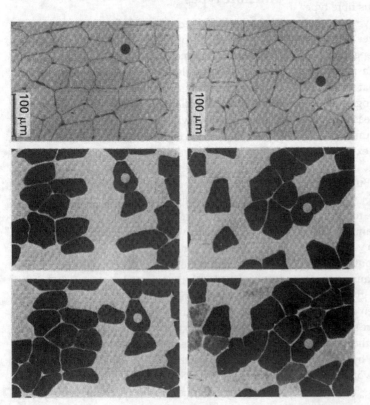

Fig. 9.7 Typical effect of 2 months of endurance training (as in Fig. 9.5) on capillary density in the human thigh muscle. The capillaries are seen in the upper sections as dark spots at the boundaries between muscle fibres (amylase–PAS staining). The histochemical muscle fibre type is indicated by the two lower sections. These are myofibrillar ATPase stains, pretreated at different pHs (the middle section at pH 4.3 and the lower one at pH 4.6). Slow-twitch (type I) fibres appear dark in both sections, whereas the fast-twitch oxidative glycolytic (type IIa) fibres appear light. Fast-twitch glycolytic (IIb) fibres appear light in the middle but dark in the lower sections. From Andersen and Henriksson (1977b); reproduced with the permission of the *Journal of Physiology (London)*.

twitch fibres has been challenged in recent years. It has been shown that (for references, see Schantz 1986):

1 Prolonged endurance training leads to the appearance of fibres intermediate between fast and slow twitch (Fig. 9.8).

2 The muscles of the dominant leg in certain types of athletes, such as badminton players, contain a significantly increased percentage of slow-twitch fibres.

3 During detraining, the percentage of fast-twitch muscle fibres increases.

Analyses of the myofibrillar protein isoform pattern within single muscle fibres are in accord with these results. Bauman *et al.* (1987) demonstrated that fast-twitch fibres containing a mixed pattern of fast and slow myofibrillar protein isoforms appeared with training. Probable reasons that fibre type transformation was not seen in early studies are: (i) the studies were too short in dura-

tion; and (ii) the muscles investigated were postural muscles and therefore relatively trained even when nominally in the pretraining state. (For a detailed discussion, see Schantz 1986.)

It is therefore reasonable to conclude that extensive endurance training will augment the percentage of slow-twitch fibres. The extent to which this occurs still remains to be determined.

It is difficult to predict the effect of endurance training on fibre size, since this depends to a large extent on the fibre size of the subjects prior to training. Trained individuals often have smaller fibre areas than untrained individuals, but the demands placed on the muscle fibre seem to determine fibre size, as illustrated by a recent human study (Kraemer *et al.* 1995). In this investigation, slow-twitch muscle fibre area decreased with endurance training, increased with strength training, but did not change when endurance training and strength training were combined.

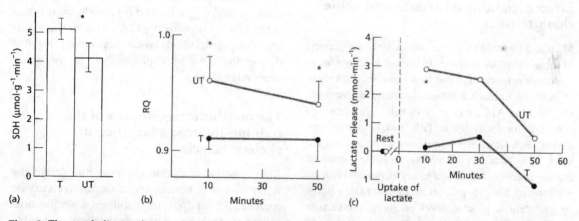

Fig. 9.8 The metabolic significance of the training-induced adaptation of human skeletal muscle. A group of subjects underwent 6 weeks of one-leg endurance training on a cycle ergometer. (a) The level of succinate dehydrogenase (SDH) was 25% higher in the well-trained (T) than in the untrained (UT) leg. Subjects performed two-leg cycle ergometer exercise at 70% of $\dot{V}_{O_{2max}}$. The energy metabolism of the two legs was analysed and compared by means of arterial and venous catheterization and muscle biopsy analyses. Catheterization allowed separate measurements of oxygen uptake ($\dot{V}_{O_2}$) and carbon dioxide production ($\dot{V}_{CO_2}$) for the two legs. The $\dot{V}_{CO_2}/\dot{V}_{O_2}$ ratio, known as the respiratory quotient (RQ), indicates the relative contributions of carbohydrate and fat to the oxidative metabolism. Carbohydrate oxidation only would result in an RQ of 1.0, whereas an RQ of 0.7 indicates that fat is the sole source of energy; (b) thus indicates that fat is a more important energy source for the trained leg than for the untrained one (the RQ value being significantly lower for the trained leg). Accompanying the greater use of carbohydrates in the untrained leg, there is a larger formation and release of lactate (c). In the trained leg, the lactate release is low and during the end of the exercise bout there is even a tendency towards an uptake of lactate from the blood. From Henriksson (1977); modified with the permission of the *Journal of Physiology (London)*.

Effects of training on muscle sensitivity to epinephrine

The effects of sympathetic hormones on muscle metabolism are exerted predominantly via adrenergic β-receptors of the β_2 subtype; these receptors are activated primarily by epinephrine. It is unclear whether endurance training is accompanied by an increase in β-receptor density (Williams *et al.* 1984; Martin *et al.* 1989; Buckenmeyer *et al.* 1990), although findings that muscle oxidative capacity normally correlates positively with β-adrenoceptor density (Williams *et al.* 1984; Plourde *et al.* 1993) support the existence of such a training effect. There is some evidence that the specific receptor subtypes differ between slow-twitch and fast-twitch muscle fibres. For example, the β_3-receptor, which is lacking the phosphorylation sites involved in receptor desensitization and downregulation, is particularly prominent in rat slow-twitch soleus muscle (see Torgan *et al.* 1995 for references).

Effect of training on muscle contractile characteristics

Muscle contractile characteristics may be influenced to some extent by training. In the rat, 8–12 weeks of treadmill running resulted in a significant increase in both the unloaded maximal shortening velocity (V_0) and the ATPase activity of soleus slow-twitch type I fibres (Schluter & Fitts 1994). In humans, slow-twitch fibres from the gastrocnemius muscle were 19% faster (V_0) in élite endurance-trained master runners than in sedentary controls (Widrick *et al.* 1996a). This adaptation may permit these fibres to maintain a greater level of force production during rapid contractions, thus reducing the athlete's reliance on more fatiguable type IIa fibres (Widrick *et al.* 1996b).

Regression of the training-induced adaptation following discontinuation of training

If training stops, the increase in oxidative capacity of a muscle induced by 2 months of endurance training is lost within 4–6 weeks (Fig. 9.5). The loss of muscle oxidative enzymes occurs faster than the decrease in muscle capillarization (Schantz *et al.* 1983) and the whole-body $\dot{V}_{O_2max}$ attained during cycle ergometry (Fig. 9.5). The time course of the decrease in muscle oxidative enzyme content agrees well with that observed on ceasing chronic stimulation in the rabbit (see above). In the latter case, however, the reversion to initial muscle capillarization and oxidative enzyme content occurs simultaneously. There has been only one detailed investigation of the enzyme changes that take place during detraining of individuals who have maintained endurance training for several years (Chi *et al.* 1983; very well trained, although not top-level athletes). The oxidative capacity of the slow-twitch fibres decreased rapidly with detraining, to the level found in untrained control subjects. However, the oxidative capacity of the fast-twitch fibres remained at an elevated level throughout the 12 weeks of detraining. One hypothesis put forward was that prolonged endurance training had changed the normal impulse pattern of fast motoneurones in the spinal cord. However, there was also a significant decrease in $\dot{V}_{O_2max}$ after 12 days of detraining (these latter data are reported by Coyle *et al.* 1984). Possibly, these individuals were kept more inactive during the detraining phase than in the study depicted in Fig. 9.5.

The metabolic significance of the training-induced adaptation of skeletal muscle

After cessation of chronic electrical stimulation, the restoration of a normal muscle oxidative enzyme content and capillarization follows a similar time course to that for the normalization of muscle endurance. This indicates that the described adaptations are of importance for the muscle's capacity to perform prolonged exercise. This is further illustrated by an investigation in which a group of subjects underwent 6 weeks of one-leg endurance training on a cycle ergometer. With one leg well trained (the level of SDH was 25% higher than in the untrained leg), the subjects then performed two-leg endurance exercise at 70% of their $\dot{V}_{O_2max}$. The energy metabolism of the two legs was analysed and compared by means of arterial and venous catheterization and muscle biopsy analysis.

There was a significantly smaller release of lactate from the trained than from the untrained leg (Fig. 9.8), and a significantly larger percentage of energy output in the trained leg was derived from fat combustion. It is well known that at the same absolute exercise intensity, trained individuals rely more on fat as an energy substrate than do untrained individuals. This is the case despite the fact that, at any given work rate, the plasma levels of free fatty acids are often lower in endurance-trained subjects (for a more detailed discussion, see Holloszy 1988). Taken together, the available evidence (including the one-leg training study) indicates that the heavier reliance on fat in endurance-trained individuals must be explained largely by local factors within the trained muscle. Such factors may include a larger utilization of intracellular or extracellular adipose tissue stores, but it is likely that the high mitochondrial oxidative enzyme content is also important in this respect. This view is supported by a rat study in which it was shown that the total amount of glycogen (muscle plus liver) remaining after an endurance treadmill test was directly proportional to the muscle's content of oxidative enzymes (Fitts *et al.* 1975). In addition to a decreased utilization of muscle glycogen, the carbohydrate-sparing effect of training also involves a decreased utilization of blood-derived glucose. In the study of Coggan *et al.* (1990) this accounted for approximately half the total post-training decrease in carbohydrate oxidation during exercise at 60% of the pretraining $\dot{V}_{O_{2max}}$. Similarly, Jansson and Kaijser (1987) found that the blood glucose extraction during exercise was considerably lower in their trained subjects (5% of total oxidative metabolism, versus 23% in untrained subjects). The low blood glucose utilization may explain why, unlike the untrained, trained subjects were able to maintain or even increase their blood glucose concentration throughout exercise. A lower utilization of blood glucose during exercise could also explain the reduced liver glycogen depletion reported earlier in trained rats (Baldwin *et al.* 1975; Fitts *et al.* 1975). Jansson and Kaijser (1987) suggested that the increased blood glucose extraction by the legs of untrained subjects was secondary

to their low muscle glycogen concentration. This would be in accord with Essén *et al.* (1977) and Gollnick *et al.* (1981), who demonstrated an inverse relationship between blood glucose extraction and muscle glycogen concentration. Figure 9.9 depicts a possible biochemical mechanism whereby a large concentration of oxidative enzymes (i.e. citric acid cycle and fat oxidation enzymes and respiratory chain components) leads to a situation where a major part of the energy supply is derived from fat metabolism, with a lower rate of lactate formation and sparing of muscle glycogen during exercise. The training-induced enhancement of muscle capillarization probably contributes to the metabolic adaptation seen in trained muscle. A conceivable mechanism for this latter effect might involve a facilitated exchange of oxygen and fatty acids.

Possible mechanisms inducing the enzyme adaptation to training

Enzymes, like other protein molecules, have a limited lifespan. They are synthesized and degraded in a continuous cycle, the biological half-life of many mitochondrial enzymes being about a week and that of glycolytic enzymes from 1 to a few days. The cellular content of any given enzyme reflects this balance between synthesis and degradation. Changes in the rate of synthesis of enzyme proteins are the most important factor explaining the enzyme changes that result from chronic stimulation or training (Booth & Holloszy 1977; Pette 1984; Williams *et al.* 1986). Changes in the rate of protein synthesis with training may be effected via both transcriptional and post-transcriptional regulation. Furthermore, the time courses of the responses of these respective pathways may differ (Neufer & Dohm 1993).

An interesting area of current research is to explore the biochemical mechanisms underlying the altered rate of enzyme synthesis, i.e. how is information on an increased need for oxidative enzymes in the muscle cell communicated to the genes? As an example, exploration has begun of interactions between training, diet and the muscle enzyme adaptations that are achieved (Helge *et al.* 1996). Suggested mediators for the increase in

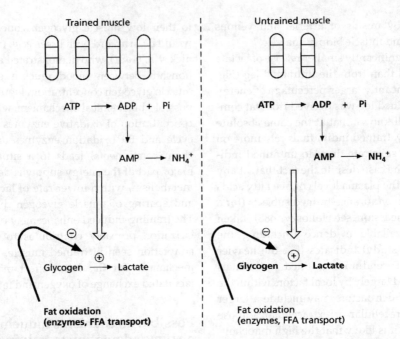

Fig. 9.9 A hypothetical biochemical mechanism whereby a large concentration of oxidative enzymes (i.e. citric acid cycle and fat oxidation enzymes and respiratory chain components) in trained muscle would lead to a greater reliance on fat metabolism, a lower rate of lactate formation and sparing of muscle glycogen during exercise. The increased content of oxidative enzymes in trained skeletal muscle is explained to a large extent by a larger mitochondrial volume (volume fraction). In the figure this is indicated schematically with mitochondrial symbols. Suppose that, in the untrained muscle, there are only half as many enzyme molecules of the citric acid cycle and half as many components of the respiratory chain (which is a reasonable assumption; see Fig. 9.4). Owing to the lower enzymatic capacity and mitochondrial volume fraction of the untrained muscle, it follows that, at a given rate of work, i.e. at a given rate of oxygen uptake, each mitochondrial unit has to be activated twice as much in the untrained muscle as in the trained one. An important component of this activation is the increased levels of the degradation products of ATP (e.g. ADP), which are the result of muscle contractions. These levels must thus be stabilized at a higher level in the untrained muscle than in the trained muscle. However, in addition to stimulating mitochondrial respiration, these ATP degradation products are also powerful stimulators of the glycolytic pathway. This would lead to a higher glycolytic rate in untrained muscle, resulting in a greater lactate release and carbohydrate oxidation. The fat oxidation rate is higher in trained muscle and the higher content of enzymes of fatty acid transport and oxidation is likely to contribute to this. An increased rate of fat oxidation leads to a more pronounced inhibition of glycolysis in the trained muscle than in the untrained muscle, where the rate of fat oxidation is lower. In concert, these factors lead to a sparing of glycogen in trained skeletal muscle during exercise. FFA, free fatty acid. After Holloszy and Booth (1976).

muscle oxidative capacity include the following: decreases in the concentration of adenosine triphosphate (ATP) or other high-energy phosphate compounds; a decreased oxygen tension; an increased sympathoadrenal stimulation of the muscle cell; substances released from the motor nerve; and calcium-induced diacylglycerol release with subsequent activation of protein kinase C. The hypothesis that a decrease in high-energy phosphate compounds is a possible mediator of the training-

induced increase in muscle oxidative capacity is strongly supported by studies where rats were fed with a creatine analogue, β-guanidinopropionic acid. This analogue, which depletes muscle stores of creatine and phosphocreatine, induced 40–50% increases in markers of muscle oxidative capacity such as cytochrome c concentration and CS activity. Similar increases were found in markers of skeletal muscle insulin sensitivity, such as the expression of the glucose transporter protein GLUT-4 and HK activity (Ren *et al.* 1993). A reduced oxygen tension seems unlikely to induce an increase in mitochondrial enzyme content, but it may influence glycolytic enzymes. This can be concluded from studies in Quechuas, natives of the Peruvian Andes, where hypoxia produced a shift from oxidative to glycolytic metabolism in slow-twitch type I fibres (Rosser & Hochachka 1993). A reduction in muscle oxidative capacity with residence at high altitude has also been reported in four out of five reported studies (see Rosser & Hochachka 1993). The role of an increased sympathoadrenal stimulation as a stimulus for oxidative enzyme synthesis is supported by the previously mentioned study in the obese Zucker rat (Torgan *et al.* 1993). On the other hand, no changes in cAMP, the β-adrenergic second messenger, have been detected up to 4 h post-exercise in rats (Sheldon *et al.* 1993).

Flux through the enzyme reaction may also be important, possibly influencing enzyme degradation. Finally, results on the enzyme 5-aminolevulinate synthase are of interest in this context. This enzyme is necessary for the synthesis of haem in skeletal muscle. Several components of the respiratory chain are haemoproteins. In training studies, the activity of this enzyme increases much earlier and to a greater extent than that of the mitochondrial enzymes. It therefore seems that a training-induced increase in the capacity of the mitochondrial respiratory chain demands an increased synthesis of haem (Town & Essig 1993).

The availability of advanced genetic techniques as well as improved cell culture systems has led to a renewed interest in this area of research, and this will probably lead to a better understanding of mechanisms whereby the skeletal muscle cell adapts to different normal and pathological states.

Acknowledgements

The author's own cited work was supported by grants from the Swedish Medical Research Council, the Karolinska Institute, the Research Council of the Swedish Sports Federation and the National Institutes of Health (USA). The author wishes to express his appreciation to Ms Christina Henriksson and Ms Anne-Britt Olrog for drawing the illustrations.

References

Allen, W.J., Mont, M.A., Talmadge, R.J., Rubenstein, A. & Edgerton, V.R. (1995) Plasticity of myonuclear number in hypertrophied and atrophied mammalian skeletal muscle fibers. *Journal of Applied Physiology* **78**, 1969–1976.

Andersen, P. & Henriksson, J. (1977a) Capillary supply of the quadriceps femoris muscle of man: adaptive response to exercise. *Journal of Physiology (London)* **270**, 677–690.

Andersen, P. & Henriksson, J. (1977b) Training induced changes in the subgroups of human type II skeletal muscle fibres. *Acta Physiologica Scandinavica* **99**, 123–125.

Baldwin, K.M., Fitts, R.H., Booth, F.W., Winder, W.W. & Holloszy, J.O. (1975) Depletion of muscle and liver glycogen during exercise. Protective effect of training. *Pflügers Archives* **354**, 203–212.

Ball-Burnett, M., Green, H.J. & Houston, M.E. (1991) Energy metabolism in human slow and fast twitch fibres during prolonged cycle exercise. *Journal of Physiology (London)* **437**, 257–267.

Baumann, H., Jäggi, M., Soland, F., Howald, H. & Schaub, M.C. (1987) Exercise training induces transitions of myosin isoform subunits within histochemically typed human muscle fibres. *Pflügers Archives* **409**, 349–360.

Bergström, J. (1962) Muscle electrolytes in man. *Scandinavian Journal of Clinical and Laboratory Investigation* **68** (Suppl.), 1–110.

Booth, F.W. & Holloszy, J.O. (1977) Cytochrome c turnover in rat skeletal muscles. *Journal of Biological Chemistry* **252**, 416–419.

Brodal, P., Ingjer, F. & Hermansen, L. (1977) Capillary supply of skeletal muscle fibres in untrained and endurance-trained men. *American Journal of Physiology* **232**, H705–H712.

Brown, M.D., Cotter, M.A., Hudlicka, O. & Vrbová, G. (1976) The effects of different patterns of muscle activity on capillary density, mechanical properties and structure of slow and fast rabbit muscles. *Pflügers Archives* **361**, 241–250.

Brown, J.M.C., Henriksson, J. & Salmons, S. (1989) Restoration of fast muscle characteristics following cessation of chronic stimulation: physiological, histochemical and metabolic changes during slow-to-fast transformation. *Proceedings of the Royal Society of London* **235**, 321–346.

Buckenmeyer, P.J., Goldfarb, A.H., Partilla, J.S., Pineyro, M.A. & Dax, E.M. (1990) Endurance training, not acute exercise, differentially alters β-receptors and cyclase in skeletal fiber types. *American Journal of Physiology* **258**, E71–E77.

Chesley, A., Heigenhauser, G.J.F. & Spriet, L.L. (1996) Regulation of muscle glycogen phosphorylase activity following short-term endurance training. *American Journal of Physiology* **270**, E328–E335.

Chi, M.M.-Y., Hintz, C., Coyle, E. *et al.* (1983) Effects of detraining on enzymes of energy metabolism in individual human muscle fibres. *American Journal of Physiology* **244**, C276–C287.

Chi, M.M.-Y., Hintz, C.S., Henriksson, J. *et al.* (1986) Chronic stimulation of mammalian muscle: enzyme changes in individual fibres. *American Journal of Physiology* 251, C633–C642.

Coggan, A.R., Kohrt, W.M., Spina, R.J., Bier, D.M. & Holloszy, J.O. (1990) Endurance training decreases plasma glucose turnover and oxidation during moderate-intensity exercise in men. *Journal of Applied Physiology* 68, 990–996.

Coyle, E.F., Martin, W.H.I., Sinacore, D.R., Joyner, M.J., Hagberg, J.M. & Holloszy, J.O. (1984) Time course of loss of adaptations after stopping prolonged intense endurance training. *Journal of Applied Physiology* 57, 1857–1864.

Dudley, G.A., Abraham, W.M. & Terjung, R.L. (1982) Influence of exercise intensity and duration on biochemical adaptations in skeletal muscle. *Journal of Applied Physiology* 53, 844–850.

Essén, B., Hagenfeldt, L. & Kaijser, L. (1977) Utilization of blood-borne and intramuscular substrates during continuous and intermittent exercise in man. *Journal of Physiology (London)* 265, 489–506.

Essén-Gustavsson, B. & Henriksson, J. (1984) Enzyme levels in pools of microdissected human muscle fibres of identified type. Adaptive response to exercise. *Acta Physiologica Scandinavica* 120, 505–515.

Fitts, R.H., Booth, F.W., Winder, W.W. & Holloszy, J.O. (1975) Skeletal muscle respiratory capacity, endurance, and glycogen utilization. *American Journal of Physiology* 228, 1029–1033.

Gollnick, P.D., Pernow, B., Essén, B., Jansson, E. & Saltin, B. (1981) Availability of glycogen and plasma FFA for substrate utilization in leg muscle of man during exercise. *Clinical Physiology Oxford* 1, 27–42.

Green, H.J., Helyar, R., Ball-Burnett, M. & Kowalchuk, N. (1992) Metabolic adaptations to training precede changes in muscle mitochondrial capacity. *Journal of Applied Physiology* 72, 484–491.

Helge, J.W., Richter, E.A. & Kiens, B. (1996) Interaction of training and diet on metabolism and endurance during exercise in man. *Journal of Physiology (London)* 492, 293–306.

Henriksson, J. (1977) Training induced adaptation of skeletal muscle and metabolism during submaximal exercise. *Journal of Physiology (London)* 270, 661–675.

Henriksson, J. & Reitman, J.S. (1976) Quantitative measures of enzyme activities in type I and type II muscle fibres of man after training. *Acta Physiologica Scandinavica* 97, 392–397.

Henriksson, J. & Reitman, J.S. (1977) Time course of changes in human skeletal muscle succinate dehydrogenase and cytochrome oxidase activities and maximal oxygen uptake with physical activity and inactivity. *Acta Physiologica Scandinavica* 99, 91–97.

Henriksson, J., Chi, M.M.-Y., Hintz, C.S. *et al.* (1986) Chronic stimulation of mammalian muscle: changes in enzymes of six metabolic pathways. *American Journal of Physiology* 251, C614–C632.

Holloszy, J.O. (1988) Metabolic consequences of endurance exercise training. In: Horton, E.S. & Terjung, R.L. (eds) *Exercise, Nutrition and Energy Metabolism*, pp. 116–131. Macmillan Publishing Co, New York.

Holloszy, J.O. & Booth, F.W. (1976) Biochemical adaptations to endurance exercise in muscle. *Annual Review of Physiology* 38, 273–291.

Ingjer, F. (1979) Effects of endurance training on muscle fibre ATPase activity, capillary supply and mitochondrial content in man. *Journal of Physiology (London)* 294, 419–422.

Jansson, E. & Kaijser, L. (1977) Muscle adaptation to extreme endurance training in man. *Acta Physiologica Scandinavica* 100, 315–324.

Jansson, E. & Kaijser, L. (1987) Substrate utilization and enzymes in skeletal muscle of extremely endurance-trained men. *Journal of Applied Physiology* 62, 999–1005.

Jolesz, F. & Sreter, F.A. (1981) Development, innervation, and activity pattern induced changes in skeletal muscle. *Annual Review of Physiology* 43, 531–552.

Komi, P.V., Viitasalo, J.T., Havu, M., Thorstensson, A. & Karlsson, J. (1976) Physiological and structural performance capacity: effect of heredity. In: Komi, P.V. (ed.) *International Series of Biomechanics*, Vol. 1A. *Biomechanics V-A*, pp. 118–123. University Park Press, Baltimore.

Kraemer, W.J., Patton, J.F., Gordon, S.E. *et al.* (1995) Compatibility of high-intensity strength and endurance training on hormonal and skeletal muscle adaptations. *Journal of Applied Physiology* 78, 976–989.

Lowry, O.H. & Passonneau, J.V. (1973) *A Flexible System of Enzymatic Analysis.* Academic Press, New York.

Martin, W.H.I., Coggan, A.R., Spina, R.J. & Saffitz, J.E. (1989) Effects of fiber type and training on β-adrenoceptor density in human skeletal muscle. *American Journal of Physiology* 257, E736–E742.

Morgan, T.E., Cobb, L.A., Short, F.A., Ross,

R. & Gunn, D.R. (1971) Effects of long-term exercise on human muscle mitochondria. In: Pernow, B. & Saltin, B. (eds) *Muscle Metabolism During Exercise*, pp. 87–95. Plenum Press, New York.

Neufer, P.D. & Dohm, G.L. (1993) Exercise induces a transient increase in transcription of the GLUT-4 gene in skeletal muscle. *American Journal of Physiology* 265, C1597–C1603.

Newsholme, E. & Leech, A. (1983) *Biochemistry for the Medical Sciences*, pp. 38–42. John Wiley & Sons, Chichester.

Petrén, T., Sjöstrand, T. & Sylvén, B. (1937) Der Einfluss des Trainings auf die Häufigkeit der Capillaren in Herz- und Skeletmuskulatur. *Arbeitsphysiologie* 9, 376–386.

Pette, D. (1984) Activity-induced fast to slow transitions in mammalian muscle. *Medicine and Science in Sports and Exercise* 16, 517–528.

Plourde, G., Rousseau-Migneron, S. & Nadeau, A. (1993) Effect of endurance training on β-adrenergic system in three different skeletal muscles. *Journal of Applied Physiology* 74, 1641–1646.

Puntschart, A., Claassen, H., Jostarndt, K., Hoppeler, H. & Billeter, R. (1995) mRNAs of enzymes involved in energy metabolism and mtDNA are increased in endurance-trained athletes. *American Journal of Physiology* 269, C619–C625.

Ren, J.-M., Semenkovich, C.F. & Holloszy, J.O. (1993) Adaptation of muscle to creatine depletion: effect on GLUT-4 glucose transporter expression. *American Journal of Physiology* 264, C146–C150.

Rosser, B.W.C. & Hochachka, P.W. (1993) Metabolic capacity of muscle fibers from high-altitude natives. *European Journal of Applied Physiology* 67, 513–517.

Salmons, S. & Henriksson, J. (1981) The adaptive response of skeletal muscle to increased use. *Muscle and Nerve* 4, 94–105.

Saltin, B. & Gollnick, P.D. (1983) Skeletal muscle adaptability: significance for metabolism and performance. In: Peachey, L.D. (ed.) *Handbook of Physiology*, Section 10, *Skeletal Muscle*, pp. 555–631. American Physiological Society, Bethesda, Maryland.

Schantz, P. (1986) Plasticity of human skeletal muscle. *Acta Physiologica Scandinavica* 128 (Suppl. 558), 1–62.

Schantz, P.G., Henriksson, J. & Jansson, E. (1983) Adaptation of human skeletal muscle to endurance training of long duration. *Clinical Physiology* 3, 141–151.

Schluter, J.M. & Fitts, R.H. (1994) Shortening velocity and ATPase activity of rat skeletal muscle fibers: effects of endurance exercise training. *American Journal of Physiology* **266**, C1699–C1713.

Sheldon, A., Booth, F.W. & Kirby, C.R. (1993) cAMP levels in fast- and slow-twitch skeletal muscle after an acute bout of aerobic exercise. *American Journal of Physiology* **264**, C1500–C1504.

Spina, R.J., Chi, M.M.Y., Hopkins, M.G., Nemeth, P.M., Lowry, O.H. & Holloszy, J.O. (1996) Mitochondrial enzymes increase in muscle in response to 7–10 days of cycle exercise. *Journal of Applied Physiology* **80**, 2250–2254.

Torgan, C.E., Etgen, G.J. Jr, Brozinick, J.T. Jr, Wilcox, R.E. & Ivy, J.L. (1993) Interaction of aerobic exercise training and clen-buterol: effects on insulin-resistant muscle. *Journal of Applied Physiology* **75**, 1471–1476.

Torgan, C.E., Etgen, G.J. Jr, Kang, H.Y. &

Ivy, J.L. (1995) Fiber type-specific effects of clenbuterol and exercise training on insulin-resistant muscle. *Journal of Applied Physiology* **79**, 163–167.

Town, G.P. & Essig, D.A. (1993) Cytochrome oxidase in muscle of endurance-trained rats: subunit mRNA contents and heme synthesis. *Journal of Applied Physiology* **74**, 192–196.

Varnauskas, E., Björntorp, P., Fahlén, M., Prerovsky, I. & Stenberg, J. (1970) Effects of physical training on exercise blood flow and enzymatic activity in skeletal muscle. *Cardiovascular Research* **4**, 418–422.

Vollestad, N.K., Vaage, O. & Hermansen, L. (1984) Muscle glycogen depletion patterns in type I and subgroups of type II fibres during prolonged severe exercise in man. *Acta Physiologica Scandinavica* **122**, 433–441.

Widrick, J.J., Trappe, S.W., Blaser, C.A.,

Costill, D.L. & Fitts, R.H. (1996a) Isometric force and maximal shortening velocity of single muscle fibers from élite master runners. *American Journal of Physiology* **271**, C666–C675.

Widrick, J.J., Trappe, S.W., Costill, D.L. & Fitts, R.H. (1996b) Force–velocity and force–power properties of single muscle fibers from élite master runners and sedentary men. *American Journal of Physiology* **271**, C676–C683.

Williams, R.S., Caron, M.G. & Daniel, K. (1984) Skeletal muscle β-adrenergic receptors: variations due to fiber type and training. *American Journal of Physiology* **246**, E160–E167.

Williams, R.S., Salmons, S., Newsholme, E.A., Kaufman, R.E. & Mellor, J. (1986) Regulation of nuclear and mitochondrial expression by contractile activity in skeletal muscle. *Journal of Biological Chemistry* **261**, 376–380.

Chapter 10

Influence of Endurance Training and Detraining on Motoneurone and Sensory Neurone Morphology and Metabolism

ROLAND R. ROY, V. REGGIE EDGERTON AND AKIHIKO ISHIHARA

Introduction

The endurance of an individual's motor performance is determined by many physiological variables, and the neural components can certainly play an important role in that performance. When and which neural components may be limiting factors in a given situation remain largely unknown. Based on a range of neuronal preparations, it appears that the physiological properties of a neurone are dependent not only on its immediate activation history, i.e. milliseconds to seconds, but also on its longer-term activation (minutes, hours and even weeks). To understand how motor performances can be sustained, we must recognize that our understanding of cellular neurophysiological properties and their changes during fatigue in reduced laboratory preparations remain far removed from the highly integrative factors influencing an athlete's behaviour, such as pain, discomfort, proprioception and motivation.

This chapter focuses on cellular events which reflect the adaptive properties of neurones to chronic elevated or reduced activation and/or loading levels, mainly in animal models. In particular, the chapter examines the properties of motoneurones and dorsal root ganglion cells that are thought to contribute to the ability of both motor and sensory neurones to sustain highly repetitive and prolonged motor tasks. An advantage of focusing on animal studies is that quantitative metabolic and morphological properties of the neuronal tissues can be collected from animals in a specific exercised or trained state. This is not feasible in humans. Since most of the experimental models investigated mimic human scenarios, e.g. exercise and spaceflight, the results from these studies provide insight into how varying activity levels may affect human motor and sensory nervous system functions that could, in turn, affect physical performance.

Understanding the relationships among motor unit recruitment, energy costs and energy replacement is an important element in determining endurance capacity. Motor units are recruited in order of 'size' as initially described by Henneman (Henneman et al. 1965). In muscles comprised of a mixture of fibre types, slow motor units generally have smaller motoneurones and axons, and fewer fibres than fast motor units. The fibres of slow motor units have higher oxidative capacities and are more fatigue resistant than the fibres in fast motor units. The recovery potential of the motor unit type is most probably also related directly to its oxidative capacity. Thus, the neuromuscular system is designed to activate small, slow fatigue-resistant units first (low force and long duration activity) and large, fast fatiguable units last (high force and short duration activity). These relationships have been previously described in detail (Burke 1981; Henneman & Mendell 1981). In addition, the plasticity of the muscle fibres to increased or decreased functional demands has been previously summarized (Pette & Vrbova 1985; Roy et al. 1991a; Edgerton & Roy 1996).

The recruitment of motor units is regulated by supraspinal and peripheral inputs to the motoneurones, i.e. the 'final common pathway'. In this chapter, we will focus on how increased or decreased input by varying activity levels and loading patterns on the neuromotor system can affect the metabolic and morphological characteristics of the motoneurones and sensory neurones. We will discuss to what extent the changes in performance associated with training can be attributed to adaptations of the motoneuronal and sensory neurone properties. Data will also be presented which address the issue of the level of control that the motoneurones have on the force, speed and fatiguability of the muscle fibres that they innervate.

Oxidative phosphorylation is the principal metabolic process that maintains a sufficient state of energy for the normal functioning of the nervous system. Several factors may drive the metabolic needs of the nervous system, but their relative importance remains unknown. Maintenance of a resting membrane potential, maintenance of cytoplasmic components, intraneuronal transport and the release and reuptake of neurotransmitters are among the functions that influence the metabolic needs of neurones (Edgerton *et al.* 1990; Chalmers *et al.* 1992b). The relative importance of each of these functions in motoneurones appears closely linked with the size principle of motor unit recruitment (Henneman *et al.* 1965; Henneman & Mendell 1981); this relationship has provided considerable insight into how the amount and pattern of activation of motor units regulate the morphological, functional and metabolic properties of the motor units. Both morphological and physiological properties related to the size principle of motor unit recruitment are significantly correlated with the mitochondrial enzyme activities of the motoneurone cell bodies. Larger motoneurones have faster axonal conduction velocities, lower input resistances, shorter afterhyperpolarization periods (Barrett & Crill 1971, 1974; Cullheim 1978; Cullheim & Ulfhake 1979; Zwaagstra & Kernell 1980; Kernell & Zwaagstra 1981) and lower oxidative enzyme activities (Penny *et al.* 1975; Sickles & McLendon 1983; Donselaar *et al.* 1986; Ishihara *et al.* 1991a,b, 1995b) than smaller motoneurones. Characterization of the adaptation-inducing events imposed on the sensorimotor networks of the spinal cord should reveal clues as to which cellular functions stimulate each specific adaptive event.

One view is that the maintenance of ionic balance is the major energy-requiring activity of a neurone (Ritchie 1967; Passonneau & Lowry 1971; Lowry 1975; Sokoloff 1984; Wong-Riley & Kageyama 1986). Based on this assumption, one might expect that the activity level (i.e. the number of action potentials) and the oxidative metabolism of a neurone would be tightly coupled. Unfortunately, one cannot make direct measurements of the activity levels of single neurones for prolonged periods *in vivo*. However, single motor unit electromyographic (EMG) recordings suggest that ~500 000 impulses per day may be generated in the frequently recruited slow oxidative motor units of the rat soleus, while as few as 3000 impulses per day may be generated by less active fast motor units in the tibialis anterior (Hennig & Lomo 1985). If we assume an action potential duration of 5 ms, this activity level implies that the most and least active motor units spend, respectively, 2.9 and 0.02% of the day in 'spiking' activity. For such neurones, activity-dependent energy requirements are unlikely to have any great total energy demand.

Accordingly, chronic increases (e.g. functional overload or exercise training) or decreases (e.g. spinal cord isolation, spinal cord transection, hindlimb unloading or spaceflight) in activation levels may neither change the total energy demand on the motoneurone significantly nor induce significant adaptations in its oxidative capacity (Roy *et al.* 1991a). Thus, it appears that factors other than activity level, and the consequent energy demands for ionic pumping, have a dominant influence on the total energy demand of the neurone, and resultant adaptive responses in cellular oxidative capacity.

Properties of motor pools and muscle units that are coupled to metabolic needs

Skeletal muscle fibres are innervated by three categories of spinal motoneurones, i.e. α, β and γ (Burke 1981). α-Motoneurones innervate the extrafusal muscle fibres. These constitute the main mass of a muscle, in which a single axon of each motoneurone branches to supply a number of muscle fibres. An α-motoneurone and the muscle fibres that it innervates constitute a motor unit. γ-Motoneurones innervate intrafusal muscle fibres, regulating the length and the tension of the intrafusal fibres of muscle spindles. The γ-motoneurones regulate the sensitivity of the spindles to a change in muscle length whether the muscle is relaxed or activated and whether it is lengthening or shortening when the muscle is activated. The motoneurones innervating a single muscle are collectively called a motor pool. α- and γ-motoneurones are intermingled in a motor pool. Each motor pool has a relatively specific topographical distribution. Segmental representation in the ventral horn of the spinal cord is associated with individual muscles and even muscle compartments (McHanwell & Biscoe 1981; Nicolopoulos-Stournaras & Iles 1983; Weeks & English 1985; Peyronnard *et al.* 1986; Balice-Gordon & Thompson 1988). Soma size is routinely used to distinguish between α- and γ-motoneurones in the ventral horn of the spinal cord. Soma diameters of 25 μm in the rat (Sickles & Oblak 1984; Swett *et al.* 1986; Ishihara *et al.* 1988) and 32.5 μm in the cat (Burke *et al.* 1977) are anatomical criteria that are used to separate the larger α- from the smaller γ-motoneurones, although there is considerable size overlap of α- and γ-motoneurones. β-Motoneurones, which innervate both extrafusal and intrafusal muscle fibres, are observed infrequently, and little is known about their metabolic properties or their recruitment patterns. The following discussion thus focuses on α- and γ-motoneurones.

Observations on the smallest motoneurones, most likely γ-motoneurones, suggest that a high oxidative potential is coupled with a high input resistance and a low threshold level (Westbury 1982). There is a higher mitochondrial density in γ- than in α-motoneurones (Ishihara *et al.* 1997a) (Fig. 10.1). This may reflect the greater tonic and higher frequency activities and oxidative enzyme levels in γ-motoneurones (Ishihara *et al.* 1988, 1991a,b, 1995a,b; cf. Johnson 1986). However, the relationship between mitochondrial density and firing frequency may not be causal, since it remains uncertain whether action potentials impose a significant metabolic demand on neurones, as discussed above (Edgerton *et al.* 1990; Chalmers *et al.* 1992b).

Another factor that may be important in determining the relative metabolic requirements of γ- and α-motoneurones may be the extent of the target

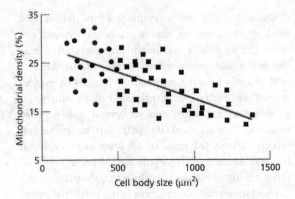

Fig. 10.1 The relationship between cell body size and mitochondrial density in neurones of the dorsolateral region of the ventral horn at the L5 spinal cord segment in four rats ($n = 57$, $r = -0.66$, $P < 0.001$). Circles, γ-motoneurones ($n = 19$); squares, α-motoneurones ($n = 38$). From Ishihara *et al.* (1997a).

field. As we have proposed for motoneurones (Edgerton *et al.* 1990; Chalmers *et al.* 1992b), the extent of the axonal tree of neurones in the dorsal root ganglion that projects to the somas and dendrites of interneurones and motoneurones may be an important determinant of the energy demands of these neurones (Willis & Coggeshall 1991). The axonal tree volume may be greater in afferent than in efferent projections. For example, a single Ia afferent from a muscle spindle anatomically projects to ~80–100% of the homonymous motoneurones and to a smaller percentage (e.g. ~40% for the cat semitendinosus) (Nelson & Mendell 1978) of heteronymous motoneurones (Henneman & Mendell 1981; Mendell *et al.* 1990). A single Ia afferent has been estimated to affect motoneurones from as many as 15 hindlimb muscles (Jankowska 1983). In addition, over 50% of all dorsospinocerebellar neurones in Clarke's column receive input from group I afferents of the gastrocnemius–soleus nerve (Osborn & Poppele 1988). These data highlight the extensiveness of Ia afferent branching. If the volume of the axonal branches is a driving factor, we would expect the metabolic cost of maintaining homeostasis within these extensive axonal projections to be greater for dorsal root ganglion neurones than for motoneurones.

Sickles and Oblak (1983) retrogradely labelled

motoneurones by exposing the muscle nerve to horseradish peroxidase; this enabled them to examine the enzyme activity of the α-motoneurones within a specific motor pool and to compare the metabolic properties of the motoneurone and the muscle fibres that it innervates. The activity of nicotinamide adenine dinucleotide diaphorase tetrazolium reductase, an oxidative marker enzyme, was determined in the motoneurones and muscle fibres of the rat tensor fascia latae (predominantly fast glycolytic fibres), the tibialis anterior (predominantly fast glycolytic and fast oxidative glycolytic fibres) and the soleus (predominantly slow oxidative fibres). The mean enzyme activity of the motoneurones in each motor pool corresponded closely with that of the muscle fibres innervated by that motor pool. This study was the first to report metabolic differences between motoneurones innervating muscles with differing fibre type compositions. Similar conclusions have now been reached in several species based on analyses of several oxidative enzymes, muscles and their motor pools (Mjaatvedt & Wong-Riley 1986; Ishihara et al. 1988, 1995a). In contrast, there is no relationship between

soma size and the activity of α-glycerophosphate dehydrogenase, a glycolytic marker enzyme, in motoneurones from some of these same motor pools (Ishihara et al. 1989).

The relationship between motoneurone properties and muscle fibre types has been examined by comparing the succinate dehydrogenase activity of motoneurones innervating the deep compared to the superficial portion of the rat tibialis anterior muscle (Ishihara et al. 1995b). The proportion of muscle fibres having a high oxidative enzyme activity increases on proceeding from the superficial (away from the tibia) to the deep (close to the tibia) portion of this muscle. The motor pool showed a large variation in enzyme activity among medium-sized motoneurones, but an inverse relationship between soma size and succinate dehydrogenase activity was evident when the total motor pool was considered. In addition, motoneurones innervating the deep portion of the rat tibialis anterior had, on average, higher succinate dehydrogenase activities than motoneurones innervating the superficial portion. Figure 10.2 depicts the size and succinate dehydrogenase activity of the motoneurones in the

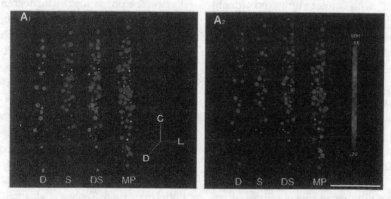

Fig. 10.2 Computerized three-dimensional reconstruction of the motor pools innervating the deep (D), superficial (S) or both (DS) portions of the left and the entire motor pool (MP) of the right tibialis anterior muscle of a representative rat. Each motoneurone is shown as a sphere which is proportional to its cross-sectional area. In A_1, DS clearly shows the intermingling of the motor pools innervating the two portions of the muscle. MP shows the distribution of the γ- (lighter shade) and α- (darker shade) motoneurones in the entire motor pool (these are colour-coded in the original paper, see reference below). In A_2, the succinate dehydrogenase (SDH) activity of each motoneurone is shaded relative to the scale on the right. This scale is a graded unit colour scale in the original paper (see reference below). The width of the vertical unit scale is equivalent to the lowest to highest SDH activities of motoneurones in the motor pools. A majority of the smaller motoneurones, presumably γ, have relatively high SDH activities. The orientation scale in A_1 shows the caudal (C), lateral (L) and dorsal (D) directions. Scale bar in A_2 = 1 mm. From Ishihara et al. (1995b).

deep, superficial and entire motor pool of the tibialis anterior in two rats. Note that the neurones seem to be dispersed randomly with respect to size and succinate dehydrogenase activity, even among neurones that project to two different muscle compartments within the tibialis anterior. Note also that this dispersion is true for the smallest neurones, the majority of which can be assumed to be γ-motoneurones. Miyata and Kawai (1992) used neuronal tracer techniques to compare the soma size and nicotinamide adenine dinucleotide diaphorase tetrazolium reductase activity of motoneurones innervating superficial (predominantly low oxidative fibres) and deep (predominantly high oxidative fibres) portions of the rat gluteus medius muscle. A higher mean enzyme activity was observed in motoneurones innervating the deep than in those innervating the superficial portion of the muscle. Again, there were no differences in the mean soma size of motoneurones innervating the two portions of the muscle. Together, these results suggest that although there is a clear link between the oxidative enzyme activities of the motoneurones in any given motor pool and the muscle fibres that they innervate, this relationship must be the result of additional factors yet to be defined and, perhaps, not closely associated with motor unit recruitment order.

Comparisons of motoneurones in relatively slow and fast muscles provide further insight into which physiological properties place significant metabolic demands on the neurone. In the α-motoneurone population, the motoneurones innervating slow muscle fibres generally have smaller cell body sizes and higher oxidative enzyme activities than motoneurones innervating fast muscle fibres (Burke et al. 1982; Ishihara et al. 1988, 1995b). Slow motor units also have the smallest number of axonal branches, since the number of muscle fibres innervated by a slow motoneurone is less than that for fast units (Burke 1981; Bodine et al. 1987). Although Asselt et al. (1993) found no difference in the mitochondrial density between slow- and fast-type neurones in the zebrafish spinal cord, the mean cell body size of slow-type neurones was smaller than that of fast-type neurones.

Fatiguability of muscles and motor units

A comparison of fatigue properties between motor units of different physiological type shows that the loss of force potential after repetitive stimulation is attributable to a loss in neuromuscular transmission only in some fast fatiguable motor units. For example, some muscle units that lose more than 80% of their force within a couple of minutes of initiation of trains of tetanic stimuli occurring every second show decreases in the single motor unit EMG amplitude accompanied by the failure of some action potentials (McDonagh et al. 1980; Hamm et al. 1989). In contrast, little or no change in electrical stimulation-induced EMG signals occurs in slow or fast fatigue-resistant motor units.

In vivo studies in normal humans show some neural limits in the ability to sustain very prolonged, but relatively low force level stimulation of motor units. Some peripheral afferent or supraspinal input to motor pools alters the firing and recruitment patterns or the preference of recruitment with prolonged activation (Tamaki et al. 1998) (Fig. 10.3). In addition, a decrease in the firing rate of motor units has been reported following prolonged, sustained and oscillatory contractions (Person & Kudina 1972). The decrement in firing frequency has been described as 'muscle wisdom', in that it provides a mechanism whereby the brain does not overstimulate motor units (Marsden et al. 1983). The potential for 'compensatory' motor unit recruitment has been demonstrated by in situ experiments in which motor units were stimulated indirectly, via descending tracts from the locomotor region of the brainstem. Under these conditions, the motor unit firing frequency increased and could compensate for a loss in the force potential of the muscle during repetitive activation (Tansey & Botterman 1996; Tansey et al. 1996). The increase in firing rate occurred similarly in all motor unit types.

In summary, the neural output generated directly by motoneurones and indirectly by interneurones shows that regular, repetitive demands can induce changes in the firing frequency of the motoneurones. These changes can be compensatory (an increase in frequency as seems to occur following

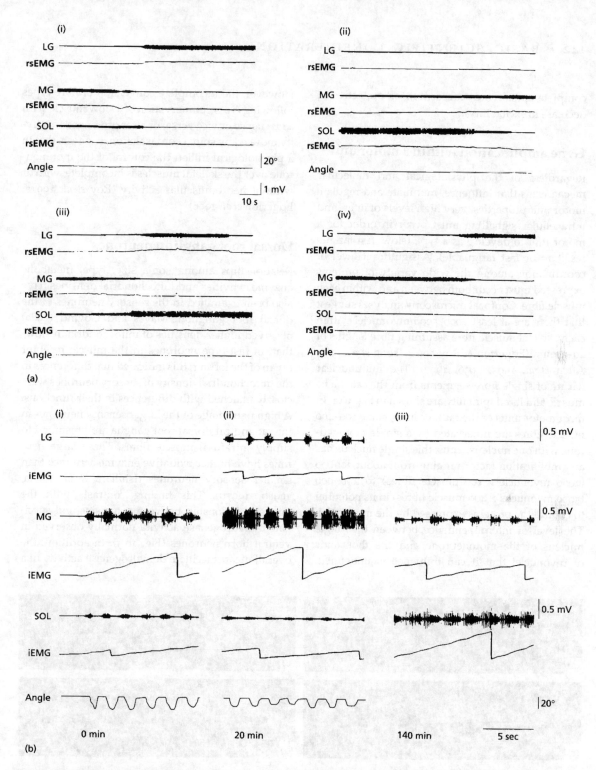

Fig. 10.3 Examples of different combinations of simultaneous electromyograph (EMG) activity from the lateral gastrocnemius (LG), medial gastrocnemius (MG) and soleus (SOL) muscles. (a) EMG and rsEMG recordings during static contractions. Note that the EMG activities are switched from MG + SOL to LG (i), SOL to MG (ii), MG + SOL to LG + SOL (iii), and MG to LG (iv) with increasing duration of the contractions. (b) EMG and integrated EMG (iEMG) recordings during concentric and eccentric plantarflexion (dynamic contractions) at ankle angles between 90° and 110° at an angular velocity of ~30°·s⁻¹. EMG activities in the MG and SOL are shown, but the LG was not active at the start of exercise (i). As the duration of the contraction is increased, the LG tends to be recruited and the MG activity increases, whereas the activity in the SOL decreases (ii). The calibration is the same for all panels in (a) and (b). Bottom line (Angle) indicates the ankle joint angle. From Tamaki *et al.* (1998).

complete spinal cord transection) or protective (a decrease in excitability).

Gene amplification within a motor unit

Regardless of the physiological and molecular mechanisms that influence, modulate and regulate motor unit properties, very high levels of inter- and intracellular signalling must occur in order for a motor unit to develop as a type (slow, fast fatigue resistant or fast fatiguable). A significant level of coordination among the wide variety of proteins expressed must occur both between and within each muscle fibre. Confocal microscopy analyses suggest that there are at least 2000–5000 myonuclei within each skeletal muscle fibre assuming fibre lengths of 20–50 mm (Edgerton & Roy 1991; Tseng *et al.* 1994; Allen *et al.* 1995, 1996, 1997). The multinuclear nature of single fibre segments from the cat soleus muscle and its adaptability are shown in Fig. 10.4. In most motor units of the rat hindlimb, some 100–400 muscle fibres are innervated by a single motoneurone with one nucleus. Thus, this single nucleus has an amplification factor ranging from about 200 000 (2000 myonuclei × 100 muscle fibres) to 2 000 000 (5000 myonuclei × 400 muscle fibres) in its potential to control the proteins expressed by the myonuclei. The level of interdependence between the single nucleus of the motoneurone and the thousands of myonuclei that it can influence is undefined.

However, the incomplete conversion of fibre types following cross-reinnervation of a slow muscle with a fast nerve or vice versa, or after prolonged inactivity induced by spinal cord isolation, suggests that in a physiological milieu the control of the motoneurone over the skeletal muscles is incomplete, with or without neuromuscular activity (Roy *et al.* 1991a; Edgerton *et al.* 1996).

Dorsal root ganglion neurones

Relationships among soma size, type, metabolic enzyme activities and mitochondrial densities have also been examined in the sensory neurones of the dorsal root ganglion. Mayes and Govind (1989) observed higher densities of mitochondria in slow- than in fast-type neurones in the muscle receptor organ of the lobster; this indicated that differences in the mitochondrial density of sensory neurones were closely matched with differences in their functions. A high percentage of the larger sensory neurones in the rat and cat dorsal root ganglia are presumed to supply intrafusal muscle fibres. These large neurones have higher oxidative enzyme activities than smaller sensory neurones (Ishihara *et al.* 1995a, 1996b, 1997b). This finding contrasts with the inverse relationship between soma size and succinate dehydrogenase activity normally observed in ventral horn neurones (Fig. 10.5). In addition, the overall mean succinate dehydrogenase activity of a

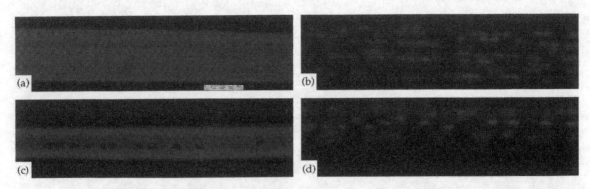

Fig. 10.4 Single fibre segments from control and 6-month spinal cord-isolated cats stained for myosin heavy chain (a and c) and myonuclei (b and d) using antislow and antifast antibodies and Hoechst 33258, respectively. (a,b) Control slow fibres; (c,d) spinal cord-isolated slow fibres. Note the smaller size and myonuclear number in the fibre segments from the spinal cord-isolated as compared to the control cats. Bar in (a) = 50 μm. Taken from a colour photograph in Allen *et al.* (1995).

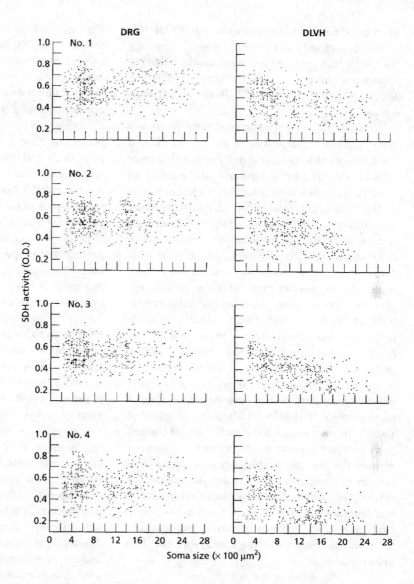

Fig. 10.5 Relationship between soma size and succinate dehydrogenase (SDH) activity of neurones in the dorsal root ganglion (DRG) and in the dorsolateral region of the ventral horn (DLVH) at spinal cord level L7 in four cats (Nos 1–4). From Ishihara *et al.* (1995a).

subpopulation of cat dorsal root ganglion neurones was significantly higher than that of a subpopulation of ventral horn neurones at the same segmental level (Ishihara *et al.* 1995a).

As might be expected from the difference in body mass between cats and rats, the mean succinate dehydrogenase activity of neurones in the dorsal root ganglia of the lumbar spinal cord is ~15% higher in rats than in cats (Ishihara *et al.* 1996b). A similar difference was reported for neurones in the ventral horn of the spinal cord; the succinate dehydrogenase activity of spinal neurones was ~25%

higher in rats than in cats (Chalmers & Edgerton 1989b). When comparisons are drawn between small and large adults of different species or between different-sized animals of the same species, the metabolic rate (oxygen consumption) per gram of body mass is inversely related to body size: smaller animals have a higher metabolic rate per gram of body mass than do larger animals (Taylor *et al.* 1970; Schmidt-Nielsen 1972; Hill 1976; Hainsworth 1981). The resting metabolic rate of the rat is about 30% higher than that of the cat (Altman & Dittmer 1971). The higher metabolic rates in motoneurones and sensory neurones in the rat than in the cat indicate that the neural tissue follows the metabolic patterns of other tissues, i.e. the oxidative capacity of neural tissues varies logarithmically and inversely with body size (Chalmers & Edgerton 1989a).

We need to identify specific sensory receptors and their location, e.g. at a specific area of the skin, at the knee or ankle joint, within a flexor or extensor muscle, etc., to gain a further understanding of which cellular functions place the greatest demands on the metabolism of dorsal root ganglion neurones. The absence of an inverse relationship between soma size and the succinate dehydrogenase activity in neurones in the dorsal root ganglia, and the wide range of succinate dehydrogenase activities may reflect specific sensory modalities, e.g. proprioception, pain, pressure, etc., each having unique metabolic demands. The differing metabolic demands may reflect the extensiveness of the axonal branching within the spinal cord, the number of action potentials and/or the type of neurotransmitters of the neurone and their means of translocating these transmitters, as has been hypothesized for motoneurones (Edgerton et al. 1990; Chalmers et al. 1992b). To understand the significance of the cell body size and the metabolic properties of sensory neurones more thoroughly, muscle-specific and sensory mode-specific neurotransmitters need to be determined. Morphological measures of the volume and length of the axonal projections to the spinal cord may also enhance the understanding of the metabolic features of the dorsal root ganglion neurones.

Plasticity of sensorimotor systems

Adaptations of the neuromotor system are multidimensional and dynamic. Removal of gravitational stimuli (chronic unloading) is in many respects the antithesis of endurance training. Thus, adaptations occurring in the microgravity environment provide a unique comparison with those occurring with increased functional demands at 1 G (see below). Functional sensorimotor adaptations induced by the prolonged absence of weight support, e.g.

during spaceflight, include the following: a sensation of tingling on the soles of the feet, a depression of maximum potentiation of spinal reflexes (although an increased sensitivity, due to a reduced threshold for the tendon tap), lower pain thresholds, altered vestibular control of posture and illusionary perceptions of roll and pitch and loads placed on the body (Edgerton & Roy 1994b, 1996). However, the magnitude and direction of these phenomena vary with the duration of spaceflight, with the time of measurement after landing and almost certainly with respect to the nature of the neuromotor tasks performed routinely during a spaceflight.

We have suggested that the integrated neuromotor response to spaceflight be considered as a gravitational unloading syndrome (GUS) (Edgerton & Roy 1996). In this model, there is a general reduction or at least severe alterations in afferent flow, particularly from the proprioceptors that respond to load-bearing and kinematics of the limb as well as from vestibular mechanisms (Magus 1924; Kozlovskaya et al. 1981). Extensive reinterpretation of the afferent signals is required to accomplish motor tasks in the changed gravitational environment, e.g. to maintain a stable posture upon re-entry to 1 G (Kenyon & Young 1986; Layne et al. 1997). These neuromotor responses to altered gravity project well beyond altered vestibular function. It seems necessary to study the neuromotor response to spaceflight using experimental designs which acknowledge that numerous parallel and interdependent adaptations are occurring concomitantly as well as sequentially. These adaptations, predominantly neural, muscular and hormonal, reflect some integrative state and level at any moment during adaptation to microgravity or subsequent return to a normal gravitational field.

Neural modulation of myosin isoforms and fibre phenotype

Since the classic cross-reinnervation experiments of Buller et al. (1960), an activity-dependent role of the motoneurone in determining the properties of a muscle have been studied extensively. A myriad of cross-reinnervation (see Edgerton et al. 1996 for a recent review) and chronic stimulation (see Jolesz & Sreter 1981; Pette & Vrbova 1985 for reviews) experiments have firmly established that the pattern and quantity of activation are among the many factors that help regulate the phenotype and functional characteristics of skeletal muscle fibres. For example, the relative expression of myosin isoforms is influenced by the degree of mechanical or weight-bearing stress that is imposed on the muscle fibres (Roy *et al.* 1991a). When the relative force demand on a mixed, fast muscle is increased (as in functional overload), the fibres hypertrophy and a selective pool of fibres increase their expression of slow and intermediate isoforms of myosin. This provides a pool of motor units that can meet gravitational demands more effectively. In contrast, if the influences of gravity and weight-bearing are reduced (as in spaceflight or hindlimb unloading), a population of fibres normally expressing predominantly slower myosin isoforms undergoes atrophy, with a down-regulation of slow myosin expression. Thus, in some muscle fibres the expression of myosin isoforms is highly plastic and responsive to the activity-related stress imposed on the fibres. Details of how the stress and strain that occur in a muscle fibre can regulate the myosin genes remain to be resolved.

Although the amount and pattern of neuromuscular activation have a strong influence on skeletal muscle fibre properties, other factors also have regulatory effects. Several lines of evidence emphasize that there is also an activity-independent neural regulation of skeletal muscle properties. For example, long-term cross-reinnervation of a slow muscle with a fast nerve or vice versa results in a conversion of muscle properties towards those normally associated with the 'crossed' nerve, although conversions are incomplete (see Edgerton *et al.* 1996 for a recent review). Similarly, after up to 2 years of inactivity induced by spinal cord isolation, the cat soleus muscle shows the expected conversion of fibres from slow to fast, but it still contains a population of slow fibres (Eldridge & Mommaerts 1981), indicating that the expression of slow phenotypic proteins is activity independent in some fibres. Although activity is reduced to zero in all fibres,

only some convert to a fast phenotype. In spinal isolated cats, cross-reinnervation of the soleus with a fast nerve causes the muscle to become faster than is the case when the soleus muscle is innervated by the soleus nerve (Roy *et al.* 1996b). The physiological motor unit types found in controls are still observed in the cat tibialis anterior after 6 months of inactivity (Pierotti *et al.* 1991, 1994) and, further, the normal interrelationships among size, succinate dehydrogenase and α-glycerophosphate dehydrogenase activity within the fibres of individual tibialis anterior motor units are unchanged following spinal cord isolation (Pierotti *et al.* 1991, 1994). Thus, a high percentage of the size and metabolic properties of skeletal muscles is independent of the levels of neuromuscular activity (Fig. 10.6).

The cat soleus, normally comprised of ~100% slow fibres, maintains a high percentage (~70%) of pure slow fibres after 4 months of inactivity (Zhong *et al.* 1998). Also, the majority of single motor units isolated are comprised exclusively of slow fibres, demonstrating a resistance to adaptation at the motor unit level (Zhong *et al.* 1997). The probability that motor units containing 100 or more fibres would remain homogeneously slow when 30% of the fibres in the muscle cross-section showed some fast myosin heavy chain expression cannot be explained by any random process that might occur in the absence of activity. It demonstrates a strong activity-independent neural influence when the motor unit is electrically silent. In motor units that had fibres expressing fast myosin heavy chains, the fibre type composition was heterogeneous, i.e. the motor unit was comprised of both slow and fast fibres. This indicates that some effect of inactivity was manifested at the motor unit level, but that this influence was not completely attributable to the silent unit.

These data indicate that differential amounts or patterns of neuromuscular activity are not essential to maintain a normal range of histochemical and physiological motor units and muscle fibre types. In addition, these studies show that cross-reinnervation can have a neural influence on muscle proteins even in the absence of neuromuscular activity.

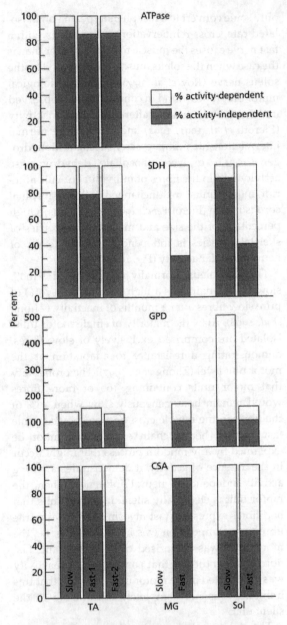

Fig. 10.6 Representation of the neuromuscular activity dependence of adenosine triphosphatase (ATPase), succinate dehydrogenase (SDH) and α-glycerophosphate dehydrogenase (GPD) activities, and cross-sectional area (CSA) in the fibres of the adult cat tibialis anterior (TA), medial gastrocnemius (MG) and soleus (Sol); 100% denotes the neuromuscular activity level in control cats. The percentage activity-independent data (black portion of the bars) are the values from 6-month spinal cord-isolated cats. The TA data are from Pierotti *et al.* (1994), the MG data from Jiang *et al.* (1991) and the Sol data from Graham *et al.* (1992). From Pierotti *et al.* (1994).

Plasticity of motor unit fatigue

The fatiguability of fast and slow muscle fibres (or properties that are related to fatiguability) seem to be affected only minimally by spaceflight or hindlimb unloading. Even during the period of most rapid atrophy of the slow soleus, fatiguability as indicated by standard tests remains relatively unaffected, as do the activities of key enzymes that probably contribute the most towards fatigue resistance. For example, after 7, 14 or 28 days of hindlimb unloading, control levels of citric acid cycle enzymes are maintained in the soleus muscle. At the same time, glycolytic enzyme activities are generally elevated and more fibres express fast myosin than before unloading (Roy *et al.* 1991a; Edgerton & Roy 1996). Neuromuscular fatiguability in response to repetitive electrical stimulation is unchanged in the soleus muscle after 28 days of hindlimb unloading or 14 days of spaceflight. In contrast, predominantly fast muscles become slightly more fatiguable after 4 weeks of unloading, reflecting a significant decrease in succinate dehydrogenase activity (Roy *et al.* 1991a; Edgerton & Roy 1996). Changes in muscle after spaceflight and hindlimb unloading that may contribute to its continued resistance to fatigue include the following: (i) a selective loss of contractile elements relative to mitochondria; (ii) a decrease in fibre size and, thus, diffusion distances from capillaries to the centre of the fibre; (iii) elevated glycolytic capacity; and (iv) elevated vascular density. Factors that might enhance fatiguability would be an increase in the number of fibres that express fast myosin types and a disassembly of contractile elements which could reduce force-generating effectiveness.

It seems likely that greater fatigue when performing daily tasks at 1 G following spaceflight may reflect the overall atrophy of muscle more than changes in the specific fatiguability of the muscle fibres. Atrophied muscles may become fatigued more easily during efforts to complete a given task because more muscle fibres and motor units will be recruited to complete the task. Further, the additional motor units recruited will be the higher threshold units that are generally more fatiguable (Edgerton & Roy 1996).

Can changes in motor unit types and muscle fibre types account for training and detraining effects?

The changes in motoneurones and motor unit types that occur by increasing or decreasing neuromuscular activity levels and the extent to which these changes contribute to changes in exercise performance can be summarized as follows. Generally, changing the activity levels of the normal neuromotor system by training or detraining results in relatively small changes in motor unit type or muscle fibre type. Furthermore, the adaptations that do occur account for a small percentage of the changes in performance associated with training or detraining. With intense training over months, some motor units will modify the type of myosin expressed in the muscle fibres. However, this will consist of a relatively small percentage of the motor units coexpressing multiple myosin isoforms with a complete conversion from fast to slow myosin (or vice versa depending on the specific type of training) occurring in a relatively small number of motor units and in relatively few muscles (Edstrom & Grimby 1986; Enoka 1997). Similarly, even with extreme disruption of motor unit activity levels as is seen following spinal cord injury, the changes in motor unit types and motoneurone properties are modest for at least a year (Edgerton et al. 1980). This is even true for the fatigue properties of muscles months after spinal cord injury (Roy et al. 1991a, 1996b, 1998). Therefore, it appears that the basic unit of the spinal neuromotor system, i.e. the motor unit, is designed with a range of specific combinations of anatomical, biochemical and physiological properties that are remarkably stable under severe and prolonged disturbances of function as can occur in some pathological states and under a wide range of functional demands. This viewpoint, however, does not imply a lack of plasticity of motor unit properties. Adaptations can occur, as discussed above, but within a general biological template for neuromotor systems having the following essential elements: (i) the smallest motor units tend to be slow and very resistant to fatigue; (ii) the moderately sized motor units tend to be fast and relatively resistant to fatigue; and (iii) the largest motor units tend to be fast and very fatiguable. Within this template, the distribution of the population of motor units in a muscle can be shifted towards one extreme or the other, but it appears that a complete conversion of phenotype rarely occurs (Edgerton et al. 1996).

Overloading of the sensorimotor systems

Gerchman et al. (1975) found an elevated oxidative capacity in the ventral horn cells of rats following 52 days of swim training, whereas Pearson and Sickles (1987) reported a reduced oxidative capacity in a motor pool innervating a mixed fast muscle following 60 days of unilateral functional overload in the rat. Although both of these models increase neural activation as determined from chronic EMG recordings (Roy et al. 1985, 1991a,b, 1992; Gardiner et al. 1986), they differ substantially in the pattern of activation and indeed are towards opposite ends of the scale in modulating the mechanical loading of the hindlimb extensor musculature. Chalmers et al. (1991) found no change in the succinate dehydrogenase activity of the cat plantaris motoneurones following 3 months of functional overload. These results may reflect what was only a modest increase in neuronal activity when considering the overall pattern of activity in a 24-h period. When cats are not stimulated to be active they remain quite inactive throughout the day and if functionally overloaded cats are not exercised periodically, muscle hypertrophy will not occur (Roy et al. 1991a). On the other hand, if functionally overloaded cats are walked on a treadmill for brief periods (2–3 min every other day) some (~60%) hypertrophy of the plantaris occurs. If the cats are exercised rigorously (running and jumping daily), the plantaris can undergo a two-fold hypertrophy (Chalmers et al. 1991, 1992a,b). These data suggest that a critical level of recruitment of the plantaris motor pool must occur for a minimal amount of time to induce hypertrophy. This interpretation also seems to apply to oxidative capacity, e.g. the oxidative capacity of functionally overloaded rat plantaris muscles is reduced unless the rats are also endurance trained (Riedy et al. 1985; Roy et al. 1999; cf. Baldwin et al. 1976). Despite the exercise-induced alterations in fibre size and oxidative capacity in the overloaded muscles, these properties are unaffected in the motoneurones (Roy *et al.* 1999).

To determine the level of coordination in succinate dehydrogenase activity between cat plantaris motoneurones and the muscle fibres that they innervate, the soleus and gastrocnemius muscles were bilaterally excised. This functionally overloaded the

plantaris muscle (Chalmers *et al.* 1991, 1992b). After 12 weeks, the muscle fibre size had doubled and the mean muscle fibre succinate dehydrogenase activity had halved, whereas the motoneurone mean succinate dehydrogenase activity and size were unaffected (Fig. 10.7). Total succinate dehydrogenase activity per cell was unchanged in both the motoneurones and muscle fibres following func-

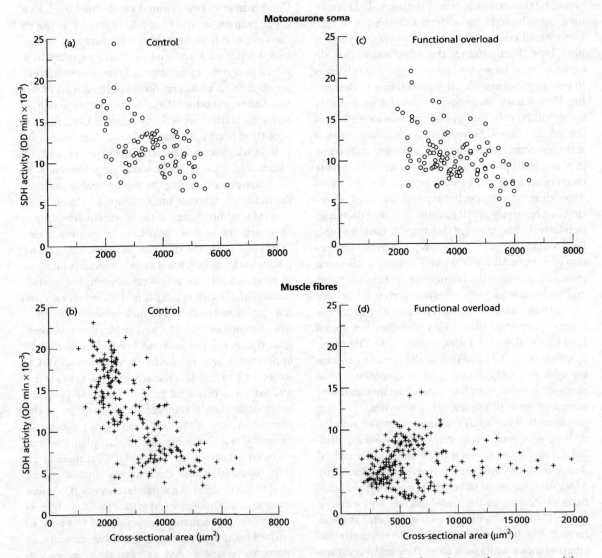

Fig. 10.7 Succinate dehydrogenase (SDH) activity versus cell cross-sectional area for plantaris control motoneurones (a) and muscle fibres (b) and functional overload (FO) motoneurones (c) and muscle fibres (d). Each point represents a single cell. Note the similarity in the shape of the control plots and the FO motoneurone plot and that the scale for the cross-sectional area of FO muscle fibres has been expanded. From Chalmers *et al.* (1991).

tional overload. These changes suggest a selective increase in contractile proteins, but little or no modulation of mitochondrial proteins in the muscle fibres, since total succinate dehydrogenase activity was unchanged following functional overload. These data also demonstrate that while mean succinate dehydrogenase activities are similar in control motoneurones and muscle fibres, mean succinate dehydrogenase activities in these two cell types can change independently. Despite an increase in neuromuscular functional activity and a large increase in the mass of the target tissue (i.e. an increase in muscle fibre size, associated with functional overload) the oxidative capacities of the involved motoneurones and muscle fibres were stressed only minimally.

Reducing the loading of sensorimotor systems

One experimental model used to reduce the demands on motoneurones is axotomy. Once a motoneurone recovers from the initial postaxotomy phase, the biosynthetic demands on the soma are greatly reduced, because 60–80% of the cytoplasmic volume is localized in the distal axonal tree and terminal branches (Edgerton *et al.* 1990). The principal modifications imposed by axotomy are an elimination of neurotransmission at the neuromuscular junction, a reduced biosynthetic demand, a decreased need for axoplasmic transport and a loss of access to neurotrophic factors such as neurotrophin-3 (NT-3) and neurotrophin-4 (NT-4) in the muscle. These modifications appear to decrease the energy demands in the soma, as reflected by a reduction in soma oxidative capacity (Kumamoto & Bourne 1963; Watson 1970).

The mechanisms by which soma metabolism is reduced following axotomy are unknown. Loss of a trophic factor from the target muscle or other peripheral tissues (e.g. Schwann cells, muscle spindles) could be a stimulus to direct the soma to support regrowth metabolically as opposed to the alternative hypothesis of missing terminals. By whatever means the soma is signalled, the decrease in succinate dehydrogenase activity after axotomy indicates a reduced energy demand.

Ventral horn neurones

Spaceflight may impose significant increases or decreases in the function of spinal cord motoneurones (see Krasnov 1994; Roy *et al.* 1996a for recent reviews). A ground-based model of spaceflight (hindlimb unloading in the rat) suggests there is a three-fold increase in the total amount of daily EMG activity of a dorsiflexor muscle (tibialis anterior) within a few days of onset of unloading and this increase persists for at least 4 weeks (Alford *et al.* 1987). The plantarflexor motor pools (soleus and medial gastrocnemius), likewise, are markedly affected, but in this case, the initial response is a marked depression in daily activity, followed by a gradual return to normal levels within about 10 days of unloading. There are no similar data on rats during spaceflight. For both dorsiflexors and plantarflexors, however, it seems highly likely that the amount, source and pattern of proprioceptive inputs to the lumbar motor pools are markedly altered by spaceflight (Krasnov 1994; Roy *et al.* 1996a). Furthermore, one might expect changes only in selected pools of neurones. A clearer understanding of the precise perturbations of an intact neuromotor system that occur during spaceflight could give unique insight into the physiological events that are apparently necessary to change the characteristics of ventral horn neurones.

A subpopulation of medium-sized ventral horn neurones at the L5 segmental level of the spinal cord showed reduced succinate dehydrogenase activity after a 14-day spaceflight. This was still present after 9 days of recovery at 1G (Ishihara *et al.* 1996a) (Fig. 10.8). Persistence of this adaptation is somewhat surprising, since the most severe behavioural changes in motor control seem to be reversed within a week after spaceflight, at least in humans (Edgerton & Roy 1994a, 1996). In another 14-day spaceflight, a population of ventral horn neurones in the upper portion of the lumbar enlargement showed an increase in the proportion of relatively small neurones with high succinate dehydrogenase activities (Jiang *et al.* 1992). Further studies are needed to elucidate how long the reduction in succinate dehydrogenase activity of medium-sized neurones continues after spaceflight and to define the specific

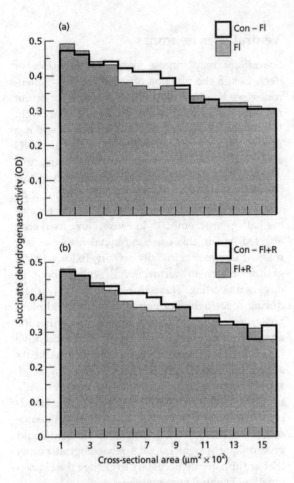

Fig. 10.8 Frequency distributions of the relationship between soma cross-sectional area and succinate dehydrogenase (SDH) activity of neurones in the dorsolateral region of the ventral horn at segmental level L5 of the spinal cord of control–flight and flight rats (a) and of control–flight + recovery and flight + recovery rats (b). The flight period was 14 days and the recovery period was 9 days. Values are based on five rats for each group. Note the decrease in SDH activity in the same bins containing medium-sized neurones in both experimental groups compared to their respective controls. OD, optical density. From Ishihara *et al.* (1996a).

population of neurones that adapt their metabolic properties. The functional consequences of these adaptations also remain undefined.

Despite significant adaptations in the soleus muscle and a reduction in the total amount of daily activation of motoneurones innervating the soleus

muscle (as determined from chronic intramuscular EMG recording during the first few days of hindlimb unloading; Alford *et al.* 1987), hindlimb unloading had no influence on the soma size and succinate dehydrogenase activity of motoneurones innervating the muscle. A lack of adaptation in spinal motoneurones following chronic increases or decreases in neuromuscular activity, i.e. electrical activation and/or mechanical loading (Roy *et al.* 1991a; Edgerton & Roy 1996; Edgerton *et al.* 1996), has been noted above. Chalmers *et al.* (1992b) observed no change in mean soma size or mean succinate dehydrogenase activity in a population of cat motoneurones after spinal cord transection or spinal cord isolation, experimental models that significantly decrease the amount of neuromuscular activity (Alaimo *et al.* 1984; Pierotti *et al.* 1991). Similarly, the soma size and succinate dehydrogenase activity of motoneurones innervating the cat plantaris muscle were unaffected following 3 months of functional overload produced by the removal of its major synergists, a process that resulted in a dramatic increase in fibre size and the proportion of high oxidative fibres (Chalmers *et al.* 1991). Further, Donselaar *et al.* (1986) found no change in the motoneurone soma succinate dehydrogenase activity of cats following 56 days of chronic antidromic electrical stimulation. Thus, it appears that motoneurones can maintain their basic properties, irrespective of chronic periods of decreased or increased activation, and that they are more resistant to change than the muscle fibres that they innervate. Moreover, the soma size and metabolic properties of motoneurones are not tightly coupled to the phenotype of the muscle fibres that they innervate when the neuromuscular system is chronically perturbed.

Combining these results with recent findings from spaceflight (see Krasnov 1994 and Roy *et al.* 1996a for reviews), it appears that spaceflight-induced adaptations cannot be associated simply with chronic non-weight-bearing of the hindlimbs. This viewpoint is supported by the fact that there are no changes in the size or the succinate dehydrogenase activity of motoneurones innervating the rat soleus muscle following 2 weeks of hindlimb unloading, despite alterations in soleus muscle fibre size similar to those observed after a similar period at zero gravity (Ishihara *et al.* 1997c). Altered supraspinal function during spaceflight, such as changes in the vestibular system, could disrupt a specific group of spinal cord neurones and contribute to the spinal plasticity that has been observed.

General morphological and physiological properties of sensory neurones

The sensory neurones located in spinal dorsal root ganglia are described as pseudounipolar neurones. They have somas that lack dendrites and they receive no synaptic endings, at least on the cell bodies (Willis & Coggeshall 1991). Contrary to the somatotopy of motoneurones in the motor pool (McHanwell & Biscoe 1981; Nicolopoulos-Stournaras & Iles 1983), there is no evidence of somatotopic organization and/or clustering of sensory neurones supplying specific muscles, with two exceptions (Baron *et al.* 1988; Peyronnard *et al.* 1990). The spinal projections of the sensory neurones, however, are somatotopically organized (Kuo *et al.* 1981; Peyronnard & Charron 1982; Ygge 1984; Peyronnard *et al.* 1986; Janjua & Leong 1987). In general, somas of neurones belonging to group I and II afferent units are relatively larger than those belonging to groups III and IV. A positive relationship exists between axonal conduction velocity and soma size for all neurones in the dorsal root ganglia ranging from the larger group I to the smaller group IV afferent units (Harper & Lawson 1985; Lee *et al.* 1986). However, there also is an extensive overlap in soma sizes and conduction velocities among neurones of different functional types.

Distinct populations of neurones in the dorsal root ganglia are characterized by a variety of different histochemical enzymes. The relationship between soma size and the activities of some of these enzymes has been investigated. For example, the smaller sensory neurones of the human cervical ganglia have a relatively higher oxidative enzyme (nicotinamide adenine dinucleotide diaphorase tetrazolium reductase and succinate dehydrogenase) activity than larger neurones (Robinson 1969).

Neurones in the dorsal root ganglia of the cat have higher succinate dehydrogenase activities than ventral horn neurones of the spinal cord at the same segmental level (Ishihara *et al.* 1995a).

Little is known about the metabolic properties of sensory neurones in the dorsal root ganglia supplying specific muscles. Although the morphology and metabolism of dorsal root ganglion neurones show some plasticity, the extent and organizational level of this plasticity remain largely undefined, particularly with respect to increased or decreased neuronal activation levels.

Dorsal root ganglia

The cross-sectional areas and succinate dehydrogenase activities of dorsal root ganglion neurones at the L5 segment were determined after 14 days of spaceflight and after 9 days of recovery in the same rats that demonstrated changes in ventral horn neurones (Ishihara *et al.* 1997b). Unlike the motoneurones, the mean succinate dehydrogenase activity of the dorsal root ganglion neurones was significantly lower in spaceflight compared to age-matched control rats. The mean succinate dehydrogenase activity of the total population of dorsal root ganglion neurones had returned to control levels 9 days after the flight. However, the mean succinate dehydrogenase activity of neurones with cross-sectional areas of between 1000 and 2000 μm^2 was 7–10% lower in both the spaceflight and the spaceflight plus recovery groups than in the corresponding control groups. The reduction in oxidative capacity of a subpopulation of sensory neurones having relatively large cross-sectional areas immediately following spaceflight and the sustained depression for 9 days after returning to a normal gravitational field suggest that the zero-gravity environment induced significant alterations in proprioceptive function (Fig. 10.9).

Although neither the type of sensory neurones affected nor the site of the receptors of the sensory neurones were determined, most rat sensory neurones belonging to groups Ia and II are large neurones with diameters exceeding 30 μm (Peyronnard *et al.* 1988) or 35 μm (Peyronnard *et al.* 1986), consistent with the interpretation that sensory receptors in

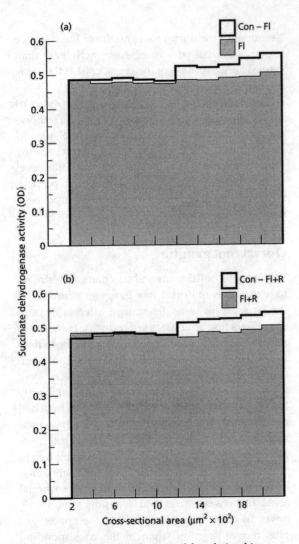

Fig. 10.9 Frequency distributions of the relationship between soma cross-sectional area and succinate dehydrogenase (SDH) activity of neurones in the dorsal root ganglia at segmental level L5 of the spinal cord of control–flight and flight rats (a) and of control–flight + recovery and flight + recovery rats (b). The flight period was 14 days and the recovery period was 9 days. Values are based on five rats for each group. Note the decrease in SDH activity in the same bins containing relatively large-sized neurones in both experimental groups compared to their respective controls. OD, optical density. Data from Table 1 in Ishihara *et al.* (1997b).

skeletal muscles could have contributed to the changes observed in the dorsal root ganglion neurones. These data are also consistent with the view that spaceflight induces changes in sensory function, and that these changes persist some days after return to a 1 G environment, as do some of the alterations in motor control (Edgerton & Roy 1994a,b, 1996; Roy *et al.* 1996a).

Adaptive response — summary

In summary, soma size and the oxidative potential of the motoneurones seem to have only limited roles in regulating the motor unit plasticity associated with chronic modulation of neuromuscular activity. The persistence of normal motoneurone properties even after extreme perturbations of neuromuscular activity could reflect the importance of multiple homeostatic mechanisms that maintain normal motor function. These data suggest that in spite of the functional interdependence of a motoneurone and the muscle fibres it innervates, the adaptations within the different components of the motor unit are not tightly coordinated. Further, it seems unlikely that the diversities of skeletal muscle fibre hypertrophy and biochemistry are closely linked to the oxidative potential and soma size of motoneurones or to their adaptability in soma size and oxidative potential.

The results summarized in this chapter provide a perspective on the adaptive potential of the neural components of the sensorimotor system, which reflect resistance to perturbation. The general stability of the oxidative potential of neurones despite marked changes in activity levels may at first seem unexpected, given the importance of oxidative metabolism to the function and survival of neurones. Given that neural survival demands a critical level of oxidative phosphorylation, perhaps the neural system is designed to function identically over a wide range of physiological and metabolic demands, assuming some threshold level of availability of oxygen and substrates. The muscles seem to operate on a graduated scale, i.e. the greater the metabolic demand over a period of weeks, the greater the metabolic enhancement in the muscle fibres. This change is coupled to the fact that more work can be accomplished by the muscle. The central nervous system, on the other hand, does not adopt this strategy. Its function remains more constant over a wide range of acceptable conditions, and it fails rapidly if these conditions are not maintained. In this sense, modest changes in the oxidative phosphorylation potential of neurones may have little functional consequence. The extraordinary functional plasticity reflected in spinal networks that generate stepping and the ability to modulate their functional properties in a highly specific use-dependent manner (Hodgson *et al.* 1994; Edgerton *et al.* 1997; de Leon *et al.* 1998a,b) suggest that other strategies are adopted by the nervous system to adapt to use, and these are not based on the potential to enhance or reduce oxidative phosphorylation.

These studies of metabolic adaptations in sensorimotor neurones lead to a number of questions. Why does a significant modification of use and loading patterns as occurs in spaceflight have such a selective and sustained effect on the oxidative phosphorylation potential of motor and sensory neurones in the spinal cord? What are the perturbations of the oxygen requirements of specific neuronal functions that could trigger this selective and sustained effect? An initial approach to these questions could be to design experiments in which the types of neurotransmitters can be identified in neurones of known targets and known physiological properties. Ideally, these experiments would be more informative when conducted under the most '*in vivo*-like' conditions.

Conclusions

1 The metabolic and morphological properties of both the motor and the sensory elements of the neural pathways associated with the hindlimbs are resistant to chronic changes in neuromuscular activity.

2 Neuromuscular fatiguability does not appear to be due to adaptations in the metabolic potential of either the motor or sensory neurones.

3 The maintenance of force during repetitive contractions is accomplished by recruitment of additional motor units and by increased firing rates of already activated motor units.

4 The neuromuscular system is designed to insure that the most fatigue-resistant motor units are preferentially recruited during tasks requiring low forces or power; larger, more fatiguable motor units are recruited only when there are demands for high forces or power.

5 The recruitment of different combinations of motor pools to perform motor tasks and the factors that determine how many motor units are needed from each motor pool to complete the intended task successfully will be a function of: (i) the skill level of the subject; (ii) the specific motor patterns that have been learned over a period of weeks or months; and (iii) the properties of the motor units recruited.

6 The number of motor units that are recruited to perform a task can change significantly if the force outputs of the motor units are changed. To compensate for muscle atrophy, for example, more motor units must be recruited to perform the same task. The additional units recruited will be more fatiguable than the population of motor units recruited initially. In contrast, if a muscle hypertrophies, i.e. muscle fibres and/or motor units increase in size and force potential, then fewer units will be recruited to perform the same task. These motor units will be less fatiguable than the population of motor units recruited prior to hypertrophy.

7 The role of sensory input in modulating motor output in normal motor performances remains largely undefined, even in animal models of physical activity.

Acknowledgements

We would like to thank all of our coworkers who have contributed significantly to the work presented in this chapter. We also thank Miss J. Kim for her assistance in preparing the figures for this chapter. A large portion of this work was supported, in part, by NIH Grant NS16333 (VRE and RRR), NASA Grant NAG-2–717 and 438 (VRE and RRR) and the National Space Development Agency of Japan (AI). All figures are reproduced from the original articles with permission from the publishers.

References

Alaimo, M.A., Smith, J.L., Roy, R.R. & Edgerton, V.R. (1984) EMG activity of slow and fast ankle extensors following spinal cord transection. *Journal of Applied Physiology* **56**, 1608–1613.

Alford, E.K., Roy, R.R., Hodgson, J.A. & Edgerton, V.R. (1987) Electromyography of rat soleus, medial gastrocnemius and tibialis anterior during hindlimb suspension. *Experimental Neurology* **96**, 635–649.

Allen, D.L., Monke, S.R., Talmadge, R.J., Roy, R.R. & Edgerton, V.R. (1995) Plasticity of myonuclear number in hypertrophied and atrophied mammalian muscle fibers. *Journal of Applied Physiology* **78**, 1969–1976.

Allen, D.L., Yasui, W., Tanaka, T. *et al.* (1996) Myonuclear number and myosin heavy chain expression in rat soleus single muscle fibers following spaceflight. *Journal of Applied Physiology* **81**, 145–151.

Allen, D.L., Linderman, J.K., Roy, R.R., Grindeland, R.E., Mukku, V. & Edgerton, V.R. (1997) Growth hormone/IGF-I and/or resistive exercise maintains myonuclear number in hindlimb unweighted muscles. *Journal of Applied Physiology* **83**, 1857–1861.

Altman, P.L. & Dittmer, D.S. (1971) *Respiration and Circulation*, pp. 460–467. Federation of American Societies of Experimental Biology, Bethesda.

van Asselt, E., de Graaf, F. & van Raamsdonk, W. (1993) Ultrastructural characteristics of zebrafish spinal motoneurons innervating glycolytic white, and oxidative red and intermediate muscle fibers. *Acta Histochimica* **95**, 31–44.

Baldwin, K.M., Martinez, O.M. & Cheadle, W.G. (1976) Enzymatic changes in hypertrophied fast-twitch skeletal muscle. *Pflügers Archives* **364**, 229–234.

Balice-Gordon, R.J. & Thompson, W.J. (1988) The organization and development of compartmentalized innervation in rat extensor digitorum longus muscle. *Journal of Physiology (London)* **398**, 211–231.

Baron, R., Janig, W. & Kollmann, W. (1988) Sympathetic and afferent somata projecting in hindlimb nerves and the anatomical organization of the lumbar sympathetic nervous system of the rat. *Journal of Comparative Neurology* **275**, 460–468.

Barrett, J.N. & Crill, W.E. (1971) Specific membrane resistivity of dye-injected cat motoneurons. *Brain Research* **28**, 556–561.

Barrett, J.N. & Crill, W.E. (1974) Specific membrane properties of cat motoneurones. *Journal of Physiology (London)* **239**, 301–324.

Bodine, S.C., Roy, R.R., Eldred, E. & Edgerton, V.R. (1987) Maximal force as a function of anatomical features of motor units in the cat tibialis anterior. *Journal of Neurophysiology* **57**, 1730–1745.

Buller, A.J., Eccles, J.C. & Eccles, R.M. (1960) Interactions between motorneurones and muscles in respect of the characteristic speeds of their responses. *Journal of Physiology (London)* **150**, 417–430.

Burke, R.E. (1981) Motor units: anatomy, physiology, and functional organization. In: Brokhart, J.M. & Mountcastle, V.B. (eds) *Handbook of Physiology*, Section 1, *The Nervous System*, Vol. 2, *Motor Control*, Part 2, pp. 345–422. American Physiological Society, Bethesda.

Burke, R.E., Strick, P.L., Kanda, K., Kim, C.C. & Walmsley, B. (1977) Anatomy of medial gastrocnemius and soleus motor nuclei in cat spinal cord. *Journal of Neurophysiology* **40**, 667–680.

Burke, R.E., Dum, R.P., Fleshman, J.W. *et al.* (1982) An HRP study of the relation between cell size and motor unit type in cat ankle extensor motoneurons. *Journal of Comparative Neurology* **209**, 17–28.

Chalmers, G.R. & Edgerton, V.R. (1989a) Marked and variable inhibition by chemical fixation of cytochrome oxidase and succinate dehydrogenase in single motoneurons. *Journal of Histochemistry and Cytochemistry* **37**, 899–901.

Chalmers, G.R. & Edgerton, V.R. (1989b) Single motoneuron succinate dehydrogenase activity. *Journal of Histochemistry and Cytochemistry* **37**, 1107–1114.

Chalmers, G.R., Roy, R.R. & Edgerton, V.R. (1991) Motoneuron and muscle fiber succinate dehydrogenase activity in control and overloaded plantaris. *Journal of Applied Physiology* **71**, 1589–1592.

Chalmers, G.C., Roy, R.R. & Edgerton, V.R. (1992a) Variation and limitations in fiber enzymatic and size responses in hypertrophied muscle. *Journal of Applied Physiology* **73**, 631–641.

Chalmers, G.R., Roy, R.R. & Edgerton, V.R. (1992b) Adaptability of the oxidative capacity of motoneurons. *Brain Research* **570**, 1–10.

Cullheim, S. (1978) Relations between cell body size, axon diameter and axon conduction velocity of cat sciatic α-motoneurons stained with horseradish peroxidase. *Neuroscience Letters* **8**, 17–20.

Cullheim, S. & Ulfhake, B. (1979) Relations between cell body size, axon diameter and axon conduction velocity of triceps surae alpha motoneurons during postnatal development in the cat. *Journal of Comparative Neurology* **188**, 679–686.

Donselaar, Y., Kernell, D. & Eerbeek, O. (1986) Soma size and oxidative enzyme activity in normal and chronically stimulated motoneurones of the cat's spinal cord. *Brain Research* **385**, 22–29.

Edgerton, V.R. & Roy, R.R. (1991) Regulation of skeletal muscle fiber size, shape and function. *Journal of Biomechanics* **24** (Suppl. 1), 123–133.

Edgerton, V.R. & Roy, R.R. (1994a) Nervous system and sensory adaptation: neural plasticity associated with chronic neuromuscular activity. In: Bouchard, C., Shephard, R.J. & Stephens, T. (eds) *Physical Activity, Fitness, and Health: International Proceedings and Consensus Statement*, 2nd edn, pp. 511–520. Human Kinetics, Champaign, IL.

Edgerton, V.R. & Roy, R.R. (1994b) Neuromuscular adaptation to actual and simulated weightlessness. In: Bonting, S.L. (ed.) *Advances in Space Biology and Medicine*, Vol. 4, pp. 33–67. JAI Press Inc, Greenwich, Connecticut.

Edgerton, V.R. & Roy, R.R. (1996) Neuromuscular adaptations to actual and simulated spaceflight. In: Fregly, M.J. & Blatteis, C.M. (eds) *Handbook of Physiology*, Section 4. *Environmental Physiology*, III, *The Gravitational Environment*, pp. 721–763. Oxford University Press, New York.

Edgerton, V.R., Goslow, G.E. Jr, Rasmussen, S.A. & Spector, S.A. (1980) Is resistance to fatigue controlled by its motoneurones? *Nature* **285**, 589–590.

Edgerton, V.R., Roy, R.R. & Chalmers, G.R. (1990) Does the size principle give insight into the energy requirements of motoneurons? In: Binder, M.D. & Mendell, L.M. (eds) *The Segmental Motor System*, pp. 150–164. Oxford University Press, New York.

Edgerton, V.R., Bodine-Fowler, S., Roy, R.R., Ishihara, A. & Hodgson, J.A. (1996) Neuromuscular adaptation. In: Rowell L.B. & Shepherd, J.T. (eds) *Handbook of Physiology*, Section 12. *Exercise: Regulation and Integration of Multiple Systems*, pp. 54–88. Oxford University Press, New York.

Edgerton, V.R., Roy, R.R., de Leon, R., Tillakaratne, N. & Hodgson, J.A. (1997) Does motor learning occur in the spinal cord? *Neuroscientist* **3**, 287–294.

Edstrom, L. & Grimby, L. (1986) Effect of exercise on the motor unit. *Muscle and Nerve* **9**, 104–126.

Eldridge, L. & Mommaerts, W.H.M. (1981) Ability of electrical silent nerves to specify fast and slow muscle characteristics. In: Pette, D. (ed.) *Plasticity of Muscle*, pp. 325–337. Walter de Gruyter, Berlin.

Enoka, R.M. (1997) Neural adaptations with chronic physical activity. *Journal of Biomechanics* **30**, 447–455.

Gardiner, P., Michel, R., Bowman, C. & Noble, E. (1986) Increased EMG of rat plantaris during locomotion following surgical removal of its synergists. *Brain Research* **380**, 114–121.

Gerchman, L.B., Edgerton, V.R. & Carrow, R.E. (1975) Effects of physical training on the histochemistry and morphology of ventral motor neurons. *Experimental Neurology* **49**, 790–801.

Graham, S.C., Roy, R.R., Navarro, C. et al. (1992) Enzyme and size profiles in chronically inactive cat soleus muscle fibers. *Muscle and Nerve* **15**, 27–36.

Hainsworth, F.R. (1981) *Animal Physiology: Adaptation in Function.* Addison-Wesley Publishing Company Inc., Massachusetts.

Hamm, T.M., Reinking, R.M. & Stuart, D.G. (1989) Electromyographic responses of mammalian motor units to a fatigue test. *Electromyography and Clinical Neurophysiology* **29**, 485–494.

Harper, A.A. & Lawson, S.N. (1985) Conduction velocity is related to morphological cell type in rat dorsal root ganglion neurones. *Journal of Physiology (London)* **359**, 31–46.

Henneman, E. & Mendell, L.M. (1981) Functional organization of motoneuron pool and its inputs. In: Brookhart, J.M. Mountcastle, V.B., Brooks V.B. & Geiger, S.R. (eds) *Handbook of Physiology*, Section 1, *The Nervous System*, Vol. II, *Motor Control*, Part I, pp. 423–507. American Physiological Society, Bethesda.

Henneman, E., Somjen, G. & Carpenter, D.O. (1965) Functional significance of cell size in spinal motoneurons. *Journal of Neurophysiology* **28**, 560–580.

Hennig, R. & Lomo, T. (1985) Firing patterns of motor units in normal rats. *Nature* **314**, 164–166.

Hill, R.W. (1976) *Comparative Physiology of Animals: an Environmental Approach.* Harper and Row Publishers, New York.

Hodgson, J.A., Roy, R.R., de Leon, R.,

Dobkin, B. & Edgerton, V.R. (1994) Can the mammalian lumbar spinal cord learn a motor task? *Medicine and Science in Sports and Exercise* **26**, 1491–1497.

Iliya, A.R. & Dum, R.P. (1988) Somatopic relations between the motor nucleus and its innervated muscle fibers in the cat tibialis anterior. *Experimental Neurology* **86**, 272–292.

Ishihara, A., Naitoh, H., Araki, H. & Nishihira, Y. (1988) Soma size and oxidative enzyme activity of motoneurones supplying the fast twitch and slow twitch muscles in the rat. *Brain Research* **446**, 195–198.

Ishihara, A., Araki, H. & Nishihira, Y. (1989) Menadione-linked alpha-glycerophosphate dehydrogenase activity of motoneurons in rat soleus and extensor digitorum longus neuron pools. *Neurochemistry Research* **14**, 455–458.

Ishihara, A., Taguchi, S., Araki, H. & Nishihira, Y. (1991a) Retrograde neuronal labeling of motoneurons in the rat by fluorescent tracers, and quantitative analysis of oxidative enzyme activity in labeled neurons. *Neuroscience Letters* **124**, 141–143.

Ishihara, A., Taguchi, S., Araki, H. & Nishihira, Y. (1991b) Oxidative and glycolytic metabolism of the tibialis anterior motoneurons in the rat. *Acta Physiologica Scandinavica* **141**, 129–130.

Ishihara, A., Roy, R.R. & Edgerton, V.R. (1995a) Succinate dehydrogenase activity and soma size relationships among cat dorsal root ganglion neurons. *Brain Research* **676**, 212–218.

Ishihara, A., Roy, R.R. & Edgerton, V.R. (1995b) Succinate dehydrogenase activity and soma size of motoneurons innervating different portions of the rat tibialis anterior. *Neuroscience* **68**, 813–822.

Ishihara, A., Ohira, Y., Roy, R.R. et al. (1996a) Influence of spaceflight on succinate dehydrogenase activity and soma size of rat ventral horn neurons. *Acta Anatomica* **157**, 303–308.

Ishihara, A., Roy, R.R. & Edgerton, V.R. (1996b) Comparison of succinate dehydrogenase activity and soma size relationships among neurons in dorsal root ganglia of rats and cats. *Brain Research* **716**, 183–186.

Ishihara, A., Hayashi, S., Roy, R.R. et al. (1997a) Mitochondrial density of ventral horn neurons in the rat spinal cord. *Acta Anatomica* **160**, 248–253.

Ishihara, A., Ohira, Y., Roy, R.R. et al. (1997b) Effects of 14 days of spaceflight and 9 days of recovery on cell body size

and succinate dehydrogenase activity of rat dorsal root ganglion neurons. *Neuroscience* **81**, 275–279.

Ishihara, A., Oishi, Y., Roy, R.R. & Edgerton, V.R. (1997c) Influence of two weeks of non-weight bearing on rat soleus motoneurons and muscle fibers. *Aviation, Space and Environmental Medicine* **68**, 421–425.

Janjua, M.Z. & Leong, S.K. (1987) Sensory, motor and sympathetic neurons forming the common peroneal and tibial nerves in the macaque monkey (*Macaca fascicularis*). *Journal of Anatomy* **153**, 63–76.

Jankowska, E. (1983) On the multiplicity of neuronal pathways from muscle spindles and tendon organs and their selection in the cat. *Journal of Physiology (Paris)* **78**, 772–774.

Jiang, B., Roy, R.R., Navarro, C., Nguyen, Q., Pierotti, D. & Edgerton, V.R. (1991) Enzymatic responses of cat medial gastrocnemius fibers to chronic inactivity. *Journal of Applied Physiology* **70**, 231–239.

Jiang, B., Roy, R.R., Polyakov, I.V., Krasnov, I.B. & Edgerton, V.R. (1992) Ventral horn cell responses to spaceflight and hindlimb suspension. *Journal of Applied Physiology* **73** (Suppl.), 107S–111S.

Johnson, I.P.A. (1986) A quantitative ultra-structural comparison of alpha and gamma motoneurons in the thoracic region of the spinal cord of the adult cat. *Journal of Anatomy* **147**, 55–72.

Jolesz, F. & Sreter, F.A. (1981) Development, innervation, and activity-pattern induced changes in skeletal muscle. *Annual Review of Physiology* **43**, 531–552.

Kenyon, R.V. & Young, L.R. (1986) M.I.T./Canadian vestibular experiments on the Spacelab-1 mission: 5. Postural responses following exposure to weightlessness. *Experimental Brain Research* **64**, 335–346.

Kernell, D. & Zwaagstra, B. (1981) Input conductance, axonal conduction velocity and cell size among hindlimb motoneurones of the cat. *Brain Research* **204**, 311–326.

Kozlovskaya, I.B., Kreidich, Y.V., Oganov, V.S. & Koserenko, O.P. (1981) Pathophysiology of motor functions in prolonged space flights. *Acta Astronautica* **8**, 1059–1072.

Krasnov, I.B. (1994) Gravitational neuromorphology. In: Bonting, S.L. (ed) *Advances in Space Biology and Medicine*, pp. 111–126. JAI Press Inc, Greenwich.

Kumamoto, T. & Bourne, G.H. (1963) Experimental studies on the oxidative enzymes and hydrolytic enzymes in spinal neurons. *Acta Anatomica* **55**, 255–277.

Kuo, D.C., Krauthamer, G.M. & Yamasaki, D.S. (1981) The organization of visceral sensory neurons in thoracic dorsal root ganglia (DRG) of the cat studied by horseradish peroxidase (HRP) reaction using the cryostat. *Brain Research* **208**, 187–191.

Layne, C.S., McDonald, P.V. & Bloomberg, J.J. (1997) Neuromuscular activation patterns during treadmill walking after space flight. *Experimental Brain Research* **113**, 104–116.

Lee, K.H., Chung, K., Chung, J.M. & Coggeshall, R.E. (1986) Correlation of cell body size, axon size, and signal conduction velocity for individually labelled dorsal root ganglion cells in the cat. *Journal of Comparative Neurology* **243**, 335–346.

de Leon, R.D., Hodgson, J.A., Roy, R.R. & Edgerton, V.R. (1998a) Full weight-bearing hindlimb standing following stand training in the adult spinal cat. *Journal of Neurophysiology* **80**, 83–91.

de Leon, R.D., Hodgson, J.A., Roy, R.R. & Edgerton, V.R. (1998b) Locomotor capacity attributable to step training versus spontaneous recovery following spinalization in adult cats. *Journal of Neurophysiology* **79**, 1329–1340.

Lowry, O.H. (1975) Energy metabolism in brain and its control. In: Ingvar, D.H. & Lassen, N.A. (eds) *Brain Work*, pp. 48–63. Academic Press, New York.

Magus, R. (1924) *Korpersfellung*, p. 540. Springer-Verlag, Berlin.

Marsden, C.D., Meadows, J.C. & Merton, P.A. (1983) 'Muscular wisdom' that minimizes fatigue during prolonged effort in man: peak rates of motoneuron discharge and slowing of discharge during fatigue. *Advances in Neurology* **39**, 169–211.

Mayes, J.I. & Govind, C.K. (1989) Higher mitochondrial density in slow versus fast lobster sensory neurons. *Neuroscience Letters* **17**, 87–90.

McDonagh, J.C., Binder, M.D., Reinking, R.M. & Stuart, D.G. (1980) Tetrapartite classification of motor units of cat tibialis posterior. *Journal of Neurophysiology* **44**, 696–712.

McHanwell, S. & Biscoe, T.J. (1981) The sizes of motoneurons supplying hindlimb muscles in the mouse. *Proceedings of the Royal Society of London (Biology)* **213**, 201–216.

Mendell, L.M., Collins, W.F. III & Koerber, H.R. (1990) How are Ia synapses distributed on spinal motoneurons to permit

orderly recruitment? In: Binder, M.D. & Mendell, L.M. (eds) *The Segmental Motor System*, pp. 308–327. Oxford University Press, New York.

Miyata, H. & Kawai, Y. (1992) Relationship between soma diameter and oxidative enzyme activity of α-motoneurons. *Brain Research* **581**, 101–107.

Mjaatvedt, A.E. & Wong-Riley, M.T.T. (1986) Double-labeling of rat α-motoneurons for cytochrome oxidase and retrogradely transported [³H]WGA. *Brain Research* **368**, 178–182.

Nelson, S.G. & Mendell, L.M. (1978) Projection of single knee flexor Ia fibers to homonymous and heteronymous motoneurons. *Journal of Neurophysiology* **41**, 778–787.

Nicolopoulos-Stournaras, S. & Iles, J.F. (1983) Motor neuron columns in the lumbar spinal cord of the rat. *Journal of Comparative Neurology* **217**, 75–85.

Osborn, C.E. & Poppele, R.E. (1988) The extent of polysynaptic responses in the dorsal spinocerebellar tract to stimulation of group I afferent fibers in gastrocnemius-soleus. *Journal of Neuroscience* **8**, 316–319.

Passonneau, J.V. & Lowry, O.H. (1971) Metabolic flux in single neurons during ischemia and anesthesia. *Current Problems in Clinical Biochemistry* **3**, 198–212.

Pearson, J.K. & Sickles, D.W. (1987) Enzyme activity changes in rat soleus motoneurons and muscle after synergist ablation. *Journal of Applied Physiology* **63**, 2301–2308.

Penny, J.E., Kukums, J.R., Taylor, J.H. & Eadie, M.J. (1975) Quantitative oxidative enzyme histochemistry of the spinal cord. Part 2. Relation of cell size and enzyme activity to vulnerability to ischaemia. *Journal of the Neurological Sciences* **26**, 187–192.

Person, R.S. & Kudina, L.P. (1972) Discharge frequency and discharge pattern of human motor units during voluntary contraction of muscle. *Electroencephalography and Clinical Neurophysiology* **32**, 471–483.

Pette, D. & Vrbova, G. (1985) Neural control of phenotypic expression in mammalian muscle fibers. *Muscle and Nerve* **8**, 676–689.

Peyronnard, J.M. & Charron, L. (1982) Motor and sensory neurons of the rat sural nerve: a horseradish peroxidase study. *Muscle and Nerve* **5**, 654–660.

Peyronnard, J.M., Charron, L.F. & Messier, J.P. (1986) Motor, sympathetic and sensory innervation of rat skeletal muscles. *Brain Research* **373**, 288–302.

Peyronnard, J.M., Charron, L., Lavoie, J., Messier, J.R. & Dubreuil, M. (1988) Carbonic anhydrase and horseradish peroxidase: double labelling of rat dorsal root ganglion neurons innervating motor and sensory peripheral nerves. *Anatomy and Embryology* **177**, 353–359.

Peyronnard, J.M., Messier, J.P., Dubreuil, M., Charron, L. & Lebel, F. (1990) Three-dimensional computer-aided analysis of the intraganglionic topography of primary muscle afferent neurons in the rat. *Anatomical Record* **227**, 405–417.

Pierotti, D., Roy, R.R., Bodine-Fowler, S., Hodgson, J. & Edgerton, V.R. (1991) Effects of chronic inactivity on the contractile properties and spatial distribution of the motor units of the cat tibialis anterior. *Journal of Physiology (London)* **444**, 175–192.

Pierotti, D.J., Roy, R.R., Hodgson, J.A. & Edgerton, V.R. (1994) Level of independence of motor unit properties from neuromuscular activity. *Muscle and Nerve* **17**, 1324–1335.

Riedy, M., Moore, R.L. & Gollnick, P.D. (1985) Adaptive response of hypertrophied skeletal muscle to endurance training. *Journal of Applied Physiology* **59**, 127–131.

Ritchie, J.M. (1967) The oxygen consumption of mammalian non-myelinated nerve fibers at rest and during activity. *Journal of Physiology (London)* **188**, 309–329.

Robinson, N. (1969) Histochemistry of human cervical posterior root ganglion cells and a comparison with anterior horn cells. *Journal of Anatomy* **104**, 55–64.

Roy, R.R., Hirota, W.K., Kuehl, M. & Edgerton, V.R. (1985) Recruitment patterns in the rat hindlimb muscle during swimming. *Brain Research* **337**, 175–178.

Roy, R.R., Baldwin, K.M. & Edgerton, V.R. (1991a) The plasticity of skeletal muscle: effects of neuromuscular activity. In: Holloszy, J. (ed.) *Exercise and Sport Sciences Reviews*, Vol. 19, pp. 269–312. Williams & Wilkins, Baltimore.

Roy, R.R., Hutchison, D.L., Pierotti, D.J., Hodgson, J.A. & Edgerton, V.R. (1991b) EMG patterns of rat ankle extensors and flexors during treadmill locomotion and swimming. *Journal of Applied Physiology* **70**, 2522–2529.

Roy, R.R., Hodgson, J.A., Chalmers, G.R., Buxton, W. & Edgerton, V.R. (1992) Responsiveness of the cat plantaris to functional overload. In: Sato, Y., Poortmans, J., Hashimoto I. & Oshida, Y. (eds) *Medicine and Sports Science: Integration of*

Medical and Sport Sciences, Vol. 37, pp. 43–51. Karger Press, Switzerland.

Roy, R.R., Baldwin, K.M. & Edgerton, V.R. (1996a) Response of the neuromuscular unit to spaceflight: what has been learned from the rat model? In: Holloszy, J. (ed.) *Exercise and Sport Sciences Reviews*, Vol. 24, pp. 399–425. Williams & Wilkins, Baltimore.

Roy, R.R., Eldridge, L., Baldwin, K.M. & Edgerton, V.R. (1996b) Neural influence on slow muscle properties: inactivity with and without cross-reinnervation. *Muscle and Nerve* **19**, 707–714.

Roy, R.R., Talmadge, R.J., Hodgson, J.A., Zhong, H., Baldwin, K.M. & Edgerton, V.R. (1998) Training effects on soleus of cats spinal cord transected (T12–13) as adults. *Muscle and Nerve* **21**, 63–71.

Roy, R.R., Ishihara, A., Kim, J.A., Lee, M., Fox, K. & Edgerton, V.R. (1999) Metabolic and morphologic stability of motoneurons in response to chronically elevated neuromuscular activity. *Neuroscience* **92**, 361–366.

Schmidt-Nielsen, K. (1972) Locomotion: energy cost of swimming, flying, and running. *Science* **177**, 222–228.

Sickles, D.W. & McLendon, R.E. (1983) Metabolic variation among rat lumbosacral α-motoneurons. *Histochemistry* **79**, 205–217.

Sickles, D.W. & Oblak, T.G. (1983) A horseradish peroxidase labeling technique for correlation of motoneuron metabolic activity with muscle fiber types. *Journal of Neuroscience Methods* **7**, 195–201.

Sickles, D.W. & Oblak, T.G. (1984) Metabolic variation among α-motoneurons innervating different muscle-fiber types. I. Oxidative enzyme activity. *Journal of Neurophysiology* **51**, 529–537.

Sokoloff, L. (1984) *Metabolic Probes of Central Nervous System Activity in Experimental Animals and Man.* Sinauer Associates, Sunderland, Massachusetts.

Swett, J.E., Wikholm, R.P., Blanks, R.H.I., Swett, A.L. & Conley, L.L. (1986) Motoneurons of the rat sciatic nerve. *Experimental Neurology* **93**, 227–252.

Tamaki, H., Kitada, K., Akamine, T., Murata, F., Sakou, T. & Kurata, H. (1998) Alternate activity in the synergistic muscles during prolonged low-level contractions. *Journal of Applied Physiology* **84**, 1943–1951.

Tansey, K.E. & Botterman, B.R. (1996) Activation of type-identified motor units during centrally evoked contractions in the cat medial gastrocnemius muscle. II. Motoneuron firing-rate modulation. *Journal of Neurophysiology* **75**, 38–50.

Tansey, K.E., Yee, A.K. & Botterman, B.R. (1996) Activation of type-identified motor units during centrally evoked contractions in the cat medial gastrocnemius muscle. III. Muscle-unit force modulation. *Journal of Neurophysiology* **75**, 51–59.

Taylor, C.R., Schmidt-Nielsen, K. & Raab, J.L. (1970) Scaling of energetic cost of running to body size in mammals. *American Journal of Physiology* **219**, 1104–1107.

Tseng, B.S., Kasper, C.E. & Edgerton, V.R. (1994) Cytoplasm-to-myonucleus ratios and succinate dehydrogenase activities in adult rat slow and fast muscle fibers. *Cell Tissue Research* **275**, 39–49.

Watson, W.E. (1970) Some metabolic responses of axotomized neurones to contact between their axons and denervated muscle. *Journal of Physiology (London)* **210**, 321–343.

Weeks, O.I. & English, A.W. (1985) Compartmentalization of the cat lateral gastrocnemius motor nucleus. *Journal of Comparative Neurology* **235**, 255–267.

Westbury, D.R. (1982) A comparison of the structures of alpha and gamma spinal motoneurones of the cat. *Journal of Physiology (London)* **325**, 79–91.

Willis, W.D. Jr & Coggeshall, R.E. (1991) Dorsal root ganglion cells and their processes. In: *Sensory Mechanisms of the Spinal Cord*, 2nd edn, pp. 47–78. Plenum Press, New York.

Wong-Riley, M.T.T. & Kageyama, G.H. (1986) Localization of cytochrome oxidase in the mammalian spinal cord and dorsal root ganglia, with quantitative analysis of ventral horn cells in monkey. *Journal of Comparative Neurology* **245**, 41–61.

Ygge, J. (1984) On the organization of the thoracic spinal ganglion and nerve in the rat. *Experimental Brain Research* **55**, 395–401.

Zhong, H., Roy, R.R., Talmadge, R.J., Grossman, E.J., Hodgson, J.A. & Edgerton, V.R. (1997) Effects of chronic inactivity on the mechanical and myosin heavy chain properties of adult cat soleus motor units. *Society for Neuroscience Abstracts* **23**, 2093.

Zhong, V., Roy, R.R., Siengthai, B. *et al.* (1998) Adaptations of cat soleus muscle fiber size and phenotype to chronic neuromuscular inactivity. *Society for Neuroscience Abstracts* **23**, 1674.

Zwaagstra, B. & Kernell, D. (1980) The duration of after-hyperpolarization in hindlimb alpha motoneurones of different sizes in the cat. *Neuroscience Letters* **19**, 303–307.

Chapter 11

Muscular Factors in Endurance

HOWARD J. GREEN

Introduction

Successful performance in a wide variety of sporting tasks often depends on the ability to perform the task repeatedly without impairment of the fundamental physical components resident in the task. The physical demands of the task may range from those requiring large expressions of force and power, encompassing the isometric or near isometric, to high velocity and involving both shortening (concentric) and lengthening (eccentric) contractions. Moreover, the task may vary in complexity, from depending primarily at one extreme on the recruitment of a single muscle group to the involvement of a wide range of synergistic muscles, both agonists and antagonists, at the other extreme. A failure of the neural system to recruit repeatedly and appropriately, both temporally and spatially, specific motor units both within and between muscles and/or a failure of the muscular system to respond adequately could lead to a rapid loss of coordination and a deterioration in task performance.

Task failure as a consequence of repetitive activity, or conversely the ability to endure and to resist fatigue, can be addressed at a number of levels of organization, including the molecular, cellular, motor unit and ultimately the systems level, where the behaviour of either the whole muscle or a group of synergistic muscles represents the primary focus. As the level of complexity increases, so do the potential mechanisms involved in failure, making the isolation of a single, unitary event problematic at best. This consideration serves to emphasize the

generally difficult nature of establishing strategies focusing on enhancing fatigue resistance in specific tasks.

This chapter concentrates on the muscle cell and the molecular events in the cell that confer contractility and mechanical function. An understanding of the molecular composition and patterns of organization of the various proteins and protein isoforms in the cell which provide for their unique mechanical properties is a necessary first step in identifying the process or processes which inhibit the cell from maintaining performance during repetitive activation. Since energy is required for muscle contraction, being able to sustain contractile activity is intimately dependent on the ability of the various metabolic pathways to supply sufficient adenosine triphosphate (ATP) and to control the accumulation of metabolic by-products (Cooke & Pate 1990; Green 1995). This type of failure, often referred to as metabolic fatigue (Green 1995), is reviewed in Chapter 9. However, the ultimate locus of the cellular impairment in contractile function resides at the level of actomyosin. Failure at this level could reflect abnormalities in the contractile proteins themselves or an inability to activate the contractile apparatus fully. The former could occur because of intrinsic, structural alterations in the proteins themselves or changes in the intracellular environment mediated by metabolic by-products. The latter cause of failure might develop because of more central inhibitory changes, such as a failure of the excitation processes leading to a decrease in the cytosolic free calcium (Ca_f^{2+}) levels (Allen et al. 1995), or changes in regulatory proteins and alterations in the response to specific Ca_i^{2+} levels (Allen *et al.* 1995). As with the contractile proteins, failure in one or more of the excitation processes may also be due to intrinsic structural changes in specific proteins or to by-product inhibition. At issue is the nature of these changes, their effect on specific mechanical functions and, equally importantly, the degree to which these processes can be adapted to resist undesirable modifications by a programme which systemically challenges their behaviour by regular exercise.

In this chapter, our objective is to provide insight into the molecular events that control the cellular response patterns to various physical demands and, where possible, to demonstrate what appears to be the limiting process when the neuromuscular system is no longer able to match performance with intent. The chapter concludes with an analysis of the interaction between metabolic and non-metabolic factors, in terms of both their impact on endurance and the putative mechanisms that are involved. Where possible, we have attempted to use studies involving human subjects. However, much of our understanding is based on animal models. A number of recent reviews on fatigue and fatigue mechanisms can be consulted for further information (Bigland-Ritchie & Woods 1984; Green 1991, 1995, 1997; Enoka & Stuart 1992; Fitts 1994; Allen *et al.* 1995).

Muscle cells—the myofibrillar system

Contractile proteins

All skeletal muscle cells possess the machinery that allows a neural signal to be translated into a mechanical response. For a mechanical response to be realized, the neural signal must ultimately be communicated to the contractile proteins, actin and myosin, and ATP must be hydrolysed to provide the energy needed by the various excitation and contraction processes when performing their respective functions.

The contractile machinery is housed in myofibrils, and specifically in the sarcomeres. A typical myofibril may contain several thousand of these organized in series (Fig. 11.1). A sarcomere, defined by a Z disc at each end, contains the regulatory (tropomyosin, troponin) and contractile (actin, myosin) proteins in the form of thick and thin filaments. The thin filaments, which are anchored to the Z discs, comprise both regulatory proteins and actin whereas the thick filament is composed essentially of myosin (Fig. 11.1). Each myosin filament appears to contain 300–400 myosin molecules; molecules are oriented in opposite directions on either side of the centre of the sarcomere. According to the sliding filament theory of muscle contraction, force is generated when actin and myosin interact and form a

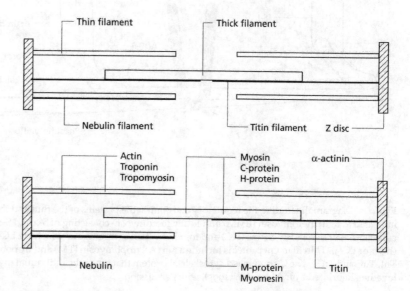

Fig. 11.1 Basic structure of the sarcomere showing major protein components of thin filament (actin, troponin, tropomyosin) and thick filament (myosin). Additional proteins are part of the cytoskeleton. Reprinted with permission from Schiaffino and Reggiani (1996).

strong binding configuration. In the process, energy is liberated and the myosin pulls the actin towards the centre of the sarcomere. Since each actomyosin interaction can only operate over a relatively short distance, significant shortening and lengthening involves myosin interacting with a succession of actin sites (Cooke 1997).

The myosin molecule plays a key role in actomyosin interaction and force generation. Each myosin molecule comprises two globular heads and a long tail (Fig. 11.2). The globular heads, which contain the ATPase, can be subdivided into a catalytic region (S-1) with specialized sites for binding to actin and the adenine nucleotides (ATP, adenosine diphosphate, ADP) and a slender neck region (S-2) that extends to the tail (Moss et al. 1995). The long tail is packed together with the tails of other myosin molecules to form the thick filament or backbone of the filament. Overall, each myosin molecule comprises two heavy chains (HC) which

contain the heads, neck region and tail, and four light chains (LC) that are divided into two classes— essential (LC-1, LC-3) and regulatory (LC-2). The essential LCs are located in close proximity to the catalytic domain, whereas the regulatory LCs are close to the coupling region between the neck and rod portion or tail (Moss et al. 1995).

During cross-bridge cycling and force generation, it appears that the myosin (M) head containing bound ATP (M.ATP) can with partial hydrolysis of the ATP (M.ADP.P_i) combine in a weak, non-force-generating state with actin (A.M.ADP.P_i). The excitation signal (Ca_f^{2+}), working through the regulatory proteins, activates the myosin ATPase, leading to release of P_i, and allowing formation of a strong binding, force-generating state (A.M.ADP). In the transition from the force-generating state to the release of ADP (A.M), rotation of the neck region occurs, using the free energy made available by P_i release; the cross-bridge is stretched, generating

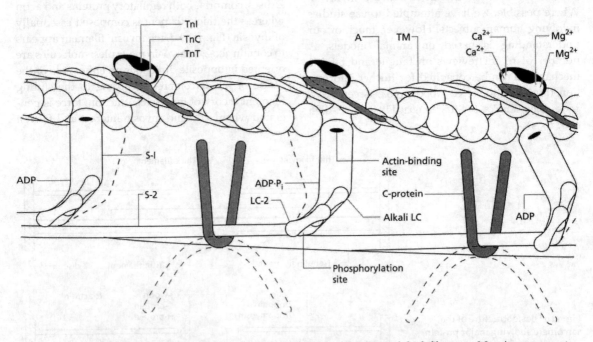

Fig. 11.2 Diagram illustrating the regulatory and contractile proteins of the thin and thick filaments. Myosin components indicated as light meromyosin (LMM) and heavy meromyosin consisting of S-2 and S-1 components. The myosin molecule consists of two heavy chains (HC) and four light chains (LC), two of which are LC-2 and two of which are alkali LCs (LC-1 or LC-3). Thin filament proteins include actin (A), tropomyosin (TM) and troponin (which contains three subunits TnI, TnC and TnT). The C-protein is a cytoskeletal protein that binds the individual myosin molecules in a filament together. Reprinted from Moss et al. (1995), with permission.

tension on the thin filament, and this results in a power stroke (Cooke 1997). The binding of ATP to the actomyosin complex (A.M.ATP) results in a rapid dissociation of the complex (Λ + M.ATP), allowing additional 'power strokes' to be initiated.

According to this model, and assuming that the force generated during each power stroke is constant, the maximal isometric force (P_0) is essentially determined by the number of cross-bridges in the muscle that are in the strong binding, force-generating state (Moss *et al.* 1995). During a concentric contraction, the maximal velocity that can be achieved at zero load (V_{max} or V_0) is determined by the rate of cross-bridge cycling, the rate at which myosin can attach to and detach from a succession of actin monomers directed towards the Z disc. Throughout this chapter, the maximal velocity of shortening is represented by both V_{max} and V_0. The two designations indicate that they were obtained by different techniques. If these contractile properties (P_0, V_{max}) cannot be sustained, failure must lie either in the molecular events involved in actomyosin cycling or in processes leading to improper signalling of the contractile proteins and an inability fully to achieve the associated and disassociated binding states. The ability to generate power is critical. Moreover, a task may require power output, the product of force times velocity, at any given velocity. Since

the force–velocity relationship is hyperbolic, the amount of curvature is important to the peak power that can be generated (Fitts & Widrick 1996).

Muscle cells differ in the rate at which they can develop force and the power that they can generate (Moss *et al.* 1995; Fitts & Widrick 1996), due to the differences in structure and composition of the myosin HC and, to a lesser extent, the myosin LC (Moss *et al.* 1995; Schiaffino & Reggiani 1996). In all, nine different HC isoforms (proteins which share the same basic function but which display variations in composition) and seven different LC isoforms (five essential and two regulatory) have been identified in skeletal muscle (Table 11.1). These isoforms are differentially expressed in different species and different muscles and at different stages of development (Schiaffino & Reggiani 1996). Of the nine different HC isoforms, only three are expressed in adult human muscle (HC-1, HC-2A and HC-2B; Table 11.1). The existence of these isoforms can be identified histochemically, using a procedure developed by Brooke and Kaiser; this procedure exploits the differences in chemical and physical properties between different HC ATPase enzymes (Staron 1991). In the Brooke and Kaiser schema, fibres that contain only HC-1 (B-slow) are labelled as Type I, whereas fibres that contain only HC-2A or HC-2B are labelled as Type IIA and Type IIB, respectively

Table 11.1 Myofibrillar proteins and protein isoforms in human skeletal muscle.

Fibre type	Heavy chain (HC)	Light chain essential (LC)	Light chain regulatory (LC)	Troponin (Tn)	Tropomyosin (TM)
Type I	2(HC-1(β-slow))	2(LC-1s)	2(LC-2s)	TnC-s	TM-αs
				TnI-s	TM-αf
				TnT-s	TM-β
Type IIA	2(HC-2A)	(LC-1f)(LC-1f)	2(LC-2f)	TnC-f	TM-αf
		(LC-3f)(LC-3f)		TnI-f	TM-αs
		(LC-1f)(LC-3f)		TnT-f	TM-β
Type IIB	2(HC-2B)	Unknown	Unknown	Unknown	
Type IC	(HC-1)(HC-2A)	Unknown	Unknown	Unknown	
Type IIC	(HC-2A)(HC-1)	Unknown	Unknown	Unknown	
Type IIAB	(HC-2A)(HC-2B)	Unknown	Unknown	Unknown	

Each myosin contains two heavy chains (HC) and four light chains (LC), two of which are essential and two of which are regulatory. Human adult muscles contain only three HC isoforms whereas muscles from other species contain an additional isoform labelled HC-2X/2D. Human HC-2B is probably HC-2X/2D. Troponin (Tn) and tropomyosin (TM) also show slow (s) and fast (f) isoforms. Several additional isoforms have been identified for TnT in other species.

(Staron 1991). Fibres may contain a mixture of the different HCs, a frequent observation following training or injury. Fibres labelled as Type IC contain both HC-1 and HC-2A, with HC-1 dominating, whereas fibres identified as IIC also contain both HC-1 and HC-2A but with HC-2A dominating (Staron & Pette 1993). Fibres may also be identified as Type IIAB based on a mixture of the HC-2A and HC-2B isoforms (Staron & Pette 1993).

An additional HC-2 isoform, HC-2X (or HC-2D), has now been identified (Schiaffino & Reggiani 1996). Current evidence suggests that this is the isoform that has been identified as HC-2B in humans (Schiaffino & Reggiani 1996). Smaller adult animals, particularly the mouse and rat, display all three HC isoforms (HC-2A, HC-2X and HC-2B). The additional isoform provides for a wider range of contractile velocities (Schiaffino & Reggiani 1996).

Myosin LCs, which are anchored between the head and stalk region, also display considerable heterogeneity. In the adult, these comprise isoforms of the alkali LCs (designated as LC-1fast, LC-3fast and LC-1slow), and of the regulatory LCs (designated as LC-2fast and LC-2slow). The regulatory LCs have also been called phosphorylatable LCs, given their ability to be phosphorylated, a property which appears essential to their effect on contractile function (Moss *et al.* 1995).

As in other muscles, selected HC and LC isoforms favourably associate with each other in adult human muscles (Tables 11.1 & 11.2). The HC-2s associate with the fast LCs, and the HC-1s with the slow LCs. Typically, myosin in a fibre could contain two HC-2A, two LC-2fast and either one LC-1fast and LC-3fast or two of either LC-1fast or LC-3fast isoforms. A typical slow muscle would contain two HC-1, two LC-1slow and two LC-2slow isoforms. The HC isoform complement of a fibre is the primary determinant of the velocity at which it can contract. Fibres that contain HC-2 are fast contracting, whereas fibres that contain HC-1 are slow contracting. For this reason, Type II fibres have been labelled as fast-twitch (FT) and Type J fibres as slow-twitch (ST).

The effects of the HC and LC isoform content on contractile properties have been studied in single fibre preparations using sensitive transducers in conjunction with electrophoresis and immunohistochemistry to determine isoform type (Moss *et al.* 1995). Observations on mouse and rat muscle indicate that when adjustment is made for cross-sectional area, little difference in P_0 exists between fast and slow fibres (Fitts & Widrick 1996). In contrast, V_{max} is three to four times greater in fast than in slow fibres (Fig. 11.3). Moreover, the curvature of the force–velocity relationship is more pronounced in slow than in fast fibres. Since power is the product of force times velocity, with peak power realized at approximately 30% P_0, fast fibres have a greater peak power because of a higher V_{max} and a less pronounced curvature in the force–velocity relationship (Moss *et al.* 1995; Fitts & Widrick 1996). Power may also be affected by the cross-sectional area of the fibre; large fibres have higher P_0 values as a

Table 11.2 Fibre type and subtype distribution and fibre areas in tissue obtained from untrained human adult female and male vastus lateralis muscle. Body mass of female volunteers averaged 60.9 kg, and that of male volunteers averaged 81.0 kg. Data from Staron *et al.* (1990) and Green *et al.* (1998b).

	Fibre type					
	I	IC	IIC	IIA	IIAB	IIB
Women						
Distribution (%)	45.0	1.0	0.5	32.5	4.8	16.2
Area (μm²)	4253			3370		2697
Men						
Distribution (%)	47.2	<1	<1	28.4	7.7	15.1
Area (μm²)	4840			6455	6065	5577

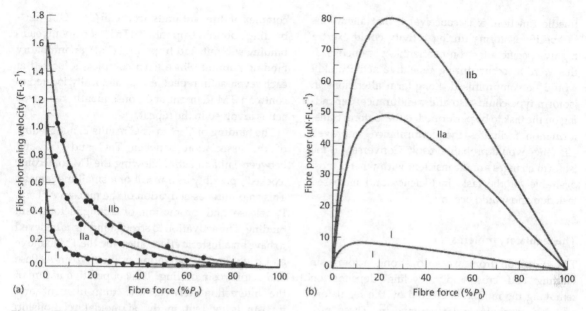

Fig. 11.3 Force–velocity (a) and power (b) characteristics of human fibre types. I, Type I; IIa, Type IIA; IIb, Type IIB. %P_0, percentage peak isometric force. Figures adapted from Fitts and Widrick (1996) with permission.

result of a greater cross-sectional area, more myofib-rils and the potential for more actin and myosin to participate in strong binding and force generation (Fitts & Widrick 1996). Type IIB fibres, which already have a high V_{max} as a consequence of their isoform composition, also have the largest fibre areas (Green 1992; Moss *et al.* 1995).

Force–velocity characteristics differ between the different fast fibre subtypes, due to differences in the myosin HC isoforms (Moss *et al.* 1995). Among the fast fibres, V_{max} is greatest in fibres containing HC-2B, followed by fibres containing HC-2X, and is least in fibres containing HC-2A (Moss *et al.* 1995; Schiaffino & Reggiani 1996).

The impact of myosin LCs on the dynamic characteristics of the fibre is less certain given the variable distribution within a given fibre. There appears to be a consensus that of the two fast alkali LCs, LC-1fast and LC-3fast, LC-3 have the greatest potentiating effect on V_{max} (Moss *et al.* 1995). Moreover, the effect is most pronounced when LC-3fast exists in combination with HC-2B (Schiaffino & Reggiani 1996). Fibres containing myosin HC-2B appear to associate preferentially with myosin LC-3fast (Schiaffino & Reggiani 1996). The effect of the

myosin regulatory LC, LC-2 on contractile characteristics appears most pronounced at submaximal levels of force production. Phosphorylation of LC-2, which occurs with activation of the fibre by a calcium-dependent process, enhances force production at force levels of 50% of P_0 and below, presumably by inducing the myosin head to develop more strong binding configurations with actin (Sweeney *et al.* 1993). This phenomenon, restricted only to FT fibres, appears to be the mechanism associated with post-tetanic potentiation. In post-tetanic potentiation, the force developed at low frequencies of stimulation is increased immediately following a tetanic contraction. Presumably, the tetanic contraction augments Ca_f^{2+}, leading to a net phosphorylation of LC-2, which persists and enhances force production following the tetanus (Sweeney *et al.* 1993).

In summary, myosin and myosin isoforms are the primary determinants of fibre contractile characteristics. The interaction between myosin and actin, leading to formation of a strong binding, acto-myosin configuration and a resultant power stroke, must be protected to sustain function. Given the role of the different HC and LC myosin isoforms in contractile function, it is conceivable that alterations in specific isoforms during activity could exert a highly specific effect on contractile parameters. If this were to occur during repetitive activity, skill would be compromised. Long-term alterations in isoform type could also affect endurance, depending on the task to be performed. If the isoform transformation facilitates the performance, improved efficiency would probably result. Conversely, if the isoform changes are inconsistent with what is most desirable for the task, inefficiency and increased task demand would occur.

The regulatory proteins

The transition from weak to strong actomyosin binding and cross-bridge cycling depends on removing the inhibition created by the regulatory proteins, troponin and tropomyosin. These proteins, which are part of the thin filament, provide the communication between the level of Ca_f^{2+} in the cytosol and the contractile proteins. With excitation, increases in Ca_f^{2+} are sensed by the troponin complex, setting up a sequence of events that leads to conformational changes in troponin, movement of tropomyosin and ultimately acceleration from weak to strong binding. Cessation of activation reduces Ca_f^{2+}, allowing the regulatory proteins to re-establish their inhibitory role and resulting in cross-bridges which are dissociated or in a weak binding state (Hochachka 1994).

The structure of the proteins and their arrangement with actin provide insight into how the regulatory proteins exert their inhibitory role. The actin consists of individual globular monomers (G-actin) formed into double helical filaments (F-actin) of a defined length. It is anchored to the Z disc, and extends inwards. A series of some 26 actin repeats (each repeat consisting of seven actin molecules) is thought to exist in a thin filament (Brandt *et al.* 1987). Tropomyosin (TM), an elongated dimeric protein also of a fixed length, lies in the groove of the actin filaments, spanning some seven individual actin monomers. Individual TM dimers show head-to-tail overlap, allowing for communication and cooperativity between segments. Troponin (Tn) is a complex of three subunits: troponin C (TnC), a Ca^{2+}-binding subunit; troponin T (TnT), a tropomyosin-binding subunit; and troponin I (TnI), an inhibitory binding subunit. Since a Tn complex is located at each seven-actin repeat, it is strategically located to control a TM filament and consequently the seven actins involved in the repeat.

The binding of Ca^{2+} to TnC results in a loosening of the association between TnC and TnI and between TnI and actin, allowing the TM to become 'cocked', possibly as a result of a small movement. This step initiates activation of the myosin ATPase, P_i release and promotion of strong actomyosin binding. The activation to strong binding is believed to have an allosteric effect, allowing the TM to move and trigger rapid activation of the myosin ATPase and actomyosin cycling. The cooperative nature of the interaction between the thin filament and myosin is evident in the sigmoidal relationship between the Ca_f^{2+} concentration (pCa) and force (Squire & Morris 1998).

Fibre types differ in the pCa–force relationship, to some degree explained by their regulatory proteins and isoforms (Schiaffino & Reggiani 1996). Type I fibres in contrast to Type II fibres need a lower concentration of Ca_f^{2+} to generate 50% of their peak isometric force (pCa 50%). Type II fibres have a much steeper pCa–force relationship (higher Hill coefficient, η). There are also differences in pCa 50% and η among the fast fibre subtypes. Type 2B fibres, in contrast to type 2A, have lower and higher values for pCa 50% and η, respectively. As with many muscle proteins, the regulatory proteins also have different isoforms, affecting the fibre force–pCa relationship. Tropomyosin has two strands, α and β, which in human skeletal muscle can exist as $\alpha\alpha$, $\beta\beta$ or $\alpha\beta$ (Schiaffino & Reggiani 1996). Isoforms of the α chain, namely TM-α fast and TM-α slow, have been isolated experimentally. However, isoforms of TM-β (TM-β fast and TM-β slow) have not yet been isolated (Schiaffino & Reggiani 1996). Both fast and slow isoforms also exist for components of the Tn complex. In the case of TnC and TnI, these have been labelled TnC-fast and TnC-slow and TnI-fast and TnI-slow, respectively (Schiaffino & Reggiani 1996). In contrast to TnC and TnI, TnT possesses multiple fast (TnT-1f, TnT-2f, TnT-3f) and slow (TnT-1s, TnT-2s) isoforms (Pette & Staron 1997). It is not clear to what extent these various TnT isoforms exist in humans.

The isoforms of the regulatory proteins associate strongly with specific myosin HC isoforms (Pette & Staron 1997). In the case of TM, the α subunit, and in particular, the TM-α fast subunit, is more pronounced in fast muscles, although both the TM-α fast and the TM-α slow subunits can be observed in slow muscles (Schiaffino & Reggiani 1996). The TnC-fast and TnI-fast subunits are also more pronounced in fast fibres, and the TnC-slow and TnI-slow subunits are more evident in slow fibres. With regard to TnT, the TnT-1s is the primary form in adult slow muscles, whereas the fast isoforms appear to associate with specific myosin HC fast isoforms (the TnT-1f and TnT-2f with HC-2X, and the TnT-3f with HC-2A) (Schiaffino & Reggiani 1996).

Differences of force–pCa relationship in the different fibre types appear to be due to the fibre-specific isoforms of both the regulatory proteins and the myosin HC (Schiaffino & Reggiani 1996). The isoforms of the regulatory protein, TnC, differ in their capacity to bind Ca^{2+} and possibly in their Ca^{2+} sensitivity. In transgenic mice, where mutants of TnC, possessing similar binding properties to TnC-fast, have been inserted, increases in cooperativity have been reported in slow but not in fast fibres (Schiaffino & Reggiani 1996). Differences in TnC isoforms have also been implicated in the differing fibre sensitivities to temperature, sarcomere length and acidity (Schiaffino & Reggiani 1996). Observations based on the natural existence of regulatory protein isoforms in different fibres have led to the hypothesis that the isoforms of TnT and TM are intimately linked to cooperativity, a relationship that might be expected given the overlapping of TM molecules that occurs in the thin filament and their association with TnT. As an example, the highest values for sensitivity (pCa 50%) and cooperativity (η) were associated with the presence of TnT-2f and TM-α fast in rabbit fast muscles (Schachat et al. 1987). The role of the myosin HC isoforms appears to originate from their effect in controlling the rate of weak to strong binding. The fast myosin HC isoforms apparently display greater cooperativity because the more rapid transition to strong binding affects thin filament responsiveness by allosteric feedback (Schiaffino & Reggiani 1996).

Differences in the force–pCa relationship between different fibre types may, in part, be responsible for differences in fatiguability (Burke et al. 1973). As an example, changes in Ca_f^{2+} would be expected to affect each fibre type differently, based on the differences in their sensitivity and cooperativity. Changes in the intracellular environment such as changes in selected metabolic by-products or in selected cations may also have a differential effect on contractility. Finally, susceptibility to intrinsic changes in the protein during repetitive activity could vary with isoform type.

Myofibrillar function and repetitive activity

There is little question that if contractile activity is sustained for sufficient time, fatigue will result and performance will be compromised. The degree to which the myofibrillar apparatus, and specifically the regulatory and contractile proteins, is involved remains controversial. Given the difficulty in distinguishing the role of specific processes in an intact muscle or muscle fibre, this is to be expected. Several experimental tactics have attempted to isolate the contribution of specific Ca_f^{2+}-dependent processes to fatigue. One approach is to measure the force–pCa relationship in single fibres undergoing repetitive activity. A rightward shift in the relationship (a reduction in force at a given Ca_f^{2+} concentration) is a well-documented effect of such activity (Allen et al. 1995). These changes could reflect an alteration in thin filament regulation of contraction or in actomyosin behaviour. The role of the contractile proteins in shifting the force–pCa relationship has been explained by examining intrinsic changes in actomyosin (myosin) ATPase activity when measured under optimal in vitro conditions prior to and following exercise. The rationale for such an approach is that if a reduction in actomyosin ATPase activity is observed, the rate of weak to strong binding should be compromised, depressing the force–velocity curve. In general, measurements performed on a rat muscle under such conditions with a predominance of either Type I or Type II fibres have failed to demonstrate alterations in enzymatic activity in response to prolonged exercise (Fitts 1994). This suggests that submaximal exercise of light to moderate intensity does not induce structural alterations in myosin HC (and myosin ATPase), regardless of isoform.

Another approach has been to use fibres that have had their sarcolemmae removed, artificially and systematically manipulating one or more metabolites in the intracellular environment to simulate heavy exercise (Cooke & Pate 1990). The accumulation of selected metabolic by-products (i.e. P_i, ADP, H^+), at least at relatively low temperatures, can induce a substantial depression of function which to some degree is specific to the different mechanical properties. Accumulation of P_i, for example, induces a major depression in P_0, but has much less effect on V_{max}. Accumulation of free ADP (ADP_f) has a minimal effect on P_0 but induces a moderate depression in V_{max}. In contrast, accumulation of H^+ substantially depresses both P_0 and V_{max}. These results demonstrate that changes in the intracellular environment, mediated by the by-products accumulated during activation of ATP-supplying pathways and by ATP hydrolysis itself, can potentially explain some causes of fatigue. Moreover, the types of mechanical property affected (P_0 and V_{max}) and their dependence on selected metabolites emphasize the role of specific biochemical steps in the actomyosin cycle (Cooke 1997). It is generally believed that the reduction in ATP (typically < 25% in human muscle with voluntary exercise, regardless of task demands) does not in itself affect actomyosin cycling or force generation (Cooke & Pate 1990). Since there is little evidence that the intrinsic properties of myosin ATPase are altered by exercise (Fitts 1994), the effects of changes in intracellular environment would appear transient, with integrity of the 'power stroke' re-established as the intracellular environment is normalized. This type of fatigue, commonly referred to as metabolic fatigue, would appear to be protective; it prevents excessive depletion of ATP and accumulation of metabolic by-products such as H^+, which might hamper cell recovery and impair viability. Nevertheless, these studies were conducted under highly unphysiological conditions, particularly in regard to temperature, and they do not demonstrate conclusively failure of the contractile proteins in the intact fibre during either voluntary or induced contractions. It is possible that sites more central to actomyosin may be more sensitive to changes in the intracellular environment; they might reduce the activation signal, thus disrupting the weak to strong binding force-generating state. Regardless of the site involved, a fundamental tactic in avoiding fatigue would seem to involve the management of by-products, either by reducing accumulation (via aerobic ATP regeneration) or by developing a greater tolerance of change in the intracellular environment.

The isoform composition of myofibrillar proteins might also be a factor in the shift of the force–pCa relationship with repetitive activity. This could occur in at least two ways. At a given level of activity, fast fibres in contrast to slow fibres may display greater alterations in the intracellular environment; for example, there might be a greater accumulation of metabolites such as H^+ and P_i (Meyer & Terjung 1979) and consequently a greater shift in cooperativity (Metzger & Moss 1987). Alternatively, because of differences in the regulatory and/or protein isoforms, a given change in one or more metabolites could elicit a greater change in one fibre type than another. Increases in H^+, for example, appear to have a greater effect on calcium affinity in fibres containing TnC-s than in fibres containing TnC-f (Metzger 1996), whereas the effect on actomyosin kinetics appears greater in fibres with myosin HC-2 than in fibres with myosin HC-1 (Moss *et al.* 1995). Similarly, accumulation of P_i appears to cause a greater depression of force in fast fibres than in slow fibres, ostensibly because of the myosin isoform composition (Metzger 1996). Care must be taken in extrapolating these effects to physiological settings. At physiological temperatures, the effects of accumulating by-products, such as H^+, do not appear as profound as at lower temperatures (Westerblad 1998).

Eccentric exercise provides the most persuasive, albeit circumstantial, evidence implicating the myofibrillar apparatus in task failure. With eccentric exercise the muscle can generate substantially greater forces with minimal disturbance of ATP levels and by-product accumulation (Evans & Cannon 1991). This type of exercise produces a profound weakness, which in the uninitiated may persist for several days (Clarkson & Tremblay 1988). The cell ultrastructure after this type of exercise shows extensive myofibrillar disorganization and damage (Lieber *et al.* 1994). Not only may actin and myosin proteins be directly altered, but there may be severe disruption of both the highly ordered array of filaments within the sarcomeres and the spatial relationship between sarcomeres, myofilaments and muscle fibres. These changes reflect damage to the cytoskeletal framework, the family of proteins responsible for stabilizing, anchoring and maintaining order within and between the various proteins and cell structures of the cell (Thornell & Price 1991). Disruption of the cytoskeletal framework has previously been noted following the generation of large forces (Lieber *et al.* 1994). Weakness mediated by disruption and damage could have important consequences for performance. Tasks requiring near-maximal force and power output would undoubtedly be compromised. Moreover, even though a task may demand submaximal force and power, the ability to recruit additional reserves of force to compensate for fatigue, either through increased firing frequency or motor unit recruitment, would be compromised. Since many tasks, particularly those with an eccentric component, can induce acute weakness, minimization of this non-metabolic effect would appear desirable to enhance endurance.

Chronic adaptations in myofibrillar function and composition

The skeletal muscle cell possesses an enormous propensity for adaptation to various challenges. If the stimulus is sufficiently severe and persistent, extensive adaptation occurs in all components of the cell including the myofibrillar proteins. The nature and magnitude of these adaptations depend on the type of contractile activity that is elicited. These adaptations may not only affect the contractile properties of the cell, such as P_0 and V_{max},

but may also alter the potential for sustained performance.

The most extreme model used to promote fibre adaptation is based on chronic contractile activity induced by low-frequency stimulation. A fast muscle, typically in the rat or rabbit, is induced to contract up to 24 h per day for up to 60 days. With this protocol, there is a near-complete transformation to Type I fibres (Pette & Staron 1997). The sequence of transformation is believed to proceed from myosin HC-2B, to HC-2X/2D to HC-2A and finally to HC-1. The shift in fast myosin HC isoforms towards HC-2A occurs relatively early in the stimulation period, whereas the shift from HC-2A to HC-1 is the most resistant to change, major shifts not being seen until late during stimulation (Pette & Staron 1997). During the transition period, multiple myosin HC isoforms may occur in a single fibre, producing fibres designated as Type IIAB, Type IIC, etc. The transformation of myosin HC isoforms is accompanied by shifts in both myosin LCs and in regulatory proteins, which occur to some degree in association with the myosin HC isoform types. Reductions in myosin HC2X/2D are accompanied by reductions in myosin LC-3f and TnT-1f and TnT-2f; increases in myosin HC-2A are coordinated with an increase in LC-1f and TnT-3f; and finally the shift to myosin HC-1 is accompanied by increases in LC-1s, LC-2s, TnT-1s, TnT-2s, TnI-s and TnC-s (Pette & Staron 1997).

Adaptations in the myofibrillar network are preceded by extensive adaptations in the potential and patterning of metabolic systems (Pette & Staron 1997). The mitochondrial potential is increased many-fold, while the high-energy phosphate system and the glycolytic system are dramatically down-regulated (Henriksson *et al.* 1986; Pette & Staron 1997). The chronically stimulated muscles also exhibit a profound increase in fatigue resistance. Much of this occurs early and has been attributed to an increase in mitochondrial potential with a predominance of oxidative phosphorylation in generating ATP for the working muscle (Pette & Staron 1997). Chronically stimulated muscles can maintain energy homeostasis with only small changes in the accumulation of metabolic by-products, unlike the response of fast muscles at the onset of stimulation

(Pette & Vrbová 1985). There is little question that the decrease in fatiguability is intimately associated with maintenance of a more stable intracellular environment, but other factors also appear important, namely development of the new isoforms observed at the regulatory and contractile protein level. These isoforms appear more resistant to the repeated insults induced by repetitive activation, retaining an ability to sustain force generation (Pette & Staron 1997). In effect, the transformed muscle becomes uniquely adapted for producing low force levels without interruption at minimal energetic cost and with minimal disturbance of the internal environment (Green *et al.* 1992b).

However, the transformation to this extreme state is not without compromise. The fibres undergo dramatic reductions in both P_0 and V_{max}. The reductions in P_0 occur primarily because of pronounced reductions in fibre cross-sectional area, and reductions in the force–frequency relationships occur because of the shift in myosin HC and LC isoforms (Pette & Staron 1997). Since the force–pCa relationship is shifted to the right, a greater Ca_f^{2+} level is needed to achieve a given percentage of peak force. Not only are fibres transformed to this extreme unable to perform tasks demanding high power outputs and high levels of isometric force, but their output is also compromised during repeated performance of the task at more moderate demands, given the inefficiency of slow fibres when performing this type of work (Crow & Kushmerick 1982; Barclay 1996).

Human adaptations to voluntary training programmes, even of the most extreme nature, are not as extensive as those observed in the fast muscle of chronically stimulated animals. In fact, changes in myofibrillar proteins are extremely modest. There is minimal evidence of significant shifts in the major fibre types, Type I and Type II, with prolonged endurance training (Fitts & Widrick 1996). Transformations that have been observed are mainly limited to fast fibre subtypes, consisting of reductions in Type IIB fibres (which represent only 10–15% of the total fibres in the untrained) and increases in Type IIAB, Type IIA and Type IIC fibres (Fitts & Widrick 1996; Pette & Staron 1997). The shift in fibre type indicated by myosin ATPase histochemistry has been confirmed with electrophoresis which has shown increases in myosin HC-2A and decreases in myosin HC-2B (Fitts & Widrick 1996). To date, few studies have addressed changes in myosin LC or the regulatory protein isoforms with prolonged voluntary exercise. One study, employing an extreme daily running programme in rats, suggested that substantial adaptations in both myosin HC and myosin LC isoforms were possible (Green *et al.* 1984).

In addition to prolonged exercise, other voluntary training models have been employed in an attempt to determine myofibrillar plasticity. High resistance training (HRT) is based on relatively few repetitions performed at near-maximal effort. With this type of training, the fibre type transitions are surprisingly similar to those which have been reported for prolonged endurance training, namely a reduction in Type IIB fibres (and myosin HC-2B), and increases in Type IIA fibres (and myosin HC-2A), with transitional fibres that contain more than one myosin HC, namely IIAB and IIC (Kraemer *et al.* 1996). Training involving high velocities and power outputs appears to have a similar effect on myosin HC isoform expression (Fitts & Widrick 1996). As with prolonged endurance training, studies completed to date have not addressed other components of the myofibrillar complex. One of the most conspicuous adaptations resulting from HRT (and which may extend in varying degrees to other types of training) is an increase in muscle fibre cross-sectional area (Kraemer *et al.* 1996).

The increase in cross-sectional area could have important consequences for muscle contractile properties and fatigue resistance. Increases in cross-sectional area would be expected to increase P_0 and to shift the force–velocity curve to the right, resulting in increased power. To some extent, the increase in power may be dampened by a reduction in Type IIB fibres (and myosin HC-2B), which are known to display a higher V_{max} than the Type IIA fibres (and myosin HC-2A) (Schiaffino & Reggiani 1996). Improved fatigue resistance could occur as a consequence of the increase in P_0 since, at any given absolute force, the relative percentage of force required is reduced; this provides a larger reserve for recruitment with voluntary repetitive contraction. There is substantial evidence that this occurs, but contradictory evidence has also been published (Fitts & Widrick 1996). The changes that occur in the neural system with HRT appear substantial, and this may explain the inability to demonstrate consistent alterations in different mechanical and endurance properties following training (Kraemer et al. 1996). Adaptations in energy-supplying systems and muscle capillarization must also not be neglected. Adaptations in these systems are particularly important in endurance performance, where an increase in the proportion of energy supplied by oxidative phosphorylation is desirable. Unlike prolonged endurance training, which increases both mitochondrial potential and capillaries per unit fibre area (Saltin & Gollnick 1983), increases in fibre area promoted by HRT have long been suspected to reduce these properties (Kraemer et al. 1996). However, an approximate 15% increase in area of the various fibre types can occur with HRT, without a reduction in either mitochondrial potential or capillary per unit fibre area (Green et al. 1998a).

At the single fibre level, training modulates the mechanical properties. In rats, prolonged treadmill training augments the V_0 by 20% in Type I fibres extracted from the soleus, an adaptation attributed to the increase in fast myosin LC isoforms, LC-1f and LC-2f (Schuler & Fitts 1994). In humans, a similar effect on V_0 in Type I fibres of the deltoid of swimmers was accompanied by a decrease of V_0 in Type II fibres (Fitts et al. 1989). Endurance training also appears to decrease P_0 in Type I fibres in humans (Fitts et al. 1989). In addition, swim training induces a rightward shift in the force–pCa relationship, resulting in a higher pCa 50% and a steeper η (Fitts et al. 1989). These studies must be interpreted in context. The human deltoid, like most other muscles, contains a mixture of Type I and Type II fibres. As a consequence, it is not clear what the contractile demands are in a given task. This contrasts with the chronic stimulated animal model, where muscles of a predominantly fast type are selected and the contractile demands do not vary (Pette & Staron 1997). Unfortunately, studies of single fibre responses to voluntary training are relatively scarce in both humans and non-humans.

Several studies have examined the effects of voluntary resistance training. Increases in P_0 can be expected (Jones & Rutherford 1987), the magnitude being greater if isometric rather than dynamic training is used. Increases in V_{max} and peak power are specific to dynamic training, with the greatest gains in torque occurring at velocities specific to the training undertaken (Caiozzo et al. 1981; Coyle et al. 1981).

Muscle cells—excitation and contraction coupling

The neural signal, once transmitted across the neuromuscular junction, must be communicated to the cell interior in order to increase Ca_f^{2+}. The collective processes involved in transmitting the signal from the muscle membrane to the cell interior are described as excitation–contraction coupling (E–C coupling).

Muscle cells have an extensive membranous network containing a phospholipid bilayer in which numerous proteins are embedded (Fig. 11.4). These proteins form a diverse and dense network of receptors, channels and transporters, allowing the selective binding and transport of ions, nutrients, metabolites and messengers across the cell membrane. Specialized proteins that provide for active transport of specific ions are also embedded in the cell membrane. In the sarcolemma and T tubules, as an example, the Na^+/K^+-ATPase can hydrolyse ATP for energy used to transport Na^+ out of the cell and K^+ into the cell, against their respective concentration gradients. The Na^+/K^+-ATPase pump is essential in excitable cells such as muscle, where the nerve impulses must result in action potentials being conducted along the sarcolemma and into the cell via the T tubules. Rapid pumping of Na^+ out of and K^+ into the cell allows the membrane potential to be re-established and repetitive action potentials to be conducted (Ewart & Klip 1995; Clausen 1996a).

The muscle cell contains a second extensive membranous network, the sarcoplasmic reticulum (SR). This functions to control the storage, release and uptake of Ca^{2+}, the messenger that regulates the myofibrillar network. The release of Ca^{2+} following

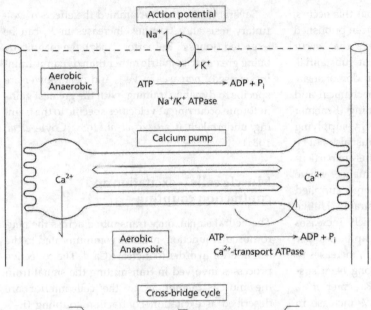

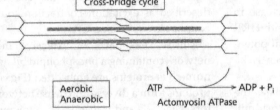

Fig. 11.4 Excitation and contraction processes in skeletal muscle fibres. The three major ATPases of the cell involved in Na$^+$/K$^+$ transport (Na$^+$/K$^+$-ATPase), sarcoplasmic reticulum Ca^{2+}-transport (Ca^{2+}-transport ATPase) and cross-bridge cycling (actomyosin ATPase) are indicated.

transmission of the excitation signal to the interior of the fibre occurs through special channels in the SR called Ca^{2+}-release or ryanodine receptors. The dramatic reduction in cytosol Ca$_f^{2+}$ that occurs when excitation is terminated and which allows relaxation to proceed, is mediated by another pump embedded in the SR membrane, namely the Ca^{2+}-ATPase. Ca^{2+} is resequestered into the SR by the Ca^{2+}-ATPase pump, which undergoes conformational changes as ATP is split and energy is released. This allows the transport of Ca^{2+} across the cell membrane into the lumen of the SR (MacLennan 1990; Martonosi 1996).

Specialized cell regions are needed to couple the excitation signal conducted in the T tubule to the Ca^{2+}-release channel of the SR if Ca$_f^{2+}$ levels are to rise and contraction is to occur. This process begins in the T tubules, where specialized proteins (dihydropyridine receptors, DHPR) communicate with the Ca^{2+}-release channel. The dominant coupling mechanism is mechanical and movements in the DHPR induced by the depolarization signal allow an unplugging of the Ca^{2+}-release channel, permitting Ca^{2+} to diffuse from the SR to the cytosol (Franzini-Armstrong & Protasi 1997).

All three processes involved in E–C coupling can compromise the muscle cell response to the neural command. In the case of P_0 and V_{max}, as examples, the peak values can only be realized if excitation processes are successful in translating the high-frequency stimulation rates into a maximal or near-maximal increase in Ca$_f^{2+}$. Where rapid and variable changes in velocity and force are required, precise control over the Ca$_f^{2+}$ transient is essential, a condition dependent on the processes controlling both SR Ca^{2+} release and Ca^{2+} uptake. There is increasing evidence that in some tasks, the onset and manifestation of fatigue occur as a result of an inappropriate Ca$_f^{2+}$ level, secondary to failure in one or more of the processes involved in E–C coupling (Allen *et al.*

1995). As with the myofibrillar ATPase, the failure could occur because of exercise-induced changes in the intracellular environment and/or intrinsic changes in protein structure.

Sarcolemma and T tubules

The Na^+/K^+ pump is a dominant mechanism for ensuring that the sarcolemma and T tubules can respond to neural commands with action potentials of high frequency, sufficient to elicit a maximal contractile response. To achieve this, the Na^+/K^+-ATPase must have a high catalytic capacity, able to hydrolyse ATP rapidly and to transport K^+ and Na^+ in and out of the cell rapidly. The maximal enzyme activity depends on the amount of protein available and the degree to which its catalytic capacity can be recruited (Ewart & Klip 1995; Clausen 1996a).

The Na^+/K^+-ATPase is a dimeric protein, containing α and β subunits, both of which are required for enzymatic activity (Ewart & Klip 1995). The α subunit, which contains binding sites for Na^+, K^+, Mg^{2+} and ATP, is recognized as the catalytic subunit, whereas the β subunit appears to be involved in assembly and membrane stabilization of the functional $\alpha\beta$ heterodimer (Ewart & Klip 1995). Increases in intracellular Na^+ and extracellular K^+ bind to the α catalytic subunit, stimulating large increases in its activity. In the process,

the bound ATP is partially hydrolysed, resulting in a charged intermediate complex. As with actomyosin ATPase, the release of P_i provides energy for conformational changes in the enzyme and the unidirectional transport of Na^+ and K^+. Sustained availability of ATP is a fundamental requirement for both Na^+/K^+ pump function and K^+/Na^+ homeostasis. A complex of other factors, operating via second messenger systems such as insulin and the catecholamines, can up-regulate pump activity acutely (Ewart & Klip 1995; Clausen 1996a). Acute contractile activity by itself can also result in a translocation of pumps for intracellular sites to the sarcolemma, leading to increased pump density and potentially increased activity and cation transport (Clausen 1996a). Collectively, these regulatory mechanisms represent accommodation phenomena following the onset of muscle contraction. They serve to protect membrane excitability and Na^+/K^+ homeostasis, conditions necessary for sustained effort.

The membrane content of Na^+/K^+-ATPase and the type of isoform varies between fibre types (Table 11.3). The content of the cation pump does not appear to be higher in fast than in slow muscles, an unexpected finding, given the higher frequency of stimulation needed to obtain a given percentage of P_0 in the fast fibres (Close 1964). But at least in rats, the activity of the pump varies with the mitochond-

Table 11.3 Na^+/K^+-ATPase content and isoform distribution in rat muscles differing in predominant fibre type composition.

	Soleus (I)	Extensor digitorum longus (IIA)	Red vastus lateralis (IIA)	White vastus lateralis (IIB)
Na^+/K^+-ATPase* ($pmol\cdot g^{-1}$ wet weight)	359	365	403	238
Isoform type†	$\alpha_1\beta_1$ $\alpha_2\beta_1$	$\alpha_1\beta_1$ $\alpha_2\beta_1$	$\alpha_1\beta_1$ $\alpha_2\beta_1$	$\alpha_2\beta_2$ $\alpha_2\beta_2$
Citrate synthase ($\mu mol\cdot min^{-1}\cdot g^{-1}$ wet weight)	12.3	9.1	11.3	4.0

Predominant fibre type composition is indicated for each muscle. Data are not available for Na^+/K^+-ATPase content and isoform distribution in human fibre types. The untrained human vastus lateralis (a muscle composed of an approximate equal percentage of Type I and Type II fibres) contains an average 339 $pmol\cdot g^{-1}$ wet weight of Na^+/K^+-ATPase.
*Data obtained from Chin and Green (1991).
†Data obtained from Hundal *et al.* (1993).

rial potential of the fibre (Chin & Green 1991). Fibres with a high oxidative potential, both Type I and Type IIA, display a much higher Na^+/K^+-ATPase content than Type IIB fibres, which typically exhibit a low oxidative potential. Fibre type differences in isoform distribution also exist. Of the three α isoforms ($\alpha_1, \alpha_2, \alpha_3$) and the three β isoforms ($\beta_1, \beta_2, \beta_3$) that have been identified, only α_1 and α_2 and β_1 and β_2 appear to be expressed in rat muscles (Ewart & Klip 1995). The α_1 and α_2 isoforms appear to be expressed in all fibre types (Type I, IIA, IIB), but β_1 is primarily expressed in high oxidative fibres, namely Type I and Type IIA and β_2 appears in Type IIB fibres which possess a low oxidative potential (Hundal et al. 1994). The distribution of β_2 in Type IIA fibres is not known. In the rat both Type I and Type IIB fibres possess $\alpha_1\beta_1$ and $\alpha_2\beta_1$ heterodimers in high density, whereas Type IIB fibres possess $\alpha_1\beta_2$ and $\alpha_2\beta_2$ in low density (Hundal et al. 1993, 1994). Studies examining isoform distribution in human muscle have yet to be performed. The only exception is for the soleus, a muscle rich in Type I fibres, where $\alpha_1\beta_1$ and $\alpha_2\beta_2$ appear to predominate (Hundal et al. 1994). It is suspected that differences in isoforms may confer different affinities for ligands such as K^+ and Na^+, allowing different kinetic responses under different intracellular conditions, but experimental evidence on this question is generally lacking for skeletal muscle (Ewart & Klip 1995).

Sarcoplasmic reticulum

The SR is an extensive membranous network that envelops the myofibrils. It is composed of a longitudinal reticulum which contains a substantial fraction of the Ca^{2+}-ATPase pumps, and terminal cisternae, the transverse portions of which contain the Ca^{2+}-release channels or ryanodine receptors (MacLennan 1990). The terminal cisternae are in close apposition to the T tubules, forming either a diad (one T tubule and one terminal cisterna) or a triad (one T tubule flanked by two terminal cisternae) at the levels of the A–I junction in the sarcomere (Ogata & Yamasaki 1997). This arrangement allows the excitation signal conducted in the T tubule to move close to the Ca^{2+}-release channels, and for the Ca_f^{2+} once released to bind quickly to the regulatory

protein, TnC. TnC, which is part of the thin filament, is located only a short distance from the site of Ca^{2+} release. The distribution of Ca^{2+}-ATPase pumps over a wide surface of the myofibril enables Ca^{2+} to be sequestered rapidly into the lumen of the SR once excitation has ceased.

The primary function of the SR is to control cytosolic Ca^{2+} levels and consequently the degree to which contractile proteins move from a weak to a strong binding, force-generating state. Disturbances in Ca^{2+} release and/or Ca^{2+} uptake could depress peak Ca_f^{2+} concentration and compromise P_0 and V_{max}. Alternatively, modifications of the kinetic behaviour of the Ca_f^{2+} transient could alter the rate at which weak to strong to weak binding occurs, causing disturbances during dynamic activity (where force and velocity must be closely coupled).

The SR Ca^{2+}-ATPase is a transmembrane protein that has special domains for binding ATP, Ca^{2+} and Mg^{2+}, as well as domains for phosphorylation and energy transduction (MacLennan 1990). Increases in cytosol Ca_f^{2+} activate the enzyme, resulting initially in a charged intermediate complex. The energy provided by the release of P_i results in a conformational change in the enzyme and, in the process, Ca^{2+} is translocated into the lumen of the SR against a concentration gradient. Two Ca^{2+} are transported per ATP hydrolysed. In vivo, the extensive distribution of Ca^{2+}-ATPase results in a rapid return of Ca_f^{2+} towards resting levels once excitation has stopped. As with Na^+/K^+-ATPase, the Ca^{2+}-ATPase is under complex regulatory control, by a variety of second messengers; this ensures that the activity of the pump is precisely regulated and the desired Ca_f^{2+} is realized.

Different fibre types differ in their content and specific composition of Ca^{2+}-ATPase (Table 11.4). In humans, the Ca^{2+}-ATPase activity is three- to fourfold higher in Type II compared to Type I fibres, resulting in similar differences in Ca^{2+} uptake (Samaha & Gergely 1965; Salviatti et al. 1982, 1983). In addition, human Type I fibres contain the SERCA 2 isoform and Type II fibres the SERCA 1 isoform (Lytton et al. 1992). To date, the functional significance of isoform types is unclear (Lytton et al. 1992). Fibre type differences in the messenger systems

Table 11.4 Characteristics of the sarcoplasmic reticulum (SR) in rat skeletal muscles of differing fibre type composition.

	Soleus (I)	Extensor digitorum longus (II)	Tibialis anterior (II)	Red vastus lateralis (II)	White vastus lateralis (II)
Ca^{2+}-release channel (ryanodine receptor)*	0.6		2.0		
Isoform	RyR1	RyR1	RyR1	RyR1	RyR1
Ca^{2+}-ATPase content (nmol·g^{-1} wet weight)†	6	40			
Ca^{2+}-ATPase activity (μmol P_i·min^{-1}·mg^{-1} protein)‡	0.220	0.683		0.550	0.711
Ca^{2+} uptake, initial rate (μmol·min^{-1}·mg^{-1} wet weight)‡	0.189	1.24		0.742	1.27
Isoform	SERCA 2a	SERCA 1b	SERCA 1b	SERCA 1b	SERCA 1b

* Data obtained from Damiani and Margreth (1994), where Ca^{2+}-release channel data based on (^{3}H) ryanodine binding (V_{max}, pmol·mg^{-1}) as measured on isolated membrane preparations.
† Data obtained from Everts *et al.* (1989).
‡ Based on data from Fitts *et al.* (1982).

controlling Ca^{2+} pump activation appear to exist (Hawkins *et al.* 1994).

The Ca^{2+}-release channel is located primarily in the terminal cisterna region. On activation, it rapidly increases Ca_f^{2+} levels in the cytosol approximately 100-fold (Rüegg 1987). The channel is embedded in the phospholipid bilayer of the membrane, with a large cytoplasmic component extruding from the membrane. The cytoplasmic component is believed to represent the mechanical link with the DHPR of the T tubules (MacLennan 1990). The Ca^{2+}-release channel also has specialized sites for binding a range of ligands such as ATP, Mg^{2+} and Ca^{2+}. Ca^{2+}-release channels in adult mammalian Type II fibres are approximately two to four times more dense than in Type I fibres (Damiani & Margreth 1994). Several other SR proteins are associated with Ca^{2+} channel function. Calsequestrin and triadin are two examples. Of the three major ryanodine isoforms that have been identified, only RyR1 appears to be distributed in both Type I and Type II adult skeletal muscles (Damiani & Margreth 1994). Differences in the SR between major fibre types closely parallel differences in myosin HC isoform composition (Damiani & Margreth 1994). The fast-contracting Type II fibres with a high V_{max} also have a well-developed SR, allowing rapid release and uptake of Ca_f^{2+} from the cytosol (Table 11.4). In contrast, the SR is not as well developed in the slow-contracting Type I fibres, and consequently the kinetics of Ca^{2+} release and sequestration are much slower (Rüegg 1987). Neither the myosin isoform composition nor the characteristics of the SR appear to influence P_0. Providing the stimulus is of sufficient duration, and data are adjusted for cross-sectional area, there are only minor differences between Type I and Type II fibres.

T tubule–SR Ca^{2+} channel interface

The coupling of the action potential in the T tubule to SR Ca^{2+} release is probably the least understood process in the chain of command linking neural activation with increases in cytosolic Ca_f^{2+}. Arguably, it is one of the most significant in fatigue. It is now commonly accepted that skeletal muscle E–C coupling involves a mechanical linkage (Lamb 1998). DHPR, located in the T tubules in close apposition to the Ca^{2+}-release channel, appear to detect the voltage charge that occurs with depolarization and generate an asymmetrical charge movement. By mechanisms as yet unknown but apparently involving a physical coupling, the charge movement in the receptor allows a rapid release of stored Ca^{2+} in the SR through the Ca^{2+}-release channel. Cessation of the activation signal results in a rapid decrease in Ca^{2+} release. Magnesium (Mg^{2+}) has a strong inhibiting effect on the Ca^{2+}-release channel, and is believed to be involved in the control of the SR Ca^{2+} channel (Lamb 1998). A number of proteins appear to be intimately involved in E–C coupling, with the protein content of each dependent on the fibre type (Sutko & Airey 1996). Triadin and calsequestrin, two proteins which function to link the DHPR to the Ca^{2+}-release channel and to bind Ca^{2+}, respectively, appear to be coordinately expressed. Both are high in Type II fibres and low in Type I fibres (Sutko & Airey 1996; Pette & Staron 1997). Only in the case of calsequestrin do isoform differences appear between fibre types (Pette & Staron 1997). In the rabbit, Type II fibres contain only the fast isoform (CaS_f) whereas slow fibres contain both a fast and slow cardiac isoform (CaS_f and CaS_s). The differences in expression of E–C coupling proteins support the contractile characteristics of the fibre. Fast-contracting fibres are able to translate the activation signal into a Ca^{2+} transient much more rapidly than slow-contracting fibres.

Excitation–contraction coupling and repetitive activity

Can muscle fatigue be identified with one or more of the processes involved in conducting the excitation signal to the cell interior and producing a Ca_f^{2+} response? Failure in any one of the various processes could conceivably account for inability of a muscle cell to sustain a particular mechanical response. One process that has received considerable attention involves the ability of the sarcolemma and T tubule system to sustain repetitive action potentials (Green 1998; McKenna 1998). A popular approach to studying fatigue at this level is to stimulate the muscle or muscle fibre artificially, either directly or via the nerve, at different frequencies of

repetitive stimulation. The electromyographic (EMG) activity and the force response are then examined. It is generally agreed that the rapid force loss that occurs, particularly at high frequencies of stimulation, is due to failure of the Na^+/K^+-ATPase, resulting in an inability to restore Na^+ and K^+ gradients across the plasma membrane (Jones 1996). It has been inferred that this type of fatigue, often alluded to as high-frequency fatigue, results in a failure of the T tubules rather than the sarcolemma (Allen *et al.* 1995). The inability to sustain action potentials at high frequency is much more pronounced in muscles containing a predominance of Type IIB fibres, which possess a low Na^+/K^+-ATPase pump density, than in the more oxidative Type I and Type IIA fibres, which have a higher pump density (Allen *et al.* 1995; Hicks *et al.* 1997).

It has been far more problematic attempting to elucidate the role of action potential failure in voluntary repetitive activity. Although disturbances in cation distribution and membrane potential have been documented (Clausen & Nielsen 1996), it is unclear whether the changes are sufficient to impair function. Moreover, with voluntary contractions, membrane excitability may be protected at least to a level where the sarcolemma and T tubule are not limiting the force generated by the muscle. Bigland-Ritchie and Woods (1984) have found that when humans exert maximal effort, the firing frequency is reduced, supposedly by afferent feedback originating in the working muscle and acting on the α motoneurone pool. In addition, rotation can occur between motor units within and between synergistic muscles (Enoka & Stuart 1992), possibly providing sufficient time to re-establish Na^+ and K^+ gradients and membrane excitability in a wide variety of tasks.

These comments notwithstanding, it would be expected that with some task demands, the activity of the Na^+/K^+-ATPase might be substantially compromised. As with myofibrillar ATPase, this could reflect direct inhibition of the enzyme by accumulating metabolic by-products, such as ADP, P_i and H^+, which would be expected to decrease the free energy of ATP hydrolysis (Korge 1995). Alternatively, intrinsic alterations in the enzyme may occur as a result of repeated activation or due to some change in the intracellular environment mediated indirectly by contractile activity. To the author's knowledge, the only study that has addressed the effect of sustained exercise on Na^+/K^+-ATPase in humans measured enzyme activity indirectly in homogenates under optimal *in vitro* conditions; this study reported a substantial reduction in maximal activity (McKenna *et al.* 1996).

Human studies are hampered because of the need for large amounts of tissue for analysis. In addition, isolation of the enriched sarcolemma fractions necessary to measure Na^+/K^+-ATPase activity directly is notoriously unreliable given the relatively small yield of sarcolemma (Clausen 1986). Preliminary evidence pointing to a time-dependent reduction in intrinsic Na^+/K^+-ATPase activity could be physiologically important. The depression in activity could reflect structural changes in the enzyme, as has been shown for SR Ca^{2+}-ATPase (Dux *et al.* 1990). The Na^+/K^+-ATPase is particularly susceptible to free radicals generated during contractile activity (Korge 1998; Kourie 1998). It is possible that the relatively high Na^+/K^+ pump concentration observed in fibres with a high oxidative potential, namely Type I and Type IIA, is a response to oxidant injury (Wendt *et al.* 1998). Given the amount of free radicals generated during sustained activity of these fibres, a high initial Na^+/K^+-ATPase content would provide a reserve, allowing a certain amount of deactivation to occur without compromising muscle excitability. Exercise-induced alterations in composition of the phospholipid membrane in which the pump is embedded could also alter pump function and efficiency by modifying fluidity and resistance to pump rotation (Green 1998).

Although this chapter has only addressed the role of the Na^+/K^+-ATPase in membrane excitability, many other proteins constituting a variety of ion channels could also be involved in maintaining membrane excitability during physical activity.

Repetitive activity disrupts Ca^{2+} cycling and depresses cytosolic Ca_f^{2+} levels (Allen *et al.* 1995). This has been demonstrated most dramatically in single mouse and frog muscle fibres, using imposed activation patterns and direct measurements of Ca_f^{2+} in the cytosol. Reductions in Ca_f^{2+} and isomet-

ric force have been demonstrated with a variety of protocols, including different force levels (using different stimulation frequencies), different stimulation durations and following eccentric contractions (Allen *et al.* 1998). In several of these protocols, the reduction in Ca_f^{2+} has been traced directly to a failure in Ca^{2+} release (Allen *et al.* 1998), whereas in other protocols, the reduction in Ca^{2+} release appears to be due to more central factors, at the level of membrane excitation and/or E–C coupling (Allen *et al.* 1998). A failure in membrane excitability and/or E–C coupling has most often been implicated in protocols employing high stimulation frequencies (Allen *et al.* 1995).

Evidence supporting a link between intrinsic disturbances in the Ca^{2+}-release channel and repetitive activity has been obtained using measurements of Ca^{2+} release measured in homogenates or enriched SR preparations *in vitro* under supposedly optimal conditions (Favero *et al.* 1993). Following prolonged submaximal exercise, as an example, Favero *et al.* (1995) reported 20–30% decreases of Ca^{2+} release in rat muscle in conjunction with a similar decrease in (^{3}H) ryanodine binding, suggesting intrinsic modification of the Ca^{2+}-release channel.

A number of studies have found that prolonged activity impairs Ca^{2+}-ATPase and consequently Ca^{2+} uptake by the SR (Byrd *et al.* 1989a,b). These effects, based on *in vitro* measurements of muscle excised after exercise, are most dramatically demonstrated with chronic electrical stimulation. Within the first few days after the onset of stimulation, reductions in Ca^{2+}-ATPase activity and Ca^{2+} uptake approximate 40–50% (Leberer *et al.* 1987; Hicks *et al.* 1997). Studies employing fluorescein isothiocyanate (FITC), a substance with a high affinity for the nucleotide binding site on the enzyme, have reported reductions in ATP following exercise, indicating structural alterations at this site (Dux *et al.* 1990; Luckin *et al.* 1991). Some studies indicate disturbances in Ca^{2+} sequestration following exercise, but exceptions exist (Green 1998). At present, interpretation of the data, particularly in animals, is problematic, given that studies using different measurement techniques have reported contradictory results (Green 1998).

The SR in the human skeletal muscle cell appears particularly susceptible to voluntary activity, a number of studies reporting reductions in Ca^{2+} sequestration with both prolonged exercise (Green *et al.* 1998b) and isometric exercise (Gollnick *et al.* 1991). Prolonged exercise also appears to impair Ca^{2+} release in humans. As with other muscle ATPases, the alterations in the Ca^{2+}-release channel and/or the Ca^{2+}-ATPase could be due to the effects of repeated activation itself, or to alterations in the intracellular environment. Increases in the metabolic by-products, H^+, P_i and ADP, are known to reduce Ca^{2+} release and to depress Ca^{2+}-ATPase activity (Zhu & Nosek 1991; Favero *et al.* 1995). The role of some metabolites such as H^+ is being challenged since, at physiological temperatures, the effects are not nearly as dramatic as when low temperatures are used (Westerblad 1998). Whether persistent changes in one or more of these by-products are responsible for the intrinsic changes in the proteins involved in Ca^{2+} release and Ca^{2+} uptake remains unknown. Possibly, the accumulation of free radicals (Korge 1998; Kourie 1998) could also induce intrinsic alterations. Both the Ca^{2+}-release channel (Brotto & Nosek 1996) and Ca^{2+}-ATPase (Dux *et al.* 1990; Luckin *et al.* 1991) can be structurally altered by exposure to free radicals.

An important issue concerns the significance of alteration in Ca^{2+} cycling on Ca_f^{2+} levels and contractility. The effect may well depend on task requirements. It is possible that a reduction in Ca^{2+} release and Ca^{2+} uptake can be accommodated without an impairment in P_0 provided the time allowed for reloading and stimulation between contractions is long enough to allow a peak Ca_f^{2+} to be realized (Zhu & Nosek 1991). Indeed, reductions in Ca^{2+} uptake occurring in conjunction with reductions in Ca^{2+} release may well be a compensatory mechanism aimed at optimizing Ca_f^{2+} levels during activation. The largest effects of alterations in SR disturbances would be expected on dynamic activity, where velocity and power of the muscle depend on rapid changes in the Ca^{2+} transient. Failure at the level of E–C coupling is being increasingly implicated in fatigue. Where depressions in cytosolic Ca_f^{2+} occur, with repetitive activity involving intermittent or low-frequency stimulation, a depression in Ca^{2+} release is most often observed (Allen *et al.* 1995). The problem could reside at the level of the

Ca^{2+}-release channel, reflecting intrinsic changes in the channel by-product inhibition secondary to the accumulation of specific metabolites or ions. Recently, attention has been focused on T tubule–SR coupling mechanisms (Lamb 1998). Increases in Mg^{2+}, which occur when metabolism is increased and particularly when ATP is reduced, appear to have an inhibitory effect at both the Ca^{2+}-release channel and the DHPR (Lamb 1998). It is unclear if metabolic by-products such as P_i and H^+ can compromise function on the T tubule side of the coupling process. Free radicals appear to have detrimental effects on both the DHPR and the Ca^{2+}-release channel and they may explain the persistent reduction in force observed at low frequencies of stimulation (Lamb 1998).

A recent study has implicated T tubule–SR coupling failure in the profound weakness that occurs with eccentric exercise in mice (Ingalls *et al.* 1998). In this study 57–75% of the reduction in P_0 could be explained by a defect at the T tubule–SR interface during 5 days of recovery.

Chronic adaptation in excitation–contraction coupling function and composition

One of the most conspicuous adaptations accompanying persistent increases in muscle activity is a rapid and pronounced increase in Na^+/K^+-ATPase content. Chronic low-frequency stimulation of rabbit fast muscle results in a dramatic up-regulation of the Na^+/K^+-ATPase pump. Increases in excess of 80% have been observed within the first 10 days of stimulation (Green *et al.* 1992a) and if stimulation persists for 20 days, a doubling of the Na^+/K^+-ATPase is seen (Hicks *et al.* 1997). A rapid up-regulation has also been reported in human muscle, increases of approximately 15% occurring within 6 days of prolonged submaximal cycle training (Green *et al.* 1993). Several studies have reported increases in pump activity in response to a variety of training regimens including prolonged submaximal exercise, sprint training and HRT (Green 1998). Prolonged submaximal exercise appears to be a much more potent stimulus for evoking increases in pump expression than HRT (Green *et al.* 1999). A variety of hormones, including insulin, glucocorticoids, catecholamines and thyroxine can also alter the long-term regulation of the Na^+/K^+-ATPase (Ewart & Klip 1995; Clausen 1996b).

The fact that the Na^+/K^+-ATPase can be altered rapidly by physical activity suggests that the pump plays a key role in controlling contractile behaviour. As emphasized, an up-regulation, although not instrumental in altering P_0 and V_{max} in unfatigued muscle, could persist in preserving excitability during repeated activity by allowing a reserve for recruitment, as part of the pump becomes inactivated. Perhaps the most dramatic evidence of this is seen with chronic low-frequency stimulation. With this model, the rapid reduction in force after the onset of stimulation is accompanied by pronounced reductions in the mass action potential (M wave), indicating a loss of membrane excitability (Hicks *et al.* 1997). As stimulation continues, force recovers. The recovery of force is accompanied by increases in M wave amplitude and Na^+/K^+-ATPase content. An increase in pump concentration may also provide a more sensitive control of K^+ and Na^+ in the cell during physical activity by increasing the Michaelis constant K_m, i.e. the concentration at half the maximal velocity of reaction, and permitting a given reaction velocity to occur at lower Na^+ and K^+ concentrations (Clausen 1996a). There is evidence that this occurs as indicated by the smaller increase in blood K^+ accumulation with exercise following training-induced increases in Na^+/K^+-ATPase (Green 1998). A higher pump concentration may also prove effective in minimizing the impact of the metabolic by-product accumulation on enzyme activity.

Cellular adaptations could also protect membrane excitability and promote fatigue resistance. Continued viability of pump activity is intimately dependent on a readily available source of ATP. Increasing evidence indicates that metabolic pathways for ATP synthesis may be compartmentalized to cell regions close to where ATP is utilized (Green 1998). Subsarcolemmal accumulations of mitochondria can be identified, ostensibly to provide ATP for the Na^+/K^+-ATPase (Korge & Campbell 1994). A pronounced up-regulation in subsarcolemmal mitochondria has been reported with training (Bizeau *et al.* 1998), an adaptation that may be beneficial in protecting ATP homeostasis when training-induced increases in Na^+/K^+ pump concentration occur. Also located close to the pump are creatine phosphokinase (CPK) and glycolytic enzymes, which appear important in ATP regeneration.

Adaptations of the signalling systems could also prove effective in protecting cation pump function. A large pump concentration may not be beneficial unless it can be fully activated. Given a complex regulatory control (Bertorello & Katz 1995), adaptations to receptors and second messengers may help to ensure maximal activation during sustained effort.

Unlike the Na^+/K^+-ATPase, the SR Ca^{2+}-ATPase is much more resistant to contractile-induced long-term regulation. Although extensive changes in protein composition have been observed with chronic low-frequency stimulation of fast muscle, adaptations only occur after 10 days of activity (Hicks *et al.* 1997). Beyond this time, a reduction in protein content and a shift towards SERCA 2a from SERCA 1a are observed (Hicks *et al.* 1997). Adaptations in the Ca^{2+}-release channel and other components of E–C coupling also occur and appear to precede changes in Ca^{2+}-ATPase protein. By 10 days of stimulation, there are parallel reductions of between 40 and 60% in the proteins of the Ca^{2+}-release channel, DHPR and triadin (Ohlendieck *et al.* 1991; Hicks *et al.* 1997). There is some evidence that a severe programme of endurance training can effect changes in SR function in rat muscles and particularly in Ca^{2+}-ATPase activity and Ca^{2+} uptake (Green *et al.* 1984), but this does not appear to be the case in humans. Neither an HRT programme, conducted for 11–12 weeks, nor a prolonged endurance programme, conducted for a similar time, altered Ca^{2+} uptake or Ca^{2+}-ATPase activity in homogenates (Green *et al.* 1995). Additional studies on humans, examining other components of SR composition and E–C coupling, particularly in the context of the functional implications, would appear to be of high priority.

Muscle cells—cytoskeletal system

Any analysis of muscle and particularly any analysis that addresses fatiguability and training would be incomplete without reference to the cytoskeletal system (Fig. 11.1). The cytoskeletal system is an elaborate network of proteins that bind to other cell proteins and protect the ultrastructural organization and assembly (Thornell & Price 1991). Two major filamentous systems have been identified, an extrasarcomeric and an intrasarcomeric. The intrasarcomeric system consists of proteins such as titin and nebulin. Titin is a long filament that is anchored to the Z line, extending to the M line of the sarcomere, where it binds to myosin. In addition to defining the length of the thick filaments, it appears to prevent overstretch (Thornell & Price 1991; Schiaffino & Reggiani 1996). Nebulin, on the other hand, extends from the Z line along the thin filament, where it is bound to actin. This protein provides structural integrity to the thin filament and also specifies the length of the thin filament (Thornell & Price 1991; Schiaffino & Reggiani 1996).

Two major extrasarcomeric proteins are desmin and dystrophin. Desmin functions primarily to link the sarcomeres together transversely, whereas dystrophin anchors the myofibrils to the plasma membrane (Thornell & Price 1991). Further details on the composition and function of the cytoskeletal network are provided in a review article (Thornell & Price 1991).

Repeated exercise, particularly if high forces are involved as in eccentric contractions, imposes strain on the various cytoskeletal proteins, resulting in myofibrillar disorganization. Force transmission both within and outside the sarcomere can become compromised, resulting in impaired fibre contractility. This is most dramatically illustrated with the eccentric model, where fibre damage to contractile and cytoskeletal components prevails (Leiber *et al.* 1996). Under such circumstances, profound weakness can occur, extending for days (Newham *et al.* 1983; Clarkson & Tremblay 1988). The cytoskeletal system appears to show considerable malleability, the results being much less imposing when the muscle is systematically exposed to eccentric-type exercise (Clarkson & Tremblay 1988).

Weakness would be expected to compromise muscle performance significantly. Where muscles are chronically weakened, not only are the peak contractile properties limited, but the ability to sustain

a given submaximal load is reduced because of a decreased potential to recruit additional force reserves and, in particular, Type II fibres, which appear most affected (Leiber & Fridén 1988). Indeed, there is probably an element of weakness due to ultrastructural changes that develop with many tasks during repetitive activity and which would impair muscle performance independent of the energy state of the cell.

Metabolic and non-metabolic interactions in fatigue

Features that most clearly differentiate the performance characteristics of the different skeletal muscle fibre types are the velocity with which they can contract, the power they can generate and the time over which a fibre can maintain a specific mechanical response without fatigue when activated repeatedly. The composition and structure of the two major fibre types, Type I and Type II, are uniquely designed to perform these respective functions. Given that the major fibre type composition in humans appears to be genetically determined, with little evidence for training-induced transformations, how can the fibres be made more fatigue resistant? The answer may well depend on the task requirements.

The fundamental adaptation that has been identified with improved endurance relates to the ATP-regenerating metabolic pathways and, specifically, the oxidative potential of the fibre (Saltin & Gollnick 1983). With appropriate training, an impressive upregulation in the potential for oxidative phosphorylation and β-oxidation can occur in both Type I and Type II fibres (Saltin & Gollnick 1983); this allows an increased regeneration of ATP by aerobic-based fat utilization processes, the amount depending on the task. By increasing the aerobic contribution to energy supply, by-product accumulation can be minimized, metabolic efficiency increased and muscle glycogen conserved (Hochachka *et al.* 1991) (Fig. 11.5). These adaptations are unquestionably critical for sustained performance during submaximal exercise (Green 1991).

Other factors also appear to be important, particularly processes involved in E–C coupling. Pro-

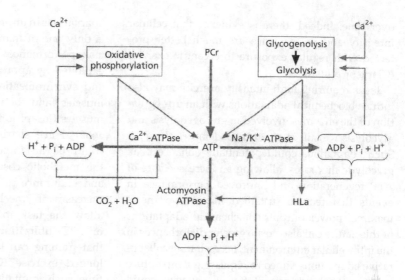

Fig. 11.5 Coordinated regulation of ATP synthesizing and ATP utilization pathways. This diagram illustrates the metabolic by-products produced by ATP hydrolysis and the inhibition of the ATPases that can result from by-product accumulation.

longed submaximal exercise appears to cause disturbances in cation cycling in terms of Na^+/K^+ gradient across the sarcolemma and T tubule, and in terms of SR Ca^{2+} cycling (Green 1998). T tubule–SR failure has also been suggested (Lamb 1998; Stephenson *et al.* 1998). These disturbances appear to be due to intrinsic changes in the proteins themselves. Although the mechanism(s) is unclear, the change does not appear to be associated with accumulation of metabolic by-products such as P_i or H^+, or to glycogen depletion, since a considerable disturbance occurs when concentrations of metabolic by-products are low and glycogen is plentiful. Possibly changes in free radical generation or a local increase in temperature are responsible (Green 1995; Korge 1998). A depression in Ca^{2+} sensitivity of the myofibrillar apparatus also indicates some alteration in the regulatory and/or contractile proteins (Allen *et al.* 1995).

Training can result in impressive increases in Na^+/K^+-ATPase, an adaptation that may be vital in protecting membrane excitability and promoting increased endurance in a variety of tasks. There is no evidence that the SR Ca^{2+}-ATPase in the Ca^{2+}-release channel can be up-regulated with voluntary training. Expression of the proteins of the SR appears to covary with the myosin HC slow and fast isoforms. Since there is little evidence that transformation of the major fibre types can occur regardless of the type

of training programme, long-term regulation of the SR with training may be unrealistic. To date, there appears to be no study that has addressed possible adaptive changes in the T tubule–Ca^{2+}-release channel interface with training.

A well-documented adaptation to regular high resistance or submaximal prolonged activity is an increase in fibre area. This could be important in increasing endurance, since it would give a greater force reserve to exploit as fatigue develops. However, beneficial effects are not entirely clear, possibly because of the 'neurospecificity' that appears to accompany training. In addition, an increase in muscle mass increases the work needed to lift the limbs against gravity. The specific nature and demands of the task should be analysed carefully before decisions are made to pursue programmes that focus on muscle hypertrophy.

The cytoskeletal system may be another area where adaptation could be induced. Given the role of the scaffold proteins in protecting cellular integrity and ultrastructure and the extensive disruption that occurs when unconditioned muscle is repeatedly subjected to large forces, adaptation of these structures could conceivably minimize the weakness that develops with this type of activity. Muscles that begin a task free of weakness or that experience little weakness after the onset of activity should be more capable of meeting task demands over time. Indeed, there is evidence that cellular integrity and performance are much better protected with regular exposure to eccentric exercise (Clarkson *et al.* 1992).

Tasks requiring high-intensity exercise may also induce biochemical adaptations with an up-regulation of the enzymes involved in glycogenolysis and glycolysis (Costill *et al.* 1979; Cadefau *et al.* 1990). Such adaptations could potentially enhance peak glycolytic flux rates, allowing an increased rate of ATP regeneration and improved performance in events that require sustained maximal or near-maximal power outputs. Biochemical adaptations of this nature can also create greater disturbances in the intracellular environment, necessitating collaborative adaptations aimed at regulating temperature increases and acidosis. Buffering capacity could conceivably be improved by increasing concentrations of proteins that remove by-products (H^+, lactate) from the cell or buffer the by-products directly.

In effect, it could be argued that the benefits of metabolic adaptations to endurance may never be fully realized without adaptations in the non-metabolic components of the cell.

Conclusions

This chapter has emphasized the role of cellular

adaptations in improving fatigue resistance, but this is only one of many levels involved in voluntary task performance. Cellular adaptations must be exploited by appropriate recruitment, rate coding and synchronization of motor units both within muscles and between agonist and antagonist muscles (Josephson 1993; Heckman & Sandercock 1996). Force sharing among synergistic muscles could be an important adaptation in allowing the metabolic costs of a task to be minimized and endurance to be emphasized (Herzog 1996). Increases in mechanical efficiency would also allow the task to be performed at lower rates of ATP utilization, and it is well established that training can lower the aerobic costs of prolonged exercise (Gaesser & Poole 1996). Over time, such adaptation could promote a more stable intracellular environment, with fuel selection directed more towards fat and less towards carbohydrate. The ability to sustain muscle glycogen appears critical to sustained performance (Green 1991).

Impressive advances in our understanding of the cellular mechanisms involved in fatigue and the manner in which fatigue alters the force–length and force–velocity characteristics of different muscles now provide an unparalleled opportunity to design innovative approaches to the management of fatigue in sport.

References

Allen, D.G., Lännergren, J. & Westerblad, H. (1995) Muscle cell function during prolonged activity: Cellular mechanisms of fatigue. *Experimental Physiology* **80**, 497–527.

Allen, G.A., Balnave, C.D., Chin, E.R. & Westerblad, H. (1998) Failure of calcium release in muscle fatigue. In: Hargreaves, M. & Thompson, M. (eds) *Biochemistry of Exercise X*, pp. 135–146. Human Kinetics, Champaign, IL.

Barclay, C.J. (1996) Mechanical efficiency and fatigue of fast and slow muscles of the mouse. *Journal of Physiology (London)* **497**, 781–794.

Bertorello, A.M. & Katz, A.I. (1995) Regulation of the Na^+-K^+ pump activity: pathways between receptors and effectors. *News in Physiological Science* **10**, 253–259.

Bigland-Ritchie, B. & Woods, J.J. (1984) Changes in muscle contractile properties and neural control during human muscle fatigue. *Muscle and Nerve* **7**, 691–699.

Bizeau, M.E., Willis, W.T. & Hazel, J.R. (1998) Differential responses to endurance training in subsarcolemmal and intermyofibrillar mitochondria. *Journal of Applied Physiology* **85**, 1279–1284.

Brandt, P.W., Diamond, M.S. & Rutchik, J. (1987) Co-operative interactors between troponin–tropomyosin units extend the length of the thin filament in skeletal muscle. *Journal of Molecular and Biological Medicine* **195**, 885–896.

Brotto, M.A.P. & Nosek, T.M. (1996) Hydrogen peroxide disrupts Ca^{2+}

release from the sarcoplasmic reticulum of rat skeletal muscle fibers. *Journal of Applied Physiology* **81**, 731–737.

Burke, R.E., Levine, D.N., Tsairis, P. & Zajac, F.E. (1973) Physiological types and histochemical profiles in motor units of the cat gastrocnemius. *Journal of Physiology (London)* **234**, 723–748.

Byrd, S.K., Bode, A.K. & Klug, G.A. (1989a) Effects of exercise of varying duration on sarcoplasmic reticulum function. *Journal of Applied Physiology* **66**, 1383–1388.

Byrd, S.K., McCutcheon, L.J., Hodgson, D.R. & Gollnick, P.D. (1989b) Altered sarcoplasmic reticulum function after high intensity exercise. *Journal of Applied Physiology* **67**, 2072–2077.

Cadefau, J., Casademonat, J., Grau, J.M. *et al.* (1990) Biochemical and histochemical adaptation to sprint training in young athletes. *Acta Physiologica Scandinavica* **140**, 341–351.

Caiozzo, V.J., Perrine, J.J. & Edgerton, V.R. (1981) Training induced alterations of the *in-vivo* force–velocity relationship of human muscle. *Journal of Applied Physiology* **51**, 750–754.

Chin, E.R. & Green, H.J. (1991) Fiber type differences in Na^+/K^+-ATPase concentration of rat skeletal muscle are related to oxidative potential. *Medicine and Science in Sports and Exercise* **23**, 523.

Clarkson, R.B. & Tremblay, I. (1988) Exercise-induced muscle damage, repair, and adaptation in humans. *Journal of Applied Physiology* **65**, 1–6.

Clarkson, P.M., Nosaka, K. & Braun, B. (1992) Muscle function after exercise-induced muscle damage and rapid adaptation. *Medicine and Science in Sports and Exercise* **24**, 512–520.

Clausen, T. (1986) Regulation of active Na^+-K^+ transport in skeletal muscle. *Physiological Reviews* **66** (3), 542–580.

Clausen, T. (1996a) The Na^+-K^+ pump in skeletal muscle: quantification, regulation and functional significance. *Acta Physiologica Scandinavica* **156**, 227–236.

Clausen, T. (1996b) Long- and short-term regulation of the Na^+-K^+ pump in skeletal muscle. *News in Physiological Science* **11**, 24–30.

Clausen, T. & Nielsen, O.B. (1996) The Na^+-K^+ pump and muscle contractility. *Acta Physiologica Scandinavica* **152**, 365–373.

Close, R.I. (1964) Dynamic properties of mammalian skeletal muscles. *Physiological Reviews* **52**, 129–197.

Cooke, R. (1997) Actomyosin interaction in striated muscle. *Physiological Reviews* **77**, 671–697.

Cooke, R. & Pate, E. (1990) The inhibition of muscle contraction by the by-products of ATP hydrolysis. In: Taylor, B. (ed.) *Biochemistry of Exercise VII*, pp. 59–72. Human Kinetics, Champaign, IL.

Costill, D.L., Coyle, E.F., Fink, W.F., Lesmes, G.F. & Witzmann, F.A. (1979) Adaptations in skeletal muscle following strength training. *Journal of Applied Physiology* **46**, 96–99.

Coyle, E.F., Feiring, D.C., Rotkis, T.C. *et al.* (1981) Specificity of power improvements through slow and fast isokinetic training. *Journal of Applied Physiology* **51**, 1437–1442.

Crow, M.T. & Kushmerick, M.J. (1982) Chemical energetics of slow and fast twitch muscles of the mouse. *Journal of General Physiology* **79**, 147–166.

Damiani, E. & Margreth, A. (1994) Charac-

terization study of the ryanodine receptor and of calsequestrin isoforms of mammalian skeletal muscles in relation to fibre types. *Journal of Muscle Research and Cell Motility* **15**, 86–101.

Dux, L., Green, H.J. & Pette, D. (1990) Chronic low-frequency stimulation of rabbit fast-twitch muscle induces partial inactivation of the sarcoplasmic reticulum Ca^{2+}-ATPase and changes in its tryptic cleavage. *European Journal of Biochemistry* **195**, 92–100.

Enoka, R.M. & Stuart, D.A. (1992) Neurobiology of muscle fatigue. *Journal of Applied Physiology* **72**, 1631–1648.

Evans, W.J. & Cannon, J.G. (1991) The metabolic effects of exercise-induced muscle damage. In: Holloszy, J.O. (ed.) *Exercise and Sport Science Reviews*, pp. 99–125. Williams & Wilkins, Baltimore.

Everts, M., Anderson, J.P., Clausen, T. & Hansen, O. (1989) Quantitative determination of Ca^{2+}-dependent Mg^{2+} ATPase from sarcoplasmic reticulum in muscle biopsies. *Biochemical Journal* **260**, 443–445.

Ewart, S.H. & Klip, A. (1995) Hormonal regulation of the Na^+-K^+-ATPase: mechanism underlying sustained changes in pump activity. *American Journal of Physiology* **269**, C295–C311.

Favero, T.G., Pessah, I.N. & Klug, G.A. (1993) Prolonged exercise reduces Ca^{2+}-release in rat skeletal muscle sarcoplasmic reticulum. *Pflügers Archives* **422**, 472–475.

Favero, T.G., Zable, A.C., Bowman, M.B., Thompson, A. & Abramson, J. (1995) Metabolic end products inhibit sarcoplasmic reticulum Ca^{2+} release and $[^3H]$ ryanodine binding. *Journal of Applied Physiology* **78**, 1665–1672.

Fitts, R.H. (1994) Cellular mechanisms of muscle fatigue. *Physiological Reviews* **74**, 49–94.

Fitts, R.H. & Widrick, J.J. (1996) Muscle mechanics: adaptations with exercise training. In: Holloszy, J.O. (ed.) *Exercise and Sport Science Reviews*, pp. 427–473. Williams & Wilkins, Baltimore.

Fitts, R.H., Courtright, J.B., Kim, D.H. & Witzmann, F.A. (1982) Muscle fatigue with prolonged exercise: contractile and biochemical alterations. *American Journal of Physiology* **242**, C65–C73.

Fitts, R.H., Costill, D.L. & Gardetto, P.R. (1989) Effect of swim exercise training on human muscle fiber function. *Journal of Applied Physiology* **66**, 465–475.

Franzini-Armstrong, C. & Protasi, F. (1997) Ryanodine receptors of striated muscles: a complex channel capable of multiple

interactions. *Physiological Reviews* **77**, 699–729.

Gaesser, G.A. & Poole, D.C. (1996) The slow component of oxygen uptake kinetics in humans. In: Holloszy, J.O. (ed.) *Exercise and Sport Science Reviews*, pp. 35–70. Williams & Wilkins, Baltimore.

Gollnick, P.D., Korge, P., Karpakka, J. & Saltin, B. (1991) Elongation of skeletal muscle relaxation during exercise is linked to reduced calcium uptake by the sarcoplasmic reticulum in man. *Acta Physiologica Scandinavica* **142**, 135–136.

Green, H.J. (1991) How important is endogenous muscle glycogen to fatigue in prolonged exercise? *Canadian Journal of Physiology and Pharmacology* **69**, 290–297.

Green, H.J. (1992) Myofibrillar composition and mechanical function in mammalian skeletal muscle. In: Shephard, R.J. (ed.) *Sports Science Reviews* **1**(1), 43–64. Human Kinetics, Champaign, IL.

Green, H. (1995) Metabolic determinants of activity induced muscular fatigue. In: Hargreaves, M. (ed.) *Exercise Metabolism*, pp. 211–256. Human Kinetics, Champaign, IL.

Green, H.J. (1997) Mechanisms of muscle fatigue in intense exercise. *Journal of Sport Sciences* **15**, 247–256.

Green, H.J. (1998) Cation pumps in skeletal muscle: potential role in muscle fatigue. *Acta Physiologica Scandinavica* **162**, 201–213.

Green, H.J., Klug, G.A., Reichmann, H., Seedorf, U., Wieher, W. & Pette, D. (1984) Exercise induced fibre type transitions with regard to myosin, parvalbumin and sarcoplasmic reticulum in muscles of the rat. *Pflügers Archives* **400**, 432–438.

Green, H.J., Ball-Burnett, M., Chin, E.R. & Pette, D. (1992a) Time dependent alterations in sarcolemma Na^+-K^+ ATPase content of low-frequency stimulated rabbit muscle. *FEBS Letters* **310**, 129–131.

Green, H.J., Düsterhöft, S., Dux, L. & Pette, D. (1992b) Metabolite patterns related to exhaustion, recovery and transformation of chronically stimulated rabbit fast-twitch muscle. *Pflügers Archives* **420**, 359–366.

Green, H.J., Chin, E.R., Ball-Burnett, M. & Ranney, D. (1993) Increases in human skeletal muscle Na^+-K^+ ATPase concentration with short term training. *American Journal of Physiology* **264**, C1538–C1541.

Green, H.J., Grange, F., Goreham, C., Shoemaker, K. & Grant, S. (1995) Failure of high resistance and submaximal exercise training to alter sarcoplasmic reticulum Ca^{2+}-ATPase in human skeletal muscle. *Medicine and Science in Sports and Exercise* **27** (Suppl.), S66.

Green, H., Dahly, A., Shoemaker, J.K., Goreham, C., Bombardier, E. & Ball-Burnett, M. (1999) Serial effects of high-resistance and prolonged endurance training on Na$^+$-K$^+$ pump concentration and enzymatic activities in human vastus lateralis. *Acta Physiologica Scandinavica* **165**, 177–184.

Green, H., Goreham, C., Ouyarg, J., Ball-Burnett, M. & Ranney, D. (1998a) Regulation of fiber size, oxidative potential and capillarization in human muscle by resistance exercise. *American Journal of Physiology* **276**, 591–596.

Green, H.J., Grange, F., Chin, C., Goreham, C. & Ranney, D. (1998b) Exercise-induced decreases in sarcoplasmic reticulum Ca^{2+}-ATPase activity attenuated by high-resistance training. *Acta Physiologica Scandinavica* **164**, 141–146.

Hawkins, C., Xu, A. & Narayan, N. (1994) Sarcoplasmic reticulum calcium pump in cardiac and slow twitch skeletal muscle but not fast twitch skeletal muscle undergoes phosphorylation by endogenous and exogenous Ca^{2+}/calmodulin-dependent protein kinase. *Journal of Biological Chemistry* **269**, 31198–31206.

Heckman, C.J. & Sandercock, T.G. (1996) From motor unit to whole muscle properties during locomotor movements. In: Holloszy, J.O. (ed.) *Exercise and Sport Science Reviews*, pp. 109–133. Williams & Wilkins, Baltimore.

Henriksson, J.M., Chi, M.Y., Hintz, C.S. *et al.* (1986) Chronic stimulation of mammalian muscle: changes in enzymes of six metabolic pathways. *American Journal of Physiology* **251**, C614–C632.

Herzog, W. (1996) Force-sharing among synergistic muscles. Theoretical considerations and experimental approaches. In: Holloszy, J.O. (ed.) *Exercise and Sport Science Reviews*, pp. 173–202. Williams & Wilkins, Baltimore.

Hicks, A., Ohlendieck, K., Göpel, S.O. & Pette, D. (1997) Early functional and biochemical adaptations to low-frequency stimulation of rabbit fast-twitch muscle. *American Journal of Physiology* **273**, C297–C305.

Hochachka, P.W. (1994) *Muscles as Molecular and Metabolic Machines.* CRC Press Inc., Boca Raton, Florida.

Hochachka, P.W., Stanley, C., Mathewson, G.O., McKenzie, D.C., Allen, P.S. & Parkhouse, W.S. (1991) Metabolic and work

efficiencies during exercise in Andean natives. *Journal of Applied Physiology* **70**, 1720–1730.

Hundal, H.S., Marette, A., Ramlal, T., Liu, Z. & Klip, A. (1993) Expression of β subunit isoforms of the Na, K-ATPase is muscle type specific. *FEBS Letters* **328**, 253–258.

Hundal, H.S., Maxwell, D.L., Ahmed, A., Darakhshan, F., Mitsumoto, Y. & Klip, A. (1994) Subcellular distribution and immunocytochemical localization of Na$^+$-K$^+$-ATPase subunit isoforms in human skeletal muscle. *Molecular and Membrane Biology* **11**, 255–262.

Ingalls, C.P., Warren, G.L., Williams, J.H., Ward, C.W. & Armstrong, R.B. (1998) E–C coupling failure in mouse EDL after *in vivo* eccentric contractions. *Journal of Applied Physiology* **85**, 58–67.

Jones, D.A. (1996) High- and low-frequency revisited. *Acta Physiologica Scandinavica* **156**, 265–270.

Jones, D.A. & Rutherford, O.M. (1987) Human muscle strength training. The effects of three different regimes and the nature of the resultant changes. *Journal of Physiology (London)* **391**, 1–11.

Josephson, R.K. (1993) Contraction dynamics and power output of skeletal muscle. *Annual Review of Physiology* **55**, 527–546.

Korge, P. (1995) Factors limiting adenosine triphosphatase function during high intensity exercise. *Sports Medicine* **20**, 215–225.

Korge, P. (1998) Factors limiting ATPase activity in skeletal muscle. In: Hargreaves, M. & Thompson, M. (eds) *Biochemistry of Exercise X*, pp. 125–134. Human Kinetics, Champaign, IL.

Korge, P. & Campbell, K.B. (1994) Local ATP regeneration is important for sarcoplasmic reticulum Ca^{2+} pump function. *American Journal of Physiology* **267**, C357–C366.

Kourie, J.I. (1998) Interaction of reactive oxygen species with ion transport mechanisms. *American Journal of Physiology* **275**, C1–C24.

Kraemer, W.J., Fleck, S.J. & Evans, W.J. (1996) Strength and power training: physiological mechanisms of adaptation. In: Holloszy, J.O. (ed.) *Exercise and Sport Science Reviews*, pp. 363–397. Williams & Wilkins, Baltimore.

Lamb, G.D. (1998) Excitation–contraction coupling and fatigue in skeletal muscle. In: Hargreaves, M. & Thompson, M. (eds) *Biochemistry of Exercise X*, pp. 99–114. Human Kinetics, Champaign, IL.

Leberer, E., Härtner, K.T. & Pette, D. (1987)

Reversible inhibition of sarcoplasmic reticulum Ca-ATPase by altered neuro-muscular activity in rabbit fast-twitch muscle. *European Journal of Biochemistry* **162**, 555–561.

Leiber, R.L., Thornell, L.E. & Fridén, J. (1996) Muscle cytoskeletal disruption occurs within the first 15 min of eccentric contractions. *Journal of Applied Physiology* **80**, 278–284.

Lieber, C.V., Schmitz, M.C., Mishra, D.K. & Fridén, J. (1994) Contractile and cellular remodelling in rabbit skeletal muscle after cyclic eccentric contractions. *Journal of Applied Physiology* **77**, 1926–1934.

Leiber, R.L. & Fridén, J. (1988) Selective damage of fast glycolytic muscle fibres with eccentric contraction of the rabbit tibialis anterior. *Acta Physiologica Scandinavica* **133**, 587–588.

Luckin, K.A., Favero, T.G. & Klug, G.A. (1991) Prolonged exercise induces structural changes in SR Ca^{2+}-ATPase of rat muscle. *Biochemical Medicine and Metabolic Biology* **46**, 391–405.

Lytton, J., Westlin, M., Burk, S.E., Shull, G.E. & MacLennan, D.H. (1992) Functional comparisons between isoforms of the sarcoplasmic or endoplasmic reticulum family of calcium pumps. *Journal of Biological Chemistry* **267**, 14483–14489.

McKenna, M.J. (1998) Role of the skeletal muscle Na$^+$-K$^+$-pump during exercise. In: Hargreaves, M. & Thompson, M. (eds) *Biochemistry of Exercise X*, pp. 71–97. Human Kinetics, Champaign, IL.

McKenna, M.J., Fraser, S.F., Li, J.L., Wang, X.N. & Carey, M.F. (1996) Impaired muscle cation regulation with fatigue. *Physiologist* **39** (5), A-79.

MacLennan, D.H. (1990) Molecular tools to elucidate problems in excitation–contraction coupling. *Biophysics Journal* **58**, 1355–1365.

Martonosi, A.N. (1996) Structure–function relationships in the Ca^{2+}-ATPase of sarcoplasmic reticulum: facts, speculations and questions for the future. *Biochimica et Biophysica Acta* **1275**, 111–117.

Metzger, J.M. (1996) Effects of troponin C isoforms on pH sensitivity of contraction in mammalian fast and slow skeletal muscle fibres. *Journal of Physiology (London)* **492**, 163–172.

Metzger, J.M. & Moss, R.L. (1987) Greater hydrogen ion induced depression of tension and velocity in skinned single fibers of rat fast then slow muscles. *Journal of Physiology (London)* **393**, 727–742.

Meyer, R.A. & Terjung, R.A. (1979) Difference in ammonia and adenylate metabolism in contracting slow and fast muscle. *American Journal of Physiology* **237**, C111–C118.

Moss, R.L., Diffee, G.M. & Greaser, M.L. (1995) Contractile properties of skeletal muscle fibers in relation to myofibillar protein isoforms. *Reviews of Physiology, Biochemistry and Pharmacology* **126**, 1–53.

Newham, D.J., McPhail, G., Mills, K.R. & Edwards, R.H.T. (1983) Ultrastructural changes after concentric and eccentric contractions. *Journal of Neurological Science* **61**, 109–122.

Ogata, T. & Yamasaki, Y. (1997) Ultra-high resolution scanning microscopy of mitochondria and sarcoplasmic reticulum in human red, white and intermediate muscle fibers. *Anatomical Record* **248**, 214–223.

Ohlendieck, K., Briggs, F.N., Lee, K.F., Wechsler, A.S. & Campbell, K.P. (1991) Analysis of excitation–contraction coupling components in chronically stimulated canine skeletal muscle. *Journal of Biochemistry* **202**, 739–747.

Pette, D. & Staron, R.S. (1997) Mammalian skeletal muscle fiber type transitions. *International Review of Cytology* **170**, 143–223.

Pette, D. & Vrbová, G. (1985) Invited review. Neural control of phenotypic expression in mammalian muscle fibers. *Muscle and Nerve* **8**, 676–689.

Rüegg, J.C. (1987) Excitation–contraction coupling in fast- and slow-twitch muscle fibers. *International Journal of Sports Medicine* **8**, 360–364.

Saltin, B. & Gollnick, P.D. (1983) Skeletal muscle adaptability: significance for metabolism and performance. In: Peachy, L.D., Adrian, R.H. & Geiger, S.R. (eds) *Handbook of Physiology. Skeletal Muscle*, pp. 551–631. Williams & Wilkins, Baltimore.

Salviatti, G., Sorenson, M. & Eastwood, A.B. (1982) Calcium accumulation by the SR in two populations of chemically skinned human muscle fibers. *Journal of General Physiology* **79**, 603–632.

Salviatti, G., Betto, R., Danieli-Betto, D. & Zeviani, M. (1983) Myofibrillar protein isoforms and sarcoplasmic reticulum Ca^{2+}-transport activity of single human muscle fibres. *Biochemical Journal* **224**, 215–225.

Samaha, F.J. & Gergely, J. (1965) Ca^{2+}-uptake and ATPase in human sarcoplasmic reticulum. *Journal of Clinical Investigation* **44**, 1425–1431.

Schachat, F.H., Diamond, M.S. & Brandt, P.W. (1987) Effect of different troponin T–tropomyosin combinations on thin filament activation. *Journal of Molecular and Biological Medicine* **198**, 551–554.

Schiaffino, S. & Reggiani, C. (1996) Molecular diversity of myofibrillar proteins: gene regulation and functional significance. *Physiological Reviews* **76**, 371–423.

Schuler, J.M. & Fitts, R.H. (1994) Shortening velocity and ATPase activity of rat skeletal muscle fibers. Effect of endurance exercise training. *American Journal of Physiology* **266**, C1699–C1713.

Squire, J.M. & Morris, E.P. (1998) A new look at thin filament regulation in vertebrate skeletal muscle. *FASEB Journal* **12**, 761–771.

Staron, R.S. (1991) Correlation between myofibrillar ATPase activity and myosin heavy chain composition in single human muscle fibers. *Histochemistry* **96**, 21–24.

Staron, R.S. & Pette, D. (1993) The continuum of pure and hybrid myosin heavy chain-based fibre types in rat skeletal muscle. *Histochemistry* **100**, 149–153.

Staron, R.S., Malicky, E.S., Leonardi, M.J., Falkel, J.E., Hagerman, F.C. & Dudley, G.A. (1990) Muscle hypertrophy and fast fiber type conversions in heavy resistance-trained women. *European Journal of Applied Physiology* **60**, 71–79.

Stephenson, D.G., Lamb, G.D. & Stephenson, G.M.M. (1998) Events of the excitation–relaxation (E–C–R) cycle in fast- and slow-twitch mamalian muscle fibres relevant to muscle fatigue. *Acta Physiologica Scandinavica* **162**, 229–245.

Sutko, J.L. & Airey, J.A. (1996) Ryanodine receptor Ca^{2+} release channels: does diversity in form equal diversity in function. *Physiological Reviews* **76**, 1027–1071.

Sweeney, H.L., Bowman, B.F. & Stull, J.T. (1993) Myosin light chain phosphorylation in vertebrate striated muscle: regulation and function. *American Journal of Physiology* **264**, C1085–C1095.

Thornell, L.E. & Price, M.G. (1991) The cytoskeleton in muscle cells in relation to function. *Biochemical Society Transactions* **19**, 1116–1120.

Wendt, C.H., Towle, H., Sharma, R. *et al.* (1998) Regulation of Na^+-K^+-ATPase gene repression by hyperoxia in MDCK cells. *American Journal of Physiology* **274**, C356–C364.

Westerblad, H. (1998) The role of pH and inorganic phosphate ions in skeletal muscle fatigue. In: Hargreaves, M. & Thompson, M. (eds) *Biochemistry of Exercise X*, pp. 149–154. Human Kinetics, Champaign, IL.

Zhu, Y. & Nosek, T.M. (1991) Intracellular milieu changes associated with hypoxia impair sarcoplasmic reticulum Ca^{2+} transport in cardiac muscle. *American Journal of Physiology* **261**, H620–H626.

Chapter 12

Endocrine Factors in Endurance

MARK S. TREMBLAY AND JENNIFER L. COPELAND

Introduction

Research in exercise endocrinology has flourished over the past 30 years, with MEDLINE™ citations for 'Exercise and Hormones' increasing from eight in 1965 to 333 in 1996 (Tremblay & Chu 1998). This increase in research has led to an improved understanding of the effect of endurance activities on the hormonal milieu. Endocrine factors have profound and diverse regulatory effects on circulatory and metabolic function both during exercise and in response to physical training. Enhanced knowledge of endocrine dynamics during exercise and in response to physical training has allowed sport scientists to monitor and tailor athlete training programmes more precisely. Unfortunately, this improved understanding has also led to more sophisticated doping practices by athletes (Kammerer 1993; Chapter 31). This chapter surveys the changes typically seen in stress hormones in response to exercise and physical training, and discusses the major metabolic consequences of these changes.

Sympathoadrenal hormones

Sympathoadrenal hormones originate from a neuroendocrine system that comprises the adrenal glands and the sympathetic nervous system. Together they control many of the functions involved in the body's response to physical stress and play a major role in the regulation of energy metabolism during exercise. This system clearly demonstrates the lack of distinction between the nervous system and the endocrine system, since the catecholamines act as hormones by stimulating receptor-mediated responses in many tissues, but they also act as neurotransmitters in the peripheral and central nervous system (Landsberg & Young 1992). Norepinephrine is the main neurotransmitter released from sympathetic nerve endings; epinephrine is secreted primarily from modified sympathetic nerve cells (chromaffin cells) in the adrenal medulla. The catecholamines activate both α- and β-adrenergic receptors; depending on the tissue and receptor sensitivity, they also regulate cardiac function, distribution of blood flow and substrate metabolism (Mazzeo 1991).

Catecholamine levels increase in response to an acute bout of endurance exercise. During dynamic activity, plasma concentrations of epinephrine and norepinephrine increase exponentially with increases in exercise intensity (Galbo 1981). Increases in catecholamine levels are related more closely to exercise intensity if the latter is expressed relative to body mass and fitness status (Galbo 1983). During graded exercise, the initial increase in catecholamines is primarily under the control of the sympathetic nervous system, but during more prolonged submaximal exercise there is a greater contribution from the adrenal gland, with a resultant decrease in the norepinephrine to epinephrine ratio (Mazzeo 1991). Hartley et al. (1972) found that norepinephrine increased in response to moderate exercise and increased further with heavy work, whereas epinephrine only increased during heavy work.

The sympathoadrenal response to exercise is both

tissue specific and intensity dependent (Mazzeo 1991). Catecholamine release can also be stimulated by reduced oxygen availability, significant increases or decreases in body temperature, decreased glucose availability, increased duration of exercise, and the mental stress of competition (Galbo 1983). Age and fitness level are other factors which can influence the catecholamine response to exercise, with older subjects and trained subjects demonstrating a blunted catecholamine response (Kohrt et al. 1993). Isometric exercise produces an amplified sympathoadrenal response.

Epinephrine and norepinephrine play a major role in metabolic control during exercise, mainly by mobilizing fuel reserves. This can occur by the direct action of catecholamines on fuel stores, but also indirectly through adrenergic inhibition or stimulation of other glucoregulatory hormones. In muscle, catecholamines directly stimulate glycogenolysis by activating glycogen phosphorylase. In the liver, they promote glycogenolysis by suppression of insulin and stimulation of glucagon (Landsberg & Young 1992). In adipose tissue catecholamines stimulate lipolysis. For more detail on cellular metabolism and endurance activity, refer to Chapter 9.

Most stress hormones exhibit a diminished acute response to exercise following endurance training. At the same absolute work rate, epinephrine and norepinephrine levels increase less with exercise in trained than in untrained individuals (Hartley et al. 1972; Lehmann et al. 1981). However, the sympathetic response at a given relative work rate may remain unchanged after training (Peronnet et al. 1981).

Winder et al. (1978) demonstrated that the catecholamine response to exercise declined after only 3 weeks of training. More recently, it has been shown that exercise-induced responses diminish following 10 days of training, after which much smaller decreases are seen (Mendenhall et al. 1994). The reduction in sympathoadrenal activity is believed to be beneficial, lowering heart rate and reducing the typical response to mental stress. However, the average daily epinephrine and norepinephrine concentrations may be much higher in trained than in untrained individuals. Dela et al. (1992) found that training did not reduce catecholamine levels during

normal daily activities, and peak catecholamine levels during exercise were much higher in trained individuals even though the response to a given absolute work rate was typically smaller than in untrained subjects.

The implications of the altered catecholamine levels during exercise are not clear. Endurance training results in a reduction of hepatic glycogenolysis and gluconeogenesis during exercise, which may be a consequence of lower catecholamine levels (Coggan et al. 1995). Muscle glycogenolysis is also reduced at a given relative work rate after training (Chesley et al. 1996). The apparent glycogen-sparing effect of lower catecholamine concentrations may account for the delayed glycogen depletion that is observed in trained subjects. However, glycogen phosphorylase is regulated by several factors in addition to hormonal mechanisms, so it is unlikely that a reduction in catecholamines is the only explanation of this training effect. Enhanced mitochondrial activity and allosteric regulation may also contribute to the decreased glycogenolysis (Chesley et al. 1996).

Pituitary and subordinate gland hormones

Adrenocorticotrophic hormone and cortisol

Cortisol is secreted from the adrenal cortex and is the predominant glucocorticoid in humans. The secretion of cortisol is regulated by the release of adrenocorticotrophic hormone (ACTH) from the anterior pituitary in a negative feedback relationship. There is a time lag between the elevation of ACTH concentrations and the subsequent increase in cortisol (Schwarz & Kindermann 1990). The secretion of ACTH is controlled by corticotrophin-releasing hormone (CRH), which is released from the hypothalamus in response to physical or emotional stress; CRH is also regulated by a negative feedback relationship with cortisol. There is a diurnal variation in the secretion of both ACTH and cortisol, with levels reaching their peak in the morning.

ACTH concentrations increase in response to both long-duration aerobic exercise and incremental, graded exercise (Schwarz & Kindermann 1990; Heitkamp *et al.* 1993). ACTH release during exercise is correlated highly with the release of β-endorphin. ACTH levels depend on the intensity and duration of exercise, and the training status of the individual (Heitkamp *et al.* 1993). In trained individuals ACTH concentrations increase significantly at 80% and 100% of $\dot{V}_{O_{2max}}$ but not at 60% of $\dot{V}_{O_{2max}}$ (Yoon & Park 1991). Heitkamp *et al.* (1993) demonstrated that ACTH concentrations increased exponentially during a marathon run. Others have shown that ACTH only increased significantly after subjects exceeded their individual anaerobic threshold (Schwarz & Kindermann 1990; Yoon & Jun 1993). Duclos *et al.* (1997) found that ACTH concentrations increased only if the exercise was intense and prolonged. ACTH levels returned to baseline within 30–60 min after short-duration exercise (Yoon & Park 1991; Heitkamp *et al.* 1993), but decreased more slowly after prolonged exercise such as a marathon run (Heitkamp *et al.* 1993).

Cortisol increases in response to a variety of exercise stimuli and is sensitive to environmental and exercise-specific stress. Stimulated by ACTH, cortisol increases with increasing exercise intensity and duration. Intense exercise increases both the rate of cortisol secretion and the rate of cortisol clearance from the plasma, whereas at lower work rates cortisol clearance increases disproportionately to secretion. Therefore, at lower work rates, plasma cortisol concentrations may actually decrease (Cashmore *et al.* 1977; Galbo 1981). Plasma cortisol increases significantly at work rates greater than 60% of $\dot{V}_{O_{2max}}$ (Galbo 1981; Yoon & Park 1991), but not during brief anaerobic exercise (Schwarz & Kindermann 1990). Duclos *et al.* (1997) found that cortisol increased only during prolonged exercise at 80% of maximum heart rate and not during brief or light exercise (50% of maximum heart rate).

There are many inconsistencies in cortisol responses to exercise, and assessment of the effects of exercise on the hypothalamic–pituitary–adrenal axis may be confounded by several factors. ACTH and cortisol secretions have a circadian rhythm, so that the cortisol response may vary depending on the time of day (Thuma *et al.* 1995). Moreover, the timing of the circadian rhythm may be influenced by training status (Wittert *et al.* 1996). There appears to be a gender difference in cortisol levels, with females tending towards higher cortisol levels during periods of intensive training (Tsai *et al.* 1991; Tyndall *et al.* 1996). In addition, the hypothalamic–pituitary–adrenal axis is responsive to emotional and psychological factors, increasing the variance in exercise-induced changes (Galbo 1983).

The metabolic consequences of the increased cortisol concentrations during exercise are not clearly defined. Cortisol increases protein breakdown, providing amino acids for hepatic glucose production. It also accelerates the mobilization of lipid stores. One of the most important functions of cortisol during exercise may be to support and enhance the action of other hormones, such as glucagon and epinephrine, in increasing glucose production (Galbo 1983).

Training generally attenuates pituitary–adrenal activation during exercise; however, for the reasons cited above, this response is quite variable. Increases in ACTH and cortisol concentrations at any given absolute work rate tend to be lower in trained than in untrained subjects (Luger *et al.* 1987). However, postexercise ACTH levels may be higher in trained than in untrained individuals (Lehmann *et al.* 1993; Duclos *et al.* 1997). There appears to be no significant difference in either recovery or basal levels of cortisol in trained versus untrained men, but ACTH concentrations are consistently higher in trained subjects (Wittert *et al.* 1996; Duclos *et al.* 1997). This indicates a change in the pituitary–adrenal relationship. It may result from a decrease in the adrenal sensitivity to ACTH, or a decrease in the sensitivity of the hypothalamic–pituitary axis to cortisol negative feedback. The former view is supported by Galbo (1983), who suggested that although physical training results in adrenal hypertrophy, cortisol secretion may still be lowered due to a decreased sensitivity to ACTH.

Some trained individuals demonstrate characteristics consistent with chronic hypercortisolism. Injections of CRH result in smaller ACTH and cortisol responses in highly trained individuals compared to moderately trained or sedentary subjects (Luger *et al.* 1987). The reduced activation of the hypothalamic–pituitary–adrenal axis is inversely proportional to the level of training; further, it appears as though there is a training threshold for these adaptations.

Thyroid hormones

The thyroid gland is controlled by thyroid-stimulating hormone (TSH), which is released from the anterior pituitary in response to hypothalamic thyrotrophin-releasing hormone (TRH). The thyroid gland secretes thyroxine (T_4) and triiodothyronine (T_3). Decreases in metabolic rate stimulate the hypothalamic–pituitary–thyroid axis. The primary action of thyroid hormones is to increase the metabolic rate of cells, although they also contribute to the maintenance of body mass; they stimulate protein synthesis and carbohydrate metabolism, and may enhance lipolysis indirectly.

TSH increases in anticipation of exercise, and continues to increase with increasing work rate, plateauing after about 40 min of exercise. This pattern, however, has not been demonstrated consistently. It is difficult to measure the influence of TSH on thyroid hormones, because the small turnover of these hormones makes acute changes hard to detect (Galbo 1983). Some have found increases of T_4 following endurance exercise (Terjung & Tipton 1971; Hackney & Gulledge 1994). In contrast, others have found no change in thyroid hormones with endurance exercise (Galbo et al. 1977a). The assessment of thyroid hormone changes after exercise is complicated by a very small turnover rate, and by the influence of factors such as body temperature, food ingestion and diurnal changes (Galbo 1983).

Endurance training has no influence on basal or postexercise levels of TSH (Lehmann et al. 1993). However, training may increase the turnover and secretion of T_4. Changes in thyroid hormones with training may be a result of changes in body composition or an increase in the sensitivity of target cells to TSH. The significance of training-induced adaptations in thyroid hormone concentrations has not yet been established. However, thyroid hormones play an important role in thermoregulation and in the mobilization of free fatty acids. Therefore, exer-

cise capacity is poor in hypothyroid individuals (Galbo 1983).

Growth hormone

Growth hormone is secreted from the anterior pituitary gland in a pulsatile fashion in response to hypothalamic growth hormone-releasing factors. Growth hormone stimulates tissue growth, promotes lipolysis and gluconeogenesis, and reduces carbohydrate metabolism (Galbo 1983). The anabolic effects of growth hormone are mediated through the production of insulin-like growth factors, which are present in most tissues (Van Wyck 1984). Hypoglycaemia, increased body temperature, hypoxia and acidosis increase growth hormone secretion at rest and during exercise (Galbo 1983; Bunt 1986).

Growth hormone increases during endurance exercise, after a brief latent period. The acute response to exercise is manifested as the intensity or duration of activity is increased (Galbo 1983; Bunt et al. 1986). Repeated bouts of aerobic exercise on a single day can augment the growth hormone response (Kanaley et al. 1997). The threshold intensity for growth hormone secretion depends on exercise duration and training history. Growth hormone levels remain elevated postexercise, and may even continue to rise if a steady state of exercise has not been achieved. Conversely, growth hormone levels following prolonged exercise like marathon running may diminish to pre-exercise values.

Resting growth hormone levels are reduced in endurance-trained athletes (Galbo 1983). However, endurance training amplifies the pulsatile release of growth hormone at rest (Weltman et al. 1992). This adaptation may be advantageous, because a pulsatile delivery of growth hormone enhances tissue responses. Peak growth hormone levels during prolonged exercise may also be increased following endurance training (Bunt 1986). Growth hormone levels at submaximal work rates are lower in trained athletes than in sedentary controls. This observation is consistent across several of the hormones discussed in this chapter; it reflects the improved ability of the body to maintain homeostasis during exercise. Because there appear to be redundancies in the function of hormones regulating substrate availability during exercise, the importance of training adaptations is not clearly understood.

Gonadotrophins and sex steroids

Chapter 49 deals in detail with reproductive changes and the endurance athlete. Plasma testosterone, oestrogen and progesterone levels increase in response to short-term aerobic and anaerobic exercise (Jurkowski et al. 1978; Jensen et al. 1991). With prolonged exercise (> 2 h), there is a consistent decrease in circulating testosterone, regardless of exercise mode (Webb et al. 1984; Kujala et al. 1990). It is unclear whether changes in luteinizing hormone or follicle-stimulating hormone induce the depressed testosterone response to prolonged exercise. There is some evidence of reduced luteinizing hormone pulse frequency and amplitude in both female (Cumming et al. 1985) and male (MacConnie et al. 1986) distance runners compared to controls. Thus, it is speculated that the mechanism for this inhibition is pituitary hyposensitivity to gonadotrophin-releasing hormone. The pulsatile release of gonadotrophins from the pituitary gland makes interpretation of venous blood samples difficult. Research on the gonadotrophin response to endurance exercise in both male and female endurance athletes has produced conflicting results and requires further research.

Many studies have demonstrated lower basal or resting levels of circulating testosterone (Hackney 1996) and oestrogen (Loucks 1994) in endurance-trained athletes. The training volume threshold at which hypogonadism develops is unknown; probably it reflects individual characteristics (training history, genetics and lifestyle habits). De Souza et al. (1994) observed lower testosterone levels in athletes running 108 km per week than in athletes running 54 km per week. Others have found similar results, though the suggested training threshold shows wide variation among different groups of athletes. The exercise dose required to induce reproductive morbidity in female endurance athletes shows similar variation. In addition to lower resting sex steroid levels, endurance-trained athletes have a blunted hormone response to short-term exercise. Because of the diverse health implications of chronically depressed sex steroid levels (decreased bone mineralization, decreased libido, decreased reproductive function, muscle atrophy, increased proteolysis and amino acid fuel utilization), this area of research has expanded significantly in recent years. Though many theories have been put forward (Loucks 1994; Hackney 1996), the aetiology of endurance training-induced hypogonadism remains unclear.

Prolactin

Prolactin is structurally similar and closely related to growth hormone. Prolactin is secreted in pulsatile fashion in response to stimuli from the hypothalamus. What differentiates prolactin release from many of the other pituitary hormones is its tonic hypothalamic inhibition by dopamine. The primary physiological functions of prolactin are to stimulate and maintain lactation. Prolactin may have metabolic effects, but research in this area is very speculative. Conflicting findings have suggested that prolactin inhibits testosterone secretion. Hodgson et al. (1983) resolved these contradictions, concluding that prolactin has a positive effect on luteinizing hormone receptors in the testis, yet chronic hyperprolactinaemia has an inhibitory effect on luteinizing hormone receptors. Research on prolactin responses to exercise and training is scarce, and it provides little insight into metabolic or circulatory regulation during endurance exercise.

β-endorphin

β-endorphin is secreted from the anterior pituitary gland, where it is synthesized from pro-opiomelanocortin, the same preprohormone as for ACTH. Not surprisingly, changes in ACTH concentration in response to exercise correlate closely with changes in circulating β-endorphin concentrations (Heitkamp et al. 1993). As with ACTH, plasma β-endorphin levels are increased after both short-term high-intensity exercise and long-duration exercise like marathon running (Yoon & Park 1991; Heitkamp et al. 1993; Goldfarb & Jamurtas 1997).

Levels return to baseline more quickly following short-term exercise than after prolonged exercise. In short-duration exercise (< 30 min) a threshold intensity, around the anaerobic threshold, must be exceeded before significant increases in β-endorphin are observed (Schwarz & Kindermann 1990; Yoon & Park 1991). Because of β-endorphin's morphine-like characteristics, it has been credited with the euphoric sensations experienced by some people following prolonged endurance exercise. However, data that substantiate this reputation of β-endorphin are still lacking (Richter & Sutton 1994).

Reported effects of training on β-endorphin levels are conflicting, with lower or unchanged resting levels; and increases, decreases or no change in exercise responses (Goldfarb & Jamurtas 1997). Lobstein and Rasmussen (1991) demonstrated lower resting plasma β-endorphin levels and lower depression scores following 8 months of fitness training. The authors speculated that changes in β-endorphin levels may have helped to mitigate non-clinical depression. The changes in β-endorphin with training and their relationship to measures of affect require further study.

Pancreatic hormones

Insulin and glucagon are two of the main glucoregulatory hormones. Insulin is secreted from pancreatic β cells. It acts to lower plasma glucose concentrations by suppressing glucose production, inhibiting lipolysis in adipose tissue and stimulating glucose uptake in the muscle. Glucagon is secreted from pancreatic α cells. It acts as a counter-regulatory hormone, activating hepatic glycogenolysis and gluconeogenesis. These hormones interact to maintain normoglycaemia and metabolic homeostasis during endurance exercise (Cryer 1992).

Insulin is one of the few hormones to show a decreased secretion during acute endurance exercise. Sympathetic stimulation of the pancreas inhibits insulin secretion when the $\dot{V}o_2$ exceeds 50% of $\dot{V}o_{2max}$ (Galbo 1983). During exercise, even the ingestion of glucose does not appear to increase insulin levels (Slentz et al. 1990). α-adrenergic blockade restores resting insulin levels, indicating that

α-adrenergic mechanisms are responsible for the exercise-induced decline in insulin concentrations (Berger et al. 1980).

The reduction of insulin concentrations during exercise theoretically results in an increased endogenous glucose production and an increased lipolysis, making more fuel available for working muscles. Although insulin levels are reduced, glucose uptake is increased during exercise. This is possible because contracting muscle is capable of glucose uptake even in the absence of insulin. Insulin and exercise have a synergistic effect on glucose uptake (Mikines et al. 1988).

Glucagon secretion increases with endurance exercise. It serves to mobilize stored glucose during prolonged exercise. Increases in glucagon are not usually seen until after 1 h or more of exercise (Galbo 1983; Mendenhall et al. 1994). This suggests that glucagon does not increase until carbohydrate stores are low, and that glucose availability is the major regulator of glucagon secretion. This speculation is supported by evidence that glucose ingestion inhibits exercise-induced increases in plasma glucagon (Galbo et al. 1977b). Although glucagon levels are reduced by glucose infusion during exercise, this does not necessarily diminish hepatic glucose output, demonstrating that sympathetic responses to exercise may play as great a role in hepatic glucose production as glucagon action (Galbo et al. 1977b). The combination of a decreased insulin secretion and an increased secretion of glucagon and epinephrine during exercise helps to regulate blood glucose during exercise.

After endurance training, insulin decreases less with an acute bout of exercise (Mendenhall et al. 1994). Basal insulin levels and glucose-stimulated insulin secretion at rest are also lower in trained individuals (Farrell et al. 1992). These changes may occur for several reasons. Both muscle tissue and liver tissue have an increased insulin sensitivity after training (Mikines et al. 1988). It has also been speculated that changes in insulin secretion may reflect changes in the β cells of the pancreas (Farrell et al. 1992). Therefore, if target tissues become more sensitive to insulin and the pancreas secretes less insulin, both the source and the target tissue are adapting to training so that less insulin is necessary to maintain normoglycaemia (Engdahl *et al.* 1995).

Glucagon responses are also altered by training. After 10 days of training, glucagon levels were significantly lower following 90 and 120 min of endurance exercise at the same absolute intensity of effort (Mendenhall *et al.* 1994). This is consistent with the notion that glucose levels control glucagon secretion, since exercise glucose levels tend to be higher in trained individuals (Galbo 1983). Endurance training reduces the rate of hepatic glycogenolysis and gluconeogenesis, sparing glycogen stores and improving performance. This may be associated with the hormonal training adaptations discussed thus far, including decreased catecholamines, decreased glucagon and a diminished decrease in insulin secretion during exercise (Coggan *et al.* 1995).

Fluid-regulating hormones

Antidiuretic hormone (ADH, vasopressin) and the renin–angiotensin–aldosterone system cooperate with neural factors in regulating blood pressure and body fluid content. During endurance exercise, fluid balance is altered significantly by fluid shifts, evaporation and sweating. ADH, secreted from the posterior pituitary gland, causes the kidneys to retain water, and stimulates vasoconstriction to elevate blood pressure. When blood flow through the kidneys is decreased, the kidneys secrete the enzyme renin. This promotes the formation of angiotensin II from already circulating proteins. Angiotensin II is a potent vasoconstrictor. It also reduces renal excretion of salt and water thereby preserving body fluid. Both renin and angiotensin II increase aldosterone secretion from the adrenal cortex. Aldosterone, in turn, promotes sodium and water retention by the kidneys.

During exercise, the sympathetic nervous system reduces renal blood flow, stimulating renin release. This provokes an increase in circulating ADH, angiotensin II and aldosterone (Galbo 1983). Freund *et al.* (1991) demonstrated that the exercise-induced increase in fluid-regulating hormones is intensity dependent, with the greatest increases observed at the highest intensities of exercise. Altenkirch *et al.*

(1990) showed that ADH, renin, aldosterone and atrial natriuretic factor (ANF) were markedly elevated immediately following a marathon run. ADH, renin and aldosterone concentrations remained high 3 h after the marathon run. It appears that fluid-regulating hormones play a role in sodium and water retention, inducing hypervolaemia during exercise and recovery (Fellmann 1992). Supporting this is evidence that the exercise response of fluid-regulating hormones is more pronounced under hyponatraemic or hypovolaemic conditions (Galbo 1983).

The decreased renal sodium and water loss that results from increases in ADH, angiotensin and aldosterone maintains body fluids during acute exercise and expands extracellular volume and plasma volume with training (Galbo 1983). However, there are no clear differences in ADH, renin or aldosterone levels between trained and untrained subjects.

Erythropoietin

Erythropoietin (EPO) is a glycoprotein hormone that originates in the kidneys. It is secreted in response to arterial hypoxia. EPO stimulates the production of red blood cells in the bone marrow, and it is regulated by feedback from the level of renal oxygenation. The relationship between EPO and endurance training is of particular interest due to the low haemoglobin concentrations associated with the 'sports anaemia' of endurance athletes.

The serum concentration of EPO is unchanged in response to an acute bout of intense, prolonged endurance exercise in trained subjects (Weight *et al.* 1992; Klausen *et al.* 1993; Remacha *et al.* 1994). Mean serum concentrations of EPO do not differ significantly between trained subjects and sedentary controls (Weight *et al.* 1992), or between iron-deficient athletes, normal athletes and sedentary controls (Remacha *et al.* 1994). These results indicate that haematological abnormalities in endurance athletes have no measurable effects on erythropoietic drive (Weight *et al.* 1992). This information may be important for the evaluation of sports anaemia and the detection of EPO abuse.

Influences confounding hormonal responses to exercise

Changes in hormone levels allow the body to adjust appropriately to numerous physiological and psychological challenges. Accordingly, many factors influence circulating hormone levels. Recent publications have detailed the numerous variables to consider when evaluating endocrine responses to exercise and training (Tremblay *et al.* 1995; Tremblay & Chu 2000). When interpreting changes in hormone levels in response to an acute bout of exercise or to a training programme, consideration should be given to standardizing or controlling for various confounding variables (Table 12.1). A lack of uniform statistical applications and data normalizing procedures have contributed to contradictory findings in exercise endocrinology (Tremblay *et al.* 1995).

Most studies in exercise endocrinology are based on venous blood samples. The limitations of this sampling procedure, particularly during endurance activities, must be recognized. First, serum or plasma analyses reflect only what is happening in the blood and not what is happening in the tissue of interest. In many cases hormonal changes in venous blood may reflect changes in the biological stimulus at the target tissue accurately, but in other cases they may not. For example, if the receptors at the target tissues are saturated, or if an increase in blood hormone levels causes a down-regulation of receptors, then changes in blood hormone levels may not reflect changes in stimulation of the target tissue. For hormones bound to plasma transporters, like steroid hormones, the dynamics between transporter availability, hormone–transporter affinity, offloading capacity in the capillary and free hormone levels also affect the cellular uptake of the hormone (Whitley *et al.* 1994).

A second consideration germane to endurance sport is the effect of changes in plasma volume. Haemoconcentration, as a consequence of fluid loss, or haemodilution, as a consequence of overhydration, will change the relative level of hormones in the blood. These changes in plasma volume may mask or amplify changes in hormone secretion, metabolism and clearance. Depending on the variable of interest, hormone levels assessed during endurance events should be corrected for changes in plasma volume, based on changes in haemoglobin and haematocrit.

Hormone doping

Many endogenous hormones can now be synthesized, utilizing recombinant DNA procedures

Table 12.1 Summary of variables important in exercise-related hormone research. Reproduced with permission from Tremblay *et al.* (1995).

Standardized conditions	Specimen collection and analysis	Exercise variables	Data manipulation and analysis/other
Temperature	Posture	Intensity	Sample size
Humidity	Circadian variation	Duration	Measurement reliability
Cigarette smoking	Pulsatile secretions	Mode	Plasma volume changes
Caffeine ingestion	Circannual variation	Muscle mass utilized	Individual versus grouped data
Alcohol consumption	Collection method	Frequency of training	Analysis procedure
Medications	Collection tubes	Exercise volume	Data normalization
Nutritional status	Storage method	Initial training status	AUC versus repeated measures
Sleeping patterns	Anticoagulant selection	Overtraining state	Error term
Psychological stress	Specimen selection	Rest periods between sets	Age
Weight fluctuation	Haemolysis	Order of exercises	Gender
Previous exercise	Analysis technique		Race
	Biological variation		Disease
	Analytical variation		

AUC, area under the curve.

Table 12.2 Summary of hormonal changes with exercise and training.

Primary source	Hormone	Physiological effects	Response to exercise	Adaptation to training	Other observations
Sympathetic nervous system and adrenal medulla	Norepinephrine and epinephrine	↑cardiac output, regulates blood flow ↑sweat rate ↑glycogenolysis ↑lipolysis	↑with exercise greater ↑ as intensity ↑	↓response at absolute work rate ↑peak levels	Norepinephrine more prominent in early exercise, epinephrine more prominent during prolonged exercise
Anterior pituitary	ACTH	Stimulates cortisol and aldosterone release	↑with exercise	↓at absolute work load ↑rest and maximal levels	Correlated with β-endorphin levels
	TSH	Stimulates production and secretion of thyroid hormones	↑with exercise	No change/unknown	Threshold intensity must be exceeded to induce a response
	Growth hormone	↑anabolism ↑FFA mobilization ↑gluconeogenesis ↓carbohydrate metabolism	↑with exercise after short sdelay ↑intensity or duration ↑response	↓resting levels ↓submaximal levels ↓peak levels	No change
	Luteinizing hormone	Promotes testosterone, oestrogen, and progesterone production and secretion	no change inconsistent findings	↓pulse frequency and amplitude	Inconsistent findings
	FSH	Promotes spermatogenesis, follicle growth and ovulation	no change inconsistent findings		Unknown
	Prolactin	Initiates/maintains lactation ↑FFA mobilization?	↑with exercise		
	β-endorphin	↓pain sensation ↑sedation and euphoria	↑with prolonged exercise ↑with intense exercise	Rest levels ↓ or no change Conflicting findings	↑with exercise intensity beyond critical threshold

Posterior pituitary	Antidiuretic hormone	Antidiuresis	↑ with increasing exercise	Conflicting findings
Testes	Testosterone	↑ anabolism ↑ androgenicity	↑ with exercise greater ↑ as intensity ↑ ↓ after prolonged exercise	↓ resting levels with endurance training ↓ postexercise if prolonged activity
Ovaries	Oestrogen and progesterone	Control menstrual cycle Promote female sex characteristics	↑ with exercise	↓ resting levels with endurance training Related to athletic amenorrhoea
Adrenal cortex	Cortisol	Glucocorticoid Promotes lipolysis and proteolysis Anti-inflammatory	↑ with exercise Greater ↑ with ↑ intensity or duration	↓ at absolute work rate No change in rest levels Confounded by many physical and psychological variables
Kidney	Aldosterone Renin Erythropoietin	Sodium and water retention ↑ angiotensin and aldosterone Red blood cell production	↑ with exercise ↑ with exercise may ↑ with exercise	Conflicting findings Conflicting findings No changes observed
Thyroid	Thyroxine and triiodothyronine	↑ metabolism	↑ free thyroxine	↑ free thyroxine at rest ↑ turnover Delayed response to TSH—large plasma pool
Pancreas	Insulin	Promotes glucose uptake by cells	↓ with exercise	↓ less with exercise ↓ basal levels ↓ at absolute work rate Insulin sensitivity improved
Pancreas	Glucagon	↑ hepatic glycogenolysis ↑ gluconeogenesis ↑ lipolysis	↑ with prolonged exercise	

ACTH, adrenocorticotrophic hormone; FFA, free fatty acid; FSH, follicle-stimulating hormone; TSH, thyroid-stimulating hormone.

(Wilson & Foster 1992). This technology has tremendously improved the ability to treat medical conditions arising from impaired endocrine function. Unfortunately, the availability of manufactured hormones has also provided athletes with the opportunity to enhance various hormone levels artificially. Hormones (or their analogues) abused in this fashion include human chorionic gonadotrophin, gonadotrophin-releasing hormone, human growth hormone, testosterone, epitestosterone and EPO (Kammerer 1993). Recently, interest in exogenous androstenedione and dehydroepiandrosterone has surged. Because these are naturally occurring hormones, laboratory detection of such hormone doping is difficult, providing unscrupulous athletes with a sense of security. Although supraphysiological doses of some of the hormones listed above have ergogenic effects, the long-term health implications of artificially altering the hormonal balance are very poorly understood. Furthermore, conclusive proof of performance-enhancing effects is lacking for many of these hormones. For details on specific doping procedures, their effects and consequences, see Chapter 31, and other detailed references (Wilson 1988; VanHelder et al. 1991; Yesalis 1993).

Summary

A summary of the primary hormones and how they change with exercise and physical training is presented in Table 12.2. In general, the endocrine system is stimulated in response to exercise. With the notable exception of insulin, the output of most hormones increases in response to an acute bout of exercise. The magnitude of the increase is related to many factors, including exercise intensity and duration, age, gender, fitness level, training status and also psychological factors. Physical training induces endocrinological adaptations. In most cases, hormonal responses to any given submaximal work rate are reduced following training. In some cases, resting and/or maximal hormone levels are also altered following exercise training, or differ between trained and untrained subjects. However, more research is necessary to understand the interplay between hormones during and following exercise, and to determine how the hormonal milieu contributes to substrate availability and delivery.

References

Altenkirch, H.U., Gerzer, R., Kirsch, K.A. et al. (1990) Effect of prolonged physical exercise on fluid regulating hormones. *European Journal of Applied Physiology* **61**, 209–213.

Berger, D., Floyd, J.C., Lampman, R.M. & Fagans, S.S. (1980) The effect of adrenergic blockade on the exercise-induced rise in pancreatic polypeptide in man. *Journal of Clinical Endocrinology* **50**, 33–39.

Bunt, J.C. (1986) Hormonal alterations due to exercise. *Sports Medicine* **3**, 331–345.

Bunt, J.C., Boileau, R.A., Bahr, J.M. & Nelson, R.A. (1986) Sex and training differences in human growth hormone during prolonged exercise. *Journal of Applied Physiology* **61**, 1796–1801.

Cashmore, G.C., Davies, C.T.M. & Few, J.D. (1977) Relationship between increases in plasma cortisol concentration and rate of cortisol secretion during exercise in man. *Journal of Endocrinology* **72**, 109–110.

Chesley, A., Heigenhauser, G.J.F. & Spriet, L.L. (1996) Regulation of muscle glycogen phosphorylase activity following short-term endurance training. *American Journal of Physiology* **270**, E328–E335.

Coggan, A.R., Swanson, S.C., Mendenhall, L.A., Habash, D.L. & Kien, C.L. (1995) Effect of endurance training on hepatic glycogenolysis and gluconeogenesis during prolonged exercise in men. *American Journal of Physiology* **268**, E375–E383.

Cryer, P.E. (1992) Glucose homeostasis and hypoglycemia. In: Wilson, J.D. & Foster, D.W. (eds) *Williams Textbook of Endocrinology*, 8th edn, pp. 1223–1253. W.B. Saunders Company, Philadelphia.

Cumming, D.C., Vickovic, M.M., Wall, S.R. & Fluker, M.R. (1985) Defects in pulsatile LH release in normally menstruating runners. *Journal of Clinical Endocrinology and Metabolism* **60**, 810–812.

Dela, F., Mikines, K.J., Von Linstow, M. & Galbo, H. (1992) Heart rate and plasma catecholamines during 24h of everyday life in trained and untrained men. *Journal of Applied Physiology* **73**, 2389–2395.

De Souza, M.J., Arce, J.C., Pescatello, L.S., Scherzer, H.S. & Luciano, A.A. (1994) Gonadal hormones and semen quality in male runners. *International Journal of Sports Medicine* **15**, 383–391.

Duclos, M., Corcuff, J.B., Rashedi, M., Fougère, V. & Manier, G. (1997) Trained versus untrained men: different immediate post-exercise responses of pituitary adrenal axis. *European Journal of Applied Physiology* **75**, 343–350.

Engdahl, J.H., Veldhuis, J.D. & Farrell, P.A. (1995) Altered pulsatile insulin secretion associated with endurance training. *Journal of Applied Physiology* **79**, 1977–1985.

Farrell, P.A., Caston, A.L., Rodd, D. & Engdahl, J. (1992) Effect of training on insulin secretion from single pancreatic beta cells. *Medicine and Science in Sports and Exercise* **24**, 426–433.

Fellmann, N. (1992) Hormonal and plasma alterations following endurance exercise: a brief review. *Sports Medicine* **13**, 37–49.

Freund, B.J., Shizuru, E.M., Hashiro, G.M. & Claybaugh, J.R. (1991) Hormonal, electrolyte, and renal responses to exercise are intensity dependent. *Journal of Applied Physiology* **70**, 900–906.

Galbo, H. (1981) Endocrinology and metabolism in exercise. *International Journal of Sports Medicine* **2**, 203–211.

Galbo, H. (1983) *Hormonal and Metabolic Adaptation to Exercise*. Georg Thieme-Verlag, New York.

Galbo, H., Hummer, L., Peterson, I., Christensen, N.J. & Bie, N. (1977a) Thyroid and testicular hormone responses to graded and prolonged exercise in man. *European Journal of Applied Physiology* **36**, 101–106.

Galbo, H., Christensen, N.J. & Holst, J.J. (1977b) Glucose induced decrease in glucagon and epinephrine responses to exercise in man. *Journal of Applied Physiology* **42**, 525–530.

Goldfarb, A.H. & Jamurtas, A.Z. (1997) Beta-endorphin response to exercise: an update. *Sports Medicine* **24**, 8–16.

Hackney, A.C. (1996) Testosterone, the hypothalamic–pituitary–testicular axis, and endurance exercise training: a review. *Biology of Sport* **13**, 85–98.

Hackney, A.C. & Gulledge, T. (1994) Thyroid hormone responses during an 8-hour period following aerobic and anaerobic exercise. *Physiological Research* **43**, 1–5.

Hartley, L.H., Mason, J.W., Hogan, R.P. *et al.* (1972) Multiple hormonal responses to graded exercise in relation to physical training. *Journal of Applied Physiology* **33** (5), 602–606.

Heitkamp, H.C.H., Schmid, K. & Scheib, K. (1993) Beta endorphin and adrenocorticotropic hormone production during marathon and incremental exercise. *European Journal of Applied Physiology* **66**, 269–274.

Hodgson, Y., Robertson, D.M. & de Kretser, D.M. (1983) The regulation of testicular function. *International Review of Physiology* **27**, 275–327.

Jensen, J., Oftebro, H., Breigan, B. *et al.* (1991) Comparison of changes in testosterone concentrations after strength and endurance exercise in well trained men. *European Journal of Applied Physiology* **63**, 467–471.

Jurkowski, J., Younglai, E., Walker, C., Jones, N.L. & Sutton, J.R. (1978) Ovarian hormone response to exercise. *Journal of Applied Physiology* **44**, 109–114.

Kammerer, R.C. (1993) Drug testing and anabolic steroids. In: C.E. Yesalis (ed.) *Anabolic Steroids in Sport and Exercise*, pp.

283–308. Human Kinetics, Champaign, IL.

Kanaley, J.A., Weltman, J.Y., Veldhuis, J.D., Rogol, A.D., Hartman, M.L. & Weltman, A. (1997) Human growth hormone response to repeated bouts of aerobic exercise. *Journal of Applied Physiology* **83**, 1756–1761.

Klausen, T., Breum, L., Fogh-Andersen, N., Bennett, P. & Hippe, E. (1993) The effect of short and long duration exercise on serum erythropoietin concentrations. *European Journal of Applied Physiology* **67**, 213–217.

Kohrt, W.M., Spina, R.J., Ehsani, A.A., Cryer, P.E. & Holloszy, J.O. (1993) Effects of age, adiposity, and fitness level on plasma catecholamine responses to standing and exercise. *Journal of Applied Physiology* **75**, 1828–1835.

Kujala, U.M., Alen, M. & Huhtaniemi, I.T. (1990) Gonadotrophin-releasing hormone and human gonadotrophin tests reveal that both hypothalamic and testicular endocrine functions are suppressed during acute prolonged physical exercise. *Clinical Endocrinology* **33**, 219–225.

Landsberg, L. & Young, J.B. (1992) Catecholamines and the adrenal medulla. In: Wilson, J.D. & Foster, D.W. (eds) *Williams Textbook of Endocrinology*, 8th edn, pp. 621–705. W.B. Saunders Company, Philadelphia.

Lehmann, M., Keul, J., Huber, G. & Da Prada, M. (1981) Plasma catecholamines in trained and untrained volunteers during graduated exercise. *International Journal of Sports Medicine* **2**, 143–147.

Lehmann, M., Knizia, K., Gastmann, U. *et al.* (1993) Influence of 6-week, 6 days per week, training on pituitary function in recreational athletes. *British Journal of Sports Medicine* **27**, 186–192.

Lobstein, D.D. & Rasmussen, C.L. (1991) Decreases in resting plasma beta-endorphin and depression scores after endurance training. *Journal of Sports Medicine and Physical Fitness* **31**, 543–551.

Loucks, A.B. (1994) Physical activity, fitness, and female reproductive morbidity. In: Bouchard, C., Shephard, R.J. & Stephens, T. (eds) *Physical Activity, Fitness, and Health*, pp. 943–954. Human Kinetics, Champaign, IL.

Luger, A., Deuster, P.A., Kyle, S.B. *et al.* (1987) Acute hypothalamic–pituitary–adrenal responses to the stress of treadmill exercise. *New England Journal of Medicine* **316**, 1309–1315.

MacConnie, S., Barkan, A., Lampman, R., Schork, M. & Beitins, I. (1986) Decreased

hypothalamic gonadotropin-releasing hormone secretion in male marathon runners. *New England Journal of Medicine* **315**, 411–417.

Mazzeo, R.S. (1991) Catecholamine responses to acute and chronic exercise. *Medicine and Science in Sports and Exercise* **23**, 839–845.

Mendenhall, L.A., Swanson, S.C., Habash, D.L. & Coggan, A.R. (1994) Ten days of exercise training reduces glucose production and utilization during moderate-intensity exercise. *American Journal of Physiology* **266**, E136–E143.

Mikines, K.J., Sonne, B., Farrell, P.A., Tronier, B. & Galbo, H. (1988) Effect of physical exercise on sensitivity and responsiveness to insulin in humans. *American Journal of Physiology* **254**, E248–E259.

Peronnet, F., Cleroux, J., Perrault, H., Cousineau, D., DeChamplain, J. & Nadeau, R. (1981) Plasma norepinephrine response to exercise before and after training in humans. *Journal of Applied Physiology* **51**, 812–815.

Remacha, A.F., Ordonez, J., Barcelo, M.J., Garcia-Die, F., Arza, B. & Estruch, A. (1994) Evaluation of erythropoietin in endurance runners. *Hematologica* **79**, 350–352.

Richter, E.A. & Sutton, J.R. (1994) Hormonal adaptation to physical activity. In: Bouchard, C., Shephard, R.J. & Stephens, T. (eds) *Physical Activity, Fitness, and Health*, pp. 331–342. Human Kinetics, Champaign, IL.

Schwarz, L. & Kindermann, W. (1990) Beta endorphin, adrenocorticotropic hormone, cortisol and catecholamines during aerobic and anaerobic exercise. *European Journal of Applied Physiology* **61**, 165–171.

Slentz, C.A., Davis, J.M., Settles, D.L., Pate, R.R. & Settles, S.J. (1990) Glucose feedings and exercise in rats: glycogen use, hormone responses, and performance. *Journal of Applied Physiology* **69** (3), 989–994.

Terjung, R. & Tipton, C.M. (1971) Plasma thyroxine and thyroid-stimulating hormone levels during submaximal exercise in humans. *American Journal of Physiology* **220**, 1840–1845.

Thuma, J.R., Gilders, R., Verdun, M. & Loucks, A.B. (1995) Circadian rhythm of cortisol confounds cortisol responses to exercise: implications for future research. *Journal of Applied Physiology* **78**, 1657–1664.

Tremblay, M.S. & Chu, S.Y. (2000) Hormonal response to exercise:

methodological considerations. In: Warren, M.P. & Constantini, N. (eds) *Sports Endocrinology*, pp. 1–30. Humana Press Inc, Totowa, NJ.

Tremblay, M.S., Chu, S.Y. & Mureika, R. (1995) Methodological and statistical considerations for exercise-related hormone evaluations. *Sports Medicine* **20**, 90–108.

Tsai, L., Johansson, C., Pousette, Å., Tegel-man, R., Carlström, K. & Hemmingsson, P. (1991) Cortisol and androgen concentrations in female and male élite endurance athletes in relation to physical activity. *European Journal of Applied Physiology* **63**, 308–311.

Tyndall, G.L., Kobe, R.W. & Houmard, J.A. (1996) Cortisol, testosterone and insulin action during intense swimming training in humans. *European Journal of Applied Physiology* **73**, 61–65.

VanHelder, W.P., Kofman, E. & Tremblay, M.S. (1991) Anabolic steroids in sport. *Canadian Journal of Sport Sciences* **16**, 248–257.

Van Wyck, J.J. (1984) Somatomedins: biologic actions and physiologic control mechanisms. In: Li, C.H. (ed.) *Growth Factors: Hormonal Proteins and Peptides*, Vol. 12, pp. 81–125. Academic Press, New York.

Webb, M.L., Wallace, J.P., Hamill, C., Hodgson, J.L. & Mashaly, M.M. (1984) Serum testosterone concentration during two hours of moderate intensity treadmill running in trained men and women. *Endocrine Research* **10**, 27–38.

Weight, L.M., Alexander, D., Elliot, T. & Jacobs, P. (1992) Erythropoietic adaptations to endurance training. *European Journal of Applied Physiology* **64**, 444–448.

Weltman, A., Weltman, J.Y., Schurrer, R., Evans, R.S., Veldhuis, J.D. & Rogol, A.D. (1992) Endurance training amplifies the pulsatile release of growth hormone: effects of training intensity. *Journal of Applied Physiology* **72**, 2188–2196.

Whitley, R.J., Meikle, A.W. & Watts, N.B. (1994) Endocrinology. In: Burtis, C.A. & Ashwood, E.R. (eds) *Tietz Textbook of Clinical Chemistry*, pp. 1645–1886. W.B. Saunders Company, Philadelphia.

Wilson, J.D. (1988) Androgen abuse by athletes. *Endocrine Reviews* **9**, 181–199.

Wilson, J.D. & Foster, D.W. (eds) (1992) *Williams Textbook of Endocrinology*, 8th edn. W.B. Saunders Company, Philadelphia.

Winder, W.W., Hagberg, J.M., Hickson, R.C., Ehsani, A.A. & McLane, J.A. (1978) Time course of sympathoadrenal adaptation to endurance exercise training in man. *Journal of Applied Physiology* **45**, 370–374.

Wittert, G.A., Livesey, J.H., Espiner, E.A. & Donald, R.A. (1996) Adaptation of the hypothalamopituitary adrenal axis to chronic exercise stress in humans. *Medicine and Science in Sports and Exercise* **28**, 1015–1019.

Yesalis, C.E. (ed.) (1993) *Anabolic Steroids in Sport and Exercise*. Human Kinetics, Champaign, IL.

Yoon, J.R. & Jun, H.S. (1993) The effects of various prolonged running on responses of plasma catecholamine, PRL, and ACTH. *Korean Journal of Sport Science* **5**, 22–32.

Yoon, J.R. & Park, S.C. (1991) Exercise intensity-related responses of β-endorphin, ACTH, and cortisol. *Korean Journal of Sport Science* **3**, 21–32.

Chapter 13

The Importance of Carbohydrate, Fat and Protein for the Endurance Athlete

TERRY E. GRAHAM

This chapter will address the importance of the three major macronutrients in the diet of endurance athletes. My goal is to integrate the importance of carbohydrates, fats and amino acids. Most reviews focus exclusively on one macronutrient and when the focus is endurance athletes, the nutrient is generally carbohydrate (CHO). This is a very artificial approach since when the intake of one nutrient, such as CHO, is altered this automatically changes the relative intake of the others. If one switches to a high CHO diet, the diet must become lower in either protein or fats or else the total energy intake is increased. It is impossible to consume a diet that is merely high CHO! The second major reason for considering the major nutrients together is that metabolically they do not act in isolation. If one alters the storage or metabolism of fat, CHO or protein, the metabolism of the other two is also affected. Altering the amount of CHO or fat that is in the diet can change the metabolism and storage of both substrates, as can the pattern of eating and exercise. However, these issues are much more important to sedentary individuals and will not be considered in this chapter. (They were recently reviewed by Graham & Adamo, 1999.) The other concepts that I will address are the short-term and long-term aspects of nutrition for the athlete. Exercise physiologists (and often coaches) tend to take a very restricted approach to nutrition, considering it to be the food intake during the few days before a competition. This short-term aspect is important, but the long-term nutrition of the athlete is also critical.

Although it is logical to examine these nutrients as a whole, due to the complexity of the topic, they are almost always investigated individually and reviewed in the same fashion. Furthermore, within each of the three major nutrients, one component is often studied by itself. CHO consists of both glucose and glycogen and nutritionally there are many forms of CHO that can be ingested. Fats consist metabolically of free fatty acids (FFAs) and triglycerides (TGs) and nutritionally there are many different fats. Similarly, proteins are tremendously varied and individual amino acids can also be ingested. It rapidly becomes apparent why the scientist studies only one portion of this area in any one study! However, for the reasons outlined above I will attempt to integrate the material in this chapter. In order to accomplish this goal, the underlying physiological regulation will be addressed only briefly.

CHO ingestion

When considering the short-term aspects of nutrition and endurance exercise, the most critical nutrient is water. This is discussed in Chapter 29. The next most immediate nutritional concern is that of CHO, because of the limited stores of CHO in the body and their critical role in prolonged, demanding exercise. Most readers are probably aware that even the body of a lean athlete contains enormous stores of fat (as TGs) and protein relative to the very modest stores of CHO. The latter are found in both muscle and liver and even together they normally account for less than 8 mJ of energy. In addition, the CHO stored in muscle is not readily available to any tissue other than that particular muscle. Thus the only CHO stores that can immediately and rapidly contribute to the blood glucose pool are those of the liver. They represent the minority of the CHO stores (approximately 90 g or 1·7 mJ). This is frequently ignored by athletes in their nutritional preparation.

CHO ingestion prior to exercise

CHO is unique among the three macronutrients in that the dietary content prior to competition is critical. Both liver and muscle glycogen are sensitive to the CHO in the diet and most athletes and coaches are very well aware of 'CHO loading' as it applies to muscle. For strenuous exercise that will last beyond approximately 30–40 min (or 15–30 min of very intense intermittent (1–5 min) activity), the ability of the athlete to maintain a high power output and withstand fatigue can be dictated by his or her pre-exercise muscle glycogen stores. If the activity is of shorter duration it is highly unlikely that CHO stores need to be enhanced. Furthermore, elevated stores could be detrimental, as the storage of CHO increases body mass (almost 3 g of water are stored with every gram of CHO) and the athlete must then carry this extra mass during the competition. The muscle glycogen stores can be enhanced by performing exercise similar to that of the competition 3–6 days prior to the event. The subsequent ingestion of large amounts of CHO ($10 g \cdot kg^{-1} \cdot day^{-1}$) for 2–3 days will ensure that the muscle CHO stores are maximal, i.e. about twice the normal resting concentration. Table 13.1 provides examples of the CHO content of various foods. Once 'supercompensation' has been achieved, the stores are quite stable. Goforth *et al.* (1997) have shown that, unless the person performs strenuous exercise, the increased muscle stores will remain elevated for at least 3–6 days. This is a nutritional manipulation that can be performed well ahead of the event and it questions the justification of the traditional high CHO meal the evening before an endurance competition in order to increase muscle CHO stores.

The benefit of such a meal has little or nothing to do with the muscles that will perform the exercise, but rather serves to augment hepatic CHO stores. It is frequently forgotten that the liver can also increase its CHO stores. Nilsson and Hultman (1974) demonstrated that the glycogen concentration of the human liver can be doubled by nutritional manipulation. Most people realize that it is critical to maintain blood glucose concentration within a normal range, both to provide the brain with its vital nutrient and also to supply the active muscles. We often lose sight of the fact that while muscle glycogen may be the major CHO metabolized during the first 30 min of exercise, as the exercise progresses, glucose oxidation increases and often becomes the dominant CHO metabolized. This glucose must be derived from one of three sources: liver glycogen, liver gluconeogenesis or ingestion of CHO during the exercise. The first source is preferred, as it can be supplied rapidly without costing energy. Gluconeogenesis (the process in which the liver synthesizes 'new' glucose from blood-borne substrates (predominantly lactate and alanine)) costs energy and its maximum rate of glucose provision is less than that of liver glycogen mobilization. If gluconeogenesis becomes the main source of blood glucose during strenuous exercise, the supply may not keep up with the demand and hypoglycaemia may limit the exercise.

Although the liver CHO can be enhanced by diet in a similar fashion to muscle stores, there are important differences that can be critical to the athlete. Muscle stores are stable over many days, but the liver stores are very dynamic. As little as 12 h of fasting (e.g. not eating after dinner, sleeping and then rising in the morning) results in the hepatic stores being reduced by up to 50% and food restriction for 24 h can essentially deplete the stores. An endurance athlete who is competing in the morning but does not eat breakfast has created a serious metabolic challenge prior to beginning the exercise. The person would be entering an exercise in which blood glucose will become a critical fuel and would begin the activity with only half the optimal storage of liver glycogen. Proper CHO provision to the brain and the active muscles will depend on the slower, metabolically costly liver gluconeogenesis and the ingestion of CHO during the activity.

The precompetition, evening CHO meal is most important for the liver, not the muscles. The precompetition breakfast is even more critical. Ideally, it should be ingested 2–4 h prior to competition and

Table 13.1 Carbohydrate (CHO)-rich foods of varying glycaemic index. Adapted from Graham and Adamo (1999).

Food group	Food item	Approximate serving size to give 50 g CHO	Glycaemic index
Breads and cereals	Cornflakes	59 g	77
	Pancakes	0.01–0.15 m	76
	Bagels	89 g	72
	White bread	201 g	70
	Whole wheat	120 g	69
	Shredded wheat	74 g	69
	Rice (white)	169 g	56
	Rice (brown)	196 g	55
	Spaghetti noodles	198 g	41
Fruit and vegetables	Raisins	78 g	64
	Banana	260 g	53
	Grapes (green)	310 g	52
	Orange	420–600 g	43
	Apple	400 g	36
	Potato (baked)	200 g	83
	Potato (boiled)	254 g	73
	Sweet potato	249 g	54
	Baked beans	485 g	48
	Chick peas	305 g	33
	Lentils	294 g	29
Dairy products	Ice cream	202 g	61
	Yogurt (sweetened)	280 g	33
	Yogurt (whole fat)	800 g	27
Snacks	Sponge cake	93 g	67
	Oatmeal cookies	79 g	55
	Potato chips	100 g	54
Liquids	Orange juice	425 ml	57
	Apple juice	425 ml	41
	Milk (skimmed)	1.1 l	32
	Milk (whole)	1.1 l	27

it should consist of easily digested, low fibre CHO. The liver particularly favours fructose, a CHO that is found predominantly in fruits. It is selectively taken up by the liver rather than muscle. However, ingestion of this CHO should be performed carefully. It is more slowly absorbed than many CHOs and in excess, can cause gastrointestinal cramps and diarrhoea. For this reason it is generally not the recommended CHO for ingestion during exercise. As with any nutritional alteration, it should first be tried outside of competition.

Traditionally, CHOs have been divided into simple (mono- and disaccharides) and complex (polysaccharides) groupings. However, this does not necessarily dictate how easily they are digested and made available for metabolism. More recently, CHOs have been described using the term glycaemic index (GI). In this approach, the ingestion of 50 g of pure glucose is given a GI of 100 and all other CHOs are rated relative to this, based on the rise in blood glucose that results from their ingestion. The GI classification does not always match that of simple versus complex CHO; some simple CHOs (e.g. fructose) have a low GI and some complex

CHOs (e.g. amylpectin) have a high GI. This classification is more practical, as it evaluates the food on the basis of its appearance in the circulation. Foods may have a different GI depending on mode of preparation and whether they are ingested with other substances (fats and proteins) that alter the CHO absorption. For example, a banana has the same CHO content (about $28 g \cdot 100 g^{-1}$) however ripe it is. However, the CHO of a green banana is virtually indigestible due to a high fibre content and it provides very little blood glucose. As it ripens, the CHO shifts from predominantly starch to predominantly sugars and from a low to a high GI. Table 13.1 gives examples of the GI of common foods. High fibre foods such as legumes (beans and lentils), green salad, raw vegetables, wholegrain breads and muesli tend to have a low GI. Similarly, the fat of dairy products results in a lower GI for these CHOs.

There is some debate as to how close to the beginning of exercise CHO should be ingested. In part this may depend on the type of CHO and the amount. It is generally recommended that ingestion be modest ($< 50 g$) in the 2 h prior to activity. The concern with ingestion close to the time of exercise is that the CHO will result in a large increase in insulin. This can impede fat mobilization, resulting in the athlete using excessive amounts of CHO and leading to early fatigue. In addition, this response can create a low blood glucose and thus cause central fatigue, i.e. fatigue resulting from alterations in the actual functioning of the brain, whereas local fatigue is the result of events within the active muscles precipitating the fatigue.

CHO ingestion during exercise

There is little that is new in this area from an applied point of view. The general recommendation is that 30–60g of CHO per hour of exercise should be ingested and this is equivalent to 500–1000 ml of most standard sport drinks. The maximum that can be absorbed is $1 g \cdot kg^{-1} \cdot h^{-1}$ and ingesting CHO above this amount can precipitate gastrointestinal problems. The GI of the CHO does not appear to be critical. It is generally recommended that the CHO be ingested as a fluid rather than a solid. This offers several advantages; it is easier to ingest fluids while exercising, solutions have the added benefit of providing water and electrolytes, most commercial sport drinks provide CHO at an optimal concentration, and solids have to be chewed and may inhibit gastric emptying, particularly if the chewing is not thorough. It is important to realize that if the athlete is ingesting CHO at a concentration greater than approximately 8%, this will inhibit gastric emptying; so sport bars and high CHO gels should be taken with a considerable amount of water. Perhaps the most important issue that is often ignored by athletes is the timing of the ingestion. It requires about 30 min for ingested liquids and CHO to enter the circulation and be of benefit. Thus, the person must anticipate the need for both water and CHO and ingest the supplement before it is required. Assuming that it is to be taken in liquid form, one cannot depend on the feeling of thirst. During exercise the athlete will dehydrate by approximately 2% of body mass before feeling thirsty. Add to this 30 min between ingestion and the actual absorption of CHO into the circulation and it is quickly apparent why the need must be anticipated and addressed early in the activity.

CHO ingestion after exercise

It has been known for decades that the ingestion of CHO postexercise is important for the recovery process. However, in the last few years there have been several developments. First, it is clear that after endurance exercise the muscle is very responsive to taking up glucose and synthesizing glycogen. This sensitivity can last up to 48 h, but during the first few hours postexercise it is independent of insulin. If rapid recovery is important, then it is critical to provide extra CHO during the first few hours postexercise. The rate of glycogen storage is most rapid during the first 4 h postexercise and it is during this time that diet is most critical. The general recommendation is that $25 g \cdot h^{-1}$ of high GI CHO be ingested during the first 4 h following exercise and $10 g \cdot kg^{-1} \cdot day^{-1}$ for the first 2 days. The appetite is often suppressed after strenuous exercise and the athlete may find it easier to drink a CHO-based sport drink (these all have a high GI). It is important that the CHO be high GI at this time, as this will result in a resynthesis rate that is twice that from low GI CHO. After the first few hours the GI of the CHO does not appear to be important.

The main advantage of this early provision of CHO is to hasten the initial phase of recovery (Adamo *et al.* 1998). If the intake of CHO is delayed, the muscle glycogen is less during the first 24 h, but after 2–3 days of recovery the glycogen concentration is not different. In situations when the activity has to be resumed within some hours (tournaments, repeated training sessions, etc.), this early CHO feeding is clearly an advantage. Generally, athletes are reluctant to ingest food soon after strenuous exercise and they may be more receptive to a CHO-rich drink. The food industry is addressing this and there are several choices available. The drink should be low in fructose and rich in high GI CHOs. There has been a report (Zawadzki *et al.* 1992) that ingesting amino acids along with the CHO is an advantage, as the amino acids may stimulate extra insulin secretion. However, others (Burke *et al.* 1995; Roy & Tarnopolsky 1998) have not confirmed this initial finding.

CHO has been suggested to enhance the administration of other putative ergogenic aids. Creatine loading has been found to be nearer optimal if the creatine is ingested with CHO (Green *et al.* 1996). However, creatine loading should be of no benefit to endurance athletes and the associated weight gain may be detrimental. There is also a report (Van Zyl *et al.* 1996) that medium-chain TG ingested with CHO may be ergogenic; this will be discussed in the next section.

Fats: ingestion and mobilization

When CHO intake is increased it is often at the expense of protein and/or fat intake. The storage of fats and the distribution of the stores will not be discussed here; the reader should refer to Chapter 24, on body composition. Fat is commonly regarded as a single substance, but in fact 'fat' consists of a wide range of substances. There are several nutritional aspects that are important to the endurance athlete. Even the lean athlete has adequate stores of TGs to promote metabolism for several weeks. Thus the intake of fats is not critical on a short-term basis.

They are stored as TGs, mainly in adipose tissue, but there are also significant stores in both muscle and in the circulation (associated with very low density lipoproteins—VLDL). Adipose tissue TGs must be 'mobilized' into the blood and carried to the active muscle as individual FFAs in order to be metabolized. The critical factors that promote mobilization are not clear, but decreasing insulin and increasing catecholamine concentrations are important humoral signals. As mentioned earlier, this is one important reason why large amounts of CHO should not be ingested close to the beginning of exercise. It has also been suggested that a prime benefit of a long warm-up is that it begins the exercise-induced decline in insulin and the associated mobilization of FFAs. It appears to take about 20 min of exercise before FFA mobilization is effective. Thus a long warm-up should make fats available for muscle metabolism early in exercise and this could also spare the limited stores of CHO. This early use of FFAs could be particularly beneficial, as the CHO stores are limited, and they also are metabolized most rapidly in the initial phase of exercise. If FFA use is enhanced at this time it could result in preservation of CHO stores.

However, it is not clear how critical such an FFA mobilization is for the élite, endurance athlete. First, such an athlete competes at a power output requiring a very high percentage of his/her aerobic power, so that the importance of FFA as a metabolic substrate is minimal. Second, endurance training results in an increase in muscle TGs and there are suggestions that trained individuals use the intramuscular stores to a greater extent (Martin *et al.* 1993). (This raises the question of the importance of warm-up with regard to adipose tissue FFA mobilization.) Third, active muscle takes up only a small portion of the FFA delivered to it and even when this is increased, there is not necessarily a parallel increased muscle uptake of FFA.

In a similar fashion, it has frequently been suggested that the ergogenic benefit of caffeine is to promote FFA mobilization (Essig *et al.* 1980). Caffeine is a potent stimulus promoting mobilization of FFA, but this action does not appear to be the critical ergogenic factor (Graham 1997). Frequently scientists have reported that caffeine does not enhance the oxidation of fats during exercise. In addition, caffeine has ergogenic effects in exercise lasting only a few minutes, when fat metabolism plays a minor role and is not limiting (Jackman *et al.* 1996).

Thus far I have referred to fat as if it were a single substance, composed of identical FFAs. The FFAs that one normally considers are long-chain fatty acids consisting of 12 or more carbon atoms. These can be either saturated or unsaturated fatty acids. Metabolically it is unimportant which type of FFA is oxidized, but from a cardiovascular health perspective the intake of saturated fats should be limited. Total fat intake as a percentage of daily food energy is 35–45% for our society, but in endurance athletes the percentage is often considerably lower. This is perceived as healthy, particularly if the fats are predominantly unsaturated. However, some athletes severely restrict their fat intake and this can result in health concerns. Athletes who avoid eating fats run the risk of creating deficiencies in fat-soluble vitamins such as A, D, E and K. In addition, there are some FFAs that are essential, i.e. the body cannot synthesize them. If an athlete has a low intake of food energy and is consciously avoiding dietary fats, the intake of essential fatty acids may be compromised. As an example, female endurance athletes are often found to have energy intakes that are much lower than expected considering their energy expenditure, and their diets tend to be high in CHO. We (Thong & Graham, unpublished) recently studied a group of female endurance runners; their daily energy intake ranged from 6 to 8 mJ and their daily fat intake was only 20–25% of total energy (39–63 g of fat per day). The amenorrhoeic athletes had the lowest energy and energy fat intakes. Female endurance athletes face several dietary concerns, including risk of deficiencies in both fat-soluble vitamins and essential fatty acids.

A current issue with regard to fats and performance is a group of compounds known as medium-chain TGs (MCTs). These are fats composed of fatty acids with 6–10 carbon atoms and derived from coconut oil. They have received attention by scientists because they are much more readily absorbed by the intestine than are the long-chain fatty acids. They are also superior to the traditional, common FFAs in that they do not impede gastric emptying,

can be delivered to tissues more rapidly and can very quickly enter cells. Thus MCTs seem to be an ideal metabolic fuel. However, they cannot be obtained in large amounts from normal food products. To obtain large amounts, one must take MCT supplements derived from coconut oil. The amount of energy available from ingestion of MCTs is limited, as ingestion of more than 30 g often causes intestinal cramping and diarrhoea. This dose of MCT contributes only about 5% of the metabolic energy expenditure during prolonged exercise. As mentioned earlier, there is one limited report (Van Zyl *et al.* 1996) that if the ingestion of MCTs was combined with a 10% CHO solution, subjects could tolerate up to 90 g of MCT during prolonged exercise and this had an ergogenic effect. This finding has not been replicated.

Short-chain fatty acids are produced by colonic fermentation of fibre and CHO and these can be absorbed and metabolized. They account for up to 6% of the metabolic fuel for basal metabolism in humans, but Alamowitch *et al.* (1996) reported that providing more of these fatty acids to the gut did not alter metabolism.

Recently there has been interest in the possibility that high fat diets could have an ergogenic effect, based on theories similar to that presented earlier of the increased availability/oxidation of fats sparing the athlete's limited CHO stores. There are few studies in this area using human subjects and a firm conclusion cannot be drawn at this time. A recent study by Helge *et al.* (1998) demonstrated that subjects on a high fat diet could have the traditional training responses that those on a high CHO diet experience, but in no way was the high fat diet shown to be superior. Such a diet could present cardiovascular health risks, but Brown and Cox (1998) have illustrated that athletes training very heavily while consuming a high (50%) fat diet for 3 months did not show any disturbance in serum lipids. It appears that strenuous training overcame the potential negative aspects of the diet. These studies have been conducted for only a few weeks. The long-term effects are unknown and high fat diets have not been shown to be superior to high CHO diets. There is no reason to endorse them at this time.

Protein and amino acid ingestion

Protein, like fat, represents an enormous body energy store, but the specific short-term intake prior to competition is not critical. As with fats, this does not mean that protein is unimportant to the endurance athlete. Protein is composed of individual amino acids. Several of these are essential and can only be obtained through the diet. The normal protein requirement for adults is 0.8–0.9 g·kg^{-1}·day^{-1}. Most Western diets supply far more protein than this requirement. Our tissues are constantly breaking down and rebuilding proteins and the gut, liver and other visceral tissues are the most active in this regard. Endurance athletes have a greater protein requirement (about 1.2–1.8 g·kg^{-1}·day^{-1}) than the sedentary individual (Tarnopolsky et al. 1988; Meredith et al. 1989). However, unless the person is avoiding protein in their diet or restricting total energy intake, their normal diet will easily supply this requirement and no supplementation is necessary.

The reasons for this increased need are not clear and the athlete does not have unique requirements for proteins or amino acids. It may seem obvious that the requirement is due to muscle repair and growth. However, many endurance athletes are not experiencing significant muscle growth and even in those who are, the rate of net gain in protein is extremely slight on a daily basis (Millward et al. 1994; Rennie et al. 1994). Furthermore, although exercise, particularly eccentric contractions, can induce muscle damage, regular repetition of the contraction patterns results in rapid adaptation and minimal damage. On the other hand, it is clear that prolonged exercise, particularly if combined with dehydration and heat stress, causes degradation of the gut and possibly the liver (Williams et al. 1996; Marshall 1998). The walls of the gastrointestinal system may become 'leaky' and bleeding can occur with no overt sensation to the athlete. The gut and liver have very high rates of protein synthesis and the increased protein needs of the athlete may be particularly related to these tissues. This does not minimize the situation, as these tissues are very critical to the athlete's health in many ways. Optimal protein nutrition may be particularly im-

portant to these organs. Fortunately when proteins are ingested the resulting amino acids are first exposed to the gut and those that are not incorporated into this tissue are delivered to the liver via the portal circulation before the muscles have the opportunity to take them up.

The protein requirements of the endurance athlete are moderately greater than normal during steady-state training; when the training volume increases (Millward et al. 1994) there is an increased protein requirement for the first 1–2 weeks, after which it returns to normal. There appear to be four categories of athlete whose protein intake needs to be monitored carefully: (i) a person who is still growing; (ii) a person who is increasing their training volume; (iii) a person who is attempting to follow a vegetarian diet but who is not careful regarding protein intake; and (iv) a person who is restricting their total energy intake. A person with any of these characteristics could become protein deficient; for example, an adolescent or young teenage female athlete who is weight conscious and who is following a vegetarian diet.

Well-balanced vegetarian diets are healthy and are not detrimental to the endurance athlete. The concern is with a person who feels that by simply eliminating meat they have a healthy vegetarian diet. Within the scope of this chapter, there are several aspects that need to be considered. Vegetarian diets can range from the vegan diet of strictly non-animal food products to 'semivegetarian' diets that may include fish and poultry. The total energy needs of an active athlete may be hard to meet as vegetarian diets tend to be high in bulk/fibre and have a low energy density. Strictly vegan diets may be low in protein or lacking in specific amino acids. Such diets should include a wide range of complementary vegetable proteins (lentils and beans, wholewheat breads, brown rice, tofu and vitamin B_{12}-fortified soy milk). Although legumes are on average 20–25% protein, only soybeans (34% protein) provide a full complement of the essential amino acids and it is generally recommended that the vegetarian consume a variety of grains and beans within a day in order to obtain a full complement of amino acids. In addition, the high fibre of the diet reduces digestibility and therefore the protein intake should be about 110% of the estimated protein requirement. For individuals who are beginning to take up a vegetarian diet, it is wise to consult a registered dietician for advice.

Moreover, individuals who eat little or no meat and have high fibre diets are susceptible to iron deficiency. This is dealt with in detail in Chapter 30. I will merely mention in passing that red meats are a particularly good source of iron, and those who eliminate this form of protein from their diet need to be particularly careful. In addition, while a high fibre diet provides health benefits, it also impedes iron absorption. This can be particularly important, because the endurance athlete appears to have greater iron requirements. It has been suggested that this is related in part to blood loss due to damage to the gut during prolonged exercise.

Amino acid supplements

The athletic world is a major target for the multitude of supplements that the food industry is marketing. Among the many products that have involved amino acids and protein are glutamine and branched-chain amino acids (BCAAs). Glutamine is purported to stimulate several metabolic processes; of particular interest for the endurance athlete are claims that it enhances immune function and stimulates protein synthesis. These claims have scientific support, but only in situations where serious trauma or disease states exist. Glutamine is found in very high concentrations relative to other amino acids in both plasma and muscle. It is not an essential amino acid; skeletal muscle produces it in abundance and releases it during exercise. Glutamine is a critical fuel for rapidly dividing cells, including those of the gut, liver and immune system. In times of trauma (infection, surgery, sepsis, etc.) there is an enormous production of glutamine from muscles to promote the actions of the immune system. This in turn results in a decreased muscle glutamine concentration, severe protein degradation and muscle wasting. Under these traumatic situations, it has been demonstrated that if glutamine infusion can maintain intramuscular glutamine, the muscle atrophy is lessened or prevented.

It is an enormous leap in logic to predict on the basis of deficiency situations that an excess in glutamine in a healthy individual will have a positive effect. There are no scientific data to support claims that ingestion of glutamine will either promote muscle protein synthesis or enhance immune function in a healthy person. Successful oral administration of glutamine is difficult to achieve. Unless a large dose ($100 \, mg \cdot kg^{-1}$) is ingested by a healthy, resting person, there is no increase in the systemic circulating concentration and even when there is an increase in concentration it is fairly transient. The gut and liver metabolize almost all of the ingested amino acid. This could be used as indirect evidence that a glutamine supplement might assist in repairing possible damage to the gut, but if ingestion does not increase the plasma concentration, it cannot help the muscles or the immune system. Furthermore, a recent study by Rohde *et al.* (1998) demonstrated that when runners ingested four doses (each $100 \, mg \cdot kg^{-1}$) of glutamine within 2 h of running a marathon, this megadose merely kept the circulating glutamine concentration constant, whereas in the control situation it declined by 20%. This could be viewed as a modest but positive effect, although the researchers followed changes in immune function and found no effects. With such results, it appears very unlikely that glutamine supplements serve any purpose for the endurance athlete.

The other amino acid supplements that have received attention are BCAAs. The three BCAAs are valine, leucine and isoleucine, which are also essential amino acids. In terms of exercise physiology they are unique, in that skeletal muscle readily oxidizes them. Although muscle has the capacity to oxidize several other amino acids, this rarely happens. Any other amino acid contribution to exercise metabolism comes from their use as a fuel of gluconeogenesis. Not only will muscle take up and oxidize BCAAs, but the liver selectively ignores them. Thus when they are ingested, they tend to pass through the portal circulation and are presented to muscle. As a substrate, they represent a very minor component (<5%) of the energy required for exercise. However, they are central to two different theories regarding fatigue. As mentioned earlier, local fatigue can be generated from within the muscle and central fatigue can originate within the brain. Ironically, one theory (Wagenmakers *et al.* 1990) suggests that BCAAs can precipitate fatigue (local) and the other (Newsholme & Blomstrand 1995) suggests that they would delay fatigue (central).

When muscle oxidizes BCAAs, it uses a compound from the Krebs cycle as a metabolic intermediate. Subsequently there are a variety of alternative metabolic steps that can be followed; most would ultimately regenerate the 'borrowed' Krebs cycle intermediate. One option would result in the intermediate being incorporated into glutamine and released into the circulation. As the duration of the exercises increases, the oxidation of BCAAs becomes greater. Wagenmakers *et al.* (1990) suggest that this removal of a key Krebs cycle intermediate will reduce the metabolic capacity of the Krebs cycle and result in metabolic fatigue. They also theorize that declining muscle glycogen availability hastens this process. However, Jackman *et al.* (1997) have shown that glycogen stores do not affect the BCAA oxidation rate and several studies have found that ingestion of BCAAs prior to exercise enhances the BCAA metabolism but does not hasten fatigue.

The BCAAs are transported into the brain by a carrier protein. Tryptophan, another amino acid, competes with the BCAAs for this same carrier. During prolonged exercise, circulating BCAA concentration tends to decline. In addition, the circulating FFA level often increases. The latter event results in an increase in free tryptophan in the circulation. Thus both the decline in BCAAs and the rise in tryptophan would increase the tryptophan/BCAA ratio. This should result in more tryptophan being transported into the brain. The potential significance of such an enhanced uptake is that tryptophan is the precursor for the neurotransmitter, serotonin. Unlike many neurotransmitters, serotonin appears to be limited by the availability of substrate. This action should increase the brain serotonin concentration, and elevated serotonin induces feelings of sleepiness and lethargy. Conversely, supplementation with BCAAs elevates their plasma concentration, lowering the tryptophan/BCAA ratio and the

brain serotonin concentration and this should delay fatigue. BCAA supplements have been marketed on this premise.

It is not possible to test human brains for serotonin levels but studies in which rats are exercised to exhaustion show that in some circumstances brain serotonin is elevated (Davis & Bailey 1997). This, of course, does not prove that the neurotransmitter caused the fatigue and it should be kept in mind that rarely would a human exercise to the complete state of exhaustion that the rats are forced to achieve. As with local fatigue, studies (Jackman *et al.* 1997; Madsen *et al.* 1996) that have elevated BCAAs by supplementation have found no effect on time to fatigue. There is little evidence that BCAA supplementation would be of benefit to the endurance athlete.

Gender

Phillips *et al.* (1993) have reported that female endurance athletes may have special needs. They found that the degree of protein oxidized during prolonged exercise was less in women than in men. However, this is a very modest amount of protein for either gender and it is not known if this means that women athletes have lower protein requirements. It is known that oestrogen is an antioxidant and Tiidus (1998) has found that oestrogen reduces the amount of oxidative damage in rats. This could result in less muscle damage in active women than in men. Tarnopolsky *et al.* (1990, 1995) have also shown that women oxidize more fat and less CHO during exercise, suggesting that glycogen stores may be less critical to women. This would be beneficial, particularly as women may have less ability to glycogen load.

The most serious nutritional concerns for female endurance athletes are associated with total energy intake. As noted when discussing CHO needs, female endurance runners are often reported to have modest energy intakes, ranging from 6 to 8 mJ per day. The total food energy ingested as each nutrient is more important than the percentage distribution among the nutrients. If the diet is high in CHO (e.g. 70% being CHO) this leaves a very modest amount of energy left for the important requirements of both fats and of protein.

These women may be lacking essential fatty acids and fat-soluble vitamins and could be protein deficient as well.

Summary

The nutrition of the endurance athlete is extremely important; traditionally one identifies CHO as the main issue. Within CHO there are many aspects that need to be addressed, ranging from amount and type of CHO ingested to optimal time for ingestion. In addition, one tends to identify muscle as the critical recipient of the CHO, but it is probably more important prior to exercise to provide CHO to enhance liver CHO stores. They are more labile and more sensitive to short periods of negative CHO balance. CHO ingestion within 4–6 h prior to exercise is important for optimal liver CHO stores.

The other macronutrients are very important but tend to receive less attention. Both fats and protein are critical in the long-term diet of the athlete. These are frequently sacrificed to the goal of enhancing CHO ingestion. In the short term of a few days this is of no concern, but in the staple diet of the athlete these nutrients need to be represented adequately. There are supplements available such as MCTs and various protein powders, and specific amino acids such as glutamine and BCAAs. There is little or no scientific evidence that these assist the athlete in any way.

Acknowledgements

The author gratefully acknowledges the assistance of Ms Farah Thong, MSc in the preparation of the manuscript and thanks both her and Heidi Neff, RD for their comments on the content of the manuscript. The scientific studies of the author have been supported by the Canadian Natural Science and Engineering Council and several of the specific studies referred to in the chapter were supported by Gatorade.

References

Adamo, K.B., Tarnopolsky, M.A. & Graham, T.E. (1998) Dietary carbohydrate and postexercise synthesis of proglycogen and macroglycogen in human skeletal muscle. *American Journal of Physiology* 275, E229–E234.

Alamowitch, C., Boillot, J., Boussairi, A. *et al.* (1996) Lack of effect of an acute ileal perfusion of short-chain fatty acids on glucose metabolism in healthy men. *American Journal of Physiology* 271, E199–E204.

Brown, R.C. & Cox, C.M. (1998) Effects of high fat versus high carbohydrate diets on plasma lipids and lipoproteins in endurance athletes. *Medicine and Science in Sports and Exercise* 30, 1677–1683.

Burke, L.M., Collier, G.R., Beasley, S.K. *et al.* (1995) Effect of coingestion of fat and protein with carbohydrate feedings on muscle glycogen storage. *Journal of Applied Physiology* 78, 2187–2192.

Davis, J.M. & Bailey, S.P. (1997) Possible mechanisms of central nervous system fatigue during exercise. *Medicine and Science in Sports and Exercise* 29, 45–57.

Essig, D., Costill, D.L. & Van Handel, P.J. (1980) Effects of caffeine ingestion on utilization of muscle glycogen and lipid during leg ergometer cycling. *International Journal of Sports Medicine* 1, 86–90.

Goforth, H.W. Jr, Arnall, D.A., Bennett, B.L. & Law, P.G. (1997) Persistence of supercompensated muscle glycogen in trained subjects after carbohydrate loading. *Journal of Applied Physiology* 82, 342–347.

Graham, T.E. (1997) The possible actions of methylxanthines on various tissues. In: Reilly, T. & Orme, M. (eds) *The Clinical Pharmacology of Sport and Exercise*, pp. 257–270. Elsevier Science BV, Amsterdam.

Graham, T.E. & Adamo, K.B. (1999) Dietary carbohydrate and its effects on metabolism and substrate stores in sedentary and active individuals. *Canadian Journal of Applied Physiology* 24, 393–415.

Green, A.L., Hultman, E., MacDonald, I.A., Sewell, D.A. & Greenhaff, P.L. (1996) Carbohydrate ingestion augments skeletal muscle creatine accumulation during creatine supplementation in humans. *American Journal of Physiology* 271, E821–E826.

Helge, J.W., Wulff, B. & Keins, B. (1998) Impact of a fat-rich diet on endurance in man: role of the dietary period. *Medicine and Science in Sports and Exercise* 30, 456–461.

Jackman, M., Wendling, P., Friars, D. & Graham, T. (1996) Metabolic, catecholamine, and endurance responses to caffeine during intense exercise. *Journal of Applied Physiology* 81, 1658–1663.

Jackman, M.L., Gibala, M.J., Hultman, E. & Graham, T.E. (1997) Nutritional status affects branch-chain oxoacid dehydrogenase activity during exercise in humans. *American Journal of Physiology* 272, E233–E238.

Madsen, K., MacLean, D.A., Kiens, B. & Christensen, D. (1996) Effects of glucose, glucose plus branched-chain amino acids, or placebo on bike performance over 100 km. *Journal of Applied Physiology* 81, 2644–2650.

Marshall, J.C. (1998) The gut as a potential trigger of exercise-induced inflammatory responses. *Canadian Journal of Physiology and Pharmacology* 76, 479–484.

Martin, W.H.I., Dalsky, G.P., Hurley, B.F. *et al.* (1993) Effect of endurance training on plasma free fatty acid turnover and oxidation during exercise. *American Journal of Physiology (Endocrinological Metabolism 28)* 265, E708–E714.

Meredith, C.N., Zackin, M.J., Fontera, W.R. & Evans, W.J. (1989) Dietary protein requirements and body protein metabolism in endurance-trained men. *Journal of Applied Physiology* 66, 2850–2856.

Millward, D.J., Bowtell, J.L., Pacy, P. & Rennie, M.J. (1994) Physical activity, protein metabolism and protein requirements. *Proceedings of the Nutrition Society* 53, 223–240.

Newsholme, E.A. & Blomstrand, E. (1995) Tryptophan, 5-hydroxytryptamine and a possible explanation for central fatigue. In: Gandevia, S.C., Enoka, R.M., McComas, A.J., Stuart, D.G., Thomas, C.K. & Pierce, P.A. (eds) *Fatigue: Neural and Muscular Mechanisms*, pp. 315–320. Plenum Press, New York and London.

Nilsson, L.H. & Hultman, E. (1974) Liver and muscle glycogen in man after glucose and fructose infusion. *Scandinavian Journal of Clinical Investigation* 33, 5–10.

Phillips, S.M., Atkinson, S.A., Tarnopolsky, M.A. *et al.* (1993) Gender differences in leucine kinetics and nitrogen balance in endurance athletes. *Journal of Applied Physiology* 75, 2134–2141.

Rennie, M.J., Bowtell, J.L. & Millward, D.J. (1994) Physical activity and protein metabolism. In: Bouchard, C., Shephard, R.J. & Stephens, T. (eds) *Physical Activity, Fitness, and Health*, pp. 432–450. Human Kinetics, Champaign, IL.

Rohde, T., Asp, S., MacLean, D.A. & Pedersen, B.K. (1998) Competitive sustained exercise in humans, lymphokine activated killer cell activity, and glutamine—an intervention study. *European Journal of Applied Physiology* 78, 448–453.

Roy, B.D. & Tarnopolsky M.A. (1998) Influence of differing macronutrient intakes on muscle glycogen resynthesis after resistance exercise. *Journal of Applied Physiology* 84, 890–896.

Tarnopolsky, M.A., MacDougall, J.D. & Atkinson, S.A. (1988) Influence of protein intake and training status on nitrogen balance and lean body mass. *Journal of Applied Physiology* 64, 187–193.

Tarnopolsky, L.J., MacDougall, J.D., Atkinson, S.A., Tarnopolsky, M.A. & Sutton, J.R. (1990) Gender differences in substrate for endurance exercise. *Journal of Applied Physiology* 68, 302–308.

Tarnopolsky, M.A., Atkinson, S.A., Phillips, S.M. & MacDougall, J.D. (1995) Carbohydrate loading and metabolism during exercise in men and women. *Journal of Applied Physiology* 78, 1360–1368.

Tiidus, P.M. (1998) Radical species in inflammation and overtraining. *Canadian Journal of Physiology and Pharmacology* 76, 533–538.

Van Zyl, C.G., Lambert, E.B., Hawley, J.A., Noakes, T.D. & Dennis, S.C. (1996) Effects of medium-chain triglyceride ingestion on fuel metabolism and cycling. *Journal of Applied Physiology* 80, 2217–2225.

Wagenmakers, A.J.M., Coakley, J.H. & Edwards, R.H.T. (1990) Metabolism of branched-chain amino acids and ammonia during exercise. Clues from McArdle's disease. *International Journal of Sports Medicine* 11, S101–S113.

Williams, B.D., Wolfe, R.R., Bracy, D.P. *et al.* (1996) Gut proteolysis contributes essential amino acids during exercise. *American Journal of Physiology* 270, E85–E90.

Zawadzki, K.M., Yaspelkis, B.B. III & Ivy, J.L. (1992) Carbohydrate–protein complex increases the rate of muscle glycogen storage after exercise. *Journal of Applied Physiology* 72, 1854–1859.

Part 2b

Psychological Aspects of Endurance Performance

Chapter 14

Psychology in Endurance Performance

JOHN S. RAGLIN AND GREGORY S. WILSON

Psychological factors such as personality and mood have long been presumed to influence success in athletics (e.g. Dudley 1888), and research on endurance athletes and performers in other sports has provided support for this contention. Studies indicate that athletes do indeed possess personality and mood profiles that differ significantly from population norms. Research also demonstrates that some of these characteristics are affected detrimentally by the stress of intense endurance training. Psychological factors such as anxiety and cognition are also associated with sport performance, but at a much more individual level. The purpose of this chapter is to provide an overview of these and other findings involving psychological research on athletes, particularly in endurance sports. Where appropriate, attention is given to methodological issues that have resulted in confusion or constrained the growth of knowledge.

Personality and athleticism: the mental health model

Although most coaches and athletes believe that personality has an impact on sport performance, conclusions reached in the research literature have been contradictory. The earliest overviews of the personality and sport research generally yielded positive findings, concluding that athletes who were successful were generally more extroverted and emotionally stable (Warburton & Kane 1966; Cooper 1969). However, reviews conducted during the following decade were nearly unanimous in declaring that the association between personality

factors and sport performance was minimal or even non-existent (Rushall 1970; Martens 1975), leading many sport psychologists to abandon the study of personality in athletes altogether. These competing perspectives were reconciled in reviews by Morgan (1978, 1980), who demonstrated that much of the research that rejected the role of personality in sport was marred by a variety of serious methodological flaws, especially concerning the appropriate use of psychological measures. Carefully executed research indicated that athletes did indeed possess unique personality traits compared to published norms for non-athletes. Morgan (1985) extended these findings by developing the 'mental health model' of sport performance. The model posits that a negative relationship exists between psychopathology and capability, such that athletes who are depressed, anxious, or possess other forms of mental illness will perform more poorly than individuals possessing average or above-average mental health. The model also has a dynamic aspect, predicting that successful athletes who develop mental health problems should experience a decline in performance.

Support for this model was yielded initially through a series of studies conducted by Morgan and colleagues (Morgan 1985), and later replicated by others (Mahoney 1989; Newcombe & Boyle 1995). Measures of personality, mood state and affect were assessed in college and élite athletes from a variety of sports, and psychological profiles were contrasted between successful and unsuccessful competitors. In other studies, psychological profiles were used to make predictions about the future success or failure of athletes vying for positions on Olympic or international teams (Morgan & Johnson 1978). The results of these studies supported the basis of the mental health model; successful athletes typically possessed lower scores for such personality factors as introversion, depression, neuroticism and trait anxiety when compared with unsuccessful competitors. Successful athletes also tended to possess comparatively healthier mood state profiles.

As measured by the 'profile of mood states' (POMS) (McNair *et al.* 1992), the combination of low scores for undesirable or negative mood factors (i.e. anger, fatigue, depression, confusion) and a high score for the desirable or positive mood factor (i.e. vigour) is commonly referred to as the *'iceberg profile'* (Morgan 1980) (Fig. 14.1). The difference in mood between successful and unsuccessful competitors was found to be most pronounced during periods in which athletes were undergoing hard training, an observation that contributed to the development of the dynamic aspect of the mental health model (Morgan & Johnson 1981). The psychological characteristics associated with successful athletes have proven stable over time. Recent longitudinal research (Morgan & Costill 1996) with a sample of élite distance runners whose psychological profiles were contrasted across a span of 20 years revealed remarkably little change in their psychological characteristics (Fig. 14.1).

The effectiveness of the mental health model in identifying successful and unsuccessful athletes has consistently exceeded chance levels of prediction. On average, from 70 to 85% of athletes could be correctly classified on the basis of psychological information. Despite this level of accuracy, Morgan (1985) cautioned against employing the mental health model in attempts to select athletes for competition. In virtually all mental health model research, some false classifications resulted. Cases in which athletes possess intermediate psychological scores preclude categorization as either successful or unsuccessful. Moreover, the level of accuracy achieved with mental health model studies is insufficient to select athletes, and there is no evidence that psychological identification models can be made more accurate (Eysenck *et al.* 1982; Vanden Auweele *et al.* 1993; Morgan 1997a). Despite this, psychological measures have been and continue to be used to select athletes for professional sport teams (Smith 1997).

Psychological responses to endurance training

Research also indicates that the mental health model

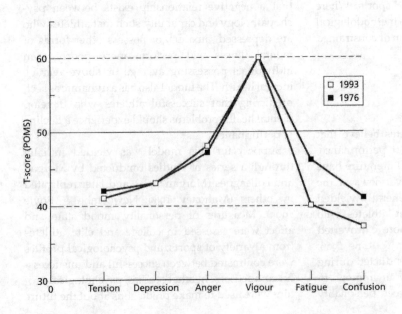

Fig. 14.1 Mood state profiles (POMS) in a sample of marathon runners tested in 1976 and 1993. Adapted from Morgan and Costill (1996).

is efficacious in a dynamic context in which the emotional health of athletes is monitored across time. Studies of over 1000 athletes in endurance sports such as swimming and running (Morgan *et al.* 1987a; Raglin 1993; O'Connor 1997) have provided considerable support for this aspect of the mental health model. Participation in long-term physical activity or sport programmes is typically associated with improvements in mental health (Morgan 1997b), but the consequences are entirely different for competitive athletes striving to achieve optimal performance. Research on sports such as swimming and distance running has consistently demonstrated that intensive endurance training is associated with mood disturbances in athletes who exhibited good mental health prior to hard training (Morgan *et al.* 1987a; Raglin *et al.* 1991). Moreover, the stress of training is closely associated with the degree of mood disturbance. As training loads are increased progressively in either volume or intensity, corresponding increases in mood disturbance develop. Athletes possessing mood state profiles one or more standard deviations better than the norm at the outset of a season typically exhibit mood disturbances such that scores often exceed the population norm at the peak of training. With reductions or tapers in training, mood disturbances typically abate. By the end of the training season, following the completion of the taper, mood profiles generally approximate those observed at the outset of training (Morgan *et al.* 1987a; Raglin *et al.* 1991). An example of this dose–response relationship is depicted in Fig. 14.2. The psychological responses to intensive endurance training do not differ significantly between men and women athletes who undergo comparable training (Morgan *et al.* 1987a; O'Connor *et al.* 1991; Raglin *et al.* 1991). Anaerobic conditioning can also significantly increase mood disturbance in non-endurance athletes, given a sufficiently intense training programme (Raglin *et al.* 1995).

Hence, mood state profiles of endurance athletes are generally healthier than those of non-athletes (Morgan 1985), but the stress of physical training routinely results in negative mood state shifts such that the values may equal or exceed population norms. This finding provides support for the dynamic aspect of the mental health model (Morgan 1985), which indicates that changes in mental health have an impact on athletic performance. Unfortunately, some reviewers of the mental health model have failed to consider the consequences of physical training on mood states in athletes, leading them to reject the mental health model on false grounds (Renger 1993; Terry 1995).

The association between mood state and training load has practical implications, given the evolution of endurance training. For example, in 1954 when Roger Bannister was preparing for his attempt at breaking the 4-min mile, he reported training approximately 30 min a day (Bannister 1989). Gunder Hägg, another world record holder in the mile of Bannister's era, had a full-time job as a firefighter and his training was restricted to a 40-min

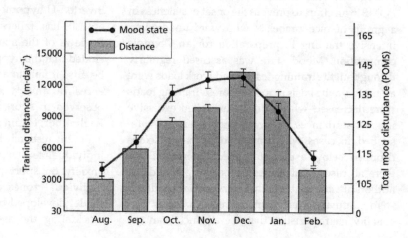

Fig. 14.2 Mood state (POMS) responses of collegiate swimmers across a season of competitive training. Adapted from Raglin (1993).

period during his lunch break (Hägg 1952). Obviously, training practices have changed dramatically over the ensuing decades, and the trend towards an ever greater volume of training continues. Unfortunately, intensive training can sometimes have detrimental consequences for the physical and mental health of the athlete. This condition, referred to as the overtraining syndrome or staleness (Chapter 34), is associated with a chronic loss of performance, possibly an increased susceptibility to infectious illness and psychological disturbances including depression (Morgan et al. 1987a; Raglin 1993; O'Connor 1997).

Staleness is not a rare event. Research indicates that between 10 and 15% of endurance athletes who undergo intensive training will develop staleness (Morgan et al. 1987a; Raglin & Wilson, 1999). The majority of athletes who develop symptoms of staleness as a result of heavy training exhibit increases in mood disturbance which exceed those observed in athletes who do not develop the disorder (Morgan et al. 1987a; O'Connor et al. 1989, 1991). Research with endurance runners and swimmers has also found that mood state changes provide a more reliable indicator of training status than commonly used physiological measures such as stress hormones (O'Connor et al. 1991; Verde et al. 1992). Observations such as these have led to proposals that mood state assessment during training may provide a means to forestall the development of staleness, and some research has examined this possibility.

Berglund and Säfström (1994) employed the POMS in an effort to prevent the onset of staleness in a group of race canoeists who were undergoing intensive training in preparation for an Olympic competition. Mood state was assessed regularly throughout the training season and work loads were adjusted on the basis of mood scores. Training loads were decreased when athletes exhibited excessive mood disturbances, whereas more training was prescribed in cases where mood disturbance scores dropped below a pre-established criterion. There were no cases of staleness in the sample, and the authors attributed this to the intervention paradigm.

To summarize, endurance athletes possess personality characteristics that are distinct from the general population. Athletes in general have positive mental health profiles and this is particularly true for successful competitors. However, the stress of intense endurance training can alter the mood state of athletes significantly, resulting in mood disturbances and, in the case of athletes who become stale, clinical depression. Some evidence indicates that the use of mood state measures to monitor and adjust training of athletes undergoing intensive training can provide a means of reducing the risk of the staleness syndrome.

Precompetition anxiety and performance

Anxiety is widely recognized as having a significant influence on performance in sport settings (Fazey & Hardy 1988; Raglin 1992; Hanin 1997). The most popular explanation for this relationship is derived from the inverted-U hypothesis (Martens 1971; Fazey & Hardy 1988; Raglin 1992). According to this explanation, moderate levels of anxiety should facilitate performance. As anxiety deviates either above or below this range, performance should deteriorate. The level of skill of an athlete and the nature of the sporting event moderate this relationship. Élite athletes should benefit from a relatively higher level of anxiety than pre-élite or inexperienced competitors. Sport events that are explosive or anaerobic in nature should benefit from a relatively higher level of anxiety compared with endurance sports. Tasks requiring fine motor control should require even lower levels of anxiety. Despite the long-standing dominance of the inverted-U hypothesis in the field of sport psychology, it has fallen under considerable criticism. Reviews of the sport anxiety literature have concluded that the hypothesis is largely invalid, in part because it fails to account for the individual differences in anxiety responses that are frequently observed in sport settings (Fazey & Hardy 1988; Raglin 1992; Hanin 1997).

Recent research has provided support for more individualized explanations of the influence of anxiety on sport performance. In particular, the 'individual zones of optimal functioning' (IZOF) model developed by Hanin (1997) is efficacious in elucidating the association between anxiety and sport performance in endurance sport athletes. The IZOF model proposes that each athlete performs better when her or his level of anxiety falls within an optimal range or zone. Unlike the inverted-U hypothesis and other group-based explanations, according to the IZOF model, optimal anxiety differs considerably across athletes, ranging from low to high depending on the individual. Moreover, neither the sport task nor the skill level predictably influence the optimal anxiety zone. Hence, even in a group of similarly skilled athletes competing in the same event, a substantial percentage of individuals should report performing best when anxiety is high, whereas other competitors will benefit from moderate or even low levels of anxiety.

Research on endurance athletes supports this prediction. In a study of élite female distance runners, Morgan *et al.* (1987b) found that 30% of the sample reported high levels of precompetition anxiety prior to their best performance. Similar findings have been noted in other studies involving track and field athletes, ranging from preadolescent (Wilson & Raglin 1997) to college-age competitors (Raglin & Turner 1993; Turner & Raglin 1996). IZOF research involving athletes from a variety of endurance and non-endurance sports indicates that between 30 and 45% of individuals perform best with high anxiety (Raglin & Hanin 1999).

The net impact of optimal anxiety on performance has also been examined. Raglin and Turner (1993) found that the performance of track and field athletes was an average of 1.5% ($P < 0.05$) better when anxiety levels fell within the optimal range determined through IZOF procedures. However, when the optimal anxiety was determined on the basis of the inverted-U hypothesis, performance was unchanged. Follow-up research (Turner & Raglin 1996) revealed that the decrement in performance was approximately equal whether anxiety was too low or exceeded optimal values, indicating that the consequences of insufficient anxiety can be as great as those of excessive anxiety.

To summarize, anxiety has a significant influence on endurance sport performance. However, its impact is more individualized than has been indicated by traditional approaches such as the inverted-U hypothesis; athletes exhibit considerable variation in the level of anxiety that is most beneficial for their performance. The IZOF model and other recently developed theories of sport anxiety do not support the traditional presumption that high levels of precompetition anxiety are uniformly detrimental to performance. In fact, popular techniques such as relaxation to lower anxiety may result in poorer levels of performance for many endurance athletes.

Psychological interventions and endurance performance

Various psychological strategies have been advocated to improve sport performance. Among these interventions, mental imagery or visualization is the most widely promoted. Yet despite the popularity of this technique, the benefits associated with imagery appear to be modest at best. A meta-analysis by Feltz and Landers (1983) concluded that 'mentally practicing a skill influences performance somewhat better than no practice at all' (p. 25). Reviews of the literature consistently indicate that the consequences of imagery are greater for tasks with a significant cognitive component, compared to sporting events in which physical capacity or strength plays a greater role (Feltz & Landers 1983; Driskell *et al.* 1994).

The mechanism by which imagery putatively enhances performance has not been identified. One popular explanation is described as the psychoneuromuscular theory. It posits that imagery of motor performance results in activity in the motor cortex and peripheral physiological changes (e.g. electromyographic activity (EMG), heart rate (HR)) that correspond to the movement which is being imagined. However, Williams *et al.* (1995) noted that 'fully convincing support for this theory remains elusive' (p. 284). Moreover, it is unclear how low-level physiological activity (e.g. EMG) would benefit endurance events where performance is limited more by physical conditioning than by fine motor skill or cognitive factors such as memorization. Despite these caveats mental imagery is still advocated for endurance sports, including distance running. In one study cited as evidence for the use of imagery for runners, Burhans *et al.* (1988) examined the effects of imagery or motivational training against a no-treatment control in adult recreational runners across 12 weeks of training. The rate of improvement in running a 2.4-km (1.5-mile) race was greatest ($P < 0.05$) after 4 weeks of training for the imagery group, but by the end of the training programme the improvement was equivalent across conditions. Unfortunately the authors did not include a placebo condition. The special attention inherent in experimental treatments (i.e. the Hawthorne effect) can alter performance significantly (Morgan 1997a), and may well account for the short-lived benefits of imagery that were noted in this study. No benefits were associated with the motivational 'psyching up' strategy and this finding is consistent with other research involving aerobic endurance activities.

Other psychological techniques such as goal setting, arousal management and cognitive self-regulation have also been promoted for athletes. Reviews of this literature have found that such methods are sometimes associated with performance improvements (Meyers *et al.* 1996), but important caveats have been acknowledged. Psychological enhancement techniques seldom include appropriate placebo conditions to determine the extent to which changes in performance are simply a consequence of the Hawthorne effect (Morgan 1997a). Research on psychological performance enhancement techniques has rarely involved élite athletes (Meyers *et al.* 1996); indeed the majority of studies have comprised 'participants with little or no proficiency with the sport task' (p. 157). Also, the endurance activities tested have generally borne little semblance to actual endurance events.

Cognitive factors during performance: association–dissociation

Research has identified some cognitive factors that have an impact on endurance performance. During competition élite men and women distance runners commonly utilize a cognitive strategy in which attention is directed inward in an attempt to monitor body signals. Endurance athletes report paying close attention to sensations such as pain, fatigue, muscle soreness, respiration and body temperature (Morgan & Pollock 1977). This tactic is described as association; it involves monitoring the feedback arising from physical exertion, and using this information to regulate pace.

Reports by élite endurance athletes competing in a variety of sports indicate their use of association. The four-time Tour de France winner, Miguel Indurain, stated he did not use heart rate monitors during competition because 'his body acts as its own monitor' (Elder 1992, p. 118). O'Connor (1992) reported that on the last day of the 1989 Tour de France race, Greg LeMond made up a 50-s deficit to win the race. LeMond instructed his race crew not to provide him with pace times or information on his competitors, because it 'would only detract from his concentration' (Swift 1989, p. 72). Ronald Da Costa, who recently set the world record in the marathon, was instructed by his coach to ignore the competition during the race and to avoid looking at his watch (Longman 1998).

In contrast, non-élite runners adopt a very different cognitive approach during competition (Morgan & Pollock 1977). These individuals use a variety of means to distract themselves from the sensations of physical exertion and discomfort, a strategy referred to as dissociation. Methods used to dissociate may range from the mundane—running at the pace of a competitor—to the exotic. Some of the more unusual reported examples of dissociation include: mentally designing and building a house, reliving one's entire education, conducting complex mathematical calculations, and out-of-body experiences where the runner enters the shadow of a competitor (Morgan 1997a). There is evidence that dissociation may lengthen the time to exhaustion in steady-state endurance tasks, but Morgan (1997a) has suggested that the use of dissociation during competition may result in subpar performance. Research has borne out this hypothesis. Stevinson and Biddle (1998) found recreational marathoners who used a dissociative strategy during a race were more likely to 'hit the wall'; they concluded that these runners were not regulating their pace adequately and underhydrating during the race. They also found that many recreational runners associated throughout the race. Descriptions of these cognitive strategies and their impact have been widely reported in running magazines, and this may account for the widespread adoption of association as a racing strategy by many recreational runners.

Some researchers have claimed that association is the 'riskier' cognitive strategy. Masters and Ogles (1998) base this contention on their finding that marathoners who routinely associate trained harder, performed better and had a higher incidence of injury than runners who relied on dissociation. However, the assumption that using association spurs harder and longer training and consequently increases the risk of injury could not be established from the cross-sectional research employed in this study. It seems feasible that more talented athletes simply must associate, just as they must train long and hard, if they are to reach their full potential.

Élite athletes do not rely exclusively on association in all situations. Research with élite distance runners has found that approximately 50% of these athletes dissociated exclusively during training, whereas none relied exclusively on dissociation during competition (Morgan et al. 1987b, 1988). It also appears that athletes differ in the degree to which they monitor body feedback accurately during physical exertion. Morgan and Pollock (1977) reported that non-élite runners tended to underrate physical exertion during treadmill running when compared with world-class distance runners. In a study of wrestlers vying for positions on the US Olympic freestyle team, Nagle et al. (1975) found that unsuccessful competitors exhibited higher exercise heart rates during standardized exercise testing compared with the wrestlers that were successful in making the team, reflecting fitness differences between the groups. However, perceived exertion ratings did not differ between successful and unsuccessful wrestlers. Morgan (1997a) has recently theorized that this finding may indicate that élite athletes are more likely to use association on a routine basis, and not simply during competition. O'Connor (1992) has suggested such differences may arise from the fact that élite athletes associate because they can afford to monitor body signals, in part because they are more capable

of enduring the discomfort of intense physical effort.

There is evidence indicating that pain tolerance is greater in athletes compared with non-athletes, and in élite compared with non-élite competitors (O'Connor 1992). It has been hypothesized that these differences reflect habituation, resulting from repeated exposure to the pain experienced during intense training (Scott & Gijsbers 1981). There is also evidence that personality factors commonly found in élite athletes are associated with enhanced pain tolerance (Eysenck et al. 1982). However, further research is needed to determine the potential contribution of these and other factors to the use of association or dissociation.

Conclusions

There is considerable interest in uncovering the factors that contribute to endurance performance. Research to date has largely centred on biological variables. There is evidence that psychological factors also impact upon endurance performance. Selected personality traits such as emotional stability are associated with success in a variety of sports. Although these findings should not be used in efforts to select athletes for competition, they underscore the impact that mental health has on performance, a fact all too often ignored when considering the needs of the athlete. Other factors such as anxiety also influence sport performance, but at a much more individual level. These findings indicate that psychological research on athletes would benefit from considering the influence of both nomothetic (i.e. 'group') and ideographic (i.e. 'individual') factors. Moreover, given the complex nature of endurance performance, a better understanding will come only when psychological and physiological variables are examined conjointly. As stated by the pioneering American sport psychologist, Coleman Griffith (1929) some 70 years ago, athletic performance involves 'the study of vexing physiological and psychological problems, many of which are distorted by the attempt to reduce them to simple terms' (p. vii). Griffith's advice retains its currency.

References

Bannister, R. (1989) *The Four-Minute Mile*. Lyons & Burford, New York.

Berglund, B. & Säfström, H. (1994) Psychological monitoring and modulation of training load of world-class canoeists. *Medicine and Science in Sports and Exercise* 26, 1036–1040.

Burhans, R.S., Richman, C.L. & Bergey, D.B. (1988) Mental imagery training: effects on running speed performance. *International Journal of Sport Psychology* 19, 26–37.

Cooper, L. (1969) Athletics, activity and personality: a review of the literature. *Research Quarterly* 40, 17–22.

Driskell, J.E., Copper, C. & Moran, A. (1994) Does mental practice enhance performance? *Journal of Applied Psychology* 79, 481–492.

Dudley, A.T. (1888) The mental qualities of an athlete. *Harvard Alumni Magazine* 6, 43–51.

Elder, D. (1992) Racing with a heart-rate monitor. *Velo News* 2(10), 118.

Eysenck, H.J., Nias, K.B.D. & Cox, D.N. (1982) Personality and sport. *Advances in Behavioral Research and Therapy* 1, 1–56.

Fazey, J. & Hardy, L. (1988) *The Inverted-U Hypothesis: a Catastrophe for Sport Psychology?* White Line Press, Leeds.

Feltz, D.L. & Landers, D.M. (1983) The effects of mental practice in the development of motor skills. *Journal of Sport Psychology* 4, 25–57.

Griffith, C.R. (1929) *The Psychology of Coaching*. Charles Scribner's Sons, New York.

Hägg, G. (1952) *Gunder Hägg's Diary — A World Champion's Experiences and Training Advice*. Tiden, Sweden.

Hanin, Y.L. (1997) Emotions and athletic performance. Individual zones of optimal functioning model. In: Seiler, R. (ed.) *European Yearbook on Sport Psychology*, Vol. 1, pp. 30–70. FEBSAC, Sant Augustin, Germany.

Longman, J. (1998) Brazilian shatters the world record. *The New York Times* 21 September, D8.

Mahoney, M.J. (1989) Psychological predictors of élite and non-élite performance in Olympic weight lifting. *International Journal of Sport Psychology* 20, 1–12.

Martens, R. (1971) Anxiety and motor behavior. *Journal of Motor Behavior* 3, 151–179.

Martens, R. (1975) The paradigmatic crisis in American sport psychology. *Sportwissenschaft* 5, 9–24.

Masters, K.S. & Ogles, B.M. (1998) The relations of cognitive strategies with injury,

motivation, and performance among marathon runners: results from two studies. *Journal of Applied Sport Psychology* 10, 281–296.

McNair, D.M., Lorr, M. & Dropplemann, L.F. (1992) *Profile of Mood States Manual*. Educational and Testing Service, San Diego, CA.

Meyers, A.W., Whelan, J.P. & Murphy, S.M. (1996) Cognitive behavioral strategies in athletic performance enhancement. In: Hersen, M., Eisler, R.M. & Miller, P.M. (eds) *Progress in Behavior Modification*, Vol. 30, pp. 137–164. Brooks/Cole, Pacific Grove, CA.

Morgan, W.P. (1978) The credulous–skeptical argument in perspective. In: Straub, W.F. (ed.) *An Analysis of Athlete Behavior*, pp. 218–227. Mouvement Publications, Ithaca, NY.

Morgan, W.P. (1980) The trait psychology controversy. *Research Quarterly* 51, 50–76.

Morgan, W.P. (1985) Selected psychological factors limiting performance: a mental health model. In: Clarke, D.H. & Eckert, H.M. (eds) *Limits of Human Performance*, pp. 70–80. Human Kinetics, Champaign, IL.

Morgan, W.P. (1997a) Mind games: the psychology of sport. In: Lamb, D.R. & Murray, R. (eds) *Optimizing Sport Peformance: Perspectives in Exercise Science and Sports Medicine*, Vol. 10, pp. 1–54. Cooper Publications, Carmel, IN.

Morgan, W.P. (1997b) *Physical Activity and Mental Health*. Taylor & Francis, Washington, DC.

Morgan, W.P. & Costill, D.L. (1996) Selected psychological characteristics and health behaviors of aging marathon runners: a longitudinal study. *International Journal of Sports Medicine* 17, 305–313.

Morgan, W.P. & Pollock, M.L. (1977) Psychologic characterization of the elite distance runner. *Annals of the New York Academy of Science* 301, 382–403.

Morgan, W.P. & Johnson, R.W. (1978) Personality characteristics of successful and unsuccessful oarsmen. *International Journal of Sport Psychology* 9, 119–133.

Morgan, W.P., Brown, D.L., Raglin, J.S., O'Connor, P.J. & Ellickson, K.A. (1987a) Psychological monitoring of overtraining and staleness. *British Journal of Sports Medicine* 21, 107–114.

Morgan, W.P., O'Connor, P.J., Sparling, P.B. & Pate, R.R. (1987b) Psychological characterization of the élite female distance

runner. *International Journal of Sports Medicine* 8 (Suppl.), 124–131.

Morgan, W.P., Costill, D.L., Flynn, M.G., Raglin, J.S. & O'Connor, P.J. (1988) Mood disturbance following increased training in swimmers. *Medicine and Science in Sports and Exercise* 20, 408–414.

Nagle, F.J., Morgan, W.P., Hellickson, R.O., Serfas, R.C. & Alexander, J.F. (1975) Spotting success traits in Olympic contenders. *Physician and Sportsmedicine* 3 (12), 31–34.

Newcombe, P.A. & Boyle, G.J. (1995) High school students' sports personalities: variations across participation level, gender, type of sport, and success. *International Journal of Sport Psychology* 26, 277–294.

O'Connor, P.J. (1992) Psychological aspects of endurance performance, In: Shephard, R. & Åstrand, P.O. (eds) *Endurance in Sport*, pp. 139–145. Blackwell Scientific Publications, Oxford.

O'Connor, P.J. (1997) Overtraining and staleness. In: Morgan, W.P. (ed.) *Physical Activity and Mental Health*, pp. 145–160. Hemisphere Publications, New York.

O'Connor, P.J., Morgan, W.P., Raglin, J.S., Barksdale, C.M. & Kalin, N.H. (1989) Mood state and salivary cortisol changes following overtraining in female swimmers. *Psychoneuroendocrinology* 14, 303–310.

O'Connor, P.J., Morgan, W.P. & Raglin, J.S. (1991) Psychobiologic effects of 3 d of increased training in female and male swimmers. *Medicine and Science in Sports and Exercise* 23, 1055–1061.

Raglin, J.S. (1992) Anxiety and sport performance. In: Holloszy, J.O. (ed.) *Exercise and Sport Sciences Reviews*, Vol. 20, pp. 243–274. Williams & Wilkins, New York.

Raglin, J.S. (1993) Overtraining and staleness: psychometric monitoring of endurance athletes. In: Singer, R.N., Murphey, M. & Tennet, L.K. (eds) *Handbook of Research in Sport Psychology*, pp. 840–850. Macmillan, New York.

Raglin, J.S. & Hanin, Y.L. (1999) Competitive anxiety. In: Hanin, Y.L. (ed.) *Emotions in Sport*, pp. 93–111. Human Kinetics, Champaign, IL.

Raglin, J.S. & Turner, P.E. (1993) Anxiety and performance in track and field athletes: a comparison of the inverted-U hypothesis with ZOF theory. *Personality and Individual Differences* 14, 163–172.

Raglin, J.S. & Wilson, G.S. (1999) Overtraining in Athletes. In: Hanin, Y.L. (ed.) *Emotions in Sport*, pp. 191–207. Human Kinetics, Champaign, IL.

Raglin, J.S., Morgan, W.P. & O'Connor, P.J. (1991) Changes in mood states during training in female and male swimmers. *International Journal of Sports Medicine* **12**, 585–589.

Raglin, J.S., Eksten, F. & Garl, F.T. (1995) Mood state responses to a pre-season conditioning program in male collegiate basketball players. *International Journal of Sport Psychology* **26**, 214–225.

Renger, R. (1993) A review of the Profile of Mood States (POMS) in the prediction of athletic success. *Journal of Applied Sport Psychology* **5**, 78–84.

Rushall, B.S. (1970) An evaluation of the relationship between personality and physical performance categories. In: Kenyon, G.S. (ed.) *Contemporary Psychology of Sport*, pp. 157–165. Athletic Institute, Chicago.

Scott, V. & Gijsbers, K. (1981) Pain perception in competitive swimmers. *British Medical Journal* **283**, 91–93.

Smith, T.W. (1997) Punt, pass, and ponder the questions. *The New York Times* 20 April, F-11.

Stevinson, C.D. & Biddle, S.J.H. (1998) Cognitive orientations in marathon running and 'hitting the wall.' *British Journal of Sports Medicine* **32**, 229–235.

Swift, E.M. (1989) LeGrand Lemond. *Sports Illustrated* **71**, 54–72.

Terry, P. (1995) The efficacy of mood state profiling with élite performers: a review and synthesis. *Sport Psychologist* **9**, 309–324.

Turner, P.E. & Raglin, J.S. (1996) Variability in precompetition anxiety and performance in college track and field athletes. *Medicine and Science in Sports and Exercise* **28**, 378–385.

Vanden Auweele, Y., DeCuyper, B., VanMele, V. & Rzenicki, R. (1993) Elite performance and personality: from description and prediction to diagnosis and intervention. In: Singer, R.N., Murphey, M. & Tennant, L.K. (eds) *Handbook of Research on Sport Psychology*, pp. 257–289. Macmillan, New York.

Verde, T., Thomas, S. & Shephard, R.J. (1992) Potential markers of heavy training in highly trained distance runners. *British Journal of Sports Medicine* **26**, 167–175.

Warburton, R.W. & Kane, J.E. (1966) Personality related to sport and physical activity. In: Kane, J.E. (ed.) *Readings in Physical Education*, pp. 61–89. P.E. Association, London, UK.

Williams, J., Rippon, G., Stone, B. & Annett, J. (1995) Psychophysiological correlates of dynamic imagery. *British Journal of Psychology* **86**, 283–300.

Wilson, G.S. & Raglin, J.S. (1997) Optimal and predicted anxiety in 9–12-year-old track and field athletes. *Scandinavian Journal of Medicine and Science in Sports* **7**, 253–258.

Part 2c

Genetic Determinants of Endurance Performance

Chapter 15

Genetic Determinants of Endurance Performance

CLAUDE BOUCHARD, BERND WOLFARTH, MIGUEL A. RIVERA,
JACQUES GAGNON AND JEAN-AIMÉ SIMONEAU

Introduction

In the language of human geneticists, performance in endurance sports and other athletic events can be conceived as complex multifactorial phenotypes. Endurance performance depends on a large number of factors, including the physique, and the biomechanical, physiological, metabolic, behavioural, psychological and social characteristics of the individual. Some of these determinants and concomitants of endurance performance are probably little influenced by our genes, but most of them are affected to a significant extent. The purpose of this chapter is to summarize the evidence accumulated to date concerning selected genetic determinants of endurance performance. Since little is known about the genetics of biomechanical, behavioural, psychological and social determinants of endurance performance, the focus of this chapter will be on physique, physiological and metabolic factors.

The fundamental questions are whether there is evidence that genetic factors contribute to the commonly observed variations in these determinants, which genes are involved, and what are the specific mutations of interest. A comprehensive response to each of these questions is beyond the present knowledge base. However, progress has been made since the first edition of this volume (Bouchard 1992), and it is reviewed here.

Firstly, the key determinants and related phenotypes are defined briefly. Secondly, the evidence for a role of genetic factors is reviewed, based on the genetic epidemiology literature, with an emphasis

on key determinants in the sedentary state and on responsiveness to exercise training. Finally, results from candidate gene studies and other molecular markers are summarized. Few genetic investigations have been undertaken to date on performance in endurance sports or endurance athletes *per se*. We must therefore rely primarily on laboratory-based research on the determinants of endurance performance phenotypes.

Phenotypes

A frequently asked question in the exercise science milieu is: what are the important determinants of endurance performance? The topic is of considerable importance, but is also highly complex, as evidenced by the large number of chapters devoted to the topic in this book. The issue also has great interest for those investigating the genetic basis of endurance performance, as studies need to focus on the most relevant determinants if an adequate understanding of the role of the genes is to be achieved. Figure 15.1 depicts the most often cited set of determinants of endurance performance. In reality, each represents a family of several factors and traits rather than a single characteristic. It is beyond the scope of this chapter to review these determinants and their contribution to endurance performance. The purpose instead is to indicate that only a fraction of these determinants are dealt with herein.

The focus of this chapter is on phenotypes of physique and body composition as well as maximal oxygen intake ($\dot{V}O_{2max}$) and some of its key affectors

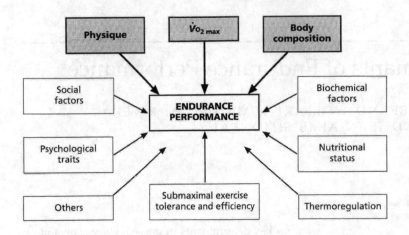

Fig. 15.1 Overview of the determinants of endurance performance. The highlighted boxes indicate the determinants that are discussed in this chapter.

including cardiovascular factors and skeletal muscle characteristics.

Briefly, $\dot{V}_{O_{2max}}$ is one of the factors limiting endurance performance (Chapter 21). $\dot{V}_{O_{2max}}$ is determined by a combination of central factors (such as cardiac output and arteriovenous oxygen differences) and peripheral influences (such as muscle capillary density and oxidative enzyme capacities). Maximal cardiac output can be twice as high in well-trained endurance athletes as in untrained subjects and the difference is mainly explained by a larger stroke volume (Saltin & Strange 1992; Mitchell & Raven 1994). The greater $\dot{V}_{O_{2max}}$ that is typical of endurance-trained subjects has also been attributed in part to an augmented maximal arteriovenous oxygen difference (Mitchell & Raven 1994; Wagner 1995). The skeletal muscle capillary bed and mitochondrial content are substantially larger in endurance-trained individuals and they favourably alter the exchange of gases, substrates and metabolites that is taking place between the systemic capillaries and the core of the muscle cell. The activities of the aerobic oxidative and lipid-metabolizing enzymes in human skeletal muscle are significantly increased with exercise training (Simoneau 1995). In addition, an increased utilization of muscle triglycerides and a greater fatty acid mobilization are observed during exercise in the trained compared with the untrained state. These factors are thought to be involved in the ability to sustain high-intensity exercise over long periods of time.

Another class of determinants relates to physique and body composition. Morphological determinants contribute only indirectly to endurance performance, but they are none the less of interest. For instance, in prolonged endurance performance, an ectomorphic physique, a low body mass for height and a low percentage of body fat may all confer an advantage. A high fat-free mass relative to total body mass is also thought to be a desirable trait for most endurance performances.

Quantitative genetic studies

In this section, we deal with the following questions. Do indicators of the capacity to perform aerobic activities show a familial concentration? What is the relative contribution of the estimated genetic effect (heritability) to the total population variation in these phenotypes? Do we have evidence for a stronger maternal or paternal influence in the transmission pattern? We review firstly the evidence for $\dot{V}_{O_{2max}}$, then for selected cardiovascular and skeletal muscle determinants of $\dot{V}_{O_{2max}}$ and finally for physique and body composition.

Maximal oxygen intake ($\dot{V}_{O_{2max}}$)

FAMILIAL RESEMBLANCE

One approach to assessing the importance of familial resemblance in relevant phenotypes is to compare the variance between families or sibships

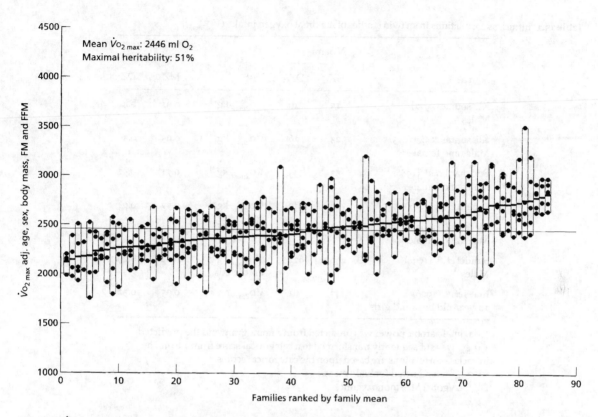

Fig. 15.2 $\dot{V}_{O_{2}max}$ adjusted for age, sex, body weight, fat mass and fat-free mass plotted by family rank. Each family is enclosed in a box, with individual data points plotted as dots and each family mean as a dash. The horizontal reference line is the group mean. Reproduced with permission from Bouchard *et al.* (1998a).

to that observed within nuclear families or sibships. However, to obtain meaningful results, one must control for relevant concomitant variables such as age, gender, body mass and body composition.

$\dot{V}_{O_{2}max}$ is characterized by a significant familial resemblance (Montoye & Gayle 1978; Lortie *et al.* 1982; Lesage *et al.* 1985). In the largest of family studies, the HERITAGE Family Study, an F ratio of 2.72 was found on comparing the between-family variance to the within-family variance for $\dot{V}_{O_{2}max}$ in the sedentary state (adjusted for age, sex, body mass and body composition). The intraclass coefficient for the familial resemblance was 0.41 (Bouchard *et al.* 1998a).

GENETIC HERITABILITY

The heritability of $\dot{V}_{O_{2}max}$ has been estimated from a few family and twin studies. Three family studies have measured $\dot{V}_{O_{2}max}$ (Lesage *et al.* 1985; Bouchard *et al.* 1986a, 1988a). Again, the most comprehensive of these is the HERITAGE Family Study in which two cycle ergometer $\dot{V}_{O_{2}max}$ tests were performed in sedentary families of Caucasian descent (Bouchard *et al.* 1998a). The maximal heritability was about 50% of the age-, sex-, body mass- and body composition-adjusted $\dot{V}_{O_{2}max}$. The concept of family lines with low and high $\dot{V}_{O_{2}max}$ phenotypes in the sedentary state is illustrated in Fig. 15.2.

Table 15.1 summarizes intraclass correlations in pairs of dizygotic (DZ) and monozygotic (MZ) twins from seven studies. The data vary in test protocol (measured or predicted aerobic power, maximal or submaximal tests), the number of twin pairs, uncontrolled age or sex effects, and differences in means or variances between twin types.

Table 15.1 Intraclass correlations from twin studies of maximal oxygen intake ($\dot{V}O_{2max}$).

Source	N pairs		Test	MZ	DZ
	MZ	DZ			
Klissouras (1971) Males	15	10	$\dot{V}O_{2max} \cdot kg^{-1}$	0.91	0.44
Klissouras et al. (1973) Males and females	23	16	$\dot{V}O_{2max} \cdot kg^{-1}$	0.95	0.36
Bouchard et al. (1986a) Males and females	53	33	$\dot{V}O_{2max} \cdot kg^{-1}$	0.71	0.51
Fagard et al. (1991)	29	19	$\dot{V}O_{2max} \cdot kg^{-1}$	0.77	0.04
Maes et al. (1993) Males and females	41	50	$\dot{V}O_{2max} \cdot kg^{-1}$	0.85	0.56
Sundet et al. (1994) Males	436	622	$\dot{V}O_{2max} \cdot kg^{-1}$ Predicted*	0.62	0.29
Maes et al. (1996) 10-year-old boys and girls	43	61	$\dot{V}O_{2max}$†	0.75	0.32

*Maximal aerobic power was predicted from a nomogram and the predicted $\dot{V}O_{2max}$ was subsequently transformed to a categorical score from 1 to 9. The intraclass correlations are based upon the categorical scores.
†$\dot{V}O_{2max}$ not adjusted for body mass.
DZ, dizygotic; MZ, monozygotic.

The intraclass correlations for MZ twins ranged from about 0.6 to 0.9, whereas correlations for DZ twins with one exception ranged from 0.3 to 0.5. The largest of the twin studies (Sundet et al. 1994) was derived from a population-based twin panel of conscripts. The data were based on predicted $\dot{V}O_{2max}$ values, which were subsequently transformed to categorical scores, from low to high maximal aerobic power, but intraclass correlations for the categorical scores were similar to those found in other twin studies (Sundet et al. 1994).

In our own study involving 27 pairs of brothers, 33 pairs of DZ twins and 53 pairs of MZ twins (Bouchard et al. 1986a), heritability of $\dot{V}O_{2max}$ per kg of body mass was about 40%. Since the correlation in DZ twins (intraclass = 0.51) was high in comparison to the brothers (intraclass = 0.41), we hypothesized that the 40% estimate was probably inflated by common environmental factors, and that the true heritability of $\dot{V}O_{2max}$ per kg of mass was more likely to lie between 25 and 40% of the adjusted phenotypic variance. In the same study, the total power

output during a 90-min maximal cycle ergometer test was also measured in 31 pairs of DZ and 33 pairs of MZ twins. The heritability for this test of endurance performance reached 60% when data were expressed per kg of body mass.

Statistical modelling tactics have been applied to estimate genetic and environmental sources of variation in $\dot{V}O_{2max}$. For example, Fagard et al. (1991) performed a path analysis of $\dot{V}O_{2max}$ in 29 MZ and 19 DZ pairs. When data were adjusted for body mass, skinfold thickness and sports participation, the heritability estimate was 66%.

Maes et al. (1996) applied structural equation modelling to data on 105 10-year-old twin pairs and their parents (97 mothers and 84 fathers) from the Leuven Longitudinal Twin Study. They quantified genetic and environmental sources of variation in several fitness components, including $\dot{V}O_{2max}$ measured during a maximal treadmill test. They observed strong assortative mating for absolute $\dot{V}O_{2max}$ ($l \cdot min^{-1}$), with a husband–wife correlation of 0.42 ($N = 79$ pairs), markedly higher than in the

HERITAGE Family Study (Bouchard *et al.* 1998a). The results did not give a straightforward indication as to which of the models best explained the data. There was clear evidence for a strong genetic component to absolute $\dot{V}_{O_{2max}}$, but the genetic influence was reduced when $\dot{V}_{O_{2max}}$ per kg of body mass was considered.

Endurance running performance has been studied in 11 inbred strains of rats (Barbato *et al.* 1998). The COP/Hsd rats were the worst performers and the DA/OlaHsd rats the best. For instance, the duration of the treadmill run reached 19.9 ± 1.8 min for COP/Hsd males and females, but it was 41.5 ± 2.2 min for the DA/OlaHsd rats. Since these inbred strains have attained a very high, if not a perfect, degree of homozygosity at all loci, such interstrain differences in endurance performance are thought to be caused mainly by genetic differences. Crossbreeding of high- and low-endurance performance strains should provide informative colonies for the identification of chromosomal areas and quantitative trait loci contributing to endurance performance. Such studies have yet to be reported.

MATERNAL EFFECTS

One familial study has suggested the likelihood of a specific maternal effect for $\dot{V}_{O_{2max}}$ per kg of mass or per kg of fat-free mass (Lesage *et al.* 1985). This hypothesis was prompted by the observation that correlations reached 0.20 and above in mother–child pairs, but were about zero in father–child pairs. In contrast, no maternal effect was found in studies of submaximal power output (Pérusse *et al.* 1987, 1988). There is also no consistent evidence that the transmission from parents to offspring is limited to one gender (boys or girls), although the additive genetic variance of absolute $\dot{V}_{O_{2max}}$ was said to be stronger in girls than boys in the Leuven Longitudinal Twin Study (Maes *et al.* 1996).

More recently, the HERITAGE Family Study (Bouchard *et al.* 1998a) has provided strong evidence for a substantial maternal heritability in $\dot{V}_{O_{2max}}$ adjusted for age, sex, body mass and body composition. About half of the maximal heritability of $\dot{V}_{O_{2max}}$ observed in the sedentary state was com-

patible with a maternal, and possibly a mitochondrial, transmission.

RESPONSE TO TRAINING

Maximal aerobic power has limited trainability in children under 10 years of age, but $\dot{V}_{O_{2max}}$ and endurance performance are clearly trainable phenotypes in older children, adolescents, young adults and older adults of both sexes (Malina & Bouchard 1991; Bouchard *et al.* 1992; Spina *et al.* 1993). There are considerable interindividual differences in the response of these phenotypes to exercise training. Among young adults, some individuals exhibit a large response, whereas others show no or minimal response; a broad range of response phenotypes lie between these extremes (Fig. 15.3). This figure depicts the individuality of response in terms of gains in $\dot{V}_{O_{2max}}$ with a standardized 20-week endurance training programme across the four clinical centres involved in the HERITAGE Family Study (Bouchard *et al.* 1999). The mean gain in $\dot{V}_{O_{2max}}$ is about $400 \, \text{ml} \, O_2 \cdot \text{min}^{-1}$ but the range extends from no gain to $1 \, l \, O_2 \cdot \text{min}^{-1}$.

What is the main cause of the heterogeneity in response to training? We believe it is related to as yet undetermined genetic characteristics. To test this hypothesis, we have performed training studies with pairs of MZ twins, the rationale being that the response pattern will vary for individuals having the same genotype (within pairs) and for subjects with differing genetic characteristics (between pairs). These results and data from the HERITAGE Family Study show that the individuality in trainability of phenotypes governing endurance performance is highly familial and primarily genetically determined.

In pairs of MZ twins, the $\dot{V}_{O_{2max}}$ response to standardized training shows six to nine times more variance between genotypes (between pairs of twins) than within genotypes (within pairs of twins) (Bouchard *et al.* 1992). The similarity of training response among members of the same MZ twin pairs is illustrated in Fig. 15.4. In this particular experiment, 10 pairs of male MZ twins were submitted to a standardized, laboratory-controlled training programme for 20 weeks. Gains in

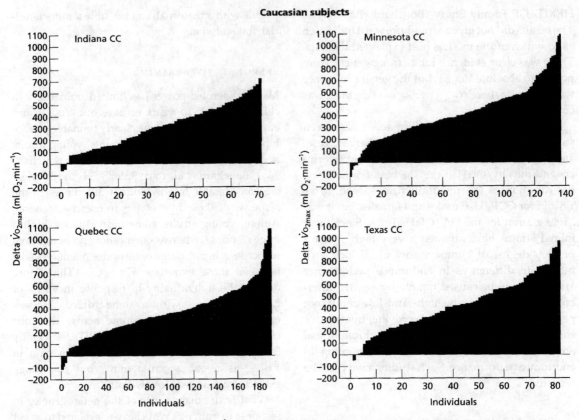

Fig. 15.3 Individual values for the increase in $\dot{V}o_{2max}$ across the four clinical centres of the HERITAGE Family Study in response to a 20-week endurance training programme. Reproduced with permission from Bouchard *et al.* (1999).

absolute $\dot{V}o_{2max}$ showed almost eight times more variance between pairs of twins than within pairs of twins (Prud'homme *et al.* 1984; Bouchard *et al.* 1990).

A related measure of aerobic performance is the total work output during a prolonged exercise bout. In six pairs of MZ twins, the total power output during a 90-min maximal cycle ergometer test was monitored before and after 15 weeks of training (Hamel *et al.* 1986). Resemblance in total power output within twin pairs was significant (intraclass r = 0.83), and the ratio of between-pairs to within-pairs variances was about 11.

The most convincing evidence for the presence of family lines in the trainability of $\dot{V}o_{2max}$ comes from the HERITAGE Family Study. The increase in $\dot{V}o_{2max}$ in 483 individuals from 99 two-generation families of Caucasian descent was adjusted for age, sex and

baseline $\dot{V}o_{2max}$. The adjusted $\dot{V}o_{2max}$ response showed 2.6 times more variance between families than within families, and the model-fitting analytical procedure yielded a maximal heritability estimate of 47% (Bouchard *et al.* 1999). The familial aggregation of the $\dot{V}o_{2max}$ response phenotype is illustrated in Fig. 15.5.

Cardiovascular determinants

Relative to their sedentary peers, endurance athletes have larger hearts, and larger stroke volumes and greater cardiac outputs during maximal exercise; they also show a resting bradycardia, and a slower heart rate at a given submaximal work rate. No genetic study on submaximal or maximal stroke volume and cardiac output has yet been reported. However, a few studies have addressed the issue

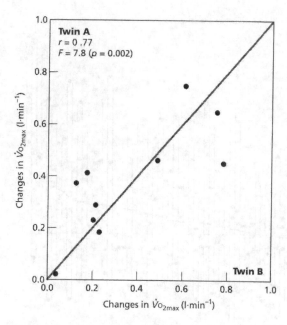

Twin A
$r = 0.77$
$F = 7.8 \ (p = 0.002)$

Fig. 15.4 Intrapair resemblance (intraclass coefficient) in 10 pairs of monozygotic twins for training changes in $\dot{V}_{O_{2max}}$ (l $O_2 \cdot min^{-1}$) after 20 weeks of endurance training. Constructed from the original data in Prud'homme *et al.* (1984).

heart structures, except left ventricular internal diameter, were significantly influenced by genetic factors, with heritability estimates ranging from 29 to 68%. The strong relationship between body size and cardiac dimensions raises the question of how much of the covariation between these two variables is explained by common genetic factors. This question was addressed in a bivariate genetic analysis of left ventricular mass and body mass in 147 MZ and 107 DZ pubertal twin pairs of both sexes (Verhaaren *et al.* 1991). Heritabilities of left ventricular mass reached 60% in males and 73% in females. After adjustment of left ventricular mass for body mass and sexual maturity, the genetic effect was reduced but remained significant, with heritabilities of 39% and 59% in males and females, respectively. Bivariate genetic analyses showed that the correlation between left ventricular mass and body mass was almost entirely of genetic origin, 90% being attributed to common genes (Verhaaren *et al.* 1991).

These studies suggest that genetic factors are important in determining cardiac dimensions under resting conditions. One study of 21 MZ and 12 DZ twin pairs considered the inheritance of cardiac changes during submaximal supine cycle exercise at a heart rate of 110 beats·min^{-1} (Bielen *et al.* 1991b). The increases of left ventricular internal diameter and fractional shortening in response to exercise showed genetic effects of 24% and 47%, respectively. The results were interpreted as indicators that adaptation of cardiac function during submaximal exercise may be partly determined by genotype (Bielen *et al.* 1991b).

of the heritability of heart size and cardiac dimensions.

Echographic measurements of cardiac dimensions in members of nuclear families suggest a familial resemblance in several ventricular dimensions (Adams *et al.* 1986; Thériault *et al.* 1986). Familial correlations among various kinds of relatives by descent and adoption were assessed for echocardiographically derived heart dimensions (Thériault *et al.* 1986). For most cardiac dimensions, correlations were significant in both biological relatives and relatives by adoption, suggesting that both genetic and environmental factors contribute to the phenotypic variance.

The inheritance of left ventricular structure has been studied in 32 MZ and 21 DZ pairs of healthy male twins (Bielen *et al.* 1991a). A path analysis model allowed the phenotypic variance to be partitioned into genetic, shared environmental and non-shared environmental components. The data were adjusted for the effects of age and body mass. All

Skeletal muscle determinants

MUSCLE FIBRE DISTRIBUTION

Skeletal muscle fibre type distribution is thought to be a significant determinant of endurance performance. Sampling variation and laboratory error variance must be taken into account when attempting to quantify the importance of genetic differences based on human muscle biopsies. For instance, repeated measurements within the adult vastus lateralis muscle indicate that sampling variability and technical error together account for about 15% of the

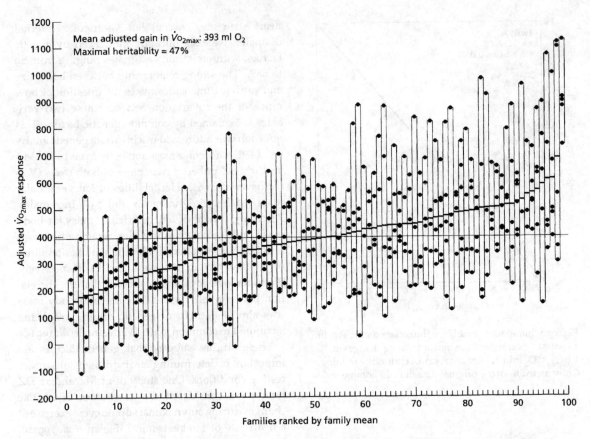

Fig. 15.5 $\dot{V}_{O_{2}max}$ response to a 20-week endurance training programme. Data are adjusted for age, sex and pretraining $\dot{V}_{O_{2}max}$ plotted by family rank. Each family is enclosed in a box, with individual data points plotted as dots and each family mean as a dash. The horizontal reference line is the group mean. Reproduced with permission from Bouchard *et al.* (1999).

variance in the proportion of type I muscle fibres (Simoneau *et al.* 1986b; Simoneau & Bouchard 1995).

Intraclass correlations for the proportion of different fibres in the vastus lateralis have been studied in 32 pairs of brothers, 26 pairs of DZ and 35 pairs of male and female MZ twins (Bouchard *et al.* 1986a). Although brothers and DZ twins share about a half of their genes by descent, comparison of the respective within-pair correlations suggests that because DZ twins experience more similar environmental circumstances than brothers separated in age, they show increased phenotypic resemblance in the proportion of type I fibres. The within-pair correlations in the proportion of type I fibres in MZ ($r = 0.55$) and DZ ($r = 0.52$) twins are reasonably close to the correlation between the proportion of type I fibres in the right and left legs of the same individual ($r = 0.67$)

(Simoneau *et al.* 1986a). Corresponding correlations indicate no genetic effect for type IIa fibres, and significant resemblance within MZ twin pairs for type IIb fibres but not for DZ twin and sibling pairs.

The variability in the percentage of type I fibres within pairs of MZ twins provides useful information on the role of non-genetic factors. The mean difference in percentage of type I fibres between a member of a MZ pair and his/her cotwin reached $9.5 \pm 6.9\%$ in the 40 pairs of MZ twins that we were able to study (Simoneau & Bouchard 1995). The difference was less than 6% in 16 pairs, between 6 and 12% in 11 pairs, between 12 and 18% in 5 pairs, and between 18 and 23% in the remaining 8 pairs. The largest pair difference of 23% was observed in three pairs, and was of the same magnitude as the largest differences when samples were taken from the right and left vastus lateralis of the same individual (Simoneau & Bouchard 1995).

These results lead to the conclusion that the genetic component accounts for about 45% of variance in the proportion of type I muscle fibres in humans (Simoneau & Bouchard 1995). A summary of genetic, environmental and methodological sources of variation in the proportion of type I fibres in human skeletal muscle is illustrated in Fig. 15.6.

The preceding results are generally consistent with animal experiments. In an inbred mouse strain, genetic factors accounted for about 75% of the variation in the proportion of type I fibres in the soleus muscle, with 95% confidence intervals ranging from 55% to 89% (Nimmo et al. 1985). In four-generation selective breeding of rats for a high percentage of type I muscle fibres in the gastrocnemius muscle, only about 17% of variance in the proportion of these fibres was genetically determined (Nakamura et al. 1993). However, the variance in the proportion of type I fibres in the gastrocnemius muscle was only about a half of that commonly observed for the vastus lateralis muscle in humans, which is a situation that may have reduced the estimated heritability.

METABOLIC PROPERTIES

There is considerable interindividual variation in

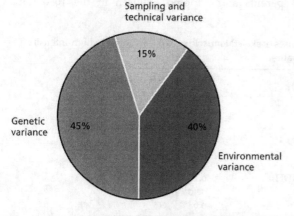

Fig. 15.6 Estimates of the sampling and technical, environmental and genetic variances for the proportion of type I fibres in human skeletal muscle. Reproduced with permission from Simoneau and Bouchard (1995).

the enzymatic activity profile of skeletal muscle. One can distinguish individuals with high and low activity levels of enzyme markers for the catabolism of different substrates in the skeletal muscle among healthy sedentary and moderately active individuals of both sexes (Simoneau & Bouchard 1989). Many factors probably contribute to interindividual differences, and it is likely that the genotype plays a role in determining the amount of protein for several important enzymes in skeletal muscle.

Data on the extent of genetic determination of enzyme marker activities in skeletal muscle are limited. Early studies, based on small samples of MZ and DZ twins (Howald 1976; Komi et al. 1977), suggested no gene-associated variation in several enzymes. However, data from larger samples of MZ ($n = 35$) and DZ ($n = 26$) twins of both sexes and pairs of biological brothers ($n = 32$) indicate significant inheritance of variation in several key enzymes of skeletal muscle (Bouchard et al. 1986b). There is significant within-pair resemblance in MZ twins for all skeletal muscle enzyme activities ($r = 0.30$–0.68), but the within-pair correlations for DZ twins and brothers suggest that variations in several enzyme activities are also related to non-genetic factors and environmental conditions. After adjusting for variation in enzyme activities associated with age and sex, genetic factors were responsible for about 25–50% of the total phenotypic variation in the activities of the regulatory enzymes of the glycolytic (phosphofructokinase—PFK) and citric acid cycle (oxoglutarate dehydrogenase—OGDH) pathways, and in the ratio of glycolytic to oxidative activities (PFK/OGDH ratio) (Bouchard et al. 1986b). Since such genetic effects could not be explained by charge variation in the enzyme molecules (Marcotte et al. 1987; Bouchard et al. 1988b), they could depend upon individual differences in transcription or translation rates.

RESPONSE TO TRAINING

Investigation of the role of the genotype in the response of skeletal muscle tissue to standardized training programmes has only just begun. Two experimental studies of the responses of young adult MZ twins to relevant training programmes provide some insights into potential genotypic contributions to the skeletal muscle training response. The studies included male and female MZ twins, and there were no sex differences in training-related gains. The effects of high-intensity intermittent training are summarized in Table 15.2. The training programme involved 15 weeks of both continuous and interval cycle ergometer work in 12 pairs of MZ twins of both sexes. Programme-related changes in fibre type proportions showed no significant within-pair resemblance. However, about 50–60% of the response of hexokinase (HK), lactate dehydrogenase (LDH), malate dehydrogenase (MDH), OGDH and the PFK/OGDH ratio to the intermittent training programme was genotype associated (Table 15.2), while about 80% of the creatine kinase (CK) training response appeared to be determined by the genotype (Simoneau *et al.* 1986a).

The second study followed six pairs of young adult MZ twins (three male and three female) through 15 weeks of endurance training on a cycle ergometer (Hamel *et al.* 1986). Genotype–training interactions were evaluated for the proportion of muscle fibres and several enzymes after 7 and 15 weeks of training. There were no significant changes in the proportions of type I and type IIa and IIb fibres. Changes in skeletal muscle enzyme activities during the first half of training were only weakly related to genotype. However, changes in the activities of PFK, MDH, 3-hydroxyacyl CoA dehydrogenase (HADH) and OGDH across the whole 15 weeks were characterized by significant within-pair

resemblance. This suggests that, early in the programme, adaptation to endurance training may be under less stringent genetic control; however, as training continues and perhaps nears maximal trainability, the response becomes more genotype dependent. Taken together, these two studies provide strong support for the notion that genetic variation accounts for some of the heterogeneity in skeletal muscle metabolic responses to exercise training.

Physique and body composition

PHYSIQUE

Physique characteristics are often assessed by somatotyping. Studies generally suggest that all three somatotype components, considered individually, are characterized by a significant genetic effect, but there is a trend for mesomorphy to exhibit a higher level of heritability than ectomorphy or endomorphy in both family and twin studies (Carter & Heath 1990; Song *et al.* 1993, 1994).

If each somatotype component is analysed with statistical control over the other two components (Song *et al.* 1993, 1994), parent–child correlations are seen to be significant for all three components, with mesomorphy again exhibiting a higher degree of covariation than the other two components. The same trend is found in full sibling correlations.

Somatotype data were obtained from foster parents and adopted children in the 1980 data

Table 15.2 Intraclass coefficients for the resemblance in responses of skeletal muscle enzyme activities to high-intensity intermittent training within monozygotic twin pairs ($N = 12$ pairs).

Enzyme	Intraclass correlation
Creatine kinase (CK)	0.82**
Hexokinase (HK)	0.59*
Phosphofructokinase (PFK)	0.38
Lactate dehydrogenase (LDH)	0.64**
Malate dehydrogenase (MDH)	0.50*
3-Hydroxyacyl CoA dehydrogenase (HADH)	0.15
Oxoglutarate dehydrogenase (OGDH)	0.50*
PFK/OGDH ratio	0.64**

Adapted from Simoneau *et al.* (1986a).
*$P < 0.05$, **$P < 0.01$.

collection phase of the Québec Family Study. The findings of adopted versus biological dyads are summarized in Table 15.3. The correlations for mesomorphy were markedly higher in the mid-parent–natural child set than in the foster mid-parent–adopted child group (Bouchard 1996). The difference between the two sets persisted and was even increased when mesomorphy was statistically adjusted for endomorphy and ectomorphy. The level of correlation for the other two components remained at 0.3–0.4 when each component was adjusted for the other two in biological relatives, but it decreased in relatives by adoption. These results imply that the level of heritability is highest for mesomorphy.

FAT-FREE MASS

There is as yet little information on the contribution of genotype to individual differences in fat-free mass (FFM). Familial data indicate a significant genetic contribution to FFM. Nine different types of relatives by descent or by adoption had their body composition estimated by underwater weighing during the Québec Family Study (Bouchard et al. 1988c). The resulting measures of body density were converted to percentages of body fat, from which estimates of FFM were obtained. Correlations for various pairs of relatives suggested a substantial contribution of biological inheritance to FFM. Path analysis (BETA) of familial resemblances indicated a total transmissible variance of 40–50% for FFM

(Bouchard et al. 1988c). The genetic component of the transmissible variance was about 30% for FFM. Subsequent commingling analysis of these data has shown that FFM was characterized by a single distribution in parents but not in the offspring (Borecki et al. 1991). Segregation analysis did not provide evidence for a major locus effect on FFM (Rice et al. 1993). Taken as a whole, these studies suggest that the genetic architecture of human variation in FFM is very complex.

FAT MASS AND PERCENTAGE BODY FAT

The contribution of genetic factors to variations in fat mass and percentage body fat has been considered in twin and family studies. In the Québec Family Study, the heritability of both phenotypes, as assessed by hydrostatic weighing, reached about 25% of the age- and sex-adjusted variance (Bouchard et al. 1988c). The latter estimate was based on nine types of relatives by descent or by adoption. In contrast, when only familial data are available, as in the HERITAGE Family Study, the heritability estimates are significantly higher. For instance, a maximal heritability coefficient of 62% was reported for the percentage of body fat in the HERITAGE Family Study cohort (Rice et al. 1997a). The few twin studies that have dealt with estimates of total body fat have also reported very high heritability coefficients (Bouchard et al. 1998b). Similar estimates have been obtained for the body mass index (BMI), i.e. the ratio of body mass (kg) relative

Table 15.3 Mid-parent–child interclass correlations for somatotype components.

Variable	Foster mid-parent–adopted child (N = 154 sets)		Mid-parent–natural child (N = 622 sets)	
Endomorphy	0.37**†	0.19*‡	0.35**†	0.41**‡
Mesomorphy	0.19*	0.02	0.41**	0.41**
Ectomorphy	0.26**	0.02	0.33**	0.32**

*P < 0.05, **P < 0.001.
†Scores adjusted for age and sex effects by generation and normalized (column 1 and 3).
‡Scores adjusted for age and sex effects and for the other two somatotype components by generation and normalized (column 2 and 4).
Reproduced with permission from Bouchard (1996).

to stature (m²): the heritability levels are quite heterogeneous, with the lowest values being obtained in adoption studies and the highest in twin study designs. In general, the largest studies which have relied on several types of relatives in the same analysis have yielded heritability estimates ranging from about 25 to 40%.

Several studies have tested the hypothesis that a major gene segregates for BMI, body fat mass and percentage body fat. Five of the 10 segregation studies of BMI provided evidence that segregation of a recessive locus with a frequency of about 0.2 accounted for 35–45% of the variance, with a multifactorial component accounting for 40–45% of the remaining variance (Bouchard *et al.* 1998b). Four segregation studies of fat mass and/or percentage body fat have been reported to date; two conducted on the Québec Family Study (Rice *et al.* 1993) and the HERITAGE Family Study (Rice *et al.* 1997b) used underwater weighing techniques, and two conducted in Mexican American families (Comuzzie *et al.* 1995) and French Caucasian families (Lecomte *et al.* 1997) used bioelectrical impedance measurements. In three of these studies (Rice *et al.* 1993; Comuzzie *et al.* 1995; Rice *et al.* 1997b), the results were very similar, suggesting that a recessive locus accounted for about a half of the phenotypic variance, with an additional quarter due to multifactorial effects.

Molecular markers

From the genetic epidemiology studies reviewed above, it appears useful to focus the search for genes and mutations on several families of phenotypes, namely endurance performance phenotypes, the determinants of endurance performance in the sedentary state and those of responsiveness to training. The genetic dissection of endurance performance phenotypes and their determinants will require a wide array of designs and technologies: case and control studies, family studies, association studies, linkage studies from genomic scans or with candidate genes, transmission disequilibrium tests, rodent transgenic models, crossbreeding studies in informative mouse or rat strains, knockout models, etc. At this time, only one linkage study has been

reported in humans, but it has dealt with a limited number of markers on one chromosome only (Gagnon *et al.* 1997). Most available reports have focused on candidate genes encoded in the nuclear DNA and on a few mitochondrial DNA sequences.

In the following sections, we review the evidence for a role of selected candidate genes and mitochondrial DNA on $\dot{V}o_{2max}$ and other relevant phenotypes. It must be recognized at the outset that it is unlikely that a single gene or a few loci will be sufficient to define the genetic component of endurance performance, its determinants and their trainability. The investigation of the molecular basis of human variation in performance and in trainability is still in its infancy. The databases necessary to undertake such studies have been or are currently being established and one can anticipate a wealth of new data in the near future.

A few reports on the topic of genetic markers and performance have appeared over the last 30 years or so. The study of élite performance by means of genetic markers was first conducted during the 1968 Olympic Games in Mexico City (deGaray *et al.* 1974). The purpose of that study was to verify if there was any association between participation in the Olympic Games as an athlete and allelic variation in single-gene blood systems. Results indicated that participation in the 1968 Olympic Games was not associated with allelic variations in red blood cell antigens or enzyme variants of red blood cells. A second effort was carried out during the 1976 Olympic Games in Montréal (Chagnon *et al.* 1984; Couture *et al.* 1986). In this study, a search for genetic markers of aerobic performance was undertaken in a group of Caucasians competing in endurance events. No significant differences between élite endurance athletes and controls were reported for genetic markers in red blood cell antigens and four red blood cell enzymes.

Angiotensin-converting enzyme (ACE) gene

It has recently been proposed that a marker in the angiotensin-converting enzyme (ACE) gene (chromosome: 17q23) has a strong influence on human physical performance (Montgomery *et al.* 1998). Two studies have reported an association between the insertion allele of the ACE insertion/deletion (I/D) polymorphism and indicators of performance. The first study was conducted with mountaineers who had a history of ascending beyond 7000 m of altitude without use of supplementary oxygen. The genotype distribution and allelic frequency of the ACE polymorphism in 25 of these mountaineers was compared with a control group of 1906 British males. A significant difference ($P < 0.003$) in allele frequency was observed between climbers and controls, with an excess of the Insertion allele and a reduced frequency of the Deletion allele in the climber group. In the second experiment, 87 out of 123 British army male recruits completed a 10-week physical training programme (Montgomery et al. 1998). Before and after training, subjects performed a repetitive elbow flexion test with a 15-kg barbell. No difference in performance time between the three ACE I/D genotypes was found at baseline. However, after training, there was an 11-fold ($P < 0.001$) improvement in muscle performance duration for the II genotype compared to the DD genotype. The same investigators had previously shown an association between ACE I/D polymorphism and changes in left ventricular mass in response to training (Montgomery et al. 1997).

The same polymorphic marker in ACE was studied in 64 Australian national rowers and 114 controls drawn from healthy volunteers and a blood bank repository. The male to female ratio was 2:1. All were Caucasians (Gayagay et al. 1998). The rowers had an excess of the ACE I allele ($P < 0.02$) and of the II genotype ($P = 0.03$). Markers for angiotensin type 1 (AT1) and type 2 (AT2) receptors were also investigated but no differences between rowers and controls were found.

It is not yet clear whether the results of these studies will be replicated or if they happened only by chance. Although these reports indicate that the I allele and the II genotype of ACE are advantageous and relate favourably to endurance performance, centenarians have been shown to carry the DD genotype more frequently at the same locus (Schachter et al. 1994).

Fifteen years ago we began investigating the genetic basis of human endurance performance using a variety of experimental strategies. In one of our initiatives, laboratories in Freiburg (Germany), Kuopio (Finland), Puerto Rico, Dallas and Québec City joined forces to study genetic differences between highly trained Caucasian élite endurance athletes (EEA) and sedentary matched controls (SC). The project is known as the GENATHLETE Study. At this time, DNA has been banked for more than 350 male EEA with maximal oxygen intake exceeding $75\,\text{ml}\,O_2\cdot\text{kg}^{-1}\cdot\text{min}^{-1}$. Sedentary male controls with a $\dot{V}_{O_{2max}}$ of less than $50\,\text{ml}\,O_2\cdot\text{kg}^{-1}\cdot\text{min}^{-1}$ are matched for the region of origin of the athletes.

ACE I/D polymorphism has been typed in 173 of the Caucasian EEA and 197 biologically unrelated Caucasian SC. The mean $\dot{V}_{O_{2max}}$ of the EEA cases reached 79.3 (SD = 3.7) whereas that of the SC cases was 34.4 (SD = 7.2). We found no differences in the distribution of the II, ID and DD genotypes between EEA and SC. Next, we grouped the EEA in three classes of $\dot{V}_{O_{2max}}$ levels: Class 1: mean $\dot{V}_{O_{2max}}$ of $77.0\,\text{ml}\,O_2\cdot\text{kg}^{-1}\cdot\text{min}^{-1}$; Class 2: mean of 82.2; and Class 3: mean of 87.2. We still could not find any difference in allelic frequencies or genotype distributions between the three classes. Finally, among the 12 EEA cases with $\dot{V}_{O_{2max}}$ greater than $85\,\text{ml}\,O_2\cdot\text{kg}^{-1}\cdot\text{min}^{-1}$, there were six II, three ID and three DD genotypes. It is noteworthy that three athletes with such a high maximal aerobic power had the DD genotype. In other words, if ACE I/D polymorphism plays any role in endurance performance, it is likely to be very marginal. One cannot rule out the possibility at this stage that ACE polymorphism is only an indirect marker of another mutation in the ACE gene or another gene in linkage disequilibrium. In brief, the GENATHLETE data do not support the conclusion that ACE polymorphism influences human endurance performance.

Erythropoietin receptor (EPOR) gene

Another attractive candidate gene is the erythropoietin receptor (EPOR) encoded on chromosome 19p1.3. There are several informative microsatellite repeats in the untranslated 5' region of the gene (Noguchi et al. 1991). A family was described a few years ago which had autosomal dominant erythrocytosis and a specific EPOR mutation, which is in linkage disequilibrium with a microsatellite marker in the 5′ region (Juvonen *et al.* 1991; de la Chapelle *et al.* 1993). The disease is benign, and most family members have reached an advanced age. In addition, one of the affected family members has won several Olympic gold medals and world championships in cross-country skiing. This observation led Longmore (1993) to hypothesize that some EPOR mutations may account for favourable genetic differences, leading to physiological advantages and allowing Olympic glory.

From a physiological point of view, an adequate oxygenation of muscle and other tissues is needed to sustain a high endurance performance. Erythropoietin, as a major regulator of erythropoiesis, influences the production of red blood cells and hence plays a key role in the regulation of oxygen transport capacity. The stimulation of erythropoiesis by erythropoietin involves interaction with its specific receptor. It is therefore conceivable that a small difference in the sequence of the EPOR gene may alter the configuration of the receptor, resulting in differences in efficiency and perhaps in adaptive capacity to exercise training. Although no data on blood erythropoietin and haemoglobin levels were available for the subjects in that particular study, the findings justify the search for EPOR gene variants and the need to perform experimental and genetic studies on the potential role of EPOR DNA sequence variations in endurance performance-related phenotypes (e.g. haemoglobin mass) or their trainability.

Wolfarth *et al.* (unpublished observations) investigated three microsatellite markers of the EPOR gene in the GENATHLETE cohort, using 215 élite endurance athletes and 201 sedentary controls. A significant difference for the number of carriers of the 185-base pair (bp) allele ($P = 0.002$) of a tetranucleotide repeat in the untranslated 5′ region of EPOR was observed, with more athletes carrying this particular fragment. A trend for a significant difference between endurance athletes and controls ($P = 0.044$) was also seen for the frequency of a 205-bp fragment. These studies need to be extended to erythropoietin and other factors influencing erythropoiesis.

Skeletal muscle-specific creatine kinase (CKMM) gene

Creatine kinase (CK) is a key enzyme in energy metabolism. It catalyses the following reaction:

phosphocreatine + MgADP + H⁺ ⇔ MgATP + creatine

There are two distinct CK mitochondrial forms (ubiquitous and sarcomeric) and two cytosolic subunits (brain and muscle) which are encoded by at least four different CK genes (Wallimann *et al.* 1992). The CKMM gene has been mapped to the q13.2–q13.3 region of chromosome 19 (Nigro *et al.* 1987). The gene extends over 17.5 kbp and contains eight exons and seven introns (Trask *et al.* 1988).

Several reports support the hypothesis that CKMM is a legitimate candidate gene to investigate in relation to endurance performance. Since CKMM activity level is two times greater in type II (fast-twitch) than in type I fibres (Yamashita & Yoshioka 1991), a low CKMM activity level is typical of the skeletal muscle of endurance athletes. An early study indicated that a CKMM protein charge variant was weakly associated with the ability to perform a 90-min endurance test (Bouchard *et al.* 1989). In addition, research on transgenic mice indicates that a low CKMM activity is associated with improved skeletal muscle resistance to fatigue (van Deursen *et al.* 1993).

More recently, a sib-pair linkage study has shown a weak genetic linkage between the CKMM locus and changes in $\dot{V}_{O_{2max}}$ (age, sex and pretraining $\dot{V}_{O_{2max}}$ adjusted) in the HERITAGE Family Study (Rivera *et al.* 1999). Siblings sharing two alleles identical by descent (IBD) at the CKMM *Nco*I locus tend to have a more similar increase in $\dot{V}_{O_{2max}}$ ($mlO_2 \cdot min^{-1}$) than sib-pairs sharing fewer alleles IBD. We cannot rule out the possibility that another gene in linkage disequilibrium with the CKMM gene could be responsible for the suggestive linkage with the responsiveness to endurance training, but there is accumulating evidence that the CKMM gene is responsible for these genetic effects.

A significant association has been reported between the CKMM genotype and the covariate-adjusted $\dot{V}_{O_{2max}}$ response to 20 weeks of endurance training in both parents and adult offspring of the HERITAGE Family Study (Rivera *et al.* 1997a). This seems the first quantification of a significant association between a DNA polymorphism in a candidate gene and $\dot{V}_{O_{2max}}$ in a training study based on a relatively large sample of biologically unrelated sedentary Caucasian adults. One-third of all homozygotes for the rare allele (CKMM *NcoI* polymorphism in the 3' untranslated region) were observed in the low responder group (lowest decile of response), whereas this genotype was not seen in any high responders (highest decile of response) (Fig. 15.7). The hypothesis of an association was verified in 80 biologically unrelated adult offspring among whom the adjusted $\dot{V}_{O_{2max}}$ response to training also differed significantly between genotypes. As in the parental generation, the homozygotes for the rare allele in the adult offspring demonstrated a lower adjusted $\dot{V}_{O_{2max}}$ response than the other two genotypes. The CKMM genotype accounted for 9 and 10% of the variance of $\dot{V}_{O_{2max}}$ response in the adult offspring and parents, respectively.

However, in the GENATHLETE cohort, the CKMM marker did not contribute to the proper classification of Caucasian males into athletes or controls (Rivera *et al.* 1997b). In light of the role of

the CKMM *NcoI* polymorphism in the training response of sedentary people (Rivera *et al.* 1997a; Rivera *et al.* 1999), this negative result suggests that the polymorphism may not contribute further once an individual is nearing the maximal trainability potential.

Mitochondrial DNA (mtDNA)

Because of the apparent maternal effect on $\dot{V}_{O_{2max}}$ (Lesage *et al.* 1985; Bouchard *et al.* 1998a), mitochondrial DNA (mtDNA) is of particular interest, as it is inherited from the maternal oocyte. The human mtDNA is a 16 569-bp circular duplex molecule that does not recombine and is self-replicative. It contains no introns. mtDNA codes for 13 of the 67 polypeptides involved in the respiratory chain and oxidative phosphorylation, plus two ribosomal and 22 transfer RNAs (tRNAs). The displacement-loop (D-loop) region is a non-coding segment that contains the promoters for transcription of heavy and light mtDNA strands, the origin of replication of the heavy strand, and conserved sequences essential for mtDNA expression (Clayton 1982; Greenberg *et al.* 1983). In addition, the mtDNA concentration is about 1.5-fold higher in endurance-trained athletes than in sedentary controls (Puntschart *et al.* 1995).

mtDNA sequence variation was investigated using restricted fragment length polymorphism (RFLP) technology in sedentary subjects submitted to endurance training (Dionne *et al.* 1991). Carriers of three mtDNA morphs, one due to a base change in the tRNA for threonine and two others caused by base substitutions in subunit 5 of the NADH dehydrogenase (MTND5) gene, had a body mass-adjusted $\dot{V}_{O_{2max}}$ in the untrained state significantly higher than that found in non-carriers. A lower response of $\dot{V}_{O_{2max}}$ to endurance training was also observed for three carriers of a variant in MTND5.

The MTND5 *NciI* polymorphism at bp 13 364, the *BamHI* marker at bp 13 470 and the D-loop *KpnI* variant at bp 16 133 were assessed in 125 endurance athletes from the GENATHLETE cohort (Rivera *et al.* 1998) and in a group of matched controls. The MTND5–*NciI* variant was found in 12.9% of the athletes and 14% of controls, and the MTND5–*BamHI*

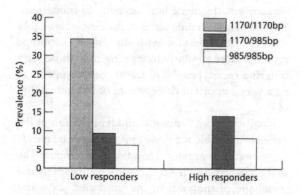

Fig. 15.7 Prevalence of CKMM *NcoI* genotype in low and high responders to training for 160 biologically unrelated sedentary Caucasian parents of the HERITAGE Family Study. The prevalence of homozygotes for the rare 1170-bp allele is at least three times that of the other two genotypes. No case of homozygotes for the rare 1170-bp allele was observed in the high responders to training. Reproduced with permission from Rivera *et al.* (1997a).

variant was observed in 12.8% of endurance athletes and 12.3% of sedentary controls. The D-loop *KpnI* mutation was found in 5.8% of athletes and in 1.6% of controls. It was concluded that these three mtDNA polymorphisms were not more prevalent in either of the two groups. However, the possibility cannot be excluded that some mtDNA variants may have functional implications in sedentary subjects and yet be no longer important in élite endurance athletes. For instance, the mitochondrial content of skeletal muscle may play a major role in sedentary subjects (i.e. those with a high content may have a higher $\dot{V}_{O_{2max}}$), whereas cardiovascular parameters or other factors may account for a significant fraction of the variance in $\dot{V}_{O_{2max}}$ between endurance athletes and sedentary people.

Specific genes and body composition

The search for genes and mutations playing a role in endurance performance and in trainability has just begun, but efforts to identify those contributing to human variation in body mass relative to height, FFM, fat mass and percentage body fat have been under way for about 10 years. It is not possible to review all relevant findings in this chapter. However, a compendium of the genes associated with these phenotypes is published every year in *Obesity Research* (Chagnon *et al.* 1998; Pérusse *et al.* 1999). A few brief comments will suffice to indicate that the number of genes identified is already high and is likely to become even larger.

For instance, the number of candidate genes shown to be associated with one of the relevant phenotypes has now reached 26 (Pérusse *et al.* 1999). The number of genes or markers linked to such phenotypes has currently attained about 15 (Pérusse *et al.* 1999). Our own Québec Family Study genomic scan initiative indicates two and potentially three genomic regions that are genetically linked to FFM (Chagnon *et al.*, unpublished observations).

Research directions and conclusions

The élite endurance athlete is an individual with a favourable profile in terms of the determinants of endurance performance. The élite athlete is also highly responsive to regular training and practice. The evidence that genes play a role in modulating the status of performance determinants in the sedentary population is accumulating slowly. The effect is generally estimated using the methods of genetic epidemiology, considering one phenotype at a time. Data are available for a variety of performance phenotypes, as well as for selected determinants, such as body size, body composition, heart size, muscle fibre type distribution, and aerobic oxidative markers of skeletal muscle metabolism, lipid mobilization from adipose cells, indicators of substrates oxidized, and others as well. The heritability of these phenotypes is generally low (25% or less) and rarely exceeds 50%. The genetic effect seems to be polygenic, and no evidence has yet been reported for single-gene effects, with the notable exception of selected body composition phenotypes.

The issue of the heterogeneity of response to regular exercise has also been examined. Evidence indicates considerable individual differences in the capacity to adapt and benefit from exercise training. The role of genes in determining the response to training has also been considered. Several training studies have been conducted with pairs of identical twins (training both members of each pair) in an attempt to understand the importance of genetic similarity and genetic heterogeneity in trainability. The message from this series of studies is reasonably coherent. Individuals with the same genotype respond more similarly to training than those with differing genotypes. Thus, the genotype appears to be a very important determinant of the trainability of $\dot{V}_{O_{2max}}$.

Finally, studies dealing with identification of the genes responsible for these apparent genetic effects have begun to appear. The task is enormous. The first reports focus on $\dot{V}_{O_{2max}}$, body composition and metabolic phenotypes in the untrained state and their responses to training. The search for genetic markers of trainability status will probably be more productive than investigation of molecular markers of the performance phenotype in the untrained state for two reasons. Firstly, the genetic effect appears to be more important when a response phenotype is considered, and secondly, the limits of adaptation become more clearly delineated when the various biological systems are challenged by the demands of regular exercise. The path to the identification of the genes and mutations is likely to be long and tortuous. For instance, we have investigated dozens of candidate genes in the context of the GENATHLETE case–control study without being able to uncover a single gene with a clear and strong effect. The list of factors examined includes genes related to erythropoietin, angiogenin, carnitive-palmitoyl-transferases, fatty acid-binding proteins, hormone-sensitive lipase, lipoprotein lipase, insulin-like growth factors and the related binding proteins, transforming growth factors, heat-shock proteins, nitric oxide synthase, tumour necrosis factors and other candidates.

Candidate gene studies and genomic scans for the identification and localization of quantitative trait loci contributing to endurance performance phenotypes are likely to yield useful information in the coming years. However, this will not be sufficient. There is a need for crossbreeding studies of informative rodent strains to provide evidence of quantitative trait loci and to delineate the mechanisms associated with these genetic signals. Such rodent studies will provide a foundation for investigation of the relevant human syntenic chromosomal regions. A variety of transgenic and knockout rodent models will also be needed if we are to understand properly the role of the genes and mutations evidenced in the human studies. These rodent models will undoubtedly foster new and innovative human molecular studies.

World-class athletes in any sport are a special breed of individuals: they are not only talented for a particular sport, but also have been willing to train and compete until world-class status is attained. Élite athletes do not happen to execute a national or world-class performance simply by chance.

Until about the middle of this century it was possible to become a national or a world-class athlete in a given athletic event without being among the most talented individuals in a nation. The selection process was less stringent, and the level of competition was not as demanding as today. With the continued expansion of the pool of young participants and competitors, and the growing sophistication of training, psychological preparation, equipment and facilities, the level of competition has increased to the point that only those individuals who are highly gifted can now expect to reach élite status. Moreover, the process is ongoing, particularly the growth in number of participants from developing countries. This will result in an expanded pool of individuals and therefore a larger array of genotypes, who potentially have the chance to test themselves in a given sport; such individuals may perhaps experience success, so that they nurture their interest and motivation to train seriously for the activity (Bouchard et al. 1997).

Although much remains to be investigated, a reasonable body of knowledge has accumulated about the physical, biomechanical, physiological, metabolic, psychological and social determinants of high-performance sport in several individual and team activities. Among these, it is fair to say that more is probably known about the determinants of endurance performance than about any other type of competitive activity. Unfortunately, the exercise science and sports medicine research domains are not particularly well funded. As a result, progress is slow. Therefore, it is not surprising that the knowledge base about the genetic and molecular foundations of human sport performance is as yet embryonic.

Even though investigation of the genetic and molecular basis of human variation in endurance performance and in trainability is still in its infancy, the resources and databases necessary to study these topics are being established and a wealth of new data can be anticipated soon.

References

Adams, T.D., Yanowitz, F.G., Fisher, G. et al. (1986) Genetics and cardiac size. In: Malina, R.M. & Bouchard, C. (eds) Sport and Human Genetics, pp. 131–145. Human Kinetics, Champaign, IL.

Barbato, J.C., Koch, L.G., Darvish, A., Cicila, G.T., Metting, P.J. & Britton, S.L. (1998) Spectrum of aerobic endurance running performance in eleven inbred strains of rats. *Journal of Applied Physiology* **85**, 530–536.

Bielen, E., Fagard, R. & Amery, A. (1991a) The inheritance of left ventricular structure and function assessed by imaging and Doppler echocardiography. *American Heart Journal* **121**, 1743–1749.

Bielen, E.C., Fagard, R.H. & Amery, A.K. (1991b) Inheritance of acute cardiac changes during bicycle exercise: an echocardiographic study in twins. *Medicine and Science in Sports and Exercise* **23**, 1254–1259.

Borecki, I.B., Rice, T., Bouchard, C. & Rao, D.C. (1991) Commingling analysis of generalized body mass and composition measures: the Québec Family Study. *International Journal of Obesity* **15**, 763–773.

Bouchard, C. (1992) Genetic determinants of endurance performance. In: Shephard, R.J. & Astrand, P.O. (eds) *Endurance in Sport*, pp. 149–159. Blackwell Scientific Publications, Oxford.

Bouchard, C. (1996) Genetic influences on human body composition and physique. In: Roche, A.F., Heymsfield, S.B. & Lohman, T.G. (eds) *Human Body Composition*, pp. 305–327. Human Kinetics, Champaign, IL.

Bouchard, C., Lesage, R., Lortie, G. *et al.* (1986a) Aerobic performance in brothers, dizygotic and monozygotic twins. *Medicine and Science in Sports and Exercise* **18**, 639–646.

Bouchard, C., Simoneau, J.A., Lortie, G., Boulay, M.R., Marcotte, M. & Thibault, M.C. (1986b) Genetic effects in human skeletal muscle fiber type distribution and enzymes activities. *Canadian Journal of Physiology and Pharmacology* **64**, 1245–1251.

Bouchard, C., Boulay, M.R., Simoneau, J.A., Lortie, G. & Perusse, L. (1988a) Heredity and trainability of aerobic and anaerobic performances. *Sports Medicine* **5**, 69–73.

Bouchard, C., Chagnon, M., Thibault, M.C., Boulay, M.R., Marcotte, M. & Simoneau, J.A. (1988b) Absence of charge variants in human skeletal muscle enzymes of the glycolytic pathway. *Human Genetics* **78**, 100.

Bouchard, C., Pérusse, L., Leblanc, C., Tremblay, A. & Thériault, G. (1988c) Inheritance of the amount and distribution of human body fat. *International Journal of Obesity* **12**, 205–215.

Bouchard, C., Chagnon, M., Thibault, M.C. *et al.* (1989) Muscle genetic variants and relationship with performance and trainability. *Medicine and Science in Sports and Exercise* **21**, 71–77.

Bouchard, C., Boulay, M.R., Dionne, F.T., Pérusse, L., Thibault, M.C. & Simoneau, J.A. (1990) Genotype, aerobic performance and response to training. In: Beunen, G., Ghesquiere, J., Reybrouck, T. & Claessens, A.L. (eds) *Children and Exercise*, pp. 124–135. Ferdinand Enke-Verlag, Stuttgart.

Bouchard, C., Dionne, F.T., Simoneau, J.A. & Boulay, M.R. (1992) Genetics of aerobic and anaerobic performances. *Exercise and Sport Sciences Reviews* **20**, 27–58.

Bouchard, C., Malina, R.M. & Pérusse, L. (1997) *Genetics of Fitness and Physical Performance*. Human Kinetics, Champaign, IL.

Bouchard, C., Daw, E.W., Rice, T. *et al.* (1998a) Familial resemblance for $\dot{V}o_{2max}$ in the sedentary state: the HERITAGE Family Study. *Medicine and Science in Sports and Exercise* **30**, 252–258.

Bouchard, C., Pérusse, L., Rice, T. & Rao, D.C. (1998b) The genetics of human obesity. In: Bray, G.A., Bouchard, C. & James, W.P.T. (eds) *Handbook of Obesity*, pp. 157–190. Dekker Inc, New York.

Bouchard, C., An, P., Rice, T. *et al.* (1999) Familial aggregation of $\dot{V}o_{2max}$ in response to exercise training: results from the HERITAGE Family Study. *Journal of Applied Physiology* **87**, 1003–1008.

Carter, J.E.L. & Heath, B.H. (1990) *Somatotyping: Development and Applications*. Cambridge University Press, Cambridge, UK.

Chagnon, Y.C., Allard, C. & Bouchard, C. (1984) Red blood cell genetic variation in Olympic endurance athletes. *Journal of Sports Sciences* **2**, 121–129.

Chagnon, Y.C., Pérusse, L. & Bouchard, C. (1998) The human obesity gene map: the 1997 update. *Obesity Research* **6**, 76–92.

de la Chapelle, A., Sistonen, P., Lehvaslaiho, H., Ikkala, E. & Juvonen, E. (1993) Familial erythrocytosis genetically linked to erythropoietin receptor gene. *Lancet* **341**, 82–84.

Clayton, D.A. (1982) Replication of animal mitochondrial DNA. *Cell* **28**, 693–705.

Comuzzie, A.G., Blangero, J., Mahaney, M.C. *et al.* (1995) Major gene with sex-specific effects influences fat mass in Mexican Americans. *Genetic Epidemiology* **12**, 475–488.

Couture, L., Chagnon, M., Allard, C. & Bouchard, C. (1986) More on red blood cell genetic variation in Olympic athletes. *Canadian Journal of Sport Sciences* **11**, 16–18.

van Deursen, J., Heerschap, A., Oerlemans, F., *et al.* (1993) Skeletal muscles of mice deficient in muscle creatine kinase lack burst activity. *Cell* **74**, 621–631.

Dionne, F.T., Turcotte, L., Thibault, M.C., Boulay, M.R., Skinner, J.S. & Bouchard, C. (1991) Mitochondrial DNA sequence polymorphism, $\dot{V}o_{2max}$ and response to endurance training. *Medicine and Science in Sports and Exercise* **23**, 177–185.

Fagard, R., Bielen, E. & Amery, A. (1991) Heritability of aerobic power and anaerobic energy generation during exercise. *Journal of Applied Physiology* **70**, 352–362.

Gagnon, J., Ho-Kim, M.A., Chagnon, Y.C. *et al.* (1997) Absence of linkage between $\dot{V}o_{2max}$ and its response to training with markers spanning chromosome 22. *Medicine and Science in Sports and Exercise* **29**, 1448–1453.

deGaray, A., Levine, L. & Carter, J.E.L. (1974) *Genetic and Anthropological Studies of Olympic Athletes*. Academic Press, New York.

Gayagay, G., Yu, B., Hambly, B. *et al.* (1998) Elite endurance athletes and the ACE I allele: the role of genes in athletic performance. *Human Genetics* **103**, 48–50.

Greenberg, B.D., Newbold, J.E. & Sugino, A. (1983) Intraspecific nucleotide sequence variability surrounding the origin of replication in human mitochondrial DNA. *Gene* **21**, 33–49.

Hamel, P., Simoneau, J.-A., Lortie, G., Boulay, M.R. & Bouchard, C. (1986) Heredity and muscle adaptation to endurance training. *Medicine and Science in Sports and Exercise* **18**, 690–696.

Howald, H. (1976) Ultrastructure and biochemical function of skeletal muscle in twins. *Annals of Human Biology* **3**, 455–462.

Juvonen, E., Ikkala, E., Fyhrquist, F. & Ruutu, T. (1991) Autosomal dominant erythrocytosis caused by increased sensitivity to erythropoietin. *Blood* **78**, 3066–3069.

Klissouras, V. (1971) Heritability of adaptive variation. *Journal of Applied Physiology* **31**, 338–344.

Klissouras, V., Pirnay, F. & Petit, J.M. (1973) Adaptation to maximal effort: genetics and age. *Journal of Applied Physiology* **35**, 288–293.

Komi, P.V., Viitasalo, J.H.T., Havu, M., Thorstensson, A., Sjodin, B. & Karlsson, J. (1977) Skeletal muscle fibres and muscle enzyme activities in monozygous and dizygous twins of both sexes. *Acta Physiologica Scandinavica* **100**, 385–392.

Lecomte, E., Herbeth, B., Nicaud, V., Rakotovao, R., Artur, Y. & Tiret, L. (1997) Segregation analysis of fat mass and fat-free mass with age- and sex-dependent effects: the Stanislas Family Study. *Genetic Epidemiology* **14**, 51–62.

Lesage, R., Simoneau, J.A., Jobin, J., Leblanc, J. & Bouchard, C. (1985) Familial resemblance in maximal heart rate, blood lactate and aerobic power. *Human Heredity* **35**, 182–189.

Longmore, G.D. (1993) Erythropoietin receptor mutations and Olympic glory. *Nature Genetics* **4**, 108–110.

Lortie, G., Bouchard, C., Leblanc, C. *et al.* (1982) Familial similarity in aerobic power. *Human Biology* **54**, 801–812.

Maes, H., Beunen, G., Vlietinck, R. *et al.* (1993) Heritability of health- and performance-related fitness: data from the Leuven Longitudinal Twin Study. In: Duquet, W. & Day, J.A.P. (eds) *Kinanthropometry IV*, pp. 140–149. Spon, London.

Maes, H.H., Beunen, G.P., Vlietinck, R.F. *et al.* (1996) Inheritance of physical fitness in 10-year-old twins and their parents. *Medicine and Science in Sports and Exercise* **28**, 1479–1491.

Malina, R.M. & Bouchard, C. (1991) *Growth, Maturation and Physical Activity.* Human Kinetics, Champaign, IL.

Marcotte, M., Chagnon, M., Côté, C., Thibault, M.C., Boulay, M.R. & Bouchard, C. (1987) Lack of genetic polymorphism in human skeletal muscles enzymes of the tricarboxylic acid cycle. *Human Genetics* **77**, 200.

Mitchell, J.H. & Raven, P.B. (1994) Cardiovascular adaptation to physical activity. In: Bouchard, C., Shephard, R.Y. & Stephens, T. (eds) *Physical Activity, Fitness, and Health*, pp. 286–301. Human Kinetics, Champaign, IL.

Montgomery, H.E., Clarkson, P., Dollery, C.M. *et al.* (1997) Association of angiotensin-converting enzyme gene I/D polymorphism with change in left ventricular mass in response to physical training. *Circulation* **96**, 741–747.

Montgomery, H.E., Marshall, R., Hemingway, H. *et al.* (1998) Human gene for physical performance. *Nature* **393**, 221–222.

Montoye, H.J. & Gayle, R. (1978) Familial relationships in maximal oxygen uptake. *Human Biology* **50**, 241–249.

Nakamura, T., Masui, S., Wada, M., Katoh, H., Mikami, H. & Katsuta, S. (1993) Heredity of muscle fibre composition estimated from a selection experiment in rats. *European Journal of Applied Physiology* **66**, 85–89.

Nigro, J.M., Schweinfest, C.W., Rajkovic, A.

et al. (1987) cDNA cloning and mapping of the human creatine kinase M gene to 19q13. *American Journal of Human Genetics* **40**, 115–125.

Nimmo, M.A., Wilson, R.H. & Snow, D.H. (1985) The inheritance of skeletal muscle fibre composition in mice. *Comparative Biochemistry and Physiology* **81A**, 109–115.

Noguchi, C.T., Bae, K.S., Chin, K., Wada, Y., Schechter, A.N. & Hankins, W.D. (1991) Cloning of the human erythropoietin receptor gene. *Blood* **78**, 2548–2556.

Pérusse, L., Lortie, G., Leblanc, C., Tremblay, A., Thériault, G. & Bouchard, C. (1987) Genetic and environmental sources of variation in physical fitness. *Annals of Human Biology* **14**, 425–434.

Pérusse, L., Leblanc, C. & Bouchard, C. (1988) Inter-generation transmission of physical fitness in the Canadian population. *Canadian Journal of Sport Sciences* **13**, 8–14.

Pérusse, L., Chagnon, Y.C., Weisnagel, J. & Bouchard, C. (1999) The human obesity gene map: the 1998 update. *Obesity Research* **7**, 111–129.

Prud'homme, D., Bouchard, C., Leblanc, C., Landry, F. & Fontaine, E. (1984) Sensitivity of maximal aerobic power to training is genotype-dependent. *Medicine and Science in Sports and Exercise* **16**, 489–493.

Puntschart, A., Claassen, H., Jostarndt, K., Hoppeler, H. & Billeter, R. (1995) mRNAs of enzymes involved in energy metabolism and mtDNA are increased in endurance-trained athletes. *American Journal of Physiology* **269**, C619–C625.

Rice, T., Borecki, I.B., Bouchard, C. & Rao, D.C. (1993) Segregation analysis of fat mass and other body composition measures derived from underwater weighing. *American Journal of Human Genetics* **52**, 967–973.

Rice, T., Daw, E.W., Gagnon, J. *et al.* (1997a) Familial resemblance for body composition measures: The HERITAGE Family Study. *Obesity Research* **5**, 557–562.

Rice, T., Després, J.P., Pérusse, L. *et al.* (1997b) Segregation analysis of abdominal visceral fat: The HERITAGE Family Study. *Obesity Research* **5**, 417–424.

Rivera, M.A., Dionne, F.T., Simoneau, J.A. *et al.* (1997a) Muscle-specific creatine kinase gene polymorphism and $\dot{V}_{O_{2max}}$ in the HERITAGE Family Study. *Medicine and Science in Sports and Exercise* **29**, 1311–1317.

Rivera, M.A., Dionne, F.T., Wolfarth, B. *et al.* (1997b) Muscle-specific creatine kinase gene polymorphisms in elite endurance athletes and sedentary con-

trols. *Medicine and Science in Sports and Exercise* **29**, 1444–1447.

Rivera, M.A., Wolfarth, B., Dionne, F.T. *et al.* (1998) Three mitochondrial DNA restriction polymorphisms in elite endurance athletes and sedentary controls. *Medicine and Science in Sports and Exercise* **30**, 687–690.

Rivera, M.A., Pérusse, L., Simoneau, J.A. *et al.* (1999) Linkage between a muscle-specific CK gene marker and $\dot{V}_{O_{2max}}$ in the HERITAGE Family Study. *Medicine and Science in Sports and Exercise* **31**, 698–701.

Saltin, B. & Strange, S. (1992) Maximal oxygen uptake: 'old' and 'new' arguments for a cardiovascular limitation. *Medicine and Science in Sports and Exercise* **24**, 30–37.

Schachter, F., Faure-Delanef, L., Guenot, F. *et al.* (1994) Genetic associations with human longevity at the APO E and ACE loci. *Nature Genetics* **6**, 29–32.

Simoneau, J.A. (1995) Adaptation of human skeletal muscle to exercise-training. *International Journal of Obesity* **19**, S9–S13.

Simoneau, J.A. & Bouchard, C. (1989) Human variation in skeletal muscle fiber type proportion and enzyme activities. *American Journal of Physiology: Endocrinology and Metabolism* **257**, E567–E572.

Simoneau, J.A. & Bouchard, C. (1995) Genetic determinism of fiber type proportion in human skeletal muscle. *FASEB Journal* **9**, 1091–1095.

Simoneau, J.A., Lortie, G., Boulay, M.R., Marcotte, M., Thibault, M.-C. & Bouchard, C. (1986a) Inheritance of human skeletal muscle and anaerobic capacity adaptation to high-intensity intermittent training. *International Journal of Sports Medicine* **7**, 167–171.

Simoneau, J.A., Lortie, G., Boulay, M.R., Thibault, M.C. & Bouchard, C. (1986b) Repeatability of fibre type and enzyme activity measurements in human skeletal muscle. *Clinical Physiology* **6**, 347–356.

Song, T.M.K., Malina, R.M. & Bouchard, C. (1993) Familial resemblance in somatotype. *American Journal of Human Biology* **5**, 265–272.

Song, T.M.K.P., Russe, L., Malina, R.M. & Bouchard, C. (1994) Twin resemblance in somatotype and comparisons with other twin studies. *Human Biology* **66**, 453–464.

Spina, R.J., Ogawa, T., Kohrt, W.M., Martin, W.H., Holloszy, J.O. & Ehsani, A.A. (1993) Differences in cardiovascular adaptations to endurance exercise training between older men and women. *Journal of Applied Physiology* **75**, 849–855.

Sundet, J.M., Magnus, P. & Tambs, K. (1994) The heritability of maximal aerobic power: a study of Norwegian twins. *Scandinavian Journal of Medicine and Science in Sports* 4, 181–185.

Thériault, G., Diano, R., Leblanc, C.P., Russe, L., Landry, F. & Bouchard, C. (1986) The role of heredity in cardiac size: an echocardiographic study on twins, brothers and sisters, and sibs by adoption. *Medicine and Science in Sports and Exercise* 18, S51.

Trask, R.V., Strauss, A.W. & Billadello, J.J. (1988) Developmental regulation and tissue-specific expression of the human muscle creatine kinase gene. *Journal of Biological Chemistry* 263, 17 142–17 149.

Verhaaren, H.A., Schieken, R.M., Mosteller, M., Hewitt, J.K., Eaves, L.J. & Nance, W.E. (1991) Bivariate genetic analysis of left ventricular mass and weight in pubertal twins (The Medical College of Virginia Twin Study). *American Journal of Cardiology* 68, 661–668.

Wagner, P.D. (1995) Muscle O_2 transport and O_2 dependent control of metabolism. *Medicine and Science in Sports and Exercise* 27, 47–53.

Wallimann, T., Wyss, M., Brdiczka, D., Nicolay, K. & Eppenberger, H.M. (1992) Intracellular compartmentation, structure and function of creatine kinase isoenzymes in tissues with high and fluctuating energy demands: the 'phosphocreatine circuit' for cellular energy homeostasis. *Biochemical Journal* 281, 21–40.

Yamashita, K. & Yoshioka, T. (1991) Profiles of creatine kinase isoenzyme compositions in single muscle fibres of different types. *Journal of Muscle Research and Cell Motility* 12, 37–44.

Part 2d

Physical Limitations of Endurance Performance

Chapter 16

Biomechanical Constraints and Economy of Movement in Endurance Performance

KEITH R. WILLIAMS

The mechanics of movement are among a number of factors that can affect an athlete's performance in endurance sports. There are mechanical factors, such as air resistance, that can reduce speed of movement from what it otherwise would be for a given metabolic cost. There are variations in movement mechanics that can influence the energy cost associated with a given power output, and thus influence performance. An inherent problem in trying to identify relationships between mechanics and performance is that generally only descriptive kinematic information can be obtained during competition. There are additional concerns due to the fact that movement patterns may be influenced by strategy or the presence of other athletes in competition, making it difficult to isolate the importance of biomechanical factors. As a result, most biomechanical studies are carried out in controlled conditions where specific movements can be simulated and specific aspects of mechanics manipulated or measured. The obvious trade-off is that it is difficult to motivate athletes to give top-level performances in a controlled situation, and what is measured in a controlled situation may differ from what occurs in competition.

Since performance conditions are difficult to reproduce under controlled conditions, mechanics are often studied in relation to other dependent measures, such as economy, the submaximal oxygen intake per unit of body mass ($\dot{V}_{O_2}$) associated with a given level of physical activity. Since energy expenditure in an endurance event can have a direct effect on performance, anything that will improve economy should have a beneficial effect on performance. If changes in movement patterns result in better economy, or if technological advances in equipment can reduce the energy needed to sustain a given level of performance, the reduced energy costs should allow an individual either to maintain a given level of performance for a longer period of time, or to raise the level of effort that can be sustained over a fixed time or distance. Other measures besides economy can and have been used to investigate relationships between mechanics and endurance performance, particularly in modelling studies where often some mechanical cost function is derived and assumed to be directly related to the corresponding metabolic energy costs (Gonzalez & Hull 1989; Gregor et al. 1991; Broker & Gregor 1994). There are exceptions to the presumed relationship between economy and performance. For example, trained cyclists consistently have preferred cadences that are higher than those that would be optimal in terms of oxygen cost (Gregor et al. 1991; Marsh & Martin 1997). In some situations, there may be criteria critical to optimization that take precedence over metabolic costs: such factors as local fatigue, localized tissue stress or maximal power in specific phases of a movement. Nevertheless, economy has proven to be a useful measure for evaluating aspects of the relationship between mechanics and endurance.

Since endurance activities typically continue for relatively long periods, a small improvement in efficiency can yield substantial benefits (Frederick 1983; Williams 1990). A 1% improvement in a world-class 10-km running event yields a 16-s faster time, putting the competitor 100 m ahead of where he or she would otherwise finish. Improvements even smaller than 1% can have an important effect on the outcome of a race. The fact that changes important to event outcome can be so small creates problems for the exercise scientist, since the small changes in movement mechanics that have an effect on economy can be very difficult to measure and to substantiate statistically. This may be especially troublesome when trying to suggest changes to élite athletes who have already optimized their movement mechanics through years of intrinsic feedback. Despite these problems, a great deal of useful information has been garnered through systematic research. This chapter explores the results of studies that have investigated the relationship between the mechanics of movement, economy and performance.

Variations in economy

The variation in economy among individuals performing at the same speed or work rate is substantial, typically exceeding 15% and sometimes being as high as 30% (Costill & Fox 1969; Conley & Krahenbuhl 1980; Williams & Cavanagh 1983; Daniels 1985). Bailey and Pate (1991) found little direct evidence that the running economy of top athletes could be improved, but they did cite manipulations of ventilation, segmental mass distribution, training status and running style as factors that showed some promise. Further complicating the issue, it appears that an individual who is economical when performing one type of physical activity may not be economical at other tasks. Daniels *et al.* (1984) measured the oxygen consumption of 13 dis-

tance runners who were performing five different physical tasks; they found that individuals were not consistently economical or uneconomical across all tasks.

Mechanical power in relation to economy

Total body mechanical power is a global measure affected by the movement of the segments of the entire body, similar in concept to the way $\dot{V}O_2$ is a systemic measure of energy expenditure for the body as a whole. It is logical to assume that mechanical power has a direct influence on energy expenditure, but strong relationships have not been found. The lack of a clear association may be due in part to difficulties in measuring mechanical power. Some, however, have argued that direct relationships between mechanical work and metabolic energy cost should not be expected, due to the complex functions that are required of muscles (Biewener 1990; Baudinette 1991).

Mechanical power is a measure of the rate of work done by the individual while performing an endurance activity. Table 16.1 indicates the relative importance of the several different types of work performed in some common endurance sports. 'Against gravity' refers to work done moving the body against gravitational forces. 'Internal segmental' is work done in moving body segments. 'Fluid resistance' is work performed to overcome air or water resistance, and is highly dependent on speed. 'Surface friction' is work performed on the body by the environment due to frictional forces at the subject–surface interface point.

Table 16.1 Components of work performed in various activities.

Type	Against gravity	Internal segmental	Fluid resistance	Surface friction
Running	M	M	m	–
Cycling	–	m	M	m
Skiing	m	M	m	M
Skating	–	M	M	m
Rowing	–	m	M	m

M, Major component; m, minor component; –, negligible component.

Measures of mechanical power

Many of the factors contributing to mechanical power were identified by early researchers such as Fenn (1930). A number of different methods have been used to measure the mechanical work involved in various sports (Winter 1979; Williams & Cavanagh 1983; Aleshinsky 1986a; van Ingen Schenau & Cavanagh 1990; Martin et al. 1993; Broker & Gregor 1994). In some cases, different methods have yielded results that show a 10-fold difference in power for a given level of effort (Williams & Cavanagh 1983). As noted by van Ingen Schenau and Cavanagh (1990), it is not yet feasible to define mechanical power completely and accurately for many activities. Despite these methodological problems, investigations into the relationship between mechanical power and economy have yielded useful information.

Efficiency ratio

Mechanical power is often used in conjunction with a measure of metabolic energy expenditure to define an efficiency ratio. This expresses the effectiveness of the conversion of metabolic energy to mechanical work. Many different measures of efficiency have been used, sometimes confusing the meaning of a specific index (Cavanagh & Kram 1985a). Although economy or power can affect an endurance performance directly, efficiency may in itself have little meaning for performance (Cavanagh & Kram 1985b; Williams 1985; van Ingen Schenau & Cavanagh 1990). For example, consider a runner who at any given speed has a high level of oxygen consumption compared to other runners; an even higher relative mechanical power results in a high efficiency ratio. We would usually regard a high efficiency ratio as desirable, but high metabolic energy costs are undesirable. The meaning of the efficiency ratio is not clear, but we might advocate trying to manipulate mechanical factors to lower metabolic energy costs. Luhtanen et al. (1990) reported that the economy of running was greatest at a speed corresponding to the aerobic threshold (where the plasma lactate concentration is $2\,\mathrm{mmol \cdot l^{-1}}$). Gross efficiency decreased with in-creasing speed and the efficiency of positive work was best at a speed slightly higher than the aerobic threshold. Although the information is interesting from a scientific standpoint, it is difficult to see how the efficiency values are relevant to performance. van Ingen Schenau and Cavanagh (1990) suggest that efficiency is more meaningful for activities where power output against an external resistance can be determined more accurately than is possible for running or walking, for instance, rowing, skating or cycling. If reducing mechanical power while maintaining a given pace leads to a reduction in the metabolic energy expenditure and improves endurance performance, then reducing power through improved technique or training would be a reasonable goal. Otherwise there may be nothing to gain by reducing power, unless it leads to other benefits such as reducing musculoskeletal strain or muscle fatigue.

Mechanical power and economy

Many studies have evaluated the pros and cons of the multitude of ways available for calculating mechanical power in human motion. However, relatively few investigators have examined the relationship between mechanical power and economy in endurance activities. Studies examining the relationship between power and economy across speeds find strong correlations between metabolic energy costs and mechanical measures of power in both running (Shorten et al. 1981; Luhtanen et al. 1990) and swimming (Toussaint et al. 1988a, 1990). In rowing, economy is linearly related to total mechanical power output as the intensity of effort (and hence speed) increases (Steinacker et al. 1984; Fukunaga et al. 1986). Since both mechanical power and economy are highly dependent on speed, these correlations are not relevant to the relationship between economy and power at a given speed. At a given running speed, several studies have shown weak trends linking a greater economy in running with lower mechanical power (Kaneko et al. 1987; Williams & Cavanagh 1987; Martin et al. 1993) or total body angular impulse (Heise & Martin 1990), but others have found no specific relationship (Norman et al. 1976; Kyröläinen et al. 1995).

It is possible that limitations in the methodology used to calculate power serve to mask a relationship between mechanical work and metabolic energy expenditure, particularly in cyclic activities such as running where little work is performed on the environment (Williams 1985; van Ingen Schenau & Cavanagh 1990; van Ingen Schenau *et al.* 1990; Martin *et al.* 1993), and in swimming where quantifying the work performed is complicated by having to account for the power needed to push the water away (Toussaint *et al.* 1990). Aleshinsky (1986b) and van Ingen Schenau and Cavanagh (1990) have suggested methods that might alleviate some of these problems, basing their equations on 'a systematic and unambiguous application of basic mechanics' (van Ingen Schenau & Cavanagh 1990). However, even these methods leave a number of problems unresolved. Many derivations of mechanical power rely on assumptions that are known to be deficient. The most often cited of these factors are: the difficulty in quantifying the influence of elastic storage and return of energy; the ability to calculate only net joint moments; limitations in accounting for the transfer of energy between body segments; a limited understanding of the role of polyarticulate muscles; and a lack of knowledge of the exact origin of positive mechanical power (Williams & Cavanagh 1983; Williams 1985; Morgan *et al.* 1989; van Ingen Schenau & Cavanagh 1990; Caldwell & Forrester 1992). Until we have a better understanding of how these factors contribute to mechanical power, the usefulness of mechanical power measures in relation to economy will remain limited.

Based on relationships across a number of species, Taylor (1994) argued that mechanical power and efficiency do not explain variations in economy, except in situations where the subject performs substantial work on the environment (as for birds in flight or mammals swimming). Taylor suggests that in cyclic activities where a primary aspect of muscle work is the need to support the body's weight, muscles will try to minimize the cost of generating force by shortening slowly. When a muscle contracts nearly isometrically, it enhances the ability to store and return strain energy which helps reduce metabolic energy costs. Others have argued that there is

sufficient evidence of concentric muscle actions in running and that the energy costs in running are higher than could be explained by predominantly isometric actions (van Ingen Schenau *et al.* 1997).

Stretch–shortening cycle and economy

The stretch–shortening cycle involving elastic tissues in the muscle, tendon and arch of the foot has long been cited as a major factor in the energetics of rhythmic activities such as running (Cavagna *et al.* 1964; Williams 1985; Ker *et al.* 1987; McMahon 1987; van Ingen Schenau & Cavanagh 1990; Alexander 1991, 1992; Taylor 1994; van Ingen Schenau *et al.* 1997), and cross-country skiing (Komi & Norman 1987). Stretch–shortening is generally not a major factor in activities such as skating or cycling, due to minimal involvement of stretch–shortening sequencing of muscle activity (di Prampero *et al.* 1976). A detailed discussion of many relevant issues involving the stretch–shortening cycle has been published in a special issue of the *Journal of Applied Biomechanics* (1997, Vol. 13). Only a few topics that relate specifically to economy will be mentioned here.

Source of stretch–shortening cycle contributions

Although work performed during the stretch–shortening cycle is often attributed to the storage and reutilization of elastic energy, other factors have been proposed as being equally, or more, important, including: increasing the time available for force production; potentiating the contractile mechanism during the concentric phase of the movement; and triggering of spinal reflexes (Bosco *et al.* 1982, 1987b; Williams 1985; van Ingen Schenau & Cavanagh 1990; van Ingen Schenau *et al.* 1997). Stretch–shortening mechanisms are used to explain the high (40–70%) efficiency rates often calculated for running (Cavagna *et al.* 1964; Heglund *et al.* 1982; Williams & Cavanagh 1983; Bosco *et al.* 1987a; Anderson 1996). There are a variety of views as to whether elastic energy can enhance work production or efficiency, but there is general agreement that economy benefits from stretch–shortening mechanisms; the mechanical work attributable to stretch–shortening sources reduces the amount of metabolic work performed by the active muscles (Williams 1985; van Ingen Schenau & Cavanagh 1990; Alexander 1991; Taylor 1994).

Stretch–shortening contributions in running and jumping

The exact influence of stretch–shortening contributions to economy is not well understood. There are indications of substantial interindividual variations in the ability to store and reuse energy (Ito *et al.* 1983; Williams & Cavanagh 1983; Aura & Komi 1986; Voigt *et al.* 1995). Heise *et al.* (1996) found significant correlations between two electromyographic (EMG) measures and running economy; they also noted trends where increased periods of coactivation were related to better economy. They hypothesized that joint stiffness may have been increased by coactivation, and this may have resulted in a greater elastic return from the muscles involved, resulting in a greater economy. Although differences in stretch–shortening cycle contributions for knee-bend and jumping activities have been examined in a variety of conditions and with different athletic groups (Asmussen & Bonde-Petersen 1974; Komi & Bosco 1978; Bosco *et al.* 1982), measurements using endurance athletes have not been extensive; existing data have usually been measured during jumping activities and the findings have then been compared with the economy during running (Luhtanen & Komi 1980; Voigt *et al.* 1995). Some have shown no relationship between economy, measures of elastic storage and return of energy (Williams & Cavanagh 1987), or no difference in mechanical efficiency between endurance-trained and power-trained athletes (Kyröläinen & Komi 1995; Kyröläinen *et al.* 1995). Others have found significant relationships, showing that greater elastic contributions, as measured in jumping activities, are associated with a greater economy in running (Bosco *et al.* 1987b; Voigt *et al.* 1995).

Dalleau *et al.* (1998) derived a measure of leg stiffness from kinematic measurements during running; they found a significant relationship, a lower energy cost being associated with greater stiffness. They further compared the resonant frequency of their spring–mass model to step frequency, finding that the further the step frequency differed from the resonant frequency, the greater the associated metabolic energy cost. Taylor (1994) proposed that to achieve maximal storage and recovery of energy, muscles should undergo only very small length changes; however, there is as yet no available evidence from experimental human studies to support this proposition. Footwear has been cited as another possible site where energy could be stored at impact and returned during the contact phase of running (McMahon 1987; Shorten 1993). Although Shorten could not eliminate the possibility that economy could be enhanced by shoe elasticity, the differences between modern running shoes in terms of elastic storage and return was too small to have a direct effect on energy expenditure; thus he concluded that it probably was not an important factor.

Training, flexibility and the stretch–shortening cycle

It is not known whether the contribution from the stretch–shortening cycle to the work performed, and the consequent savings of metabolic energy, can be improved by training. Suggestions that flexibility training enhances the ability to store elastic energy (Wilson *et al.* 1991, 1992) have been criticized as incorrect if the benefits of the stretch–shortening cycle come not from storing and returning energy, but from an increase in the time available to generate force (Goubel 1997; van Ingen Schenau *et al.* 1997). Several studies have examined the influence of lower extremity flexibility on economy. One study found that increases in flexibility after a period of flexibility training were associated with improved running economy (Godges *et al.* 1989), but other similar studies have shown superior economy in individuals with less flexibility (Gleim *et al.* 1990; Craib *et al.* 1996), with increased contributions from stored elastic energy cited as the likely mechanism. Further work is needed to investigate how training-induced changes in stretch–shortening contributions might improve the economy of effort.

Relationships between economy and body size

Measures of submaximal energy cost $\dot{V}_{O_2}$ are usually expressed relative to body mass ($ml \cdot kg^{-1} \cdot min^{-1}$), but often an influence of size on economy remains after this simple scaling to body mass. In running, moderate correlations suggest that greater economy is associated with a greater body mass (Williams & Cavanagh 1986; Williams *et al.* 1987; Bergh *et al.* 1991; Bourdin *et al.* 1993; Anderson 1996), although other studies have reported no relationship (Helgerud 1994). Taylor (1994) reported that the cost of running per unit of body mass in different animal species decreased with body size across an 850-fold range of body mass. $\dot{V}_{O_{2max}}$ shows a similar relationship with body mass to that found for submaximal $\dot{V}_{O_2}$ (Bergh *et al.* 1991; Bergh & Forsberg 1992). The greater economy found in heavier runners may thus confer no advantage, since they may be operating at the same percentage of $\dot{V}_{O_{2max}}$ as lighter runners. Several investigators have suggested that oxygen consumption should be scaled to body mass raised to the two-thirds or three-quarters power, rather than to full body mass (Bergh & Forsberg 1992; Martin & Morgan 1992; Svedenhag & Sjodin 1994; Brisswalter *et al.* 1996).

The inverse relationship between economy and body mass may be due to differences in mass distribution among body segments (Cavanagh & Kram 1985b; Bailey & Pate 1991; Pate *et al.* 1992), but studies of animals with very different distribution of limb mass have shown little difference in energy consumption (Taylor 1994). Studies that add loads to the extremities during running do show increased energy costs, indicating the potential for a mass distribution effect (Catlin & Dressendorfer 1979; Martin 1985), but no effect from actual differences in mass distribution among athletes has yet been demonstrated.

Swain (1994) found that smaller cyclists were at a disadvantage due to their size; the energy cost due to frontal drag, when expressed relative to body mass, is greater for smaller cyclists, and the rela-

tively higher $\dot{V}_{O_{2max}}$ found in smaller individuals is not enough to compensate for this disadvantage. Additionally, he concluded that the heavier cyclist had an advantage in hilly cycling since the mass of the bicycle was relatively smaller than for a smaller cyclist. In rowing, smaller rowers may again have a slight disadvantage, due to the dependence of drag coefficients on scale (Sanderson & Martindale 1986). The metabolic cost of swimming is increased by greater body size and surface area, and is decreased by increased buoyancy (Costill *et al.* 1985; Chatard *et al.* 1990, 1991).

There is some indication that longer segment lengths are associated with better economy in running (Walt & Wyndham 1973; Williams & Cavanagh 1986; Svedenhag & Sjodin 1994; Brisswalter *et al.* 1996), but others have found no relationship (Williams *et al.* 1987; Pate *et al.* 1992; Svedenhag & Sjodin 1994). Economy is also significantly related to arm length in swimming, longer-armed swimmers using significantly more oxygen than those with shorter arms (in height-matched groups) (Chatard *et al.* 1990, 1991). In contrast, swimming performance bears no relationship to body height or mass in men, and in women faster performances are correlated with greater height and mass and less body fat (Siders *et al.* 1993).

Relationships between economy and biomechanical measures

Speed, stride length and cadence

Many studies have shown a general linear relationship between economy and speed in running (Daniels 1985; Morgan *et al.* 1989; Daniels & Daniels 1992), and a linear relationship between economy and work rate in ergometer cycling (Davies 1980a). In activities where viscous air or fluid resistance is a major factor, submaximal oxygen costs increase with speed in a curvilinear fashion; for example in cycling (Davies 1980a; McCole *et al.* 1990), skating (di Prampero *et al.* 1976) and swimming (Toussaint *et al.* 1988a). Of primary interest is how biomechanical factors influence economy at a given speed. Stride length (SL) is one of the most studied variables in distance-running biomechanics (Walt &

Wyndham 1973; Cavanagh & Williams 1982; Cavanagh & Kram 1989; Bailey & Messier 1991). There appears to be no relationship between economy and the freely chosen SL among individuals at any given speed of running (Svedenhag & Sjodin 1994; Brisswalter *et al.* 1996), but there is an SL that is most economical for an individual at a given speed of running; this usually coincides with the one freely chosen (Hogberg 1952; Cavanagh & Williams 1982; Powers *et al.* 1982; Cavagna *et al.* 1997). Bailey and Messier (1991) found no changes in the SL or $\dot{V}O_2$ of novice runners after a 7-week training period; yet Morgan *et al.* (1994) demonstrated that it was possible to train runners to choose an SL closer to the one predicted as optimal, with a concomitant lowering of $\dot{V}O_2$.

In contrast, the preferred cadence of experienced cyclists is typically greater than that predicted as the most economical (Hagberg *et al.* 1981; Gregor *et al.* 1991; Faria 1992; Marsh & Martin 1997), indicating that the choice of cadence is governed by factors other than economy. Gonzalez and Hull (1989) predicted a minimum for their mechanical cost function at a pedalling rate of 115 r.p.m. for an average-sized person, and Redfield and Hull (1986) proposed that competitors might minimize net joint moment preferentially over metabolic energy cost. Swain and Wilcox (1992) found greater economy at faster cadences when cycling uphill, but the only cadences tested were 41 and 82 r.p.m.

Kinematic and kinetic measures

A variety of measures of running mechanics have been identified as being related to greater economy, but there are many inconsistencies, with a variable being related in one or more studies but not in others. A greater running economy has been associated with: less extension at the hip and greater extension at the knee during toe-off, more dorsiflexion and a greater decrease and subsequent increase in forward velocity during support (Williams *et al.* 1987); a higher first vertical force peak, a greater angle of the shank with the vertical at footstrike, less plantar flexion at toe-off, greater forward trunk lean and a lower minimum velocity of a point on the knee during foot contact (Williams & Cavanagh

1987); longer support time, lower medially directed ground reaction force, greater extension of the hip and knee at toe-off and a faster horizontal velocity of a point on the heel at footstrike (Williams & Cavanagh 1986); and less arm movement (Anderson & Tseh 1994). Until more consistent relationships are established, these findings should not be used as the basis for trying to alter a competitor's mechanics to improve their economy of movement.

Technique

In cross-country skiing, economy is affected by both the type of skis used and skiing technique (Hoffman & Clifford 1990; Hoffman 1992). A diagonal stride typically has the highest oxygen cost; in comparison a V1 skate, marathon skate and kick double-pole technique reduce the metabolic cost by 16%, and a double-pole technique results in a 26% lower cost. Others have found that the traditional diagonal stride technique has greater metabolic costs than skating techniques (Zupan & Sheperd 1988; Sabiene *et al.* 1989). Chatard *et al.* (1990, 1991) noted that if coaches evaluated swimmers as showing a preference for using their arms rather than their legs they had a 12% lower oxygen cost.

Relationships between economy and equipment

Equipment used by athletes, including footwear, clothing and vehicles directly involved in the sport (e.g. bicycles, boats) can affect the economy of movement in many different ways. Factors related to drag forces will be covered in a later section. The mass of clothing is not usually a factor, since typically it does not add substantially to overall body mass (Stevens 1983). Footwear, however, can affect economy in two different ways. The heavier the shoes worn, the greater the submaximal energy costs, with significant increases in $\dot{V}O_2$ coming from an increase as little as 75 g per shoe (Catlin & Dressendorfer 1979; Frederick *et al.* 1984). The increased metabolic costs are thought to be due to the greater muscular forces needed to accelerate and decelerate the foot segment during leg movements, as when other weights are added to the extremities (Martin 1985). Cushioning in shoes significantly affects economy: shoes that provide more cushioning can lower energy cost by as much as 2.6% (Frederick et al. 1983b). A second study showed a lower, but still significant, saving of $0.4\,ml\cdot kg^{-1}\cdot min^{-1}$ (Frederick et al. 1983a). There are no significant differences in energy costs between running on cement, an all-weather track surface or a cinder track (Pugh 1970; Bonen et al. 1974), although an indoor track tuned to the stiffness characteristics of the lower extremities of runners may enhance performance (McMahon & Greene 1979).

A number of variables related to the bicycle affect both economy and generation of power during cycling (Faria 1992). An optimal crank length of $0.15-0.18\,m$ has been reported (Hull & Gonzalez 1988; Kyle 1994), but others have not found a clear relationship of economy to crank length (Carmichael et al. 1982; Conrad & Thomas 1983). There is also an optimal seat height, usually expressed as a percentage of one of several measures of leg length (e.g. 105% of inseam length) (Norden-Snyder 1977; Gonzalez & Hull 1989). Gonzalez and Hull (1989) developed a model that determined the cadence, crank arm length, seat tube angle, seat height and longitudinal foot position on the pedal that would minimize a mechanical cost function for a given size of rider. No metabolic results were given to show how the mechanical cost function corresponded to metabolic energy consumption.

Economy and external resistance forces

Anything that produces a force that opposes forward movement during an endurance activity will increase metabolic energy costs and limit performance. The major factor in many events is fluid resistance, but in a sport such as cycling additional resistive forces come from rolling resistance and internal friction in the cycling machinery (Gregor et al. 1991; Capelli et al. 1993). In skating and skiing there are also frictional forces that oppose forward movement (van Ingen Schenau 1982; Frederick 1992). In aquatic sports there is resistance due to both water and air, but the resistance is much less for air than for water (e.g. in rowing air resistance is 10% of the drag due to water) (Sanderson & Martindale 1986). Fluid resistance causes fluctuations in speed from 3.5 to $5.5\,m\cdot s^{-1}$ in single sculling, causing rowers to do 5% more work than if a constant velocity could be maintained (Sanderson & Martindale 1986).

Drag forces resulting from fluid resistance can be represented by the following equation:

$$F = 0.5\,C_d A \rho v^2$$

where C_d is the drag coefficient, A is the projected frontal area, ρ is the density of the fluid and v is the relative fluid velocity (di Prampero et al. 1976; Davies 1980a,b; van Ingen Schenau 1982; Frohlich 1985; Sanderson & Martindale 1986; Gregor et al. 1991; Péronnet et al. 1991; Capelli et al. 1993; van Ingen Schenau et al. 1994). Anything that changes any of the variables on the right side of this equation has an effect on drag and thus affects economy.

Work done to overcome fluid resistance

The greater the relative fluid velocity, the greater the effect on the economy of movement. Pugh (1970) found that the extra oxygen consumed while running on a treadmill against a wind increased with the square of wind velocity. He estimated the overall energy cost of overcoming air resistance in track running to be approximately 8% at a typical distance speed of $6\,m\cdot s^{-1}$ and 16% at a sprint speed ($10\,m\cdot s^{-1}$). Davies (1980b) predicted a somewhat smaller effect (7.8% at $10\,m\cdot s^{-1}$, 4% at $6\,m\cdot s^{-1}$, and 2% at marathon speeds). In cycling, skiing and skating the energy cost due to air resistance is proportional to the velocity squared (Davies 1980a; van Ingen Schenau 1982; Capelli et al. 1993), but since these sports occur at much higher speeds than for running, the relative proportion of the total work required to overcome air resistance is higher, as much as 80–90% in cycling (Kyle 1979).

Pugh (1970) estimated that the net energy cost to overcome air resistance in middle-distance events at the 1968 Olympic Games in Mexico City (2270m) would be reduced by approximately 1.9% due to the lower air resistance at altitude. Péronnet et al. (1991)

developed an equation to predict the combined influence at altitude of reduced air resistance due to decreased air density and reduced maximal aerobic power due to the decreased partial pressure of oxygen. Since aerodynamic energy cost is only a minor component of the total energy cost, the relatively greater reduction in aerobic power resulted in poorer distance-running performances at altitude. Their equations predict an increase in performance times of 7% for a marathon run and 4% for a 1500-m run at Mexico City's altitude, despite the beneficial effects of reduced air resistance.

Wind speed and direction

The benefits of a tail wind do not match the extra energy costs of running or cycling into the wind (Davies 1980b; Frohlich 1985; van Ingen Schenau et al. 1994). This is important for performances on oval tracks or 'out-and-back' race courses, leading Davies to conclude that it would be difficult for an athlete to achieve a best performance on a windy day. Swain (1997) modelled the influence of hills and wind on oxygen cost and predicted a performance improvement by adopting a strategy of slightly increasing power when going uphill or against the wind and slightly reducing power when going downhill or with the wind. In contrast, a model for skating (van Ingen Schenau 1982) suggested performance would be enhanced by skating at constant power rather than trying to keep speed as constant as possible. Hatsell (1974) modelled energy expenditure for running on a circular track on a windy day, finding an optimum strategy that varied speed depending on wind direction, with acceleration beginning when the wind was directly in the face of the runner and deceleration starting when the wind was at his or her back.

Variations in body position can markedly reduce aerodynamic drag, in turn reducing metabolic energy costs (van Ingen Schenau 1982; Spring et al. 1988; Faria 1992). Changing from an upright position to a crouched racing posture can reduce frontal area by 30% or more (Faria & Cavanagh 1978; Spring et al. 1988), and cycling with elbow-rest handlebars reduces drag even more (Kyle 1994). Gnehm et al. (1997) found an increase in oxygen consumption

when cycling with aerodynamic handlebars on a stationary bicycle, but concluded that the approximate increase of 9 W in $\dot{V}O_2$ due to the changed body position would be outweighed by the predicted 100 W savings due to reduced drag when on the track. Body position also affects skating; air friction in skating is related to knee angle and trunk-lean angle (van Ingen Schenau 1982). In swimming, Toussaint et al. (1988a,b) found a difference in drag force between males and females, due partly to a higher projected frontal area in the males.

Clothing and equipment

Smooth tight-fitting racing clothing reduces drag by 8–30% in cycling (Gregor et al. 1991; Faria 1992; Kyle 1994) and 7–10% in skating at speeds higher than 6–7 m·s⁻¹ (van Ingen Schenau 1982). Aerodynamic helmets also reduce drag. Kyle (1994) estimated that a cyclist using a good aerodynamic racing helmet would have a substantial advantage over an equal opponent using a standard helmet. An aerodynamic design of frames and/or wheels can also reduce drag, leading to improvements in economy of 5–7% at typical cycling speeds (McCole et al. 1990; Capelli et al. 1993; Kyle 1994). Capelli et al. (1993) tied this to an approximate 3% improvement in performance for an aerodynamic versus a traditional bicycle. Kyle (1986) simulated differences in equipment, clothing and riding positions for the top two riders in the 1989 Tour de France. The increased air resistance of Fignon's standard bicycle with standard handlebars, unzipped jersey, no helmet and ponytail resulted in a simulated 1.5-min disadvantage compared to LeMond's more aerodynamic profile over the 24-km final time trial; this figure was not far from the actual 58-s difference in race times.

The energy costs of swimming can be affected by swimsuit design. Use of a form-fitting torso suit can reduce oxygen costs (Starling et al. 1995), and the use of a triathlon wetsuit reduced drag by 14%, leading to a predicted 5% increase in swimming speed (Toussaint et al. 1989). The primary effect of this suit is a decrease in the surface area presented to the water, due to the buoyancy provided by the suit.

Shielding

Running, skiing, cycling or skating behind other competitors provides shielding from air resistance, reducing both drag and metabolic costs (Kyle 1979; Frohlich 1985; Spring *et al.* 1988; Faria 1992). McCole *et al.* (1990) found an 18% reduction in metabolic cost for drafting behind one rider at $32 km \cdot h^{-1}$, and as much as a 40% reduction in $\dot{V}o_2$ for riders at the back of a pack of eight cyclists travelling at $40 km \cdot h^{-1}$. Similar results have been found in other studies (Kyle 1979). Running in a pack is predicted to reduce air resistance from 40 to 80%, depending on how close one runner follows another; this can lower oxygen costs by 3–6% (Pugh 1971; Kyle 1979). Drag is reduced by 16–23% when following 1–2 m behind another skater (van Ingen Schenau 1982).

Concluding comments

Mechanical factors have important influences on both economy and performance, and mechanics also affect other areas not covered in this review, such as susceptibility to injury and fatigue. The assumption is usually made that individuals will self-optimize their movement patterns in ways that are most beneficial to performance. However, no one factor can be optimized in isolation. A low $\dot{V}o_2$ is not important if a runner ignores musculoskeletal signs of stress and sustains an injury that keeps him or her from competing. At the same time that efforts are made to minimize metabolic energy costs, there must be adaptations to deal effectively with fatigue,

to keep tissue stresses within acceptable limits, and to put the athlete in a psychological state where he or she can put forth an optimal performance. Any efforts to manipulate mechanics in an effort to improve performance should also consider the effects these manipulations may have on other factors important to performance.

There are many indications that athletes at both élite and subélite levels are very good at optimizing mechanics in terms of economy of movement (Cavanagh & Williams 1982; Williams 1990; Morgan & Craib 1992). Humans can adapt to changes in movement patterns very quickly, but a high level of optimization probably results from years of fine-tuning mechanics. Several investigators have trained subjects over a period of weeks, using feedback aimed at improving mechanics and lowering economy; they have found no significant changes in submaximal oxygen consumption (Petray & Krahenbuhl 1985; Messier & Cirillo 1989; Miller *et al.* 1990). Such studies indicate that optimizing mechanics is not a simple matter, and is probably the result of a long adaptation process.

All athletes strive to find ways to get an edge on their competitors, and a full evaluation of the mechanics of movement related to their sport has the potential to identify subtle changes that might enhance performance. As we learn more about mechanics in relation to economy, musculoskeletal stress and performance, and find how best to apply this knowledge to athletes at all levels of skill, the fine-tuning of biomechanical factors related to movement has the potential to become a very important part of an athlete's training regimen.

References

Aleshinsky, S.Y. (1986a) An energy 'sources' and 'fractions' approach to the mechanical energy expenditure problem. I. Basic concepts, description of the model, analysis of a one-link system movement. *Journal of Biomechanics* **19**, 287–293.

Aleshinsky, S.Y. (1986b) An energy 'sources' and 'fractions' approach to the mechanical energy expenditure problem. V. The mechanical energy expenditure reduction during motion of

the multi-link system. *Journal of Biomechanics* **19**, 311–315.

Alexander, R.M. (1991) Energy-saving mechanisms in walking and running. *Journal of Experimental Biology* **160**, 55–69.

Alexander, R.M. (1992) A model of bipedal locomotion on compliant legs. *Philosophical Transactions of the Royal Society of London. Series B: Biological Sciences* **338**, 189–198.

Anderson, T. (1996) Biomechanics and

running economy. *Sports Medicine* **22**, 76–89.

Anderson, T. & Tseh, W. (1994) Running economy, anthropometric dimensions and kinematic variables (abstract). *Medicine and Science in Sports and Exercise* **26**, S170.

Asmussen, E. & Bonde-Petersen, F. (1974) Apparent efficiency and storage of elastic energy in human muscles during exercise. *Acta Physiologica Scandinavica* **92**, 537–545.

Aura, O. & Komi, P.V. (1986) The mechanical efficiency of locomotion in men and women with special emphasis on stretch–shortening cycle exercises. *European Journal of Applied Physiology* **55**, 37–43.

Bailey, S.P. & Messier, S.P. (1991) Variations in stride length and running economy in male novice runners subsequent to a seven-week training program. *International Journal of Sports Medicine* **12**, 299–304.

Bailey, S.P. & Pate, R.R. (1991) Feasibility of improving running economy. *Sports Medicine* **12**, 228–236.

Baudinette, R.V. (1991) The energetics and cardiorespiratory correlates of mammalian terrestrial locomotion. *Journal of Experimental Biology* **160**, 209–231.

Bergh, U. & Forsberg, A. (1992) Influence of body mass on cross-country ski racing performance. *Medicine and Science in Sports and Exercise* **24**, 1033–1039.

Bergh, U., Sjödin, B., Forsberg, A. & Svedenhad, J. (1991) The relationship between body mass and oxygen uptake during running in humans. *Medicine and Science in Sports and Exercise* **23**, 205–211.

Biewener, A.A. (1990) Biomechanics of mammalian terrestrial locomotion. *Science* **250**, 1097–1103.

Bonen, A., Gass, G.C., Kachadorian, W.A. & Johnson, R.R. (1974) The energy cost of walking and running on different surfaces. *Australian Journal of Sports Medicine* **6**, 5–11.

Bosco, C., Tarkka, I. & Komi, P.V. (1982) Effect of elastic energy and myoelectrical potentiation of triceps surae during stretch–shortening cycle exercise. *International Journal of Sports Medicine* **3**, 137–140.

Bosco, C., Montanari, G., Ribacchi, R. *et al.* (1987a) Relationship between the efficiency of muscular work during jumping and the energetics of running. *European Journal of Applied Physiology* **56**, 138–143.

Bosco, C., Montanari, G., Tarkka, I. *et al.* (1987b) The effect of pre-stretch on mechanical efficiency of human skeletal muscle. *Acta Physiologica Scandinavica* **131**, 323–329.

Bourdin, M., Pastene, J., Germain, M. & Lacour, J.R. (1993) Influence of training, sex, age and body mass on the energy cost of running. *European Journal of Applied Physiology* **66**, 439–444.

Brisswalter, J., Legros, P. & Durand, M. (1996) Running economy, preferred step length correlated to body dimensions in elite middle distance runners. *Journal of Sports Medicine and Physical Fitness* **36**, 7–15.

Broker, J.P. & Gregor, R.J. (1994) Mechanical energy management in cycling: source relations and energy expenditure. *Medicine and Science in Sports and Exercise* **26**, 64–74.

Caldwell, G.E. & Forrester, L.W. (1992) Estimates of mechanical work and energy transfers: demonstration of a rigid body power model of the recovery leg in gait. *Medicine and Science in Sports and Exercise* **24**, 1396–1412.

Capelli, C., Rosa, G., Butti, F., Ferretti, G., Veicsteinas, A. & di Prampero, P.E. (1993) Energy cost and efficiency of riding aerodynamic bicycles. *European Journal of Applied Physiology* **67**, 144–149.

Carmichael, J.K.S., Loumis, J.L. & Hodgson, L. (1982) The effect of crank length on oxygen consumption and heart rate when cycling at a constant power output (abstract). *Medicine and Science in Sports and Exercise* **14**, 162.

Catlin, M.J. & Dressendorfer, R.H. (1979) Effect of shoe weight on the energy cost of running. *Medicine and Science in Sports and Exercise* **11**, 80.

Cavagna, G.A., Saibene, F.P. & Margaria, R. (1964) Mechanical work in running. *Journal of Applied Physiology* **19**, 249–256.

Cavagna, G.A., Mantovani, M., Willems, P.A. & Musch, G. (1997) The resonant step frequency in human running. *Pflügers Archives* **434**, 678–684.

Cavanagh, P.R. & Kram, R (1985a) The efficiency of human movement—a statement of the problem. *Medicine and Science in Sports and Exercise* **17**, 304–308.

Cavanagh, P.R. & Kram, R. (1985b) Mechanical and muscular factors affecting the efficiency of human movement. *Medicine and Science in Sports and Exercise* **17**, 326–331.

Cavanagh, P.R. & Kram, R. (1989) Stride length in distance running: Velocity, body dimensions, and added mass effects. *Medicine and Science in Sports and Exercise* **21**, 467–479.

Cavanagh, P.R. & Williams, K.R. (1982) The effect of stride length variation on oxygen uptake during distance running. *Medicine and Science in Sports and Exercise* **14**, 30–35.

Chatard, J.C., Lavoie, J.M. & Lacour, J.R. (1990) Analysis of determinants of swimming economy in front crawl. *European Journal of Applied Physiology* **61**, 88–92.

Chatard, J.C., Lavoie, J.M. & Lacour, J.R. (1991) Energy cost of front-crawl swimming in women. *European Journal of Applied Physiology* **63**, 12–16.

Conley, D.L. & Krahenbuhl, G.S. (1980) Running economy and distance running performance of highly trained athletes. *Medicine and Science in Sports and Exercise* **12**, 357–360.

Conrad, D.P. & Thomas, T.R. (1983) Bicycle crank arm length and oxygen consumption in trained cyclists. *Medicine and Science in Sports and Exercise* **15**, 111.

Costill, D.L. & Fox, E.L. (1969) Energetics of marathon running. *Medicine and Science in Sports and Exercise* **1**, 81–86.

Costill, D.L., Kovaliski, J., Porter, D., Fielding, R. & Ding, D. (1985) Energy expenditure during front crawl swimming: predicting success in middle distance events. *International Journal of Sports Medicine* **6**, 266–270.

Craib, M.W., Mitchell, V.A., Fields, K.B., Cooper, T.R., Hopewell, R. & Morgan, D.W. (1996) The association between flexibility and running economy in sub-élite male distance runners. *Medicine and Science in Sports and Exercise* **28**, 737–743.

Dalleau, G., Belli, A., Bourdin, M. & Lacour, J.R. (1998) The spring–mass model and the energy cost of treadmill running. *European Journal of Applied Physiology* **77**, 257–263.

Daniels, J.T. (1985) A physiologist's view of running economy. *Medicine and Science in Sports and Exercise* **17**, 332–338.

Daniels, J. & Daniels, N. (1992) Running economy of elite male and elite female runners. *Medicine and Science in Sports and Exercise* **24**, 483–489.

Daniels, J.T., Scardina, N.J. & Foley, P. (1984) $\dot{V}O_{2submax}$ during five modes of exercise. In: Bachl, N., Prokop, L. & Sucket, R. (eds) *Proceedings of the World Congress on Sports Medicine*, pp. 604–615. Urban & Schwartzenberg, Vienna.

Davies, C.T.M. (1980a) Effect of air resistance on the metabolic cost and performance of cycling. *European Journal of Applied Physiology* **45**, 245–254.

Davies, C.T.M. (1980b) Effects of wind assistance and resistance on the forward motion of a runner. *Journal of Applied Physiology* **48**, 702–709.

Faria, I.E. (1992) Energy expenditure, aerodynamics and medical problems in cycling. An update. *Sports Medicine* **14**, 43–63.

Faria, I. & Cavanagh, P.R. (1978) *The Physiology and Biomechanics of Cycling.* John Wiley and Sons, New York.

Fenn, W.O. (1930) Work against gravity and work due to velocity changes in running. *American Journal of Physiology* **93**, 133–461.

Frederick, E.C. (1983) Extrinsic biomechanical aids. In: Williams, M. (ed.) *Ergogenic Aids in Sport*, pp. 323–339. Human Kinetics, Champaign, IL.

Frederick, E.C. (1992) Mechanical constraints on Nordic ski performance. *Medicine and Science in Sports and Exercise* **24**, 1010–1014.

Frederick, E.C., Clarke, T.C., Hansen, J.L. & Cooper, L.B. (1983a) The effects of shoe cushioning on the oxygen demands of running. In: Nigg, B. & Kerr, B. (eds) *Biomechanical Aspects of Sports Shoes and Playing Surfaces*, pp. 107–114. University of Calgary, Calgary.

Frederick, E.C., Howley, E.T. & Powers, S.K. (1983b) Lower O_2 cost while running in air cushion type shoes. *Medicine and Science in Sports and Exercise* **12**, 81–82.

Frederick, E.C., Daniels, J.R. & Hayes, J.W. (1984) The effect of shoe weight on the aerobic demands of running. In: Bachl, N., Prokop, L. & Sucket, R. (eds) *Proceedings of the World Congress on Sports Medicine*, pp. 616–625. Urban & Schwartzenberg, Vienna.

Frohlich, C. (1985) Effect of wind and altitude on record performance in foot races, pole vault, and long jump. *American Journal of Physics* **53**, 726–730.

Fukunaga, T., Matsuo, A., Yamamoto, K. & Asami, T. (1986) Mechanical efficiency of rowing. *European Journal of Applied Physiology* **55**, 471–475.

Gleim, G.W., Stachenfeld, N.S. & Nicholas, J.A. (1990) The influence of flexibility on the economy of walking and jogging. *Journal of Orthopaedic Research* **8**, 814–823.

Gnehm, P., Reichenbach, S., Altpeter, E., Widmer, H. & Hoppeler, H. (1997) Influence of different racing positions on metabolic cost in elite cyclists. *Medicine and Science in Sports and Exercise* **29**, 818–823.

Godges, J.J., Macrae, H., Londgon, C. & Tinberg, C. (1989) The effects of two stretching procedures on hip range of motion and gait economy. *Journal of Orthopaedic and Sports Physical Therapy* **7**, 350–357.

Gonzalez, H. & Hull, M.L. (1989) Multivariable optimization of cycling biomechanics. *Journal of Biomechanics* **22**, 1151–1161.

Goubel, F. (1997) Series elasticity behavior during the stretch–shortening cycle. *Journal of Applied Biomechanics* **13**, 439–443.

Gregor, R.J., Broker, J.P. & Ryan, M.M.

(1991) The biomechanics of cycling. In: Holloszy, J.O. (ed.) *Exercise and Sport Science Reviews*, Vol. 19, pp. 1127–1169. Williams & Wilkins, Baltimore.

Hagberg, J.M., Mullin, J.P., Giese, M.D. & Spitzangel, E. (1981) Effect of pedalling rate on submaximal exercise responses of competitive cyclists. *Journal of Applied Physiology* **51**, 477–481.

Hatsell, C.P. (1974) A note on jogging on a windy day. *IEEE Transactions on Biomedical Engineering*, pp. 428–429.

Heglund, N.C., Fedak, M.A., Taylor, C.R. & Cavagna, G.A. (1982) Energetics and mechanics of terrestrial locomotion. IV. Total mechanical energy changes as a function of speed and body size in birds and mammals. *Journal of Experimental Biology* **97**, 57–66.

Heise, G.D. & Martin, P.E. (1990) Interrelationships among mechanical power measures and running economy. *Medicine and Science in Sports and Exercise* **22**, S22.

Heise, G.D., Morgan, D.W., Hough, H. & Craib, M. (1996) Relationships between running economy and temporal EMG characteristics of bi-articular leg muscles. *International Journal of Sports Medicine* **17**, 128–133.

Helgerud, J. (1994) Maximal oxygen uptake, anaerobic threshold and running economy in women and men with similar performance levels in marathons. *European Journal of Applied Physiology* **68**, 155–161.

Hoffman, M. (1992) Physiological comparisons of cross-country skiing techniques. *Medicine and Science in Sports and Exercise* **24**, 1023–1032.

Hoffman, M.D. & Clifford, P.S. (1990) Physiological responses to different cross country skiing techniques on level terrain. *Medicine and Science in Sports and Exercise* **22**, 841–848.

Hogberg, P. (1952) How do stride length and stride frequency influence the energy output during running? *Arbeitsphysiologie* **14**, 437–441.

Hull, M. & Gonzalez, H. (1988) Bivariate optimization of pedaling rate and crank arm length in cycling. *Journal of Biomechanics* **21**, 839–849.

van Ingen Schenau, G.J. (1982) The influence of air friction in speed skating. *Journal of Biomechanics* **21**, 449–458.

van Ingen Schenau, G.J. & Cavanagh, P.R. (1990) Power equations in endurance sports. *Journal of Biomechanics* **23**, 865–881.

van Ingen Schenau, G.J., van Woensel, W.W., Boots, P.J., Snackers, R.W. & de

Groot, G. (1990) Determination and interpretation of mechanical power in human movement: application to ergometer cycling. *European Journal of Applied Physiology* **61**, 11–19.

van Ingen Schenau, G.J., de Koning, J.J. & de Groot, G. (1994) Optimisation of sprinting performance in running, cycling and speed skating. *Sports Medicine* **17**, 259–275.

van Ingen Schenau, G.J., Bobbert, M.F. & de Haan, A. (1997) Does elastic energy enhance work and efficiency in the stretch–shortening cycle? *Journal of Applied Biomechanics* **13**, 389–415.

Ito, A., Komi, P.V., Sjödin, B., Bosco, C. & Karlsson, J. (1983) Mechanical efficiency of positive work in running at different speeds. *Medicine and Science in Sports and Exercise* **15**, 299–308.

Journal of Applied Biomechanics. (August 1997) Volume 13, Part 3. Human Kinetics Publishers, Champaign, IL.

Kaneko, M., Matsumoto, M., Ito, A. & Fuchimoto, T. (1987) Optimum step frequency in constant speed running. In: Jonsson, B. (ed.) *Biomechanics X-B*, pp. 803–897. Human Kinetics, Champaign, IL.

Ker, R.F., Bennett, M.B., Bibby, S.R., Kester, R.C. & Alexander, R.M. (1987) The spring in the arch of the human foot. *Nature* **325**, 147–149.

Komi, P.V. & Bosco, C. (1978) Utilization of stored elastic energy in leg extension muscles by men and women. *Medicine and Science in Sports and Exercise* **10**, 261–265.

Komi, P.V. & Norman, R.W. (1987) Preloading of the thrust phase in cross-country skiing. *International Journal of Sports Medicine* **8** (Suppl. 1), 48–54.

Kyle, C.R. (1979) Reduction of wind resistance and power output of racing cyclists and runners traveling in groups. *Ergonomics* **22**, 387–397.

Kyle, C.R. (1986) Mechanical factors affecting the speed of a cycle. In: Burke, E. (ed.) *Science of Cycling*, pp. 123–136. Human Kinetics, Champaign, IL.

Kyle, C.R. (1994) Energy and aerodynamics in bicycling. *Clinics in Sports Medicine* **13**, 39–73.

Kyröläinen, H. & Komi, P.V. (1995) Differences in mechanical efficiency between power- and endurance-trained athletes while jumping. *European Journal of Applied Physiology* **70**, 36–44.

Kyröläinen, H., Komi, P.V. & Belli, A. (1995) Mechanical efficiency in athletes during running. *Scandinavian Journal of Medicine and Science in Sports* **5**, 200–208.

Luhtanen, P. & Komi, P.V. (1980) Force–, power–, and elasticity–velocity relationships in walking, running, and jumping. *European Journal of Applied Physiology* **44**, 279–289.

Luhtanen, P., Rahkila, P., Rusko, H. & Viitasalo, J.T. (1990) Mechanical work and efficiency in treadmill running at aerobic and anaerobic thresholds. *Acta Physiologica Scandinavica* **139**, 153–159.

Marsh, A.P. & Martin, P.E. (1997) Effect of cycling experience, aerobic power, and power output on preferred and most economical cycling cadences. *Medicine and Science in Sports and Exercise* **29**, 1225–1232.

Martin, P.E. (1985) Mechanical and physiological responses to lower extremity loading during running. *Medicine and Science in Sports and Exercise* **17**, 427–433.

Martin, P.E. & Morgan, D.W. (1992) Biomechanical considerations for economical walking and running. *Medicine and Science in Sports and Exercise* **24**, 467–474.

Martin, P.E., Heise, G.D. & Morgan, D.W. (1993) Interrelationships between mechanical power, energy transfers, and walking and running economy. *Medicine and Science in Sports and Exercise* **25**, 508–515.

McCole, S.D., Claney, K., Conte, J.-C., Anderson, R. & Hagberg, J. (1990) Energy expenditure during bicycling. *Journal of Applied Physiology* **68**, 748–753.

McMahon, T.A. (1987) The spring in the human foot. *Nature* **325**, 108–109.

McMahon, T.A. & Greene, P.R. (1979) The influence of track compliance on running. *Journal of Biomechanics* **12**, 893–904.

Messier, S.P. & Cirillo, K.J. (1989) Effects of a verbal and visual feedback system on running technique, perceived exertion and running economy in female novice runners. *Journal of Sports Science* **7**, 113–126.

Miller, T.A., Milliron, M.J. & Cavanagh, P.R. (1990) The effect of running mechanics feedback training on running economy. *Medicine and Science in Sports and Exercise* **22**, S17.

Morgan, D.W. & Craib, M. (1992) Physiological aspects of running economy. *Medicine and Science in Sports and Exercise* **24**, 456–461.

Morgan, D.W., Martin, P.E. & Krahenbuhl, G.S. (1989) Factors affecting running economy. *Sports Medicine* **7**, 310–330.

Morgan, D., Martin, P., Craib, M., Caruso, C., Clifton, R. & Hopewell, R. (1994) Effect of step length optimization on the aerobic demand of running. *Journal of Applied Physiology* **77**, 245–251.

Norden-Snyder, K.S. (1977) The effect of bicycle seat height variation upon oxygen consumption and lower limb kinematics. *Medicine and Science in Sports and Exercise* **9**, 113–117.

Norman, R.W., Sharratt, M.T., Pezack, J.C. & Noble, E.G. (1976) Re-examination of the mechanical effifficiency of horizontal treadmill running. In: Komi, P.V. (ed.) *Biomechanics V-B. International Series on Biomechanics*, pp. 87–93. University Park Press, Baltimore.

Pate, R.R., Macera, C.A., Bailey, S.P., Bartoli, W.P. & Powell, K.E. (1992) Physiological, anthropometric, and training correlates of running economy. *Medicine and Science in Sports and Exercise* **24**, 1128–1133.

Péronnet, F., Thibault, G. & Cousineau, D.L. (1991) A theoretical analysis of the effect of altitude on running performance. *Journal of Applied Physiology* **70**, 399–404.

Petray, C.K. & Krahenbuhl, G.S. (1985) Running training, instruction on running technique, and running economy in 10-year-old males. *Research Quarterly for Exercise and Sport* **56**, 251–255.

Powers, S.K., Hopkins, P. & Ragsdale, M.R. (1982) Oxygen uptake and ventilatory responses to various stride lengths in trained women. *American Corrective Therapy Journal* **36**, 5–8.

di Prampero, P.E., Cortili, G., Mognoni, P. & Saibene, F. (1976) Energy cost of speed skating and efficiency of work against air resistance. *Journal of Applied Physiology* **40**, 584–591.

Pugh, L.G.C.E. (1970) Oxygen intake in track and treadmill running with observations on the effect of air resistance. *Journal of Physiology (London)* **207**, 823–835.

Pugh, L.G.C.E. (1971) The influence of wind resistance in running and walking and the mechanical efficiency of work against horizontal or vertical forces. *Journal of Physiology (London)* **213**, 255–276.

Redfield, R. & Hull, M.L. (1986) On the relation between joint moments and pedalling rates at constant power in bicycling. *Journal of Biomechanics* **19**, 317–329.

Sabiene, F., Cortill, G., Roi, G. & Colombini, A. (1989) The energy cost of level cross-country skiing and the effect of the friction of the ski. *European Journal of Applied Physiology* **58**, 791–795.

Sanderson, B. & Martindale, W. (1986) Towards optimizing rowing technique. *Medicine and Science in Sports and Exercise* **18**, 454–468.

Shorten, M.R. (1993) The energetics of running and running shoes. *Journal of Biomechanics* **26** (Suppl. 1), 41–51.

Shorten, M.R., Wootton, S. & Williams, C. (1981) Mechanical energy changes and the oxygen cost of running. *Engineering in Medicine* **10**, 213–217.

Siders, W.A., Lukaski, H.C. & Bolonchuk, W.W. (1993) Relationships among swimming performance, body composition and somatotype in competitive collegiate swimmers. *Journal of Sports Medicine and Physical Fitness* **33**, 166–171.

Spring, E., Savolainen, S., Erkkilä, J., Hämäläinen, T. & Pihkala, P. (1988) Drag area of a cross-country skier. *International Journal of Sport Biomechanics* **4**, 103–113.

Starling, R.D., Costill, D.L., Trappe, T.A., Jozsi, A.C., Trappe, S.W. & Goodpaster, B.H. (1995) Effect of swimming suit design on the energy demands of swimming. *Medicine and Science in Sports and Exercise* **27**, 1086–1089.

Steinacker, J.M., Marx, T.R. & Mars, U. (1984) The oxygen consumption and work efficiency for rowing (abstract). *International Journal of Sports Medicine* **5**, 287–288.

Stevens, E.D. (1983) Effect of the weight of athletic clothing in distance running by amateur athletes. *Journal of Sports Medicine and Physical Fitness* **23**, 185–190.

Svedenhag, J. & Sjodin, B. (1994) Body-mass-modified running economy and step length in elite male middle- and long-distance runners. *International Journal of Sports Medicine* **15**, 305–310.

Swain, D.P. (1994) The influence of body mass in endurance bicycling. *Medicine and Science in Sports and Exercise* **26**, 58–63.

Swain, D.P. (1997) A model for optimizing cycling performance by varying power on hills and in wind. *Medicine and Science in Sports and Exercise* **29**, 1104–1108.

Swain, D.P. & Wilcox, J.P. (1992) Effect of cadence on the economy of uphill cycling. *Medicine and Science in Sports and Exercise* **24**, 1123–1127.

Taylor, C.R. (1994) Relating mechanics and energetics during exercise. *Advances in Veterinary Science and Comparative Medicine* **38A**, 181–215.

Toussaint, H.M., Beelen, A., Rodenburg, A. et al. (1988a) Propelling efficiency of front-crawl swimming. *Journal of Applied Physiology* **65**, 2506–2512.

Toussaint, H.M., de Groot, G., Savelberg, H.H.C.M., Vervoorn, K., Hollander, A.P. & van Ingen Schenau, G.J. (1988b) Active drag related to velocity in male and female swimmers. *Journal of Biomechanics* **21**, 435–438.

Toussaint, H.M., Bruinink, L., de Coster, R. et al. (1989) Effect of a triathlon wet suit on drag during swimming. *Medicine and Science in Sports and Exercise* **21**, 325–328.

Toussaint, H.M., Knops, W., de Groot, G. & Hollander, A.P. (1990) The mechanical efficiency of front crawl swimming. *Medicine and Science in Sports and Exercise* **22**, 402–408.

Voigt, M., Bojsen-Mller, F., Simonsen, E.B. & Dyhre-Poulsen, P. (1995) The influence of tendon Youngs modulus, dimensions and instantaneous moment arms on the efficiency of human movement. *Journal of Biomechanics* **28**, 281–291.

Walt, W.H.V.D. & Wyndham, C.H. (1973) An equation for prediction of energy expenditure of walking and running. *Journal of Applied Physiology* **34**, 559–563.

Williams, K.R. (1985) The relationship between mechanical and physiological energy estimates. *Medicine and Science in Sports and Exercise* **17**, 317–325.

Williams, K.R. (1990) Relationships between distance running biomechanics and running economy. In: Cavanagh, P.R. (ed.) *Biomechanics of Distance Running*, pp. 271–305. Human Kinetics, Champaign, IL.

Williams, K.R. & Cavanagh, P.R. (1983) A model for the calculation of mechanical power during distance running. *Journal of Biomechanics* **16**, 115–128.

Williams, K.R. & Cavanagh, P.R. (1986) Biomechanical correlates with running economy in elite distance runners. *Proceedings of the North American Congress on Biomechanics*, Vol. 2, pp. 287–288. American Society of Biomechanics, Montreal, Canada.

Williams, K.R. & Cavanagh, P.R. (1987) Relationship between distance running mechanics, running economy, and performance. *Journal of Applied Physiology* **63**, 1236–1245.

Williams, K.R., Cavanagh, P.R. & Ziff, J.L. (1987) Biomechanical studies of elite female distance runners. *International Journal of Sports Medicine* **8**, 107–118.

Wilson, G.J., Wood, G.A. & Elliott, B.C. (1991) Optimal stiffness of series elastic component in a stretch–shorten cycle activity. *Journal of Applied Physiology* **70**, 825–833.

Wilson, G.J., Elliott, B.C. & Wood, G.A. (1992) Stretch shorten cycle performance enhancement through flexibility training. *Medicine and Science in Sports and Exercise* **24**, 116–123.

Winter, D.A. (1979) A new definition of mechanical work done in human movement. *Journal of Applied Physiology* **46**, 79–83.

Zupan, M. & Sheperd, T.A. (1988) Physiological responses to Nordic tracking and skating in elite cross-country skiers (abstract). *Medicine and Science in Sports and Exercise* **20**, S81.

Chapter 17

Endurance in Hot and Cold Environments

GARY W. MACK AND ETHAN R. NADEL

Introduction

Athletic performance in an endurance event may be limited by an inability to generate energy at a sufficient rate to meet the energy requirements of contracting skeletal muscles. We typically define this scenario as fatigue. However, it is clear that the fatigue that develops during maximal voluntary muscle contraction differs from that which develops during prolonged exercise in a hot or cold environment. The aetiology of fatigue during prolonged exercise in hot or cold environments is more complex and reflects the impact of changes in body temperature on energy balance and cellular function, especially on cells within the central nervous system. This chapter describes the impact of hot and cold environmental conditions on the physiology of exercise and the contribution of these environments to an early onset of fatigue that limits endurance performance.

One definition of fatigue during prolonged exercise (for example, loss of pace during a marathon race) is that the metabolic cost of maintaining a constant pace becomes greater than that which can be sustained entirely by aerobic metabolism. A consequence is that there is an increased reliance on anaerobic energy production as time progresses. This view of fatigue defines an individual's maximal ability to generate energy aerobically (maximal aerobic power, $\dot{V}_{O_{2max}}$) as:

$$\dot{V}_{O_{2max}} = [HR_{max}] \times [SV_{max}] \times [(a-v)O_{2max}]$$

where $\dot{V}_{O_{2max}}$ = maximal aerobic power (ml $O_2 \cdot min^{-1}$); HR_{max} = maximal heart rate (beats·min^{-1}); SV_{max} = maximal cardiac stroke volume (ml blood·beat^{-1}); and $(a-v)O_{2max}$ = maximal oxygen extraction (ml $O_2 \cdot$ml blood^{-1}).

Any decrease in HR_{max}, SV_{max} or $(a-v)O_{2max}$ during prolonged exercise will reduce maximal aerobic power and will ultimately lead to a decrement in performance. For example, a sequestration of blood volume in peripheral blood vessels below the heart during exercise in the heat will cause a decrease in central blood volume that will limit SV_{max}, and thereby $\dot{V}_{O_{2max}}$. Body heating and/or cooling during exercise will affect the determinants of $\dot{V}_{O_{2max}}$ and thus contribute to an early onset of fatigue. Changes in body temperature during exercise also impact on the development of fatigue through several mechanisms, including an influence on cellular energy metabolism (i.e. altering fuel utilization and thus the rate of lactate production by skeletal muscles), or through a disruption of normal cellular function (i.e. an excessive tissue temperature causing cell damage). Environmental temperature is linked to endurance performance through its impact on body temperature. Thus, in the following pages, we provide a brief explanation of temperature regulation and heat exchange during exercise and their impact on performance.

The physiology of temperature regulation

Humans and other homeothermic animals maintain body core temperature through a balance of heat production and heat loss, using a number of different physiological processes. These include the metabolic production of heat, the transfer of this heat from the body core to its surface and the physical processes of heat transfer from the body surface to the surrounding environment. The overall concept can be summarized by a simple heat balance equation that states:

Heat production		Heat losses			Heat storage
$(M-W)$	$=$	$\pm R$	$\pm C$	$+E$	$\pm S$

where M is metabolism, W is external work, R is radiation, C is convection, E is evaporation and S is storage.

Heat production represents the free energy released during the metabolism of fuels such as carbohydrates, proteins, fats and alcohol. At rest, the rate of heat production is about the same as that generated by a normal 60 W light bulb. Heat production may be augmented by an increase in metabolism, especially in skeletal muscle. This is illustrated by the augmented metabolic rate seen during increased rates of muscle contraction associated with exercise or shivering. During exercise, the rate of oxidation of fuels in skeletal muscle increases dramatically, in order to provide the energy necessary for the processes of contraction and relaxation. The rate of oxygen consumption by skeletal muscle can increase from about $1.5\,\text{ml}\,O_2 \cdot \text{min}^{-1} \cdot \text{kg}^{-1}$ in the resting state to as much as $150\,\text{ml}\,O_2 \cdot \text{min}^{-1} \cdot \text{kg}^{-1}$ during heavy exercise. During moderately intense exercise, the rate of heat production may exceed 1000 W. Such high levels of metabolic heat production can be maintained throughout prolonged activity, such as a marathon run. The metabolic response to cold exposure includes shivering. Shivering thermogenesis may reach levels of 500–700 W. The maximal level of shivering thermogenesis is determined by several factors, including an individual's maximal aerobic capacity and total muscle mass (Toner & McArdle 1996).

The majority of the heat generated within the human body must be convected from the inner core to the skin's surface via the circulation. Local blood flow and the temperature difference between the delivered blood and the muscle primarily govern the transfer of heat from the skeletal muscle to the core (see also Chapters 7 & 8). At rest, arterial blood temperature is about 37°C and muscle temperature

is between 33 and 35°C. Heat flows down a temperature gradient. Resting heat transfer is low, because of low blood flow, and its direction is from arterial blood to the muscle. During the early stages of exercise the temperature gradient between arterial blood and muscle reverses and local blood flow increases. Thus, this convective process removes heat from the muscle and transfers it to the body core. The blood is then directed towards the skin, where heat can be transferred to the environment by one of several mechanisms. A hallmark response of the human thermoregulatory system is its enormous ability to increase blood flow to the skin.

The second stage in the process involves the transfer of heat from the skin surface to the environment. Figure 17.1 illustrates the routes of heat transfer from the body core to the environment and important factors that determine transfer rates. Heat is transferred from the skin to the environment by convection, radiation and evaporation. The rates of heat transfer from the skin to the environment by convection and radiation are functions of the heat transfer coefficients (h_c and h_r) and temperature differences between the skin and the environment; these rates of transfer are under physiological control only in so far as the changes in skin blood flow determine changes in the average skin temperature. Both h_r and h_c depend on the body surface area available for exchange with the environment. The value of h_r is constant, but the value of h_c varies directly with the air or water velocity (Nishi & Gagge 1970) and differs dramatically between air and water environments (Rapp 1971; Nadel et al. 1974a). The combined coefficient can vary five-fold between resting conditions in still air and when running or cycling on a breezy day, and the rate of heat transfer by convection varies accordingly. However, on a very hot day, when the difference between skin and ambient temperature is small, the ability to transfer heat from the skin to the environment is likewise small and of minimal importance in dissipating the thermal load imposed by vigorous exercise.

During exposure to ambient temperatures > 20°C, the primary avenue of heat loss is the evaporation of sweat. The efficiency of the evaporative route of heat transfer depends on both physiological and

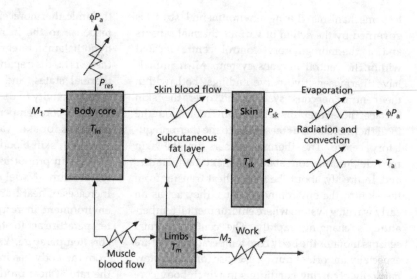

Fig. 17.1 Routes of heat transfer from the body core to the environment and the important factors that determine transfer rates. M, metabolic rate (M_1, at rest; M_2, during exercise); P, pressure; T, temperature.

environmental factors. The rate of evaporation depends upon the evaporative heat transfer coefficient and the partial pressure gradient of water vapour between skin and the environment. Air movement influences the heat transfer coefficient, and heat transfer is enhanced by increased wind speed. The water vapour pressure at the skin is a function of sweating rate and is therefore under physiological control. Each gram of water evaporated from the skin surface removes about 2.5 kJ of energy from the body. The sweat glands of a physically fit individual can deliver sweat to the skin surface at a rate of 30 g·min^{-1}, so nearly all of the heat produced during heavy exercise could be dissipated by evaporation under ideal conditions. If the environmental humidity is high, the skin-to-environment water vapour pressure gradient cannot be increased to any great extent and the evaporative rate will be low. This explains why excessive heat storage becomes inevitable during prolonged exercise on a hot, humid day.

During exercise on a cool day (ambient temperature < 20°C) the rate of heat production is still sufficiently great to cause body core temperature to rise and the potential problem remains the risk of hyperthermia rather than hypothermia. The main environment that presents a cold stress during prolonged exercise, and therefore a legitimate risk of hypothermia, is water. During water immersion the radiative and evaporative components of heat loss are minimal and heat transfer occurs primarily by convective mechanisms. Because of its thermal properties, water has a much greater heat transfer coefficient than air, and it also provides practically no insulation at its interface with the skin surface. Thus, the heat that reaches the skin surface from the body core is transferred rapidly to the water and skin temperature rapidly approaches that of water temperature. As in an air environment, the heat flux from the body surface is a function of both the heat transfer coefficient and the skin-to-environment temperature gradient. Thus, the actual rate of heat flow from the body core to the water can only be minimized if the resistance to heat flow from the core to the skin surface is large. This can be accomplished by maximal constriction of the skin vasculature, an autonomic response to body cooling. Protection is more effective in fat than in thin individuals, because fat is relatively underperfused and has a thermal conductivity about a half that of muscle and a third that of blood. Thus, the relative thickness of the subcutaneous fat layer is the primary determinant of heat flow from the body to the water. Keatinge (1960) recognized this years ago and his view has been confirmed in subsequent studies involving submaximal swimming (Holmér & Bergh 1974).

Physiological control of heat production and heat

loss mechanisms during environmental stress is governed by the action of various thermal sensors and a thermoregulatory control centre located within the central nervous system. All mammals have thermosensitive nerve endings, both within the central nervous system and over the skin surface; these receptors relay information about the local thermal status at these sites to the thermoregulatory centre. The thermal sensors on the skin provide information about ambient temperature and, indirectly, about the rate of heat transfer from the skin to the environment. Thus, they act as an early warning system where environmental temperature is changing rapidly. The central thermal sensors monitor the body core temperature; they are especially important during exercise (one of the few naturally occurring conditions in which body core temperature is driven upward) and during immersion in cold water (one of the few naturally occurring conditions in which body core temperature is driven downward).

The primary organs that enable humans to control the rates of heat transfer from the body core to the environment are the smooth muscles of the arterioles in the skin blood vessels and the sweat glands. Skin blood vessels control heat conductance from the core to the skin and sweat glands secrete an ultrafiltrate of plasma onto the skin surface, thereby providing a substrate for evaporative cooling of the skin. In cases of body cooling, skeletal muscles can produce heat above that generated by basal metabolism by undergoing involuntary shivering contractions.

The central nervous system centre that integrates temperature regulation lies in the preoptic anterior hypothalamus. This centre constantly evaluates sensory information from peripheral and central thermal sensors, comparing this information with an idealized thermal state. In conditions when these differ, the thermoregulatory centre induces changes in physiological activity that modify heat transfer and act to restore the ideal thermal state.

With this background, it becomes easy to describe the thermoregulatory events that occur during exercise. As heat is transferred from the contracting muscles to the body core during the first minutes of exercise, body core temperature rises and the hypo-thalamic thermoreceptors increase their activity in response to the increased local temperature. The hypothalamic integration centre determines that there is a discrepancy between actual and ideal thermal states, and it increases efferent nervous system activity to the organs of heat dissipation. As the body core temperature rises, the threshold temperatures for skin vasodilatation and sweating are exceeded; skin blood flow and sweating rates then increase in proportion to the increase in body core temperature (Nadel *et al.* 1971; Wenger *et al.* 1975). Increases of heat transfer from the body core to the environment in response to the rising body core temperature act to attenuate the rate of rise in body core temperature. When the rate of heat transfer from the body has increased sufficiently to balance the rate of heat production in the body, the rate of heat storage becomes zero. The body core temperature remains elevated at this new steady-state level until some further perturbation occurs. These events are depicted in Fig. 17.2 and are described in more detail by Stitt (1979).

The new steady-state body core temperature is not regulated at its elevated level, but has merely attained that elevated level as a consequence of: (i) a temporary imbalance between the rates of heat production in the body and heat dissipation from the body; and (ii) a lag in the heat dissipation response to the increase in body core temperature. Physical training increases the sensitivity of the sweating rate–internal temperature relationship and decreases the internal temperature threshold for sweating (Nadel *et al.* 1974b); it thus allows the attainment of a new, steady state at a lower internal temperature than when in the untrained state. This offers a somewhat greater margin of safety between operating and limiting temperatures, as well as placing a lower demand on the peripheral circulation during exercise.

Exercise in the heat

The ability to deliver an adequate blood flow to the contracting skeletal muscles and to the skin under conditions when both require a high flow rate, such as during prolonged heavy exercise in a warm or humid environment, depends largely on the body's

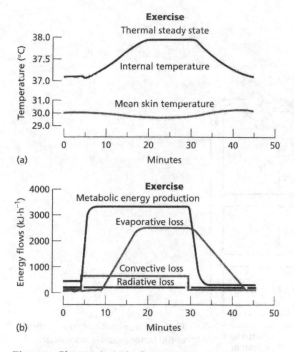

Fig. 17.2 Changes in (a) body temperature and (b) energy (heat) flows during exercise. A thermal steady state occurs when the rate of heat loss balances the rate of heat production. The absolute rise in internal temperature depends on the 'quickness' of the heat loss response.

ability to maintain an adequate central blood volume; this provides for the maintenance of an adequate cardiac filling pressure and stroke volume. During mild-intensity exercise or during exercise in a cool environment, the heart has no difficulty in providing an adequate output to meet the demands of both muscle and skin (Rowell *et al.* 1966; Nadel *et al.* 1979). The muscle blood flow requirement remains relatively low and the heart meets the combined demand easily. In a cool environment, the demand of the thermoregulatory system for blood flow to the skin is modest, and again the heart easily meets the combined blood flow requirement. However, during moderately heavy exercise in a warm environment, the combined demands from skin and muscle are great and the ability of the heart to meet these demands becomes increasingly compromised. The increased skin blood flow is accompanied by an increased blood volume in the capacious skin veins below the level of the heart;

this reduces the central blood volume, the cardiac filling pressure and therefore the cardiac stroke volume. The effect is magnified when the internal temperature is high (Fig. 17.3). Although the muscle pump serves to aid the return of blood to the heart in such circumstances, the first reflex line of defence against a falling central venous pressure appears to be an increase in forearm vascular resistance (Johnson *et al.* 1974; Tripathi *et al.* 1989), which serves to reduce the volume of blood in the dependent veins. The regulated arterial pressure decreases when the uncompensated fall in central venous pressure becomes even greater; cardioacceleration occurs and thus compensates for the decrease in cardiac stroke volume, restoring cardiac output and arterial blood pressure if exercise is conducted in the semirecumbent position (Nadel *et al.* 1979), but not in the upright position (when the hydrostatic pressure head is greater (Rowell *et al.* 1966)). In the upright position, when the effects of gravity on a dilated cutaneous circulation are greatest, a heart rate increase of 20 beats·min^{-1} is insufficient to compensate for the decreased cardiac stroke volume; the cardiac output is about 1.5 l·min^{-1} less during heavy exercise in the heat than during comparable exercise in a cool environment (Rowell *et al.* 1966), despite a major redistribution of blood flow away from relatively inactive organs (Rowell *et al.* 1965). The maximal cardiac stroke volume is also likely to be decreased in these circumstances (Rowell 1983), and thus $\dot{V}_{O_{2max}}$ and performance should be reduced by an equivalent proportion.

Prolonged exercise in the heat presents the body with a more complex problem. Not only is the ability to maintain an adequate cardiac stroke volume threatened by the displacement of a portion of the blood volume towards the periphery, but the continuous loss of body water due to sweat production decreases the body water content, including the water content of the intravascular compartment. Under such conditions, a relative restriction of cutaneous blood flow develops (Mack *et al.* 1988; Mack 1998), presumably in response to a low-pressure stimulus on the filling side of the heart. The progressive fall in cardiac stroke volume ceases at the point of relative vasoconstriction in the skin (Nadel *et al.*

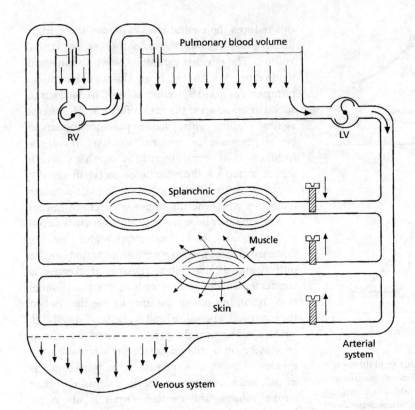

Pulmonary blood volume

RV

LV

Splanchnic

Muscle

Skin

Arterial
system

Venous system

Fig. 17.3 Schematic representation of the factors associated with the pooling of blood in veins below heart level. LV, left ventricle; RV, right ventricle.

1979). The consequence of a relative restriction in skin blood flow is that an optimal rate of heat transfer can no longer occur. In our 1979 study, the exercising volunteer subjects continued to store heat at a rate of 0.1°C per minute, a storage that would limit exercise due to hyperthermia if continued for more than a few minutes.

The more serious effects of prolonged exercise in the heat are due to the progressive hypovolaemia that accompanies dehydration. In actuality, the intravascular fluid compartment is defended reasonably well during dehydration, since the hyperosmolality that develops as water leaves the vascular compartment tends to draw water into the vessels from the interstitial and intracellular fluid compartments (Nose *et al.* 1988). None the less, hypovolaemia induces an upward shift in the internal temperature threshold for cutaneous vasodilatation and reduces the maximal cutaneous blood flow (Nadel *et al.* 1980); these responses increase the operating temperature, due to a reduction in the maximal rate of heat transfer from the body

core to the skin. These changes combined with the lower maximal cardiac stroke volume due to the lower central blood volume are likely to reduce $\dot{V}_{O_{2max}}$ and the ability to prolong exercise at a high intensity.

The question whether blood flow to the active skeletal muscles can be maintained at appropriate rates during prolonged exercise in the heat remains open. If muscle blood flow is compromised, the rate of delivery of fuels and oxygen may become inadequate to meet the muscle's requirements, and fatigue will occur. Brown *et al.* (1982) claimed, from measurements of the relative rates of blood lactate accumulation during intense exercise in cool and hot conditions, that muscle blood flow might be lower in the heat. This confirmed observations of lower muscle blood flow in sheep exercising in the heat compared with responses in cool conditions (Bell *et al.* 1983). However, as noted above (Rowell *et al.* 1965), hepatic blood flow becomes progressively reduced during exercise in the heat and a reduced clearance of lactate by the liver rather than greater muscle lactate production may explain its more rapid rate of accumulation. Savard *et al.* (1988) reported that muscle blood flow was not reduced during exercise in the heat. They induced a heat load by using a water-perfused suit to clamp skin temperature at an artificially high level. Although it is not yet clear to what extent the decrease in cardiac output during upright, submaximal exercise in the heat (Rowell *et al.* 1966) is reflected by a reduction in muscle blood flow, it is clear that the onset of fatigue occurs earlier.

Is there an upper critical level of body temperature that limits endurance performance? Limitations to exercise performance during heat stress can be related to perceived 'discomfort' in three general categories: circulatory, muscle and thermal. Circulatory discomfort has been clearly outlined in the earlier portion of this chapter. It relates to the impact of heat on the determinants of maximal aerobic capacity. A volume of literature is accumulating that indicates an influence of tissue temperature on energy metabolism. Specifically, muscle discomfort may arise during exercise in the heat due to a faster rate of muscle glycogen depletion and a faster rise in plasma lactate concentration. In addition, as muscle temperature rises above 40.5°C the motor nerve excitation needed to produce a given force is increased. A high skin or body core temperature can generate thermal discomfort and impact performance. Rectal temperatures in the range of 38.9–41.7°C have been reported for marathon runners who successfully finished races without developing a heat-related illness (Adams *et al.* 1975; Maron *et al.* 1977). Higher values have been reported for competitive events involving running or cycling (rectal temperature > 42°C), but these cases were associated with circulatory collapse and heat exhaustion. In controlled laboratory studies, MacDougall *et al.* (1974) showed that the treadmill run time to exhaustion was shorter with added heat stress (higher skin temperature), but that running was terminated at about the same rectal temperature (an average of 39.4°C with a range of 38.8–40.3°C). Over a range of environmental temperatures from 10 to 30°C (excluding high humidity conditions) the rise in body core temperature depends primarily on exercise intensity, with little influence from ambient temperature (Saltin *et al.* 1968). Nielsen *et al.* (1993) showed that endurance capacity increased following heat acclimatization when heat-dissipating mechanisms were enhanced. Heat acclimatization reduced the rate of rise in body core temperature, but exhaustion before and after acclimatization corresponded to the same body core temperature (about 39.7°C). Animal studies have defined a body core temperature of around 40.4°C as the threshold temperature for developing risk of heatstroke. The integrated time–body temperature relationship above this threshold provides an index for predicting morbidity and mortality during hyperthermia. As body core temperature exceeds 39.2°C, strain on the human body becomes considerable. The observation that some athletes can complete the final 10 km of a marathon with core temperatures of around 41.7°C suggests that the upper temperature limit must vary, based upon an individual's level of physical fitness or state of heat acclimatization.

Exercise in the cold

As mentioned earlier, cold ambient conditions are not usually an issue in so far as exercise performance or fatigue is concerned. The one environment that presents an overall cold stress during exercise is water. To evaluate the driving force for heat loss to the water and the difference in this drive between resting and exercising conditions, Nadel *et al.* (1974a) made measurements of heat flow and skin temperature while immersed and during swimming. The heat transfer coefficient from the skin to the water was increased three-fold during swimming (independently of the swimming speed, to our surprise). Absolute values were close to those predicted from theoretical analyses (Rapp 1971) and copper manikin studies (Witherspoon *et al.* 1971). In fact, exercise in cold water may contribute to a drop in rectal temperature due to the impact of body movement on the rate of heat loss. However, knowledge of the heat transfer coefficient does not allow prediction of the rate of development of hypothermia. The latter depends on the product of the transfer coefficient (elevated during swimming) and the skin-to-water temperature gradient (narrowed during swimming), as well as the rate of heat production (elevated during swimming) and the core-to-skin heat conductance (also elevated during swimming). Thus, for any given individual there is a water temperature at which the heat conserved via insulation and circulatory adjustments and the heat generated by exercise do not offset the heat transfer in cold water and, in this situation, hypothermia develops.

Primary hypothermia occurs when the environmental conditions overwhelm the normal thermoregulatory mechanisms and core temperature decreases. As body core temperature decreases, alterations in physiological function will eventually limit performance. Bergh and Ekblom (1979) showed that body cooling in water was accompanied by a decline of peak aerobic power and $\dot{V}_{O_{2max}}$. The impact of hypothermia on physiological function is graded with the decrease in body core temperature. A decrease in tissue temperature (such as muscle) and a general decrease in body core temperature cause central nervous system dysfunction and impair skeletal muscle excitation–contraction coupling. For example, at a body core temperature of 34–35°C, muscle coordination is impaired and individuals report feeling tired and apathetic (Pozos et al. 1996). Thus, one might suggest that a core temperature of 35°C represents a critical lower limit of body core temperature that should be avoided in order that eventual decrements in performance do not occur. If we look at cold water endurance events we see that channel swimmers have reported rectal temperatures of 34–38.3°C during prolonged (≈18h) exposure to water as cold as 16°C (Pugh

et al. 1960). Thus, some individual variation in the lower critical temperature must exist, similar to that seen with the highest tolerable body core temperature. A decrease in performance in hypothermic athletes is the consequence of several factors, including an increased viscosity of skeletal muscle (requiring greater forces to overcome), an increased resistance to maximal blood flow (reducing maximal oxygen delivery) and a reduced maximal nerve conduction velocity (limiting the ability to transmit signals for repeated contractions).

Conclusions

The environment places many limits on the ability to perform an endurance task. This chapter describes the limits imposed by thermal characteristics. Limits imposed by clothing have not been discussed; clothing imposes a barrier to optimal convective and evaporative cooling in a warm environment and offers insulation against excessive convective and evaporative cooling in a cold environment. The effects of hyperthermia and hypothermia on performance generally occur via their direct impact on cellular function and indirectly via their influence on the body's ability to transfer oxygen from the environment to the contracting skeletal muscles. Excessive body heating during exercise reduces the effectiveness of the circulatory system by limiting the heart's ability to deliver blood flow at the required rates to skin and muscle. Excessive body cooling during exercise is much more unusual than excessive heating, but is a real risk during exercise in water.

References

Adams, W.C., Fox, R.H., Fry, A.J. & MacDonnald, I.C. (1975) Thermoregulation during marathon running in cool, moderate, and hot environments. *Journal of Applied Physiology* **38**, 1030–1037.

Bell, A.W., Hales, J.R.S., King, R.B. & Fawcett, A.A. (1983) Influence of heat stress on exercise-induced changes in regional blood flow in sheep. *Journal of Applied Physiology* **55**, 1916–1923.

Bergh, U. & Ekblom, B. (1979) Physical performance and peak aerobic power at dif-

ferent body temperatures. *Journal of Applied Physiology* **46**, 885–889.

Brown, N.J., Stephenson, L.A., Lister, G.L. & Nadel, E.R. (1982) Relative anaerobiosis during heavy exercise in the heat. *Federation Proceedings* **41**, 1677.

Holmér, I. & Bergh, U. (1974) Metabolic and thermal response to swimming in water at varying temperatures. *Journal of Applied Physiology* **37**, 702–705.

Johnson, J.M., Rowell, L.B., Niederberger, M. & Eisman, M.M. (1974) Human splanchnic and forearm vasoconstrictor

responses to reductions of right atrial and aortic pressures. *Circulation Research* **34**, 515–524.

Keatinge, W.R. (1960) The effects of subcutaneous fat and of previous exposure to cold on the body temperature, peripheral blood flow and metabolic rate of men in cold water. *Journal of Physiology (London)* **153**, 166–178.

MacDougall, J.D., Reddan, W.G., Layton, C.R. & Dempsey, J.A. (1974) Effects of metabolic hyperthermia on performance during heavy prolonged exercise.

Journal of Applied Physiology **36**, 538–544.

Mack, G.W. (1998) Baroreceptor modulation of thermoregulatory function in humans. In: Nose, H., Nadel, E.R. & Morimoto, T. (eds) *The 1997 Nagano Symposium of Sports Sciences*, pp. 297–305. Cooper Publishing Group, Carmel, IN.

Mack, G., Nose, H. & Nadel, E.R. (1988) Role of cardiopulmonary baroreflexes during dynamic exercise. *Journal of Applied Physiology* **65** (4), 1827–1832.

Maron, M.B., Wagner, J.A. & Horvath, S.M. (1977) Thermoregulatory responses during competitive marathon running. *Journal of Applied Physiology* **42**, 909–914.

Nadel, E.R., Bullard, R.W. & Stolwijk, J.A.J. (1971) Importance of skin temperature in the regulation of sweating. *Journal of Applied Physiology* **31**, 80–87.

Nadel, E.R., Holmer, I., Bergh, U., Astrand, P.-O. & Stolwijk, J.A.J. (1974a) Energy exchanges of swimming man. *Journal of Applied Physiology* **36**, 465–471.

Nadel, E.R., Pandolf, K.B., Roberts, M.F., Wenger, C.B. & Stolwijk, J.A.J. (1974b) Mechanisms of thermal adaptation to exercise and heat. *Journal of Applied Physiology* **37**, 515–520.

Nadel, E.R., Cafarelli, E., Roberts, M.F. & Wenger, C.B. (1979) Circulatory regulation during exercise in different ambient temperatures. *Journal of Applied Physiology* **46**, 430–437.

Nadel, E.R., Fortney, S.M. & Wenger, C.B. (1980) Effect of hydration state on circulatory and thermal regulations. *Journal of Applied Physiology* **49**, 715–721.

Nielsen, B., Hales, J.R., Strange, S., Christensen, N.J., Warberg, J. & Saltin, B. (1993) Human circulatory and thermoregulatory adaptations with heat acclimation and exercise in a hot, dry environment. *Journal of Physiology (London)* **460**, 467–485.

Nishi, Y. & Gagge, A.P. (1970) Direct evaluation of convective heat transfer coefficient by naphthalene sublimation. *Journal of Applied Physiology* **29**, 603–609.

Nose, H., Mack, G.W., Shi, X. & Nadel, E.R. (1988) Role of osmolality and plasma, during rehydration in humans. *Journal of Applied Physiology* **65**, 325–331.

Pozos, R.S., Iaizzo, P.A., Danzl, D.F. & Mills, W.T.J. (1996) Limits of tolerance to hypothermia. In: Fregly, M.J. & Blatteis, C.M. (eds) *Handbook of Physiology*, Vol 1. *Environmental Physiology*, pp. 557–578. Oxford University Press, New York.

Pugh, L.G.C.E., Edholm, O.G., Fox, R.H. *et al.* (1960) A physiological study of channel swimming. *Clinical Science* **19**, 257–273.

Rapp, G.M. (1971) Convection coefficients of man in a forensic area of thermal physiology. *Journal of Physiology (Paris)* **63**, 392–396.

Rowell, L.B. (1983) Cardiovascular adjustments to thermal stress. In: Shepherd, J.M. & Abboud, F.M. (eds) *Handbook of Physiology: the Cardiovascular System III*, pp. 967–1023. The American Physiological Society, Bethesda, MD.

Rowell, L.B., Blackmon, J.R., Martin, R.H., Mazzarella, J.A. & Bruce, R.A. (1965) Hepatic clearances of indocyanine green in man under thermal and exercise stresses. *Journal of Applied Physiology* **20**, 384–394.

Rowell, L.B., Marks, H.J., Bruce, R.A., Conn, R.D. & Kusumi, F. (1966) Reductions in cardiac output, central blood volume and stroke, with thermal stress in normal men during exercise. *Journal of Clinical Investigation* **43**, 1801–1816.

Saltin, B., Gagge, A.P. & Stolwijk, J.A.J. (1968) Muscle temperature during submaximal exercise in man. *Journal of Applied Physiology* **25**, 679–688.

Savard, G.K., Nielsen, B., Laszczynska, I., Larsen, B.E. & Saltin, B. (1988) Muscle blood flow is not reduced in humans during moderate exercise and heat stress. *Journal of Applied Physiology* **64**, 649–657.

Stitt, J.T. (1979) Fever versus hyperthermia. *Federation Proceedings* **38**, 39–43.

Toner, M.M. & McArdle, W.D. (1996) Human thermoregulatory responses to acute cold stress with special reference to water. In: Fregly, M.J. & Blatteis, C.M. (eds) *Handbook of Physiology*, Vol. 1. *Environmental Physiology*, pp. 379–398. Oxford University Press, New York.

Tripathi, A., Mack, G.W. & Nadel, E.R. (1989) Peripheral vascular reflexes elicited during lower body negative pressure. *Aviation, Space and Environmental Medicine* **60**, 1187–1193.

Wenger, C.B., Roberts, M.F., Stolwijk, J.A.J. & Nadel, E.R. (1975) Forearm blood flow during body temperature transients produced by leg exercise. *Journal of Applied Physiology* **38**, 58–63.

Witherspoon, J.M., Goldman, R.F. & Breckenridge, J.R. (1971) Heat transfer coefficients of humans in cold water. *Journal of Physiology (Paris)* **63**, 459–462.

PART 3

MEASUREMENTS IN ENDURANCE SPORT

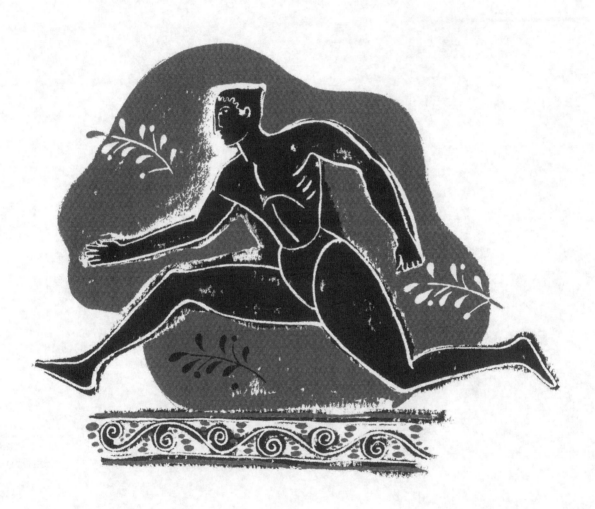

Chapter 18

Factors to be Measured

PER-OLOF ÅSTRAND

Competitive sport is the classical test of physical fitness and performance. Under such conditions the performance may be measured objectively in metres and centimetres, and in time down to hundredths of seconds in some events. In sport shooting, there is the point system. In gymnastics, figure skating and diving, the skill is judged subjectively. From a scientific point of view we have the inevitable question: why does one athlete perform better than others in one particular type of competition? Figure 18.1 presents a simple effort to break down an analysis of physical performance into some basic components. If, without exception, élite athletes in one event have a high maximal oxygen intake, the event is apparently very demanding aerobically; that is the case in rowers, for whom the oxygen intake in litres per minute is critical. In events such as middle- and long-distance running, the aerobic power, expressed in $ml\,kg^{-1}\,min^{-1}$ (or $ml\,kg^{-0.75}\cdot min^{-0.75}$; the most relevant exponent is so far not known), must be high. In endurance events, aerobic processes dominate. Figure 18.2 is an effort to summarize the factors that should be considered when analysing the aerobic demands of various events and the individual's potential to perform well. There are precise methods of measuring the aerobic power, because for each litre of oxygen consumed in the cells about 20 kJ is yielded for the resynthesis of adenosine triphosphate (ATP) (range 19.7–21.2 kJ, depending on the relative proportions of carbohydrate and free fatty acids that are metabolized). Unfortunately, we have no good methods for quantifying anaerobic power accurately. However, this is not a dramatic handicap when endurance is being considered.

Most of the measurements related to physiological and behavioural aspects of sports are made under standardized conditions in laboratories. Under field conditions, measurements can be very difficult, and sophisticated studies are more or less impossible to carry out during important competitions. Therefore, the question is to what extent can we extrapolate our knowledge from laboratory studies to field conditions? Is there a risk that we generalize too much? There is a specificity in the human response to a particular exercise and in the effects of training. For example, two identical twins were top swimmers, but one of the sisters gave up training. Some years later their maximal oxygen intakes were measured both when they were running on a treadmill and when they were swimming in a flume. On that occasion they both were students in physical education and were well trained. The sister who also undertook intensive swimming training attained the same maximal aerobic power when running as when swimming, $3.6\,l\,min^{-1}$. Her sister, now not swim-trained, reached a similar maximum when running, $3.6\,l\,min^{-1}$ but achieved only $2.8\,l\,min^{-1}$ when swimming (Holmér & Åstrand 1972). Unfortunately, we cannot explain the nature of the specificity of training. We have access to telemetric systems to transmit signals triggered by heart rate, blood pressure and muscle activity which do not bother subjects. There are efforts to construct lightweight equipment to follow pulmonary ventilation and oxygen intake under field conditions (Chapter 19), but inevitably the subject becomes restricted. For analyses of blood and muscle specimens we must 'go under the skin', which sometimes worries athletes. Cycle ergometers and treadmills have now been supplemented by

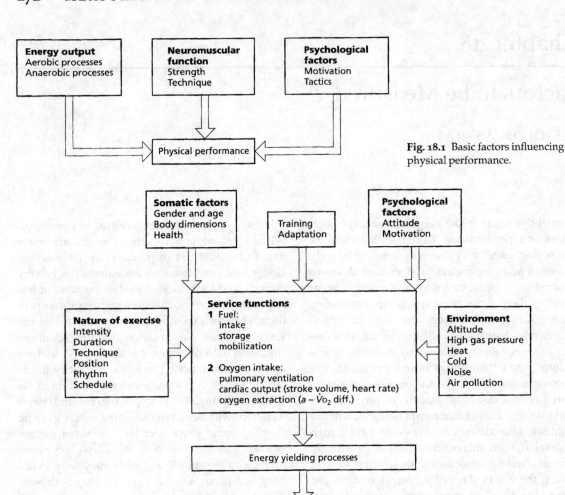

Fig. 18.1 Basic factors influencing physical performance.

Fig. 18.2 Factors influencing the power and capacity for aerobic muscular activity. From Åstrand and Rodahl (1986), with permission.

equipment for simulated rowing, canoeing, swimming and skiing (see Chapter 19). Computerized methods have been developed for the study of locomotion and body composition.

There is a danger in using equipment that produces printed data because of the tendency to believe in figures obtained from computers. For example, undue reliance is placed on sophisticated (but at times inaccurate) methods available for the measurement of oxygen intake. Of key importance for reliability is calibration of the apparatus. Too many laboratory workers have forgotten how to analyse a gas chemically, using a Haldane or a Scholander apparatus.

References

Åstrand, P.-O. & Rodahl, K. (1986) *Textbook of Work Physiology*. McGraw-Hill, New York.

Holmér, I. & Åstrand, P.-O. (1972) Swimming training and maximal oxygen uptake. *Journal of Applied Physiology* 33, 510–513.

Chapter 19

Sport-Specific Testing in Laboratory and Field

ANTONIO DAL MONTE, MARCELLO FAINA AND GIOVANNI MIRRI

To reach high-level performance in sport it is not sufficient to have genetically suited athletes; it is also essential that natural talent is appropriately enhanced through an adequate training process. In fact, the evolution of sport performance observed in the last half century has essentially been determined by physiological and biomechanical changes, including central and peripheral adaptations induced by severe, and particularly by specific, training programmes.

This hypothesis has been confirmed by several authors (Holmér *et al.* 1974; Tesch & Karlsson 1985; Pelliccia *et al.* 1991). To quote one of the most significant pieces of research on this topic, Holmér and Åstrand (1972) studied two female homozygotic twins, only one of whom had undertaken specific training in swimming. The results of the study were as follows.
- Both girls had an identical oxygen intake in a maximal treadmill test.
- The girl swimmer was able to reach an oxygen intake that was a little higher than her twin in a swimming test in which the propulsive action was produced by only the lower limbs.
- The girl swimmer achieved double the oxygen intake of her sister when both girls underwent a maximal test in which only the upper limbs produced the propulsive effort.

The acquisition of appropriate laboratory data is more and more important in order to verify the specificity of the functional adaptation attained by athletes, relative to the different sport disciplines to be performed. This in turn implies a need for more specific and more sophisticated methodology. Such tests are essential in order to monitor the effect of a specific training programme longitudinally, and to verify whether the results eventually obtained approach the predetermined targets.

The development of a more specific and precise method of evaluating the longitudinal adaptations induced by highly specific sport and training is one aspect of the research activity that has been carried out for the last 30 years by the Physiology and Biomechanics Department of the Institute of Sports Science (ISS) of the Italian National Olympic Committee. This institute also applies specific testing in cross-sectional studies, in order to assess the 'specific model of the athletes excelling in each sport'. To succeed in this task, two fundamental branches of research have been followed:
1 the development of specific ergometers; and
2 the devising, designing, realization and testing of highly sophisticated systems for measuring the physiological and biomechanical characteristics of athletes directly in the field.

Definition of specific ergometry

By sport-specific ergometry (Dal Monte 1975, 1989; Dal Monte & Lupo 1989; Dal Monte *et al.* 1996), we imply a multidisciplinary science-based evaluation of the athlete in conditions that simulate, as closely as possible, a competition or phases of training similar to competitions. In particular, the following parameters must be considered.
- The type of sport.
- The spatial position of the athlete's body.

• The frequency of movement used during the competition.

• The duration of testing in order to simulate the energy sources used by the athlete in her or his performance.

• The kinds of stress that the athlete will experience during competition.

The first prototypes of specific ergometers were constructed by the ISS about 30 years ago. Some of these ergometers are unique designs and are able to reproduce almost exactly the typical movements of athletes during competition.

Types of ergometer

Among the ergometers currently used in the ISS laboratory are treadmills, cycle ergometers, kayak ergometers, ergometers for the Canadian canoe and an ergometer pool (high-speed flume) for the testing of competitors in aquatic sports (swimming, swimming with flippers, wind-surfing, canoeing and diving activities).

The treadmill is used to evaluate athletic disciplines connected with running or speed walking (500–10000-m events, marathon runs, etc.). The cycle ergometer is used almost exclusively for the evaluation of cyclists; the aim is to study the limits of strength, power and endurance shown by the

cyclist when using her or his typical movement patterns.

In order to simulate the kayak canoeing movement, several ergometers were produced, but in this chapter we will describe only two of them. The first (Fig. 19.1) is the most recent in a series of specific ergometers designed to be utilized only by kayakers. The second, which has an isokinetic basis, can be utilized for a large variety of movements; it will be described later. The specific kayak ergometer is based on a metal frame with a fixed central shaft, from which originates a pair of angled simulated paddles. The height of the central shaft can be varied through an electric mechanism; in addition, the seat is sliding, as is the footrest, in order to adapt the equipment to all sizes of athlete. Resistance is offered by an electromagnetic brake, able to measure efforts up to 900 W: the power developed is independent of the speed of operation (revolutions per minute, r.p.m.), which can vary between 40 and 140 r.p.m. In front of the athlete, there is quite a complex digital display, able to monitor such parameters as r.p.m., power developed, heart rate, duration of test and the simulated distance covered. The system is interfaced with a personal computer integrated with a dedicated software system. Kayakers can be evaluated in a more sophisticated way using the Dalmex 240 apparatus, described in the section

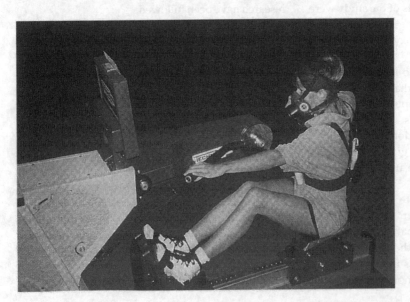

Fig. 19.1 Ergometer for kayak canoe, designed and used at the Department of Physiology and Biomechanics of the Institute of Sports Science of the Italian National Olympic Committee (CONI), in Rome.

on isokinetic equipment. A specific form of ergometer has also been constructed for the Canadian canoe (Fig. 19.2) so that the athlete can maintain the same knee position as when paddling the canoe.

For rowing, different types of ergometer are available. In the Gjessing–Nilsen type (Dal Monte 1983) the support bearing the athlete (footrest and trolley) and the movement pattern reproduce the action of rowing, but the handle is fastened to the edge of a sliding pole and thus can effect only a sagittal or longitudinal movement, whereas in normal rowing the oar moves by rotating in the rowlock. The resistance of the oar during its passage through the water is simulated by means of a brake, linked to a belt rolled around a pulley. The 'Concept II' (Fig. 19.3) is another kind of ergometer; the handle of the paddle is similar to that of the Gjessing–Nilsen design. It is connected to a chain; this actuates a free wheel, shaped in the form of a centrifugal air turbine. The resulting air brake can absorb the energy produced by the athletes when they are tested. In this equipment, there is a seat and a footrest whose kinematic

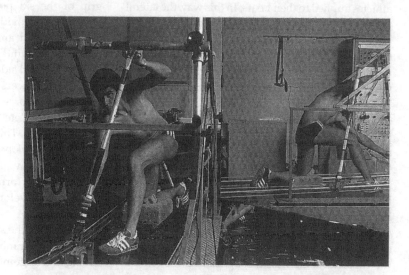

Fig. 19.2 Ergometer for laboratory reproduction of specific kinetics of the Canadian canoe.

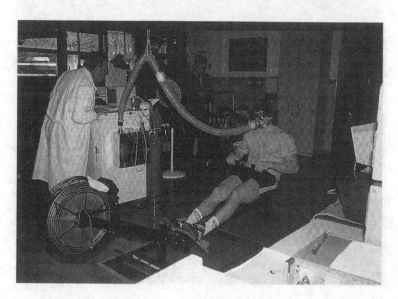

Fig. 19.3 Concept II rowing ergometer.

movement reproduces only the longitudinal movement of the rowing boat. The equipment is linked to a computer, and is able to calculate several parameters relating to the power output and the amount of energy produced by the athletes using scull or oar.

In the rowing ergometers designed by Dal Monte, the aim was to reproduce fully the appropriate kind of boat (scull and oar) movements, including not only longitudinal but also lateral movements, i.e. the rotating action of the upper limbs and, in the case of the oar speciality, the torsion of the trunk that athletes applied to their boats. In this way, the lateral movements of the arms and the torsion of the trunk were mimicked, so that the normal movement of scull or oar was reproduced precisely. The equipment initially included a hydraulic brake in order to measure the efforts of the athletes. The most recent design is based on a special kit able to adapt a type of commercial equipment (Fig. 19.4), the 'Rowrace', produced by Technogym (Italy); originally, this had more or less the same movement pattern as the Gjessing–Nilsen and 'Concept II' ergometers, but the incorporation of more sophisticated equipment has transformed the 'Rowrace' ergometer into a highly specific rowing simulator. As with the previously described hydraulic airbrake ergometer, the equipment became a real simulator because it had the capacity to transform longitudinal movement into the movement pattern performed by the athlete when in a boat. The special leverage adopted in the kit can also reproduce the specific technical act of the actual stroke in the water, in which the first part of the stroke encounters a greater resistance than the last part of the movement.

A specific ergometer has also been constructed for cross-country skiing (Fig. 19.5). This device is installed on a treadmill; the ski poles are placed in two tracks, one on each side of the treadmill belt. The ski poles slide on the tracks, and a linear force-measuring transducer is located close to the hand-grip of the ski pole. During the pushing phase, resistance is provided by a mechanical brake linked to a belt rolled around a pulley. The athlete uses roller-skis mounted in two tracks (each 2 m in length) to avoid sideways deviations during testing. Linear transducers are fitted to the ski bindings to measure the force developed on the skis. During testing, the athlete 'skis' on the inclined treadmill at various speeds. This method allows calculation of:

• the total work performed by the subject in raising her or his body while skiing on the treadmill;
• the work performed by the upper limbs; and
• the force developed by both the upper and lower limbs.

To improve the study of aquatic sport disciplines such as swimming, sailing, wind-surfing and diving, an ergometer pool (Dal Monte 1989) or

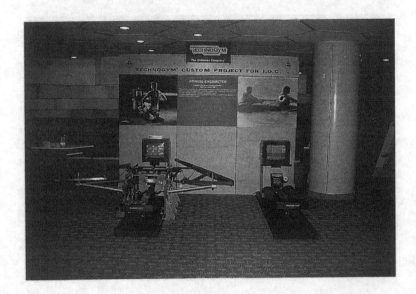

Fig. 19.4 Ergometers to reproduce the specific kinetics of rowing in the laboratory. On the right, the commercial item, on the left the kit to transform it into a real rowing simulator ergometer.

flume was built in our department. Some of the characteristics of this flume are quite original (Fig. 19.6). The water surface of 6.70 × 3 m has a frontal section of 3 m × 1.5 m. The fluid is driven by four propellers, each 0.7 m in diameter, coupled to a 170-kW marine piston engine. A lateral wall of the flume

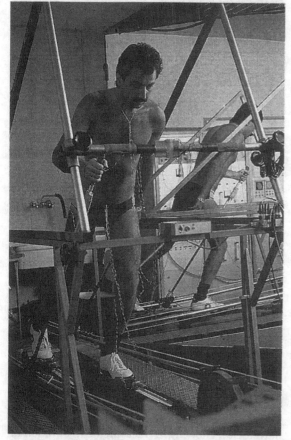

Fig. 19.5 Ergometer for simulating cross-country skiing. The apparatus allows for the measurement of power and force produced by each limb (arms and legs) using linear vertical displacement transducers applied to the ski rollers and on the ski poles.

is constructed from transparent glass, with a large window (2 m × 1 m) to allow observation. Through this porthole it is possible to observe the underwater movement of the athlete, as well as the bottom of the boats, oars or paddles. Observations can also be made by television or high-speed cameras. The hydrodynamics of the flume have been designed to ensure a uniformity of water speed at all points in a transverse section. The flume can operate over a wide range of speeds, from $0.3\,m\cdot s^{-1}$ to about $6\,m\cdot s^{-1}$. The flume is also used with special additional devices to study surface and underwater drag (for sailing and other types of racing boats, scale models are used).

An isokinetic ergometer (Dal Monte & Lupo 1989) (Fig. 19.7) is extremely versatile. It allows work to be performed in vertical, prone, recumbent and seated positions, and it offers the possibility of checking the upper and lower limbs separately or in conjunction. When it is utilized on all four limbs at the same time, the alternation of movement between the upper and lower limbs, or 'amble' movements of the upper and lower limbs can be studied. This type of ergometer is currently used to check the performance of cyclists and kayakers whose body positions can be exactly reproduced. During rehabilitation, it allows the measurement of peak force or power or average power in a single or a series of movements. The equipment can test parameters for the right and left limbs simultaneously and force–velocity relationships can be recorded automatically over an extremely wide range of speeds, from 0 to 240 r.p.m. This equipment may be considered an 'active' isokinetic device, because it is furnished with a very powerful engine whose speed cannot be varied by the active effort or the negative resistance of the athlete. The speed of movement does not represent the maximal speed at which the athlete can work, but depends on the intrinsic speed of the equip-

Fig. 19.6 Diagram of high-speed swimming flume used at the Department of Physiology and Biomechanics of the Institute of Sports Science of CONI.

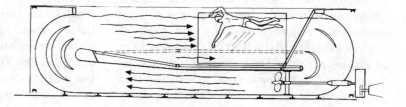

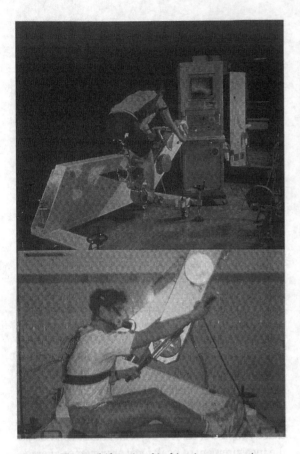

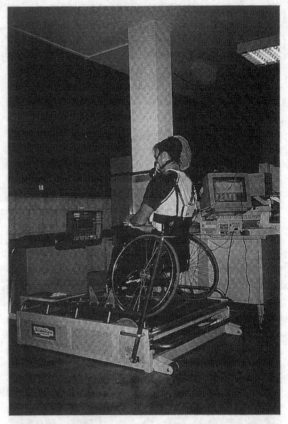

Fig. 19.7 The 'multifunctional isokinetic ergometer' makes it possible to test lower and upper limbs separately and simultaneously at constant speed, power and torque. Power and force exerted during the test can be illustrated by power–velocity and force–velocity curves.

Fig. 19.8 Ergometer to check disabled athletes in their wheelchairs.

ment, both in the pedals and in the arm movements. This particular equipment can work, if required, at an angular speed three times greater than any other isokinetic commercial equipment. This allows tests to be performed at a speed comparable to that reached in all kinds of competitions. Aerobic or anaerobic metabolism can be studied with this ergometer, according to which working protocol is adopted. The device can also work at constant torque or at constant mechanical power. This ergometer is invaluable not only as a means of exploring the muscular and articular characteristics of athletes, but also when organizing their training programme. The equipment can be used directly as a training device, to improve the athlete's capability

to produce force at low speed of movement, or to stimulate neuromuscular conduction in order to improve high-speed muscular recruitment. The device can also be used to induce passive movements. The engine of the equipment produces the movement, allowing a measurement of internal viscous forces or, if required, an evaluation of eccentric forces. After effort, such passive movement helps the athletes recover more rapidly.

Figure 19.8 illustrates a new ergometer designed to check athletes with disabilities while they are sitting in their own wheelchairs (Palmieri 1990), which (in the case of athletes) are quite specifically shaped. A ramp allows the principal traction wheels of the wheelchair to be positioned on a large-diameter roller. The athletes are then in a good position to check their performance, because the inertia of the equipment is identical to that encountered on the normal track. The latest version of this equipment is equipped with a very sophisticated dedicated computer to record all relevant mechanical data, i.e. the required power, the speed and other parameters that must be compared to physiological and biomechanical characteristics.

Wind tunnel

Our institute has also constructed a treadmill in a wind tunnel (Dal Monte 1988). The total dimensions of the tunnel are 9×18 m, and the test chamber is 5 m long, 3 m high and 3.2 m wide. This device allows us to study the aerodynamic drag on the human body, vehicles and equipment at full scale. The treadmill belt, which moves at the same speed as the air, can reproduce the 'ground' effect and permit aerodynamic studies on moving, wheeled vehicles. Many endurance and speed sports have been studied in the wind tunnel, particularly cycling, skiing, bobsleighing, ice- and roller-skating (Fig. 19.9). Aerodynamic factors are a key consideration in cycling, and attempts have always been made to reduce the air drag caused by the characteristics of the cyclist–bicycle combination. In this context, new bicycles or body positions to reduce the size of the frontal cross-section, and thus the air drag, have been studied and clear aerodynamic benefits demonstrated (Fig. 19.10). However, these advantages have had to fit in with a progressive adaptation of riding technique and an optimal training programme in order to achieve top performances (Fig. 19.11) (for instance, two gold medals in individual pursuit events in the Atlanta Olympic Games, 1996).

Higher speed wind-tunnel studies have also been carried out on race vehicles and equipment such as bob-sleighs, racing motor-boats, go-karts, downhill skis, roller- and ice-skates, and crash helmets. The position of athletes during take-off from the ski-jumping board has also been explored (Dal Monte & Faina 1999).

The introduction of these modern ergometers has allowed the development of very high power outputs in the laboratory and intensities of effort quite similar to those that occur in actual sport competitions. Longitudinal repetition of the tests has also provided a reliable and reproducible methodology for monitoring the specific adaptations induced by training programmes. As long ago as 1975, the use of a specific kayak ergometer showed (Dal Monte & Lupo 1989; Dal Monte & Mirri 1996) that top-level competitors could use their upper limbs to develop a larger oxygen intake than that which could be produced on the treadmill using the lower limbs (Table 19.1).

Sometimes the results are less satisfactory and the specific ergometer may not give reliable informa-

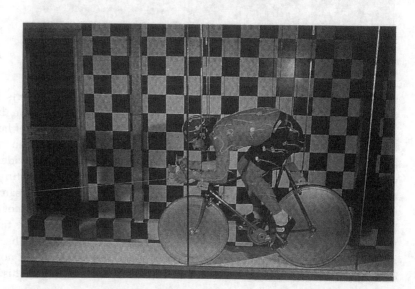

Fig. 19.9 The bicycle and the cyclist carried out an aerodynamic evaluation in the wind tunnel of the Department of Physiology and Biomechanics of the Institute of Sports Science of CONI. The wool threads, which permit visualization of air turbulence, are visible.

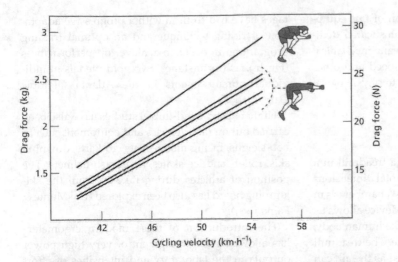

Fig. 19.10 Wind resistance at different cycling speeds for the classic cycling position and the new Dal Monte position. The new Dal Monte position was tested with four different configurations.

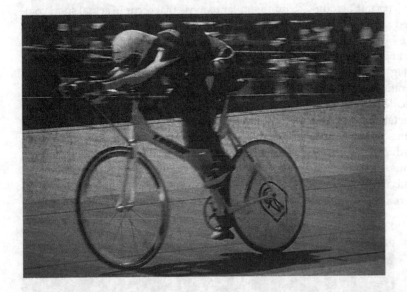

Fig. 19.11 Antonella Bellutti, gold medallist in female individual pursuit at the Atlanta Olympic Games, 1996. In her performance she adopted the Dal Monte position studied in the wind tunnel of the Institute of Sports Science of CONI.

tion on the condition of top athletes. This may mean that the supposedly specific ergometers are not really as specific as they should be; in fact (Dal Monte & Lupo 1989), among athletes who practise a given sport, some are perfectly adapted to the ergometer, but others cannot reproduce in the laboratory test the power that they develop on the field (Fig. 19.12). Moreover, in some sports it is not possible to build an ergometer that can really simulate with sufficient precision the type and intensity of movement performed by the athletes (Squadrone et al. 1994).

In several sports, the classical method of physiological evaluation thus remains testing on the field: measurements of heart rate and/or oxygen intake. Improvements in electronic, miniaturized pulsemeters now provide quite good estimates of average cardiac expenditures on large groups of athletes performing the same kind of sport. However, this methodology is not sufficiently accurate to evaluate the small changes that athletes develop in longitudinal studies. The heart rate does not always depend on the work rate, nor is it closely correlated with the cardiac output: this is particularly evident in sports

Table 19.1 Comparison between the metabolic and cardiac parameters in one middle-distance runner and one kayaker utilizing the treadmill or kayak simulator. From Dal Monte (1975).

	Middle-distance runner (age 21; height 1.725 m; weight 58 kg)		Kayaker (age 25; height 1.84 m; weight 80 kg)	
	Treadmill	Kayak ergometer	Treadmill	Kayak ergometer
Maximum speed or total work performed	$22 \, km \cdot h^{-1}$	13 kJ	$16 \, km \cdot h^{-1}$	105 kJ
Maximum heart rate (beats·min^{-1})	210	166	174	188
$\dot{V}_{Emax}$ (l·min^{-1})	126.8	58.1	131.2	130.0
$\dot{V}_{O_{2}max}$ (l·min^{-1})	4.045	2.303	4.516	4.814
$\dot{V}_{CO_{2}max}$ (l·min^{-1})	4.045	1.898	4.737	5.023
RER	1.00	0.82	1.04	1.02
$\dot{V}_{O_{2}} \, ml \cdot kg^{-1} \, min^{-1}$	69.74	39.70	56.46	61.42

RER, respiratory exchange ratio.

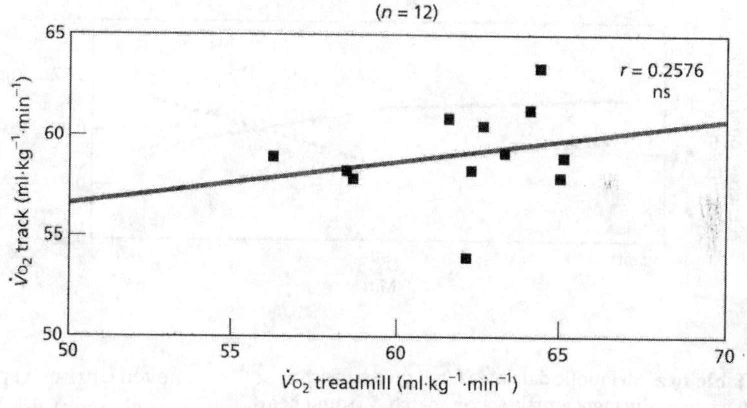

Fig. 19.12 Energy cost of running at 17.5 km·h^{-1} on the track and on the treadmill in 12 high-level middle-distance runners. There is a lack of correlation between the data, suggesting a lack of adaptation to the treadmill.

with large and rapid variations in speed and work rate. The heart rate can be influenced by several extraneous factors, such as variations in the percentage and kind of muscle mass activated by the exercise. In some sports, such as car racing, the heart rate depends more on emotional factors than on metabolic involvement. Therefore, the energy expenditure is not always correlated to heart rate, although it usually is in sports characterized by submaximal, cyclic and constant work rates. Recent developments in miniaturized wireless telemetry now allow not only the heart rate, but also the ventilation and oxygen intake to be transmitted to a recording

station. One important contribution in this field was the development of a very reliable, miniaturized, low weight (800 g) mixing-chamber metabolimeter, the K2 COSMED (Dal Monte et al. 1989). This has now been refined as the K4RQ (Faina et al. 1996) version, which allows the measurement of carbon dioxide (CO_2) production. The small dimensions and flexibility of this equipment facilitate field studies (Dal Monte & Faina 1999) on athletes and the vehicles they use in almost all sport disciplines (Figs 19.13 & 19.14; Table 19.2).

The K4RQ can be coupled to a kit (Dalaqua) that allows the measurement of physiological parame-

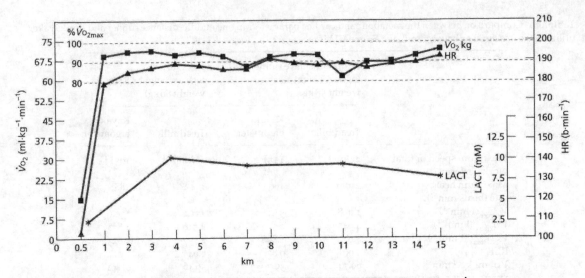

Fig. 19.13 Metabolic data measured on a young rider during an individual time trial cycling race. $\dot{V}O_2$ and heart rate were detected by the K4RQ metabolimeter (Cosmed, Italy). HR, heart rate; LACT, lactate concentration.

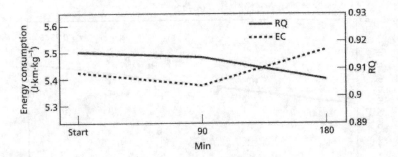

Fig. 19.14 Energy cost of competitive walking measured at the beginning, middle and conclusion of a 3-h race in five top-level walkers by the K4RQ metabolimeter. EC, energy cost; RQ, respiratory quotient.

Table 19.2 Metabolic data measured on a subject (sweeper) during a female soccer match. $\dot{V}O_2$ and heart rate (HR) were detected by the K4RQ metabolimeter (Cosmed, Italy).

	Mean	SD	Range
$\dot{V}O_2$ (ml·kg^{-1}·min^{-1})	32.9	11.4	14.6–55.9
$\dot{V}O_2$ (% $\dot{V}O_{2max}$)	54.3	18.8	24.1–92.2
Lactate (mM)	3.05	1.47	1.41–4.28
HR (beats·min^{-1})	155.2	14.4	116–184
HR (% HR$_{max}$)	83	7.7	62–98.4

ters in swimming (in a swimming pool or in a swimming flume) and in other activities performed below the water surface. The device (Fig. 19.15) (Dal Monte *et al.* 1994), built of carbon fibre, is extremely light and flexible, so that it does not disturb athletes

even during a sport as complex as swimming (Faina *et al.* 1997). Its buoyancy in the water is perfectly balanced, so that it does not interfere with the buoyancy of the athlete. The dead space between the mouth and the valve system is only about 15 ml. All submerged parts of the equipment are hydrodynamically shaped and the internal airways offer an extremely low air flow resistance. The dependent part of the equipment incorporates a miniaturized closed circuit pump, which eliminates the water and saliva that can accumulate during very prolonged tests. The pump circuit does not alter respiratory minute volumes.

The latest improvement of the K4 (the K4b^2) measures oxygen intake breath by breath, allowing a more reliable study of oxygen kinetics. It is quite interesting to study kinetics under actual competi-

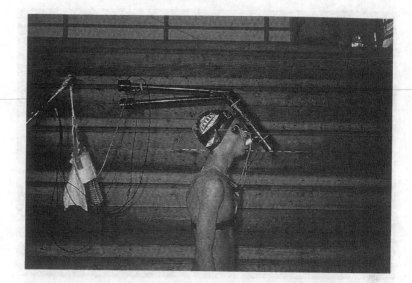

Fig. 19.15 The telemetric miniaturized metabolimeter (K4RQ, Cosmed, Italy) can be adapted for swimming through utilization of a specially designed respiratory tube. This device has a low dead space and a hydrodynamic shape.

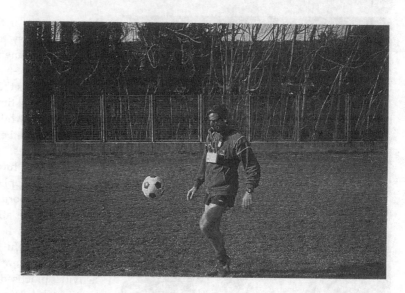

Fig. 19.16 K4b² metabolimeter used in the field to evaluate breath-by-breath oxygen intake kinetics. Note that the equipment does not disturb the athlete's movements.

tive conditions. Current research is examining the onset and the slow component of $\dot{V}_{O_2}$ in endurance and aerobic–anaerobic sports (Fig. 19.16), as well as the O_2 kinetics in alternate sport disciplines during actual performance (Fig. 19.17). Initial data (Faina *et al.* 1998) have shown that among junior high-level rowers there are no significant differences in the speed of onset of oxygen intake between a race simulated in a boat or on a rowing ergometer (Table 19.3). Breath-by-breath equipment has been utilized very recently (Faina *et al.* 1999) to study the slow component of oxygen kinetics at high alti-

tude (5050 m) (Fig. 19.18). Even under such exceptional conditions, characterized by a severe reduction in air density, the device gave valid and reliable data, allowing a comparison of the adaptation of subjects to muscular activities inside and outside the laboratory; this work was carried out at the Italian permanent high-altitude laboratory, 'Piramide', situated high in the Himalayan mountains.

Improvements in equipment to test athletes in the field have influenced the evaluation not only of physiological but also of biomechanical parameters.

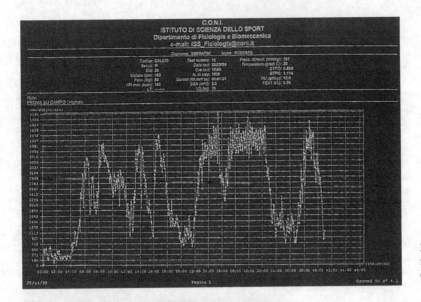

Fig. 19.17 $\dot{V}O_2$ measured by K4b^2 metabolimeter on a soccer player during a specific field test.

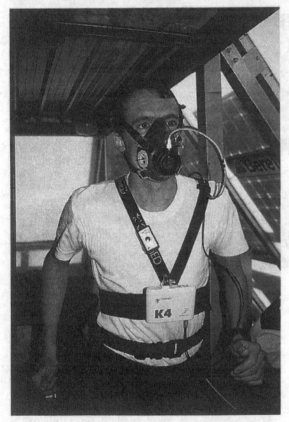

Fig. 19.18 The K4b^2 metabolimeter was used to study, breath by breath, the effect of extreme hypoxia due to low atmospheric pressure at 5050 m above sea-level ('Piramide' high altitude laboratory of Italian National Council of Research (CNR) on Mount Everest).

Measurement of the latter requires methods that are simple, easy to utilize and do not disturb the athlete's movement. Specific examples include the portable torque-meter utilized in cycling as well as the optical bars that measure a runner's flight time and the contact time (Figs 19.19 & 19.20) of the foot on the terrain while an athlete is on the track. These parameters can be studied in parallel with physiological variables.

Present and future studies of the athlete's physiology and applied biomechanics seem to place increasing importance on a monitoring system that can follow the athlete during his or her specific training and, when possible, during competition. This is very useful for athletes and coaches, but from the point of view of the pure scientist, the testing activities practised on the field cannot be performed under standardized conditions. Variations in temperature, humidity, wind direction and intensity and mechanical characteristics of the terrain, etc. affect the precision and the comparability of the results obtained in both cross-sectional and longitudinal studies.

In conclusion, even if the improvement in field tests represents a new frontier for athletic evaluation, it cannot be considered a substitute for standardized, reproducible and reliable tests that can be conducted only in well-equipped laboratories.

Table 19.3 High-level junior rowers: comparison of the onset of $\dot{V}o_2$ measured in a race simulated on a boat and in a race simulated on a rowing ergometer. There was no difference in the onset of $\dot{V}o_2$ (as shown by comparing the time constants), but the peak blood lactate concentration was higher on the ergometer than in the boat.

	$\dot{V}o_2$ peak (ml·kg^{-1}·min^{-1})	Heart rate peak (beats·min^{-1})	Lactate peak (mM)	Strokes (min^{-1})	τ (s)	$\dot{V}o_{2bas}$ (ml·min^{-1})	A (ml·min^{-1})	r
Laboratory	64.70 (±2)	184 (±1.9)	12.6 (±1.3)	35.5 (±1.9)	25.4 (±5.6)	584 (±55.2)	4517 (±260)	0.74 (±0.04)
Field	64.64 (±5)	179 (±4.3)	8 (±1.6)	36.2 (±1.9)	23.4 (±1.7)	749 (±24.2)	4487 (±604)	0.76 (±0.09)
P	0.916	0.116	0.028	0.180	0.916	0.027	0.753	0.465

τ, time constant of the monoexponential curve fitting the onset of $\dot{V}o_2$; $\dot{V}o_{2bas}$, basal value of $\dot{V}o_2$ before the test; A, increment of $\dot{V}o_2$ above $\dot{V}o_{2bas}$ during the test ($\dot{V}o_2 = \dot{V}o_{2bas} + A[1 - e^r/\tau]$); r, coefficient of the monoexponential curve.

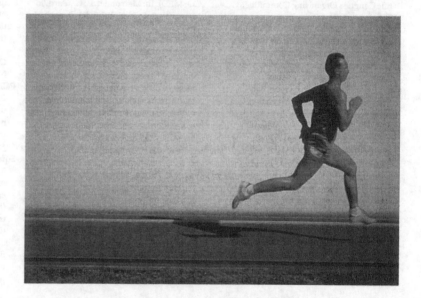

Fig. 19.19 The optical apparatus used to measure the contact time and flight time during running.

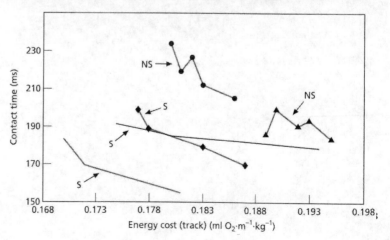

Fig. 19.20 Correlation between the energy cost and contact time on the ground during running in five middle-distance runners. NS, non-significant; S, significant $P < 0.05$.

References

Dal Monte, A. (1975) Metodologia della valutazione funzionale specifica negli atleti praticanti attività sportive di media e lunga durata. (Methodology of specific functional evaluation of long- and middle-distance athletes.) *Medicina Dello Sport* 28, 323–353.

Dal Monte, A. (1983) *La Valutazione Funzionale dell'Atleta. (The Functional Evaluation of Athletes.)* Sansoni Editore, Florence.

Dal Monte, A. (1988) A new Wind Tunnel for research in sport. In: *Proceedings of Olympic Congress on New Horizons of Human Movement*. Seoul Olympic Scientific Congress Organising Committee, Seoul, p. 308.

Dal Monte, A. (1989) Exercise testing and ergometers. In: Dirix, A., Knuttgen, H.G. & Tittel, K. (eds) *The Olympic Book of Sports Medicine*, pp. 121–150. Blackwell Scientific Publications, Oxford.

Dal Monte, A. & Faina, M. (1999) *Valutazione dell'atleta*. (Evaluation of Athlebe). UTET, Turin.

Dal Monte, A. & Lupo, S. (1989) Specific ergometry in the functional assessment of top class sportsmen. *Journal of Sports Medicine and Physical Fitness* 29, 4–8.

Dal Monte, A., Faina, M., Leonardi, L.M., Todaro, A., Guidi, G. & Petrelli, G. (1989) Il consumo massimo di ossigeno in telemetria. (Maximal oxygen intake measured by telemetric equipment.) *Rivista di Cultura Sportiva CONI* 15, 35–44.

Dal Monte, A., Sardella, F., Alippi, B., Faina, M. & Manetta, A. (1994) A new respiratory valve system for measuring oxygen uptake during swimming. *European Journal of Applied Physiology* 69, 159–162.

Dal Monte, A., Mirri, G. & Faina, M. (1996) The specificity in testing top level athletes. In: Marconnet, P., Gaulard, J., Margaritis, I. & Tessier, F. (eds) *Proceedings of the 1st Annual Congress of the European College of Sports Science*, pp. 96–97. SICA Imprimerie, Nice.

Faina, M., Pistelli, T., Franzoso, G., Petrelli, G. & Dal Monte, A. (1996) Validity and reliability of a new telemetric portable system with CO_2 analyser (K4RQ COSMED). In: Marconnet, P., Gaulard, J., Margaritis, I. & Tessier, F. (eds) *Proceedings of the 1st Congress of the European College of Sports Science*, pp. 572–573. SICA Imprimerie, Nice.

Faina, M., Billat, V., Squadrone, R., De Angelis, M., Koralszein, J.P. & Dal Monte, A. (1997) Anaerobic contribution to the time exhaustion at the minimal exercise intensity at which maximal oxygen uptake occurs in elite cyclists, kayakists and swimmers. *European Journal of Applied Physiology* 76, 13–20.

Faina, M., De Angelis, M. & Aguillar, F. (1998) Comparison of $\dot{V}o_2$ kinetics at onset of actual and laboratory simulated rowing performance. In: Sargeant, A.J. & Siddons, H. (eds) *Proceedings of the 3rd Congress of the European College of Sport Science*, p. 279. Health Care Development, Liverpool.

Faina, M., Mirri, G.B., Felici, F. & Rosponi, A. (1999) Comparison between $\dot{V}o_2$ slow component at sea level and at high altitude. In: *Proceedings of 46th Annual Meeting of ACSM*, Med Sc Sp Ex, 31,5 (supplement), S182, nr. 813.

Holmér, J. & Åstrand, P.O. (1972) Swimming training and maximal oxygen uptake. *Journal of Applied Physiology* 33, 510–513.

Holmér, J., Lundin, A. & Eriksson, B.O. (1974) Maximum oxygen uptake during swimming and running by elite swimmers. *Journal of Applied Physiology* 36, 711–714.

Palmieri, V. (1990) Biomeccanica di un ergometro specifico per la valutazione del disabile in carrozzina. (Biomechanics of an ergometer for the specific evaluation of the disabled wheelchair athletes.) In: Zeppili, P. & Palmieri, V. (eds) *Proceedings of the 8th Congress 'Campioni Oltre L'handicap'*, pp. 35–38. Litostampa Nomentana, Rome.

Pelliccia, A., Maron, B.J., Spataro, A., Proshan, M.A. & Spirito, P. (1991) The upper limit of physiologic cardiac hypertrophy in highly trained elite athletes. *New England Journal of Medicine* 324, 295–301.

Squadrone, R., Gallozzi, C., Pasquini, G. & Mattioli, M.L. (1994) Il controllo dell'allenamento in velocisti di alto livello: esperienze di valutazione della forza. (Monitoring training of élite sprinters: evaluation of muscular force.) *Rivista di Cultura Sportiva CONI* 30, 18–35.

Tesch, P.A. & Karlsson, J. (1985) Muscle fiber type and size in trained and untrained muscle of elite athletes. *Journal of Applied Physiology* 59, 1716.

Chapter 20

Assessment of Environmental Extremes and Competitive Strategies

KENT B. PANDOLF AND ANDREW J. YOUNG

Introduction

The environmental extremes of heat, cold, high terrestrial altitude and air quality each pose a threat to the endurance performance of competitive athletes. This chapter, which primarily concerns the environmental extremes of heat and cold, describes proper assessment of the particular environment, when competition should be modified and, if appropriate, when competition should be curtailed. In addition, competitive strategies are presented for each of the environmental extremes which should help optimize athletic performance.

Environmental heat stress

Heat stress assessment

Proper assessment of a hot environment should generally consider ambient temperature, humidity, wind velocity and radiant heat, in order to characterize the level of environmental heat stress imposed on the athlete. One index of environmental heat stress which may have application for competitive athletic endurance performance is the wet bulb globe temperature (WBGT). For outdoor environments with a solar load, WBGT = $0.7 T_{wb(n)} + 0.2 T_g + 0.1 T_{db}$, where $T_{wb(n)}$ is the temperature of the naturally convected wet bulb which incorporates a wetted sensor exposed to natural air movement, T_g is the temperature of a black globe thermometer 0.15 m in diameter, and T_{db} is the dry bulb temperature. Portable WBGT meters are simple to operate,

available commercially, and offer a digital display of the WBGT index.

The American College of Sports Medicine (ACSM) has published a position stand on heat illnesses during distance running, based in part on the WBGT index (American College of Sports Medicine 1996). For instance, when WBGT is greater than 28°C (82°F, very high risk), ACSM suggests that athletic competition should be curtailed or rescheduled until a lower WBGT is prevalent. When the WBGT is at or below 28°C, ACSM proposes the use of large signs to alert athletic participants and officials to the existing risk of heat stress. These signs should be placed at the start of the event and at key points along the event course. High risk is associated with a WBGT of 23–28°C (73–82°F), while moderate risk is represented by a WBGT of 18–20°C (65–73°F) and low risk by a WBGT of below 18°C (65°F). These WBGT values are appropriate for athletes dressed in running shorts, shoes and a T-shirt, while different clothing systems would necessitate further adjustments in the WBGT values associated with each level of risk. Finally, ACSM recommends that all athletic competition, where heat stress is prevalent, should begin in the early morning (before 0800 h) or in the evening (after 1800 h) to lessen the effects of the solar load and air temperature.

Other alternatives to WBGT are the wet globe temperature (WGT) and the newly developed modified discomfort index (MDI). The WGT is measured from a Botsball which incorporates the T_{db}, T_{wb} and solar load into a single reading from a mechanical dial thermometer. WBGT = 0.8 × Botsball reading (WGT) + 0.2 × T_{db} + 0.7°C (or 1.3°F). Unfortunately,

287

the relationship between the WBGT and the Botsball reading is not constant and substantial variation is reported between the WGT and the WBGT (Bricknell 1996). The MDI = $0.75\,T_{wb} + 0.30\,T_{db}$, and it is highly correlated ($r^2 = 0.92$–0.95) with WBGT over a wide range of environmental conditions involving a large ($n = 8500$) sample size (Moran & Pandolf 1999). Although further validation appears necessary, the MDI is easier to calculate and use than the WBGT, and the calculated MDI values fall into the same four categories (very high risk, high risk, moderate risk and low risk) that are used for WBGT.

WBGT, WGT and MDI are easily measured indices, but they are empirically based and not rationally derived from heat transfer theory. Examples of rationally derived environmental indices for quantifying human heat strain and endurance performance are the heat stress index (HSI) and effective temperature (ET*). The various environmental heat stress indices are discussed in detail elsewhere (Gonzalez 1988; Gagge & Gonzalez 1996).

Competitive strategies

During exercise in the heat, human thermoregulation is known to be influenced primarily by exercise–heat acclimatization state (Wenger 1988; Sawka et al. 1996), level of aerobic fitness (Armstrong & Pandolf 1988; Sawka et al. 1996), hydration level (Sawka & Pandolf 1990; Sawka et al. 1996) and clothing worn (Gonzalez 1987). In addition, competitors with a previous history of heat illness such as heat-stroke will generally display greater exercise–heat intolerance than those not so predisposed. A discussion of heat illnesses and their influence on human exercise performance is beyond the scope of this chapter, but has been previously reviewed in detail (Pandolf 1995; Hales et al. 1996) (see also Chapter 40).

EXERCISE–HEAT ACCLIMATIZATION

The classical physiological adjustments during exercise–heat acclimatization are a potentiated sweating response, reduced heart rate and lowered skin and rectal temperatures, while exercise–heat tolerance is greatly improved (Sawka et al. 1996; Pandolf 1998). For both hot–dry and hot–humid environments, nearly complete exercise–heat acclimatization occurs after 7–10 days of exposure. However, about two-thirds to three-quarters of the physiological acclimatization responses and improvements in performance are developed within 4–6 days (Pandolf 1998). Regular heavy exercise in the heat is the most effective method for developing heat acclimatization (Wenger 1988; Sawka et al. 1996). Daily 100-min bouts of exercise are optimal for inducing the heat acclimatization process. Competitive athletes who expect to participate in an event involving heat stress should acclimatize/train in the hot environment for at least 5 days prior to participation, in order to help maximize their performance (Pandolf 1998).

Table 20.1 reviews the actions of exercise–heat

Table 20.1 Actions of exercise–heat acclimatization. From Montain et al. (1996).

Thermal comfort—improved	Exercise performance—improved
Core temperature—reduced	*Metabolic rate*—lowered
Sweating—improved	*Cardiovascular strain*—reduced
Onset—earlier	Heart rate—lowered
Rate—higher	Stroke volume—increased
Distribution—improved (tropic)	Blood pressure—better defended
Hidromeiosis—reduced (tropic)	
	Fluid balance—improved
Skin blood flow—increased	Thirst—improved
Onset—earlier	Electrolyte loss—reduced
Flow—higher	Total body water—increased
	Plasma volume—increased and better defended

acclimatization from a recent report (Montain *et al.* 1996). As noted earlier, body core temperature is reduced while cardiovascular strain is lessened through a lowered heart rate, increased stroke volume and a better-defended blood pressure. Although this is somewhat debatable, metabolic rate has been shown by some to be lowered after acclimatization. Sweating is generally thought to become more effective in dissipating heat through an earlier onset, higher rate and, in humid environments, a more uniform distribution and an increased resistance to hidromeiosis. Skin blood flow is increased earlier with attainment of a higher flow. Fluid balance is improved through an increased thirst, reduced electrolyte loss, increased total body water and increased and better-defended plasma volume. No single cause/action can explain this adaptive process; exercise–heat acclimatization probably results from the interplay of many mechanisms.

Heat acclimatization gradually decays or is lost if it is not maintained by repeated exercise–heat exposure (Sawka *et al.* 1996). Lower heart rate is one of the more rapid changes during heat acclimatization, but heart rate also reverts more rapidly than the other improvements in thermoregulatory responses as acclimatization is lost. The published literature indicates considerable variability of opinion concerning the rate of decay or loss of exercise–heat acclimatization (Sawka *et al.* 1996; Pandolf 1998). Nevertheless, retention of the benefits of heat acclimatization appears to persist longer for dry compared to humid heat, and high levels of aerobic fitness also seem to be associated with greater retention of heat acclimatization (Pandolf 1998).

AEROBIC FITNESS

Researchers generally agree that a high aerobic fitness achieved through endurance training reduces the physiological strain during exercise in the heat (Armstrong & Pandolf 1988; Sawka *et al.* 1996). Figure 20.1 presents findings from different hot climates (hot–humid (a); hot–dry (b)) and shows that maximal oxygen intake accounts for 42–46% of the variability in core temperature after 3 h of exercise in the heat, or the heat acclimatization day for a

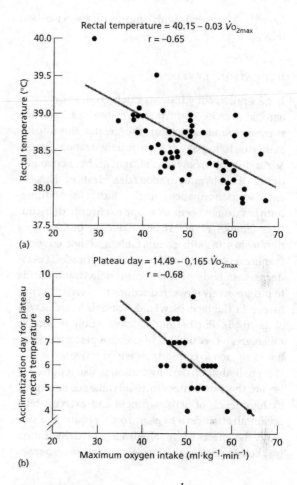

Fig. 20.1 The relationship between $\dot{V}o_{2max}$ and rectal temperature in a hot–humid environment (a), or between $\dot{V}o_{2max}$ and the acclimatization day for a plateau in rectal temperature during dry-heat exposure (b). From Armstrong and Pandolf (1988).

plateau in core temperature. However, an increase in aerobic fitness by endurance training must be associated with significant elevations in core temperature during training in order to improve exercise–heat tolerance (Armstrong & Pandolf 1988). It has also been hypothesized that high aerobic fitness is a major factor limiting decay and facilitating rapid reacclimatization of individuals after they have stopped exercising in the heat (Pandolf 1998). Endurance athletes should be at peak levels of aerobic fitness in order to maximize the potential benefits associated with improved exercise–heat tolerance.

HYDRATION LEVEL

In general, hypohydration or dehydration degrades aerobic exercise performance in the heat, and the warmer the environment, the greater the impairment due to hypohydration or dehydration (Sawka & Pandolf 1990; Sawka et al. 1996). There is no evidence that hypohydration/dehydration benefits exercise performance in the heat. In addition, humans do not seem to adapt to chronic dehydration (Sawka et al. 1996). Exercise performance diminishes in both comfortable and hot environments even at marginal levels of dehydration (1–2% decrease in body mass). Greater dehydration leads to progressively larger reductions in exercise performance in the heat (Sawka & Pandolf 1990; Sawka et al. 1996). Furthermore, dehydration results in much greater reductions of exercise performance in hot compared to comfortable environments.

Hypohydration or dehydration is also reported to negate the core temperature advantages conferred by high levels of aerobic fitness and exercise–heat acclimatization (Sawka et al. 1996). Figure 20.2 displays the effects of hypohydration or dehydration (5% body mass loss) on core temperature responses

of the same individuals when unacclimatized or heat acclimatized during exercise in both hot–dry and hot–wet environments. Exercise–heat acclimatization is shown to lower core temperature responses when a person is euhydrated (not dehydrated). However, when they are hypohydrated or dehydrated, similar core temperature responses are found regardless of acclimatization state (Sawka et al. 1998). Thus, the core temperature penalty resulting from dehydration is greater for heat-acclimatized than for unacclimatized individuals. Endurance athletes should be encouraged to avoid becoming dehydrated during events in hot environments and should aim for their body weight loss not to exceed 2%.

Recent studies on the thermoregulatory effects of hyperhydration or increased total body water during exercise–heat exposure have reported somewhat conflicting results. One study showed that glycerol/water hyperhydration significantly improved an individual's ability to thermoregulate during exercise in the heat (Lyons et al. 1990). However, more recent studies have reported similar body core temperatures and sweating rates for glycerol and water hyperhydration, whether given before exercise in a comfortable environment, or as rehydration beverages during exercise in warm and hot climates (Latzka et al. 1997, 1998). The preponderance of evidence now suggests that hyperhydration provides no thermoregulatory advantage over euhydration during exercise in the heat (see also Chapter 29).

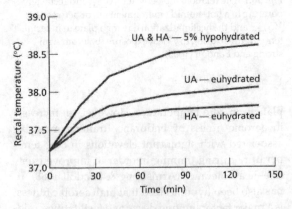

Fig. 20.2 Rectal temperature responses during exercise–heat exposure in euhydrated and hypohydrated (5% body mass loss) individuals both before (UA) and after (HA) being exercise–heat acclimatized. From Sawka et al. (1998).

CLOTHING

Proper clothing helps to optimize the endurance performance of a competitive athlete in the heat (Gonzalez 1987). For hot environments, the proper clothing ensemble must allow evaporative heat transfer, but it should also be lightweight and afford solar protection. Light-coloured clothing is preferred during endurance exercise in the heat. In general, synthetic materials have most of the thermal advantages of materials made of natural fibres such as cotton, and most synthetic fabrics do not harbour microorganisms.

Endurance athletes should select their clothing

for performance in hot environments with a view to compensating for the air temperature, relative humidity and solar load.

Cold stress

Assessing cold stress

Many people exercise indoors during winter to avoid the cold, but competitive endurance athletes often continue training outdoors throughout winter, and some endurance events such as Nordic ski contests involve prolonged exposure to very low temperatures. Excessive body heat loss during cold exposure can result in hypothermia (a decrease in body core temperature below 35°C), frostbite (freezing of body tissues, typically the skin of the extremities) or other serious cold injuries (reviewed in detail elsewhere (Bracker 1992)). Winter weather usually poses less of a health risk than summer heat for well-equipped endurance athletes who are training or competing outdoors. Modern cold weather clothing is more than adequate to protect against the effects of cold (Gonzalez 1995) except when insulation is degraded by rain or heavy sweating. Additional protection is provided by the body's primary physiological responses to cold, peripheral vasoconstriction (which limits body heat loss) and muscular shivering (which increases body heat production) (Young et al. 1998b). Furthermore, even though muscle blood flow increases during exercise, overriding cold-induced vasoconstriction and facilitating heat flux from core to skin, the metabolic heat production during high-intensity endurance exercise in cold air is generally sufficient to maintain thermal balance and body temperature (Young et al. 1998b). Nevertheless, under some conditions, athletes exercising outdoors in cold weather may risk local cold injury or impair performance.

COLD AIR AND WIND CHILL

The principal cold stress determinants during outdoor events in cold weather are air temperature and wind speed. Most body heat loss during cold exposure occurs via conductive and convective mechanisms, so when ambient temperature is colder than body temperature, the thermal gradient favours body heat loss. Wind (or relative air movement as in downhill skiing) exacerbates heat loss by facilitating convection at the body surface (Santee et al. 1988). No single cold stress index integrates the effective stress from both of these factors in terms of the potential for body heat loss, but the wind chill index (WCI) has achieved popular acceptance and is widely reported (Siple & Passel 1945).

The WCI purports to integrate the potential stress arising from wind and air temperature by estimating their combined cooling effects (Siple & Passel 1945). WCI formulae allow cooling power for various combinations of air temperature and wind speed to be expressed as equivalent chill temperature, or the temperature of 'calm' air that would result in the same heat flow through bare skin as different combinations of air temperature and wind speed. Typically, wind chill equivalent tables are divided into zones reflecting the relative risk of freezing tissue injuries ('little danger' $\geq -30°C \geq$ 'increasing danger' $\geq -58°C \geq$ 'great danger') (Gonzalez 1986).

In the absence of a better tool, these tables are useful for guiding decisions regarding the need to cancel outdoor activities, but, as with the WBGT, the limitations to this approach should be appreciated. The wind chill concept is sound, but the equation for calculating WCI appears flawed in its physical and physiological rationale, and the tables overestimate wind effects, while underestimating air temperature effects (Danilesson 1996). Although widely reported and broadly accepted as an overall cold stress index, wind chill temperatures are really rather specific in their correct application, only estimating the danger of cooling the exposed flesh of sedentary persons. Wind chill effects are greatly reduced by wearing windproof clothing (Gonzalez 1995) and exercising strenuously (Young et al. 1998b). Finally, wind chill tables provide no meaningful estimate of the risk of hypothermia.

Thus, wind chill tables probably somewhat exaggerate the risk of cold injury during endurance competition, and events in which participants are properly dressed and maintain high metabolic rates need not be cancelled due to wind chill alone. Prudence does warrant increased safety surveillance of competitors when equivalent chill temperatures fall below −30°C, since injured or fatigued athletes may be unable to sustain high metabolic rates and the high skin temperatures (T_{sk}) that would protect them from wind chill. Wind chill effects may actually constitute a greater danger to non-exercising spectators and competition officials than to competitors.

Water has a much higher thermal capacity than air; therefore, heat conduction away from the skin is more rapid when clothing is wet than when it is dry (Gonzalez 1988). With an air temperature of 5°C, heat loss in wet clothes may be double that in dry (Kaufman & Bothe 1986). Even so, heat loss predictions (Stolwijk & Hardy 1977) indicate that the core temperature (T_c) of an average-sized individual performing high-intensity endurance exercise (600 W) in an air temperature of 5°C and continuous rain will not fall below 35°C for at least 7 h. In this situation, fatigue rather than body cooling would limit performance. Also, the heat loss prediction for a properly clothed athlete performing a Nordic ski event at −35°C for 1 h at a high exercise intensity suggests that T_c will remain above 37°C and T_{sk} will remain above 25°C.

COLD WATER

During exercise in water, skin heat conductance can be 70 times greater than during comparable exercise in air at the same temperature (Gonzalez 1988). Thus, marathon swimmers and triathletes can experience considerable body heat loss even in relatively mild water temperatures. However, individuals vary considerably with respect to the water temperature that can be tolerated without experiencing a decline in T_c during exercise. Anthropomorphic factors, exercise type, metabolic rate, aerobic power and water temperature all interact in a complex manner to determine the net thermal balance between heat production and heat loss during cold water immersion (Toner & McArdle 1988; Young et al. 1998b). Safe limits for allowable water immersion duration as a function of water temperature can be formulated based on observations of survival times following accidental immersion (Molnar 1946). More conservative limits are indicated when

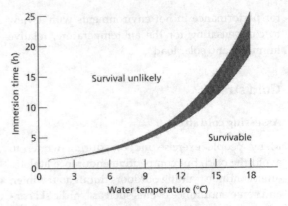

Fig. 20.3 Estimated survival time during immersion in water of varying temperature. The upper margin of the curve defining the boundary between the temperature–duration conditions thought 'survivable' from those considered 'survival unlikely' was derived from actual human survival time data collated by Molnar (1946), whereas the lower margin of the curve was derived using a thermoregulatory model developed by Tikuisis and Frim (1994) to predict immersion duration required for rectal temperature to fall to 30°C.

a physiological model of human thermoregulation is used to predict survival times (Tikuisis & Frim 1994). Figure 20.3 illustrates both approaches to establishing water temperature safety limits for aquatic events. However, in both cases, the limits are defined by the expected time to death due to hypothermia or drowning due to the inability to maintain consciousness or sustain useful physical activity, and this approach may be too liberal for athletic competition.

Performance factors

ANTHROPOMORPHIC FACTORS

Body size and shape, as well as the amount and distribution of body fat, all influence heat loss. Individuals having a small surface area relative to body mass and a thick layer of subcutaneous fat are best able to resist body cooling (Young et al. 1996). Figure 20.4 shows how fat thickness influences an individual's maximal tissue insulation. Fat individuals tolerate lower temperatures with less shivering and

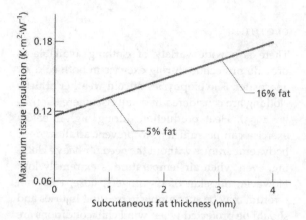

Fig. 20.4 Relationship between body fat and maximal tissue insulation during immersion in cold water (Hong 1973).

smaller declines in core temperature than people who are lean; this difference is especially pronounced in cold water (Toner & McArdle 1988). For athletic performance on land, any thermoregulatory advantage of extra body fat and a low surface area to mass ratio is negated by the increased cardiovascular and biomechanical stress of carrying excess weight. Long-distance swimmers whose body fat content is 5% or less, however, have a third less insulation compared to swimmers whose body fat content is 16% or more, and they are at a distinct thermoregulatory disadvantage during prolonged events in cool water (Young et al. 1996).

Most women have a greater body fat content and a thicker layer of subcutaneous fat than men of comparable age or body mass; thus women have a greater maximal tissue insulation than men. Despite this, women may not have any thermoregulatory advantage over men during cold exposure, at least in terms of maintaining normal heat balance (McArdle et al. 1984a; Gonzalez 1988, Young et al. 1996, 1998b). For example, when men and women of equivalent body mass are compared, the women's greater fat content enhances insulation, but their smaller lean body mass limits their capacity for heat production. The women also begin an event with a smaller total body heat content, and have a lesser thickness of muscle (which itself confers some insulation). This disparity may be inconsequential

under conditions where metabolism is low. However, in severely cold conditions that stimulate maximal shivering, a limited thermogenic capacity may allow women's core temperature to decline more rapidly than men's. If, on the other hand, women and men of equivalent subcutaneous fat thickness are compared, the women have a greater surface area and smaller total body mass than men. Although their insulation is equivalent, the women's smaller body mass contains less body heat initially, and with cold exposure their larger surface area allows more convective heat flux; therefore body temperature falls more rapidly for any given thermal gradient and metabolic rate (McArdle et al. 1984b). In addition, women's greater fat content may retard rewarming following cold exposure (Giesbrecht & Bristow 1995).

PHYSICAL TRAINING

It is unclear whether exercise training and a high level of physical fitness confer some physiological advantage that improves cold tolerance. Cross-sectional comparisons have indicated that aerobically fit persons maintain warmer skin temperatures than less fit persons during cold exposure (Bittel et al. 1988). Although a warmer skin during cold exposure might improve comfort and protect against peripheral cold injury, any such advantage comes at the expense of an increased body heat loss; this must be offset by a higher rate of metabolic heat production, or else core temperature will fall. The warmer skin temperatures of fit subjects during cold exposure appear to be attributable to a thinner layer of subcutaneous fat than that found in less fit individuals (Bittel et al. 1988). Since the low body fat content of highly trained endurance athletes is a consequence of both chronic endurance training and genetic selection, cross-sectional comparisons cannot really address how endurance training affects thermoregulation. Longitudinal investigations indicate that 8–9 weeks of endurance training strengthens the cutaneous vasoconstrictor response to cold, leading to a more rapid decline in T_{sk} during exposure to cold water (Kollias et al. 1972; Young et al. 1995). Such an adaptation might provide some thermoregulatory advantage for persons exposed to cold. However, the primary thermoregulatory advantage of a high aerobic fitness level is that it allows a higher exercise intensity; thus, a greater metabolic heat production can be sustained during endurance competition in the cold.

Overtraining might compromise an endurance athlete's cold tolerance. Chronic exercise performed without adequate recovery between sessions can lead to exertional fatigue. An anecdotal association between exertional fatigue and susceptibility to hypothermia is frequently reported, although physiological mechanisms remain undefined. Two recent studies (Thompson & Hayward 1996; Weller *et al.* 1997) of the effects of prolonged fatiguing exercise on maintenance of thermal balance in the cold both showed that as fatigue develops, the intensity of exercise that can be sustained declines; thus, metabolic heat production declines and thermal balance during cold exposure is compromised. With respect to more direct effects on thermoregulation, a recent study indicates that exertional fatigue combined with sleep deprivation may delay the onset of shivering (Young *et al.* 1998a).

HYDRATION

Even in cold environments, exercise-induced sweating occurs and, although sweating may be less, ventilatory fluid loss can be more pronounced during exercise in the cold than in warm conditions. Cold exposure can also induce a diuresis (Freund & Young 1996). Athletes competing in cold environments thus need to drink sufficient fluid to offset these losses and avoid the dehydration-associated performance impairments that ensue as fluid deficits exceed 2% of body mass. However, in cold weather, thirst is blunted, and persons sometimes restrict fluid intake to minimize the need to urinate outdoors (Freund & Young 1996). Hypohydration can impair endurance performance in the cold via the same mechanisms as in hot environments, and may additionally increase susceptibility to peripheral cold injuries. Hypohydration does not appear to impair shivering during whole-body cold exposure, but it may impair vasoconstrictor responses to cold, if exposures are prolonged or severe (O'Brien *et al.* 1998).

CLOTHING

There is a wide variety of clothing available to provide protection during exercise in both cold air and water. The biophysics of cold weather athletic clothing are considered in detail elsewhere (Gonzalez 1995). Heat production during high-intensity exercise can be sufficient to prevent a fall in deep body temperature without the need for heavy clothing, even when air temperature is extremely low. However, the skin of the fingers, nose, ears and scrotum may be susceptible to freezing injuries and should be protected when wind chill conditions are extreme. Athletes dressed for optimal performance during their events may be inadequately protected from cold before starting, or when exercise ceases due to fatigue, injury or completion of the event.

COLD ACCLIMATIZATION

Humans experience physiological adaptations to chronic cold exposure; some of these may improve comfort during cold exposure, and others may facilitate maintenance of normal body temperatures (Young 1996). However, the magnitude of the effects of these acclimatization influences on overall thermal balance during exercise is not large (Young 1996; Young *et al.* 1996).

High altitude

Assessment of the environment

Assessing high-altitude stress is relatively simple. As altitude increases, barometric pressure decreases, resulting in a reduction in the partial pressure of oxygen in inspired air. This hypoxia is the cause of the performance impairments experienced when persons who normally live in low-altitude regions ascend to high elevations. The magnitude of hypoxia is easily assessed by measuring barometric pressure or inspired oxygen pressure, but this is not usually necessary. For one thing, the International Civil Aviation Organization has promulgated a standardized relationship between barometric pressure and terrestrial altitude (Ward *et al.* 1995). Although local weather fluctuations and gravitational effects can cause the 'standardized' and measured barometric pressure to vary somewhat, these variations have little significance for performance below 3000 m, where most endurance competitions take place. Furthermore, investigators usually describe the effects of altitude on performance according to the elevation above sea-level, a figure which can be obtained from a map, rather than as a function of barometric pressure.

Performance at high altitude

Detailed reviews of the effects of high-altitude exposure on humans are published elsewhere (Chapter 41; Young & Young 1988; Young & Reeves 1998). The principal physiological factor relevant for endurance exercise performance when people living near sea-level ascend higher is the decline in atmospheric oxygen pressure, which reduces O_2 diffusion across the lung into blood; this in turn causes the arterial O_2 pressure (P_aO_2), O_2 saturation of haemoglobin (S_aO_2) and arterial O_2 content (C_aO_2) to fall (Grover *et al.* 1986). As a result, maximal O_2 intake ($\dot{V}O_{2max}$) declines with ascent. In addition, a higher cardiac output ($\dot{Q}$) is required to achieve O_2 delivery requirements for a given intensity of steady-state submaximal exercise at altitude compared to sea-level.

The reduction in $\dot{V}O_{2max}$ and increased cardiovascular strain associated with elevated $\dot{Q}$ during submaximal exercise are the two key mechanisms degrading aerobic work capacity and endurance performance in unacclimatized lowlanders on arrival at high altitude (Fulco *et al.* 1998). Figure 20.5 shows the decrements in $\dot{V}O_{2max}$ measured in 67 different investigations at different altitudes. The most important factor determining the decline in $\dot{V}O_{2max}$ at high altitude is the elevation ascended. The decrement in $\dot{V}O_{2max}$ experienced by lowland residents ascending to high altitudes may be measurable at elevations as low as 600 m, but between 600 m and 1000 m the decrement is small and variable. However, between 1000 and 6000 m, the $\dot{V}O_{2max}$ decreases approximately linearly with altitude by about 8–10% per 1000 m ascended. Above 6300 m, the rate of decline is even more pronounced.

The significance of the altitude-induced reduction

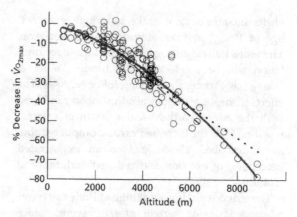

Fig. 20.5 Effects of reduced partial pressure of oxygen at high altitude on maximal oxygen intake ($\dot{V}O_{2max}$) expressed as a percentage of $\dot{V}O_{2max}$ at sea-level. Solid line represents regression line calculated by Fulco *et al.* (1998) based on mean reductions measured at different altitudes and reported by 67 different investigators; dashed and dotted lines represent similar regressions calculated using smaller numbers of measurements by Buskirk (1969) (dashed) and Grover *et al.* (1986) (dotted). Modified from Fulco *et al.* (1998).

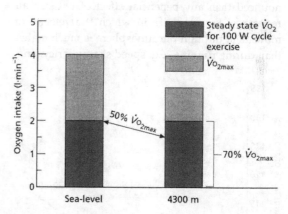

Fig. 20.6 Effects of high altitude on the relationship between absolute power output for cycle exercise, oxygen intake ($\dot{V}O_{2max}$) and the relative exercise intensity (% $\dot{V}O_{2max}$). From Young and Young (1988).

in $\dot{V}O_{2max}$ for submaximal endurance exercise is illustrated in Fig. 20.6. Neglecting the effects of reduced air density at high altitude (which may be significant for certain types of exercise, as discussed below), exercise at a given intensity or power output (e.g. running at a given velocity) at high altitude elicits the same oxygen intake, but a higher percentage of $\dot{V}_{O_{2max}}$ at high altitude than at sea-level. Therefore, muscle glycogen use and lactate accumulation will be accelerated at altitude (Young & Young 1988; Young 1990; Young & Reeves 1998). The effects of these physiological adjustments combined with the added cardiovascular strain of exercise resulting from the increased cardiac output requirement described above lead to an exaggerated perception of exertion and reduced endurance at altitude.

The reduced air density at high altitude can prove advantageous for certain athletic events, since objects move through the atmosphere with less resistance (Fulco *et al.* 1998). This can contribute to an improved performance in short-duration, high-velocity running events, e.g. sprinting, where the small aerobic component of the activity is little compromised by hypoxia. However, as illustrated in Fig. 20.7, the compromising effect of hypoxia on the large aerobic component of longer-duration, lower-velocity endurance running events is more pronounced than any beneficial effect of reduced air resistance. For activities in which the velocity of movement through the atmosphere is much higher than during running, e.g. speed skating or cycling,

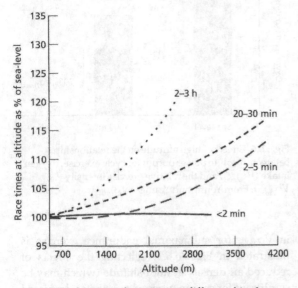

Fig. 20.7 Performance decrements at different altitudes for running and swimming events lasting for different durations. Redrawn from Fulco *et al.* (1998).

the reduced air resistance may again allow performance to improve over sea-level norms, even when the aerobic component of the activity is high.

Competitive strategies

ACCLIMATIZATION

High-altitude illnesses can compromise endurance capacity over and above impairments attributable to the direct physiological effects of acute hypoxia. The illnesses, which are reviewed elsewhere (Chapter 41; Malconian & Rock 1988; Tom *et al.* 1994), not only impair endurance performance, but can also be life threatening. Rapid ascent and intense exercise may increase susceptibility to or exacerbate the symptoms of high-altitude illnesses. Young adult males may be particularly at risk of high-altitude pulmonary oedema. The occurrence and severity of altitude illnesses diminish with acclimatization, especially if acclimatization is combined with staging (stops at intermediate altitude). Athletes ascending to high altitude should stop for 24 h upon reaching 2500 m, and a 24-h stop should be allowed for every additional 600 m ascended (Malconian & Rock 1988). Acute mountain sickness, the most common altitude illness at moderate elevations (< 5000 m), usually resolves after 3–7 days spent at altitude, whereas the more serious altitude illnesses (e.g. high-altitude pulmonary or cerebral oedema) require immediate descent (Tom *et al.* 1994).

Ventilatory and cardiovascular adaptations becoming evident after 3–8 days at moderate altitude permit some improvement in endurance, and after 3 weeks of acclimatization, metabolic adaptations develop which further contribute to improved endurance (Young & Young 1988; Young 1990). Although altitude acclimatization enables improvement in endurance, sea-level capacity will not be restored (Young & Young 1988; Young & Reeves 1998).

TRAINING

Similarities between altitude acclimatization and physical training have long led athletes and coaches to think that training at high altitude is advantageous for sea-level competition. Recently, some scientific evidence has been reported to support this contention. Levine and Stray-Gundersen (1997) reported that élite distance runners who lived for 4 weeks at a moderately high altitude (2500 m) and participated in a training regimen at a somewhat lower elevation (1250 m) exhibited an improvement in both performance (faster 5-km run times) and $\dot{V}o_{2max}$, while runners who lived at sea-level and followed the same training regimen did not. The authors attributed the enhanced training effect to a 9% expansion of erythrocyte volume induced by altitude acclimatization. A third group of runners who lived at 2500 m while training at that altitude rather than at a somewhat lower elevation also experienced the expansion of erythrocyte volume, but not the enhanced training effect. The third group of athletes were unable to sustain the same intensity of exercise training as was being undertaken at sea-level or at the lower altitude. Subsequent studies by these researchers demonstrated that a significant number of individuals were 'non-responders' who failed to exhibit the expansion of plasma volume shown by 'responders' under the same altitude and training conditions (Chapman *et al.* 1998).

Physical training at sea-level does not lessen the decrement in $\dot{V}o_{2max}$ at altitude. On the contrary, those with the highest maximal aerobic power appear to experience the greatest reductions in $\dot{V}o_{2max}$ at altitude (Fulco *et al.* 1998). For lowlanders competing at high altitude, the principal concern is how to maintain their fitness while acclimatizing. Increased emphasis on high-intensity 'interval'-type training may offset reductions in endurance training and allow muscle power to be maintained.

Air quality

In addition to the environmental extremes of heat, cold and high altitude, poor air quality or air pollution is another environmental stressor which can affect human endurance performance (Chapter 42; Pandolf 1988; Folinsbee 1995a,b). Air pollutants have been categorized as primary or secondary. Primary pollutants include carbon monoxide, sulphur and nitrogen dioxide, and primary particulates. Secondary pollutants result from interactions between primary pollutants and include ozone, peroxyacetyl nitrate and certain aerosols. Of these various air pollutants, carbon monoxide, sulphur dioxide and ozone may warrant particular concern for the exercising athlete (Folinsbee 1995a,b).

Primary pollutants

Carbon monoxide (CO) does not appear to impair submaximal exercise performance at carboxy-haemoglobin (COHb) levels below 15%; however, breathing CO significantly affects maximal exercise performance when COHb exceeds about 4% (Folinsbee 1995a). In general, healthy athletes performing high-intensity submaximal exercise should not have problems with normal outdoor levels of sulphur dioxide (SO_2) (Folinsbee 1995b). The threshold level of SO_2 which affects submaximal exercise performance is between 1.0 and 3.0 ppm; however, insufficient research has been reported concerning this pollutant and maximal exercise performance (Pandolf 1988). Asthmatic athletes are about 10 times more sensitive to SO_2 than non-asthmatic athletes and SO_2 levels of only 0.40 ppm can result in pulmonary dysfunction in individuals with asthma (Folinsbee 1995a,b). No research has yet evaluated the impact of nitrogen dioxide (NO_2) on maximal exercise performance, but NO_2 exposure does not seem to affect submaximal exercise performance adversely (Pandolf 1988; Folinsbee 1995b). The physiological effects of primary particulate exposure have not been studied during exercise in athletes.

Secondary pollutants

While ozone (O_3) exposure does not appear to alter submaximal exercise performance at light to moderate exercise intensities, exposure to O_3 for 1 h at 0.18 ppm can limit performance during heavy exercise, primarily due to severe respiratory discomfort and alterations in pulmonary function (Folinsbee 1995b). Submaximal and maximal exercise performance are not altered dramatically during peroxyacetyl nitrate exposure (Pandolf

1988). The sulphate aerosols, sulphuric acid and the nitrate aerosols produce minimal adverse effects during exercise relative to some of the other pollutants when tested separately.

Environmental stressor interactions

Performance of submaximal or maximal exercise can be expected to suffer under the combined stressors of excessive heat, humidity and poor air quality (Pandolf 1988). The interactive effects of breathing cold polluted air may increase the degree of exercise-induced bronchospasm and adversely affect exercise performance in susceptible individuals such as asthmatic athletes (Folinsbee 1995a). The adverse effects of certain pollutants such as CO may be enhanced during exercise at high altitude, due to a greater degree of hypoxaemia (Folinsbee 1995a).

Air quality assessment

The rate and severity of air pollution episodes are influenced by environmental and meteorological factors, and by time of day (Pandolf 1988). Primary pollutants such as carbon monoxide and the nitrogen oxides display daily peaks associated with peak traffic conditions. They reach their highest levels in midwinter. Secondary pollutants such as ozone have a distinctive pattern related to sunlight, with peak daily values in the afternoon, and peak seasonal values in the summer or early autumn. In addition to sunlight, other meteorological factors known to influence air quality adversely are a low wind speed and inversion of the normal vertical temperature gradient.

Historic air pollution episodes have led to development of public guidelines to help assess the potential health problems associated with poor air quality (Pandolf 1988). In turn, certain nations such as the United States have developed national average air quality standards relative to many of the more important air pollutants (carbon monoxide, ozone, sulphur dioxide, total suspended particulates, etc.). When poor air quality is expected, officials associated with athletic endurance events should contact sources such as the US Environmental Protection Agency for information about pending air quality to aid in their decisions concerning the curtailment or delay of competition.

Disclaimer and distribution statements

The views, opinions and/or findings in this chapter are those of the authors, and should not be construed as an official Department of the US Army position, policy or decision, unless so designated by other official documentation.

Approved for public release; distribution is unlimited.

References

American College of Sports Medicine (1996) Heat and cold illnesses during distance running. *Medicine and Science in Sports and Exercise* **21**, i–x.

Armstrong, L.E. & Pandolf, K.B. (1988) Physical training, cardiorespiratory physical fitness and exercise–heat tolerance. In: Pandolf, K.B., Sawka, M.N. & Gonzalez, R.R. (eds) *Human Performance Physiology and Environmental Medicine at Terrestrial Extremes*, pp. 199–226. Benchmark Press, Indianapolis.

Bittel, J.H.M., Nonott-Varly, C., Livecchi-Gonnot, G.H., Savourey, G.L.M.J. & Hanniquet, A.M. (1988) Physical fitness and thermoregulatory reactions in a cold environment in men. *Journal of Applied Physiology* **65**, 1984–1989.

Bracker, M.D. (1992) Environmental and thermal injury. *Clinics in Sports Medicine* **11**, 419–436.

Bricknell, M.C.M. (1996) Heat illness—a review of military experience (part 2). *Journal of the Royal Army Medical Corps* **142**, 34–42.

Buskirk, E.R. (1969) Decrease in physical working capacity at high altitude. In: Hegnauer, A.H. (ed.) *Biomedicine of High Terrestrial Elevations*, pp. 204–222. US Army Research Institute of Environmental Medicine, Natick, MA.

Chapman, R.F., Stray-Gundersen, J. & Levine, B.D. (1998) Individual variation in altitude training. *Journal of Applied Physiology* **85**, 1448–1456.

Danilesson, U. (1996) Windchill and the risk of tissue freezing. *Journal of Applied Physiology* **81**, 2666–2673.

Folinsbee, L.J. (1995a) Exercise and air pollution. In: Torg, J.S. & Shephard, R.J. (eds) *Current Therapy in Sports Medicine*, 3rd edn, pp. 574–577. Mosby, St. Louis.

Folinsbee, L.J. (1995b) Heat and air pollution. In: Pollock, M.L. & Schmidt, D.H. (eds) *Heart Disease and Rehabilitation*, 3rd edn, pp. 327–342. Human Kinetics, Champaign, IL.

Freund, B. & Young, A.J. (1996) Environmental influences on body fluid balance during exercise: cold exposure. In: Buskirk, E. & Puhl, S.M. (eds) *Body Fluid Balance*, pp. 159–181. CRC Press, New York.

Fulco, C.S., Rock, P.B. & Cymerman, A. (1998) Maximal and submaximal exercise performance at altitude. *Aviation, Space, and Environmental Medicine* **69**, 793–801.

Gagge, A.P. & Gonzalez, R.R. (1996) Mechanisms of heat exchange: biophysics and physiology. In: Fregly, M.J. & Blatteis, C.M. (eds) *Handbook of Physiology*, Section 4. *Environmental Physiology*, pp. 45–84. Oxford University Press, New York.

Giesbrecht, G.G. & Bristow, G.K. (1995) Influence of body composition on rewarming from immersion hypothermia. *Aviation, Space, and Environmental Medicine* **66**, 1144–1150.

Gonzalez, R.R. (1986) Work in the north: physiological aspects. *Arctic Medical Research* **44**, 7–17.

Gonzalez, R.R. (1987) Biophysical and physiological integration of proper clothing for exercise. In: Pandolf, K.B. (ed.) *Exercise and Sport Sciences Reviews*, pp. 261–295. Macmillan, New York.

Gonzalez, R.R. (1988) Biophysics of heat transfer and clothing considerations. In: Pandolf, K.B., Sawka, M.N. & Gonzalez, R.R. (eds) *Human Performance Physiology and Environmental Medicine at Terrestrial Extremes*, pp. 45–95. Benchmark Press, Indianapolis.

Gonzalez, R.R. (1995) Biophysics of heat exchange and clothing: applications to sports physiology. *Medicine, Exercise, Nutrition, and Health* **4**, 290–305.

Grover, R.F., Weil, J.V. & Reeves, J.T. (1986) Cardiovascular adaptation to exercise at high altitude. In: Pandolf, K.B. (ed.) *Exercise and Sport Sciences Reviews*, pp. 269–302. Macmillan, New York.

Hales, J.R.S., Hubbard, R.W. & Gaffin, S.L. (1996) Limitation of heat tolerance. In: Fregly, M.J. & Blatteis, C.M. (eds) *Handbook of Physiology*, Section 4. *Environmental Physiology*, pp. 285–355. Oxford University Press, New York.

Hong, S.K. (1973) Pattern of cold adaptation in women divers of Korea (Ama). *Federation Proceedings* **32**, 1614–1622.

Kaufman, W.C. & Bothe, D.J. (1986) Wind chill reconsidered, Siple revisited. *Aviation, Space, and Environmental Medicine* **57**, 23–26.

Kollias, J., Boileau, R. & Buskirk, E.R. (1972) Effects of physical condition in man on thermal responses to cold air. *International Journal of Biometeorology* **16**, 389–402.

Latzka, W.A., Sawka, M.N., Montain, S.J. *et al.* (1997) Hyperhydration: thermoregulatory effects during compensable exercise–heat stress. *Journal of Applied Physiology* **83**, 860–866.

Latzka, W.A., Sawka, M.N., Montain, S.J. *et al.* (1998) Hyperhydration: tolerance and cardiovascular effects during uncompensable exercise–heat stress. *Journal of Applied Physiology* **84**, 1858–1864.

Levine, B.D. & Stray-Gundersen, J. (1997) 'Living high–training low': effect of moderate-altitude acclimatization with low-altitude training on performance. *Journal of Applied Physiology* **83**, 102–112.

Lyons, T.P., Riedesel, M.L., Meuli, L.E. & Chick, T.W. (1990) Effects of glycerol-induced hyperhydration prior to exercise in the heat on sweating and core temperature. *Medicine and Science in Sports and Exercise* **22**, 477–483.

McArdle, W.D., Magel, J.R., Gergley, T.J., Spina, R.J. & Toner, M.M. (1984a) Thermal adjustment to cold-water exposure in resting men and women. *Journal of Applied Physiology* **56**, 1565–1571.

McArdle, W.D., Magel, J.R., Spina, R.J., Gergley, T.J. & Toner, M.M. (1984b) Thermal adjustment to cold-water exposure in exercising men and women. *Journal of Applied Physiology* **56**, 1572–1577.

Malconian, M.K. & Rock, P.B. (1988) Medical problems related to altitude. In: Pandolf, K.B., Sawka, M.N. & Gonzalez, R.R. (eds) *Human Performance Physiology and Environmental Medicine at Terrestrial Extremes*, pp. 545–563. Benchmark Press, Indianapolis.

Molnar, G.W. (1946) Survival of hypothermia by men immersed in the ocean. *Journal of the American Medical Association* **131**, 1046–1050.

Montain, S.J., Maughan, R.J. & Sawka, M.N. (1996) Heat acclimatization strategies for the 1996 Summer Olympics. *Athletic Therapy Today* **1**, 42–46.

Moran, D.S. & Pandolf, K.B. (1999) Wet Bulb Globe Temperature (WBGT)—to what extent is GT essential? *Aviation, Space, and Environmental Medicine* **70**, 480–484.

O'Brien, C., Young, A.J. & Sawka, M.N. (1998) Hypohydration and thermoregulation in cold air. *Journal of Applied Physiology* **84**, 185–189.

Pandolf, K.B. (1988) Air quality and human performance. In: Pandolf, K.B., Sawka, M.N. & Gonzalez, R.R. (eds) *Human Performance Physiology and Environmental Medicine at Terrestrial Extremes*, pp. 591–629. Benchmark Press, Indianapolis.

Pandolf, K.B. (1995) Avoiding heat illness during exercise. In: Torg, J.S. & Shephard, R.J. (eds) *Current Therapy in Sports Medicine*, 3rd edn, pp. 578–582. Mosby, St. Louis.

Pandolf, K.B. (1998) Time course of heat acclimation and its decay. *International Journal of Sports Medicine* **19**, S157–S160.

Santee, W.R., Gonzalez, R.R. & Sawka, M.N. (1988) Characteristics of the thermal environment. In: Pandolf, K.B., Sawka, M.N. & Gonzalez, R.R. (eds) *Human Performance Physiology and Environmental Medicine at Terrestrial Extremes*, pp. 1–43. Benchmark Press, Indianapolis.

Sawka, M.N. & Pandolf, K.B. (1990) Effects of body water loss on exercise performance and physiological functions. In: Gisolfi, C.V. & Lamb, D.R. (eds) *Perspectives in Exercise Science and Sports Medicine: Fluid Homeostasis During Exercise*, Vol. 3, pp. 1–38. Benchmark Press, Indianapolis.

Sawka, M.N., Wenger, C.B. & Pandolf, K.B. (1996) Thermoregulatory responses to acute exercise–heat stress and heat acclimation. In: Fregly, M.J. & Blatteis, C.M. (eds) *Handbook of Physiology*, Section 4. *Environmental Physiology*, pp. 157–185. Oxford University Press, New York.

Sawka, M.N., Latzka, W.A., Matott, R.P. & Montain, S.J. (1998) Hydration effects on temperature regulation. *International Journal of Sports Medicine* **19**, S108–S110.

Siple, P.A. & Passel, C.R. (1945) Measurements of dry atmospheric cooling in sub freezing temperatures. *Proceedings of the American Philosophical Society* **89**, 177–199.

Stolwijk, J.A.J. & Hardy, J.D. (1977) Control of body temperature. In: Lee, D.H.K., Falk, H.L., Murphy, S.D. & Geiger, S.R. (eds) *Handbook of Physiology*, Section 9. *Reactions to Environmental Agents*, pp. 45–68. American Physiological Society, Bethesda.

Thompson, R.L. & Hayward, J.S. (1996) Wet–cold exposure and hypothermia: thermal and metabolic responses to prolonged exercise in rain. *Journal of Applied Physiology* **81**, 1128–1137.

Tikuisis, P. & Frim, J. (1994) Prediction of survival time in cold air. *DCIEM Technical Report 94–29*. Defence and Civil Institute of Environmental Medicine, North York, Ontario.

Tom, P.A., Garmel, G.M. & Auerbach, P.S. (1994) Environment-dependent sports emergencies. *Sports Medicine* **78**, 305–325.

Toner, M.N. & McArdle, W.D. (1988) Physiological adjustments of man to the cold. In: Pandolf, K.B., Sawka, M.N. & Gonzalez, R.R. (eds) *Human Performance Physiology and Environmental Medicine at Terrestrial Extremes*, pp. 361–399. Benchmark Press, Indianapolis.

Ward, M.P., Milledge, J.S. & West, J.B. (1995) *High Altitude Medicine and Physiology*. University of Pennsylvania Press, Philadelphia.

Weller, A.S., Millard, C.E., Stroud, M.A., Greenhaff, P.L. & MacDonald, I.A. (1997) Physiological responses to a cold, wet, and windy environment during prolonged intermittent walking. *American Journal of Physiology* **272**, R226–R233.

Wenger, C.B. (1988) Human heat acclimatization. In: Pandolf, K.B., Sawka, M.N. & Gonzalez, R.R. (eds) *Human Performance Physiology and Environmental Medicine at Terrestrial Extremes*, pp. 153–197. Benchmark Press, Indianapolis.

Young, A.J. (1990) Energy substrate utilization during exercise in extreme environments. In: Pandolf, K.B. & Hollozsy, J.O.

(eds) *Exercise and Sport Sciences Reviews*, pp. 66–117. Williams & Wilkins, Baltimore.

Young, A.J. (1996) Homeostatic responses to prolonged cold exposure: human cold acclimatization. In: Fregley, M.J. & Blatteis, C.M. (eds) *Handbook of Physiology, Section 4. Environmental Physiology*, pp. 419–438. Oxford University Press for the American Physiological Society, New York.

Young, A.J. & Reeves, J.T. (1998) Human adaptation to high terrestrial altitude. In: Burr, R.E. & Pandolf, K.B. (eds) *Textbook of Military Medicine*, Part III. *Disease and the Environment*. Volume: *Medical Aspects of Deployment to Harsh Environments*. Office of the Surgeon General, Department of the Army, and Borden Institute, Washington, DC, in press.

Young, A.J. & Young, P.M. (1988) Human acclimatization to high terrestrial altitude. In: Pandolf, K.B., Sawka, M.N. & Gonzalez, R.R. (eds) *Human Performance Physiology and Environmental Medicine at*

Terrestrial Extremes, pp. 497–543. Benchmark Press, Indianapolis.

Young, A.J., Sawka, M.N., Levine, L. *et al.* (1995) Metabolic and thermal adaptations from endurance training in hot or cold water. *Journal of Applied Physiology* **78**, 793–801.

Young, A.J., Sawka, M.N. & Pandolf, K.B. (1996) Physiology of cold exposure. In: Marriott, B.M. & Carlson, S.J. (eds) *Nutritional Needs in Cold and in High-Altitude Environments*, pp. 127–147. National Academy Press, Washington, DC.

Young, A.J., Castellani, J.W., O'Brien, C. *et al.* (1998a) Exertional fatigue, sleep loss and negative energy balance increase susceptibility to hypothermia. *Journal of Applied Physiology* **85**, 1210–1217.

Young, A.J., Castellani, J.W. & Sawka, M.N. (1998b) Human physiological responses to cold exposure. In: Nose, H., Morimoto, T. & Nadel, E.R. (eds) *The 1997 Nagano Symposium on Sports Sciences*, pp. 273–286. Cooper Publishing Group, Carmel, IN.

Chapter 21

Maximal Oxygen Intake

ROY J. SHEPHARD

Significance of maximal oxygen intake

The maximal oxygen intake, or maximal aerobic power, is a measure of the body's ability to transport oxygen from the ambient air to the exercising muscles. It is thus one of the more important determinants of endurance performance (Shephard 1994). Indeed, if international performers in events such as cross-country skiing are compared with the general population (Table 21.1; Neumann 1988), their maximal oxygen intakes (with occasional male values of 85–90 ml·kg^{-1}·min^{-1}) are four to five standard deviations above the norm for a healthy young man (48 ± 8 ml·kg^{-1}·min^{-1}). In events of 1-min duration, 50% or more of the energy needs of the body may be satisfied by anaerobic metabolism, but if all-out activity is continued for 5 min, 80% of the required energy can be derived from aerobic metabolism, and with 60 min of effort, as much as 98% of metabolism may be aerobic.

The term maximal oxygen intake is usually applied to an effort that can be sustained for no more than a few minutes. It is a peak rate of working, or power, rather than a capacity. However, in sports of very long duration, interest also focuses on the oxygen consumption that a competitor can maintain for 30 min or longer. This value is somewhat smaller than the aerobic power, and can reasonably be described as the aerobic capacity.

Criteria of maximal oxygen intake

The principle adopted for the direct measurement of maximal oxygen intake is simple. The intensity of some type of large muscle effort is increased, either in a stepwise, progressive fashion, or through a series of individual tests of graded intensity, until a 'plateau' of oxygen intake is reached (Fig. 21.1). The 'plateau' has been defined arbitrarily as an increase in oxygen consumption of less than 150 ml·min^{-1} or 2 ml·kg^{-1}·min^{-1} in response to a further increase in the intensity of effort (for example, a further 1% increase in treadmill gradient at a consistent speed of running) (Shephard et al. 1968; Weiner & Lourie 1981).

The demonstration of an oxygen consumption plateau is thought to imply that the individual who is being tested has reached a central limitation of effort — that is to say that, under the particular conditions of measurement, the heart is unable to develop a larger maximal cardiac output, and is thus responsible for the plateauing of oxygen transport. However, in practice, a proportion of subjects halt an intended maximal test because of peripheral symptoms such as muscle weakness, pain or fatigue, despite the strong urgings of the investigator, and in many subjects (particularly children and older adults) a satisfactory oxygen consumption plateau cannot be demonstrated. There may then be attempts to evaluate the 'quality' of the observed effort (Shephard 1994; Howley et al. 1995) in terms of such subsidiary criteria of maximal performance as the peak heart rate (preferably at least 220 – the individual's age in years), the peak respiratory gas exchange ratio (carbon dioxide output/oxygen intake, a measure of metabolic acidosis, preferably higher than 1.10) and the peak blood lactate (preferably at least 10–12 mmol·l^{-1} in

Table 21.1 Typical values of maximal oxygen intake in various sports. From Neumann (1988).

Type of event	Maximal oxygen intake ($ml \cdot kg^{-1} \cdot min^{-1}$)	
	Men	Women
Endurance sports		
Long-distance running	75–80	65–70
Cross-country skiing	75–78	65–70
Biathlon	75–78	–
Road cycling	70–75	60–65
Middle-distance running	70–75	65–68
Skating	65–72	55–60
Orienteering	65–72	60–65
Swimming	60–70	55–60
Rowing	65–69	60–64
Track racing	65–70	55–60
Canoeing	60–68	50–55
Walking	60–65	55–60
Games		
Football (soccer)	50–57	–
Handball	55–60	48–52
Ice hockey	55–60	–
Volleyball	55–60	48–52
Basketball	50–55	40–45
Tennis	48–52	40–45
Table tennis	40–45	38–42
Combative sports		
Boxing	60–65	–
Wrestling	60–65	–
Judo	55–60	50–55
Fencing	45–50	40–45
Power sports		
Sprint (200 m track)	55–60	45–50
Sprint track and field (100 m, 200 m)	48–52	43–47
Long jump	50–55	45–50
Competition consisting of several events (decathlon, septathlon)	60–65	50–55
Nordic combination (15-km ski-walking and ski-jumping)	60–65	–
Weightlifting	40–50	–
Discus throwing, shot-putting	40–45	35–40
Javelin throwing	45–50	42–47
Pole vaulting	45–50	–
Ski-jumping	40–45	–
Technical/acrobatic sports		
Downhill skiing (Alpine disciplines)	60–65	48–53
Figure skating	50–55	45–50
Gymnastics	45–50	40–45
Rhythmic gymnastics	–	40–45
Sailing	50–55	45–50
Shooting	40–45	35–40

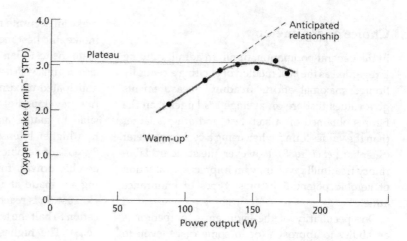

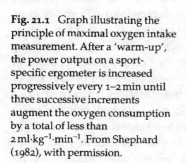

Fig. 21.1 Graph illustrating the principle of maximal oxygen intake measurement. After a 'warm-up', the power output on a sport-specific ergometer is increased progressively every 1–2 min until three successive increments augment the oxygen consumption by a total of less than $2\,ml\cdot kg^{-1}\cdot min^{-1}$. From Shephard (1982), with permission.

young adults and around $8\,mmol\cdot l^{-1}$ in older individuals). There have been claims that, particularly in children (Armstrong *et al.* 1996) and the elderly (Thomas *et al.* 1987), non-plateau values are as stable and reproducible criteria of the individual's aerobic potential as clear-cut plateaux, and that the peak oxygen consumption thus determined cannot be increased further by a deliberate 'supramaximal' effort (Armstrong *et al.* 1996).

The oxygen consumption per unit volume of active muscle is at least as large for arm as for leg work. However, demonstration of a centrally limited plateau of oxygen consumption depends on the activation of a large muscle volume (Sol & Sinning 1980; Shephard *et al.* 1988). Thus plateaux are rarely demonstrated during arm exercise, and they are also seen much less frequently during cycle ergometry (which is heavily dependent on the force developed by the quadriceps) than in uphill treadmill running (a task where the effort is widely distributed over the major muscle groups of the body).

Although information on peak oxygen transport is more satisfying if a plateau has been reached, many authors maintain that peak values without a clear plateau are still sufficiently consistent to be used in the management of athletes.

Preparations for a test of maximal aerobic power

The commonly recommended schedule of pre-parations for the measurement of maximal aerobic power include 24 h of rest, an overnight fast and a room temperature of 22°C (Shephard *et al.* 1968; Andersen *et al.* 1971; Weiner & Lourie 1981; Shephard 1994). It may be difficult to persuade a top athlete to accept 24 h of total rest, and indeed the state of the body would then be unrepresentative of normal conditions for that individual. However, the investigator should insist that the athlete perform a lighter than average workout on the day preceding a maximal test. Some laboratories may also lack air conditioning. There is no strong evidence that a room temperature higher than 22°C has any direct influence on the results of a brief maximal oxygen intake test, although prolonged heat exposure, with resultant salt, mineral and water depletion, can have a negative effect upon test scores. If the room is hot, the comfort of the test subject can be improved by the use of a well-placed fan. Often, the heat loss thus achieved is equivalent to a 2°C decrease in room temperature.

Test scores vary somewhat with the time of day (Shephard 1984). The largest values are observed in the morning (when central blood volume has been maximized by a night of recumbency). The time of testing should thus be noted carefully, and when possible it should be matched to the anticipated time of competition. Cigarette smoking, overindulgence in alcohol and a recent viral infection are other factors that can have a negative influence on test scores.

Choice of ergometer

In the general population, uphill treadmill running is regarded as the best method of eliciting a centrally limited maximal effort. Treadmill measurements give values that are on average 4% larger than the figures obtained on a step test, and are 7% larger than the values found when using a cycle ergometer (Shephard *et al.* 1968). However, the standard laboratory treadmill gives only an imprecise evaluation of aerobic potential in most types of endurance athlete.

One peculiarity of the endurance competitor is an ability to approach (or in some cases, even to exceed) the treadmill maximal oxygen consumption while performing the specific sport for which they have been trained. Thus Verstappen *et al.* (1982) compared eight runners with eight cyclists. When exercising on the cycle ergometer, the cyclists obtained the same score as they had achieved on the treadmill, but in the case of the runners the treadmill aerobic power was 14% larger than that seen on a cycle ergometer. Differences between the two modes of exercise largely disappear if the cycle ergometer is equipped with toe clips (Tanaka *et al.* 1987). A variety of specialized devices such as swimming flumes, rowing ergometers and kayaking ergometers have been devised to allow athletes to reach peak effort in a sport-specific manner (see Chapter 19). In some instances, the competitor has been tested by exhaling into a Douglas bag or metabolic cart during a simulated competition, or the oxygen consumption during peak effort has been estimated by backwards extrapolation of data collected immediately following competition. More recently, there has also been some success with devices such as the COSMED telemeter, a portable device that uses a simplified calculation to estimate oxygen consumption from transmitted signals of ventilation and expired oxygen concentrations (Lucia *et al.* 1993).

Irrespective of the choice of ergometer, there has been much discussion concerning an appropriate test protocol. The results are surprisingly similar for continuous and discontinuous tests, and for progressive tests with slow and rapid ramp functions (Fairshter *et al.* 1983). If the intent is simply to make an accurate measurement of maximal oxygen intake, the best recommendation seems to approximate the test plan for a normal healthy adult; exercise begins with a 3-min 'warm-up' at 60–70% of the anticipated maximal oxygen intake. From the heart rate developed at this intensity of effort, it is possible to gauge and to move relatively precisely to a higher intensity of exercise that will demand 85–90% of aerobic power. After 2 min at 85–90% of aerobic power, further small increments of loading are made at 1–2 min intervals until subjective exhaustion is reached, or there is some clinical indication to halt the test (Andersen *et al.* 1971; Shephard 1994). The highest oxygen consumptions are attained if the test duration falls within the range 8–17 min (Buchfuhrer *et al.* 1983). An effective test can thus be achieved with a minimum investment of time if the investigator aims to reach both a plateau of oxygen consumption and subjective exhaustion over 9–11 min of heavy exercise (Andersen *et al.* 1971; Buchfuhrer *et al.* 1983; Shephard 1994).

If constraints of time require the concurrent estimation of ventilatory threshold (Chapter 22), the warm-up is based upon 3 min of loadless operation of the ergometer. An attempt is then made to reach both an oxygen consumption plateau and subjective exhaustion, using from nine to 11 small and equal increments of effort, applied at 1-min intervals.

If a true central limitation of effort is reached, the athlete will commonly show a greying of the complexion and some loss of postural control. There may also be feelings of nausea, a confused response to questioning and impending loss of consciousness. Depending on the circumstances of the test, the investigator must be prepared to offer physical support (particularly in treadmill testing, where unattended subjects have sometimes suffered unpleasant cuts and abrasions from falling against the moving parts of the machine).

A sudden cessation of maximal effort can lead to collapse from a pooling of blood in the dilated vessels of the lower limbs, and it is advisable to allow a gentle cool-down of at least 1 min following completion of the formal test. This precaution is particularly important if the test has been performed in a warm environment.

Use of ancillary equipment

If resources permit, it is desirable to use an automated measuring system such as the Sensor-Medics/Horizon metabolic cart or the Jaeger Ergostat to provide on-line monitoring of oxygen consumption. These devices incorporate an infrared detector to measure carbon dioxide concentrations, a paramagnetic or electrochemical oxygen sensor, and a turbine or screen flowmeter for the determination of respiratory minute volume. The data thus generated are fed to a computer and oxygen consumption is displayed or printed out at 20–30-s intervals. The investigator thus gains a semicontinuous indication of progress towards an oxygen consumption plateau. Some investigators (for example, Miles et al. 1994) have found substantial differences in results between different designs of metabolic cart, but Unnithan et al. (1994) noted that values obtained with the most popular device (the Sensor-Medics cart) agreed closely with an older and well-accepted technology (Douglas bag measurements).

If a laboratory is less lavishly equipped, it is quite possible to obtain valid metabolic data by collecting expired gas samples in Douglas bags at 1-min intervals. The volume of expired gas is subsequently measured, using a carefully calibrated gasmeter or Tissot spirometer, and the expired gas concentrations are determined chemically, by Lloyd-Haldane or Scholander apparatus.

A continuous electrocardiogram provides a check on the safety of the test, and allows an accurate counting of heart rates. In sedentary individuals, it is customary to monitor at least three chest leads (for instance, CM-2, CM-4 and CM-6) during an exercise test (Fig. 21.2). The neutral lead is fixed to the back of the neck, one lead is secured to the manubrium sterni, and the exploring electrodes are placed in the V-2, V-4 and V-6 positions. However, in a young and healthy adult who has little risk of developing myocardial ischaemia, a single (CM-5) lead is adequate for most exercise tests. Some ingenuity in the placement of the electrodes may be needed in order to avoid electrical interference from muscle action potentials, particularly if the subject is operating a type of ergometer that requires rhythmic arm

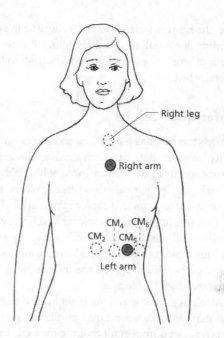

Fig. 21.2 Diagram illustrating the recommended placement of electrocardiography electrodes for an exercise test involving leg exercise. The lead marked 'right arm' is attached over the manubrium sterni, and the lead marked 'right leg' is attached to the nape of the neck. The lead labelled 'left arm' is attached 7–10 cm to the left of the midline, in the fifth interspace (CM-5 recording). From Shephard (1977), with permission.

movements. A wandering baseline is usually an indication of poor electrode contact or inadequate preliminary abrasion of the skin. Abnormalities of heart rhythm may develop early in the recovery period, and it is thus wise to continue monitoring both the subject and the electrocardiogram for at least 5 min after exercise has ceased.

The systemic blood pressure should be measured at 1-min intervals throughout a progressive maximal exercise test. A standard sphygmomanometer allows systolic readings to be auscultated with reasonable confidence, and it can be assumed that the diastolic readings (which are hard to detect during vigorous exercise) remain relatively constant. Failure of the mean systemic blood pressure to rise with work rate implies that the subject has difficulty in sustaining cardiac stroke volume during vigorous exercise. This situation is particularly likely if maximal oxygen intake has been surpassed and the heart is starting to fail. A decline in systolic reading of more than 10 mmHg with a further increment of work rate is an urgent indication to halt an exercise test.

Safety precautions

Exercise testing has a very low morbidity and mortality, even in patients with cardiac disease. The great majority of athletes are extremely healthy individuals, and in their case the risks of exercise testing are even lower than in a clinical population. Nevertheless, it is important to look for and observe both relative and absolute contraindications to exercise testing (Tables 21.2 & 21.3), and to discontinue a test if any of the widely agreed warning signs or symptoms are noted (Table 21.4).

At all ages, there is a very slight risk that exercise may provoke ventricular fibrillation or cardiac arrest, and it is important that the investigator who is conducting the test is familiar with procedures for cardiac resuscitation. Emergency equipment should always be available to deal with such a contingency. There is no need for a physician to be present when testing a symptom-free athlete who is under the age

Table 21.2 Relative contraindications to exercise testing, based on the recommendations of the American College of Sports Medicine. From American College of Sports Medicine (1991), with permission.

Relative diastolic blood pressure over 120 mmHg or resting systolic pressure over 200 mmHg
Moderate valvular heart disease
Digitalis or drug effect
Electrolyte abnormalities such as hypokalaemia or hypomagnesia
Fixed-rate artificial pacemaker
Frequent or complex ventricular ectopic beats
Ventricular aneurysm
Cardiomyopathy, including hypertrophic cardiomyopathy
Uncontrolled metabolic disease (such as diabetes, thyrotoxicosis or myxoedema)
Any serious systemic disorder or chronic disease (such as mononucleosis, hepatitis or AIDS)
Neuromuscular, musculoskeletal or rheumatoid disorders that are exacerbated by exercise
Advanced or complicated pregnancy

Table 21.3 Absolute contraindications to maximal exercise testing, based on the recommendations of the American College of Sports Medicine. From American College of Sports Medicine (1991), with permission.

Recent complicated myocardial infarction
Unstable angina
Uncontrolled ventricular dysrhythmia
Uncontrolled atrial dysrhythmia which compromises cardiac function
Acute congestive heart failure
Severe aortic stenosis
Suspected or known dissecting aneurysm
Active or suspected myocarditis or pericarditis
Thrombophlebitis or intracardiac thrombi
Recent systemic or pulmonary embolus
Acute infection
Third degree atrioventricular block
Significant emotional distress (psychosis)
A recent significant change in the resting electrocardiogram suggestive of myocardial infarction or other acute cardiac events

Table 21.4 Indications to halt a maximal exercise test, based on the recommendations of the American College of Sports Medicine. From American College of Sports Medicine (1991), with permission.

Subject requests to stop
Failure of the monitoring system
Progressive angina (stop at 3+ or earlier on a scale of 1+ to 4+)
Four millimetres (0.4 mV) horizontal or downsloping ST segmental depression or elevation
Sustained supraventricular tachycardia
Ventricular tachycardia
Exercise-induced left bundle branch block
Any significant drop (20 mmHg) in systolic blood pressure, or failure of the systolic blood pressure to rise with an increase in exercise load
Light-headedness, confusion, ataxia, pallor, cyanosis, nausea or signs of severe peripheral circulatory insufficiency
Excessive blood pressure rise; systolic >250 mmHg; diastolic >120 mmHg
R on T premature ventricular complexes
Unexplained bradycardia—pulse rate more than 25 beats·min^{-1} below age-adjusted normals in absence of beta blockade
Onset of second or third degree heart block
Multifocal premature ventricular complexes
Increasing ventricular ectopy

of 40 years, but for older competitors, medical coverage is a wise precaution.

The inherent risk of myocardial infarction is less for most types of endurance athlete than for the general population, but contrary to the views of Bassler (1977), regular endurance activity such as marathon running does not confer a total immunity from coronary vascular disease (Winget *et al.* 1994; Goodman 1995). Indeed, because most athletes are high achievers, they may continue a test in the face of symptoms that would halt the effort of a sedentary person.

Possible use of submaximal tests

Partly because of fears that maximal tests have a greater tendency to provoke cardiac arrest, and partly because of a desire to eliminate the supposed discomfort of all-out effort, much research has been directed to possible submaximal indicators of aerobic potential.

The usual theoretical basis of submaximal test procedures has been the relationship between oxygen consumption (or the equivalent power output) and heart rate (Shephard 1994). Contrary to expectations of the Conconi test (Chapter 22), a roughly linear plot is obtained from 50% to near 100% of maximal oxygen intake. Unfortunately, because of some lability in the heart rate during submaximal exercise, slight departures from a linear heart rate/oxygen consumption relationship and substantial interindividual variations in maximal heart rate at any given age, heart rate-based predictions of maximal oxygen intake show a coefficient of variation of 10–15% relative to directly measured values. Predicted values may have some application in determining the aerobic potential of large populations under difficult field conditions (Shephard & Rode 1995), and they may allow a rough assessment of changes in the condition of an individual from week to week. On the other hand, it is hardly useful to predict that the maximal oxygen intake of a cross-country skier is $68\,ml\cdot kg^{-1}\cdot min^{-1}$ if the 95% confidence limits of the prediction extend from 88 to $48\,ml\cdot kg^{-1}\cdot min^{-1}$!

Other methods of predicting maximal oxygen intake have been based upon intensity-related changes in the respiratory gas exchange ratio; this ratio increases progressively as maximum effort is approached. Unfortunately, such predictions are no more precise than estimates based on the heart rate observed during submaximal exercise (Shephard 1975).

Possible use of field tests

Given that a substantial part of the large maximal oxygen intake of the endurance competitor may be inherited rather than developed through rigorous training (Chapter 15), one potential approach to national athletic success is to search extensively through the entire population in an attempt to discover unusually well-endowed candidates. The number of individuals to be tested in such a search precludes the use of any sophisticated laboratory procedures, and the question thus arises as to whether a simple field test can provide an approximate measure of oxygen transport which is sufficiently accurate for preliminary screening. In the general adult population, the standard error of estimates of maximal oxygen intake, based on walking speed over a distance of 1.6–2 km, is typically 9–15% (Kline *et al.* 1987; McCutcheon *et al.* 1990; Oja *et al.* 1991). However, precision can be increased by the introduction of terms relating to body mass index (Cureton *et al.* 1995), age and gender (Kline *et al.* 1987).

The most obvious approach for a potential competitor is to measure the times achieved in an actual or a simulated athletic event. For example, runners can be compared in terms of the times that they take to cover a fixed distance, or the distance covered in a fixed time. An immediate difficulty is that athletic selection is being made at ever younger ages, and the relationship between performance times and oxygen transport is not very close, particularly in young children (Table 21.5). Much depends on the sport-specific skill of the individual and on an appropriate choice of pace rather than upon peak oxygen transport. Indeed, cynics have suggested that timed trials of running or swimming add little information that could not have been obtained from age, body mass and skinfold thicknesses.

If mass testing is contemplated, it is further quite

Table 21.5 Some reported coefficients of correlation between the directly measured maximal oxygen intake and running speed. After data collected by Disch *et al.* (1975) and Shephard (1982). See Shephard (1982) for details of references.

Subjects	*n*	Authors	Coefficients of correlation with $\dot{V}o_{2max}$
402 m			
College males	35	Wiley & Shaver (1972)	−0.22
College males	11	Ribisl & Kachadorian (1969)	−0.31
549 m			
Boys, 10 years	20	Larivière *et al.* (1974)	−0.58
Boys, 12–13 years	30	Metz & Alexander (1970)	−0.67
Boys, 14–15 years	30	Metz & Alexander (1970)	−0.27
Boys, grade 9	9	Doolittle & Bigbee (1968)	−0.62
Faculty and staff	87	Falls *et al.* (1966)	−0.64
Sedentary men	141	Drake *et al.* (1968)	−0.27
805 m			
Boys, 10 years	20	Larivière *et al.* (1974)	−0.37
College males	11	Ribisl & Kachadorian (1969)	−0.67
Physical education majors	10	Kearney & Byrnes (1974)	−0.30
College males	11	Byrnes & Kearney (1974)	−0.73
Physical education majors	11	Byrnes & Kearney (1974)	−0.04
Cross-country runners	11	Byrnes & Kearney (1974)	−0.42
1610 m			
College males	25	Wiley & Shaver (1972)	−0.29
College males	11	Ribisl & Kachadorian (1969)	−0.79
College males	11	Byrnes & Kearney (1974)	−0.72
Physical education majors	11	Byrnes & Kearney (1974)	−0.25
Cross-country runners	11	Byrnes & Kearney (1974)	−0.51
3220 m			
College males	11	Ribisl & Kachadorian (1969)	−0.85
College males	25	Wiley & Shaver (1972)	−0.47
Older males	24	Ribisl & Kachadorian (1969)	−0.86
4830 m			
College males	35	Wiley & Shaver (1972)	−0.43
8050 m			
Cross-country runners	17	Kearney & Byrnes (1974)	−0.38
9-min run			
Boys, 9–12 years	25	Coleman (1974)	0.82
Girls, 9–12 years	25	Coleman (1974)	0.71
12-min run			
Boys, 9–12 years	25	Coleman (1972)	0.82
Boys, 10 years	20	Larivière *et al.* (1974)	0.44
Boys, 11–14 years	17	Maksud & Coutts (1971)	0.65
Boys, grade 9	9	Doolittle & Bigbee (1968)	0.90
Girls, 9–12 years	25	Coleman (1974)	0.71
College males	7	Kearney & Byrnes (1974)	0.80
Physical education majors	10	Kearney & Byrnes (1974)	0.64
Cross-country runners	17	Kearney & Byrnes (1974)	0.28
Adult males	115	Cooper (1968a)	0.90
College females	30	Burris (1970)	0.74
College females	36	Katch *et al.* (1973)	0.67

difficult to standardize the conditions of measurement. Indoor running times, for example, may suffer from overheated rooms or the need to make repeated turns in order to cover the required distance. Outdoor measurements are not only susceptible to differences of environmental temperature and humidity, but also face problems from wind, rain and changing track or ground conditions.

Performance times may help to identify talented youngsters, but they provide an even less satisfactory measure of a person's underlying aerobic potential than do submaximal laboratory tests.

Interpretation of test results

In the general population, the reproducibility of maximal oxygen intake data depends very much on the care that has been taken in calibrating the test equipment, and the success of the observer in motivating subjects to an all-out, centrally limited maximal effort. But even assuming careful technique and good motivational skills on the part of the investigator, there remains an unavoidable intraindividual test-to-test variation in scores of 4–5%.

When testing the aerobic power of endurance athletes, the results are often no more precise or consistent. A competitor may be reluctant to give an all-out effort, fearing that this will impair performance in an upcoming contest. Moreover, in many cases the generality of the measured aerobic power is compromised by differences in the pattern of exercise between that required to operate the test ergometer and normal competition. For example, there are considerable differences between any of the strokes used in normal swimming and the type of exercise that is possible on a swim-bench or a tethered swimming device. Likewise, a rowing machine provides only a limited simulation of the competitor's experience when exercising in a racing shell. Even a cycle ergometer differs from a racing bicycle in terms of gearing, use of toe clips, saddle and handlebar configuration and posture (sitting versus standing exercise). It is thus optimistic to assume that the test-to-test variation in measurements will be any less for athletes than the 4–5% cited for the general population.

Interindividual differences in mechanical efficiency also limit the closeness of match between maximal oxygen intake and an athlete's competitive times. Given that most races are decided by margins much smaller than 4–5%, measurements of peak oxygen transport can allow only a very crude ranking of competitors. If the treadmill maximal oxygen intake is substantially larger than the sport-specific measurement, this may indicate a need for the athlete to concentrate his or her training upon local muscular development. However, if both treadmill and sport-specific values are low, then a general development of the cardiorespiratory system should be attempted. If both the treadmill and the sport-specific values are high, but performance is poor, the implication is that the coach should concentrate upon improving mechanical and technical skills.

In the general population, measured gains of maximal oxygen intake are sometimes used to encourage an individual to continue training. If an athlete is showing substantial gains in peak oxygen transport, the laboratory findings can be exploited for a similar purpose. But as a peak of conditioning is approached, the physiological gains are likely to be disappointingly small relative to the effort that the athlete is investing in training. The data thus have only limited motivational value for most high-performance competitors.

Overtraining may be associated with a decrease in maximal oxygen intake, but again the day-to-day margin of error in test data is sufficiently large that oxygen transport measurements cannot provide as sensitive an index of overtraining as would simple measurements of performance times, serum enzyme levels and assessments of mood state.

The measurement of maximal oxygen intake has other possible uses. Sometimes, it has served to monitor the recovery of function following injury or illness. It also provides the denominator for such indices as ventilatory threshold (Chapter 22). Finally, it may help in establishing an appropriate intensity of training sessions, and the grouped data for an entire team may be useful in evaluating the response to novel methods of training.

Acknowledgement

Dr Shephard's studies are supported in part by research grants from the Defence and Civil Institute of Environmental Medicine, Toronto, ON.

References

American College of Sports Medicine (1991) *Guidelines for Graded Exercise Testing and Exercise Prescription*, 4th edn. Lea & Febiger, Philadelphia.

Andersen, K.L., Shephard, R.J., Denolin, H., Varnauskas, E. & Masironi, R. (1971) *Fundamentals of Exercise Testing*. World Health Organization, Geneva.

Armstrong, N., Welsman, J. & Winsley, R. (1996) Is peak $\dot{V}o_2$ a maximal index of children's aerobic fitness? *International Journal of Sports Medicine* 17, 356–359.

Bassler, T.J. (1977) Marathon running and immunity to atherosclerosis. *Annals of the New York Academy of Science* 301, 579–592.

Buchfuhrer, M.J., Hansen, J.E., Robinson, T.E., Sue, D.Y., Wasserman, K. & Whipp, B.J. (1983) Optimizing the exercise protocol for cardiopulmonary assessment. *Journal of Applied Physiology* 55, 1558–1564.

Cureton, K.J., Sloniger, M.A., O'Bannon, J.P., Black, D.M. & McCormack, W.P. (1995) A generalized equation for prediction of $\dot{V}o_{2peak}$ from 1 mile run/walk performance. *Medicine and Science in Sports and Exercise* 27, 445–451.

Disch, J., Frankiewicz, R. & Jackson, A. (1975) Construct validation of distance run tests. *Research Quarterly* 46, 169–176.

Fairshter, R.D., Walters, J., Salness, K., Fox, M., Minh, V.D. & Wilson, A.F. (1983) A comparison of incremental exercise tests during cycle and treadmill ergometry. *Medicine and Science in Sports and Exercise* 15, 549–554.

Goodman, J.M. (1995) Exercise and sudden cardiac death: etiology in apparently healthy individuals. *Sports Science Reviews* 4 (2), 14–30.

Howley, E., Bassett, D.R. & Welch, H.G. (1995) Criteria for maximal oxygen uptake: review and commentary. *Medicine and Science in Sports and Exercise* 27, 1292–1301.

Kline, G.M., Porcari, J.P., Hintermeister, R. *et al.* (1987) Estimation of $\dot{V}o_{2max}$ from a one-mile track walk, gender, age and body weight. *Medicine and Science in Sports and Exercise* 19, 253–259.

Lucia, A., Fleck, S.J., Gotshall, R.W. & Kearney, J.T. (1993) Validity and reliability of the Cosmed K2 instrument. *International Journal of Sports Medicine* 14, 380–386.

McCutcheon, M.C., Sticha, S.A., Giese, M.D. & Nagle, F.J. (1990) A further analysis of the 12-minute run prediction of maximal aerobic power. *Research Quarterly* 61, 280–283.

Miles, D.S., Cox, M.H. & Verde, T. (1994) Four commonly utilized metabolic systems fail to produce similar results during submaximal and maximal testing. *Sports Medicine, Training and Rehabilitation* 5, 189–198.

Neumann, G. (1988) Special performance capacity. In: Dirix, A., Knuttgen, H.G. & Tittel, K. (eds) *The Olympic Book of Sports Medicine*, Vol. 1, pp. 97–108. Blackwell Scientific Publications, Oxford.

Oja, P., Laukkanen, R., Pasanen, M., Tyry, T. & Vuori, I. (1991) A 2km walking test for assessing the cardiorespiratory fitness of healthy adults. *International Journal of Sports Medicine* 12, 356–362.

Shephard, R.J. (1975) Respiratory gas exchange ratio and the prediction of aerobic power. *Journal of Applied Physiology* 38, 402–406.

Shephard, R.J. (1977) *Endurance Fitness*, 2nd edn. University of Toronto Press, Toronto.

Shephard, R.J. (1982) *Physiology and Biochemistry of Exercise*. Praeger Publications, New York.

Shephard, R.J. (1984) Sleep, biorhythms and human performance. *Sports Medicine* 1, 11–37.

Shephard, R.J. (1994) *Physical Activity,*

Fitness and Health. Human Kinetics, Champaign, IL.

Shephard, R.J. & Rode, A. (1995) *The Health Consequences of 'Modernization'*. Cambridge University Press, London.

Shephard, R.J., Allen, C., Benade, A.J.S. *et al.* (1968) The maximum oxygen intake: An international reference standard of cardiorespiratory fitness. *Bulletin of the World Health Organization* 38, 757–764.

Shephard, R.J., Bouhlel, E., Vandewalle, H. & Monod, H. (1988) Muscle mass as a factor limiting physical work. *Journal of Applied Physiology* 64, 1472–1479.

Sol, N. & Sinning, W.E. (1980) Physiological responses of arm and leg work adjusted for active muscle. *Medicine and Science in Sports and Exercise* 12, 116.

Tanaka, K., Nakadomo, F. & Moritani, T. (1987) Effects of standing cycling and the use of toe stirrups on maximal oxygen uptake. *European Journal of Applied Physiology* 56, 699–703.

Thomas, S.G., Cunningham, D.A., Rechnitzer, P.A., Donner, A.P. & Howard, J.H. (1987) Protocols and reliability of maximal oxygen uptake in the elderly. *Canadian Journal of Sport Sciences* 12, 144–151.

Unnithan, V.B., Wilson, J., Buchanan, D., Timmons, J.A. & Paton, J.V. (1994) Validation of the Sensor-Medics (S2900Z) metabolic cart for pediatric exercise testing. *Canadian Journal of Applied Physiology* 19, 472–479.

Verstappen, F.T.J., Huppertz, R.M. & Snoeckx, L.H.E.H. (1982) Effect of training specificity on maximal treadmill and bicycle ergometer exercise. *International Journal of Sports Medicine* 3, 43–46.

Weiner, J.S. & Lourie, J.A. (1981) *Handbook of Practical Biology*. Academic Press, London.

Winget, J.F., Capeless, M.A. & Ades, P.A. (1994) Sudden death in athletes. *Sports Medicine* 18, 375–383.

Chapter 22

Anaerobic Metabolism and Endurance Performance

ROY J. SHEPHARD

Introduction

The tolerance of lactate accumulation in both the exercising muscles and the bloodstream has a substantial influence on an individual's ability to sustain a large oxygen intake (the aerobic capacity) and thus overall performance in competitions of long duration. In this chapter, we will review some fundamental concepts of anaerobic metabolism and muscular endurance, and will then examine in more detail the topics of blood lactate accumulation, the anaerobic threshold and acid–base balance in the context of the endurance performer.

Fundamental concepts of anaerobic metabolism

The classical viewpoint

The classical viewpoint of the exercise physiologist was that a person could pursue physical activity in an aerobic mode until the intensity of effort was sufficient to elicit the maximal oxygen intake (Margaria *et al.* 1963). However, beyond this ceiling the intensity of effort became 'supramaximal', and there was a sudden transition to anaerobic metabolism. According to this viewpoint, the endurance athlete would only draw upon anaerobic energy resources and accumulate significant quantities of lactate during the initial jockeying for position, and the final sprint to the finish line.

The validity of the classical hypothesis plainly depends on: (i) a rapid increase of oxygen transport to a steady-state level that matches energy demands at the onset of exercise; (ii) a uniform and adequate perfusion of the active muscles once a steady state is attained; (iii) a uniform metabolic demand by the various muscle fibres engaged in performance of the activity; and (iv) the absence of any oxygen deficit during the subsequent metabolic drift (Barstow *et al.* 1993). None of these conditions are fully satisfied in practice.

Current concepts

Current observers recognize that the concentration of lactate found in the circulating blood during vigorous exercise is not tightly linked to the immediate extent of anaerobic metabolism. Rather, it represents a balance between the recent rate of lactate production (mainly in poorly oxygenated muscles) and its rate of metabolism in other better-oxygenated tissues.

The end result of these two competing processes is a less-than-sharp transition from aerobic metabolism to the stage of lactate accumulation. Lactate first appears in the arterial blood in significant quantities at an intensity of effort somewhere between 50 and 70% rather than 100% of maximal oxygen intake. The precise threshold varies, depending on the type of exercise that is being performed. At higher intensities of effort, lactate accumulates progressively, and during all-out ('supramaximal') effort the athlete quickly reaches the highest tolerated arterial lactate concentration ($11–15\,\text{mmol·l}^{-1}$ in young adults, less in children (Gaul *et al.* 1995), women (Bovens *et al.* 1993) and older adults (Shephard 1997)).

Benefits of limiting lactate accumulation

During an endurance competition, the athlete attempts to regulate the intensity of her or his effort so that the rate of lactate metabolism matches its rate of production, and blood levels are held below a figure of about $4\,mmol\cdot l^{-1}$ (Farrell *et al.* 1979).

Four primary arguments suggest the wisdom of such tactics.

1 Firstly, from a metabolic viewpoint, anaerobic activity is extremely inefficient. During aerobic metabolism, each molecule of glucose phosphate generates 39 molecules of adenosine triphosphate (ATP). In contrast, if there is an incomplete breakdown of carbohydrate to lactate (Shephard 1982), only three molecules of ATP are generated. Nevertheless, much of the remaining unspent chemical energy can be recouped if the lactate is metabolized to carbon dioxide and water elsewhere in the body, or is used as a substrate for hepatic gluconeogenesis.

2 Secondly, triglycerides cannot be metabolized anaerobically. If anaerobic mechanisms are needed to fuel physical activity (for instance, when climbing a hill during a marathon run), the performance at this stage of competition depends largely on the remaining reserves of carbohydrate. If anaerobic work has been performed unnecessarily, these reserves may be depleted prematurely (Chapter 13).

3 Thirdly, the intramuscular accumulation of hydrogen ions, and possibly also of lactate (Hogan *et al.* 1995), quickly inhibits key enzymes in the glycolytic chain (phosphorylase and phosphofructokinase). Energy release from carbohydrate is halted, and this causes weakness and pain in the active muscles (Shephard 1982), with a progressive decline in muscle power.

4 Finally, the progressive build-up of hydrogen ions in the bloodstream stimulates a vigorous hyperventilation. This is distressing for the individual, and it diverts a substantial fraction of the available cardiac output from the limbs to meet the metabolic needs of the chest muscles (Chapter 5).

Markers of competitive performance

As discussed below, the intensity of effort at which lactate begins to accumulate is influenced by such factors as the individual's dominant fibre type,

muscle capillarity and event-specific training. Nevertheless, the threshold for any given event remains a fairly consistent fraction of maximal oxygen intake from one person to another. Thus, the determination of maximal oxygen intake provides a useful guide to the likely pace that can be tolerated without lactate accumulation in events that last from 5 to 30 min.

In shorter events, performance is quite closely correlated with the size of the peak oxygen deficit (Weyand *et al.* 1994), much of which is accumulated in the first minute of exercise. If endurance effort continues for longer than 20–30 min, the maximal oxygen intake again becomes progressively less important as a determinant of successful performance. Competitive results over running distances of 5–42 km are often correlated more closely with measurements of blood lactate concentration than with maximal oxygen intake determinations (Table 22.1; Jacobs 1986; Iwaoka *et al.* 1988; Loats & Rhodes 1993).

Influence of training

The well-trained competitor is characterized by an ability to perform a specific athletic skill for a long period at an above-average fraction of maximal oxygen intake, without apparent fatigue (Bunc & Leso 1993).

This feature of the successful athlete seems to reflect in part a strengthening of the muscles in the active limbs. Further, the performance yielded by a given oxygen transport improves progressively as training enhances the individual's movement skills. For these reasons, competitive results may show a continuing improvement in endurance performance, despite a stagnation of training-induced gains in peak oxygen transport (Williams *et al.* 1967; Heck *et al.* 1985; Henritze *et al.* 1985).

Muscular endurance

Lactate accumulation and muscular endurance

Muscular endurance is normally expressed as the ratio of the peak force currently generated by a given muscle relative to the peak force that the same muscle can develop during a single brief effort.

Endurance may be considered with respect to

Table 22.1 Coefficients of correlation of maximal oxygen intake and blood lactate variables with endurance performance. From Jacobs (1986), with permission (see original paper for details of references).

Type of performance	Coefficient of correlation		Reference
	Maximal oxygen intake	Lactate	
4.2.2-km run	0.91	0.98	Farrell et al. (1979)
19.3-km run	0.91	0.97	
15.0-km run	0.89	0.97	
9.7-km run	0.86	0.96	
3.2-km run	0.83	0.91	
90-km run	n.s.	0.93	Jooste et al. (1981)
10-km run	0.75	0.84	Kumagi et al. (1982)
6.2-km run	0.49	0.84	
5-km run	0.46	0.95	
Race walking	0.62	0.94	Hagberg & Coyle (1983)
30-km run	0.71	0.76	Lehmann et al. (1983)
21.1-km run	0.81	0.88	Williams & Nute (1983)
10-km run	Lower	>0.89	Allen et al. (1985)

n.s., not significant.

either the rate of decay of force during a single, prolonged isometric contraction, or the progressive reduction in force which is seen during a series of rhythmically repeated maximal contractions. In each of these situations, the decrement of force over time probably reflects, at least in part, a local accumulation of lactate, with an inhibition of glycolysis and a failure to regenerate ATP within the active muscle fibres (Shephard 1982; Tesch & Wright 1983; Chapter 23). The overall loss of force at any given time thus depends on the proportion of muscle fibres in which lactate concentrations exceed the ceiling compatible with continued contractile function.

Muscle function in very prolonged events

Activities that continue for longer than 1 h are performed mainly by slow-twitch muscle fibres (Chapter 23). In such prolonged events, muscle endurance becomes limited by factors other than lactate accumulation, particularly a depletion of intramuscular glycogen reserves (Hultman 1971; Chapter 13). Muscle biopsy reveals a progressive loss of glycogen from individual muscle fibres. The depletion of local stores is virtually complete after 90–120 min.

Further physical activity then depends on the output of growth hormone, cortisol and catecholamines (Shephard & Sidney 1975; Galbo 1992), and on the capacity of these products to mobilize alternative fuels (glucose, released by the breakdown of liver glycogen; amino acids, released by the proteolysis of muscle tissue; and triglycerides, mobilized by the lipolysis of depot fat) (Shephard 1984). The bloodstream carries the alternative metabolites (glucose and fatty acids) to the exercising muscle, but the rate of transfer across the muscle membrane and on to the mitochondria is not rapid enough to sustain the performance observed at the beginning of an event (Lloyd 1966). Athletes speak of 'hitting the wall'.

Effects of hypoglycaemia

Despite an increase in hepatic gluconeogenesis, the decrease of blood glucose concentration over a contest such as an ultramarathon run can be sufficient to cause a clinically significant hypoglycaemia. This has negative effects on cerebral function (Noakes *et al.* 1985). The deterioration in cerebration is particularly important in sports such as orienteering, where quick tactical decisions are required.

Hypoglycaemia also causes weakness at points in a race where anaerobic effort is required (for example, the cyclist who must exert near-peak muscle force when climbing a steep hill), since anaerobic metabolism depends on an adequate supply of carbohydrate.

Response to training

The training of muscular endurance influences performance positively in several ways.

1 Firstly, if the muscles required for a specific activity are strengthened, they can perform their task while contracting at a smaller fraction of their maximal voluntary force. Perfusion of the active muscles is then more readily sustained, and there is no occasion for recourse to the anaerobic activity that would cause lactate accumulation and a progressive decrease of peak muscle force.

2 Secondly, an increase of peripheral vascular conductance results from the increase in bulk of the active muscle (see Chapter 7). There is usually quite a close correlation between lean body mass and maximal oxygen intake (Davies & van Haaren 1973). Nevertheless, in many endurance sports, muscle hypertrophy has the practical disadvantage of increasing total body mass, and thus the load that must be transported against gravity (Shephard 1982).

3 Thirdly, endurance training increases the activity of aerobic enzymes in the muscles that have been conditioned (Holloszy 1973; Chapters 11 and 23). This facilitates a continuation of aerobic metabolism at low partial pressures of oxygen, and also encourages the metabolism of fat, with a resultant sparing of intramuscular glycogen.

4 Fourthly, the size of intramuscular glycogen stores is greater in well-trained individuals than in those who are not accustomed to endurance activity.

Because training acts largely upon specific muscle groups, the response is specific to the type of training which has been undertaken and to the main muscle groups that have been involved in the activity (Hoffmann *et al.* 1993).

Blood lactate

Practical value of data

Measurements of blood lactate can help the coach, trainer and sports physician in several ways.

Such measurements provide a simple method of identifying those individuals who are well suited to distance competition in terms of capillary density (Tesch *et al.* 1981; Jacobs *et al.* 1983), muscle enzyme activity (Sjödin *et al.* 1982) and the proportion of slow-twitch fibres that are activated during exercise (Farrell *et al.* 1979; Tesch *et al.* 1981). Those individuals who have the characteristics predisposing to a good performance in events such as marathon races can operate at very close to their maximal oxygen intake before lactate accumulates in significant quantities (Costill 1972; Neumann 1983).

The determination of blood lactate levels immediately following training activities is a useful method of regulating the intensity of conditioning (Stegmann & Kindermann 1982; Jacobs 1986; Bishop & Martino 1993). Such measurements help to define a level of endurance training or a running pace which is just below the threshold where substantial accumulation of lactate would occur (Sjödin *et al.* 1982; Stegmann & Kindermann 1982). A regimen at this intensity is well suited to the unfit individual with a poor exercise tolerance. Further, because the training response tends to be intensity specific, and athletes are vulnerable to overtraining, it may be a useful intensity to adopt in much of the training of an endurance competitor (Pelayo *et al.* 1996).

Lactate data can also contribute to the design of an interval training plan, the length of recovery intervals being adjusted to ensure that there is no more than a modest accumulation of lactic acid in the working muscles or the circulating blood (Tesch & Wright 1983; Yates *et al.* 1983).

Methods of measurement

The critical variable that limits sustained endurance performance is usually the intramuscular rather than the arterial lactate concentration, but unfortunately it is not possible to collect muscle biopsy specimens on a frequently repeated basis. Inferences are thus based on blood lactate concentrations, or their surrogates.

If only a small number of data points are needed, it is acceptable to collect specimens of arterial blood. However, arterial sampling is difficult to arrange in the field, and when evaluating athletes the practical choice is between 'arterialized' capillary and venous blood. If a peripheral venous catheter is inserted into the median antecubital vein, modern enzymatic techniques (Maughan 1982; Karlsson et al. 1983) allow frequent and fairly rapid determinations of blood lactate (although Jacobs et al. (1985) have questioned the necessity of such detail, arguing that the necessary information for the effective management of an endurance athlete can be obtained from a single measurement of blood lactate during submaximal exercise).

Venous sampling has the disadvantage of imposing a time lag between the release of lactate from the exercising muscles and its sampling in the bloodstream (Yoshida et al. 1982; Yeh et al. 1983). Nevertheless, this problem is more significant for those who are engaged in a brief all-out effort than for contestants who are completing a marathon run over a period of several hours.

If the activity involves the leg muscles, but blood is being collected from the antecubital vein, the lactate formed in the legs traverses the capillary beds of both the lungs and the forearm before it is collected. This may result in a substantial decrease of lactate concentrations relative to arterialized capillary blood specimens (Yoshida et al. 1982; Orok et al. 1989; El-Sayed et al. 1993; Reaburn & Mackinnon 1990).

Arterialized capillary blood samples are collected following application of a chemical vasodilator or hot water to the ear lobe or the fingertip. It is important to cleanse the skin thoroughly prior to sampling, since substantial amounts of lactate are secreted by the sweat glands (Pilardeau et al. 1988). Care must also be taken to avoid squeezing the finger or the ear, since this could dilute the sample of capillary blood with extracellular fluid.

If either finger puncture or venepuncture is repeated frequently, it becomes unpopular with the athlete. Chicharro et al. (1995) have thus argued that salivary lactate determinations provide an adequate substitute when regulating the intensity of normal training sessions.

Because of slow sarcolemmal transport (Chapter 3), blood lactate concentrations peak 1–5 min following a brief bout of exhausting exercise. The timing of blood sampling is critical to the interpretation of lactate data for such activities (Bishop & Martino 1993). Unfortunately, the time at which peak concentrations are reached varies widely from one person to another.

Finally, it is important to note the type of specimen which has been examined. There can be analytical discrepancies of around 10% between plasma or saliva and whole blood following a bout of vigorous exercise. This is due, at least in part, to an incomplete equilibration of lactate across the erythrocyte membranes (Foxdal et al. 1994; Lormes et al. 1995).

Patterns of blood lactate accumulation during exercise

The original hypothesis of a sudden transition from aerobic to anaerobic metabolism as the intensity of exercise approached 100% of maximal oxygen intake was built around a limited database (Margaria et al. 1963). More precise and more extensive measurements have since demonstrated that lactate begins to accumulate in arterial blood at intensities of effort ranging from 50 to 70% of maximal oxygen intake, depending on the type of exercise that is being performed and the proportion of the skeletal musculature that has been activated (Shephard et al. 1968, 1988). Some authors have coined the term 'anaerobic threshold' for the relative intensity of effort where lactate begins to accumulate (Wasserman et al. 1973), although in fact there is a gradual transition rather than a clear-cut threshold intensity where lactate begins to be produced in substantial quantities.

During a progressive laboratory test, the intensity of effort at which an increase in blood lactate concentration is first observed depends on the ramp function that has been chosen (Hughson & Green

1982; Campbell *et al.* 1989; von Duvillard & Hagan 1994) (Fig. 22.1), the type of ergometer that is used and the person's familiarity with this particular form of exercise. There is also a substantial inter-individual variation.

If steady-state effort is pursued at 60–70% of maximal oxygen intake, it is common for the blood lactate to rise at first, but to return towards resting values as exercise continues (Kay & Shephard 1969). This may reflect an anaerobic on-transient during the first 30–60 s of exercise, with a subsequent improvement in muscle perfusion as systemic blood pressure rises and the body warms up. By manipulating the intensity of effort, a loading can usually be found where the blood lactate remains constant to within $0.5 \, mmol \cdot l^{-1}$ (McLellan & Jacobs 1993; Urhausen *et al.* 1993). But if exercise is performed at a slightly larger fraction of maximal oxygen intake (80–90%), lactate concentrations rise progressively until the subject is exhausted (Kay & Shephard 1969; Tegtbur *et al.* 1993).

If exercise is continued for 30 min or longer, a slow upward drift of oxygen consumption is seen. Both this drift and the related decline in power output of the muscles are associated with lactate accumulation (Capelli *et al.* 1993).

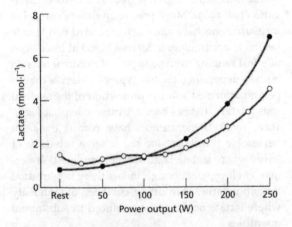

Fig. 22.1 Influence of ramp function on the relationship between power output and blood lactate readings. A comparison of two cycle ergometer tests with load increments of 25 (open circles) and 50 (closed circles) $W \cdot min^{-1}$. From Jacobs (1986), with permission.

The rate of return to resting lactate levels following exercise is facilitated by a continuation of low-intensity activity into the recovery period (Thiriet *et al.* 1993; Francaux *et al.* 1995; Ahmaidi *et al.* 1996). The recovery process becomes slower as the duration of exercise is extended (Freund *et al.* 1990).

Underlying mechanisms

The increase in blood lactate concentration during exercise is a complex phenomenon (Brooks 1985, 1987; Davis 1985), dependent on the many factors that influence the input and egress of lactic acid to and from the muscles (Zouloumian & Freund 1981) and the circulation (Eldridge 1975; Jacobs 1986).

Intramuscular lactate concentrations are affected by both the overall rate of pyruvate metabolism (a factor that is independent of local oxygen partial pressures: Huckabee 1958; Jobsis & Stainsby 1968; Connett *et al.* 1984; Durkot *et al.* 1995) and the extent of any local hypoxia in the muscle fibres. The nature of the physical activity undertaken may be such that one muscle group is operating at a large fraction of its maximal force, and therefore lacks adequate perfusion. A second muscle group, contracting less vigorously, remains able to function aerobically. Capillary perfusion is also non-uniform within a given muscle, and enzyme activities differ from one fibre to another; such differences allow one fibre to function aerobically, while another resorts to anaerobic metabolism. Lactate can then diffuse from anaerobically contracting fibres and be metabolized by fibres that are still operating aerobically within the same muscle (Mazzeo *et al.* 1982).

The blood concentration of lactate depends strongly on its rate of diffusion from the muscle fibre into the bloodstream. This is a relatively slow process (Chapter 3). At normal temperatures, peak blood concentrations may be reached 1–5 min after a brief maximal effort such as a standard laboratory maximal oxygen intake measurement, but the time lag may be even longer if exercise is performed in a cold environment (Bergh & Ekblom 1979; Blomstrand *et al.* 1984).

During a typical large muscle endurance activity, the function of key glycolytic enzymes becomes inhibited when the local intramuscular lactate concentration reaches 30–40 mmol·l⁻¹. The corresponding peak blood concentration does not usually exceed 10–15 mmol·l⁻¹, although it can rise 20–30% higher if arterial buffering is increased by bicarbonate administration (Hirakoba *et al.* 1993). The large concentration gradient from muscle to blood reflects slow diffusion across the sarcolemmal membrane, and arterial values as high as 30 mmol·l⁻¹ may be reached with some types of interval training (Hermansen & Stensvold 1972). The ratio of intramuscular to blood lactate concentration and the corresponding accumulated oxygen deficit (Green & Dawson 1993) are influenced by the total volume of muscle that is functioning anaerobically (Weyand *et al.* 1993; Jensen-Urstad *et al.* 1994), by the activity of a lactate transport protein in the sarcoplasmal membrane (McCullagh & Bonen 1995), and by the circulating blood volume (Shephard *et al.* 1988).

Other factors influencing blood lactate levels include the extent of any initial warm-up (Mitchell & Huston 1993), a decrease (Koistinen *et al.* 1995) but not an increase (Sadowsky *et al.* 1995) in the ambient partial pressure of oxygen, the proportion of carbohydrate in the diet and thus the extent of glycogen reserves (Jansson 1980; Maughan & Poole 1981; Greenhaff *et al.* 1988), the predominant type of muscle fibre that has been activated (Ivy *et al.* 1980), the extent of tissue buffering and thus the rate of diffusion of hydrions from the muscles into the bloodstream (Hughson & Green 1982), and the rate of pyruvate dehydrogenation (Mercier *et al.* 1994). The rate of lactate metabolism is an important consideration. The accumulated lactate may be metabolized in better-oxygenated muscle fibres, in other muscle groups that are contracting less vigorously, and in the liver (Shephard 1984). The speed of lactate clearance depends strongly on the blood flow carrying lactate away from the active muscles, particularly postexercise (Boileau *et al.* 1983). Other moderating influences include the rate of excretion of lactic acid by the kidneys and the sweat glands (Lamont 1987). Lactate removal following vigorous exercise is facilitated by a continuation of moderate activity during the recovery period (Taoutaou *et al.* 1996), but is unaffected by environmental temperature (Oyono-Enguelle *et al.* 1993; Falk *et al.* 1995).

Practical applications

Under competitive conditions, the rate of lactate production varies throughout the event (Boulay *et al.* 1997). For instance, a distance cyclist may have to exert a much greater force on the pedals when ascending a rise than when covering level ground or travelling downhill. Lactate thus accumulates during the climb, to be metabolized during the subsequent descent.

There are many potential situations where the accumulation of lactate can influence physical performance, but its maximal contribution to endurance performance is relatively small. There are practical difficulties in translating lactate into an equivalent quantity of oxygen delivery (Rieu *et al.* 1988), or a corresponding accumulated deficit in oxygen supply. But if data are expressed in such terms, DiPrampero (1971) has suggested that anaerobic metabolism can generate the equivalent of a total oxygen delivery of 70 ml·kg⁻¹ in an average person. During the first minute of sustained activity, this would satisfy some 50% of metabolic requirements in an endurance athlete with a maximal oxygen intake of 70 ml·kg⁻¹·min⁻¹. The accumulated oxygen deficit remains an important determinant of performance in events lasting as long as 5 min (for example, a 4000-m cycle race, Craig *et al.* 1993). However, if this same contribution (an oxygen equivalent of 70 ml·kg⁻¹) were to be distributed uniformly over a 1-h event, the anaerobic component of metabolism would drop to less than 1%.

The speed that an athlete can sustain for a given time without becoming fatigued (the critical power) is plainly related to his or her anaerobic capacity (Hill & Smith 1993). There is a close relationship between an athlete's speed at the traditional anaerobic threshold (a blood lactate of 4 mmol·l⁻¹) and the speed adopted during competition (Bonifazi *et al.* 1993), although Clingeleffer *et al.* (1994) found that in absolute terms the critical power was somewhat greater than the power output observed at a blood lactate of 4 mmol·l⁻¹.

Maffulli *et al.* (1994) point out that most of the gains in endurance performance of top-level competitors in recent years have been due not to increases in maximal oxygen intake, but rather to an ability to exploit a larger fraction of maximal oxygen intake. Training at a blood lactate concentration of 3–5 mmol·l^{-1} (Sjödin *et al.* 1982; Hurley *et al.* 1984) or a rate of lactate accumulation of 0.086 mmol·m^{-1}·min^{-1} (Borch *et al.* 1993) seem optimal tactics in terms of developing a good tolerance of anaerobic effort. Casaburi *et al.* (1995) found that, if a comparable total amount of work was performed, the training response was just as great at intensities that avoided any substantial accumulation of lactate, as at higher intensities, where a significant lactate accumulation occurred.

Anaerobic threshold

The basic concept

The concept of the anaerobic threshold has revolved largely around the search for a bloodless indicator of lactate accumulation. Such a measure would be very helpful, particularly in monitoring the intensity of athletic training sessions. However, there has been much controversy as to both the existence (Hughson *et al.* 1987) and the definition of such a threshold (Brooks 1985, 1987; Davis 1985).

The basic idea, described originally by Jervell (1929) and Owles (1930), but popularized by Wasserman *et al.* (1973), is straightforward enough. If a person engages in a task of progressively increasing intensity, a point is reached where effort can no longer be sustained by aerobic means. Anaerobic metabolism supervenes. The blood lactate concentration begins to rise, and if respiratory variables are being plotted against work rate, a disproportionate increase of ventilation is seen. The literature on this topic is unfortunately rather confusing, different authors describing similar (but not necessarily identical) phenomena by such terms as anaerobic threshold, the aerobic/anaerobic threshold, the onset of blood lactate accumulation (OBLA), the onset of plasma lactate accumulation, the lactate threshold, the lactate turning point, the maximal steady state, critical power, the individual anaerobic threshold, excess lactate and aerobic capacity (Jacobs 1986; Green 1994; Beneke 1995; Billat 1996; Stockhausen *et al.* 1996).

Wasserman *et al.* (1973) proposed the use of a continuous, ramp function ergometer test. At the anaerobic threshold, the ventilatory equivalent for oxygen (which to this point had been decreasing) began to increase again. Because of more vigorous ventilation, the oesophageal pressure–time integral also showed a breakpoint (Formanek *et al.* 1993), and the respiratory gas exchange ratio began to increase rapidly, although the ratio of ventilation to carbon dioxide output continued to fall.

The turning point of the ventilatory equivalent for oxygen (the respiratory minute volume needed to deliver a litre of oxygen) is probably the easiest method of identifying the anaerobic threshold from work-rate–ventilation curves (Reinhard *et al.* 1979; Davies *et al.* 1986). However, it is important that the exercise test begin at a low enough initial power output to accommodate the occasional individual who shows a turnpoint as low as 35–40% of maximal oxygen intake (McLellan 1987).

If the search is concentrated on finding a disproportionate increase in ventilation or carbon dioxide output (Langill & Rhodes 1992) relative to work rate, the breakpoint tends to occur at a higher power output (Beaver *et al.* 1986). Some observers who have made a detailed analysis of the ventilatory record (McLellan 1987) suggest that this constitutes a second breakpoint.

First and second breakpoints

Authors who identify two breakpoints in the ventilation curve argue that the first reflects an increase of ventilation in proportion to oxygen consumption; this is sometimes termed the ventilatory threshold or the aerobic threshold (Ribeiro *et al.* 1985). It may indicate a local intramuscular accumulation of lactate or other metabolites in some of the more poorly perfused muscle fibres (what Antonutto & DiPrampero 1995 have termed 'unevenly aerobic' conditions), without any substantial increase in blood lactate concentration (Systrom *et al.* 1990).

The second breakpoint then coincides with an accelerated accumulation of lactate in the bloodstream (Ahmaidi *et al.* 1993). A further possible factor is an increasing recruitment of fast-twitch muscle fibres as the intensity of effort is increased and/or slow-twitch fibres become fatigued (Helal *et al.* 1987; Matieka & Duffin 1994); in support of this last suggestion, there is a parallel, non-linear increase of electromyographic (EMG) discharge at the lactate threshold (Chwalbinska-Moneta *et al.* 1994; Cabrera & Chizeck 1996).

It has been claimed that the ventilatory threshold corresponds to a blood lactate concentration of $2\,mmol\cdot l^{-1}$, and that the relationship between the ventilatory threshold and blood lactate concentration persists over the course of an interval training programme (Burke *et al.* 1994). Other investigators object that the correspondence between the ventilatory threshold and the hypothetical blood lactate level is not only poor (Davis *et al.* 1983; Aunola & Rusko 1984), but is likely to be coincidental rather than causal (Hagberg 1984; Neary *et al.* 1985; Gaesser & Poole 1986; Loats & Rhodes 1993). A particularly telling argument is that the breakpoint can still be detected in patients with McArdle's disease, where enzyme deficiencies preclude the production of lactate (Riley *et al.* 1993). Further, in healthy individuals any apparent relationship between ventilatory threshold and blood lactate concentrations can be altered by such tactics as a β-adrenergic-induced vasoconstriction in the tissues that normally metabolize lactate and/or a stimulation of cAMP-dependent glycolysis (Fleck *et al.* 1993; McGuiggin & Schneider 1993; Weltman *et al.* 1994; Hambrecht *et al.* 1995).

If the observer identifies two thresholds, then the second breakpoint is termed the 'anaerobic threshold'. It is argued that, at this intensity of effort, the blood lactate concentration begins to rise more steeply, ventilation becomes disproportionate to carbon dioxide output and arterial Pco_2 falls (Ribeiro *et al.* 1985). With the usual ramp function exercise test, the second breakpoint is said to correspond to an arterial lactate concentration of about $4\,mmol\cdot l^{-1}$. However, it remains unclear whether the rising blood lactate concentration or a peripheral neurogenic drive is responsible for the observed hyperventilation (Hagberg *et al.* 1982; Dempsey *et al.* 1985).

One and sometimes two breakpoints can be identified fairly readily during a large muscle task such as cycling or treadmill running. If subjects perform a progressive test of predetermined ramp profile, and a search is made for a single breakpoint, then the findings for a given large muscle activity seem quite reproducible, not only in adult endurance athletes, but also in children (where peak lactate levels are substantially lower, Tolfrey & Armstrong 1995), and even in sedentary patients with a very low aerobic power. Readings are consistent from one day to another and from one observer's assessment of the data to another (Kavanagh *et al.* 1990).

It becomes much harder to locate any clear breakpoint during small muscle activity, when the rise of blood lactate concentration is always quite small (Shephard *et al.* 1988). The identification of breakpoints can sometimes be facilitated by plotting data in logarithmic format (Beaver *et al.* 1985), or by determining the point at which there is a maximal deviation from a linear relationship (the D_{max} approach, Cheng *et al.* 1992). However, for practical management of an athlete it may be enough to identify the maximal steady-state work intensity from one or two data points (for example, Billat *et al.* 1994). Enthusiasts maintain that a determination of ventilatory threshold provides at least as good (Fernhall *et al.* 1996) and sometimes a better indication of endurance performance than the measurement of maximal oxygen intake (Zacharogiannis & Farrally 1993; Loftin & Warren 1994). Moreover, a decrease in ventilatory threshold is correlated with the development of fatigue in events such as an Olympic triathlon (De Vito *et al.* 1995). Likewise, in debilitated individuals, a measure of the absolute ventilatory threshold may provide a better method of assessing aerobic fitness than attempts to carry a maximal exercise test through to voluntary exhaustion.

Morton *et al.* (1994) have argued that, at least in large muscle activity, there is statistical justification for fitting two breakpoints to the ventilation–work-rate curve. However, sceptics note that the identification of even a single breakpoint can be quite subjective, with a poor reproducibility (Jones & Doust 1995). They reason that the accuracy of the ventilation curve rarely warrants an attempt at fitting two breakpoints. Further, they point out that the particular shape of curve that is observed in any given experimental or athletic situation depends heavily upon the ratio of active muscle mass to blood volume (Beneke & von Duvillard 1996), and the intensity–time profile for the exercise under evaluation (Hughson & Green 1982; Campbell *et al.* 1989; Foxdal *et al.* 1996).

Measurement options

When the anaerobic function of an athlete is being investigated, the measurement of ventilation and/or the maximal accumulated oxygen deficit (Friedmann *et al.* 1996) plainly have attractions relative to more invasive approaches such as the repeated collection of blood samples. Investigators have thus persisted in their search for an ideal method of identifying both ventilatory and anaerobic thresholds. The values thus obtained have been used in both functional assessment and the regulation of training, in athletes and sedentary patients alike (Stegmann & Kindermann 1982; Jacobs 1986; Friedmann *et al.* 1996).

It is nevertheless inconvenient to breathe through a tightly fitting facemask or mouthpiece during an athletic event, and interest has thus been aroused by suggestions that—at least for purposes of regulating training—an analogous breakpoint can be detected by a simple measure of heart rate (Snyder *et al.* 1994), a rating of perceived exertion (Steed *et al.* 1994), or a plot of breathing frequency (Cheng *et al.* 1992) or heart rate against power output or oxygen consumption (Conconi *et al.* 1982; Droghetti *et al.* 1985; Bunc *et al.* 1995). Other options are to teach the athlete the perceptions associated with a blood lactate of 2.5 or 4 mmol·l^{-1} (Stoudemire *et al.* 1996), or to seek a breakpoint in plots of double-product (heart rate × systolic pressure) (Riley *et al.* 1997) or transcutaneous carbon dioxide pressure against work rate (Liu *et al.* 1995). Finally, Foster *et al.* (1995) have argued that a determination of relative velocity (the actual pace of running as a percentage of the velocity attained at maximal oxygen intake) offers a bloodless method of regulating training intensity that is almost as effective as frequent lactate determinations.

The plot of heart rate against power output (the Conconi test) has been the most widely advocated alternative to blood lactate or ventilatory measurements (Ballarin *et al.* 1996; Conconi *et al.* 1996). It is easy to envisage how an increasing hydrion concentration can cause a disproportionate hyperventilation. However, the theoretical basis of the Conconi test is less certain (Thorland *et al.* 1994). The heart rate–power output relationship is influenced by changes of stroke volume, arteriovenous oxygen difference, core temperature and catecholamine concentrations as the intensity of exercise is increased, and interindividual differences in these several variables militate against successful application of the Conconi principle (Hofmann *et al.* 1994). Nevertheless, a theoretical explanation can possibly be found in an added respiratory pumping of blood, an irradiation of impulses from the respiratory or the vasomotor centres, or a stimulation of the vasomotor centre from peripheral muscular chemoreceptors as anaerobic effort supervenes.

In an apparent direct contradiction of the hypothesis of Conconi and associates, some observers (for instance, Åstrand 1960) have suggested that there is a linear relationship between heart rate and power output over the range from 50 to 100% of maximal oxygen intake. Thus, the concept of a disproportionate tachycardia at the anaerobic threshold has yet to gain wide credence (Ribeiro *et al.* 1985; Kuipers *et al.* 1988; Francis *et al.* 1989).

Acid–base balance

From the viewpoint of muscle function, the critical location for an acid–base determination is within the working muscle fibre. There is some evidence that intramuscular buffering can be enhanced by an appropriate training programme (Weston *et al.* 1997). However, for practical reasons, observations are generally limited to the acid–base balance in the blood.

Measurements can be made using the micro-Åstrup apparatus, a specialized device that can equilibrate blood with known concentrations of carbon dioxide in oxygen, determining the resultant pH. Graphic manipulation of the data yields estimates of pH, P_{CO_2}, HCO_3^-, base excess and standard bicarbonate reserve (Comroe 1974).

There are problems in interpreting both base

excess and standard bicarbonate levels during athletic competition, since the measurements assume a fixed body core temperature of 37°C. During prolonged exercise, there may be substantial departures from this assumed temperature, due to either hyperthermia or hypothermia.

Blood pH

Under normal resting conditions, the blood pH is in the range 7.33–7.45. During long-distance running, there is commonly a decrease to 7.15–7.25 (a somewhat smaller change than is usual in sprint competitions). The more rapidly the normal resting values are restored after exercise, the less the residual fatigue that the competitor experiences.

Base excess

The total buffer base of whole blood is the sum of buffer anions (the bicarbonate in plasma and red blood cells, haemoglobin, plasma protein, and the phosphate content of plasma and red blood cells). Lactate competes with carbon dioxide for the buffering offered by the NH_2-terminal valine of β-globin in deoxygenated haemoglobin (Böning et al. 1993). The base excess relative to standard normal values can be computed using the Siggard–Andersen nomogram. The estimate is based on two of total plasma CO_2, pH and Pco_2 (Comroe 1974). For example, with an arterial pH of 7.4 and a Pco_2 of 5.3 kPa (40 mmHg), the base excess is zero. However, if a lactate-related bicarbonate loss has brought about a lower pH at this carbon dioxide pressure, a negative base excess is calculated.

Base excess values show a high correlation with blood lactate, and Keul et al. (1969) suggested that the blood lactate concentration ($mmol·l^{-1}$) could be estimated as (0.54 – base excess/1.25). The decrease of base excess incurred over the course of an athletic event represents an overall deficit of 'alkaline radicals', associated with the bloodstream accumulation of not only lactic acid, but also pyruvic acid, ketoacids and fatty acids. A good performer on a standard cycle ergometer shows only about a half of the decrease in base excess that is seen in a poor performer.

Standard bicarbonate

The standard bicarbonate, or alkaline reserve, provides a second measure of any metabolic acidosis. It may be defined as the bicarbonate concentration observed at a standard temperature of 37°C and a standard CO_2 pressure of 5.3 kPa (40 mmHg). Normal resting values range from 22 to 26 $mmol·l^{-1}$, but values can drop as low as 15 $mmol·l^{-1}$ following exhausting exercise (Shephard 1984).

Some 95% of the decrease in standard bicarbonate induced by all-out exercise is attributable to an accumulation of lactic acid and pyruvic acid, with the remaining 5% of change being caused by an accumulation of free fatty acids. The impact of lactate accumulation on performance depends essentially on the related change of hydrion concentration. The critical intramuscular pH for an inhibition of glycolysis is around 7.0. Likewise, the impact of a rising blood lactate concentration on ventilatory function depends on the arterial acid–base balance.

Modifications of acid–base balance

Buffering capacity can increase during adaptation to carbon dioxide retention (a compensated respiratory acidosis). This has traditionally been described in submariners (Schaefer et al. 1971), but it can also arise through repeated underwater exploration using self-contained underwater breathing apparatus. In contrast, the hyperventilation associated with living at high altitudes leads to a progressive loss of carbon dioxide from the body, with a compensating adjustment of buffering by the kidneys. A normal resting pH is restored, but the person concerned now has a poor tolerance of anaerobic activity, because the loss of bicarbonate buffering does not compensate fully for the altitude-induced increase in haemoglobin level (Shephard 1982; Chapter 41).

Acetazolamide, a carbonic anhydrase inhibitor, is used to treat the symptoms of respiratory alkalosis seen in mountaineers at very high altitudes (see Chapter 41). The athlete who prepares for endurance competition by altitude training will also develop the hyperventilation-related handicap of a reduced serum bicarbonate concentration (see

Chapter 41). Banister and Woo (1976) suggested the possibility of simulating altitude training by having teams rebreathe through long tubes during their practices. Finnish athletes have also experimented with the effects of living in houses where the ambient oxygen concentration is deliberately reduced. 'Tube breathing' has the advantage that subjects are presented simultaneously with a combination of hypoxia and hypercarbia. In theory, haemoglobin formation is then stimulated without the disadvantage of reducing bicarbonate reserves. However, in practice the technique is rather clumsy, and experience to date has not suggested any great gains in performance from tube breathing, possibly because the tubes are only used for a short period each day.

A further potential option is to modify the acid–base balance by the deliberate ingestion of bicarbonate preparations. This is plainly a form of doping, although because of the prevalence of bicarbonate in the human body, it is extremely difficult to detect such an abuse. Observations have shown that such an approach can speed the transfer of lactate from muscle to blood (McNaughton et al. 1991; Linderman & Gosselink 1994; Chapter 41), thus increasing the speed of a short-distance run by a substantial 3%, although the dosage and timing of bicarbonate ingestion are critical to such an advantage (Wilkes et al. 1983). To the author's knowledge, there have been no studies of the impact of bicarbonate doping upon endurance performance, although a number of investigators have demonstrated improved running speeds over distances of up to 800 m. If a sufficient dose of a bicarbonate preparation (at least $0.3 \, \mathrm{g \cdot kg^{-1}}$ body mass) were to be given at an appropriate point before or during a race, it might serve to counter some of the adverse effects of lactate accumulation, although it would also have the adverse effect of causing acute gastric discomfort (Horswill et al. 1988).

Acknowledgement

The studies of Dr Shephard are supported in part by research grants from the Defence and Civil Institute of Environmental Medicine, Toronto, ON.

References

Ahmaidi, S., Hardy, J.M., Varray, A., Collomp, K., Mercier, J. & Préfaut, C. (1993) Respiratory gas exchange indices used to detect the blood lactate accumulation threshold during an incremental exercise test in young athletes. *European Journal of Applied Physiology* 66, 31–36.

Ahmaidi, S., Granier, P., Taotaou, Z., Mercier, J., Dubouchard, H. & Préfaut, C. (1996) Effects of active recovery on plasma lactate and anaerobic power following repeated intensive exercise. *Medicine and Science in Sports and Exercise* 28, 450–456.

Antonutto, G. & DiPrampero, P.E. (1995) The concept of lactate threshold. *Journal of Sports Medicine and Physical Fitness* 35, 6–12.

Åstrand, I. (1960) Aerobic work capacity in men and women with special reference to age. *Acta Physiologica Scandinavica* 49 (Suppl. 169), 1–92.

Aunola, S. & Rusko, H. (1984) Reproducibility of aerobic and anaerobic thresholds in 20–50-year-old men. *European Journal of Applied Physiology* 53, 260–266.

Ballarin, E., Sudhues, U., Borsetto, C. et al.
(1996) Reproducibility of the Conconi test: test repeatability and observer variations. *International Journal of Sports Medicine* 17, 520–524.

Banister, E.W. & Woo, W. (1976) Effects of simulated altitude training on aerobic and anaerobic power. *European Journal of Applied Physiology* 38, 55–69.

Barstow, T.J., Casaburi, R. & Wasserman, K. (1993) O_2 uptake kinetics and the O_2 deficit as related to exercise intensity and blood lactate. *Journal of Applied Physiology* 75, 755–762.

Beaver, W.L., Wasserman, K. & Whipp, B.J. (1985) Improved detection of lactate threshold during exercise using a log–log transformation. *Journal of Applied Physiology* 59, 1936–1940.

Beaver, W.L., Wasserman, K. & Whipp, B.J. (1986) A new method for detecting anaerobic threshold by gas exchange. *Journal of Applied Physiology* 60, 2020–2027.

Beneke, R. (1995) Anaerobic threshold, individual anaerobic threshold, and maximal lactate steady state in rowing. *Medicine and Science in Sports and Exercise* 27, 863–867.

Beneke, R. & von Duvillard, S.P. (1996) Determination of maximal lactate steady state response in selected sports events. *Medicine and Science in Sports and Exercise* 28, 241–246.

Bergh, U. & Ekblom, B. (1979) Physical performance and peak aerobic power at different body temperatures. *Journal of Applied Physiology* 46, 885–889.

Billat, V. (1996) Use of blood lactate measurements for prediction of exercise performance and for control of training. Recommendations for long-distance running. *Sports Medicine* 22, 157–175.

Billat, V., Dalmay, F., Antonini, M.T. & Chassain, A.P. (1994) A method for determining the maximal steady state of blood lactate concentration from two levels of submaximal exercise. *European Journal of Applied Physiology* 69, 196–202.

Bishop, P. & Martino, M. (1993) Blood lactate measurement in recovery as an adjunct to training. Practical considerations. *Sports Medicine* 16, 5–13.

Blomstrand, E., Bergh, U., Essén-Gustavsson, B. & Ekblom, B. (1984) Influence of low muscle temperature on muscle metabolism during intense dynamic exercise. *Acta Physiologica Scandinavica* **120**, 229–236.

Boileau, R.A., Misner, J.E., Dykstra, G.L. & Spitzer, T.A. (1983) Blood lactic acid removal during treadmill and bicycle exercise at various intensities. *Journal of Sports Medicine and Physical Fitness* **23**, 159–167.

Bonifazi, M., Martelli, G., Marugo, L., Sardella, F. & Carli, G. (1993) Blood lactate accumulation in top level swimmers following competition. *Journal of Sports Medicine and Physical Fitness* **33**, 13–18.

Böning, D., Schünemann, H.J., Maasen, N. & Busse, M.W. (1993) Reduction of oxylabile CO_2 in human blood by lactate. *Journal of Applied Physiology* **74**, 710–714.

Borch, K.W., Ingjer, F., Larsen, S. & Tomten, S.E. (1993) Rate of accumulation of blood lactate during graded exercise as a predictor of 'anaerobic' threshold. *Journal of Sports Sciences* **11**, 49–55.

Boulay, M.R., Simoneau, J.-A., Lortie, G. & Bouchard, C. (1997) Monitoring high-intensity endurance exercise with heart rate and thresholds. *Medicine and Science in Sports and Exercise* **29**, 125–132.

Bovens, A.M.P.M., van Baak, M.A., Vrencken, J.G.P., Wijnen, J.A.G. & Verstappen, F.T.J. (1993) Maximal heart rates and plasma lactate concentrations observed in middle-aged men and women during a maximal cycle ergometer test. *European Journal of Applied Physiology* **66**, 281–284.

Brooks, G.A. (1985) Anaerobic threshold: review of the concept and directions for future research. *Medicine and Science in Sports and Exercise* **17**, 22–31.

Brooks, G.A. (1987) Lactate production during exercise: oxidizable substrate versus fatigue agent. In: Macleod, D., Maughan, R., Nimmo, M., Reilly, T. & Williams, C. (eds) *Exercise — Benefits, Limits and Adaptations*. E. & F.N. Spon, London.

Bunc, V. & Leso, J. (1993) Ventilatory threshold and work efficiency during exercise on a cycle and rowing ergometer. *Journal of Sports Sciences* **11**, 43–48.

Bunc, V., Hofmann, P., Leitner, H. & Gaisl, G. (1995) Verification of the heart rate threshold. *European Journal of Applied Physiology* **70**, 263–269.

Burke, J., Thayer, R. & Belcamino, M. (1994) Comparison of effects of two interval training programmes on lactate and ventilatory thresholds. *British Journal of Sports Medicine* **28**, 18–21.

Cabrera, M.E. & Chizeck, H.J. (1996) On the existence of a lactate threshold during incremental exercise: a systems

analysis. *Journal of Applied Physiology* **80**, 1819–1828.

Campbell, M.E., Hughson, R. & Green, H. (1989) Continuous increase in blood lactate concentration during different ramp exercise protocols. *Journal of Applied Physiology* **66**, 1104–1107.

Capelli, C., Antonutto, G., Zamparo, P., Girardis, M. & di Prampero, P.E. (1993) Effects of prolonged cycle ergometer exercise on maximal muscle power and oxygen uptake in humans. *European Journal of Applied Physiology* **66**, 189–195.

Casaburi, R., Storer, T.W., Sullivan, C.S. & Wasserman, K. (1995) Evaluation of blood lactate elevation as an intensity criterion for exercise training. *Medicine and Science in Sports and Exercise* **27**, 852–862.

Cheng, B., Kuipers, H., Snyder, A.C., Keizer, H.A., Jeukendrup, A. & Hesselink, M. (1992) A new approach for the determination of ventilatory and lactate thresholds. *International Journal of Sports Medicine* **13**, 518–522.

Chicharro, J.L., Calvo, F., Alvarez, J. *et al.* (1995) Anaerobic threshold in children: determination from saliva analysis in field tests. *European Journal of Applied Physiology* **70**, 541–544.

Chwalbinska-Moneta, J., Hänninen, O. & Penttila, I. (1994) Relationships between EMG and blood lactate accumulation during incremental exercise in endurance- and speed-trained athletes. *Clinical Journal of Sports Medicine* **4**, 31–38.

Clingeleffer, A., McNaughton, L.R. & Davoren, B. (1994) The use of critical power as a determinant for establishing the onset of blood lactate accumulation. *European Journal of Applied Physiology* **68**, 182–187.

Comroe, J.H. (1974) *Physiology of Respiration*, 2nd edn. Year Book Publishers, Chicago.

Conconi, F., Ferrari, M., Ziglio, P.G., Droghetti, P. & Codeca, L. (1982) Determination of the anaerobic threshold by a non-invasive field test in runners. *Journal of Applied Physiology* **52**, 869–873.

Conconi, F., Grazzi, G., Casoni, I. *et al.* (1996) The Conconi test: methodology after 12 years of application. *International Journal of Sports Medicine* **17**, 509–519.

Connett, R.J., Gayeski, T.E. & Honig, C.R. (1984) Lactate accumulation in fully aerobic, working dog gracilis muscle. *American Journal of Physiology* **246**, H120–H128.

Costill, D.L. (1972) Physiology of marathon running. *Journal of the American Medical Association* **221**, 1024–1029.

Craig, N.P., Norton, K.I., Bourdon, P.C. *et al.* (1993) Aerobic and anaerobic indices contributing to track endurance cycling performance. *European Journal of Applied Physiology* **67**, 150–158.

Davies, C.T.M. & van Haaren, J.P.M. (1973) Maximum aerobic power and body composition in healthy East African older male and female subjects. *American Journal of Physical Anthropology* **39**, 395–401.

Davies, S.F., Iber, C., Keene, S.A., McArthur, C.D. & Path, M.J. (1986) Effect of respiratory alkalosis during exercise on blood lactate. *Journal of Applied Physiology* **61**, 948–952.

Davis, J.A. (1985) Anaerobic threshold: review of the concept and directions for future research. *Medicine and Science in Sports and Exercise* **17**, 6–18.

Davis, J.A., Caiozoo, V.J., Lamarra, N. & Ellis, J.F. (1983) Does the gas exchange anaerobic threshold occur at a fixed blood lactate concentration of 2 or 4 mM? *International Journal of Sports Medicine* **4**, 89–93.

Dempsey, J.A., Vidruk, E.H. & Mitchell, G.S. (1985) Pulmonary control systems in exercise: update. *Federation Proceedings* **44**, 2260–2270.

De Vito, G., Bernardi, M., Sproviero, E. & Figura, F. (1995) Decrease of endurance performance during Olympic triathlon. *International Journal of Sports Medicine* **16**, 24–28.

DiPrampero, P.E. (1971) Anaerobic capacity and power. In: Shephard, R.J. (ed.) *Frontiers of Fitness*, pp. 155–173. C.C. Thomas, Springfield, IL.

Droghetti, P., Borsetto, C., Casoni, I. *et al.* (1985) Noninvasive determination of the anaerobic threshold in canoeing, cross-country skiing, cycling, roller, and ice skating, rowing and walking. *European Journal of Applied Physiology* **53**, 299–303.

Durkot, M.J., De Garavilla, L., Caretti, D. & Francesconi, R. (1995) The effects of dichloroacetate on lactate accumulation and endurance in an exercising rat model. *International Journal of Sports Medicine* **16**, 167–171.

von Duvillard, S.P. & Hagan, R.D. (1994) Independence of ventilation and blood lactate responses during graded exercise. *European Journal of Applied Physiology* **68**, 298–302.

Eldridge, F.L. (1975) Relationship between turnover rate and blood concentration of lactate in exercising dogs. *Journal of Applied Physiology* **39**, 231–234.

El-Sayed, M.S., George, K.P., Wilkinson, D., Mullan, N., Fenoglio, R. & Flannigan, J. (1993) Fingertip and venous blood lactate concentration in response to graded treadmill exercise. *Journal of Sports Sciences* **11**, 139–143.

Falk, B., Einbinder, M., Weinstein, Y. *et al.* (1995) Blood lactate concentration following exercise: effects of heat exposure and of active recovery in heat acclimatized subjects. *International Journal of Sports Medicine* **16**, 7–12.

Farrell, P.A., Wilmore, J.H., Coyle, E.F., Billing, J.E. & Costill, D.L. (1979) Plasma lactate accumulation and distance running performance. *Medicine and Science in Sports and Exercise* **11**, 338–344.

Fernhall, B., Kohrt, W., Burkett, L.N. & Walters, S. (1996) Relationship between the lactate threshold and cross-country run performance in high school male and female runners. *Pediatric Exercise Science* **8**, 37–47.

Fleck, S.J., Lucia, A., Storms, W.W., Wallach, J.M., Vint, P.F. & Zimmerman, S.D. (1993) Effects of acute inhalation of albuterol on submaximal and maximal $\dot{V}O_2$ and blood lactate. *International Journal of Sports Medicine* **14**, 239–243.

Formanek, D., Wanke, T., Lahrmann, H., Rauscher, H., Popp, W. & Zwick, H. (1993) Inspiratory muscle performance relative to the ventilatory threshold in healthy subjects. *Medicine and Science in Sports and Exercise* **25**, 1120–1125.

Foster, C., Crowe, M.P., Houm, D. *et al.* (1995) The bloodless lactate profile. *Medicine and Science in Sports and Exercise* **27**, 927–933.

Foxdal, P., Sjödin, B., Sjödin, A. & Ostman, B. (1994) The validity and accuracy of blood lactate measurements for prediction of maximal endurance running capacity. Dependency of analyzed blood media in combination with different designs of the exercise test. *International Journal of Sports Medicine* **15**, 89–95.

Foxdal, P., Sjödin, A. & Sjödin, B. (1996) Comparison of blood lactate concentrations obtained during incremental and constant intensity exercise. *International Journal of Sports Medicine* **17**, 360–365.

Francaux, M., Jacqmin, P., de Welle, J.M. & Sturbois, X. (1995) A study of lactate metabolism without tracer during passive and active postexercise recovery in humans. *European Journal of Applied Physiology* **72**, 58–66.

Francis, K.T., McClatchen, P.R., Sumsion, J.R. & Hansen, D.E. (1989) The relationship between anaerobic threshold and heart rate linearity during cycle ergometry. *European Journal of Applied Physiology* **59**, 273–277.

Freund, H., Oyono-Enguéllé, S., Heitz, A. *et al.* (1990) Comparative lactate kinetics after short and prolonged submaximal exercise. *International Journal of Sports Medicine* **11**, 284–288.

Friedmann, B., Siebold, R. & Bärtsch, P. (1996) Vergleich der anaeroben Leistungsfähigkeit von 400 m- und Langstreckenläufern unter Anwendung unterschiedlicher Messmethoden. (Comparison of anaerobic capacity determined by different methods in 400 m- and long-distance runners.) *Deutsche Zeitschrifte für Sportmedizin* **47**, 379–390.

Gaesser, G.A. & Poole, D.C. (1986) Lactate and ventilatory thresholds: disparity in time course of adaptations to training. *Journal of Applied Physiology* **61**, 999–1004.

Galbo, H. (1992) Exercise physiology: humoral function. *Sport Science Reviews* **1** (1), 65–93.

Gaul, C.A., Docherty, D. & Cicchini, R. (1995) Differences in anaerobic performance between boys and men. *International Journal of Sports Medicine* **16**, 451–455.

Green, S. (1994) A definition and systems view of anaerobic capacity. *European Journal of Applied Physiology* **69**, 168–173.

Green, S. & Dawson, B. (1993) Measurement of anaerobic capacities in humans. Definitions, limitations, and unsolved problems. *Sports Medicine* **15**, 312–327.

Greenhaff, P.L., Gleeson, M. & Maughan, R.J. (1988) Diet-induced metabolic acidosis and the performance of high intensity exercise in man. *European Journal of Applied Physiology* **57**, 254–259.

Hagberg, J.M. (1984) Physiological implications of the lactate threshold. *International Journal of Sports Medicine* **5**, 106–109.

Hagberg, J.M., Coyle, E.F., Carroll, J.E., Miller, J.M., Martin, W.H. & Brooke, M.H. (1982) Exercise hyperventilation in patients with McArdle's disease. *Journal of Applied Physiology* **52**, 991–994.

Hambrecht, R.P., Niebauer, J., Fiehn, E. *et al.* (1995) Effect of an acute beta-adrenergic blockade on the relationship between ventilatory and plasma lactate threshold. *International Journal of Sports Medicine* **16**, 219–224.

Heck, H., Mader, A., Hess, G., Mücke, S., Müller, R. & Hollmann, W. (1985) Justification of the 4 mmol/l lactate threshold. *International Journal of Sports Medicine* **6**, 117–130.

Helal, J.N., Guezennec, C.Y. & Goubel, F. (1987) The aerobic–anaerobic transition: reexamination of the threshold concept including an electromyographic approach. *European Journal of Applied Physiology* **56**, 643–649.

Henritze, J., Weltman, A., Schurrer, R.L. & Barlow, K. (1985) Effects of training at and above the lactate threshold on the lactate threshold and maximal oxygen intake. *European Journal of Applied Physiology* **54**, 84–88.

Hermansen, L. & Stensvold, I. (1972) Production and removal of lactic acid during exercise in man. *Acta Physiologica Scandinavica* **86**, 191–201.

Hill, D.W. & Smith, J.C. (1993) A comparison of methods of estimating anaerobic work capacity. *Ergonomics* **36**, 1495–1500.

Hirakoba, K., Maruyama, A. & Misaka, K. (1993) Effect of acute sodium bicarbonate ingestion on excess CO_2 output during incremental exercise. *European Journal of Applied Physiology* **66**, 536–541.

Hoffmann, J.J., Loy, S.F., Shapiro, B.I. *et al.* (1993) Specificity effects of run versus cycle training on ventilatory threshold. *European Journal of Applied Physiology* **67**, 43–47.

Hofmann, P., Pokan, R., Preidler, K. *et al.* (1994) Relationship between heart rate threshold, lactate turn point and myocardial function. *International Journal of Sports Medicine* **15**, 232–237.

Hogan, M.C., Gladden, B., Kurdak, S.S. & Poole, D.C. (1995) Increased [lactate] in working dog muscle reduces tension independent of pH. *Medicine and Science in Sports and Exercise* **27**, 371–377.

Holloszy, J.O. (1973) Biochemical adaptations to exercise: aerobic metabolism. *Exercise and Sport Sciences Reviews* **1**, 45–71.

Horswill, C.A., Costill, D.L., Fink, W.J. *et al.* (1988) Influence of sodium bicarbonate on sprint performance: relationship to dosage. *Medicine and Science in Sports and Exercise* **20**, 566–569.

Huckabee, W.E. (1958) Relationships of pyruvate and lactate during anaerobic metabolism. II. Exercise and formation of O_2 debt. *Journal of Clinical Investigation* **37**, 255–271.

Hughson, R. & Green, H. (1982) Blood acid–base and lactate relationships studied by ramp work tests. *Medicine and Science in Sports and Exercise* **14**, 297–302.

Hughson, R.L., Weisiger, K.H. & Swanson, G.D. (1987) Blood lactate concentration increases as a continuous function in progressive exercise. *Journal of Applied Physiology* **62**, 1975–1981.

Hultman, E. (1971) Muscle glycogen stores and prolonged exercise. In: Shephard, R.J. (ed.) *Frontiers of Fitness*. C.C. Thomas, Springfield, IL.

Hurley, B.F., Hagberg, J.M., Allen, W.K. *et al.* (1984) Effect of training on blood lactate levels during submaximal exercise. *Journal of Applied Physiology* **56**, 1260–1264.

Ivy, J.L., Withers, R.T., van Handel, P.J., Elger, D.H. & Costill, D.L. (1980) Muscle respiratory capacity and fiber type as determinants of the lactate threshold. *Journal of Applied Physiology* **48**, 523–527.

Iwaoka, K., Hatta, H., Atomi, Y. & Miyashita, M. (1988) Lactate, respiratory compensation thresholds, and distance running performance in runners of both sexes. *International Journal of Sports Medicine* **9**, 306–309.

Jacobs, I. (1986) Blood lactate: implications for training and sports performance. *Sports Medicine* **3**, 10–25.

Jacobs, I., Schéle, R. & Sjödin, B. (1983) A single blood lactate determination as an indicator of cycle ergometer endurance capacity. *European Journal of Applied Physiology* **50**, 355–364.

Jacobs, I., Schéle, R. & Sjödin, B. (1985) Blood lactate vs exhaustive exercise to evaluate aerobic fitness. *European Journal of Applied Physiology* **54**, 151–155.

Jansson, E. (1980) Diet and muscle metabolism in man. *Acta Physiologica Scandinavica* (Suppl) **487**, 1–24.

Jensen-Urstad, M., Svedenhag, J. & Sahlin, K. (1994) Effect of muscle mass on lactate formation during exercise in humans. *European Journal of Applied Physiology* **69**, 189–195.

Jervell, O. (1929) Milchsäureuntersuchungen in Blut bei Nephriditien. *Acta Medica Scandinavica* **72**, 262–273.

Jobsis, F. & Stainsby, W. (1968) Oxidation of NADH during contractions of circulated skeletal muscle. *Respiration Physiology* **4**, 292–300.

Jones, A.M. & Doust, J.H. (1995) Lack of reliability in Conconi's heart rate deflection point. *International Journal of Sports Medicine* **16**, 541–544.

Karlsson, J., Jacobs, I., Sjodin, B. *et al.* (1983) Semiautomatic blood lactate assay: experiences from an exercise laboratory. *International Journal of Sports Medicine* **4**, 52–55.

Kavanagh, T.J., Mertens, D.J., Myers, M.G., Baigrie, T. & Shephard, R.J. (1990) Assessment of patients with congestive failure: ventilatory threshold or aerobic power determination? *Proceedings of the International Congress of Cardiology*, Manila, C1656.

Kay, C. & Shephard, R.J. (1969) On muscle strength and the threshold of anaerobic work. *Internationale Zeitschrift für Angewandte Physiologie* **27**, 311–328.

Keul, J., Doll, E. & Keppler, D. (1969) *Muskelstoffwechsel*. J.A. Barth, Munich.

Koistinen, P., Takala, T., Martikkala, V. &

Leppäluoto, J. (1995) Aerobic fitness influences the response of maximal oxygen uptake and lactate threshold in acute hypobaric hypoxia. *International Journal of Sports Medicine* **16**, 78–81.

Kuipers, H., Keizer, H.A., DeVries, T., van Rijthoven, P. & Wijts, M. (1988) Comparison of heart rate as a non-invasive determinant of anaerobic threshold with the lactate threshold when cycling. *European Journal of Applied Physiology* **58**, 303–306.

Lamont, L.S. (1987) Sweat lactate secretion during exercise in relation to women's aerobic capacity. *Journal of Applied Physiology* **62**, 194–198.

Langill, R.H. & Rhodes, E.C. (1992) Comparison of the lactate and ventilatory responses during a progressive intensity test. *Australian Journal of Science and Medicine in Sport* **24**, 100–102.

Linderman, J.K. & Gosselink, K.L. (1994) The effects of sodium bicarbonate ingestion on exercise performance. *Sports Medicine* **18**, 75–80.

Liu, Y., Steinacker, J.M. & Stauch, M. (1995) Does the threshold of transcutaneous partial pressure of carbon dioxide represent the respiratory compensation point or anaerobic threshold? *European Journal of Applied Physiology* **71**, 326–331.

Lloyd, B.B. (1966) Presidential address, Section 1. (Physiology and Biochemistry) In: *Advancement of Sciences*, pp. 515–530. British Association for the Advancement of Sciences, London.

Loats, C.E.R. & Rhodes, E.C. (1993) Relationship between the lactate and ventilatory thresholds during prolonged exercise. *Sports Medicine* **15**, 104–115.

Loftin, M. & Warren, B. (1994) Comparison of a simulated 16.1-km time trial, $\dot{V}O_{2max}$ and related factors in cyclists with different ventilatory thresholds. *International Journal of Sports Medicine* **15**, 498–503.

Lormes, W., Steinacker, J.M. & Stauch, M. (1995) Laktatbestimmung mittels ACCUSPORT und vollenzymatisch-photometrisch bei leistungsdiagnostichem Mehrstufentest und bei Langzeitbelastungen. (A new lactate measurement system (ACCUSPORT) in comparison to a common lactate test combination.) *Deutsche Zeitschrift für Sportmedizin* **46**, 3–11.

McCullagh, K.J.A. & Bonen, A. (1995) L(+)-lactate binding to a protein in rat skeletal muscle plasma membranes. *Canadian Journal of Applied Physiology* **20**, 112–124.

McGuiggin, M.E. & Schneider, D.A. (1993) Plasma cyclic AMP and blood lactate responses to incremental cycling in untrained male subjects. *International Journal of Sports Medicine* **14**, 362–367.

McLellan, T.M. (1987) The anaerobic threshold: concept and controversy. *Australian Journal of Science and Medicine in Sport* **19**, 3–8.

McLellan, T. & Jacobs, I. (1993) Reliability, reproducibility and validity of the individual anaerobic threshold. *European Journal of Applied Physiology* **67**, 125–131.

McNaughton, L., Curtin, R., Goodman, G., Perry, D., Turner, B. & Showell, C. (1991) Anaerobic work and power output during cycle ergometer exercise: effects of bicarbonate loading. *Journal of Sports Sciences* **9**, 151–160.

Maffulli, N., Testa, V. & Capasso, G. (1994) Anaerobic threshold determination in master endurance runners. *Journal of Sports Medicine and Physical Fitness* **34**, 242–249.

Margaria, R., Cerretelli, P., DiPrampero, P.E., Massari, C. & Torelli, G. (1963) Kinetics and mechanisms of oxygen debt contraction in man. *Journal of Applied Physiology* **18**, 371–377.

Matieka, J.H. & Duffin, J. (1994) The ventilation, lactate and electromyographic thresholds during incremental exercise tests in normoxia, hypoxia and hyperoxia. *European Journal of Applied Physiology* **69**, 110–118.

Maughan, R.J. (1982) A simple, rapid method for the determination of glucose, lactate, pyruvate, alanine, 3-hydroxybutyrate and acetoacetate on a single 20 µl blood sample. *Clinica Chimica Acta* **122**, 231–240.

Maughan, R.J. & Poole, D.C. (1981) The effects of glycogen loading regimen on the capacity to perform anaerobic exercise. *European Journal of Applied Physiology* **46**, 211–219.

Mazzeo, R.S., Brooks, G.A., Budinger, T.F. & Schoeller, D.A. (1982) Pulse injection, ^{13}C tracer studies of lactate metabolism in humans during rest and two levels of exercise. *Biomedicine and Mass Spectrometry* **9**, 310–314.

Mercier, B., Granier, P., Mercier, J., Anselme, F., Ribes, G. & Préfaut, C. (1994) Effects of 2-chloropropionate on venous plasma lactate concentration and anaerobic power during periods of incremental intensive exercise in humans. *European Journal of Applied Physiology* **68**, 425–429.

Mitchell, J.B. & Huston, J.S. (1993) The effect of high- and low-intensity warm-up on the physiological responses to a standardized swim and tethered swimming performance. *Journal of Sports Sciences* **11**, 159–165.

Morton, R.H., Fukuba, Y., Banister, E.W., Walsh, M.L., Kenny, C.T.C. & Cameron,

B.J. (1994) Statistical evidence consistent with two lactate turnpoints during ramp exercise. *European Journal of Applied Physiology* **69**, 445–449.

Neary, P.J., MacDougall, J.D., Bachus, R. & Wenger, H.A. (1985) The relationship between lactate and ventilatory thresholds: coincidental or cause and effect? *European Journal of Applied Physiology* **54**, 104–108.

Neumann, G. (1983) Metabole Regulation bei Langzeitausdauerleistungen. *Medizin und Sport* **23**, 169.

Noakes, T.D., Nathan, M., Irving, R.A. *et al.* (1985) Physiological and biochemical measurements during a 4-day surf–ski marathon. *South African Medical Journal* **67**, 212–216.

Orok, C.J., Hughson, R.L., Green, H.J. & Thompson, J.A. (1989) Blood lactate responses in incremental exercise as predictors of constant load performance. *European Journal of Applied Physiology* **59**, 2262–2267.

Owles, W.H. (1930) Alterations in the lactic acid content of the blood as a result of light exercise and associated changes in the CO_2 combining power of the blood and in the alveolar CO_2 pressure. *Journal of Physiology (London)* **69**, 214–237.

Oyono-Enguelle, S., Heitz, A., Marbach, J., Ott, C., Pape, A. & Freund, H. (1993) Heat stress does not modify lactate exchange and removal abilities during recovery from short exercise. *Journal of Applied Physiology* **74**, 1248–1255.

Pelayo, P., Mujika, I., Sidney, M. & Chatard, J.-C. (1996) Blood lactate recovery measurements, training and performance during a 23-week period of competitive swimming. *European Journal of Applied Physiology* **74**, 107–113.

Pilardeau, P.D., Lavie, F., Vaysse, J. *et al.* (1988) Effect of different work-loads on sweat production and composition in man. *Journal of Sports Medicine and Physical Fitness* **28**, 247–252.

Reaburn, P.R.J. & Mackinnon, L.T. (1990) Blood lactate response in older swimmers during active and passive recovery following maximal sprint swimming. *European Journal of Applied Physiology* **61**, 246–250.

Reinhard, U., Müller, P.H. & Schmülling, R.M. (1979) Determination of anaerobic threshold by the ventilation equivalent in normal individuals. *Respiration* **38**, 36–42.

Ribeiro, J.P., Fielding, R.A., Hughes, V., Black, A., Bochese, M.A. & Knuttgen, H.G. (1985) Heart rate break point may coincide with the anaerobic and not the aerobic threshold. *International Journal of Sports Medicine* **6**, 220–224.

Rieu, M., Duvallet, A., Scharapan, L., Thieulart, L. & Ferry, A. (1988) Blood lactate accumulation in intermittent supramaximal exercise. *European Journal of Applied Physiology* **57**, 235–242.

Riley, M., Nicholls, D.P., Nugent, A.-M. *et al.* (1993) Respiratory gas exchange and metabolic responses during exercise in McArdle's disease. *Journal of Applied Physiology* **75**, 745–754.

Riley, M., Maehara, K., Porszasz, J. *et al.* (1997) Association between the anaerobic threshold and the break-point in the double product/work rate relationship. *European Journal of Applied Physiology* **75**, 14–21.

Sadowsky, S., Dwyer, J. & Fischer, A. (1995) Failure of hyperoxic gas to alter the arterial lactate anaerobic threshold. *Journal of Cardiopulmonary Rehabilitation* **15**, 114–121.

Schaefer, K.E., Bond, G.F., Mazzone, W.F., Carey, C.R. & Dougherty, J.H. (1971) Carbon dioxide retention and metabolic changes during prolonged exposure to high pressure environment. *Aerospace Medicine* **39**, 1206–1215.

Shephard, R.J. (1982) *Physiology and Biochemistry of Exercise.* Praeger Publications, New York.

Shephard, R.J. (1984) *Biochemistry of Physical Activity.* C.C. Thomas, Springfield, IL.

Shephard, R.J. (1997) *Physical Activity, Aging and Health.* Human Kinetics, Champaign, IL.

Shephard, R.J. & Sidney, K.H. (1975) Effects of physical exercise on plasma growth hormone and cortisol levels in human subjects. *Exercise and Sport Sciences Reviews* **3**, 1–30.

Shephard, R.J., Allen, C., Benade, A.J.S. *et al.* (1968) Standardization of submaximal exercise tests. *Bulletin of the World Health Organization* **38**, 765–776.

Shephard, R.J., Bouhlel, E., Vanderwalle, H. & Monod, H. (1988) Anaerobic threshold, muscle volume and hypoxia. *European Journal of Applied Physiology* **58**, 826–832.

Sjödin, B., Schéle, R., Karlsson, J., Linnarsson, D. & Willensten, R. (1982) The physiological background of onset of blood lactate accumulation (OBLA). In: Komi, P.V. (ed.) *Exercise and Sport Biology*, pp. 43–56. Human Kinetics, Champaign, IL.

Snyder, A.C., Woulfe, T., Welsh, R. & Foster, C. (1994) A simplified approach to estimating the maximal lactate steady state. *International Journal of Sports Medicine* **15**, 27–31.

Steed, J., Gaesser, G.A. & Weltman, A. (1994) Rating of perceived exertion and blood lactate concentration during submaximal running. *Medicine and Science in Sports and Exercise* **26**, 797–803.

Stegmann, H. & Kindermann, W. (1982) Comparison of prolonged exercise tests at the individual anaerobic threshold of 4 mmol/l. *International Journal of Sports Medicine* **3**, 105–110.

Stockhausen, W., Huber, G., Maier, J.B., Tinsel, J. & Keul, J. (1996) Ein einzeitiges Verfahren zur Bestimmung des maximalen Laktat-Steady-State auf dem Fahrradergometer. *Deutsche Zeitschrift für Sportmedizin* **46**, 291–302.

Stoudemire, N.M., Wideman, L., Pass, K.A., McGinnes, C.L., Gaesser, G.A. & Weltman, A. (1996) The validitiy of regulating blood lactate concentration during running by ratings of perceived exertion. *Medicine and Science in Sports and Exercise* **28**, 490–495.

Systrom, D.M., Kanarck, D.J., Kohler, S.J. & Kazemi, H. (1990) ^{31}P nuclear magnetic resonance spectroscopy study of the anaerobic threshold in humans. *Journal of Applied Physiology* **68**, 2060–2066.

Taoutaou, Z., Granier, P., Mercier, B., Mercier, J., Ahmaidi, S. & Préfaut, C. (1996) Lactate kinetics during passive and partially active recovery in endurance and sprint athletes. *European Journal of Applied Physiology* **73**, 465–470.

Tegtbur, U., Busse, M.W. & Braumann, K.M. (1993) Estimation of an individual equilibrium between lactate production and catabolism during exercise. *Medicine and Science in Sports and Exercise* **25**, 620–627.

Tesch, P.A. & Wright, J.E. (1983) Recovery from short term intense exercise; its relation to capillary blood supply and blood lactate concentration. *European Journal of Applied Physiology* **52**, 98–103.

Tesch, P.A., Sharp, D.S. & Daniels, W.L. (1981) Influence of fiber type composition and capillary density on onset of blood lactate accumulation. *International Journal of Sports Medicine* **2**, 252–255.

Thiriet, P., Gozal, D., Wouassi, D., Oumarou, T., Gelas, H. & LaCour, J.R. (1993) The effect of various recovery modalities on subsequent performance, in consecutive supramaximal exercise. *Journal of Sports Medicine and Physical Fitness* **33**, 118–129.

Thorland, W., Podolin, D.A. & Mazzeo, R.S. (1994) Coincidence of lactate threshold and HR-power output threshold under varied nutritional status. *International Journal of Sports Medicine* **15**, 301–304.

Tolfrey, K. & Armstrong, N. (1995) Child–adult differences in whole blood lactate responses to incremental treadmill exercise. *British Journal of Sports Medicine* 29, 196–199.

Urhausen, A., Coen, B., Weiler, B. & Kindermann, W. (1993) Individual anaerobic threshold and maximum lactate steady-state. *International Journal of Sports Medicine* 14, 134–139.

Wasserman, K., Whipp, B.J., Koyal, S.N. & Beaver, W.L. (1973) The anaerobic threshold and respiratory gas exchange during exercise. *Journal of Applied Physiology* 35, 236–243.

Weltman, A., Wood, C.M., Womack, C.J. *et al.* (1994) Catecholamine and blood lactate responses to incremental rowing and running exercise. *Journal of Applied Physiology* 76, 1144–1149.

Weston, A.R., Myburgh, K.H., Lindsay, F.H., Dennis, S.C., Noakes, T.D. & Hawley, J.A. (1997) Skeletal muscle buffering capacity and endurance performance after high intensity interval training by well-trained cyclists. *European Journal of Applied Physiology* 75, 7–13.

Weyand, P.G., Cureton, K.J., Conley, D.S. & Higbie, E.J. (1993) Peak oxygen deficit during one- and two-legged cycling in men and women. *Medicine and Science in Sports and Exercise* 25, 584–591.

Weyand, P.G., Cureton, K.J., Conley, D.S., Sloniger, M.A. & Liu, Y.L. (1994) Peak oxygen deficit predicts sprint and middle-distance track performance. *Medicine and Science in Sports and Exercise* 26, 1174–1180.

Wilkes, D., Gledhill, N. & Smyth, R. (1983) Effect of acute induced metabolic alkalosis on 800-m racing times. *Medicine and Science in Sports and Exercise* 15, 277–280.

Williams, C.G., Wyndham, C.H., Kok, R. & von Rahden, M.J. (1967) Effect of training on maximum oxygen intake and anaerobic metabolism in man. *Internationale Zeitschrift für Angewandte Physiologie* 24, 18–23.

Yates, J.W., Gladden, L.B. & Cresanta, M.K. (1983) Effects of prior dynamic leg exercise on static effort of the elbow flexors. *Journal of Applied Physiology* 55, 891–896.

Yeh, M.P., Gardner, R.M., Adams, T.D., Yanowitz, F.G. & Crappo, R.O. (1983) 'Anaerobic threshold': problems of determination and validation. *Journal of Applied Physiology* 55, 1178–1186.

Yoshida, T., Takeuchi, N. & Suda, Y. (1982) Arterial versus venous blood lactate increase in the forearm during incremental bicycle exercise. *European Journal of Applied Physiology* 50, 87–93.

Zacharogiannis, E. & Farrally, M. (1993) Ventilatory threshold, heart rate deflection point and middle distance running performance. *Journal of Sports Medicine and Physical Fitness* 33, 337–347.

Zouloumian, P. & Freund, H. (1981) Lactate after exercise in man. III. Properties of the compartment model. *European Journal of Applied Physiology* 46, 135–147.

Chapter 23

Metabolism in the Contracting Skeletal Muscle

JAN HENRIKSSON

Major metabolic pathways of the muscle cell: an overview

Introduction

Ultimately, endurance performance depends on metabolism in the contracting muscles. Muscle metabolism is a broad concept, including all of the chemical reactions that take place in the muscle cell. An important part of muscle metabolism is the uptake of fuels from the blood and their subsequent degradation to yield energy in a form that can be used by the muscle cell, for example to perform contractile work or to build new cellular material in a continuous cycle of degradation and synthesis. Muscle metabolism further includes: (i) the hepatic mobilization of glucose from glycogen; and (ii) the mobilization of fatty acids from triglycerides in the adipose tissue, together with the transport of these compounds to the muscle.

The metabolic processes are regulated by a complicated chemical interaction between the body's different organs. The muscle cell is unique in the sense that its metabolic rate can vary over a very wide range, increasing more than 200 times from rest to maximal exercise. The major portion of this increase is due to processes related to the production of chemical energy for the contracting filaments. The most important principles of energy metabolism in skeletal muscle also apply to most of the other tissues in the body. For most chemical compounds in the body, the net turnover is zero, i.e. their degradation over a given period of time equals their resynthesis. Only a limited number of compounds constitute quantitatively important reactants and products in the net metabolic equation. The total body metabolism can thus be simplified as consisting of a rather small number of biochemical pathways that have a significant impact on the cellular metabolic equilibrium. These include:

1 the complete oxidation of carbohydrates, fats (and proteins);
2 the net transformation of carbohydrates into fats and of proteins into carbohydrates (gluconeogenesis) and fats;
3 the net formation of ketoacids (acetoacetic acid and β-hydroxybutyric acid) from fatty acids (liver only);
4 the net formation of lactic acid from carbohydrates (glucose), the pathway known as anaerobic glycolysis; and
5 the oxidation of alcohol which, during times of alcohol intake, may make up a significant portion of the body's metabolism and partly replace the oxidation of carbohydrates and fats.

The storage polysaccharide glycogen is channelled into glycolysis by two enzymatic steps (glycogen phosphorylase and phosphoglucomutase), a feeder pathway which is correctly termed glycogenolysis. In this chapter, however, in order to avoid confusion, the term glycogenolysis is avoided and instead glycolysis is used to mean both glycolysis from glucose and glycolysis from glycogen. The initial steps in the oxidation of alcohol occur almost exclusively in the liver. This is likely to explain why the maximal turnover of alcohol is not increased by physical exercise, despite the fact that its hepatic degradation product, acetic acid, is transported to skeletal muscle and other organs for final oxidation. For the contracting muscle, only pathways 1, 4 and gluconeogenesis are of quantitative importance. These biochemical pathways, as well as the energy exchange between adenosine triphosphate and phosphocreatine, are discussed in the following section.

Muscle metabolism: general principles

The muscle cell obtains its energy by degrading carbohydrates and fats to smaller molecules. As a result of this degradation, part of the energy stored in carbohydrate and fat molecules is released and used by the cell to cover its energy demands. Proteins, the third large group of organic compounds, are not normally used as a fuel by skeletal muscles. This makes sense physiologically, since proteins constitute the building blocks of the cells in the body. This is especially true of skeletal muscle cells, due to their high content of the contractile proteins (myosin and actin). However, in situations where the body's energy supply is compromised, such as in long-term starvation, proteins (including those derived from muscle tissue) will be used as a fuel in the energy metabolism of muscle.

All energy originates from the sun. The chlorophyll of green plants traps solar energy in the photosynthetic process, where carbon dioxide is combined with water to yield carbohydrate (starch and sucrose) (see Fig. 23.1). Carbohydrates and proteins contain approximately 17 kJ of energy per gram, whereas fats contain more than twice as much: $39 kJ \cdot g^{-1}$ (corresponding to $29 kJ \cdot g^{-1}$ of adipose tissue). From an energy point of view, fat is thus by far the best storage fuel (Fig. 23.2). One drawback, however, is that once transformed to fat for storage, carbohydrates and proteins cannot be re-formed. On the other hand, it has become clear that in humans the transformation of carbohydrates and proteins into fat occurs to a much smaller extent than was previously thought. The reason is that *de novo* lipogenesis is an energetically expensive process, which is suppressed when the diet contains more than 10–15% of its energy as fat. The fat stores of the body therefore originate almost exclusively from dietary fat and the composition of fatty acids in

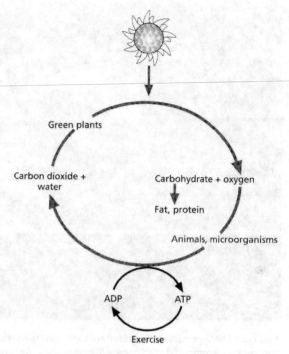

Fig. 23.1 Schematic view of the cycle of carbon compounds in nature. The chlorophyll of the green plants traps solar energy in the photosynthetic process. In this process, carbon dioxide is combined with water to yield carbohydrate (starch and sucrose), with the formation of oxygen. Solar energy is thus incorporated into these carbohydrates, and is 'transferred' to fats and proteins when a part of the carbohydrate is used in the synthesis of these compounds in plants or animals. In cells of animals and microorganisms, oxygen is utilized in the combustion of carbohydrates and fats (and proteins), whereby carbon dioxide and water are re-formed. The energy thus released permits the synthesis of adenosine triphosphate (ATP), the cell-specific energy source. ADP, adenosine diphosphate.

adipose tissue will reflect the dietary intake of the different fatty acids (Åstrup & Flatt 1996).

Humans can synthesize 10 of the 20 amino acids from which proteins are formed. The remaining amino acids belong to the group of 'essential' amino acids, which must be ingested via the diet.

Another product of photosynthesis is oxygen. The circle is closed when, in muscle and other cells, oxygen is utilized in the combustion of carbohydrates, fats (and proteins), whereby carbon dioxide and water are re-formed (Fig. 23.1). For further

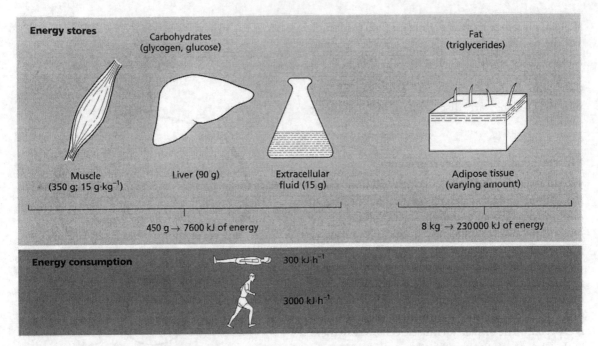

Fig. 23.2 The approximate magnitude of the largest body stores of carbohydrates and fat. The energy content of these compounds is compared with energy consumption at rest and during relatively intense exercise ($\dot{V}o_2 = 2.5\,l\cdot min^{-1}$).

study, the reader is referred to standard textbooks of biochemistry and physiology.

Enzyme-catalysed reactions

In cellular energy metabolism, fats and carbohydrates are degraded by successive small steps. Each step (reaction) is made possible (catalysed) by one enzyme. Enzymes are small proteins, one specific enzyme existing for each of the thousands of chemical reactions that occur in the body. Without these biological catalysts, all chemical reactions would proceed very slowly at body temperature. Different chemical processes occur in a specific number of steps. For example, the degradation of glucose to lactate requires 10 enzyme steps (reactions) (see Fig. 23.3).

The ultimate goal of the energy metabolism in muscle is to release the energy bound in the carbohydrate and fat molecules. Therefore, it is to be expected that most reactions occur with a release of energy, the energy content of the product being less

than that of the substrate. Such reactions are termed exergonic. There are also several reactions (Fig. 23.3) where energy must be added in order for the reaction to occur (endergonic reactions, e.g. A→B, C→D) and other reactions with little or no energy exchange (e.g. B→C, J→Z). The cell can make use of the energy released in reactions only where there is a large energy loss (in Fig. 23.3, steps F→G and I→J). In other reactions involving an energy loss, the liberated energy cannot be used by the cell and is released as heat instead (in Fig. 23.3, steps D→E, E→F, G→H). The generated heat, although a by-product, contributes to the normal body temperature of homeothermic species.

How cells make use of the liberated energy

In reaction steps with a sufficiently large energy release, the liberated energy is used to synthesize a cell-specific, energy-rich compound, adenosine triphosphate (ATP). ATP is of paramount importance, since it is the only form of energy the cell can

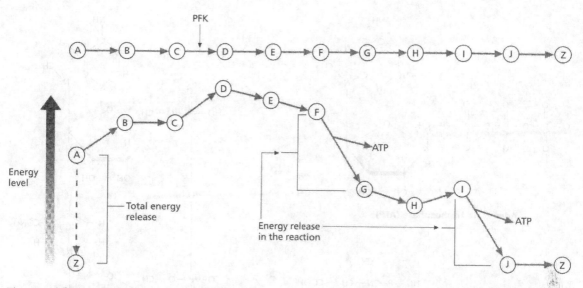

Fig. 23.3 Schematic illustration of the chemical reactions involved in the glycolytic pathway. A symbolizes glucose, J pyruvate and Z lactate. Each arrow symbolizes one chemical reaction (one enzyme step). The letters B–I represent metabolic intermediates between glucose and pyruvate. 6-Phosphofructokinase, PFK, the rate-limiting enzyme of glycolysis, catalyses the reaction C→D. The energy contents of the different compounds are indicated at the bottom of the figure. In reactions where there is a large energy loss, the released energy is utilized in the resynthesis of adenosine triphosphate (ATP). From McMurray (1983), modified with permission.

use directly. The structure of the ATP molecule is illustrated in Fig. 23.4. The three phosphate groups are an important feature of this molecule. These are bound with high-energy chemical bonds. This means that their formation involves the utilization of a large amount of energy, but also that much energy is liberated when the bond is broken (hydrolysed).

In order to bind a phosphate group to ADP, adenosine diphosphate, to give rise to ATP, approximately 70 J·g⁻¹ of ADP or 5 × 10–20 J per molecule of ADP are required. If less energy than this is liberated in a specific reaction, no ATP can be produced at this step, and all of the liberated energy is released as heat. When the muscle is activated, the outermost phosphate group of the ATP molecule is cleaved off enzymatically, liberating energy for the contracting filaments (see Fig. 23.1). ATP is stored in each muscle cell, but in an amount sufficient only for a few seconds of intense contraction. Thus, for the muscle to continue contracting, it is essential that ATP should be resynthesized continuously from ADP at a very high rate. Over 24 h, the total mass of the ATP produced and consumed in the human body generally exceeds body mass.

Major metabolic pathways of the muscle cell: an overview

The cell utilizes four major metabolic pathways to degrade and obtain energy from fats and carbohydrates. These are glycogenolysis/glycolysis, the fatty acid degradation system (β-oxidation), the citric acid cycle and the respiratory chain (Fig. 23.5). A metabolic pathway, or enzyme system, is a group of enzymes that catalyse a consecutive chain of reactions. One such enzyme system, anaerobic glycolysis, is illustrated in Fig. 23.3. The enzymes of a specific metabolic pathway are often located close to each other in the same cellular compartment.

Each cell in the body is delineated by a cell membrane, inside which are many different organelles such as the nucleus, the mitochondria and the sarcoplasmic reticulum. In skeletal muscle cells, the most abundant structures in the cytoplasm are the contractile filaments, myosin and actin, which

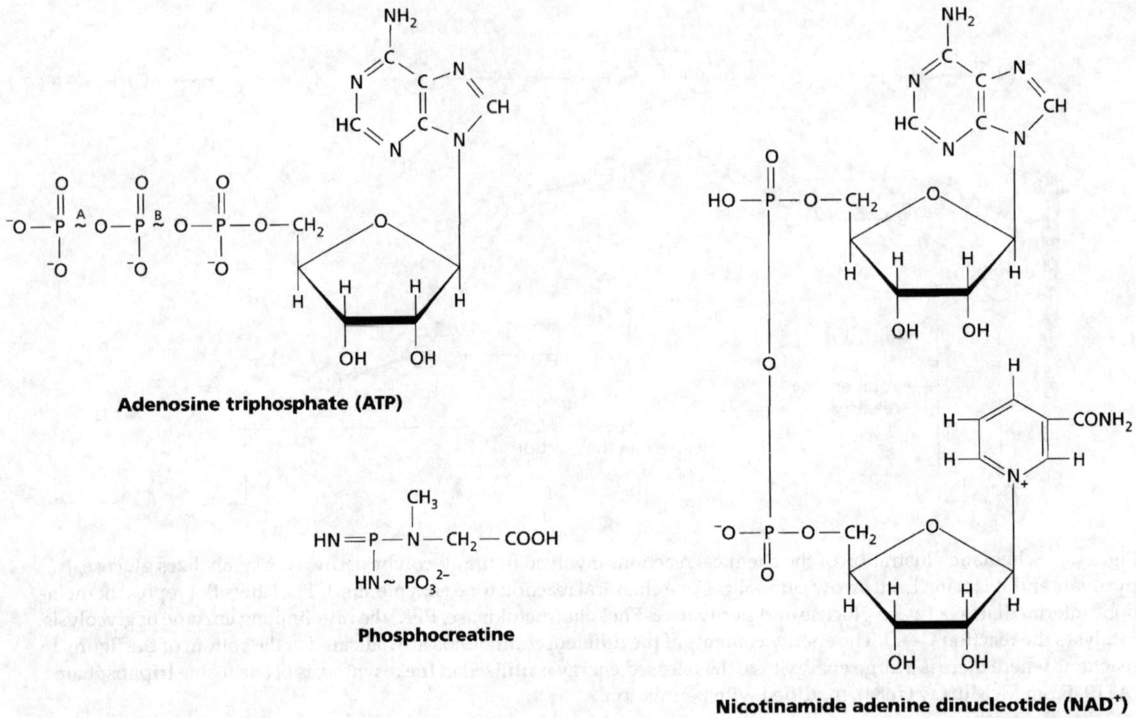

Adenosine triphosphate (ATP)

Phosphocreatine

Nicotinamide adenine dinucleotide (NAD⁺)

Fig. 23.4 Three key substances in the cellular energy metabolism: adenosine triphosphate (ATP), nicotinamide adenine dinucleotide (NAD^+) and phosphocreatine. ATP contains two phosphate groups bound by high-energy bonds (A and B). (The bond of the innermost phosphate group contains less energy.) The energy released when these bonds are hydrolysed is the only form of energy that can be used directly by the cell. When bond A is hydrolysed, ATP is converted to adenosine diphosphate (ADP). The cleaving of the next phosphate group (bond B) converts ADP to adenosine monophosphate (AMP). ATP is subsequently resynthesized from ADP (or AMP) via the energy which is released in the cellular degradation of carbohydrates and fats. ATP may also be resynthesized from ADP, using energy liberated by cleavage of the high-energy phosphate group of phosphocreatine (PO_3^{2-}). The function of NAD^+ is to take up electrons (and hydrogen), which are released at several points in the cellular degradation of carbohydrates and fats (and proteins). These are incorporated in the NAD^+ molecule in the lower nitrogen-containing ring, resulting in the conversion (reduction) of NAD^+ to NADH. NADH subsequently donates its electrons to the mitochondrial respiratory chain. The electron flow in the respiratory chain represents the body's most important energy source in producing ATP (three molecules of ATP per molecule of NADH). Note the similarity between the configuration of the ATP and NAD^+ molecules; both are termed nucleotides. ~ symbolizes a high-energy bond.

in concert with several other proteins execute the contractile activity. The glycolytic enzymes are located in the cytoplasm, close to the contractile filaments. Thus, the ATP produced via the glycolytic pathway is formed near the site of its use. Part of the muscle store of ATP and phosphocreatine is likewise in close proximity to the contractile filaments.

The other three major metabolic pathways in muscle energy metabolism (fatty acid β-oxidation,

the citric acid cycle and the respiratory chain) are, unlike glycolysis, strictly aerobic. Most of the enzymes of aerobic metabolism are localized in one specific cellular organelle, the mitochondrion. The fatty acid β-oxidation enzymes are arranged in the inner space of the mitochondria (the matrix), whereas many enzymes of the citric acid cycle and the components of the respiratory chain are situated on the inner mitochondrial wall. Thus, the substrates for the aerobic pathways, such as fatty acids

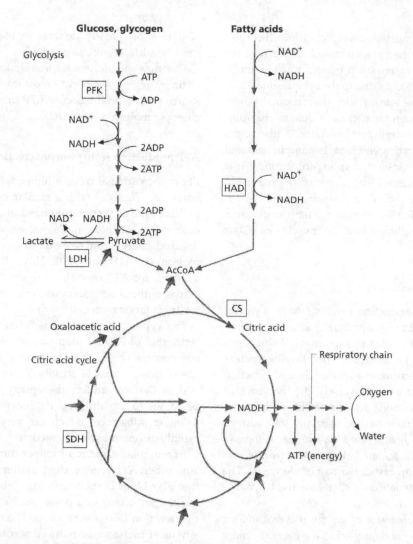

Fig. 23.5 The major metabolic pathways in muscle energy metabolism. Each arrow in the figure designates a chemical reaction, i.e. one enzyme step; the metabolic intermediates are illustrated only as the empty space between arrows. Enzymes, the levels of which are commonly used as a measure of the capacity of their respective meta-bolic pathways, are indicated: 6-phosphofructokinase (PFK) and lactate dehydrogenase (LDH) of glycolysis; 3-hydroxyacyl CoA dehydrogenase (HAD) of the fatty acid β-oxidation pathway; and citrate synthase (CS) and succinate dehydrogenase (SDH) of the citric acid cycle. The proteins enter this system when their building blocks, the amino acids, are degraded either to different metabolic intermediates in glycolysis and the citric acid cycle or to AcCoA (acetyl coenzyme A) (see the large arrows). The figure indicates that in each of two steps of glycolysis, two molecules of ATP are formed. This is explained by the fact that the glucose molecule (which contains six carbon atoms) is split to yield two three-carbon units in the step following the PFK reaction. There is a cost of one additional ATP molecule to phosphorylate glucose. To increase clarity, the diagram omits the two molecules of carbon dioxide and the GTP (guanosine triphosphate) molecule which are formed in the citric acid cycle. Large arrows, entry of amino acids.

and pyruvate, must be transported into the mitochondria from the cytoplasm and, conversely, the ATP produced in aerobic processes must be transported from mitochondria to the cytoplasmic site of use. This is one reason why the maximal power is lower in the aerobic pathways than in anaerobic glycolysis. The transport of fatty acids across the mitochondrial membrane is complicated and involves their transient coupling to carnitine. It is furthermore believed that a specific plasma membrane fatty acid-binding protein (FABPPM) is involved in facilitated transport of fatty acids across the plasma membrane into the muscle cell (Glatz et al. 1998).

Oxidation–reduction

Oxidation and reduction reactions have a central position in cellular metabolism. Oxidation is chemically defined as a release of electrons. Reduction is its counterpart, i.e. an electron uptake. The reactant that receives electrons in a specific chemical reaction will be reduced and, conversely, the reactant that donates the electrons will be oxidized. In many oxidation–reduction (redox) reactions, the electrons are released or incorporated via hydrogen atoms (a proton with an associated electron) or hydride ions (a proton with an associated pair of electrons). The term dehydrogenation is therefore used synonymously with oxidation.

The major substrates of energy metabolism, for example glucose and fatty acids, are generally more reduced than their degradation products, such as carbon dioxide and water. They therefore have a greater tendency to release electrons (and hydrogen). Thus the entire degradation of carbohydrates and fats to carbon dioxide and water is often termed oxidation. The central cellular substance in redox reactions is the compound NAD^+, nicotinamide adenine dinucleotide (see Fig. 23.4). NAD^+ functions as an electron carrier. This means that it can easily take up or release electrons and hydrogen. At several points in the cellular degradation of carbohydrates and fats, hydride ions are released from the metabolic intermediates and taken up by NAD^+, and a proton is liberated into the medium (see Fig. 23.5). In this process NAD^+ is reduced to NADH.

NADH subsequently donates its electrons to the mitochondrial respiratory chain.

The flow of electrons through the respiratory chain represents the body's most important energy source for the production of ATP (three ATP molecules per molecule of NADH).

ATP production from phosphocreatine

Phosphocreatine also has a high-energy phosphate bond (see Fig. 23.4) with a similar energy content to that of the corresponding bond in the ATP molecule. When this bond is cleaved enzymatically, the released energy can be used to resynthesize one molecule of ATP from ADP. This is the fastest way available for ATP resynthesis in the cell, because it occurs without activation of the carbohydrate and fat degradation systems.

The cellular store of phosphocreatine is three times that of ATP; if used up completely, the two compounds would yield sufficient energy for 5–10 s of intense muscle activity. There is no cellular system that can utilize the energy derived from phosphocreatine directly. Its function is that of a 'buffer substance' which can resynthesize ATP rapidly during muscle contraction.

In muscular exercise of longer duration than 5–10 s, other ATP-regenerating systems must come into play. None of the remaining systems, however, has the same maximal power as the phosphocreatine reaction (McGilvery 1975). The exercise intensity must therefore be reduced accordingly. Below, these other ATP-regenerating systems (anaerobic glycolysis, carbohydrate oxidation and fat oxidation) are described in order of decreasing maximal power.

ATP production from glycolysis

GENERAL BACKGROUND

In glycolysis, glucose or glycogen molecules are broken down to pyruvate (or lactate) (Fig. 23.5). If glucose is the starting substance of glycolysis, the net gain is two ATP molecules per molecule of glucose consumed. If the starting substance is glycogen, the gain per molecule of glucose is three molecules of ATP. In one of the glycolytic reactions, hydride ions are released to NAD^+ (Fig. 23.5), which is transformed into NADH. The cellular content of NAD^+ is sufficient for only a few seconds of maximal glycolytic activation. Therefore, a prerequisite for glycolytic energy production is that NADH continuously releases its electrons and hydrogen in order to re-form NAD^+.

This release may occur in two different ways. The most advantageous is the release of electrons and protons to the mitochondrial respiratory chain, with the subsequent formation of three molecules of ATP per molecule of NADH. This demands in turn an adequate cellular supply of oxygen, since the respiratory chain is strictly aerobic. In this situation, the glycolytically formed pyruvate is transported from the cytoplasm into the mitochondrion to be converted to acetyl coenzyme A (acetyl CoA), and further degraded in the citric acid cycle (Fig. 23.5).

When the oxygen supply is inadequate, for instance during intense exercise or when the glycolytic rate is high, part of the NAD^+ is re-formed via an alternative mechanism. This involves the transfer of electrons and hydrogen from NADH to pyruvate $(C_3H_4O_3)$, which is then transformed into lactate $(C_3H_6O_3)$. No ATP is regenerated in this reaction, but NAD^+ is re-formed, thus enabling continued ATP production via the glycolytic pathway.

The formation of lactate as a consequence of an insufficient oxygen supply can be readily understood, but why does a high glycolytic rate also lead to an increased production of lactate? The probable reason is that, in this situation, the cytoplasmic NADH concentration must be set at a higher level in order to establish a sufficiently high driving pressure for the transport of cytoplasmic NADH into the mitochondrial respiratory chain. This is necessary because a high glycolytic rate results in more NADH having to be transported into the mitochondrion. An increased cytoplasmic NADH content automatically leads to more pyruvate being converted to lactate (see Fig. 23.5).

The two causes of lactate formation are closely linked, since a relative lack of oxygen automatically leads to a high glycolytic rate in the muscle cell. The drawbacks of lactic acid formation are: (i) that the possibility of obtaining ATP from NADH in the respiratory chain is not utilized; and (ii) that the pH is gradually reduced, leading to impaired muscle function. Part of the lactate formed in muscles during intense exercise is released to the bloodstream and is subsequently taken up by the liver or by other muscles. A large part, however, remains in the muscle, where one portion follows the opposite route, i.e. it is utilized to resynthesize glucose and glycogen. A large portion is subsequently reconverted to pyruvate and further degraded in the citric acid cycle.

The energy yield is the same whether the degradation of glycogen goes directly via pyruvate into the mitochondrion or makes a 'detour' to lactate first. The importance of the latter route is illustrated by the fact that, following a bout of intense exercise, lactate disappearance occurs markedly faster if a subject continues to exercise at a lower intensity rather than remaining completely at rest. The exercise intensity most suitable for this purpose has been found to be one demanding approximately 40% of the person's $\dot{V}O_{2max}$ (see references in Åstrand & Rodahl 1986).

ANAEROBIC GLYCOLYSIS

In this pathway (Figs 23.3 & 23.5), where glycogen is gradually converted to lactate without the participation of oxygen, ATP is regenerated from ADP, at a rate of about one-third to one-half of that of the phosphocreatine reaction (McGilvery 1975). The high rate of ATP regeneration in anaerobic glycolysis is due to the fact that the mitochondrial oxidative processes need not be activated. The price for this independency of oxygen is lactate, or more correctly H^+, accumulation, which gradually fatigues the muscle.

The starting point of this pathway is glycogen. Glycogen, essentially a branched chain of glucose molecules, is stored in skeletal muscle in varying amounts, normally between 15 and $25\,g\cdot kg^{-1}$ muscle (see Fig. 23.2; see also Chapter 13). In glycolysis, about 1 kJ of energy is released per gram of glycogen degraded. Roughly half of this amount is used to resynthesize ATP; the remaining half is released as heat.

AEROBIC GLYCOLYSIS (CARBOHYDRATE OXIDATION)

Anaerobic glycolysis constitutes the main source of energy in intense exercise of relatively short duration (under 2 min). Longer exercise periods require that the main energy delivery occurs through aerobic processes. Carbohydrate oxidation occurs without the accumulation of lactate and accompanying protons and is therefore tolerated longer by the muscle cell. In addition, a much larger portion of the stored glycogen is utilized for ATP formation.

The power of aerobic glycolysis is about half of that in anaerobic glycolysis. In a given muscle, the two processes occur simultaneously; in one fraction of the muscle aerobic metabolism may dominate, while other muscle cells, due to their enzyme characteristics and blood supply, may derive a large part of their energy supply from anaerobic metabolism. The lower the intensity of exercise, the more aerobic metabolism predominates.

The aerobic degradation of carbohydrates is limited by the cellular supply of glycogen. It has been shown that 10–20 km of running is sufficient to deplete the muscle store of glycogen (Saltin & Karlsson 1971). The capacity to exercise at 70–80% of maximal oxygen intake thus depends largely on the pre-exercise store of muscle glycogen (Bergström et al. 1967). The muscle glycogen content varies; it can be markedly increased by a diet rich in carbohydrates and is decreased following fasting and muscular exercise (Bergström et al. 1967; Saltin & Hermansen 1967).

HYPOGLYCAEMIA AS A CAUSE OF FATIGUE

Which factor is likely to limit endurance at exercise intensities lower than those at which the muscle stores of glycogen are the major limiting factor? Paradoxically, in this situation also, fatigue may be related to a lack of carbohydrates—in this case a lack of blood glucose. Although the predominant energy supply, for instance during moderate running, may be derived from fat combustion, there is always some increase in the rate of muscle glucose oxidation. The carbohydrate needed for this purpose is derived from muscle glycogen as well as from an increased uptake of glucose from the blood.

Blood glucose is regulated by the liver, which releases glucose in an amount that should balance the amount used by the different tissues of the body. The liver normally possesses a glycogen store of about 90 g, plus some capacity for *de novo* glucose synthesis (gluconeogenesis). The increased glucose uptake by the exercising muscles may, if continued for several hours, deplete the liver's glycogen stores, and the rate of gluconeogenesis may not be sufficient to avert hypoglycaemia. This rapidly affects the function of the brain and nervous system, since these organs are normally restricted to blood glucose as their energy substrate. Due to a feeling of weakness and dizziness, the individual is forced to stop exercise, or may continue exercising only after ingesting glucose (Pruett 1971; see also Chapter 29).

If the rate of exercise is sufficiently low, the point where liver glucose production becomes limiting is never reached. Possible causes of fatigue under these conditions include changes in the membrane potential of the muscle cell, leading to impaired excitability (Sjögaard 1990; see also Chapters 9 and 10).

ATP production from fatty acid degradation

Free fatty acids, originating from the adipose tissue and taken up by muscle cells, or originating from intramuscular stores of triglycerides, are transported into the mitochondria for further degradation. Transport across the mitochondrial wall requires that the fatty acids are bound to carnitine. Inside the mitochondria, the fatty acids are degraded stepwise to acetyl CoA, the same final product as in aerobic glycolysis (Fig. 23.5). The most abundant fatty acids give rise to eight or nine molecules of acetyl CoA. The degradation, termed β-oxidation, requires four enzymes. No ATP is directly formed in this pathway; large amounts of NADH are generated instead.

Continued operation of the β-oxidation pathway requires the regeneration of NAD^+ from NADH by the respiratory chain. However, there is no anaerobic alternative available, as is the case for glycolysis.

β-oxidation is therefore strictly oxygen dependent, and all ATP regeneration occurs in the respiratory chain. Acetyl CoA constitutes the common degradation product of carbohydrates, fats and, to some extent, proteins (Fig. 23.5).

In spite of the body's large supply of adipose tissue, fatty acid combustion is not always an appropriate fuel for contracting skeletal muscle. The reason is that the energy released per unit time is only about half of that of aerobic glycolysis (McGilvery 1975). This may be explained by the comparatively low enzymatic capacity of the free fatty acid transport and oxidation pathways. The practical consequence of this is that, when the carbohydrate stores are depleted, it is not possible to continue at the same pace. To avoid or delay a slowing of pace, the pre-exercise carbohydrate stores may be increased by consuming a diet rich in carbohydrates. The maximal pace that it is possible to maintain with predominantly fat oxidation varies with the muscle enzymatic capacity for fat combustion as well as the muscle capillarization. The effect of training on these systems is described in Chapter 9.

The citric acid cycle and the respiratory chain

The citric acid cycle and respiratory chain are central pathways in the metabolism of muscle and other cells (Fig. 23.5). The starting point is acetyl CoA, which reacts with oxaloacetic acid, the final product of the citric acid cycle, to give rise to citric acid. Then follows a circle of eight enzymatic reactions, the last one ending with a regeneration of oxaloacetic acid. Two carbon atoms, equivalent to the carbon content of acetyl CoA, have by then disappeared as carbon dioxide in the expired air. In addition, one molecule of ATP and four molecules of NADH have been formed. The latter molecules are oxidized in the respiratory chain, which results in the generation of three molecules of ATP per molecule of NADH.

The respiratory chain consists of iron-containing proteins, so-called cytochromes. The first cytochrome of the chain is reduced by NADH, regenerating NAD^+. This cytochrome reduces the following cytochrome, and so on. The last cytochrome in the chain (cytochrome a) finally reduces oxygen brought to the muscle cell via the blood. Thus, in this step, oxygen combines with the electrons and hydrogen contained in the hydride ion originally incorporated in NADH, plus the proton released to the medium when NADH was formed. The product of this reaction is water.

The flow of electrons along the respiratory chain represents an energy source, which is utilized at three locations along the chain to regenerate ATP from ADP and inorganic phosphate. The final degradation of acetyl CoA in the citric acid cycle and the ensuing reactions in the respiratory chain are by far the cell's largest energy source. By way of comparison, anaerobic glycolysis (glycogen→lactate) yields less than 10% of the amount of energy released when pyruvate, instead of being converted to lactate, is converted to acetyl CoA and subsequently metabolized in the citric acid cycle and the respiratory chain.

How to determine the metabolic capacity of skeletal muscle

The capacity of a metabolic pathway is decided mainly by the amount of pathway enzymes contained in the cell. In this context, some enzymes are more important than others: these have been termed rate-limiting or flux-generating enzymes. Such an enzyme has a low activity and constitutes a bottleneck in a pathway. Generally, however, as was discussed in Chapter 9, it is possible to obtain a good estimation of the cellular capacity of a specific metabolic pathway by measuring the maximal activity of any one of its enzymes. Enzymes commonly used as a measure of the capacity of their respective metabolic pathway are indicated in Fig. 23.5.

Intracellular signalling

In the last decade it has become apparent that physical activity and other types of cellular stress, as well as cellular stimulation by hormones and growth factors, lead to the activation of intracellular signalling pathways in the skeletal muscle cell. The best known signalling pathway is that involving the insulin receptor, insulin receptor substrate-1 and phosphatidylinositol-3 kinase. This pathway results in a number of reactions involved in metabolic regulation in muscle, e.g. glucose transport and the degradation and resynthesis of glycogen during and after physical activity (Goodyear & Kahn 1998). Another important pathway is the mitogenic signalling pathway, involving a family of protein kinases called the mitogen-activated protein kinases (MAPK) (Seger & Krebs 1995). This pathway is strongly activated by exercise (Goodyear & Kahn 1998) and is likely to be important in muscle adaptation.

Elucidation of the mechanisms involved in the different signalling pathways and their physiological importance is one of the most active research areas in muscle physiology today. This research utilizes a technique known as Western blotting, which involves electrophoresis through acrylamide gels for protein separation, identification of proteins by antibodies (immunoblotting) and densitometric quantification of protein bands, visualized by enhanced chemiluminescence (ECL) or by radioiodine-based techniques. Some of these methods are briefly described in the methodological section of this chapter.

The study of muscle metabolism during exercise in humans

Due to its large mass and high exercise energy expenditure, skeletal muscle dominates metabolism in the exercising body. Muscle metabolism can therefore be studied indirectly via analyses of blood samples or expired air.

Lavoisier, in 1789, was the first to use oxygen ('air vital') intake measurements in an attempt to quantify the aerobic combustion of foodstuffs in muscle induced by exercise (Séguin & Lavoisier 1862). Lavoisier, who might be called the first exercise physiologist, was active in Paris during the latter part of the 18th century. In the latter part of the 19th century, improved techniques allowed a more accurate determination of oxygen intake and carbon dioxide production. In concert with the development of ergometers, such as the cycle ergometer, these techniques made possible a more precise quantification of the relationship between exercise intensity and aerobic metabolism.

During that period several groups used the respiratory quotient, RQ, to estimate the relative extent to which carbohydrates and fats contributed to exercise metabolism. RQ is the ratio of the body's carbon dioxide production to its oxygen consumption. Proteins had been excluded as an important fuel for the exercising muscle by Pettenkofer and Voit (1866), who estimated protein combustion by measuring the urinary nitrogen output. The pitfalls of determining the true RQ, lactate (H^+) formation and hypo- or hyperventilation, were already known at that time and could be avoided. The question as to whether carbohydrate alone, or fat and carbohydrate combined, delivered the energy for muscular work was, however, left unanswered for many decades.

The matter was first resolved through the experiments of Benedict and Cathcart (1913), Krogh and Lindhard (1920) and Hohwü Christensen and Hansen (1939). RQ determination of expired air or across the exercising muscles (arteriovenous differences of oxygen and carbon dioxide) is still one of the most widely used methods in muscle metabolic research.

Biochemical determinations in muscle

At the beginning of the 20th century a new line of research was introduced, that of muscle biopsy analysis. On the basis of biochemical determinations, Fletcher and Hopkins (1907), using an improved technique for extracting substances from isolated muscle, were able to show that lactic acid is formed from glycogen stored in the muscle. In the years before and after the Second World War, new methods were developed with a sensitivity and precision not previously seen. As early as 1935, a method was described for the determination of glucose-6-phosphate dehydrogenase, based on absorption in the near-ultraviolet wavelength range, as the pyridine nucleotide NADPH was produced (Negelein & Haas 1935). This represented a new analytical approach, that of enzymatic analysis. Greengard (1956) was the first to describe fluorometric pyridine nucleotide methods (Fig. 23.6), which now allow the measurement of almost every substance and enzyme of biological interest (Lowry

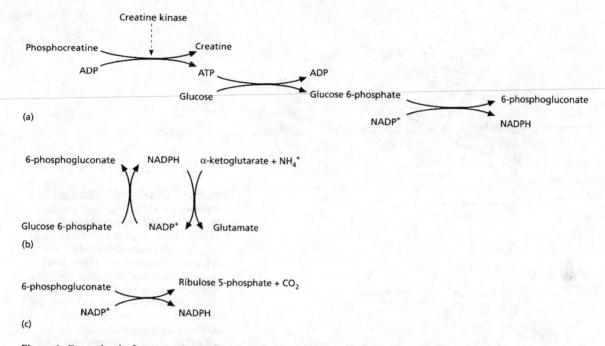

Fig. 23.6 Example of a fluorometric pyridine nucleotide method for measuring enzymes or metabolites in muscle samples or fragments of muscle fibres. It is applicable to any substance that can be made to oxidize or reduce NAD^+ or $NADP^+$, directly or indirectly. In the example shown, phosphocreatine or creatine kinase is measured by the NADPH formed in (a). In the case of creatine kinase, enough NADPH is produced to be measured by means of its own fluorescence. However, for phosphocreatine, considerable amplification may be necessary, because 20 ng dry muscle fibre contains only about 2 pmol of phosphocreatine, whereas the creatine kinase found in the same quantity of muscle can break down 2000 times this amount of phosphocreatine in 1 h. Fortunately, amplification is easy: the excess $NADP^+$ is destroyed with NaOH and heat, and the sample is added to a reagent with components which can carry out the rapidly repeating enzymatic cycle shown in (b). After a sufficient number of cycles, the enzymes are killed with heat or alkali and the 6-phosphogluconate is measured by the fluorescence of the NADPH formed from extra $NADP^+$ in the final enzymatic step (c). The amplification that can be achieved in this way is rather impressive. Cycling rates of up to 30 000 times per hour can be obtained by using high levels of two enzymes (in this case glutamic and glucose-6-phosphate dehydrogenase). By incubating for long periods, an overall amplification of 400 000 times may be achieved (Lowry & Passonneau 1972; Chi *et al.* 1978).

& Passonneau 1972). During the last two decades, the pyridine nucleotide methods have to a large extent been replaced by other methods, which allow the determination of other compounds, are faster or more sensitive or allow the determination of many metabolites in each assay. The enzymatic techniques are likely to remain an essential tool, however, for example in the determination of the maximal activity of several muscle enzymes (Chapter 9) and in association with techniques for the study of single muscle cells (Fig. 23.7, Fig. 9.3) (Lowry & Passonneau 1972; Essén *et al.* 1975).

For metabolite analyses of muscle homogenates, chromatographic techniques have largely replaced the enzymatic techniques. The basis of chromatography is the partition of compounds between two immiscible phases, one stationary phase (for example, a solid, a gel, or a liquid or solid/liquid mixture that is immobilized) and one mobile phase (liquid or gaseous) flowing over or through the stationary phase. Different compounds can be separated, based on their different partition coefficients between the two phases. The most commonly used chromatographic technique is high-performance

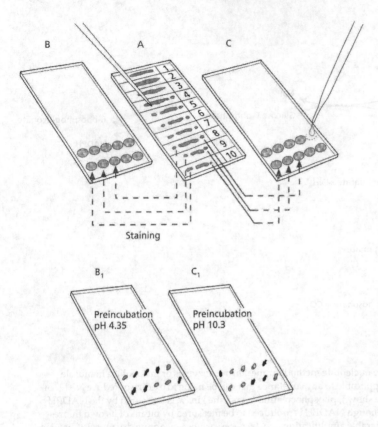

Staining

Preincubation
pH 4.35

Preincubation
pH 10.3

Fig. 23.7 Schematic illustration of a myofibrillar ATPase staining procedure for fibre type determination of individual muscle fibres. Single muscle fibre fragments (1–10) are dissected from freeze-dried biopsy specimens and two small pieces are cut off from the ends. Each of these is placed in a drop of water (B, C) that is allowed to evaporate. The result is shown on staining for myofibrillar ATPase after preincubation at different pH values (B_1, C_1). The type-identified fibre fragment (A) is subsequently used for biochemical analysis. From Essén *et al.* (1975), modified with permission.

liquid chromatography (HPLC). This method utilizes a stationary phase which is attached to an inert support packed into a glass or metal column. The mobile phase passes through the column, normally by the use of a pumping system. Different compounds distribute themselves within a distinct band in the effluent and can be analysed continuously by a detector, normally utilizing ultraviolet-visible spectrophotometry, fluorescence or electrochemical detection.

Each separated compound is represented by a peak on a chart recorder. Quantification is accomplished by comparing the area of the peaks to the corresponding areas of separately analysed standard samples of known concentration. HPLC can be used for the analysis of a wide variety of compounds; examples are purine nucleotides (e.g. ATP, ADP, adenosine), glycolytic intermediates, amino acids and catecholamines. Immunochemical techniques, such as radioimmunoassay (RIA) or enzyme-linked immunosorbent assay (ELISA),

may be used for the quantification of hormones and steroids with extreme specificity and high sensitivity.

Bioluminescence assays (see Campbell & Simpson 1979) utilize the firefly luciferase reaction, where the enzyme catalyses the oxidation of luciferin in an ATP-dependent reaction. The emitted light, being proportional to the ATP content of the solution, is the measured variable. In principle, all the enzymes and metabolites involved in ATP interconversion reactions may be assayed with very high sensitivity with this method.

Capillary electrophoresis (CE) (see Kennedy *et al.* 1989) involves electrophoresis of samples in very narrow-bore tubes. CE yields high-resolution analysis of a wide spectrum of biological molecules in small sample volumes.

Proteins and phosphorylated proteins, such as those involved in intracellular signalling, may be determined by Western blot. A protein solution, such as a muscle homogenate, is first subjected to a sodium dodecyl sulphate polyacrylamide gel electrophoresis (SDS-PAGE). This separates the denatured proteins according to molecular mass. Since the polyacrylamide gels are very fragile, the proteins are then transferred with electricity to a membrane made of nitrocellulose or nylon. These membranes are then incubated with antibodies specific for the protein or phosphorylated protein that is being measured. The antibodies carry a specific 'labelling', which enables detection on a photographic film, with subsequent quantification in a densitometer (Walker 1994). SDS-PAGE may also be used for the quantification of the muscle composition of myosin heavy chains (MHC) or myosin light chains (MLC) (Aagaard & Andersen 1998).

Molecular biology techniques are increasingly being used in skeletal muscle research. This work also involves gel electrophoresis, with transfer of DNA or RNA from the gel on to nitrocellulose paper. The technique is called Southern blot when DNA is transferred and Northern blot when the transferred molecules are RNA. A common approach in this type of research is the isolation of the mRNA transcribed from a specific gene, since quantification gives information about how the genetic machinery of the muscle cell reacts to a physiological perturbation such as a bout of exercise. This work involves the enzyme reverse transcriptase, which synthesizes a DNA strand complementary to the mRNA. The DNA strand can be copied repeatedly in the polymerase chain reaction (PCR), providing the amplification necessary for subsequent quantification (Boffey 1994).

Concurrent with the rapid development of new analytical methods, new techniques have become available for the subcellular fractionation of muscle and the measurement of transport phenomena across the muscle cell membrane.

Catheterization and radioactive technique in humans

Up until the 1950s, all detailed studies of the metabolic processes involved in cellular energy metabolism in skeletal muscle were restricted to experimental animals or *in vitro* systems. A methodological development of decisive importance for the extension of these studies to humans was the introduction of the catheterization technique by Seldinger (1953). With this technique, small intravenous catheters could be introduced subcutaneously and directed via the circulatory system to almost any organ in the body (Fig. 23.8). Catheterization has enabled researchers to study the importance of substrates stored in the muscle cells relative to substrates brought to the muscle cells by the bloodstream. Measurements of arteriovenous differences for substances such as glucose, free fatty acids, lactate and pyruvate in resting and exercising muscles, as well as in the liver and other organs, have been important in elucidating the fate of such metabolites (see Pernow & Saltin 1971).

Quantitative data on the flux of various substances across different muscle beds have required methods for the determination of local blood flow. The product of blood flow and the arteriovenous difference for a given compound indicates the uptake or release of that compound over unit time. The dye dilution technique has proven a reliable method for the determination of blood flow in the liver (Bradley *et al.* 1945) and the extremities (Wahren 1966; Jorfeldt & Wahren 1971; Wahren & Jorfeldt 1973). Thermodilution is an alternative method which has been used to estimate blood flow in exercising muscle (Jorfeldt *et al.* 1978; Andersen & Saltin 1985).

Another very important development has been the use of labelled compounds, notably ^{14}C or ^3H compounds. Tracer techniques have been used to investigate the metabolism of free fatty acids and glucose in human muscle, both at rest and during exercise (see Hagenfeldt 1975; Searle 1976; references in Pernow & Saltin 1971), as well as protein turnover (Smith & Rennie 1996). A small amount of radioactive isotope, for instance ^{14}C- or ^3H-labelled glucose, equivalent to a few weeks of the normal background cosmic radiation, is infused intravenously. From determinations of the specific activity of the compound in the blood, its total turnover in the body can be determined. It is also possible to study the different degradation pathways of a compound by measuring the specific activity of its metabolites. The use of stable isotopes to label metabolic tracers has markedly increased the feasibility of radioactive techniques in humans

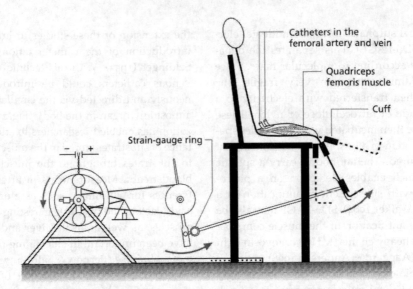

Fig. 23.8 A one-leg model for the study of metabolic regulation in skeletal muscle. One of the subject's legs is attached to a cycle ergometer in such a way that, during exercise, only the quadriceps femoris muscle is activated. Exercise is performed by pulling a rod attached to both the ankle of the subject and the crank of a modified Krogh cycle ergometer. The flywheel momentum returns the relaxed leg. Detailed study of metabolic processes is made possible by arterial and venous catheterization and muscle biopsy analysis. Quantitative data on the flux of various substances are obtained by blood flow determinations, using thermodilution or dye dilution techniques. To minimize the sampling of blood from tissues other than active muscle, the circulation to the lower leg is occluded with a pressure cuff. From Andersen and Saltin (1985).

(Smith & Rennie 1996). However, quantification of the flux through different metabolic pathways is hampered by the inevitable exchange of isotopes that occurs within the tissues (Landau 1986; Sahlin 1987).

The muscle biopsy technique

The use of a needle technique to obtain muscle biopsy specimens was described by Charrière and Duchenne (1865) more than 100 years ago. Reintroduction of the technique by Bergström (1962) opened a new field of research in human physiology. Together with the catheterization technique described above, biopsy has been used extensively over the past four decades, and it has led to an indepth understanding of the metabolic processes occurring in exercised muscle.

The Bergström needle (Fig. 23.9) is 3–5 mm in diameter, the outer cylinder having a small window close to the tip of the needle. After anaesthetizing the skin and the tissue immediately above the muscle fascia (for example, with 1 ml of 1% lido-

caine), a small incision (approximately 5 mm in length) is made, extending through the muscle fascia. When the needle is inserted into the muscle, tissue bulges into the needle window and can be cut by the sharp edge of the inner cylinder. The piece of muscle thus obtained generally weighs 20–100 mg. Larger samples may be obtained by attaching a suction device to the needle (Edwards *et al.* 1983), or by replacing the needle with a Weil–Blakesley conchotome (Fig. 23.9, Henriksson 1979). The latter is an alligator forceps, which is as easy to use as the biopsy needle, and has therefore replaced it in many laboratories. Several other biopsy needles are also in current use (Nichols *et al.* 1968; Siperstein *et al.* 1968; Young *et al.* 1978).

The needle or conchotome technique is important because, unlike surgical biopsy, it allows repeated sampling from the same muscle. Moreover, subjects need not restrict physical activity after a biopsy has been performed. The lateral aspect of the thigh muscle has been the most common biopsy site for both physiological and clinical studies, but biopsies have been performed in many other muscles,

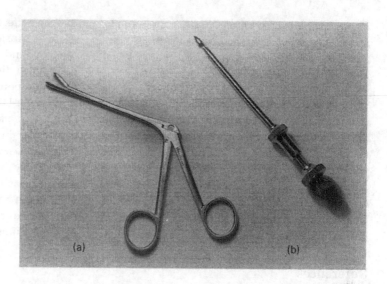

Fig. 23.9 The Weil–Blakesley conchotome (a) and the Bergström biopsy needle (b). The length of the needle is 0.14 m.

(a)

(b)

including the deltoid, biceps and triceps brachii, gastrocnemius, soleus and tibialis anterior muscles. For a more detailed description of the procedure, the reader is referred to the review by Edwards *et al.* (1980). Methods applied to and results obtained by the biopsy technique have been reviewed by Saltin and Gollnick (1983).

Newer techniques for the study of muscle metabolism

During the past two decades, nuclear magnetic resonance (NMR) spectroscopy has become available at many university centres. It is a completely atraumatic technique, and allows a continuous study of muscle metabolism (see Shulman 1983). The method is based on the fact that atomic nuclei with an odd number of nucleons (protons and neutrons) have an intrinsic magnetism that makes each of such nuclei a magnetic dipole. Such nuclei include the proton (H-1), the carbon-13 nucleus (C-13, 1.1% of all carbon atoms) and the phosphorus-31 nucleus (P-31).

Metabolites containing these nuclei can be measured after two types of field have been applied to the tissue. One is a strong magnetic field, which causes the nuclear dipoles to align either with the field (less energy stored) or against it. The other field consists of electromagnetic radiation in the radiofrequency portion of the spectrum; at a given magnetic field strength, each nucleus will 'flip' over in the magnetic field, absorbing radiophotons (resonating) when the field has a certain frequency. The precise resonance frequency differs for a given nucleus, depending on which other chemical groups are bound to it. Different compounds can be localized and quantified on the basis of the 'chemical shift' in the frequency of resonance.

To date, most NMR studies of human muscle metabolism have been conducted with P-31 (for references, see Wilkie *et al.* 1984), but because of the ubiquitous presence of carbon, C-13 NMR looks particularly promising for future research. The latter technique has to date been used mainly for the quantification of hepatic and skeletal muscle glycogen concentrations (Laurent *et al.* 1998; Petersen *et al.* 1998). A novel C-13 NMR method has furthermore made possible the determination of muscle intracellular concentrations of glucose (Cline *et al.* 1998). Recently, non-invasive determinations of skeletal muscle lactate concentrations have been performed by H-1 NMR spectroscopy (Mercier *et al.* 1998).

Other new and important techniques in muscle metabolic research include positron emission tomography (PET) and microdialysis. With PET, extremely short-lived isotopes may be injected into the bloodstream and their behaviour in specific tissues (uptake, release, metabolism, receptor binding) can be studied by an external camera (see

Phelps *et al.* 1986). PET has been used, for example, to measure skeletal muscle protein synthesis rates, free fatty acid uptake rates, skeletal muscle blood flow and glucose uptake rates.

The microdialysis technique (Delgado *et al.* 1972; Ungerstedt & Pycock 1974) utilizes a hollow catheter continuously perfused with physiological fluid. The microdialysis catheter can be viewed as an 'artificial blood vessel' inserted into the tissue, where diffusion of chemical substances occurs in the direction of the lowest concentration. Constituents of the muscle extracellular space can be collected for analysis, and foreign compounds may be added to the extracellular space via the dialysis catheter so that their effect on the muscle cell can be monitored. At low perfusion rates, the interstitial concentration of compounds such as glucose and lactate can be determined directly by analysing the concentration of the compound in the dialysate outflow (Rosdahl *et al.* 1998). Use of the microdialysis ethanol technique also allows the determination of nutritive blood flow in skeletal muscle and adipose tissue (Hickner *et al.* 1992).

It is likely that the microdialysis technique will be used increasingly to study how skeletal muscle metabolism and blood flow are influenced by and regulated during different types of exercise and physical training.

References

Aagaard, P. & Andersen, J.L. (1998) Correlation between contractile strength and myosin heavy chain isoform composition in human skeletal muscle. *Medicine and Science in Sports and Exercise* **30**, 1217–1222.

Andersen, P. & Saltin, B. (1985) Maximal perfusion of skeletal muscle in man. *Journal of Physiology (London)* **366**, 233–249.

Åstrand, P.-O. & Rodahl, K. (1986) *Textbook of Work Physiology*, 3rd edn. McGraw-Hill, New York.

Astrup, A. & Flatt, J.P. (1996) Metabolic determinants of body weight regulation. In: Bouchard, C. & Bray, G.A. (eds) *Regulation of Body Weight. Biological and Behavioral Mechanisms*. Life Sciences Research Report 57, pp. 193–210. John Wiley & Sons, Chichester.

Benedict, F.G. & Cathcart, E.P. (1913) *Muscular Work*. Carnegie Institute of Washington, Publication no. 187.

Bergström, J. (1962) Muscle electrolytes in man. *Scandinavian Journal of Clinical and Laboratory Investigation* **14** (Suppl. 68), 1–110.

Bergström, J., Hermansen, L., Hultman, E. & Saltin, B. (1967) Diet, muscle glycogen and physical performance. *Acta Physiologica Scandinavica* **71**, 140–150.

Boffey, S. (1994) Molecular biology techniques. In: Wilson, K. & Walker, J. (eds) *Principles and Techniques of Practical Biochemistry*, 4th edn, pp. 110–161. Cambridge University Press, London.

Bradley, S.E., Ingelfinger, F.J., Bradley, G.P. & Curry, J.J. (1945) The estimation of hepatic blood flow in man. *Journal of Clinical Investigation* **24**, 890–897.

Campbell, A.K. & Simpson, J.S.A. (1979) Chemi- and bio-luminescence as an analytical tool in biology. In: Kornberg, H.L., Metcalfe, J.C., Northcote, D.H., Pogson, C.I. & Tipton, K.F. (eds) *Techniques in the Life Sciences, Biochemistry*—Vol. B2/II. *Techniques in Metabolic Research*, Part II, B 213, pp. 1–56. Elsevier/North-Holland Scientific Publishers, Ireland.

Charrière, M. & Duchenne, G.B. (1865) Emporte pièce histologique. *Bullétin de l'Académie de Médécine* **30**, 1050–1051.

Chi, M.M.-Y., Lowry, C.V. & Lowry, O.H. (1978) An improved enzymatic cycle for nicotinamide-adenine dinucleotide phosphate. *Analytic Biochemistry* **89**, 119–129.

Cline, G.W., Jucker, B.M., Trajanoski, Z., Rennings, A.J. & Shulman, G.I. (1998) A novel ^{13}C NMR method to assess intracellular glucose concentration in muscle, *in vivo. American Journal of Physiology* **274**, E381–E389.

Delgado, J.M.R., Defeudis, F.V., Roth, R.H., Ryugo, D.K. & Mitruka, B.K. (1972) Dialytrode for long term intracerebral perfusion in awake monkeys. *Archives Internationales de Pharmacodynamie Thérapeutique* **198**, 9–21.

Edwards, R., Young, A. & Wiles, M. (1980) Needle biopsy of skeletal muscle in the diagnosis of myopathy and the clinical study of muscle function and repair. *New England Journal of Medicine* **302**, 261–271.

Edwards, R.H.T., Round, J.M. & Jones, D.A. (1983) Needle biopsy of skeletal muscle: a review of 10 years experience. *Muscle and Nerve* **6**, 676–683.

Essén, B., Jansson, E., Henriksson, J.,

Taylor, A.W. & Saltin, B. (1975) Metabolic characteristics of fibre types in human skeletal muscle. *Acta Physiologica Scandinavica* **95**, 153–165.

Fletcher, W.M. & Hopkins, F.G. (1907) Lactic acid in amphibian muscle. *Journal of Physiology (London)* **35**, 247–309.

Glatz, J.F., Van Breda, E. & Van der Vusse, G.J. (1998) Intracellular transport of fatty acids in muscle. Role of cytoplasmic fatty acid-binding protein. *Advances in Experimental Medicine and Biology* **441**, 207–218.

Goodyear, L.J. & Kahn, B.B. (1998) Exercise, glucose transport, and insulin sensitivity. *Annual Reviews of Medicine* **49**, 235–261.

Greengard, P. (1956) Determination of intermediary metabolites by enzymic fluorimetry. *Nature (London)* **178**, 632–634.

Hagenfeldt, L. (1975) Turnover of individual free fatty acids in man. *Federation Proceedings* **34**, 2246–2249.

Henriksson, K.G. (1979) 'Semi-open' muscle biopsy technique. A simple outpatient procedure. *Acta Neurologica Scandinavica* **59**, 317–323.

Hickner, R.C., Rosdahl, H., Borg, I., Ungerstedt, U., Jorfeldt, L. & Henriksson, J. (1992) The ethanol technique of monitoring local blood flow changes in rat skeletal muscle: implications for microdialysis. *Acta Physiologica Scandinavica* **146**, 87–97.

Hohwü Christensen, E. & Hansen, O. (1939) I. Zur Metodik der Respiratorischen Quotient-Bestimmungen in Ruhe und bei Arbeit. II. Untersuchungen über die Verbrennungsvorgänge bei langdauernder, schwerer Muskelarbeit. III. Arbeitsfähigkeit und Ernährung. *Skandinavisches Archives für Physiologie* **81**, 137–171.

Jorfeldt, L., Juhlin-Dannfelt, A., Pernow, B. & Wassén, E. (1978) Determination of human leg blood flow: a thermodilution technique based on femoral venous bolus injection. *Clinical Science* **54**, 517–523.

Kennedy, R.T., Oates, M.D., Cooper, B.R., Nickerson, B. & Jorgenson, J.W. (1989) Microcolumn separations and the analysis of single cells. *Science* **246**, 57–63.

Krogh, A. & Lindhard, J. (1920) The relative value of fat and carbohydrate as source of muscular energy. *Biochemical Journal* **14**, 290–363.

Landau, B.R. (1986) A potential pitfall in the use of isotopes to measure ketone body production. *Metabolism* **35**, 94.

Laurent, D., Petersen, K.F., Russell, R.R., Cline, G.W. & Shulman, G.I. (1998) Effect of epinephrine on muscle glycogenolysis and insulin-stimulated muscle glycogen synthesis in humans. *American Journal of Physiology* **274**, E130–E138.

Lowry, O.H. & Passonneau, J.V. (1972) *A Flexible System of Enzymatic Analysis.* Academic Press, New York.

McGilvery, R.W. (1975) The use of fuels for muscular work. In: Howald, H. & Poortmans, J.R. (eds) *Metabolic Adaptation to Prolonged Physical Exercise*, pp. 12–30. Birkhäuser-Verlag, Basel.

McMurray, W.C. (1983) *Essentials of Human Metabolism*, 2nd edn. Lippincott, Philadelphia.

Mercier, B., Granier, P., Mercier, J. *et al.* (1998) Noninvasive skeletal muscle lactate detection between periods of intense exercise in humans. *European Journal of Applied Physiology* **78**, 20–27.

Negelein, E. & Haas, E. (1935) Über die Wirkungsweise des Zwischenferments. *Biochemische Zeitung* **282**, 206–220.

Nichols, B.L., Hazlewood, C.F. & Barnes, D.J. (1968) Percutaneous needle biopsy of quadriceps muscle: potassium analysis in normal children. *Journal of Pediatrics* **72**, 840–852.

Pernow, B. & Saltin, B. (1971) *Muscle Metabolism During Exercise.* Proceedings of a Karolinska Institute Symposium held in Stockholm, Sweden, September 6–9, 1970. Plenum Press, New York.

Petersen, K.F., Laurent, D., Rothman, D.L., Cline, G.W. & Shulman, G.I. (1998) Mechanism by which glucose and insulin inhibit net hepatic glycogenoly-

sis in humans. *Journal of Clinical Investigation* **101**, 1203–1209.

Pettenkofer, M. & Voit, C. (1866) Untersuchungen über den Stoffverbrauch des normalen Menschen. *Zeitschrifte für Biologie* **2**, 537.

Phelps, M., Mazzeota, J. & Schelbert, H. (eds) (1986) *Positron Emission Tomography. Principles and Application for the Brain and Heart.* Raven Press, New York.

Potter, B.J., Sorrentino, D. & Berk, P.D. (1989) Mechanisms of cellular uptake of free fatty acids. *Annual Review of Nutrition* **9**, 253–270.

Pruett, E.D.R. (1971) *Fat and Carbohydrate Metabolism in Exercise and Recovery, and its Dependence Upon Work Load Severity.* Institute of Work Physiology, Oslo.

Rosdahl, H., Hamrin, K., Ungerstedt, U. & Henriksson, J. (1998) Metabolite levels in human skeletal muscle and adipose tissue studied with microdialysis at low perfusion flow. *American Journal of Physiology* **274**, E936–E945.

Sahlin, K. (1987) Lactate production cannot be measured with tracer techniques. *American Journal of Physiology* **252**, E439–E440.

Saltin, B. & Gollnick, P.D. (1983) Skeletal muscle adaptability: significance for metabolism and performance. In: Peachey, L.D., Adrian, P.H. & Geiger, S.R. (eds) *Handbook of Physiology*, Section 10. *Skeletal Muscle*, pp. 555–631. American Physiological Society, Bethesda, MD.

Saltin, B. & Hermansen, L. (1967) Glycogen stores and prolonged severe exercise. In: Blix, G. (ed.) *Nutrition and Physical Activity*, p. 32. Almqvist & Wiksell, Uppsala.

Saltin, B. & Karlsson, J. (1971) Muscle glycogen utilization during work of different intensities. In: Pernow, B. & Saltin, B. (eds) *Muscle Metabolism During Exercise*, pp 289–299. Plenum Press, New York.

Searle, G.L. (1976) The use of isotope turnover techniques in the study of carbohydrate metabolism in man. In: Besser, G.M., Bierich, J.R., Bondy, P.K., Daughaday, W.H., Franchimont, P. & Hall, R. (eds) *Clinics in Endocrinology and Metabolism*, Vol. 5, No. 3. *Disorders of Carbohydrate Metabolism Excluding Diabetes*, pp. 783–804. W.B. Saunders, London.

Seger, R. & Krebs, E.G. (1995) The MAPK signaling cascade. *Federation of American Societies of Experimental Biology* **9**, 726–735.

Séguin, A. & Lavoisier, A.L. (1862) *Oeuvres*

de Lavoisier, Vol. II, p. 688 (*Mémoires de l'Académie des Sciences 1789*, p. 185). Académie des Sciences, Paris.

Seldinger, S.I. (1953) Catheter replacement of the needle in percutaneous arteriography. A new technique. *Acta Radiologica (Stockholm)* **39**, 368–376.

Shulman, R.G. (1983) NMR spectroscopy of living cells. *Scientific American* **248**, 86–93.

Siperstein, M.D., Unger, R.H. & Madison, L.L. (1968) Studies of muscle capillary basement membranes in normal subjects, diabetic, and prediabetic patients. *Journal of Clinical Investigation* **47**, 1973–1999.

Sjögaard, G. (1990) Exercise-induced muscle fatigue: the significance of potassium. *Acta Physiologica Scandinavica* **140** (Suppl.), 593.

Smith, K. & Rennie, M.J. (1996) The measurement of tissue protein turnover. *Baillières Clinical Endocrinology and Metabolism* **10**, 469–495.

Ungerstedt, U. & Pycock, C. (1974) Functional correlates of dopamine neurotransmission. *Bulletin Schweiz für Akademische Medizin Wissenschaft* **1278**, 1–13.

Wahren, J. (1966) Quantitative aspects of blood flow and oxygen uptake in the human forearm during rhythmic exercise. *Acta Physiologica Scandinavica* **67** (Suppl.), 269.

Wahren, J. & Jorfeldt, L. (1973) Determination of leg blood flow during exercise in man: an indicator-dilution technique based on femoral venous dye infusion. *Clinical Science and Molecular Medicine Supplement* **42**(2), 135–146.

Walker, J.M. (1994) Electrophoretic techniques. In: Wilson, K. & Walker, J. (eds) *Principles and Techniques of Practical Biochemistry*, 4th edn, pp. 425–461. Cambridge University Press, London.

Widegren, U., Jiang, X.J., Krook, A. *et al.* (1998) Divergent effects of exercise on metabolic and mitogenic signaling pathways in human skeletal muscle. *FASEB Journal* **12**, 1379–1389.

Wilkie, D.R., Dawson, M.J., Edwards, R.H.T., Gordon, R.E. & Shaw, D. (1984) ^{31}P NMR studies of resting muscle in normal human subjects. In: Pollock, G.H. & Sugi, H. (eds) *Contractile Mechanisms in Muscle*, pp. 333–347. Plenum Publishing, New York.

Young, A., Wiles, C.M. & Edwards, R.H.T. (1978) University College Hospital muscle-biopsy needle. *Lancet* **ii**, 1285.

Chapter 24

Body Composition of the Endurance Performer

SCOTT GOING AND VERONICA MULLINS

Introduction

Body size, structure and composition are separate yet interrelated aspects of the body that contribute to what has been defined as physique. Body size refers to the volume, mass, length and surface area of the body, whereas body structure refers to the distribution or arrangement of body parts such as the skeleton and muscle–fat distribution. Body composition, the third aspect of physique, refers to the amounts of the various constituents in the body. Body composition is the major focus of this chapter, although it is important to recognize that each aspect of physique and their interplay are important determinants of athletic success.

A variety of indirect methods have been used to describe the body composition of athletes. This chapter begins with a brief overview of models and selected methods and their assumptions, since an understanding of these issues is essential to the valid interpretation of available data. The relationship of physique to performance is also reviewed, and this is followed by descriptions of the body composition of male and female endurance athletes in comparison to other athletic groups and the general population.

Body composition models

The human body comprises more than 30 major components at the atomic, molecular, cellular, tissue-system and whole-body levels of body composition (Wang *et al.* 1992). Direct measurement

of body composition in living humans is not feasible, so various models for indirect estimation of the constituents of the body have been developed. The two-component chemical model has been the primary one used in the study of the relationship between body composition and athletic performance. This model divides the body into fat mass and fat-free mass (FFM). Fat is a molecular-level component, not to be confused with fat cells or adipose tissue, which are cellular and tissue-system components of body composition. In the two-component chemical model, the fat component has historically included all lipids, and all other body constituents are included in the FFM. In more complex three- or four-component chemical models, the FFM is subdivided into its major constituents: water, mineral and protein (Boileau & Lohman 1977).

Methods based on multicomponent models give more valid and accurate estimates of composition, but they are more time consuming and expensive, and have rarely been applied in descriptive studies of athletes.

Body composition assessment

Criterion methods

Although the application of many experimentally derived methods is limited to a laboratory setting, an understanding of these criterion methods and their limitations is important, since field methods can be no more accurate than the criterion methods on which they are based.

TWO-COMPONENT MODELS AND METHODS

The three most widely applied criterion methods for dividing the body into fat mass and FFM are densitometry, dilution of deuterated water and potassium (^{40}K) spectroscopy. These methods and others based on the two-component body composition model are similar in the sense that they rely upon a known and stable relationship between the compartment of interest (FFM) and the measured body constituent. For example, when FFM is estimated using deuterated water, the total body water (TBW) is first estimated by determining the dilution of a small ingested volume (10–30 ml) of isotopically labelled water as it spreads throughout the much larger volume of body water. FFM is then calculated from TBW on the basis of the average water content of FFM, which in an average non-athletic individual is assumed to be about 73% (Brozek et al. 1963). Similarly, FFM can be calculated from total body potassium (K) which can be estimated by measuring the amount of naturally occurring radioactive ^{40}K in the body (Forbes 1987; Flynn et al. 1989) or the total exchangeable potassium in the body (Forbes 1987). Once the mass of total body potassium is known, it can be divided by the average mass of potassium in a kilogram of FFM to estimate FFM. Thus, in average non-athletic adult males, FFM = total body potassium in grams (g)/2.66 (g·kg^{-1}); in adult females, the denominator is 2.55 (Forbes 1987). The validity and accuracy of both isotope dilution and potassium spectroscopy methods for estimating body composition depend largely on the appropriateness of the identified conversion constants for the individual in whom they are applied. Unfortunately, the constants assumed for the sedentary population do not apply very well to endurance athletes.

Densitometry is based on the relationship between whole-body density (D_b) and the respective densities of the body compartments, regardless of how they are defined (Behnke & Wilmore 1974). The general principle is that density varies inversely with the percentage of body fat (%BF), i.e.

$$FM = f(1/D) \qquad (1)$$

where FM (fat mass) is the ether-extractable lipid fraction of body mass and f is the function describing the relationship between fat and density. To derive simple, useful solutions of Equation 1, an additional assumption is required, i.e. that the respective densities of the two compartments (FM and FFM) are constant from one person to another. The well-known Siri (1956) and Brozek et al. (1963) formulae represent the simplest solutions of Equation 1. In these equations, %BF is calculated from total body density (D_b), and assumed densities of 0.9 for the fat (Fidanza et al. 1953) and 1.1 for the fat-free constituents (Brozek et al. 1963) according to the equation

$$1/D_b = FM/d_{FM} + FFM/d_{FFM} \qquad (2)$$

where $1/D_b$ is body mass (set equal to unity) divided by body density (D_b), and FM/d_{FM} and FFM/d_{FFM} are the fractions of body mass that are fat and fat free divided by their respective densities. The density of adult human body fat is relatively constant within and among individuals at 0.9 kg·m^{-3}. In the simplest chemical model, FFM is composed primarily of water, protein and mineral compartments and d_{FFM} (1.1 kg·m^{-3}) is derived from the proportions of water, protein and mineral divided by constant values for their densities (Lohman 1992):

$$1/d_{FFM} = W/d_W + P/d_P + M/d_{Mf} \qquad (3)$$

where W, P and M are the fractions of the FFM that consist of water, protein and mineral, respectively. Thus, for d_{FFM} to be constant, the proportions of water, protein and minerals must be constant or they must vary in such a way that d_{FFM} does not change.

In the densitometric approach, any deviation of D_b is assumed to be due to the addition of body fat. However, it is clear from a number of studies that the chemical composition of FFM is not constant. Rather, there is considerable variation among individuals, and predictable changes in FFM constituents occur with growth, maturation and ageing (Lohman 1992). Long-term specialized training may also alter FFM composition, e.g. by increasing muscle and bone mass (Modlesky et al. 1996). Conversely, in some sports, competitors may have less than average muscle and bone mass. Deviations from the assumed chemical composition of the FFM result in under- or overestimation of body fat by hydrodensitometry, depending on whether the d_{FFM} is greater than or less than the assumed density of 1.1. Thus, %BF may be overestimated in individuals with lower than average bone mass and higher than average muscle mass and underestimated in individuals with higher than average bone mass and lower than average muscle mass.

The estimates of body composition for any group of athletes must be interpreted with these potential errors in mind. Estimates from field techniques such as skinfold thicknesses and circumferences must also be interpreted cautiously, since the errors in the densitometric method are passed on to the simpler field methods when they are validated against this criterion method. For example, in a female runner with lower than average bone mass the predicted %BF value would be higher than her actual value (Bunt et al. 1990), since the criterion method would overestimate her actual body fat.

MULTIPLE-COMPONENT MODELS AND METHODS

Because of the limitations in the two-component model, multicomponent approaches have been developed in which two or more constituents of the FFM are measured in the criterion method. Such methods can provide a more accurate estimate of body composition than the two-component approach (Siri 1961; Lohman 1992).

A four-component model of body composition can be derived when the FFM is divided into its primary constituents of water, protein and mineral:

$$1/D_b = FM/d_{FM} + W/d_W + P/d_P + M/d_M \qquad (4)$$

where FM/d_{FM} is the fraction of the total body mass that consists of fat divided by the density of that fat mass, and W/d_W, P/d_P and M/d_M are the fractions of FFM consisting of water, protein and mineral, divided by their respective densities. Three-component models can also be derived by combining two constituents of the FFM into one component. For example, if the protein and mineral fractions of FFM are combined, then:

$$1/D_b = FM/d_{FM} + W/d_W + S/d_S \qquad (5)$$

where S/d_S represents the non-aqueous (solids) fraction of FFM divided by its density. This approach is useful as a criterion method when it is expected that the body-water fraction of the FFM will vary from the designated biological constant of 0.73. Variation in body water accounts for the largest proportion of variance in d_{FFM} in the general population (Siri 1961).

A second three-component model can be derived by combining water and protein to form the lean soft tissue (LST) fraction of FFM:

$$1/D_b = FM/d_{FM} + M/d_M + LST/d_{LST} \qquad (6)$$

This approach is useful when it is expected that the mineral fraction of FFM will deviate from the designated constant of 6.8% (Brozek et al. 1963), which is possible in some groups of sports competitors, e.g. swimmers, amenorrhoeic runners and bodybuilders.

Multiple-component models are useful to minimize the potential errors in estimates of %BF associated with variability in FFM composition. The ideal laboratory procedure is to combine measures of body density with measures of body water and bone mineral and to estimate body composition using an equation based on a four-component model of body composition. This approach eliminates the need for assumptions regarding the proportionalities among the constituents of the FFM and it provides the best criterion estimate of body composition against which to validate field methods. Alternatively, body density can be combined with measures of body water or bone mineral and estimates of body fat based on three-component models can be derived. Although more accurate than the two-component equations, these equations do assume a constant protein to mineral ratio (Equation 5) or protein to water ratio (Equation 6), and individual deviations from the assumed ratios introduce errors, albeit less than for the two-component model. Whether body water or bone mineral should be measured depends on which constituent is likely to vary most within the population being studied, which is influenced by the age, sex and race of the athlete, and the type of training performed.

Dual-energy X-ray absorptiometry (DXA), a relatively new technique, is based on a three-component model. It is capable of resolving body mass into its fat, lean and mineral components without an estimate of body density. Thus, DXA is relatively unaffected by the variation in FFM water and mineral fractions that confounds hydrodensitometry and other methods based on the two-component model. Studies to date have shown DXA to give reliable and accurate estimates of bone and soft tissue composition (Lohman 1996). DXA is likely to be very useful in future studies of athletes.

Field methods

Because of the time and expense involved in most laboratory methods, many descriptive studies have used simpler field methods such as anthropometry and bioelectric impedance analysis. Historically, field methods have predicted body density from equations validated against underwater weighing and then body composition has been estimated from density by traditional equations. Although this approach may give accurate estimates of body density, substantial errors can occur when density is converted to %BF using prediction equations based on two-component models such as the Brozek and Siri equations (Siri 1956; Brozek et al. 1963). It is better to use equations based on three- or four-component models, in which %BF is estimated directly from anthropometric measurements; unfortunately, few such equations have as yet been published, with the notable exceptions of equations for children and adolescents (Slaughter et al. 1988) and for older men and women (Williams et al. 1992).

An alternative approach is to estimate %BF from density alone, using modifications of the Siri equation derived from estimates of FFM composition in the population of interest. Using average estimates of water and mineral fractions of the FFM for a given age to estimate d_{FFM}, Lohman (1989) has derived two-component equations for use in children and adolescents. These equations make it possible to use densitometry as a criterion method in children. Unfortunately, there has been no systematic attempt to define the water and mineral fractions of the FFM in different groups of sports

participants; thus, estimation of %BF from density becomes relatively inaccurate because of variability in FFM composition and density. A better description of the contributions of water and mineral to FFM in different groups of competitors should be an important focus for future research, so that population-specific equations can be developed. This will allow more accurate estimation of body composition in athletes, using both densitometry and also the more acces-sible field techniques.

Body composition and performance

Although levels of %BF and FFM for sports participants influence successful performance within a sport, athletic performance cannot be accurately predicted solely on the basis of body composition. All the components of physique (body size, structure and composition) are significant determinants of competitive success. Each component is related to performance in a logical and predictable way. More massive individuals, for example, have an advantage over their lighter counterparts when an activity demands that the inertia of another body or an external object must be overcome. Less massive individuals have the advantage when the goal is to propel the body, especially over moderate to long distances, as in marathons and triathlons. Taller individuals with longer levers (limbs) have the advantage in jumping and throwing events because of their higher centre of gravity, and in some running events because of their longer stride length, whereas shorter individuals have the advantage when the body must be rotated around an axis as in diving and tumbling events.

Fat mass and performance

Evidence from athletes of various ages has demonstrated an inverse relationship between fat mass and performance of physical activities requiring translocation of the body mass, either vertically, as in jumping, or horizontally, as in running (Boileau & Lohman 1977; Pate et al. 1989; Malina 1992). Excessive fatness is detrimental to these types of activities, because it adds mass to the body without additional ability to produce force. Because acceleration is proportional to force, but inversely proportional to mass, excess fat at a given level of force application will result in slower changes in velocity and direction. Excess fatness also increases the metabolic cost of physical activities requiring movement of the total body mass (Buskirk & Taylor 1957). Thus, in most performances involving movement of the body mass, a relatively low %BF would be advantageous both mechanically and metabolically (Boileau & Lohman 1977).

Cross-sectional data indicate that %BF is inversely related to aerobic power ($\dot{V}_{O_{2max}}$) expressed relative to body mass and is also inversely related to distance-running performance (Cureton 1992). Only a few experimental studies have investigated the effect of altered body composition on physical performance. Cureton and coworkers conducted three experiments on the effects of artificially increasing body mass on the physiological response to exercise and physical performance capabilities (Cureton et al. 1978a,b; Cureton & Sparling 1980; Sparling & Cureton 1983). Data from these studies demonstrated that the running performance of fit, normal-weight individuals decreased when they wore a weight belt and shoulder harness. Their performances were similar to those of obese individuals with similar FFM and body mass.

In contrast, adequate amounts of appropriately distributed fat mass are advantageous in sports in which the absorbing of force or momentum is important, and in sports where buoyancy is an issue. For example, long-distance swimmers are likely to benefit from a relatively high fat mass because of the contributions of fat to thermal insulation and buoyancy (Sinning 1985).

Fat-free mass and performance

Successful performance in activities such as throwing, pushing and weightlifting, each of which requires the application of force against external objects, is positively related to the absolute amount of FFM and therefore to body size (Boileau & Lohman 1977; Harman & Frykman 1992). However, a large FFM and body size may adversely affect performance requiring translocation of the body mass,

such as in running, jumping or rotation of the body about an axis, as in gymnastics or diving. In other activities, such as cycling and swimming, in which the weight is not self-supported or buoyancy is a factor, a larger FFM may be an advantage, or at least not a disadvantage.

The FFM is better correlated with performance than is %BF, if performance is measured by such indices as maximal aerobic power, treadmill run time, 12-min run distance, or the ability to push, carry and exert torque (Harman & Frykman 1992). Based on their data, Harman and Frykman suggested that military recruits should be required to meet standards for both minimum FFM and maximum %BF. For most sports, high ratios of FFM to fat mass at a given body mass are associated with better performances, although too little body fat can result in deterioration of both health and physical performance (Sinning & Wilson 1984; Wilmore 1992). Minimum %BF values compatible with health and physical performance are estimated to be 4–6% fat in males and 8–10% in females (Lohman 1992).

Bone mass and performance

Skeletal mass and density are not as highly related to performance as are FFM and %BF, since bone accounts for only a small fraction (3–4%) of body mass. Nevertheless, a predictable relationship reflects requirements of the athlete's sport. Endurance athletes in weight-bearing sports (for example, runners and race walkers) require sufficient skeletal mass and density to withstand the repetitive, moderate impact forces characteristic of their sports, but not so much as to add greatly to the total mass that must be transported. Strength and power athletes require greater bone mineral density (BMD) than endurance athletes, to endure the high loads and impact forces (jumpers, volleyball players) sustained in training and competition. Endurance athletes engaged in non-weight-bearing sports (cycling, rowing and swimming) require less BMD than athletes in weight-bearing sports, although BMD may be similar or even higher at muscle attachment sites where high pulling forces are regularly sustained.

Body composition of endurance athletes

It is widely believed by competitors and coaches that there is an ideal body mass and body composition for any given sport. There must be an optimal value above which or below which performance is negatively affected. Nevertheless, many factors contribute to competitive success making the optimal combination of body fat mass and FFM difficult to define. As a result, recommendations concerning body mass and body composition are usually based on average %BF and FFM values obtained from samples of élite performers in various sports (Sinning & Wilson 1984; Wilmore 1992). Such findings generally support relationships between the various components of composition and performance as described above, but there is considerable overlap in body fat, FFM and bone content among various groups of athletes, attesting to the importance of other factors influencing competitive success. This point cannot be overemphasized. There is considerable individual variation in body composition. Not all athletes are capable of achieving the theoretical ideal values, and the performance (and health) of some athletes may suffer if they are forced to make the attempt. Moreover, the errors inherent in assessment techniques must be considered when interpreting available data and defining optimal levels. For these reasons, it is more appropriate to specify a range of ideal values rather than the average.

Percentage fat of endurance athletes

Tables 24.1 and 24.2 summarize %BF values and FFM of female and male competitors in various

Table 24.1 Body composition of élite female endurance athletes.

Sport	n	Age (years)	Height (m)	Body mass (kg)	%BF	FFM (kg)	FFM/ HT	Technique	Reference
Distance running	10	20.5	1.65	50.8	14.8	43.28	26	UWW	Bartlett et al. (1984)[c]
	15	27.6	1.61	47.2	14.3	40.45	25	UWW	Graves et al. (1987)[a]
	2	23.0	1.67	56.7	20.8	44.91	27	UWW	Cureton et al. (1978a,b)[e]
	10	43.8	1.62	53.8	18.3	43.95	27	UWW	Vaccaro et al. (1981)[b]
	11	32.4	1.69	57.2	15.2	48.51	29	UWW	Wilmore et al. (1977)[a]
	42	25.0	1.67	54.3	16.9	45.12	27	UWW	Wilmore et al. (1977)[a]
Weighted average		27.9	1.65	53.1	16.3	44.42			
Swimming	4	—	1.66	53.1	16.3	44.42	30	UWW	Wilmore et al. (1977)[b]
	10	19.5	—	63.9	19.2	51.63	—	UWW	Sprynarova & Parizcova (1969)[b]
Weighted average		—	—	63.0	18.6	51.30			
Rowing	40	23.0	—	68.0	14.0	58.48	—	Skinfolds	Hagerman et al. (1979)[b]
Cross-country skiers	10	20.2	1.63	55.9	15.7	47.12	29	Skinfolds	Haymes & Dickinson (1980)[b]
Cycling	7	—	1.68	61.3	15.4	51.86	31	UWW	Burke (1980)[b]
Triathlon	6	31.3	1.68	56.4	14.8	48.05	29	UWW	O'Toole et al. (1987)[a]
	3	—	—	—	12.6	—	—	UWW	Holly et al. (1986)[a]
Weighted average		—	—	—	14.1	—			
Soccer	10	24.7	1.69	62.2	22.3	48.33	29	Skinfolds	Jenson & Larson (1993)[b]
	14	25.4	1.66	59.6	21.1	47.02	28	Skinfolds	Davis (1995)[b]
	12	20.3	1.65	59.5	19.7	47.78	29	Skinfolds	Rico-Sanz (1998)[c]
Weighted average		23.5	1.66	60.3	21.0	47.64			

%BF, percentage fat; FFM/HT, fat-free mass (kg) divided by height (m).
a, world class/Olympic; b, national; c, collegiate; d, élite; e, trained.

Table 24.2 Body composition of élite male endurance athletes.

Sport	n	Age (years)	Height (m)	Body mass (kg)	%BF	FFM (kg)	FFM/HT	Technique	Reference
Distance running	114	26.1	1.76	64.2	7.5	59.39	34	Skinfolds	Costill *et al.* (1970)[b]
	41	26.2	1.77	66.2	8.4	60.64	34	Skinfolds	Rusko *et al.* (1978)[d]
	99	27.3	1.74	62.4	1.4	61.53	35	Bone diameter	Hirata (1966)[a]
	34	25.3	1.72	59.8	−0.5	60.10	35	Bone diameter	De Garay *et al.* (1974)[a]
	10	—	1.76	63.1	5.0	59.95	34	UWW	Pollock (1977)[d]
	8	—	1.77	62.1	4.3	59.43	34	UWW	Pollock (1977)[d]
	4	27.8	1.81	69.0	9.4	62.51	34	UWW	Cureton *et al.* (1978)[e]
Weighted average		—	1.75	63.4	4.7	60.37			
Swimming	450	20.4	1.79	74.1	12.1	65.13	36	Bone diameter	Hirata (1966)[a]
	66	19.2	1.80	72.1	9.0	65.61	37	Bone diameter	De Garay *et al.* (1974)[a]
	13	21.8	1.82	79.1	8.5	72.38	40	UWW	Sprynarova & Parizcova (1969)[d]
Weighted average		20.3	1.79	74.0	11.6	65.37			
Rowing	357	25.0	1.86	82.2	14.1	70.61	38	Bone diameter	Hirata (1966)[a]
	85	24.3	1.85	82.6	15.4	69.88	38	Bone diameter	De Garay *et al.* (1974)[a]
	503	23.0	—	88.0	11.0	78.32	—	Skinfolds	Hagerman *et al.* (1979)[b]
	120	21.0	—	71.0	8.5	64.97	—	Skinfolds	Hagerman *et al.* (1979)[b]
Weighted average		23.5	—	83.7	12.1	73.56			
Cross-country skiers	10	22.7	1.76	73.2	7.9	67.42	38	Skinfolds	Haymes & Dickinson (1980)[b]
Cycling	12	—	1.80	67.1	8.8	61.20	34	UWW	Burke (1980)[b]
	8	—	1.80	70.8	8.4	64.85	36	UWW	Burke (1980)[b]
Weighted average		—	1.80	68.6	8.6	62.66			
Triathlon	8	30.5	1.79	74.7	9.9	67.30	38	UWW	O'Toole *et al.* (1987)[a]
	4	—	—	—	7.1	—	—	UWW	Holly *et al.* (1986)[a]
Weighted average		—	—	—	9.0	—			
Canoeing	13	20.1	1.80	76.3	10.4	68.36	38	UWW	Vaccaro *et al.* (1984)[a]
	8	23.7	1.82	79.6	12.4	69.73	38	Skinfolds	Rusko *et al.* (1978)[d]
Weighted average		21.5	1.81	77.6	11.2	68.88			
Soccer	12	20.6	1.79	72.5	9.1	65.90	37	Skinfolds	Kirkendahl (1985)[b]
	12	23.5	1.79	75.8	10.8	67.61	38	Skinfolds	Kirkendahl (1985)[b]
	12	22.5	1.79	76.2	9.9	68.66	38	Skinfolds	Kirkendahl (1985)[b]
	99	25.4	1.78	74.5	9.2	67.65	38	Skinfolds	Thkmakidis (1991)[d]
	78	26.8	1.80	76.6	11.8	67.56	38	Skinfolds	Vos (1980)
Weighted average		25.4	1.79	75.3	10.3	67.57			

%BF, percentage fat; FFM/HT, fat-free mass (kg) divided by height (m).
a, world class/Olympic; b, national; c, collegiate; d, élite; e, trained.

endurance sports. As in the general population, male endurance athletes have a lower %BF and a higher FFM than their female counterparts. Both male and female endurance athletes have lower %BF levels than the average young, healthy adult, for whom %BF ranges from approximately 15% to 22% in males and 22% to 28% in females (Lohman 1992). Male endurance runners, averaging 4.7%, have the lowest %BF, followed by cyclists (8.6%), triathletes (9.0%) and soccer players (10.3%) (Table 24.2). Of the female endurance athletes, rowers have the lowest %BF at 14.0%, followed by triathletes

(14.1%), cyclists (15.4%) and cross-country skiers (15.7%) (Table 24.1). As noted above, excess fatness is detrimental to these types of activities, because it adds mass to the body without contributing to force production, and it increases the metabolic cost of physical activity.

The ratio of male to female %BF in the general population is about 0.63. A comparison of male and female athletes participating in the same sport shows considerable variation in this ratio by sport. The male to female %BF ratio is considerably lower than the general population in runners (0.29), followed by soccer players (0.49), cross-country skiers (0.50), cyclists (0.56), swimmers (0.62) and triathletes (0.64). In rowers (0.86) the ratio is considerably higher than in the general population, showing that %BF values of male and female rowers are more similar than in other groups. Male rowers have higher %BF compared to other groups whereas female rowers have the lowest %BF of the female endurance athletes.

The ranges of %BF observed in female and male athletes participating in various endurance sports, along with ranges for other non-endurance athletes, are illustrated in Figs 24.1 and 24.2. As would be expected, endurance athletes who would benefit the most from a low body mass have the lowest %BF (Hirata 1966; De Garay et al. 1974; Fleck 1983; Thor-

land et al. 1983; Clarkson et al. 1985; Berg et al. 1990; Houtkooper et al. 1992; Wilmore 1992; Houtkooper & Going 1994). Nevertheless, there is considerable overlap, and most groups of athletes have a relatively low %BF and a high fraction of FFM. Long-distance swimmers represent one group of endurance athletes who may benefit from a relatively high fat mass, because of the contributions of fat to thermal insulation and buoyancy (Sinning 1985); however, they are lean relative to the general population, values averaging 21% in women (Table 24.1) and 11% in men (Table 24.2). In some studies, extremely low (<3% BF) or negative %BF values have been reported (Hirata 1966; De Garay et al. 1974). These non-physiological levels illustrate the errors that can occur when methods and models are applied in groups for whom the underlying assumptions are not valid.

There is relatively little information on the body composition of sports participants who are less than 18 years of age. Employing two-component hydrodensitometric models, Malina and Bouchard (1991) and Fleck (1983) compared %BF estimates for young sports competitors and non-competitors. The young sports participants as a group had lower %BF levels than non-participants of the same age and gender. Those studied included age-group swimmers, runners, gymnasts, tackle football players and

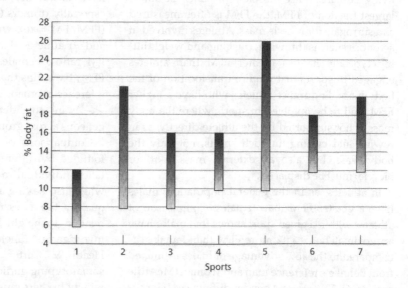

Fig. 24.1 Reported ranges of percentage body fat levels measured in élite female athletes in various sports. Key: 1, body-building; 2, cycling, heptathlon, pentathlon, triathlon, track/field: running events; 3, ballet, gymnastics, orienteering, rowing, skating; 4, basketball, canoeing, kayaking, fencing, horse racing; 5, racquetball, skiing, soccer, swimming, synchronized swimming, tennis, volleyball, weightlifting; 6, baseball, softball, ice hockey, field hockey; 7, golf, track/field: field events. Adapted from Houtkooper and Going (1994).

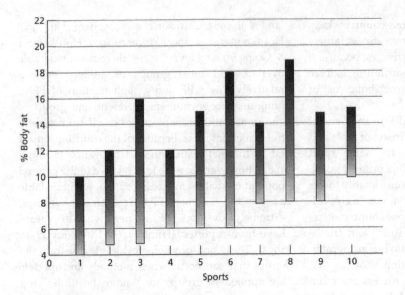

Fig. 24.2 Reported ranges of percentage body fat levels measured in élite male athletes in various sports. Key: 1, bodybuilding, marathon running, track/field: running events; 2, cross-country skiing, cycling, gymnastics, orienteering, skating, triathlon, weightlifting; 3, wrestling; 4, basketball, canoeing, kayaking, horse racing, swimming; 5, racquetball, rowing, soccer, tennis; 6, rugby football; 7, baseball, softball, fencing; 8, ice hockey, field hockey, track/field: field events; 9, skiing, ski-jumping, volleyball; 10, golf. Adapted from Houtkooper and Going (1994).

wrestlers. The range of %BF values for girls was 13–23% and for boys it was 4–15%. These values should be interpreted with due consideration for the prediction error inherent in estimates of body composition.

Fat-free mass of endurance athletes

Accurate assessment of muscle mass is difficult in living humans. Since muscle represents the single largest fraction of FFM, the FFM is often measured as a surrogate for muscle mass. Athletes involved in activities such as throwing, pushing and weightlifting typically have a greater FFM than athletes engaged in sports that require translocation of the body mass. Endurance athletes who have a higher FFM tend to be involved in sports where the body mass is not supported by the athlete directly, as in rowing and cycling; in such sports, not only the body mass, but also an external mass (skiff or bicycle) must be displaced.

In athletes, as in the general population, males have a greater FFM than females. Comparison of athletes within a given sport shows that males have approximately 21–43% more FFM than females, as compared to the 40% advantage of males estimated from Behnke's reference man and woman (McArdle *et al.* 1996). The greatest gender differences (favour-

ing males) were observed for cross-country skiers (43%), soccer players (42%), triathletes (40%) and runners (36%), with smaller differences observed between male and female cyclists (21%), rowers (26%) and swimmers (27%). Based on the reference man and woman, males have approximately 5–6 times more FFM than fat whereas in women the ratio is about 2.5–3.0. Although there is considerable variation across studies, male endurance athletes have considerably higher ratios than reference man, especially runners (FFM/FM = 10–20) and cyclists (FFM/FM = 10), with swimmers (~8), rowers (~7) and triathletes having somewhat lower FFM/FM ratios. Female endurance athletes also have FFM/FM ratios that are somewhat higher than the reference woman, although values (ranging from ~3–6) are considerably lower and more homogeneous across groups than in males.

Comparisons of FFM among athletes are confounded by differences in average height, since a taller individual may have a higher absolute FFM while also having a lower mass for height. Consequently, the assessment of musculoskeletal size in relation to height has been proposed by several investigators (Sheldon *et al.* 1954; Parnell 1958; Heath & Carter 1967). While evidence from somatotyping indicates that athletic groups vary widely in their musculoskeletal size, the method is

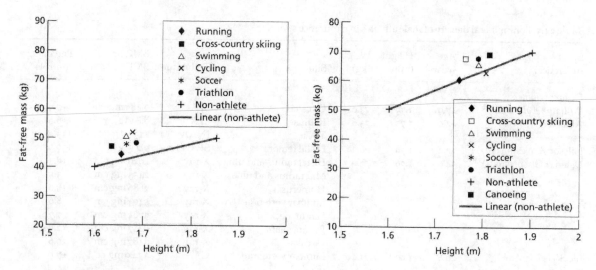

Fig. 24.3 Deviation from regression of fat-free mass on height measured in élite female athletes from various sports; running, cross-country skiing, swimming, cycling, soccer, triathlon. Regression line for non-athletic women calculated from equation: $y = FFM = 51.4(Ht) - 41.8$. Adapted from Slaughter and Lohman (1979).

Fig. 24.4 Deviation from regression of fat-free mass on height measured in élite male athletes from various sports; running, cross-country skiing, canoeing, cycling, soccer, triathlon, swimming. Regression line for non-athletic men calculated from equation: $y = FFM = 71.9(Ht) - 63.9$. Adapted from Slaughter and Lohman (1979).

very indirect. A more direct estimate of musculoskeletal size can be obtained from FFM as measured by densitometry or some other technique, and expressed relative to standing height (Slaughter & Lohman 1979). Using the ratio FFM/height, one can compare athletes of different statures and ascertain the importance of FFM relative to height for a particular sport.

The FFM/height ratios for female and male endurance athletes relative to the general population are shown in Figs 24.3 and 24.4. Typically, endurance athletes of both sexes have more FFM per unit height than their non-athletic counterparts. Male ($34-35\,kg\cdot m^{-2}$) and female ($25-29\,kg\cdot m^{-2}$) runners have the lowest FFM/height ratios among endurance athletes because in running a low %BF and a low FFM/height ratio are advantageous. Male rowers ($38\,kg\cdot m^{-2}$) and female cyclists ($31\,kg\cdot m^{-2}$) who must generate higher forces than distance runners have the highest FFM/height ratios.

Bone mineral mass and density

With the development of techniques such as computed tomography, photon absorptiometry and

DXA, it is now possible to measure bone mineral mass and density accurately. Although a number of studies of athletes have been reported, systematic characterization of the skeletal status of athletes has yet to be undertaken. By necessity, most studies have examined convenience samples of a limited number of athletes. Few studies have compared athletic groups using the same technology and protocol.

The bone mineral content (BMC) and BMD for male and female endurance athletes are shown in Tables 24.3 and 24.4. With the possible exception of swimmers, endurance athletes, like other athletes, have BMDs that are usually greater than age-matched, non-athletic controls. A wide range of BMDs is evident. Differences across studies are due in part to sampling differences in both athletic and non-athletic groups. Other factors potentially contributing to differences among studies include variation in training history, and nutritional, hormonal and pharmacological factors. Unfortunately these factors are often not reported and not controlled.

Whether endurance athletes have more or less bone mass or density than controls depends in large part on the athletic group and the skeletal site that is

Table 24.3 Bone mineral density of male athletes in endurance sports.

Sport (reference)	Age (years)	Height (m)	Weight (kg)	Site	Technique	BMC or BMD	Percentage controls
Distance runners							
Williams et al. (1984)[a,b]	47.9	1.79	73.0	Os calcis	SPA	$0.485\,mg\cdot cm^{-3}$	+0.5
Aloia et al. (1978)[a,b]	42.0	1.75	73.6	Radius	SPA	$0.840\,g\cdot cm^{-2}$	+6.3
				TBCa	INAA	1175.0 g	+15.2
Nilsson & Westlin (1971)[d]	22.2	1.79	66.2	Distal femora	SPA	$0.235\,g\cdot cc^{-1}$	+39.9
Dalen & Olsson (1974)[a,b]	54.6	1.76	73.0	Distal radius and ulna	X-ray	$2029\,mg\cdot cm^{-1}$	18.5
				Mid radius and ulna	X-ray	$2455\,mg\cdot cm^{-1}$	5.5
				Humerus	X ray	$2886\,mg\cdot cm^{-1}$	19.0
				Lumbar vertebrae (L3)	X-ray	$5404\,mg\cdot cm^{-1}$	8.6
				Femur, neck	X-ray	$3764\,mg\cdot cm^{-1}$	7.7
				Femur, shaft	X-ray	$6457\,mg\cdot cm^{-1}$	12.5
				Os calcis	X-ray	$3487\,mg\cdot cm^{-1}$	20.6
Block et al. (1986)[b]	26.8	1.80	71.2	Lumbar vertebrae (L1–L2)	CT	$172.9\,mg\cdot cc^{-1}$	+7.0
Bennell et al. (1997)[b,d]	20.7	1.79	67.2	Whole body	DXA	2.534 g	−0.2
				Upper limb	DXA	$0.881\,g\cdot cm^{-2}$	−0.3
				Lumbar spine	DXA	$1.095\,g\cdot cm^{-2}$	+4.2
				Femur	DXA	$1.333\,g\cdot cm^{-2}$	+7.2
				Tibia and fibula	DXA	$1.205\,g\cdot cm^{-2}$	+8.6
				Foot	DXA	$1.206\,g\cdot cm^{-2}$	+16.2
Swimmers							
Nilsson & Westlin (1971)[d]	17.9	1.83	75.4	Distal femora	SPA	$0.226\,g\cdot cc^{-1}$	+34.5
Orwoll et al. (1989)[b]	60	1.79	79	Proximal radius	SPA	$0.84\,g\cdot cm^{-2}$	+3.7
				Vertebrae (T12–L1)	CT	$123\,mg\cdot cm^{-3}$	13.9

Abbreviations: SPA, single photon absorptiometry; INAA, *in vivo* neutron activation analysis; X-ray, X-ray densitometry; CT, computed tomography; DXA, dual-energy X-ray absorptiometry.
a, master's level; b, club sports, regional and national competitions; c, college varsity; d, élite national and international competitions.

assessed. Exercise has a local rather than a systemic effect on bone. Thus, endurance athletes may have a similar whole-body bone mineral mass and density to controls while having significant regional differences that vary according to the stimuli placed on the bone. In runners and athletes in other weight-bearing sports, the BMD is often high relative to controls at distal appendicular sites (tibia, fibula, distal femur) but not at axial sites, since the impact forces from ground contact are attenuated as they are transmitted through the skeleton. In athletes in non-weight-bearing sports (e.g. swimmers, cyclists and rowers) BMD is often similar to controls and less than competitors in weight-bearing sports, although at some muscle attachment sites where large forces are consistently exerted BMD may

be higher than in controls. Differences among athletic groups may also be due to differences in body size and composition which are often not adequately controlled; body mass, body fat and FFM are significant correlates of bone mineral mass and density (Reid et al. 1992a,b).

The optimal stimulus for increasing BMC and BMD in humans is not known. Animal studies suggest that strains that are high in rate and magnitude, and of abnormal distribution, but not necessarily long in duration, are best for inducing new bone formation (O'Connor & Lanyon 1982; Lanyon & Rubin 1984; Rubin & Lanyon 1984, 1985). In humans, repetitive activities that induce strains below the minimum effective strain for bone remodelling would not stimulate bone formation as effec-

Table 24.4 Bone mineral density of female athletes in endurance sports.

Sport (reference)	Age (years)	Height (m)	Body mass (kg)	Site	Technique	BMC or BMD	Percentage controls
Distance runners							
Brewer et al. (1983)[a,b]	37.7	1.66	54.5	Radius	SPA	0.905 g·cm^{-1}	+4.7
				Finger	X-ray	0.245 mmAlmm·bone^{-1}	−12.4
				Os calcis	X-ray	0.236 mmAlmm·bone^{-1}	−6.4
Taaffe et al. (1997)[c,d]	19.5	1.68	54.9	Lumbar spine	DXA	0.991 g·cm^{-2}	−11.0
				Femur, neck	DXA	0.917 g·cm^{-2}	−5.6
				Whole body	DXA	1.060 g·cm^{-2}	−3.3
Snead et al. (1992)	30.8	1.65	58.7	Lumbar spine	DPA	1.145 g·cm^{-2}	+0.4
				Femur, neck	DPA	0.974 g·cm^{-2}	0.0
Bennell et al. (1997)[b,c]	20.8	1.65	58.0	Whole body	DXA	2.082 g	+2.5
				Upper limb	DXA	0.775 g·cm^{-2}	+1.2
				Lumbar spine	DXA	1.036 g·cm^{-2}	+1.6
				Femur	DXA	1.190 g·cm^{-2}	+6.0
				Tibia and fibula	DXA	1.094 g·cm^{-2}	+7.9
				Foot	DXA	1.011 g·cm^{-2}	+13.6
Wolman et al. (1991)[d]	26	1.64	50.9	Femur, shaft	DPA	1.51 g·cm^{-2}	+7.8
Swimmers							
Jacobsen et al. (1984)	18–22			Distal radius	SPA	0.436 g·cm^{-2}	+2.6
				Midradius	SPA	0.713 g·cm^{-2}	+0.4
				Metatarsal	SPA	0.565 g·cm^{-2}	+10.4
				Lumbar vertebrae	DPA	1.319 g·cm^{-2}	−2.7
Taaffe et al. (1997)[c,d]	19.0	1.74	66.5	Lumbar spine	DXA	1.111 g·cm^{-2}	+1.6
				Femur, neck	DXA	0.882 g·cm^{-2}	+1.3
				Whole body	DXA	1.069 g·cm^{-2}	−0.1
Dook et al. (1997)[a,b]	46.00	1.66	65.7	Whole body	DXA	1.06 g·cm^{-2}	+3.9
				Arm	DXA	0.71 g·cm^{-2}	+6.0
				Leg	DXA	1.11 g·cm^{-2}	+5.7
Lee et al. (1995)[c]	18.98	1.69	61.8	Whole body	DXA	1.13 g·cm^{-2}	−1.8
				Lumbar spine	DXA	1.20 g·cm^{-2}	+2.6
				Femur, neck	DXA	0.99 g·cm^{-2}	−5.3
				Pelvis	DXA	1.10 g·cm^{-2}	−3.5
				Right arm	DXA	0.96 g·cm^{-2}	+2.1
				Right leg	DXA	1.20 g·cm^{-2}	−2.4
Orwoll et al. (1989)[b]	55	1.66	64	Proximal radius	SPA	0.67 g·cm^{-2}	+1.5
				Vertebrae (T12–L1)	CT	129 mg·cm^{-3}	+1.6
Orienteers							
Heinonen et al. (1993)[b]	23.3	1.69	59.3	Lumbar spine	DXA	1.068 g·cm^{-2}	−0.3
				Femur, neck	DXA	1.000 g·cm^{-2}	+1.7
				Distal femur	DXA	1.320 g·cm^{-2}	+4.7
				Patella	DXA	1.091 g·cm^{-2}	+3.2
				Tibia	DXA	1.151 g·cm^{-2}	+4.2
				Calcaneus	DXA	0.699 g·cm^{-2}	+4.1
				Distal radius	DXA	0.352 g·cm^{-2}	+0.6

(Continued)

Table 24.4 (*Continued*)

Sport (reference)	Age (years)	Height (m)	Body mass (kg)	Site	Technique	BMC or BMD	Percentage controls
Cross-country skiers							
Heinonen *et al.* (1993)[b]	21.3	1.69	61.6	Lumbar spine	DXA	$1.072\,\mathrm{g \cdot cm^{-2}}$	0.0
				Femur, neck	DXA	$1.035\,\mathrm{g \cdot cm^{-2}}$	+5.3
				Distal femur	DXA	$1.321\,\mathrm{g \cdot cm^{-2}}$	+4.8
				Patella	DXA	$1.080\,\mathrm{g \cdot cm^{-2}}$	+2.2
				Tibia	DXA	$1.139\,\mathrm{g \cdot cm^{-2}}$	+3.2
				Calcaneus	DXA	$0.694\,\mathrm{g \cdot cm^{-2}}$	+3.4
				Distal radius	DXA	$0.348\,\mathrm{g \cdot cm^{-2}}$	−0.6
Cyclists							
Heinonen *et al.* (1993)[b]	24.0	1.66	61.8	Lumbar spine	DXA	$1.067\,\mathrm{g \cdot cm^{-2}}$	−0.4
				Femur, neck	DXA	$1.288\,\mathrm{g \cdot cm^{-2}}$	−2.1
				Distal femur	DXA	$1.288\,\mathrm{g \cdot cm^{-2}}$	+2.1
				Patella	DXA	$1.068\,\mathrm{g \cdot cm^{-2}}$	+1.0
				Tibia	DXA	$1.094\,\mathrm{g \cdot cm^{-2}}$	−0.9
				Calcaneus	DXA	$0.654\,\mathrm{g \cdot cm^{-2}}$	−2.6
				Distal radius	DXA	$0.368\,\mathrm{g \cdot cm^{-2}}$	+5.1

Abbreviations: SPA, single photon absorptiometry; X-ray, X-ray densitometry; CT, computed tomography; DXA, dual-energy X-ray absorptiometry.
a, master's level; b, club sports, regional and national competitions; c, college varsity; d, élite national and international competitions.

tively as activities that require lifting heavy loads or enduring high-impact loads (Frost 1997). The results of studies comparing BMD at different sites among athletic groups support this notion both in men (Fig. 24.5) and in women (Fig. 24.6). Strength-trained athletes and athletes who sustain high-impact loads in training and competition (gymnasts, skaters, basketball and volleyball players) typically have greater BMC and BMD than endurance athletes (Nichols *et al.* 1994); this difference is seen in older as well as younger adults. Among endurance athletes, runners typically have a higher BMD than swimmers; cyclists and rowers seem to have intermediate values, although this conclusion may depend on the bone site that is assessed (Kirk *et al.* 1989; Risser *et al.* 1990; Wolman 1990; Fehling *et al.* 1995; Heinonen *et al.* 1995).

Although studies of athletic groups favour strength and power over endurance training for improving BMD, cross-sectional studies must be interpreted cautiously. The weightlifters used in most studies have come from highly selected groups and therefore are not very suitable for comparison against normal populations. Moreover, anabolic steroid use could be a confounding variable; this may increase bone mass, and not all investigators have screened for steroid use. Body mass is another confounding variable, although differences persist in studies which have adjusted for body mass (Heinonen *et al.* 1993).

Although it is tempting to attribute differences in BMD between athletes and controls to specialized training, the effect of self-selection must not be minimized. The heritability of bone density may be as high as 70–80% (Pocock *et al.* 1987; Bouchard *et al.* 1997). Moreover, the BMD differences reported between athletes and controls are often much greater than the gains achieved in most successful longitudinal training studies (Drinkwater 1994a,b; Chilibeck *et al.* 1995), where increases in bone mass average about 1–2% per year. One might presume that at this rate of change, large differences could develop over years of training, but there are no prospective, long-term studies to support this

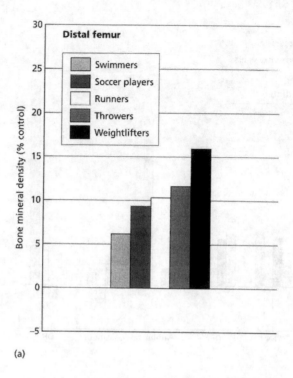

(a)

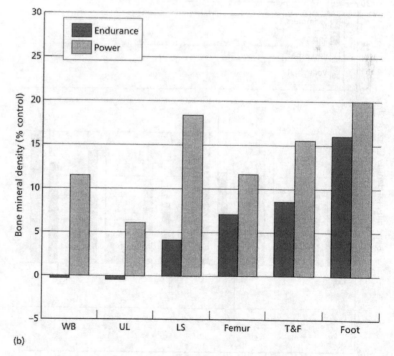

(b)

Fig. 24.5 Bone mineral density (BMD) in male athletes as a percentage of sedentary control values. Data in (a) from Nilsson and Westlin (1971) and in (b) from Bennell *et al.* (1997). LS, lumbar spine; T & F, tibia and fibula; UL, upper limb; WB, whole body.

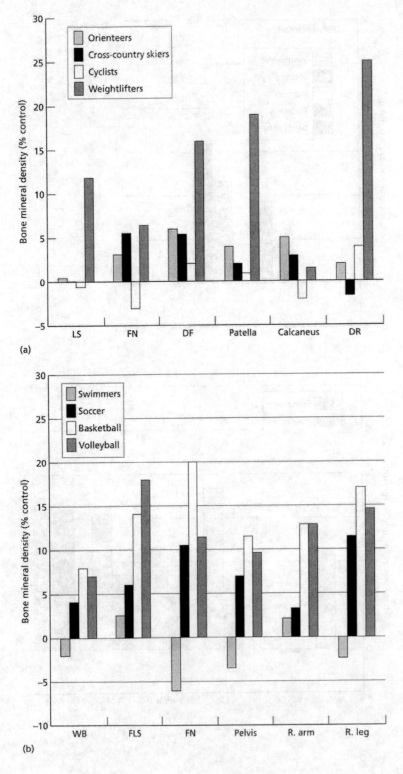

(a)

(b)

Fig. 24.6 Bone mineral density (BMD) in female athletes as a percentage of sedentary control values. Data in (a) from Heinonen *et al.* (1993), in (b) from Lee *et al.* (1995) and in (c) from Heinrich *et al.* (1990). DF, distal femur; DR, distal radius; FN, femur neck; LS, lumbar spine; MR, midradius.

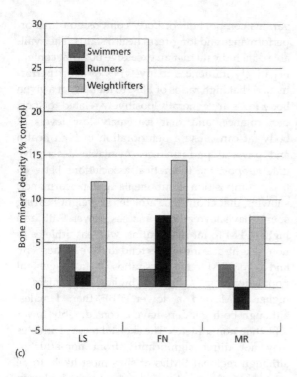

Fig. 24.6 (*Continued*)

point of view. Nevertheless, over a competitive season, gymnasts (Taaffe *et al.* 1997) and other power athletes (Bennell *et al.* 1997) have shown significant increases in BMD relative to controls. Thus, training regimens contribute to differences between athletes and non-athletes, although much less so than is suggested by cross-sectional comparisons. The greater bone width and BMD in the dominant arm versus the non-dominant arm in tennis players also supports a significant response to training (Jones *et al.* 1977; Huddleston *et al.* 1980; Montoye *et al.* 1980; Haapasalo *et al.* 1996).

No study has attempted to define the exercise dose–bone response relationship, but there may be a range of exercise intensities that stimulate bone formation, with higher intensities having a negative effect on bone density. Male runners (20–45 years of age), for example, who ran 24–32 km per week had a significantly greater lower leg BMD than those running 8–16 km per week (MacDougall *et al.* 1992), but BMD tended to decrease in runners with a training mileage greater than 32 km per week. In another

study, lumbar BMD was significantly lower in young male runners with a training mileage averaging 92 km per week than in non-runners (Bilanin *et al.* 1989). It was hypothesized that the high weekly mileage may have resulted in lowered testosterone and increased cortisol levels, with a catabolic effect on bone. Thus, moderate training loads may affect bone density positively, whereas extreme amounts of training have detrimental effects, with altered hormonal responses overriding the load-induced stimulus to bone formation.

A hormonal mechanism may also be responsible for reduced BMD in female endurance athletes who engage in a high volume of training to the point that oestradiol and prolactin levels fall.

Oligomenorrhoeic and amenorrhoeic athletes have a lower BMD than their eumenorrhoeic teammates (Drinkwater *et al.* 1984; Linnell *et al.* 1984; Marcus *et al.* 1985). First observed in the spine (Drinkwater *et al.* 1984; Marcus *et al.* 1985), a significantly lower BMD has now been demonstrated at multiple skeletal sites (Myburgh *et al.* 1993; Rencken *et al.* 1996). Grimston *et al.* (1993) showed that female runners with a low BMD had an altered calciotrophic hormone response to a calcium load administered before a treadmill run, such that the parathyroid hormone response (which increases bone resorption) was increased, and the calcitonin response (which inhibits bone resorption) was decreased. These responses are opposite to the changes observed in non-runners and runners with normal BMD. Although women who resume a normal menstrual cycle regain some bone (Drinkwater *et al.* 1986; Lindberg *et al.* 1986), women with a history of menstrual irregularities have a lower vertebral density than women who have always had regular periods (Drinkwater *et al.* 1990; Cann *et al.* 1998). Not only does the higher incidence of stress fractures reported for oligomenorrhoeic and amenorrhoeic athletes place their future as athletes at risk, but if the bone loss proves irreversible, they may be at risk of premature osteoporosis.

Problems of extreme leanness

Although available data must be interpreted with the limitations of indirect methods in mind, it appears that many endurance athletes have a low body mass and levels of %BF that are at or near the minimal levels (5%BF for males and 12%BF for females) compatible with good health (Lohman 1992). Further attempts to lose weight and lower %BF may place the athlete at risk of substrate depletion, chronic fatigue, a deterioration in performance and increased susceptibility to both minor and major illnesses and injuries (Sinning & Wilson 1984; Wilmore 1992). The critical level of weight loss is poorly defined, and it is probably reached only rarely in sport. Nevertheless, weight-loss goals must be realistic, carefully monitored and based on ranges associated with high-level performance, rather than an absolute goal. Athletes who habitually strive to reach or maintain a body mass or %BF goal that is inappropriate are at risk of developing an eating disorder. Although the exact prevalence is difficult to estimate, it has been suggested that the prevalence of eating disorders in female athletes at the élite or world-class level may be as high as 50% in some endurance sports such as middle- and long-distance running (Chapter 36; Wilmore & Bergfeld 1978; Wilmore 1992). Such competitors are at high risk of developing a triad of interrelated disorders that include anorexia nervosa or bulimia nervosa, menstrual dysfunction and bone demineralization (Wilmore 1992; Arena *et al.* 1995). The long-term consequences of the triad are not well established.

Conclusions

A considerable amount of research has focused on the development of methods and models to measure body composition more accurately and reliably, but newer methods have not been applied systematically to the description of the body composition of athletes. Moreover, few experimental data are available to describe the relationships of the various components of body composition to sport performance and long-term health status. The available data indicate that an excessive body fat content negatively influences many types of sport performance, that high ratios of FFM to fat mass at a given body mass are generally positively related to sport performance, and that extremely low levels of body fat can cause a deterioration in both health and physical performance. Available descriptive data support the theoretical associations between body composition components and performance, showing that endurance athletes in weight-bearing sports have lower body masses, lower %BF and higher FFM to fat mass ratios, whereas athletes in non-weight-bearing sports tend to have higher %BF and lower FFM to fat mass ratios. As in the general population, males have a higher body mass, a higher FFM and a lower %BF than females, although both genders have a considerably lower %BF than non-athletes. The skeletal mass of athletes may not differ significantly from non-athletes, although regional BMDs at sites most likely to be stressed by the sport regimen tend to be higher in athletes.

Given the limitations of available methods for assessment of body composition and the influence of factors other than body composition on athletic success, it is not reasonable to define optima of %BF and FFM for participants in different sports. However, it is feasible to define ranges of %BF or FFM associated with top performance in a given sport and these ranges can be used to establish training goals for body mass and body composition that are compatible with good performance and health.

Considering the strong positive relationship between performance and a high ratio of FFM to fat mass at a given body mass, more emphasis should be placed on defining optimal ranges for these relationships in endurance athletes.

References

Aloia, J.F., Cohn, S.H., Babu, T., Abesamis, C., Kalici, N. & Ellis, K. (1978) Skeletal mass and body composition in marathon runners. *Metabolism* 27, 1793–1796.

Arena, B., Maffulli, N., Maffulli, F. &

Morleo, M.A. (1995) Reproductive hormones and menstrual changes with exercise in female athletes. *Sports Medicine* 19 (4), 278–287.

Bartlett, H.L., Mance, M.J. & Buskirk, E.R.

(1984) Body composition and expiratory reserve volume in female gymnasts and runners. *Medicine and Science in Sports and Exercise* 16 (3), 311–315.

Behnke, A.R. & Wilmore, J.H. (1974) *Evalu-*

ation and Regulation of Body Build and Composition. Prentice Hall, Englewood Cliffs, NJ.

Bennell, K.L., Malcolm, S.A., Khan, K.M. et al. (1997) Bone mass and bone turnover in power athletes, endurance athletes, and controls, a 12-month longitudinal study. Bone 20 (5), 477–484.

Berg, K., Latin, R.W. & Baechle, T. (1990) Physical and performance characteristics of NCAA Division I football players. Research Quarterly for Exercise and Sport 61 (4), 395–401.

Bilanin, J.E., Blanchard, M. & Russek-Cohen, E. (1989) Lower vertebral bone density in male long distance runners. Medicine and Science in Sports and Exercise 21, 66–70.

Block, J.E., Genant, H.K. & Black, D. (1986) Greater vertebral bone mineral mass in exercising young men. Western Journal of Medicine 145, 39–42.

Boileau, R.A. & Lohman, T.G. (1977) The measurement of human physique and its effect on physical performance. Orthopedic Clinics of North America 8, 563–581.

Bouchard, C., Malina, R.M. & Perusse, L. (1997) Genetics of Fitness and Physical Performance. Human Kinetics, Champaign, IL.

Brewer, V., Meyer, B.M., Keele, M.S., Upton, S.J. & Hagan, R.D. (1983) Role of exercise in prevention of involutional bone loss. Medicine and Science in Sports and Medicine 15 (6), 445–449.

Brozek, J., Grande, F., Anderson, J.T. & Keys, A. (1963) Densitometric analysis of body composition. Revision of some quantitative assumptions. Annals of the New York Academy of Sciences 110, 113–140.

Bunt, J.C., Going, S.B., Lohman, T.G., Heinrich, C.H., Perry, C.D. & Pamenter, R.W. (1990) Variation in bone mineral content and estimated body fat in young adult females. Medicine and Science in Sports and Exercise 22, 564–569.

Burke, E.R. (1980) Physiological characteristics of competitive cyclists. Physician and Sportsmedicine 8 (7), 78–84.

Buskirk, E. & Taylor, H.L. (1957) Maximal oxygen intake and its relation to body composition with special reference to chronic physical activity and obesity. Journal of Applied Physiology 11, 72–78.

Cann, C.E., Cavanaugh, D.J., Schnurpfiel, K. & Martin, M.C. (1998) Menstrual history is the primary determinant of trabecular bone density in women. Medicine and Science in Sports and Exercise 20, S59.

Chilibeck, P.D., Sale, D.G. & Webber, C.E.

(1995) Exercise and bone mineral density. Sports Medicine 19 (2), 103–122.

Clarkson, P.M., Freedson, P.S., Keller, B., Carney, D. & Skrinar, M. (1985) Maximal oxygen uptake, nutritional patterns and body composition of adolescent female ballet dancers. Research Quarterly for Exercise and Sport 56, 180–184.

Costill, D.L., Bowers, R. & Kramer, W.F. (1970) Skinfold estimates of body fat among marathon runners. Medicine and Science in Sports and Exercise 2, 93–95.

Cureton, K.J. (1992) Effects of experimental alterations in excess weight on physiological responses to exercise and physical performance. In: Marriott, B.M. & Grumstrup-Scott, J. (eds) Body Composition and Physical Performance: Applications for the Military Services, pp. 71–88. National Academy Press, Washington, DC.

Cureton, K.J. & Sparling, P.B. (1980) Distance running performance and metabolic responses to running in men and women with excess weight experimentally equated. Medicine and Science in Sports and Exercise 12, 288–294.

Cureton, K.J., Sparling, P.B., Evans, B.W., Johnson, S.M., Kong, U.D. & Purvis, J.W. (1978a) Effect of experimental alterations in excess weight on aerobic capacity and distance running performance. Medicine and Science in Sports and Exercise 15, 218–223.

Cureton, K.J., Sparling, P.B., Evans, B.W., Johnson, S.M., Kong, U.D. & Purvis, J.W. (1978b) Effects of experimental alterations in excess weight on aerobic capacity and distance running. Medicine and Science in Sports and Exercise 10, 194–198.

Dalen, N. & Olsson, K.C. (1974) Bone mineral content and physical activity. Acta Orthopedica Scandinavica 45, 170–174.

Davis, J.M. (1995) Carbohydrates, branched-chain amino acids, and endurance: the central fatigue hypothesis. International Journal of Sport Nutrition 5, S29–S38.

De Garay, et al. (1974) Genetic and Anthropometrical Studies of Olympic Athletes. Academic Press, New York.

Dook, J.A., James, C., Henderson, N.K. & Price, R.I. (1997) Exercise and bone mineral density in mature female athletes. Medicine and Science in Sports and Exercise 29, 291–296.

Drinkwater, B.L. (1994a) Physical activity, fitness, and osteoporosis. In: Bouchard, C., Shephard, R.J. & Stephens, T. (eds) Physical Activity, Fitness, and Health, pp. 724–736.

Drinkwater, B.L. (1994b) C. H. McCloy Research Lecture: Does physical activity play a role in preventing osteoporosis. Research Quarterly for Exercise and Sport 65, 197–206.

Drinkwater, B.L., Nilson, K., Chesnut, C.H. III, Bremner, W.J., Shainholtz, S. & Southworth, M.B. (1984) Bone mineral content of amenorrheic and eumenorrheic athletes. New England Journal of Medicine 311, 277–281.

Drinkwater, B.L., Nilson, K., Ott, S. & Chestnut, C.H. III (1986) Bone mineral density after resumption of menses in amenorrheic women. Journal of the American Medical Association 256, 380–382.

Drinkwater, B.L., Bruenmer, B. & Chesnut, C.H. III (1990) Menstrual history as a determinant of current bone density in young athletes. Journal of the American Medical Association 263, 545–548.

Fehling, P.C., Alekel, L., Clasey, J., Rector, A. & Stillman, R.J. (1995) A comparison of bone mineral densities among female athletes in impact loading and active loading sports. Bone 17, 205–210.

Fidanza, F.A., Keys, A. & Anderson, J.T. (1953) Density of body fat in man and other animals. Journal of Applied Physiology 6, 252–256.

Fleck, S.J. (1983) Body composition of elite American athletes. American Journal of Sports Medicine 11, 398–403.

Flynn, M.A., Nolph, G.B., Baker, A.S., Martin, W.M. & Krause, G. (1989) Total body potassium in aging humans: a longitudinal study. American Journal of Clinical Nutrition 50, 713–717.

Forbes, G.B. (1987) Human Body Composition. Growth, Aging, Nutrition and Activity. Springer-Verlag, New York.

Frost, H.M. (1997) Why do marathon runners have less bone than weight lifters. A vital biomedical view and explanation. Bone 20, 183–189.

Graves, J.E., Pollock, M.L. & Sparling, P.B. (1987) Body composition of elite distance runners. International Journal of Sports Medicine 8, 96–102.

Grimston, S.K., Tanguay, K.E., Bundberg, C.M. et al. (1993) The calciotropic hormone response to changes in serum calcium during exercise in female long distance runners. Journal of Clinical Endocrinology and Metabolism 76, 867–872.

Haapasalo, H., Sievanen, H., Kannus, P., Heinonen, A., Oja, P. & Vuori, I. (1996) Dimensions and estimated mechanical characteristics of the humerus after long-term tennis loading. Journal of Bone and Mineral Research 11, 864–872.

Hagerman, F.C., Hagerman, F.R. & Mickelson, T.C. (1979) Physiological profile of elite rowers. *Physician and Sportsmedicine* 7, 74–83.

Harman, E.A. & Frykman, P.N. (1992) The relationship of body size and composition to the performance of physically demanding military tasks. In. Marriott, B.M. and Grumstrup-Scott, J. (eds) *Body Composition and Physical Performance: Applications for the Military Services*, pp. 105–118. National Academy Press, Washington DC.

Haymes, E.M. & Dickinson, A.L. (1980) Characteristics of elite male and female ski racers. *Medicine and Science in Sports and Exercise* 12, 153–158.

Heath, B.H. & Carter, J.E.L. (1967) A modified somatotype method. *American Journal of Physical Anthropology* 27, 57–74.

Heinonen, A., Oja, P., Kannus, P. *et al.* (1993) Bone mineral density of female athletes in different sports. *Journal of Bone and Mineral Research* 23, 1–14.

Heinonen, A., Oja, P., Kannus, P. *et al.* (1995) Bone mineral density in female athletes representing sports with different loading characteristics of the skeleton. *Bone* 17, 197–203.

Heinrich, C.H., Going, S.B., Pamenter, R.W., Perry, C.D., Boyden, T.W. & Lohman, T.G. (1990) Bone mineral content of cyclically menstruating female resistance and endurance trained athletes. *Medicine and Science in Sports and Exercise* 22 (5), 558–563.

Hirata, K. (1966) Physique and age of Tokyo Olympic champions. *Journal of Sports Medicine and Physical Fitness* 6, 207–222.

Holly, R.G., Barnard, R.J., Rosenthal, M., Applegate, E. & Pritikin, N. (1986) Triathlete characterization and response to prolonged strenuous competition. *Medicine and Science in Sports and Exercise* 18, 123–127.

Houtkooper, L.B. & Going, S.B. (1994) Body composition: How should it be measured? Does it affect sports performance? *Sports Science Exchange* 7 (5). Gatorade Sports Science Institute.

Houtkooper, L., Aldag, L., Hall, M., Myers, B., Going, S. & Lohman, T.G. (1992) Nutritional status of elite female heptathletes. *Medicine and Science in Sports and Exercise* 24, S184.

Huddleston, A.L., Rockwell, D., Kulund, D.N. & Harrison, R.B. (1980) Bone mass in lifetime athletes. *Journal of the American Medical Association* 244, 1107–1109.

Jacobsen, P.C., Beaver, W., Grubb, S.A., Taft, T.N. & Talmage, R.V. (1984) Bone density in women: college athletes and older athletic women. *Journal of Orthopaedic Research* 2, 328–332.

Jenson, K. & Larson, B. (1993) Variations in physical capacity in a period including supplemental training of the national Danish soccer team for women. In: Reilly, T., Clarysand, J. & Stibbe, A. (eds) *Science and Football II*, pp. 114–117. E. & F.N. Spon, London.

Jones, H.H., Priest, J.D., Hayes, W.C., Technor, C.C. & Nagel, D.A. (1977) Humeral hypertrophy in response to exercise. *Journal of Bone and Joint Surgery* 59A, 204–208.

Kirk, S., Sharp, C.F., Elbaum, N. *et al.* (1989) Effect of long-distance running on bone mass in women. *Journal of Bone and Mineral Research* 4, 515–522.

Kirkendahl, D.T. (1985) The applied sports science of soccer. *Physician and Sportsmedicine* 13 (4), 53–59.

Lanyon, L.E. & Rubin, C.T. (1984) Static vs dynamic loads as an indulgence on bone remodeling. *Biomechanics* 17, 897–905.

Lee, E.J., Long, K.A., Risser, W.L., Poindexter, H.B.W., Gibbons, W.E. & Goldzieher, J. (1995) Variations in bone status of contralateral and regional sites in young athletic women. *Medicine and Science in Sports and Exercise* 27, 1354–1361.

Lindberg, J.S., Powell, M.R., Hunt, M.M., Ducey, D.E. & Wade, C.E. (1986) Increased vertebral bone mineral in response to reduced exercise in amenorrheic runners. *Western Journal of Medicine* 146, 39–42.

Linnell, S.L., Stager, J.M., Blue, P.W. *et al.* (1984) Bone mineral contents and menstrual regularity in female runners. *Medicine and Science in Sports and Exercise* 16, 343–348.

Lohman, T.G. (1989) Assessment of body composition in children. *Pediatric Exercise Science* 1, 19–30.

Lohman, T.G. (1992) In: *Advances in Body Composition Assessment*. Monograph Number 3. Human Kinetics, Champaign, IL.

Lohman, T.G. (1996) Dual energy X-ray absorptiometry. In: Roche, A.F., Heymsfield, S.B. & Lohman, T.G. (eds) *Human Body Composition*, pp. 63–78. Human Kinetics, Champaign, IL.

McArdle, W.D., Katch, F.I. & Katch, V.L. (1996) *Energy, Nutrition, and Human Performance. Exercise Physiology*, pp. 543–545. Williams & Wilkins, Baltimore, MD.

MacDougall, J.D., Webber, C.E., Martin, J. *et al.* (1992) Relationship among running mileage, bone density, and serum testosterone in male runners. *Journal of Applied Physiology* 73, 1165–1170.

Malina, R.M. (1992) Physique and body composition. Effects on performance and effects on training, semistarvation, and overtraining. In: Brownell, K.D., Rodin, J. & Wilmore, J.H. (eds) *Eating, Body Weight, and Performance in Athletes*, pp. 94–114. Lea & Febiger, Philadelphia.

Malina, R.M. & Bouchard, C. (1991) Characteristics of young athletes. In: *Growth, Maturation and Physical Activity*, pp. 443–463. Human Kinetics, Champaign, IL.

Marcus, R., Cann, C., Madvig, P. *et al.* (1985) Menstrual function and bone mass in elite women distance runners. *Annals of Internal Medicine* 102, 158–163.

Modlesky, C.M., Cureton, K.J., Prion, B.M., Sloniger, M.A. & Rowe, D.A. (1996) Density of the fat-free mass and estimates of body composition in male weight trainers. *Journal of Applied Physiology* 80, 2085–2096.

Montoye, H.J., Smith, E.L., Fardon, D.F. & Howley, E.T. (1980) Bone mineral in senior tennis players. *Scandinavian Journal of Sports Sciences* 2, 26–32.

Myburgh, K.H., Bachrach, L.K., Lewis, B., Kent, K. & Marcus, R. (1993) Low bone mineral density at axial and appendicular sites in amenorrheic athletes. *Medicine and Science in Sports and Exercise* 25, 1197–1202.

Nichols, D.L., Sanborn, C.F., Bonnick, S.L., Ben-Ezra, V., Gench, B. & DiMarco, N.M. (1994) The effects of gymnastics training on bone mineral density. *Medicine and Science in Sports and Exercise* 26, 1220–1225.

Nilsson, B.E.R. & Westlin, N.E. (1971) Bone density in athletes. *Clinical Orthopedics* 77, 179–182.

O'Connor, J.A. & Lanyon, L.E. (1982) The influence of strain rate on adaptive bone remodeling. *Journal of Biomechanics* 15, 767–781.

Orwoll, E.S., Ferar, J., Oviatt, S., McClung, M.R. & Huntington, K. (1989) The relationship of swimming exercise to bone mass in men and women. *Archives of Internal Medicine* 149, 2197–2200.

O'Toole, M.L., Hillee, D.B., Crosby, L.D. & Douglas, P.S. (1987) The ultraendurance triathlete: a physiological profile. *Medicine and Science in Sports and Exercise* 19, 45.

Parnell, R.W. (1958) *Behavior and Physique*, pp. 134. Edward Arnold Ltd., London.

Pate, R.R., Slentz, C.A. & Katz, D.P. (1989) Relationships between skinfold thickness and performance of health related fitness test items. *Research Quarterly for Exercise and Sport* 60, 183–189.

Pocock, N.A., Eisman, J.A., Hopper, J.L.,

Yeates, M.G., Sanbrook, P.N. & Eberl, S. (1987) Genetic determinants of bone mass in adults: a twin study. *Journal of Clinical Investigation* **80**, 706–710.

Pollock, M.L. (1977) Body composition of elite class distance runners. *Annals of the New York Academy of Sciences* **301**, 361–370.

Reid, I.R., Plank, L.D. & Evans, M.C. (1992a) Fat mass is an independent determinant of whole body bone density in premenopausal women but not in men. *Journal of Clinical Endocrinology and Metabolism* **75**, 775–782.

Reid, I.R., Ames, A., Evan, M.C. et al. (1992b) Determinants of total body and regional bone mineral density in normal postmenopausal women. *Journal of Clinical Endocrinology and Metabolism* **75**, 775–782.

Rencken, M.L., Chesnut, C.H. III & Drinkwater, B.L. (1996) Bone density at multiple skeletal sites in amenorrheic athletes. *Journal of the American Medical Association* **276**, 238–240.

Rico-Sanz, J. (1998) Body composition and nutritional assessments in soccer. *International Journal of Sport Nutrition* **8**, 113–123.

Risser, W.L., Lee, E.J., Leblanc, A., Poindexter, H.B.W., Risser, J.M.H. & Schneider, V. (1990) Bone density in eumenorrheic female college athletes. *Medicine and Science in Sports and Exercise* **22**, 570–574.

Rubin, C.T. & Lanyon, L.E. (1984) Regulation of bone formation by applied dynamic loads. *Journal of Bone and Joint Surgery* **66**, 397–402.

Rubin, C.T. & Lanyon, L.E. (1985) Regulation of bone mass by mechanical strain magnitude. *Calcified Tissue International* **37**, 411–417.

Rusko, H., Havu M. & Karvinen, E. (1978) Aerobic performance capacity in athletes. *European Journal of Applied Physiology* **38**, 151–159.

Sheldon, W.H., Dupertuis, C.W. & McDermott, E. (1954) *Atlas of Men*, pp. 357. Harper and Brothers, New York.

Sinning, W.E. (1985) Body composition and athletic performance. In: Clarke, D.H. & Eckert, H.M. (eds) *Limits of Human Performance*, pp. 45–56. Human Kinetics, Champaign, IL.

Sinning, W.E. & Wilson, J.R. (1984) Validity of 'generalized' equations for body composition analysis in women athletes. *Research Quarterly for Exercise and Sports* **55**, 153–160.

Siri, W.E. (1956) The gross composition of the body. *Advances in Biology, Medicine and Physiology* **4**, 239–280.

Siri, W.E. (1961) Body composition from fluid spaces and density. Analysis of methods. In: Brozek, J. & Henschel, A. (eds) *Techniques for Measuring Body Composition*, pp. 223–244. National Academy of Science, Washington DC.

Slaughter, M.H. & Lohman, T.G. (1979) An objective method for measurement of musculo-skeletal size to characterize body physique with application to the general population. *Medicine and Science in Sports and Exercise* **12**, 170–174.

Slaughter, M.H., Lohman, T.G., Boileau, R.A. et al. (1988) Skinfold equations for estimation of body fatness in children and youth. *Human Biology* **60**, 709–723.

Snead, D.B., Weltman, A., Weltman, J.Y. et al. (1992) Reproductive hormones and bone mineral density in women runners. *Journal of Applied Physiology* **72**, 2149–2156.

Sparling, P.B. & Cureton, K.J. (1983) Biological determinants of sex difference in 12 min run performance. *Medicine and Science in Sports and Exercise* **15**, 218–222.

Sprynarova, S. & Parizcova, J. (1969) Comparison of the functional circulatory and respiratory capacity in girl gymnasts and swimmers. *Journal of Sports Medicine and Physical Fitness* **9**, 165–172.

Sprynarova, S. & Parizcova, J. (1979) Functional capacity and body composition in weight lifters, swimmers, runners, and skiers. *International Zeitschrift fur Angewandte Physiologie* **29**, 184–194.

Taaffe, D.R., Robinson, T.L., Snow, C.M. & Marcus, R. (1997) High-impact exercise promotes bone gain in well-trained female athletes. *Journal of Bone and Mineral Research* **12**, 255–260.

Thorland, W.G., Johnston, G.O., Housh, T.J. & Refsell, M.J. (1983) Anthropometric characteristics of elite adolescent competitive swimmers. *Human Biology* **55**, 735–748.

Vaccaro, P., Morris, A.F. & Clarke, D.H. (1981) Physiological characteristics of masters female distance runners. *Physician and Sportsmedicine* **9** (7), 105–108.

Vaccaro, P., Gray, P.R., Clarke, D.H. & Morris, A.F. (1984) Physiological characteristics of world class white-water slalom paddlers. *Research Quarterly for Exercise and Sports* **55**, 206–210.

Vos, J.A. (1980) Physiological comparison between Dutch soccer players and other teamsmen. In: Vecchiet, L. (ed.) *Proceedings of the 1st International Congress on Sports Medicine Applied to Football*, pp. 695–701. D. Guanillo, Rome.

Wang, Z., Pierson, R.N. & Heymsfield, S.B. (1992) The five level model: a new approach to organizing body composition research. *American Journal of Clinical Nutrition* **56**, 19–28.

Williams, D.P., Going, S.B., Lohman, T.G., Hewitt, M.J. & Haber, A.E. (1992) Estimation of body fat from skinfold thicknesses in middle-aged and older men and women: a multiple component approach. *American Journal of Human Biology* **4**, 595–605.

Williams, J.A., Wagner, J., Wasnich, R. & Heilbrun, L. (1984) The effect of long-distance running upon appendicular bone mineral content. *Medicine and Science in Sports and Exercise* **16** (3), 223–227.

Wilmore, J.H. (1992) Body weight standards and athletic performance. In: Brownell, K.D., Rodin, J. & Wilmore, J.H. (eds) *Eating, Body Weight, and Performance in Athletes*, pp. 315–329. Lea & Febiger, Philadelphia.

Wilmore, J.H. & Bergfeld, J.A. (1978) A comparison of sports. Physiological and medical aspects. In: Strauss, R.H. (ed.) *Sports Medicine and Physiology*, pp. 353–372. W.B. Saunders, Philadelphia.

Wilmore, J.H., Brown, C.H. & Davies, J.A. (1977) Body physique and composition of women distance runners. *Annals of the New York Academy of Sciences* **301**, 764–776.

Wolman, R.L. (1990) Bone mineral density levels in elite female athletes. *Annals of the Rheumatic Diseases* **49**, 1013–1016.

Wolman, R.L., Faulmann, L., Clark, P., Hesp, R. & Harries, M.G. (1991) Different training patterns and bone mineral density of the femoral shaft in elite, female athletes. *Annals of the Rheumatic Diseases* **50**, 487–489.

Chapter 25

Personality Structure of the Endurance Performer

LARRY M. LEITH

Over the years, athletes have continued to become faster, stronger, more technically advanced and capable of greater feats of endurance. In consequence, coaches and practitioners must scramble to keep up with developments having the potential to give their athletes a margin of advantage. This is particularly evident in the field of sport psychology, since success in high-level sports has been estimated to be 10–20% physiological and 80–90% psychological (Kozar & Lord 1983). Intuitively, the dominance of psychological factors makes sense, since all athletes at the élite level are at an optimal fitness level and are technically flawless. It therefore becomes important to look at psychological factors that may be responsible for ultimate victory. In this chapter, we consider the role of personality structure as a determinant of success in endurance sports.

In the present context, personality is defined as 'that pattern of characteristic thoughts, feelings, and behaviours that distinguishes one person from another and that persists over time and situations' (Phares 1991, p.4). Traditionally, personality research has generated a great deal of controversy. Morgan (1980) identified the most basic concern as the *credulous versus sceptical argument*. He implied that researchers were generally polarized on the issue of the credibility of personality research. On one side, some researchers believe that positive and accurate predictions of sport performance can be made from personality profiles based on measured traits (the credulous perspective). The opposite viewpoint maintains that the value of personality assessment in predicting athletic success is limited (the sceptical perspective). Although this controversy has generated a substantial amount of research, it has done little to clarify those times when personality testing could prove to be of value. A second debate has revolved around the *state–trait controversy*. At issue are the relative merits of assessing personality states versus personality traits. For a more thorough discussion of this argument, refer to Leith's (1992) chapter in the first edition of *Endurance in Sport* (Shephard & Åstrand 1992).

Regardless of recent controversy, the issue of personality assessment of endurance athletes warrants serious consideration. In this chapter, we: (a) look at the most popular assessment techniques; (b) examine completed research with direct relevance to this chapter; and (c) indicate the implications of these findings for the training and performance of endurance athletes.

Measuring personality

This section identifies and discusses briefly various techniques used for assessing personality. Cox (1998) and Wann (1997) have identified three basic classes of personality measurement techniques. These are: (i) rating scales; (ii) unstructured projective tests; and (iii) structured questionnaires. Each of these categories is briefly examined, but particular emphasis is placed on the questionnaire method. This method is highlighted because of its demonstrated objectivity, validity and reliability (Whiting *et al.* 1973; Wann 1997; Cox 1998).

Rating scales

Rating scales typically involve the participation of a judge or judges who are asked to observe an individual in a particular situation. The judges usually use a scale or checklist that has been predesigned for maximum objectivity. If the assessors have been well trained and the checklist is used properly, the results can be fairly reliable and objective.

Rating scales are applied in two types of situation: the *interview* and *observation of performance*. In an interview, the judge systematically asks the subject numerous open-ended questions that have been designed to ascertain personality traits and general first impressions. Several interviews are usually necessary to gain impressions of underlying motives (the core of personality). If it is carried out properly, this technique can provide valid and reliable results, although the ultimate data depend largely upon the skill and sensitivity of the judge/interviewer.

The second method of rating involves the observation of a subject during a particular performance situation. Such observations can be effective if the observer is highly trained and if the checklist is well designed and planned. In most cases, the checklist would identify specific behaviours and traits that the observer would attempt to witness. As a final step, these traits and behaviours would be rated in terms of their strength and their clarity.

Because every situation is different, specific rating scales are required and no standard instrument is available that can be administered across various settings. For this reason, the average sports physician or coach is well advised to focus on some of the more structured personality assessment techniques outlined below.

Unstructured projective procedures

Projective techniques typically allow subjects to reveal their innermost feelings and motives through their approach to a series of unstructured tasks. This form of personality assessment is used predominantly by clinical psychologists, and it remains synonymous with a psychoanalytical approach to personality theory. Proponents of this methodology assume that if subjects perceive that there are no right or wrong answers, they are likely to be open and honest in their responses.

Several unstructured tests have been developed over the years. They include the *Rorschach ('ink-blot') test* (Saranson 1954), the *thematic apperception test* (Tompkins 1947), the *sentence completion test* (Holsopple & Miale 1954), and the *house–tree–person test* (Buck 1948). The most commonly used unstructured projective procedure is the Rorschach test. A brief discussion of this procedure follows.

The test material contains 10 cards, with an 'ink-blot' printed on each card. The cards are presented systematically to the subject, who is then encouraged to describe what he or she sees on the card. The tester keeps a verbatim record of the subject's responses, also noting any spontaneous remarks or emotional reactions. After all the cards have been viewed, the tester questions the subject about the associations which she or he has made with each card. Early research by sport psychologists suggested that this procedure lacked objectivity, reliability and validity (Ryan 1981), but more recent opinion (Weiner 1994) concludes that the test is psychometrically sound, with verifiable test/retest reliability and criterion and construct validity. However, the test must be administered by highly trained clinical psychologists in order to yield accurate and reliable results. For this reason, the procedure is not recommended for consideration by the sports medicine practitioner unless a clinical psychologist is available for testing (Kroll 1976; LeUnes & Nation 1989; Wann 1997; Cox 1998).

Structured questionnaires

The structured questionnaire is a paper-and-pencil test in which the subject is asked to answer specific true–false or Likert scale-type statements. A relatively large number of questionnaire-type personality inventories are now available. Some have been designed for the diagnosis of psychopathologies, but others have been developed for use with the normal population. In the athletic environment, four tests have been used almost exclusively. These are the *Minnesota multiphasic personality inventory (MMPI)*, the *Cattell sixteen personality factor* questionnaire (16PF), the *athletic motivation inventory (AMI)*, and the *profile of mood states (POMS)*. Each of these tests will now be briefly examined. For a more complete description of available personality inventories, along with their psychometric properties, the reader is referred to Ostrow (1996).

MINNESOTA MULTIPHASIC PERSONALITY INVENTORY (MMPI)

The MMPI (Hathaway & McKinley 1943) was originally designed to provide objective assessment of the major personality characteristics that affect personal and social adjustment in persons with disabling psychological abnormalities. Twelve scales are included in the modern test version. These include hypochondriasis (Hs), depression (D), hysteria (Hy), psychopathic deviation (Pd), masculinity–femininity (Mf), paranoia (Pa), psychasthenia (Pt), schizophrenia (Sc), hypomania (Ma), lying (L), validity (F) and correction (K). The MMPI contains more than 500 questions intended to assess the aforementioned personality factors. Although the test was originally designed for the evaluation of abnormal subjects, it can and has been used in the normal population. For the most part, however, its use is restricted to the clinical setting. Some of the questions appear bizarre to healthy individuals, it takes rather long to complete and it is not highly recommended for use in the athletic population.

CATTELL SIXTEEN PERSONALITY FACTOR QUESTIONNAIRE (16PF)

The 16PF (Cattell *et al.* 1980) is considered to be the most sophisticated paper-and-pencil test of personality currently available. Development of the test involved the use of factor analysis to isolate 16 different and supposedly orthogonal personality-type dichotomies such as humble–assertive, relaxed–tense, conservative–experimenting, undisciplined–controlled and trusting–suspicious. Each of these 16 dichotomies identifies what Cattell *et al.* (1980) refer to as *source traits*, or first-order traits of personality. These traits are deeply ingrained in an individual's personality make-up. Additionally, Cattell believes that the 16 source traits can be reduced to four *surface*, or second-order traits. The

surface traits of anxiety, tough-mindedness, extroversion and independence each represent a cluster of several source traits that relate to learned behaviour (Fredenburgh 1971). This distinction implies that source traits are fundamental structures of personality, while surface traits are learned.

In terms of reliability and validity, there is little doubt that the Cattell 16PF is the best test to be used for the personality testing of athletes (Cox 1998). Test/retest reliability averages 0.80, and empirical validation data include average profiles for more than 50 occupational groups and about the same number of psychiatric syndromes. It is also the test that has been utilized most often in the athletic environment. For this reason, it deserves serious consideration by the sports science practitioner.

THE ATHLETIC MOTIVATION INVENTORY (AMI)

The AMI (Tutko & Richards 1971) was designed to measure a number of personality traits that appeared to be related more directly to high athletic achievement, including drive, aggression, determination, responsibility, leadership, self-confidence, emotional control, mental toughness, coachability, conscience development and trust. These factors were supposedly derived, in a modified form, from the Cattell 16PF (Cattell *et al.* 1980) and the Jackson personality research form (Ogilvie *et al.* 1971).

Several researchers quickly questioned both the reliability and the validity of the AMI (Rushall 1973; Martens 1975; Corbin 1977; Vealey 1992). However, the real concern of sport psychologists is that the developers of the test suggested that the AMI could predict athletic success (Cox 1998). A study by Davis (1991) supports this concern; he found that less than 4% of the variance between scout rankings and the on-ice performance of hockey players could be attributed to AMI scores. For this reason, most researchers in sport psychology avoid use of the AMI.

THE PROFILE OF MOOD STATES (POMS)

Earlier in the chapter, the state–trait controversy was introduced. Proponents of the state approach have conducted most of their personality research using the POMS questionnaire (McNair *et al.* 1971). The POMS is not the only state measure of personality and mood, but over the last 10 years, it has certainly been the most commonly used instrument (Snow & LeUnes 1994). The original POMS was a 65-item unipolar inventory that measured six elements of affect: depression, anxiety, anger, vigour, fatigue and confusion. For ease of administration in the sport environment, three different short versions of the test have been developed. These include a 37-item short form introduced by Schacham (1983), a 40-item version proposed by Grove and Prapavessis (1992), and a 27-item test by Terry *et al.* (1996) that was designed specifically for children.

The interactive relationship between personality traits and mood states has been documented by Prapavessis and Grove (1994a,b). These studies report that when athletes are categorized as high or low on a particular personality trait, they also differ significantly on selected mood states. Another interesting finding is that mood states measured immediately prior to an athletic contest are not strong predictors of actual performance. In contrast, mood states measured immediately after the event are highly predictive of athletic performance. Immediately following competition, successful performers score lower in the negative moods of depression, anger and tension than do their unsuccessful counterparts (Renger 1993; Meyers *et al.* 1994; Hassmen & Bomstrand 1995). Unfortunately, it is difficult to determine if these mood differences preceded or were caused by the event outcome. A meta-analysis by Rowley *et al.* (1995) tends to support the aforementioned research, concluding that a small but significant difference exists between successful and unsuccessful athletes in terms of reported mood states (POMS). It therefore appears that the POMS has potential for use by the sports science practitioner.

Personality and sport performance

Now that we have examined the most popular methods of personality assessment, it is important to consider the results of completed research utilizing these measurement techniques. The majority of investigations have focused on three particular themes: comparing athletes and non-athletes, comparing athletes from different sports, and comparing athletes differing in skill levels.

Comparisons between the personalities of athletes and non-athletes

One of the most common research themes in sport personality concerns the extent to which athletes and non-athletes differ in their personality structures. A literature review by Morgan (1980) concluded that athletes were more stable and extroverted than their peers. An earlier review by Cooper (1969) had reported that athletes were also more competitive, dominant, self-confident and achievement-orientated than non-athletes. Similar findings were reported by Butt and Cox (1992). In addition, athletes have been found to be psychologically more well adjusted (Cooper 1969; Snyder & Kivlin 1975; LeUnes & Nation 1982) and often display higher levels of self-esteem than non-athletes (Trujilo 1983; Mahoney 1989; Kamal *et al.* 1995; Marsh *et al.* 1995). Research has also revealed that, compared with non-athletes, athletes hold more conservative political views (Rehberg & Schafer 1968), are more authoritarian (LeUnes & Nation 1982), and demonstrate higher levels of persistence (Lufi & Tenenbaum 1991).

Although these various differences between athletes and non-athletes have been well documented, Vealey (1992) suggests that a clear pattern has yet to emerge. Athletes may be more likely than non-athletes to possess certain personality traits, but a composite personality pattern indicative of athletes has yet to be identified. This is not surprising when one considers that the research has been conducted across such a wide range of sports.

Comparisons of personality between athletes from different sports

Although certain inter-sport differences have been reported (Singer 1969; Geron *et al.* 1986; Sadalla *et al.* 1988; Cox *et al.* 1993), Cratty (1989) notes that only a few consistencies have emerged. Moreover, these consistencies are far from surprising. Firstly, participants in individual sports tend to be less anxious and emotional as well as more introverted than team sports participants. Secondly, participants in sports that demand aggression tend to be more aggressive than athletes in non-aggressive sports. However, other investigators have contradicted both of these conclusions (Colley *et al.* 1985) or have found no differences between different sports (Wann & Lingle 1994; Andre & Holland 1995). Thus, more research is required before we can arrive at a definitive understanding of personality differences between participants in different types of sports.

Comparisons of personality between athletes of differing skill levels

One of the most popular lines of research examining athletes of differing skill levels involves the measurement of mood profiles. Studies utilizing the POMS questionnaire have consistently found differences of mood profile between successful and unsuccessful athletes (Morgan & Pollock 1977; Morgan 1979, 1980, 1985; LeUnes & Nation 1982; Morgan *et al.* 1988). These studies support the notion that successful athletes have a more positive mood profile than unsuccessful athletes. They score lower on tension, depression, anger, fatigue and confusion, but are higher in vigour. This pattern has been termed the *iceberg profile*.

However, a few studies have not supported the notion of an iceberg profile (Miller & Miller 1985; Craighead *et al.* 1986; Daiss *et al.* 1986). In addition, two studies have questioned the magnitude of differences between successful and unsuccessful competitors (Renger 1993; Terry 1995). To put this in perspective, a meta-analysis of 33 studies utilizing the POMS supported the iceberg profile, although differences between successful and unsuccessful athletes were very small (Rowley *et al.* 1995). In fact, mood state accounted for less than 1% of the athletes' performances. It therefore appears that three conclusions can be drawn. Firstly, the iceberg profile is a real and significant phenomenon. Secondly, differences of profile between athletic categories are not as large as was once perceived. Thirdly, situational factors such as event duration and type of sport may influence the magnitude of differences in mood profile (Terry 1995). This last point has direct

relevance for the sports science practitioner who is working with endurance athletes. It is discussed at more length in the following section.

Implications for sports science practitioners

What implications and recommendations can be gleaned from sport personality research? The following suggestions are offered to provide the sports science practitioner with specific guidelines for use in endurance sports.

1 One of the first decisions practitioners usually feel obliged to make is whether to subscribe to a *state* or *trait* perspective on personality assessment. Although this is in line with traditional reasoning, it might not be the most productive approach in the context of competitive sport. Perhaps a better tactic is to consider the basic tenets of the *interactional theory* of personality assessment. The interactionist approach suggests that one must take into consideration not only the individual's characteristics, but also situational factors specific to the particular environment in which the athlete must perform. The practitioner endorsing this viewpoint is less likely to make simple, absolute predictions concerning the relationship between personality and behaviour. An interactionist approach highlights the dynamic relationship between trait measures, state measures and the sport-specific environment. This perspective recognizes the value of both trait and state assessments, and the advisability of sport- and/or situation-specific research. The remaining implications provide some direction for the sports science practitioner who wishes to proceed in this direction.

2 Most experts would agree that the Cattell 16PF provides the most sophisticated, reliable and valid trait personality assessment currently available for use with athletes. In terms of endurance athletes, the source traits categorized as *assertive, self-sufficient* and *controlled* all appear to be factors which would load on success in endurance athletes. One might expect athletes with higher scores on these factors to experience more long-term success in endurance sport. In addition, the surface traits labelled as *tough-minded* and *independent* represent learned

characteristics that would prove invaluable in both training and competing in endurance sport. Although research has yet to prove or refute this hypothesis, it is tempting to suggest that athletes scoring higher on these source and surface traits may indeed have an advantage in attaining élite levels of performance. Athletes with lower scores on these same traits may require special coaching and training.

3 The POMS is by far the most consistently used state measure of personality and mood. When one looks at the six elements of mood as measured in the POMS, it appears that the subscales of *vigour* and *fatigue* have the most relevance to the endurance performer. Earlier in the chapter it was pointed out that élite athletes consistently score higher on the vigour dimension than do their less successful counterparts, although the magnitude of differences has been questioned. Further, situational factors, such as event duration and sport type may affect the magnitude of differences. This observation has particular relevance for contestants in endurance events. It seems likely that endurance athletes will score significantly higher than athletes who are involved in other types of sport, even at the élite level. The type and duration of endurance events make vigour a valuable commodity. Similarly, one would expect scores on fatigue to be significantly lower among endurance competitors, since participation in endurance events necessitates an ability to handle prolonged energy expenditure. For these reasons, the sports science practitioner would be justified in considering the use of these two subscales of the POMS scale as screening or training tools.

4 The ambitious practitioner should also consider the development of behaviour observation rating scales that are specific to a particular endurance sport. In this manner, it would become progressively more possible to categorize athlete responses that are consistently related to success in a given event. With continued use, it would also be possible to establish norms across a variety of skill levels. Once these and other psychometric properties have been developed, the rating scale could be used to predict future athletic success, and also to provide specific direction for development of the individual competitor. Used in this manner, individual scores on the instrument could provide an actual training tool.

5 Finally, regardless of the type of personality assessment technique that is chosen by the sport science practitioner, it is strongly recommended that an appropriately trained and licensed sport psychologist be involved in any scale development, test administration or interpretation of results. This will not only satisfy conditions of test copyright in certain cases, but will also ensure that the measurement process is performed in the most appropriate and valid manner.

References

Andre, T. & Holland, A. (1995) Relationship of sport participation to sex role orientation and attitudes toward women among high school males and females. *Journal of Sport Behavior* **18**, 241–253.

Buck, J.N. (1948) The H–T–P technique: a qualitative and quantitative scoring manual. *Journal of Clinical Psychology* (monograph, Suppl. 5), October.

Butt, D.S. & Cox, D.N. (1992) Motivational patterns in Davis Cup, University and recreational tennis players. *International Journal of Sport Psychology* **23**, 1–13.

Cattell, R.B., Eber, H.W. & Tatsuoka, M.M. (1980) *Handbook for the Sixteen Personality Factor Questionnaire (16PF)*. Institute for Personality and Ability Testing, Champaign, IL.

Colley, A., Roberts, N. & Chipps, A. (1985) Sex-role identity, personality, and participation in team and individual sports by males and females. *International Journal of Sport Psychology* **16**, 103–112.

Cooper, L. (1969) Athletics, activity, and personality: a review of the literature. *Research Quarterly* **40**, 17–22.

Corbin, C.B. (1977) The reliability and internal consistency of the motivation rating scale and the general trait rating scale. *Medicine and Science in Sports* **9**, 208–211.

Cox, R.H. (1998) *Sport Psychology: Concepts and Applications*. WCB McGraw-Hill, New York.

Cox, R.H., Qui, Y. & Liu, Z. (1993) Overview of sport psychology. In:

Singer, R.N. Murphey, M. & Tennant, L.K. (eds) *Handbook of Research on Sport Psychology*, pp. 3–31. Macmillan, New York.

Craighead, D.J., Privette, G., Vallianos, F. & Byrkit, D. (1986) Personality characteristics of basketball players, starters and non-starters. *International Journal of Sport Psychology* **17**, 110–119.

Cratty, B.J. (1989) *Psychology in Contemporary Sport*. Prentice Hall, Englewood Cliffs.

Daiss, S., LeUnes, A.D. & Nation, J. (1986) Mood and locus of control of a sample of college and professional football players. *Perceptual and Motor Skills* **63**, 733–734.

Davis, H. (1991) Criterion validity of the athletic motivation inventory: Issues in professional sport. *Journal of Applied Sport Psychology* **3**, 176–182.

Fredenburgh, G.A. (1971) *The Psychology of Personality and Adjustment*. Benjamin-Cummings, Menlo Park, CA.

Geron, E., Furst, D. & Rotstein, P. (1986) Personality of athletes participating in various sports. *International Journal of Sport Psychology* **17**, 120–135.

Grove, J.R. & Prapavessis, H. (1992) Preliminary evidence for the reliability and validity of an abbreviated profile of mood states. *International Journal of Sport Psychology* **23**, 93–109.

Hassmen, P. & Bomstrand, E. (1995) Mood state relationships and soccer team performance. *Sport Psychologist* **9**, 297–308.

Hathaway, S.R. & McKinley, J.C. (1943) *Manual for the Minnesota Multiphasic Personality Inventory*. Psychological Corporation, New York.

Holsopple, J.Q. & Miale, G.R. (1954) *Sentence Completion*. Charles C. Thomas, Springfield.

Kamal, A.F., Blais, C., Kelly, P. & Trand, K. (1995) Self-esteem attributional components of athletes versus nonathletes. *International Journal of Sport Psychology* **26**, 189–195.

Kozar, B. & Lord, R. (1983) Psychological considerations for training the elite athlete. In: Hall, E. & McIntyre, M. (eds) *Proceedings of the United States Olympic Academy VII*, pp. 78–96. Texas Tech University, Lubbock.

Kroll, W. (1976) Current strategies and problems in personality assessment of athletes. In: Fisher, A.C. (ed.) *Psychology of Sport*, pp. 371–390. Mayfield, Palo Alto.

Leith, L.M. (1992) Personality and endurance performance: the state–trait controversy. In: Shephard, R.J. & Åstrand, P.O. (eds) *Endurance in Sport*, pp. 256–260. Blackwell Scientific Publications, Oxford.

LeUnes, A. & Nation, J. (1982) Saturday's heroes: A psychological portrait of college football players. *Journal of Sport Behavior* **5**, 139–149.

LeUnes, A. & Nation, J. (1989) *Sport Psychology: an Introduction*. Nelson-Hall, Chicago.

Lufi, D. & Tenenbaum, G. (1991) Persistence among young male gymnasts. *Perceptual and Motor Skills* **72**, 479–482.

McNair, D., Lorr, M. & Droppleman, L. (1971) *Manual for the Profile of Mood States*. Educational and Industrial Testing, San Diego.

Mahoney, M.J. (1989) Psychological predictors of élite and non-élite performance in

Olympic weightlifting. *International Journal of Sport Psychology* **20**, 1–12.

Marsh, H.W., Perry, C., Horsely, C. & Roche, L. (1995) Multidimensional self-concepts of élite athletes: how do they differ from the general population? *Journal of Sport and Exercise Psychology* **17**, 70–83.

Martens, R. (1975) *Social Psychology and Physical Activity*. Harper & Row, New York.

Meyers, M.C., Sterling, J.C., Treadwell, S., Bourgeois, A. & LeUnes, A. (1994) Psychological skills of world-ranked female tennis players. *Journal of Sport Behavior* **17**, 156–165.

Miller, B.P. & Miller, A.J. (1985) Psychological correlates of success in élite sportswomen. *International Journal of Sport Psychology* **16**, 289–295.

Morgan, W.P. (1979) Prediction of performance in athletics. In: Klavora, P. & Daniel, J.V. (eds) *Coach, Athlete, and the Sport Psychologist*, pp. 172–186. Human Kinetics, Champaign, IL.

Morgan, W.P. (1980) The trait psychology controversy. *Research Quarterly for Exercise and Sport* **51**, 50–76.

Morgan, W.P. (1985) Selected psychological factors limiting performance: a mental health model. In: Clarke, D. & Eckert, H. (eds) *Limits of Human Performance*, pp. 70–80. Human Kinetics, Champaign, IL.

Morgan, W.P. & Pollock, M.L. (1977) Psychological characterization of the élite distance runner. *Annals of the New York Academy of Science* **301**, 382–403.

Morgan, W.P., O'Connor, P.J., Ellickson, K.A. & Bradley, P.W. (1988) Personality structure, mood states, and performance in élite male distance runners. *International Journal of Sport Psychology* **19**, 247–263.

Ogilvie, B.C., Johnsgard, K. & Tutko, T.A. (1971) Personality: effects of activity. In: Larson, L.A. (ed.) *Encyclopedia of Sport Sciences and Medicine*, pp. 225–233. Macmillan, New York.

Ostrow, A.C. (ed.) (1996) *Directory of Psychological Tests in the Sport and Exercise Sciences*. Fitness Information Technology Inc., Morgantown.

Phares, E. (1991) *Introduction to Personality*. Harper-Collins, New York.

Prapavessis, H. & Grove, R. (1994a) Personality variables as antecedents of precompetitive mood states. *International Journal of Sport Psychology* **25**, 81–99.

Prapavessis, H. & Grove, R. (1994b) Personality variables as antecedents of precompetitive mood state temporal

patterning. *International Journal of Sport Psychology* **25**, 347–365.

Rehberg, R.A. & Schafer, W.E. (1968) Participation in interscholastic athletics and college expectations. *American Journal of Sociology* **73**, 732–740.

Renger, R. (1993) A review of the Profile of Mood States (POMS) in the prediction of athletic success. *Journal of Applied Sport Psychology* **5**, 8–84.

Rowley, A.J., Landers, D.M., Kyllo, L.B. & Etnier, J.L. (1995) Does the iceberg profile discriminate between successful and less successful athletes? A meta-analysis. *Journal of Sport and Exercise Psychology* **17**, 185–199.

Rushall, B.S. (1973) The status of personality research and application in sports and physical education. *Journal of Sports Medicine and Physical Fitness* **13**, 281–290.

Ryan, F. (1981) *Sports and Psychology*. Prentice Hall, Englewood Cliffs.

Sadalla, E.K., Linder, D.E. & Jenkins, B.A. (1988) Sport preference: a self-presentational analysis. *Journal of Sport and Exercise Psychology* **10**, 214–222.

Saranson, S.B. (1954) *The Clinical Interaction with Special Reference to Rorschach*. Harper, New York.

Schacham, S. (1983) A shortened version of the Profile of Mood States. *Journal of Personality Assessment* **47**, 305–306.

Shephard, R.J. & Åstrand, P.O. (eds) (1992) *Endurance in Sport*. Blackwell Scientific Publications, Oxford.

Singer, R.N. (1969) Personality differences between and within baseball and tennis players. *Research Quarterly* **40**, 582–587.

Snow, A. & LeUnes, A. (1994) Characteristics of sports research using profile of mood states. *Journal of Sports Behavior* **17**, 207–211.

Snyder, E.E. & Kivlin, J.E. (1975) Women athletes and aspects of psychological well-being and body image. *Research Quarterly* **46**, 191–199.

Terry, P. (1995) The efficacy of mood state profiling with élite performers: a review and synthesis. *Sport Psychologist* **9**, 309–324.

Terry, P., Keohane, L. & Lane, H. (1996) Development and validation of a shortened version of the profile of mood states suitable for use with young athletes. *Journal of Sports Sciences* **14**, 49.

Tompkins, S.S. (1947) *The Thematic Apperception Test: The Theory and Technique of Interpretation*. Grune & Stratton, New York.

Trujilo, C.M. (1983) The effect of weight training and running exercise intervention programs on the self-esteem of college women. *International Journal of Sport Psychology* 14, 162–173.

Tutko, T.A. & Richards, J.W. (1971) *Psychology of Coaching*. Allyn & Bacon, Boston.

Vealey, R.S. (1992) Personality and sport: a comprehensive view. In: Horn, T.S. (ed.) *Advances in Sport Psychology*, pp. 25–59. Human Kinetics, Champaign, IL.

Wann, D.L. (1997) *Sport Psychology*. Prentice Hall, Upper Saddle River.

Wann, D.L. & Lingle, S.E. (1994) Comparison of team and individual sports participants' tendencies to join groups. *Perceptual and Motor Skills* 79, 833–834.

Weiner, I.B. (1994) Rorschach assessment. In: Maruish, M.E. (ed.) *The Use of Psychological Testing for Treatment Planning and Outcome Assessment*, pp. 249–278. Erlbaum, Hillsdale, NJ.

Whiting, H.T., Hardman, K., Hendry, L.B. & Jones, M.G. (1973) *Personality and Performance in Physical Education and Sport*. Kimpton, London.

Chapter 26

Perception of Effort During Endurance Training and Performance

BRUCE J. NOBLE AND JOHN M. NOBLE

Introduction

Competitive endurance performance requires considerable physical effort and that effort is in the conscious awareness of the participant. Whether effort awareness can be called a human sense (Sherrington 1900) and whether it can be measured (James 1890) were debated over much of the first half of the twentieth century. However, with the establishment of Stevens' power law (Stevens 1957), and its application to more than two dozen sensory dimensions (Stevens & Galanter 1957), human effort responses are now known to be related predictably to stimulus intensity. Borg (1961) published the first practical scale to measure perception of physical effort. This scale, known variously as the 'Borg Scale' or 'RPE scale', for rating of perceived exertion, has been studied and applied widely in a variety of clinical and sports settings.

Although the difference between sensation and its perception may be obvious to most people, defining each will serve as a useful starting point. Sensation is a passive activation of a specific class of sense organ (Bartley 1970), without conscious awareness. For example, the body can detect a slight change in core body temperature during a marathon event without awareness on the part of the runner. Detection serves to maintain physiological homeostasis. Perception, on the other hand, is an active process in which many internal and external inputs are organized in the cerebral cortex. Students of effort perception have attempted to develop a theoretical understanding of the process by which a multitude of effort-related inputs are detected,

mediated and organized into a report of effort intensity.

The purpose of this chapter is modest but complex. The complexity lies in the multifactorial nature of the perceptual process during endurance activity and our incomplete understanding of that process. Our modest intent is to review literature that bears upon, but is not necessarily directly related to, the process by which effort is perceived during endurance activity. In addition, practical applications of the process to endurance training and competition are discussed. Our understanding of such applications depends heavily on extrapolation of the scientific data and informed speculation, due to a dearth of research in this area.

Psychophysiological model of perceived effort

The earliest attempt to model exercise perceptual responses was undertaken by Kinsman and Weiser (1976). The underlying assumption is instructive. Kinsman and Weiser assumed that exercise 'symptoms have their genesis in known or as yet unidentified physiological changes occurring during work'. Symptoms were said to arise from the physiological substrata, termed the subordinate level, producing a conscious awareness of effort at an ordinate level. This in turn led to a subjective report at the supraordinate level. These authors also postulated a role for psychological factors, specified as 'motivation' and 'task aversion', in the setting of effort perceptions. However, they made it clear that these factors were secondary to physiological processes. We recognize that the genesis of felt effort lies in muscular contraction, with all of the biological implications therein. Where we depart from Kinsman and Weiser is in the notion that psychological factors only operate in response to the physiological substrata. We are more inclined to agree with the parallel processing hypothesis of Levanthal and Everhart (1979). The latter is more inclusive and capable of accounting for pre-existing traits that may moderate perceptual reports of effort. That is to say, certain factors operate as independent inputs at the preconscious level, not only as influences modulating physiological sensation. They are factors not dependent on muscular contraction or the resulting physiological response, and they may exert their effect even before movement begins.

In the Noble–Robertson model (Noble & Robertson, 1996) (Fig. 26.1), stimuli from the physiological substrata serve as a major attribution source for the setting of effort perception. Sensory signals arise from both central respiratory–metabolic sources and peripheral influences in exercising muscle. In parallel to physiological inputs, we find contributions from psychological and performance sources. These sources may include, but are not limited to, mood states, personality type, competitive strategy and audience-related factors. In addition, feedback from symptoms, such as sweating and laboured breathing, contribute to the setting of an effort rating. Integration of the vast array of inputs takes place in the cerebral cortex. Little is known about the exact mechanisms involved. However, in the case of physiological stimuli, we do know that as the motor cortex responds to muscle tension demands,

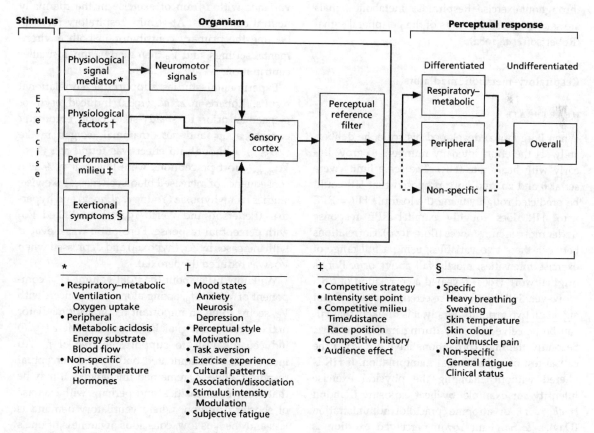

Fig. 26.1 Noble–Robertson psychophysiological model.

a copy of motor commands is relayed to the sensory cortex (Cafarelli 1982), providing continuously updated information.

Physiological inputs to the perception of effort

Ekblom and Goldbarg (1971) made the first attempt to categorize physiological inputs. Their research, which involved several perturbations of the effort report, showed two broad explanatory factors, central and local. Central factors were said to emanate from cardiopulmonary inputs, whereas local factors comprised stimuli arising from exercising muscles and joints. Current refinement of this two-factor model utilizes the terms 'respiratory–metabolic' and 'peripheral' mediators (Noble & Robertson 1996). Peripheral signals are primary under most circumstances and they remain so throughout exercise. Respiratory–metabolic signals are said to act as amplifiers of the peripheral signal (Robertson et al. 1982).

Respiratory–metabolic mediators

HEART RATE

When Borg (1962) developed his scale, he deliberately set the effort intensity numbers to grow linearly with heart rate (HR). The scale limits were set at 6 and 20, and Borg proposed that HR could be predicted roughly using the formula HR = RPE × 10. HR does roughly parallel RPE response under most circumstances (Borg 1970). Correlations between these two variables, using a full range of exercise intensities, mostly fall above 0.70. Borg's original work (1962) revealed a correlation of 0.85. However, HR has been rejected as a significant signal on two grounds. Firstly, it is unlikely that HR can be perceived directly during intense exercise. Secondly, the high correlations have not stood the causal test of experimental manipulation. If HR is altered without changing the physical exercise intensity, for example, by heat exposure (Pandolf et al. 1972), or atropine/practolol administration (Davies & Sargeant 1979), perceived exertion is unchanged. Generally, RPE responds to the work

performed rather than the HR response (Pandolf et al. 1972).

VENTILATION

Ventilation ($\dot{V}_E$) seems a likely contributor to setting of the perceptual report, since respiratory demand is so closely linked with physical effort and its symptomatology. Likewise, ventilatory symptomatology is available to conscious awareness, especially during high-intensity exercise. An early research paper utilized a multiple regression approach to determine the contributions of eight respiratory–metabolic variables to the RPE (Noble et al. 1973b). With exercise durations of 5 and 15 min, conducted in both neutral and hot environments, $\dot{V}_E$ was the leading contributor to the regression model (correlation coefficient, $R = 0.56–0.75$). Ventilation contributed as much as 56% of the explained variance with 15 min of exercise in the thermally neutral conditions. At 30 min, respiratory rate (f_B) became the primary contributor in both environmental settings, and $\dot{V}_E$ then made a much smaller contribution.

Experimental studies support the correlational results. Robertson et al. (1982) induced erythrocythaemia prior to steady-state cycle ergometer exercise at 45 and 70% maximal oxygen intake ($\dot{V}_{O_{2max}}$). Although no effect was found at 45% of $\dot{V}_{O_{2max}}$, effort perceptions were lower at 70% as a consequence of increased blood cell mass. Likewise, studies using hypoxia (Young et al. 1982) and hyperoxia (Pederson and Welch 1977) have linked $\dot{V}_{O_2}$ with perceptual response. Perception was elevated with increases in $\dot{V}_{O_2}$ (hypoxia) and depressed when $\dot{V}_{O_2}$ was reduced (hyperoxia).

We know little about the tidal volume (V_T) component of $\dot{V}_E$, but f_B, acting alone or in concert with $\dot{V}_E$, seems to be an important respiratory mediator of the perceptual signal. Robertson and Metz (1986) induced alkalosis to support the role of f_B. An increase in pH augmented both f_B and perceptual response while V_T remained unchanged. It may be that at lower intensities, and perhaps with exercise of shorter duration, where ventilatory demand is less and the f_B is low, conscious awareness of one's breathing is not the primary focus of attention, i.e.

perceptions are low. But at high exercise intensities $\dot{V}_E$ and f_B cannot be ignored, and perceptions of effort are augmented.

METABOLIC RATE

It is axiomatic that metabolic rate rises with exercise intensity, as do $\dot{V}_E$ and perceptual intensity. Since metabolic rate, expressed as oxygen consumption, is a product of $\dot{V}_E$ and the respiratory exchange ratio, i.e. carbon dioxide production ($\dot{V}\text{CO}_2$) divided by oxygen utilization ($\dot{V}\text{O}_2$), the perceptual roles of $\dot{V}\text{O}_2$ and $\dot{V}\text{CO}_2$ have been widely studied. Like HR, $\dot{V}\text{O}_2$ is highly correlated with effort perceptions (Noble & Robertson 1996). When $\dot{V}\text{O}_2$ is manipulated by factors such as air temperature (Noble *et al.* 1973a), or rate of pedalling (Pandolf & Noble 1973), no causation of effort perceptions is revealed. However, when $\dot{V}\text{O}_2$ is expressed as a percentage of maximum aerobic power, correspondence with RPE is demonstrated. Robertson *et al.* (1982) showed this when comparing perceptions in normoxic and hypoxic environments. Absolute $\dot{V}\text{O}_2$ was unrelated to RPE. Since aerobic power is reduced under hypoxic conditions, $\dot{V}\text{O}_2$ was alternatively expressed as a percentage of the $\dot{V}\text{O}_{2\text{max}}$ measured in each environment. With this adjustment, a clear relationship to perceived effort could be demonstrated. Most studies have confirmed relative $\dot{V}\text{O}_2$ as a mediator of the perceptual signal, but some inconsistencies have been found. For example, some authors have proposed that the onset of blood lactate accumulation (OBLA) is a more consistent reference point when comparing the perceptual response of individuals differing in aerobic power, e.g. gender and training differences (DeMello *et al.* 1987). For a complete discussion of this topic, see Noble and Robertson (1996).

CARBON DIOXIDE PRODUCTION

Further support for respiratory metabolic mediators can be found in experiments which have manipulated carbon dioxide production ($\dot{V}\text{CO}_2$). In one experiment, subjects inspired hypercapnic gas mixtures while exercising at various intensities. At the highest intensity (71% $\dot{V}\text{O}_{2\text{max}}$) and the strongest

hypercapnic mixture (3.5% CO_2), ventilatory minute volume was greatly increased compared to normocapnic conditions. RPE also tended to be higher with hypercapnia. These data suggest a mediating role for $\dot{V}\text{CO}_2$ in the ventilation/RPE relationship. This view is supported by Robertson *et al.* (1986) who used sodium bicarbonate (NaHCO$_3$) to reduce the necessity for buffering H ions, with a consequent decrease in CO_2 production. The suppression of $\dot{V}_E$ during high-intensity exercise was accompanied by a significant reduction in perceptual responses. It may well be that the $\dot{V}_E$/RPE relationship, mentioned above, is secondary to alterations in $\dot{V}\text{CO}_2$ which, in turn, are influenced by antecedent changes in pH.

LACTIC ACID

Because lactic acid (HLa) production can be discussed in terms of its effect both on pulmonary ventilation and on the muscle itself, it will be discussed as both a possible respiratory–metabolic and a peripheral mediator. 'It is always tempting to implicate the accumulation of lactic acid with increasing perceptual intensity' (Noble 1986). Like other respiratory–metabolic variables, there are strong correlations between lactate and perceptual response (Pandolf 1983). In contrast to the linear HR and $\dot{V}\text{O}_2$ responses lactate, $\dot{V}_E$ and $\dot{V}\text{CO}_2$ demonstrate curvilinear responses. The latter three variables are physiologically linked to the buffering of H ions, driving exponential increases in $\dot{V}\text{CO}_2$ and $\dot{V}_E$ when exercise is conducted above the lactate threshold. (Successful endurance performance probably occurs above the lactate threshold, if the intensity is not so high as to exceed the body's ability to buffer lactate successfully.) The work of Noble *et al.* (1983) supports this hypothesis, but Pederson and Welch (1977) found no correspondence between lactate and perceptual responses.

SUMMARY

There seems good evidence that respiratory–metabolic variables mediate the perceptual signal, especially at higher exercise intensities. The threshold for this contribution is located some where between 45% and 75% of $\dot{V}O_{2max}$ (Noble & Robertson 1996). Peripheral muscular factors are the dominant contributors to the perceptual signal at all exercise intensities. Likewise, the relative $\dot{V}O_2$ response is proportional to effort perceptions, especially at higher exercise intensities. Robertson's integrative model (1982) proposes $\dot{V}O_2$ as the other significant component of the respiratory–metabolic mediating system. However, its contribution is subject to exercise intensity, i.e. having limited potency below 50% of $\dot{V}O_{2max}$, moderate potency between 50% and 70%, and substantial potency above 70%. Carbon dioxide output, elevated in response to the need for buffering HLa above the lactate threshold and a driving force for increases in $\dot{V}_E$, is likewise an important contributor to the respiratory–metabolic signal.

Peripheral mediators

Noble et al. (1973a) examined the perceptual and metabolic responses to walking and running at various speeds. As walking speed increases a point is reached where running would normally commence. On average, this occurs at 4.5–5 km·h⁻¹. HR and $\dot{V}O_2$ show that when speeds exceed 8 km·h⁻¹ it is metabolically more efficient to run rather than walk. The point at which running is perceived as easier is a speed of about 6.5 km·h⁻¹. The difference (6.5 versus 8.0 km·h⁻¹) indicates a discrepancy between perceptual and metabolic efficiency. Some factor other than metabolic response is clearly at work. Neuromuscular difficulty with gait at high walking speeds, reflected in a higher RPE, precedes the need to change the mode of movement from a purely metabolic perspective. Thus, peripheral factors, those that incorporate all sensations and physiological factors occurring in the working limbs, including auxiliary support sites in the trunk and torso, seem more important to setting the perceptual response than metabolism. This view is supported by recent research which found that compared to general ratings peripheral ratings were more highly related to both aerobic endurance and the ability to sustain high cycling intensities (Garcin et al. 1998a). The following is a brief summary of research relating to the influence of peripheral mediators on perceived exertion.

METABOLIC ACIDOSIS

The role that pH shifts may play has already been discussed relative to lactate response and ventilatory regulation. We can also examine this factor as it relates to peripheral muscle. We need to distinguish the role of HLa per se from its influence on pH. Further, we need to examine whether muscle acidosis can be predicted effectively by measuring lactate levels in the blood. Noble et al. (1983) compared muscle and blood lactate levels during a continuous, progressive exercise protocol. Whereas blood lactate and perceptual values increased with the square of the exercise intensity, muscle lactate had an approximately cubic exponent. It is not surprising that a lactate concentration gradient exists between muscle and blood samples (see Chapter 3), but even though muscle lactate rises more acutely above the lactate threshold, perceptual ratings seem more closely related to the blood lactate values.

Correlational studies generally support the role of blood lactate as a peripheral indicator, but this may be because lactate and perception share a common high correlation with exercise intensity. Attempts to find a causal link have been unsuccessful (Pandolf 1983).

The hypothesized mechanism for the role of pH lies in its effects on contractility and energy metabolism in skeletal muscle (Kostka & Cafarelli 1982). Muscle fatigue brings an increase in motor unit recruitment and firing frequency (Kostka & Cafarelli 1982) and this response is monitored by the sensory cortex (McCloskey et al. 1983). Thus, one would expect perceptual intensity to rise as motor unit recruitment increases.

The work of Robertson et al. (1986) supports pH as a factor, since bicarbonate ingestion raised the pH and lowered the RPE. Likewise, when blood acidity was decreased, RPE was increased (Kostka & Cafarelli 1982). In both cases, the effect remained unnoticed until the lactate threshold had been reached. One finding that argues against a role for pH, of relevance to the endurance performer, is that longer duration exercise increased perceptual ratings even when pH was normalized (Poulus et al. 1974). The jury is still out on the role of blood lactate per se but blood pH shows considerable promise as a mediator of effort perceptions.

MUSCLE FIBRE TYPE

Studies examining the role of muscle fibre type have been both limited and conflicting. A causal link is theoretically attractive as the onset of muscle fatigue, secondary to metabolic acidosis, occurs sooner in fast-twitch (FT) than in slow-twitch (ST) fibres. As force production declines with fatigue, more motor units are recruited, thus increasing the signal to the sensory cortex (Kostka & Cafarelli 1982; Noble *et al*. 1983). Noble *et al*. (1983) reported that perceptions were greater in subjects with a higher percentage of FT fibres. Likewise, Tesch (1980) found that lactate accumulation was greater in high FT subjects who engaged in short-term high-intensity exercise. Endurance-trained athletes with high ST percentages may, by virtue of their training or genetics, have a resistance to the high rates of lactate production which would otherwise augment perceptual ratings. However, Lollgen *et al*. (1980) found no relationship between fibre type and effort perception.

MUSCLE BLOOD FLOW

Continuous muscle contraction requires an uninterrupted blood flow. Perceptual ratings of handgrip exercise were increased when limb blood flow was occluded experimentally (Cain & Stevens 1973; Stevens & Krimsley 1977). This effect appears to be limited to the later stages of exercise and is related to increased metabolic acidosis.

SUBSTRATE AVAILABILITY

The availability of carbohydrate (CHO) and free fatty acids (FFA), the substrates exclusively used in endurance activity at 60–90% of $\dot{V}O_{2max}$, should be examined for their possible contributions to effort perception (Noble 1986). Fatigue of skeletal muscle is seldom observed during low-intensity exercise and substrate availability is rarely an issue. At high intensities and 'over time, the depletion of CHO fuel sources trigger muscular fatigue, causing the termination of endurance exercise' (Noble & Robertson 1996). This would include endurance events lasting an hour or more. Several studies support CHO as a factor. We will only report one

example. Carbohydrate supplementation prior to exhaustive arm exercise was compared to a placebo trial (Robertson *et al*. 1990). Subjects maintained higher blood glucose levels, exercised longer, and reported lower exertional ratings with CHO supplementation. Since CHO is a principal substrate for central nervous system function, CHO depletion may serve as an important perceptual signal. Other authors have not supported the role of glucose supplementation (Foster *et al*. 1979), and research has not supported the role of FFA in effort perception. One criticism of CHO research is that FFA needs to be monitored along with blood glucose to appreciate the energy substrate dynamics fully.

SUMMARY

Irrefutably supportable peripheral inputs to the effort sense are elusive. Definite but ethereal factors in the periphery seem to be the predominant inputs across the full range of exercise intensities. Even though lactate concentration rises in parallel with perceptual ratings, this probably reflects the high correlation these two variables share with exercise intensity. Likewise, it is possible that blood lactate readings do not predict muscle lactate levels reliably. Although blood pH changes secondary to increases in HLa show some promise as a mediating variable, the jury is still out. Fibre type and muscle blood flow are also theoretically attractive possibilities, but much more evidence is required. Blood glucose seems supportable, especially for prolonged exercise above the lactate threshold; however, future experiments where glucose is manipulated need to control for the influence of FFA, a variable that may have an important influence when glucose is depleted (Noble & Robertson 1996).

Non-specific mediators

A number of non-specific mediators have been identified recently (Noble & Robertson 1996). The reader is referred to Noble and Robertson (1996) for a complete review. Such factors as catecholamine secretion, β-endorphin levels, body and skin temperatures, and exercise-induced pain have all been studied. A few of these variables are known to affect or be affected by endurance performance. Rudolph and McAuley (1998) compared cortisol levels in male cross-country runners and non-runners before, during and after 30 min of exercise at 60% $\dot{V}_{O_{2max}}$. Cortisol concentration increased continuously over the exercise period. Postexercise cortisol was positively related to exercise perceptions.

Core body temperature (T_c) was not related to perceptual ratings, probably because T_c is influenced more by the relative metabolic rate than by ambient temperature (Nadel 1980). On the other hand, skin temperature (T_s) decreased along with effort perceptions following 4 weeks of endurance training, suggesting a possible mediating role for T_s (Pivarnik & Senay 1986). Since core body temperature did not increase significantly in the same subjects, T_c was not considered supportable as a mediator.

Endurance activity can be accompanied by sensations emanating from muscles and supporting joint structures. Leg pain parallels leg and chest effort perceptions over a wide spectrum of exercise intensities (Noble *et al.* 1983). This relationship may not be causal, however, leading us to be cautious in our conclusions but very interested in what variables might be precursors to pain, e.g. muscle ischaemia and lactic acid concentration.

Psychological inputs to effort perception

Exercise scientists have been interested in the relative contributions of physiological and psychological factors to the mediation of perceived effort for 25 years. Morgan (1973) stated, based on the correlation between HR and RPE (R Square = 0.67), that 'a portion of the unexplained variance (33%) must be dependent upon factors of a psychometric nature'. A recent investigation showed that three out of seven psychosocial variables entered in a regression analysis explained 4–10% of the total variance in RPE (Yu 1998). Psychological factors contributed most at lower intensities and least at higher intensities of effort.

Experimental studies support the contribution of psychological factors to perception of effort. Several authors have proposed theoretical psychophysiological models (Noble 1986; Robertson & Metz 1986;

Noble & Robertson 1996). Theory supports a parallel processing model (Levanthal & Everhart 1979) to account for intra- and interindividual variability in perceptual ratings. Strictly physiological modelling (Kinsman & Weiser 1976) characterizes the perceptual process as sequential. Sequential models are additive. Thus, psychological factors are seen as modulators of experienced physiological sensations (Noble & Robertson 1996). Parallel processing posits that psychological factors alter sensory cues prior to their entering the sensory cortex (Noble & Robertson 1996). Support for parallel modelling is based partly on the work of Morgan (1976), who found that the hypnotic suggestion of hard exercise increased effort perceptions even though physiological responses remained at levels appropriate to exercise intensity. Moreover, it appears that dispositional traits, like personality, may influence perceptual ratings (Morgan 1973). Dispositional traits, factors embedded in one's temperament, are present prior to exercise and can begin exerting their influence before exercise commences.

Role of situational factors

EXPECTED DURATION

Rejeski and Ribisl (1980) found that one's expectation of exercise duration can alter perceptions. Subjects exercised in two trials. In one, they exercised for 20 min. In the second trial, they were told that they would exercise for 30 min, but the exercise was terminated after only 20 min. RPE was depressed in the second trial, even though the physiological response did not change.

SELF-PRESENTATION

Self-presentation theory asserts that 'in social situations, individuals typically attempt to present themselves in a socially desirable manner by appearing attractive, competent, and honest' (Baumeister 1982). Subjects who display high self-presentation rate effort as less severe than low self-presentation subjects (Boucher *et al.* 1988). The self-presentation outcome may depend on the intensity of social information. Subjects riding a cycle ergometer at

50% $\dot{V}O_{2max}$ rated their effort as less intense when coupled with a coactor, who was presumed to be riding at the same exercise intensity although in fact it had been halved (Hardy *et al.* 1986). No difference was observed when the coactor rode at 75% $\dot{V}O_{2max}$. It seems that the effect disappears when social information is high, as in the latter condition. In a related experiment, the same authors found self-presentation was also affected by exercise intensity. A coactor effect was found at 25 and 50% $\dot{V}O_{2max}$ but not at 75% $\dot{V}O_{2max}$. Social influence seems less salient when physiological cues are at a high level. Further, social influence may be less effective in highly trained athletes (Sylva *et al.* 1990). These authors suggested that athletic subjects were more attuned to physiological cues when evaluating perceptual intensity.

ATTENTIONAL FOCUS

Studies of attentional focus hypothesize that sensory cues from one source may dampen the influence of another source (Noble & Robertson 1996). One experiment compared a condition that promoted internal focus, breathing, with a condition where attention was concentrated on external stimuli, street sounds (Pennebaker & Lightner 1980). Fatigue was greater during the breathing condition. This supports the view that concentration on external factors may attenuate the perception of effort. Pennebaker and Lightner (1980) also compared perception during a walk/jog on an 1800-m cross-country course with nine 200-m walk/jog laps around a field. Faster times were recorded on the cross-country course, but perception did not differ between conditions. The authors concluded that the more stimulating cross-country course dampened perceptual response. These data would seem to indicate that an external focus would be beneficial. However, this does not seem the case with élite marathoners (Morgan & Pollock 1977) who, by virtue of training or genetic predisposition, prefer an internal mental focus.

Further, an active attentional focus, solving mathematical problems, significantly lowered perceived exertion compared to a passive focus, i.e. music, or a control condition (Johnson & Siegel 1987). Presumably, the solving of mathematical problems diverts focus from incoming sensory information. Light music was an effective suppressor of exercise symptoms during light exercise, but not during high-intensity exercise (Boucher & Trenske 1990). This warns us of the possible pitfalls of generalizing data across an entire spectrum of exercise intensities. It is likely that physiological stimuli at higher intensities are so concentrated that external sources of information are overridden.

Some studies have found that perception is unrelated to attentional focus (Franks & Myers 1984; Wrisberg *et al.* 1988; Fillingim *et al.* 1989; Copeland & Franks 1991). However, because methodological flaws were identified in these studies, it is tentatively concluded that attentional focus is a mediator of effort perception.

CONTRIBUTIONS ACROSS EXERCISE INTENSITIES

'Physiological factors have more saliency at high exercise intensities, whereas psychological factors have greater import at light and moderate intensities' (Noble & Robertson 1996). Much more work is needed in this area, but a recent experiment (Yu 1998) supports and extends the contention of non-collinearity. A multiple regression analysis that used anaerobic threshold (AT) to identify exercise intensity revealed the following five physiological variables ($\dot{V}O_2$, HR, $\dot{V}_E$, respiratory gas exchange ratio (RER) and HLa) and three psychological variables (physical self-efficacy, self-presentation and neuroticism) all contributed significantly to the regression model (see Table 26.1).

SUMMARY

Most athletes affirm the role of psychosocial factors in sport and can offer anecdotes of incidents where exercise felt either more or less demanding. It is more difficult to design experiments that can tease out such effects, if they truly exist. Nevertheless, 'it should be obvious that manipulation of one's attention as well as social environment can have a profound effect on perception of exertion' (Noble & Robertson 1996). Likewise, there is growing support

Table 26.1 Contribution of psychological and physiological factors to perception of effort at selected intensities of exercise.

	20% below AT (%)	AT (%)	20% above AT (%)
Psychological contribution	10	6	4
Physiological contribution	14	43	57

AT, anaerobic threshold.

for the notion that psychological factors are more salient at lower exercise intensities, when cues from physiological sensations are less potent.

Role of dispositional factors

Whether one's disposition, i.e. temperament, is a function of heredity or a developmental process, humans possess more or less permanent traits that guide patterns of behaviour. One such trait is personality.

PERSONALITY

Personality has been specifically defined and measured for much of the 20th century, beginning with the work of Carl Jung (1921). Jung identified two personality types, introversion and extroversion. Introverts focus their attention internally, whereas extroverts are oriented more to external objects. Using the Eysenck Personality Inventory (EPI), Morgan (1973) found that university-aged extroverts rated exercise conducted across several intensities as less intense than introverts. Additionally, Morgan (1973) found a high correlation ($R = 0.70$) between a preferred 30-min exercise intensity and extroversion; extroverts selected a higher level of preferred exercise. Extroverts also had a higher pain tolerance (Morgan & Costill 1972). These results were not confirmed in 16-year-old boys, using an age-adjusted instrument (Williams & Eston 1986). This promising variable needs to be studied further in postuniversity subjects, using refined and standardized measurement techniques (Dishman et al. 1991). Morgan's personality data (1973) belie the contention that an internal focus may afford an advantage to élite endurance athletes (Morgan &

Pollock 1977); however, high-level performance capacity may be a special case.

NEUROSIS

Neurotic individuals are characterized by emotional instability and hyperreactivity. Morgan (1981) found that neuroticism was negatively related to perceptions of effort ($R = -0.69$) reported at the end of a 30-min moderate-intensity exercise bout. In the same study, trait anxiety was highly correlated with RPE. It does not seem reasonable that subjects with high neuroticism or high anxiety would rate effort as low. We suspect that the exercise intensity may have been too low to stimulate a neurotic or anxiety response. Morgan (1973) studied the same variables using short-term high-intensity exercise, and he found positive correlations. He states that such a result 'makes sense at an intuitive level since one would expect the influence of personality structure to be greatest where discomfort and pain are encountered'. If his view is correct, these variables respond differently from other psychometric variables, which appear to exert their greatest effect at lighter intensities.

STIMULUS INTENSITY MODULATION

Subjects can be classified with regard to their tendency to modulate stimulus intensity (Petrie 1967). 'Augmenters' exaggerate stimuli whereas 'reducers' minimize the effects of discomfort. Weiser et al. (1973) additionally characterized reducers as 'extroverted, active, and likely to have participated in athletics' whereas augmenters tended to be 'introverted, less active, and less likely to have participated in athletics'. When these two groups were compared across several exercise intensities, augmenters rated effort significantly higher than reducers (Robertson *et al.* 1977).

FIELD DEPENDENCE/INDEPENDENCE

Those who are characterized as field independent, or internally oriented, have been hypothesized to increase perception of exertion, consistent with the hypotheses reported above. However, this could not be confirmed experimentally (Robertson *et al.* 1978). These findings may be related to the choice of exercise intensity and/or subject population.

LOCUS OF CONTROL

Those who display an internal locus of control believe they can influence outcomes with their behaviour, and they are more adept at using available information. In contrast, those with an external locus of control place emphasis on outside forces, such as chance and other people, and are said to be less able to process information. Kohl and Shea (1988), manipulating expected work intensity and duration, hypothesized that those with an external locus would rate exertion as higher under both conditions. Experimental results, however, were inconclusive. In a related study, individuals with internal and external loci were compared, while both cycling and treadmill running (Koivula & Hassmen 1998). Those with external loci rated cycling exercise as demanding significantly more effort, but no intergroup differences were discovered for treadmill running. Although this construct still interests investigators in theory, it has not been well substantiated in fact.

SELF-EFFICACY

Bandura (1977) defined self-efficacy as the belief or conviction that one has the capability to engage successfully in a course of action sufficient to satisfy the situational demands. One would predict that those with high self-efficacy would 'approach more challenging tasks, put forth more effort, and persist longer in the face of obstacles, barriers, and aversive or stressful stimuli' (McAuley & Courneya 1992).

It is hypothesized that highly efficacious subjects would rate effort as less severe than those with low self-efficacy. This hypothesis was confirmed by McAuley and Courneya (1992).

COGNITIVE STRATEGIES

Morgan and Pollock (1977) identified a concept known as cognitive style in a group of élite marathoners and recreational long-distance runners. Cognitive style consists of two divergent mental strategies, association and dissociation. In association, attention is centred on internal stimuli. Focusing on distractive thoughts is characteristic of the dissociation style. Élite runners were found to use the association style, keeping in touch with changing internal sensations, while recreational runners were more apt to dissociate. An increase of training increased associative thinking in experienced marathoners (Schomer 1986). Jones and Cale (1989) also observed that as perceived exertion increased over the course of a 16.9-km run, more associative thinking was used. The cognitive style data seem to contradict the attentional focus results, where an internal focus led to higher effort ratings. The benefit of associative cognition may lie in a greater awareness of internal states, and thus a fine tuning of necessary adjustments. Likewise, greater awareness may enhance one's ability to push through painful sensation.

SUMMARY

Those identified as extroverts, stimulus intensity reducers, highly self-efficacious and associative thinkers rate exercise as less intense than their paired opposites. Multiple regression studies (Yu 1998) have found significant contributions from self-efficacy, self-presentation and neuroticism at all levels of exercise, below, at and above the AT. Contributions were greatest at lower intensities and least at higher intensities.

Measurement issues

The measurement of perceptual effort is deceptively simple. It usually requires only an uncomplicated number scale with attached expressions. It thus appears that anyone can use the scales without instruction. However, an understanding of some basic principles of scaling can help the practitioner and researcher do a better job of both administration and interpretation.

The first publication devoted to the practical scaling of perceived exertion appeared in the early 1960s (Borg 1961). The early scale reflected its correlation with the human HR range (see Fig. 26.2). Variously called the Borg Scale, or RPE scale, this 15-grade instrument was found to be both reliable (Skinner *et al.* 1973) and valid (Stamford 1976). Other so-called category scales have been developed and also have provided reliable and valid assessments of perceived effort. Hogan *et al.* (1980) developed a 7-grade scale for materials handling tasks and a group at the University of Pittsburgh generated a 9-grade scale that is highly correlated with the RPE scale (Stamford & Noble 1974). In 1982, Borg reasoned that since some variables like blood lactate and pulmonary ventilation did not increase linearly with exercise intensity, there was a need for a new scale that rose as a power function of exercise intensity (Borg 1982). This scale, named the CR-10 (category ratio) scale, has 10 grades with attached expressions, such as 'strong', 'very strong'

and 'extremely strong' placed against numbers 5, 7 and 10 to force a curvilinear response. Although the 15-grade RPE scale has been most widely used, the scale selected should match the experimental purpose, which in research settings may mean developing a whole new scale.

Prior to laboratory or field use of a scale, the concept of perceived exertion should be defined in the context of that setting. It is also important to anchor the scale at the extremes of the perceptual range, maximal and minimal effort. One procedure is to anchor it with personal experience, either provided or remembered. For instance, the bottom of the Borg Scale, 6, can be anchored by asking an athlete to remember the smallest effort ever experienced in a certain event. 'That remembered feeling we will call 6.' For the top of the scale, 20, a memory of the most exhausting feeling ever experienced in the same event can be recalled. 'That remembered feeling we will call 20.' In laboratory situations it is sometimes useful to have the subject actually experience each end of the scale by walking easily (6) and running at maximum effort (20).

Likewise, it is important to inform each person who is using a scale what they should be monitoring. Usually it is sufficient to call for an overall response, i.e. take every sensation into consideration with a so-called Gestalt rating. In other instances, it may be appropriate to ask for only those sensations coming from the torso, i.e. sensations of respiratory–metabolic origin, or attend only to the feelings in the arms and shoulders, in order to assess peripheral factors in swimming. The instruction should fit the purpose. In differentiated measurement, the subject is instructed to differentiate those sensations that are respiratory–metabolic in origin from those that are strictly peripheral. The overall rating is an undifferentiated rating.

Assuming that you have no reason to believe the subject is answering dishonestly, any number that is reported should be accepted. An athlete may respond with a 17 when the same exercise has always been rated previously as 15. This may indicate some underlying problem that needs to be corrected. Questions are always welcomed. Noble and Noble (1998) and Borg (1998) provide extensive discussions of measurement issues.

Rating of Perceived Exertion (RPE)	
6	
7	Very, very light
8	
9	Very light
10	
11	Fairly light
12	
13	Somewhat hard
14	
15	Hard
16	
17	Very hard
18	
19	Very, very hard
20	

Fig. 26.2 Borg's rating of perceived exertion (RPE) scale.

Practical application of perceived effort to endurance performance and training

Performance

GENERAL NOTION OF
PERCEPTION/ENDURANCE RELATIONSHIP

Endurance performance is maintained via a variety of internal and external inputs. These inputs are monitored as perceptions that allow the performer to assess the intensity of muscular effort selectively. The ideal performance plan would match monitored effort with strategic effort objectives, i.e. match actual against planned pace. If effort expenditures are above the training-based goal, one risks overexertion. Sensed effort can be influenced by fatigue, previous experience, motivation, personality, competitive strategies and situational circumstances. Through endurance training, the performer can become increasingly aware of effort status, and therefore more in control of the current status/goal equation. Many complicating elements create special control problems for the endurance performer. Some modifying factors are based on unconscious processes, such as the role one's personality plays in decisions about effort expenditure. Level of fatigue, previous experience, motivation, competitive strategies and environmental conditions can also exert an effect. The performer, and scientists who study these problems, are dealing with a constantly changing landscape of inputs over a relatively long time.

Few studies elaborate the relationship between perception of effort and endurance performance/training. However, those who have studied these issues have contributed exemplary information, from which we can construct a tentative model of how perception of exertion modifies, and is modified by, endurance exercise.

LONG-DURATION RESPONSE

In the early 1970s, a group from the University of Pittsburgh monitored a recreational marathoner during the Mechanicsburg, Pennsylvania Marathon (unpublished). Heart rate and perceived exertion were recorded at 13.2, 22.8, 32.4 and 42.1 km. While HR remained stable at 140 beats·min^{-1}, RPE rose continually from 13 at 13.2 to 19 at 42.1 km. Because this was not a laboratory experiment, pace was not controlled, but split times revealed a relatively constant pace. What factors explained this perceptual augmentation, and could it be duplicated under experimental conditions?

Morgan (1973) studied this question, using a paradigm in which subjects rode a cycle ergometer at a controlled submaximal intensity (100 W) for 30 min. Heart rate plateaued at 115 beats·min^{-1}, whereas RPE rose from 9.5 at 5 min to 14 at 30 min. Other authors confirmed these findings during shorter-duration (15-min) exercise bouts (Borg & Johansson 1986). It seems that RPE begins to rise in the first 2 min of exercise (Johansson 1986). Heart rate is not a good predictor of RPE during endurance activity.

Johansson (1986) studied well-trained subjects over 50 min of cycling. Participants cycled at 50 W for 20 min, rested for 5 min, then continued for 30 min at both 100 W and 200 W. Exercise intensity was estimated to be 20%, 33% and 60% $\dot{V}O_{2max}$. Perceived effort accelerated negatively over time for both the 50 W and 200 W conditions. The HLa response at 200 W plateaued at 3.5 mmol·l^{-1} after 10 min. Although anaerobic threshold (AT) was not measured, it is common to use 4.0 mmol·l^{-1} as a standard reference point for HLa accumulation (Chapter 22). Therefore we can conjecture that the 200 W exercise intensity did not exceed the AT. It would not be surprising to find the AT above 60% $\dot{V}O_{2max}$ (200 W) or that any increase in lactate production was easily buffered in well-trained subjects. Thus, we can suggest that for exercise durations of 50 min, HLa is unlikely to predict the rise in RPE.

Pandolf et al. (1984) found that the overall RPE during arm crank exercise increased continually over 60 min at an absolute intensity demanding a $\dot{V}O_2$ of 1.6 l·min^{-1}. When the same subjects cycled with their legs for 60 min at the same absolute exercise intensity, a near steady-state RPE response was observed after 40 min. RPE increased continuously over 45 min of treadmill exercise at 75% $\dot{V}O_{2max}$ (Casal & Leon 1985).

Marathoners were asked to run on a treadmill

for 3 h, at a race pace established from previous performances (Bell 1975). Subjects began to withdraw from the protocol during the last hour; thus, the most reliable data were recorded over the first 2 h. Perceived exertion increased significantly, from approximately 9 at 15 min to 17.5 after 120 min of running. Oxygen consumption plateaued at $2.7 l \cdot min^{-1}$ while blood glucose decreased significantly. Glucose depletion was implicated in the increased RPE over time. In a glucose supplementation trial, RPE still increased, but to a lesser extent. It seems that the preponderance of evidence supports a progressive increase in perception of effort when exercise is conducted continuously for 15–120 min, at various intensities from 20 to 85% of $\dot{V}o_{2max}$, and across several modes of exercise (arm crank, cycle and treadmill).

EXERCISE INTENSITY AND DURATION

The work of Johansson (1986) suggests an influence of exercise intensity on perceived effort during prolonged activity. This experiment utilized Borg's CR-10 Scale (Borg 1982). Perceptual responses displayed a family of gradually increasing exponential curves as exercise intensity rose. Thirty-minute values were approximately 1.5 for 50 W, 3.5 for 100 W and 5.5 for 200 W. Thus, effort perceptions not only increased over time, but also increased as a function of exercise intensity. Skrinar et al. (1983) examined this question in women who had trained for 6–8 weeks over distances increasing from 32 to 80 km per week. In a 1-h treadmill run at 60%, 70% and 80% of $\dot{V}o_{2max}$ (20 min each), peak overall RPE increased significantly, to 10.3, 12.9 and 16.1 with rising exercise intensity. At 80% of $\dot{V}o_{2max}$ these trained subjects reached ratings above 15 ('hard') after only 20 min of exercise. Some cumulative effect from the previous 40 min of exercise may have occurred, even though the RPE responses to the 60% and 70% bouts were only 'light' to 'somewhat hard'. As with the previous studies, HLa differed significantly between intensities, although absolute values were not reported. Garcin et al. (1998b) recently confirmed the gradual increase in RPE during cycle exercise to exhaustion at 60%, 73% and 86% of $\dot{V}o_{2max}$.

MUSCLE MASS

The role of muscle mass in endurance exercise is of special interest to those engaged in triathlon competition, where swimming, a lower muscle mass activity, is coupled with running and cycling, both of which involve a larger muscle mass. Arm and leg exercise were compared with arm crank and cycle ergometers (Pandolf 1986). When energy expenditure was equated between the two exercise modes ($\dot{V}o_2 = 1.61 l \cdot min^{-1}$), effort was perceived to be lower in the high muscle mass activity, cycling. One can expect different perceptual experiences when arm and leg exercise are compared at the same absolute metabolic intensity, since more motor units are needed to elicit the same $\dot{V}o_2$ when arm cranking. Additionally, arm effort (peripheral) in swimming is known to exceed the effort perceived from respiratory–metabolic cues; thus the performer should pay close attention to peripheral cues when monitoring performance fatigue (Noble & Allen 1984).

HOLDING RPE CONSTANT

What happens when we try to perform at a constant RPE? This is one way of conceiving a strategic performance plan. The plan would be based on feeling, not pace, assuming that one could monitor perception successfully and adjust pace to modulate that perception. Ulmer (1986) conceived of a training plan in which a programme of effort perception would be preplanned before competition. The idea was that during competition, the plan could be modulated, depending on conditions, position of competitors and personal judgements of the difference between the degree of exhaustion and the distance/time remaining. This system depends on feedback from the environment, competition and self. Ulmer asked 11 runners to run 400 m and 1500 m at constant RPE levels of 8, 13 and 18. In addition, a race-pace maximum performance was monitored at each distance. These distances can hardly be considered endurance performances, but they illustrate an important principle of race tactics. Running times were monitored every 100 m, in order to evaluate pace. In the 400-m trials, running pace declined over the distance at all perception levels and at maximum effort. The average velocity declined successively from maximum effort down through the RPE = 8 trial, showing the validity of such a technique. With the rapid build-up of fatigue, downward adjustments in pace were necessary to keep a constant perceptual state. In contrast, pace for the 1500-m trials plateaued after the first 500–800 m, depending on the physical intensity level. Similar results were reported for cycling and swimming. Ulmer concluded that athletes can perform at given RPE set points. A useful competitive tactic would thus be to design a performance using a particular set point, making adjustments as circumstances demand.

PACE STRATEGY

Ariyoshi *et al.* (1979) studied 10 middle- and long-distance runners, examining responses to running 1400 m at three separate paces: fast/slow, gradually decreasing pace; slow/fast, gradually increasing pace; and a steady-state pace. All runs were completed in 4 min, representing an average velocity of 350 m·min^{-1}. Oxygen consumption plateaued after 2 min in all three trials. The slow/fast pace required a significantly lower $\dot{V}O_2$ than the fast/slow trial for the first 2 min. Perceptions did not differ between the slow/fast and steady-state trials. However, RPE was significantly lower for the final 2 min of the fast/slow method, compared to the slow/fast method. Maximum lactate production was significantly lower for the fast/slow pace. The authors concluded that their results validated coaches' beliefs, showing that the fast/slow method was superior. An explanation of this was based on the more rapid attainment of near-maximum $\dot{V}O_2$ levels and the recruitment of FT fibres early and ST fibres later. We encourage researchers to engage in these more practical studies to uncover the interaction of perception of effort and race tactics under endurance-distance conditions.

INTERACTION OF VARIOUS PHYSIOLOGICAL INDICES

The aforementioned studies bring us to the difficult matter of explaining the interaction of various physiological indices and the perception of effort in endurance performances. We will try to integrate information delineated in earlier sections with a few studies that have used long-duration experimental trials. The question of HR seems relatively clear. Although HR rises with the increase in exercise intensity, it remains relatively constant during long-duration work. Thus, HR is not a limiting factor either for perceptual effort, which rises with duration, or for the performance *per se*. The same pattern seems to hold for absolute $\dot{V}O_2$. Lactic acid accumulation, although often highly correlated with effort perceptions, is probably not a contributing factor until exercise intensities exceed the AT, and even then, any contribution would not appear until the buffering mechanisms could no longer maintain a constant pH. Endurance runners with high ATs can perform at very high metabolic levels without significant effects from lactate production.

SUBSTRATE AVAILABILITY

As mentioned earlier, Bell (1975) asked trained marathoners to run on the treadmill for 3 h at race pace. Blood glucose was manipulated by providing a supplemental glucose drink in one trial and a placebo in another. Although blood glucose decreased in both performances, especially in the second hour, the decrease was significantly less in the supplementation trial. Likewise, RPE was significantly lower with the administration of a glucose drink. These data, coupled with results that show the advantages of carbohydrate diet enhancement (Bergstrom *et al.* 1967), speak to the role that blood glucose plays in perception of effort and, of equal importance, they indicate that RPE reflects the performance decline. Bell's results are supported by other investigators (Burgess *et al.* 1990; Robertson *et al.* 1990).

Effort perceptions are related more to glucose levels than to lipid metabolism. In fact, FFA is known to increase while blood glucose is decreasing (Coyle *et al.* 1986). This occurs in the face of rising perceptual ratings during prolonged activity. Thus, it is likely that the availability of carbohydrate is critical to both continued exercise and the perception of that exercise. In contrast, lipids are rarely depleted and are not implicated (Noble & Robertson 1996).

IMPACT OF PSYCHOLOGICAL FACTORS

Few studies have looked specifically at the impact of psychological factors during prolonged performance. However, some designs have utilized exercise durations that might constitute endurance performance, and they may provide important insights and/or provide direction for future research. Rejeski and Ribisl (1980) evaluated the role of expected duration. The first trial that lasted 20 min was compared with a subsequent trial where subjects were told they would be exercising for 30 min but the exercise was terminated after only 20 min. Subjects suppressed RPE under these conditions. Whether this result was caused by the use of a dissociative mental strategy or by the duration of exercise itself, the perception changed even though physiological variables did not. The practical significance of this data for endurance performers is unclear, but the results support the view that more than physiology can drive perceptual response.

Expected performance was hypothesized to play a role in the modulation of effort perceptions during longer-term exercise (Zohar & Spitz 1981). Subjects were asked to ride a cycle ergometer as fast as possible, keeping in mind that they were expected to complete 45 min of exercise. Subjects were asked to rate their effort and their expected performance every 3 min. Expected performance for the subsequent 3-min period was based on feedback from the previous 3-min period. Subjects received either no feedback from previous performance, partial feedback, or full feedback. Expected and actual performance ran parallel and basically unchanged throughout the 45 min for the full and partial feedback groups. As is normal for longer-duration exercise, the RPE accelerated negatively over time. In the no feedback group, expected performance fell as exertion rose, so that a −0.90 correlation was observed. Perceived effort grew similarly between the three treatments; thus, falling expectations in the no feedback trial did not affect RPE any differently. Heart rate remained relatively unchanged through-

out the 45-min period in all three conditions. Since none of the feedback methods were found to be useful, the practice of providing split times may not be effective, at least with regard to modulating RPE. One can speculate that the high intensity used in this study limited the value of feedback, but evidence on this point is lacking. The work of Yu (1998) and Hardy *et al.* (1986) suggests that psychological factors are less salient at high exercise intensities.

Although Morgan and Pollock (1977) did not deal with perceived exertion, they addressed the important question of awareness strategies used by élite and non-élite marathoners during long-distance competition. Élite runners used an associative strategy, whereby they focused on body signals and could modulate race pace. Non-élite runners, on the other hand, used a dissociative strategy to maintain pace.

It is likely that runners use both strategies, but that one or the other predominates. From a perceptual point of view, dissociation is self-limiting and possibly injurious, whereas association utilizes awareness to facilitate performance. Not focusing on the body during intense heat is certainly not recommended. An awareness of body sensations may lead to an adaptive reduction of pace. Schomer (1987) suggested the use of a 'mental strategy training program' to optimize adaptation to long-distance running. He found that superior marathoners did not necessarily use associative strategies predominantly, despite the advantages of doing so. Schomer (1986) also found that more intense training was related to greater use of association. It appears that awareness strategies can be manipulated through training.

Further confirmation of the pliability of association was provided by Jones and Cale (1989). As perceived effort increased over a 16.8-km run, more association was used. Perhaps the physiological input becomes so strong that no other attentional focus is possible.

SUMMARY

The data indicate that perception of effort begins to increase fairly quickly after the start of endurance activity, probably within the first 2 min. This increase continues with a negative acceleration throughout performances that last 2 h and probably beyond. Since the curves are intensity dependent, performers whose activity lasts 4 or 5 h most likely have flatter slopes after the initial rise. More research is needed on longer-duration response patterns. Generally, we can say that HLa accumulation does not play a role in the rise of perceived effort when exercise intensity is below the AT, 13 units on the Borg Scale for women and 14 for men (Purvis & Cureton 1981); nor is it important above the AT until lactate buffering cannot keep up with production. Since a rating of 16 is associated with 90% $\dot{V}_{O_{2max}}$ (Noble & Robertson 1996) it is doubtful that performances above this level could be sustained. Successful performance is often a matter of pushing the edge of one's buffering system delicately. This metabolic balancing act may be achieved better by planning tactics that modulate pace by holding RPE constant, a method that has proven feasible. Heart rate and oxygen consumption are circumstantially linked, but perceived effort generally follows physical work rather than these metabolic markers. Blood glucose availability seems to be implicated in the setting of the perceptual report, especially after 1 h; thus glucose supplements may be advisable. Free fatty acids, in contrast, do not seem to be factors. Thus attempts to enhance them (e.g. by administering caffeine) probably will not produce a positive effect (Casal & Leon 1985). Hard research data are sparse regarding psychological contributions to effort perceptions during long-duration activity. Data suggest that psychological variables are less salient at the high exercise intensities commonly used by élite endurance athletes. The mental strategy known as association, which is preferable in long-duration activity where pace regulation depends so much on internal awareness, appears to be trainable.

Training

In this section we will discuss how the Borg Scale and similar perceptual measures can be utilized in training for endurance activity. Although one can be put off at first by unfamiliarity with the Borg Scale numbers (6–20) this difficulty is quickly overcome.

Of special importance to the effectiveness of the scale is the utility of the adjective/adverbial expressions attached to alternate numbers. These expressions have tremendous face value, especially above 10. Iteration of the number/expression pairs is instructive: 11—fairly light; 13—somewhat hard; 15—hard; 17—very hard; and 19—very, very hard (see Fig. 26.2). Experience with hundreds of subjects using the scale in testing and field situations, as well as matching ratings with physiological values, reveals several important practical insights. After 11 or 12 ('fairly light') on the Borg Scale, respiratory–metabolic variables have risen to a level that is readily noticed by the subject/performer— perhaps not the variables *per se*, but the physical effort required and certain secondary symptomatology. Most training, especially among recreational exercisers, occurs between 12 and 15 ('hard') on the scale, with 14 found to be a preferred level (Noble & Robertson 1996). These numbers can be raised a little for competitive endurance training, perhaps to 15–18 on harder workout days. Practical experience with endurance performers indicates that maintenance of hard effort (15) over a long period of time is possible, but most exercisers are less able to sustain levels much above 15.

ANAEROBIC THRESHOLD AS A
PRESCRIPTION MARKER

The AT is reached when RPE reaches 13 (women) or 14 (men) on the Borg Scale (Purvis & Cureton 1981) and this level is unaffected by training status (DeMello *et al.* 1987). Thus, the AT has been proposed as an important marker for the prescription of training intensity. Exercising above the AT would result in the accumulation of lactate which may affect comfort or necessitate lowering exercise intensity. Both training and competition can be conceived as a matter of regulating effort precisely, so that one stays at or just below the AT in recreational exercisers, or pushes into the anaerobic zone for possible training effects and competitive advantage in competitive athletes. It is possible to buffer HLa to maintain a steady pH above the AT, but going too far can be limiting (Noble 1986). The training zone for enhancing aerobic power and capacity is thought to lie between an RPE of 12 and 15, corresponding to 50% and 85% of $\dot{V}O_{2max}$ (Noble & Robertson 1996). Exercising at an RPE of 16 is associated with 90% of $\dot{V}O_{2max}$ which may push the exerciser beyond a point where pH is buffered effectively. Some exercisers, by virtue of either training or genetics, can exercise at a very high percentage of aerobic power before reaching the AT, i.e. greater than 13 or 14 on the scale. Frank Shorter, former élite American marathoner, could run at high percentages of his $\dot{V}O_{2max}$ without experiencing lactate overload (Noble 1986).

TRAINING CHANGES

If perception of effort is linked to physiological response it would be logical to assume that when physiological variables are altered with training, RPE would be similarly affected. Interpretation of training studies, however, is affected by whether data are expressed in absolute terms, the same $\dot{V}O_2$ level, or relative terms, the same percentage of $\dot{V}O_{2max}$, i.e. corrected for training increases in aerobic power. Endurance training should promote decreases in RPE when comparisons are made at absolute submaximal exercise intensities.

On the other hand, no change should be observed with relative intensity comparisons, i.e. RPE follows the physical load (Noble & Robertson 1996). Since increased aerobic power post-training demands a higher physical intensity in a relative comparison, RPE increases in post-training tests to levels approximating the pretraining level. Although RPE would not decrease in this scenario, the mere fact that the same value was achieved at a higher exercise intensity signifies a training effect. Two studies have supported the first half of this hypothesis, regarding absolute comparisons (Docktor & Sharkey 1971; Pandolf et al. 1975).

An early training study found significant increases in $\dot{V}O_{2max}$ after 8 weeks of cross-country running (Ekblom & Goldbarg 1971). When data were compared at absolute levels of submaximal $\dot{V}O_2$, RPE was significantly reduced. At equivalent percentages of $\dot{V}O_{2max}$ the authors reported, and have been widely quoted as saying, that RPE was unchanged by training. Re-examination of these data by the authors of the present chapter revealed

that, in fact, only at 100% intensity was there no clear difference. A significant reduction in RPE was found at 25%, 50% and probably 75% of $\dot{V}O_{2max}$. Ekblom and Goldbarg's data again support the absolute comparison aspect of the above hypothesis, but not the relative comparison feature.

Another study found the exact opposite of the results predicted by the above hypothesis. Following the training of men and women aged 60–70 years, Sidney and Shephard (1977) reported that RPE did not change at standard cycle ergometer loads, but that it was augmented at relative loads. When these subjects were compared to a group of younger subjects, RPE was found to be independent of both age and gender at relative exercise intensities. Still, the lower muscle mass typical of older exercisers would make relative post-training comparisons difficult to sustain.

Skrinar et al. (1983) trained women who progressed from 32 to 80 km weekly in a 6–8-week training programme. They reported a significant drop in overall RPE at 60%, 70% and 80% of $\dot{V}O_{2max}$. These data, also, do not support the relative comparison aspect of the above hypothesis. Another notable finding in this study involves the so-called differentiated perceptual responses. Overall and respiratory–metabolic reports changed significantly, but the peripheral reports did not. The authors speculated that the peripheral factor may be less susceptible to training.

Three out of four reviewed studies that made absolute comparisons before and after training reported a decrease in RPE, which seems to support the hypothesis. However, the three studies that measured training changes in RPE on a relative basis did not support the hypothesis. Additionally, two of these investigations reported decreases in RPE, whereas one found an increase. These differences may be a function of the age of the subjects and/or training intensities and durations.

Urhausen et al. (1998) evaluated perceptions of effort over a 19-month period in trained cyclists and triathletes. Ratings of perceived exertion were significantly impaired during overtraining, when compared to times when the athletes were not overtrained.

Training studies present complex logistical problems, especially if they are designed with appropriate controls. Pandolf *et al.* (1975) were the only investigators to use a control comparison group, and they only evaluated absolute changes. No standard ergometer was used in the training studies, i.e. some employed a cycle ergometer, whereas others used treadmills. Relative intensity levels were not standardized among investigations. Different exercise regimens were applied using several intensities and durations of training. Much more standardization and better controls are mandatory before we can evaluate hypotheses about training and perceptual responses adequately.

A practical point to be made concerning training studies is that absolute ratings may have greater utility to those who are training. Relative values are essential when comparisons are made between exercise modes, ages and genders. However, it is often more interesting for both the recreationist and the athlete to receive absolute exercise data when pre- and post-training changes are compared. The differences in absolute data that are often observed make the training efforts seem worthwhile. To report no change in relative values has a negative psychological effect. It can also be argued that there is a certain unfairness in relative comparisons. Trained subjects have to work harder during the post-training testing in order to reach the required $\%\dot{V}_{O_{2max}}$. This may place an undue strain on sites in and around the working muscles, making the comparison metabolically equal but not equal in peripheral stress.

INTERVAL VERSUS CONTINUOUS TRAINING

Endurance athletes have occasion to include shorter, more intense interval training into their workouts. It would seem reasonable that, given the same power output, interval training with its higher exercise intensities would be perceptually more intense than training at a continuous pace. This hypothesis has been tested and confirmed (Edwards *et al.* 1972). Perception, $\dot{V}_{O_2}$, HR and HLa were all higher with interval workouts, even though the training dose, measured in total work output, was held constant. Higher RPEs can be tolerated during shorter inter-

val bouts of training, as the glycolytic metabolic system and FT fibres are being challenged. This stimulus differs from the aerobic system and the ST fibres utilized in less intense, longer-duration exercise.

TRAINING SUMMARY

The training zone for achieving improvements in endurance lies between 12 and 15 on the RPE scale, equivalent to 50% and 85% of $\dot{V}_{O_{2max}}$. Élite competitors may be able to push their RPEs above 15 during continuous training, but they risk going above the point where HLa can be buffered effectively. With interval training, it is possible to tolerate higher RPE levels because of their shorter duration. Data support the use of absolute exercise intensity comparisons for evaluating RPE changes following training. The value of relative exercise intensity comparisons is less clear.

Conclusions

A psychophysiological model has been described, based on a parallel processing paradigm with four input sources: physiological signals, psychological factors, performance milieu elements and exertional symptoms. Physiological signals and psychological factors exert their influence in parallel, prior to integration in the cerebral cortex. Physiological signals are derived from three sources: respiratory–metabolic mediators, peripheral mediators and non-specific physiological sources. Psychological factors are grouped into those that are situational in nature and those that are disposition related.

Respiratory–metabolic mediators have their greatest effect at higher exercise intensities. Pulmonary ventilation is a major mediator in this category. Relative oxygen consumption ($\%\dot{V}_{O_{2max}}$) has a strong link with perceptual ratings as well.

Peripheral mediators dominate at all levels of exercise intensity. Potential variables include pH, fibre type and muscle blood flow. The availability of blood glucose appears to be a strong contributor, especially after 1 h of endurance activity. Possible non-specific mediators include hormonal regulation, temperature regulation and pain reactivity.

Situational psychological factors that may be linked to effort perception during endurance activity are expected duration, self-presentation and attentional focus. Psychological contributions appear to decline as physiological signals increase at the higher exercise intensities. Personality, stimulus intensity modulation, self-efficacy and associative mental strategies are promising dispositional factors.

Physiological and psychological factors are both known contributors to the perception of effort. Psychological contributions are highest at low exercise intensities and physiological contributions exert their greatest influence at higher exercise intensities.

The Borg Scale provides a reliable and valid method for assessing effort perception. It is recommended that scale users receive: a clear definition of effort perception and description of scale use; a definitional description or behavioural experience of the limits of the perceptual range; and instruction

as to what to monitor, whether an overall sense of effort and/or differentiated effort.

RPE increases with exercise duration, beginning as early as 1 or 2 min, and increasing with a negative acceleration. Blood glucose supplements should be considered, especially after 1 h, because they reduce perception of effort. Use of an associative mental strategy is recommended, and it seems that this factor is trainable.

Endurance training should be performed at an RPE of 12–15, equivalent to 50–85% of $\dot{V}O_{2max}$. RPE at the AT is about 13 for women and 14 for men, and it appears to be unaffected by the state of training. If training and performance RPE rise above 15, the trainee/performer is flirting with lactate accumulation that cannot be buffered sufficiently to regulate pH. The use of RPE to regulate and evaluate training provides a mixed picture. Changes can be found when RPE is compared on an absolute basis ($\dot{V}O_2$) but it is unclear whether changes can be demonstrated by using relative values ($\%\dot{V}O_{2max}$).

References

Ariyoshi, M., Tanaka, H., Kanamori, K. et al. (1979) Influence of running pace upon performance: Effects upon oxygen intake, blood lactate, and rating of perceived exertion. *Canadian Journal of Applied Sports Science* 4, 210–213.

Bandura, A. (1977) Self-efficacy: toward a unifying theory of behavioral change. *Psychological Review* 84, 191–215.

Bartley, S.H. (1970) The homeostatic and comfort perceptual systems. *Journal of Psychology* 75, 157–162.

Baumeister, R.F. (1982) A self-presentational view of social phenomena. *Psychological Bulletin* 91, 3–26.

Bell, C.W. (1975) *Perceptual, biochemical, and physiological responses in long term work, an investigation of the influence of glucose ingestion.* Unpublished doctoral dissertation, University of Pittsburgh.

Bergstrom, J., Hermansen, L., Hultman, E. et al. (1967) Diet, muscle glycogen, and physical performance. *Acta Physiologica Scandinavica* 71, 140.

Borg, G. (1961) Perceived exertion in relation to physical work load and pulse rate. *Kungliga Fysiografiska Sallskapets i Lund Forhandlinger* 31, 105–115.

Borg, G. (1962) *Physical Performance and Perceived Exertion.* Gleerup, Lund, Sweden.

Borg, G. (1970) Perceived exertion as an indicator of somatic stress. *Scandinavian Journal of Rehabilitation Medicine* 2, 92–98.

Borg, G. (1982) Psychophysical bases of perceived exertion. *Medicine and Science in Sports and Exercise* 14, 377–381.

Borg, G. (1998) *Borg's Perceived Exertion and Pain Scales.* Human Kinetics, Champaign, IL.

Borg, G. & Johansson, S.E. (1986) The growth of perceived exertion during a prolonged bicycle ergometer test at a constant workload. In: Borg, G. & Ottoson, D. (eds) *The Perception of Exertion in Physical Work*, pp. 47–55. Macmillan, London.

Boucher, S. & Trenske, M. (1990) The effects of sensory deprivation and music on perceived exertion and affect during exercise. *Journal of Sport and Exercise Psychology* 12, 167–176.

Boucher, S., Fleischer-Curtian, L. & Gines, S. (1988) The effects of self-presentation on perceived exertion. *Journal of Sport and Exercise Psychology* 10, 270–280.

Burgess, M., Robertson, R., Davis, J. & Norris, J. (1990) RPE, blood glucose, and carbohydrate oxidation during exercise: Effects of glucose feedings. *Medicine and Science in Sports and Exercise* 23, 353–359.

Cafarelli, E. (1982) Peripheral contribu-

tions to the perception of effort. *Medicine and Science in Sports and Exercise* 14, 382–389.

Cain, W. & Stevens, J. (1973) Constant effort contractions related to the electromyogram. *Medicine and Science in Sports and Exercise* 5, 121–127.

Casal, D. & Leon, A. (1985) Failure of caffeine to affect substrate utilization during prolonged running. *Medicine and Science in Sports and Exercise* 17, 174–179.

Copeland, B. & Franks, B. (1991) Effects of types and intensities of background music on treadmill endurance. *Journal of Sports Medicine and Physical Fitness* 31, 100–103.

Coyle, E., Coggan, A., Hemmert, M. & Ivy, J. (1986) Muscle glycogen utilization during prolonged strenuous exercise when fed carbohydrate. *Journal of Applied Physiology* 61, 165–172.

Davies, C. & Sargeant, A. (1979) The effects of atropine and practolol on the perception of exertion during treadmill exercise. *Ergonomics* 22, 1141–1146.

DeMello, J., Cureton, K., Boineau, R. & Singh, M. (1987) Ratings of perceived exertion at the lactate threshold in trained and untrained men and women. *Medicine and Science in Sports and Exercise* 19, 354–362.

Dishman, R., Graham, R., Holly, R. & Tieman, J. (1991) Estimates of type A behavior do not predict perceived exertion during graded exercise. *Medicine and Science in Sports and Exercise* 23, 1276–1282.

Docktor, R. & Sharkey, B. (1971) Note on some physiological and subjective reactions to exercise and training. *Perceptual and Motor Skills* 32, 233–234.

Edwards, R., Melcher, A., Hesser, C., Wigerbtz, O. & Ekelund, L. (1972) Physiological correlates of perceived exertion in continuous and intermittent exercise with the same average power output. *European Journal of Clinical Investigation* 2, 108–114.

Ekblom, B. & Goldbarg, A. (1971) The influence of physical training and other factors on the subjective rating of perceived exertion. *Acta Physiologica Scandinavica* 83, 399–406.

Eston, R.G. & Williams, J.G. (1986) Exercise intensity and perceived exertion in adolescent boys. *British Journal of Sports Medicine* 20, 27–30.

Fillingim, R., Roth, D. & Haley, W. (1989) The effects of distraction on the perception of exercise-induced symptoms. *Journal of Psychosomatic Research* 33, 241–248.

Foster, C., Costill, D. & Fink, W. (1979) Effects of pre-exercise feedings on endurance performance. *Medicine and Science in Sports and Exercise* 11, 1–5.

Franks, B. & Myers, B. (1984) Effects of talking on exercise tolerance. *Research Quarterly for Exercise and Sport* 55, 237–241.

Garcin, M., Vautier, J., Vandewalle, H. & Monod, H. (1998a) Ratings of perceived exertion (RPE) as an index of aerobic endurance during local and general exercises. *Ergonomics* 41, 1105–1114.

Garcin, M., Vautier, J., Vandewalle, H., Wolff, M. & Monod, H. (1998b) Ratings of perceived exertion (RPE) during cycling exercises at constant power output. *Ergonomics* 41, 1500–1509.

Hardy, C., Hall, E. & Prestholdt, P. (1986) The mediational role of social influence in the perception of exertion. *Journal of Sport Psychology* 8, 88–104.

Hogan, J., Ogden, G., Gebhardt, D. & Fleishman, E. (1980) Reliability and validity of methods for evaluating perceived physical effort. *Journal of Applied Psychology* 65, 672–679.

James, W. (1890) *Principles of Psychology*. Holt, New York.

Johansson, S.-E. (1986) Perceived exertion, heart rate and blood lactate during prolonged exercise on a bicycle ergometer.

In: Borg, G. & Ottoson, D. (eds) *The Perception of Exertion in Physical Work*, pp. 57–68. Macmillan, London.

Johnson, J. & Siegel, D. (1987) Active vs. passive attentional manipulation and multidimensional perceptions of exercise intensity. *Canadian Journal of Sport Sciences* 12, 41–45.

Jones, J. & Cale, A. (1989) Changes in mood and cognitive functioning during long distance running—an exploratory investigation. *Physical Education Reviews* 12, 78–83.

Jung, C. (1921) *Psychological Types*. Princeton University Press, Princeton, NJ.

Kinsman, R. & Weiser, P. (1976) Subjective symptomatology during work and fatigue. In: Simonson, E. & Weiser, P. (eds) *Psychological Aspects and Physiological Correlates of Work and Fatigue*, pp. 336–405. Charles C. Thomas, Springfield, IL.

Kohl, R. & Shea, C. (1988) Perceived exertion: influences of locus of control and expected work intensity and duration. *Journal of Human Movement Studies* 15, 225–272.

Koivula, N. & Hassmen, P. (1998) Central, local, and overall ratings of perceived exertion during cycling and running by women with an external and internal locus of control. *General Psychology* 125, 17–29.

Kostka, C. & Cafarelli, E. (1982) Effect of pH on sensation and vastus lateralis electromyogram during cycling exercises. *Journal of Applied Physiology* 52, 1181–1185.

Levanthal, H. & Everhart, D. (1979) Emotion, pain and physical illness. In: Izard, C. (ed.) *Emotions in Personality and Psychopathology*. Plenum Press, New York.

Lollgen, H., Graham, T. & Sjoggard, G. (1980) Muscle metabolites, force, and perceived exertion bicycling at varying pedal rates. *Medicine and Science in Sports and Exercise* 12, 345–351.

McAuley, E. & Courneya, K. (1992) Self-efficacy relationships with affective and exertion responses to exercise. *Journal of Applied Social Psychology* 22, 312–326.

McCloskey, D., Gandevia, S., Potter, E. & Colebatch, J. (1983) Muscle sense and effort: motor commands and judgements about muscular contractions. *Advances in Neurology* 39, 151–167.

Morgan, W. (1973) Psychological factors influencing perceived exertion. *Medicine and Science in Sports and Exercise* 5, 97–103.

Morgan, W. (1976) Hypnotic perturbation

of perceived exertion: Ventilatory consequences. *American Journal of Clinical Hypnosis* 18, 182–190.

Morgan, W. (1981) C. H. McCloy research lecture: Psychophysiology of self-awareness during vigorous physical activity. *Research Quarterly for Exercise and Sport* 52, 385–427.

Morgan, W. & Costill, D. (1972) Psychological characteristics of the marathon runner. *Journal of Sports Medicine and Physical Fitness* 12, 42–46.

Morgan, W. & Pollock, M. (1977) Psychological characteristics of élite runners. *Annals of the New York Academy of Science* 301, 382–403.

Nadel, E. (1980) Circulatory and thermal regulations during exercise. *Federation Proceedings* 39, 1491–1497.

Noble, B. (1986) *Physiology of Exercise and Sport*. Times Mirror/Mosby, St. Louis, MO.

Noble, B. & Allen, J. (1984) Perceived exertion in swimming. *Swimming Technique* 21, 11–15.

Noble, B. & Noble, J. (1998) Perceived exertion: the measurement. In: Duda, J. (ed.) *Advances in Sport and Exercise Psychology Measurement*, pp. 351–359. Fitness Information Technology, Inc., Morgantown, WV.

Noble, B. & Robertson, R. (1996) *Perceived Exertion*. Human Kinetics, Champaign, IL.

Noble, B., Metz, K., Pandolf, K., Bell, C., Cafarelli, E. & Sime, W. (1973a) Perceived exertion during walking and running II. *Medicine and Science in Sports and Exercise* 5, 116–120.

Noble, B., Metz, K., Pandolf, K. & Cafarelli, E. (1973b) Perceptual responses to exercise: a multiple regression study. *Medicine and Science in Sports and Exercise* 5, 104–109.

Noble, B., Borg, G., Jacobs, I., Ceci, R. & Kaiser, P. (1983) A category-ratio perceived exertion scale: Relationship to blood and muscle lactates and heart rate. *Medicine and Science in Sports and Exercise* 15, 523–528.

Noble, B., Kraemer, W., Allen, J., Plank, J. & Woodward, L. (1986) The integration of physiological cues in effort perception: Stimulus strength vs. relative contribution. In: Borg, G. & Ottoson, D. (eds) *The Perception of Exertion in Physical Work*, pp. 83–96. Macmillan, London.

Pandolf, K. (1983) Advances in the study and application of perceived exertion. *Exercise and Sport Sciences Reviews* 11, 118–158.

Pandolf, K. (1986) Local and central factor contributions in the perception of effort during physical exercise. In: Borg, G. & Ottoson, D. (eds) *The Perception of Effort in Physical Work*, pp. 97–110. Macmillan, London.

Pandolf, K. & Noble, B. (1973) The effect of pedalling speed and resistance changes on perceived exertion for equivalent power outputs on the bicycle ergometer. *Medicine and Science in Sports and Exercise* 5, 132–136.

Pandolf, K., Cafarelli, E., Noble, B. & Metz, K. (1972) Perceptual responses during prolonged work. *Perceptual and Motor Skills* 35, 975–985.

Pandolf, K., Burse, R. & Goldman, R. (1975) Differentiated ratings of perceived exertion during physical conditioning of older individuals using leg weight loading. *Perceptual and Motor Skills* 40, 563–574.

Pandolf, K., Billings, D., Drolet, L., Pimetal, N. & Sawka, M. (1984) Differential ratings of perceived exertion and various physiological responses during prolonged upper and lower body exercise. *European Journal of Applied Physiology* 53, 5–11.

Pederson, P. & Welch, H. (1977) Oxygen breathing, selected physiological variables and perception of effort during submaximal exercise. In: Borg, G. (ed.) *Physical Work and Effort*, pp. 385–400. Pergamon Press, New York.

Pennebaker, J. & Lightner, J. (1980) Competition of internal and external information in an exercise setting. *Journal of Personality and Social Psychology* 39, 165–174.

Petrie, A. (1967) *Individuality in Pain and Suffering*. University of Chicago Press, Chicago.

Pivarnik, J. & Senay, L. (1986) Effect of endurance training and heat acclimation on perceived exertion during exercise. *Journal of Cardiopulmonary Rehabilitation* 6, 499–504.

Poulus, A., Docter, H. & Westra, H. (1974) Acid–base balance and subjective feelings of fatigue during physical exercise. *European Journal of Applied Physiology* 33, 207–213.

Purvis, J. & Cureton, K. (1981) Ratings of perceived exertion at the anaerobic threshold. *Ergonomics* 24, 295–300.

Rejeski, W. & Ribisl, P. (1980) Expected task duration and perceived effort: an attributional analysis. *Journal of Sport Psychology* 2, 227–236.

Robertson, R. & Metz, K. (1986) Ventilatory precursors for central signals of perceived exertion. In: Borg, G. & Ottoson, D. (eds) *The Perception of Exertion in Physical Work*, pp. 111–121. Macmillan, London.

Robertson, R., Gillespie, R., Hiatt, E. & Rose, K. (1977) Perceived exertion and stimulus intensity modulation. *Perceptual and Motor Skills* 45, 211–218.

Robertson, R., Gillespie, R., McCarthy, J. & Rose, K. (1978) Perceived exertion and the field-independence-dependence dimension. *Perceptual and Motor Skills* 46, 495–500.

Robertson, R., Gilcher, R., Metz, K. *et al.* (1982) Effect of induced erythrocythemia on hypoxia tolerance during physical exercise. *Journal of Applied Physiology* 53, 490–495.

Robertson, R., Falkel, J., Drash, A. *et al.* (1986) Effect of blood pH on peripheral and central signals of perceived exertion. *Medicine and Science in Sports and Exercise* 18, 114–122.

Robertson, R., Stanko, R., Goss, F., Spina, R., Reilly, J. & Greenwalt, K. (1990) Blood glucose extraction as a mediator of perceived exertion during prolonged exercise. *European Journal of Applied Physiology* 61, 100–105.

Rudolph, P. & McAuley, E. (1998) Cortisol and affective responses to exercise. *Journal of Sports Science* 16, 121–128.

Schomer, H. (1986) Mental strategies and the perception of effort of marathon runners. *International Journal of Sports Psychology* 17, 41–59.

Schomer, H. (1987) Mental strategy training programme for marathon runners. *International Journal of Sports Psychology* 18, 133–151.

Sherrington, C. (1900) The muscle sense. In: Schafer, E. (ed.) *Textbook of Physiology*. Pentland, Edinburgh and London.

Sidney, K. & Shephard, R. (1977) Perception of exertion in the elderly, effects of aging, mode of exercise, and physical training. *Perceptual and Motor Skills* 44, 999–1010.

Skinner, J., Hustler, R., Bergsteinova, V. & Buskirk, E. (1973) The validity and reliability of a rating scale of perceived exertion. *Medicine and Science in Sports and Exercise* 5, 97–103.

Skrinar, G., Ingram, S. & Pandolf, K. (1983) Effect of endurance training on perceived exertion and stress hormones in women. *Perceptual and Motor Skills* 57, 1239–1250.

Stamford, B. (1976) Validity and reliability of subjective ratings of perceived exertion during work. *Ergonomics* 19, 53–60.

Stamford, B. & Noble, B. (1974) Metabolic cost and perception of effort during bicycle ergometer work performance. *Medicine and Science in Sports and Exercise* 6, 226–231.

Stevens, S. (1957) On the psychophysical law. *Psychological Review* 64, 153–181.

Stevens, S. & Galanter, E. (1957) Ratio scales and category scales for a dozen perceptual continua. *Journal of Experimental Psychology* 54, 377–411.

Stevens, J. & Krimsley, A. (1977) Build-up of fatigue in static work: Role of blood flow. In: Borg, G. (ed.) *Physical Work and Effort*, pp. 145–156. Pergamon, New York.

Sylva, M., Byrd, R. & Mangum, M. (1990) Effects of social influence and sex on rating of perceived exertion in exercising élite athletes. *Perceptual and Motor Skills* 70, 591–594.

Tesch, P. (1980) Muscle fatigue in man with special reference to lactate accumulation during short term intense work. *Acta Physiologica Scandinavica* (Suppl.) 480, 5–31.

Ulmer, H. (1986) Perceived exertion as a part of a feedback system and its interaction with tactical behavior in endurance sports. In: Borg, G. & Ottoson, D. (eds) *The Perception of Exertion in Physical Work*, pp. 317–326. Macmillan, London.

Urhausen, A., Gabriel, H., Weiler, B. & Kindermann, W. (1998) Ergometric and psychological findings during overtraining: a long-term follow-up study in endurance athletes. *International Journal of Sports Medicine* 19, 114–120.

Weiser, P., Kinsman, R. & Stamper, D. (1973) Task specific symptomatology changes resulting from prolonged submaximal bicycle riding. *Medicine and Science in Sports and Exercise* 5, 79–85.

Wrisberg, C., Franks, B., Birdwell, M. & High, D. (1988) Physiological and psychological responses to exercise with an induced attentional focus. *Perceptual and Motor Skills* 66, 603–618.

Young, A., Cymerman, A. & Pandolf, K. (1982) Differentiated ratings of perceived exertion are influenced by high altitude exposures. *Medicine and Science in Sports and Exercise* 14, 223–228.

Yu, M. (1998) *Perceived exertion: integration of psychological and physiological factors*. Unpublished doctoral dissertation, Purdue University.

Zohar, D. & Spitz, G. (1981) Expected performance and perceived exertion in a prolonged physical task. *Perceptual and Motor Skills* 52, 975–984.

PART 4

PRINCIPLES OF ENDURANCE PREPARATION

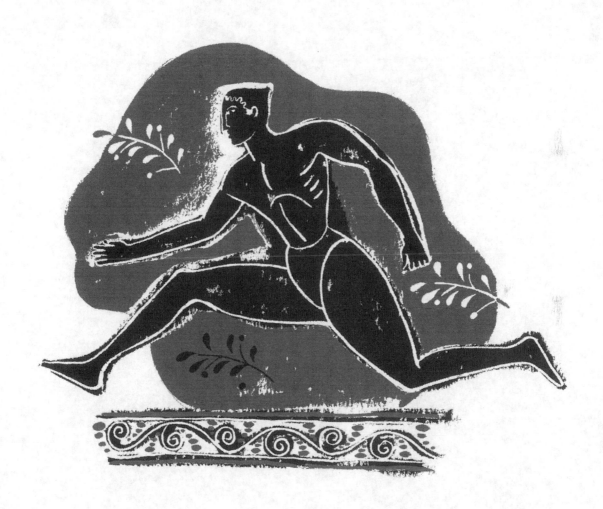

Chapter 27

Influences of Biological Age and Selection

PER-OLOF ÅSTRAND

Chronological versus biological age

Chronological age is not a good reference point for the analysis of biological data, particularly in the case of children and teenagers. However, in physical activity programmes young people are nearly always teamed against each other by chronological age.

It is an inevitable evolutionary consequence that individuals within a species differ from each other in many ways. Tanner (1980) has established the general framework of biological age. The most reliable criterion for assessing biological age is skeletal or bone age. However, the method of establishing bone age is quite complicated: it needs special apparatus (X-ray) and is time consuming. More readily applicable methods are measurements of physical characteristics such as body height and mass at least twice a year, and observations on the development of secondary sex characteristics, such as breasts, pubic hair and time of first menstruation in girls, and genital and pubic hair in boys. Figure 27.1 gives an example of the growth of height in one boy.

During the first years of life, the child grows rapidly, followed by a slower growth rate for about a 10-year period. Then comes a second spurt, when (in northern Europe and North America) the increase in height is, on average, about 0.08 m per year for girls, and about 0.1 m for boys. A girl's first menstruation normally occurs shortly after this accelerated growth period, with a time lag of about 1 year. The development of the secondary sex characteristics for both girls and boys is also related to this adolescent growth spurt, which is described as the age at peak height velocity (PHV age). A peak body mass velocity is usually observed some months later. Results from a Swedish longitudinal study are presented in Fig. 27.2 (Lindgren 1978). The PHV age occurred as early as 9.5 years for one girl, but was delayed until the age of 15 years for another. In the boys' group, one had his adolescent growth spurt at the age of 11 years, but another had his as late as 17 years. The PHV age was, on average, at an age of 12 years for girls and 2 years later for boys. At the age of about 13 years, the majority of the girls were already 'young women', while the boys were still children. In this study the PHV ages varied around 5 chronological years within each gender and the total variation was at least 7 chronological years (Fig. 27.2). The greatest interindividual variation in biological age was observed between the chronological ages of 12 and 14 years. Table 27.1 illustrates the quite dramatic interindividual difference in body size and maximal aerobic power in 13-year-old girls and boys.

The characterization of an individual on the basis of calendar age may be practical, but it is biologically unsound. However, an alternative basis of classification is not easy to find. At any rate, it is important to be aware of the problem. Because the adolescent growth spurt has a profound effect on physical performance, it is not only unfair, but may even be harmful, to group children athletically according to calendar age. An individual who has developed early may be at the top of his or her class athletically for a period of time, causing the parents and coach to overestimate his or her athletic talent.

397

In time, his or her classmates may catch up, only to show that the early success was not due to talent, but was simply a matter of early maturation. For a relatively long period, the early maturer may achieve success and be held in high esteem by her or his peers. In contrast, the late maturer is left behind in relation to athletic success in events where body size is important. It may be traumatic to find one is a champion one year, but only an average athlete the next; the interest in sports may be lost.

As an individual ages, the genetic code may have more of an effect than environment and lifestyle on the function of key systems that are important for physical performance. However, a change in lifestyle can definitely modify the 'biological age', either upward or downward, at almost any chronological age.

Early specialization in sports

The early maturer who eventually becomes a 'retired athlete' might have specialized in one or two events but have had real talent for another event which she or he never tried. There are anecdo-

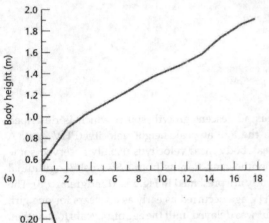

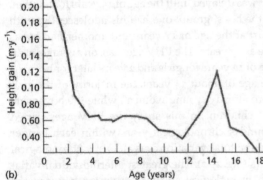

Fig. 27.1 The growth in height of a French boy recorded by his father De Montbeillard, 1759–1777: (a) shows the gradual gain during an 18-year period; (b) shows the height gain each year. Note the accelerated growth at about the age of 14–15 years ('peak height velocity'). From Tanner (1962), with permission.

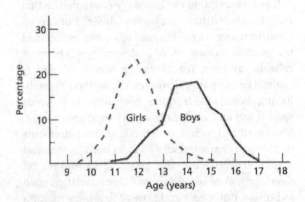

Fig. 27.2 Distribution of age at peak height velocity for girls ($n = 358$) and boys ($n = 373$). Modified from Lindgren (1978).

Table 27.1 Range of scores (R) in height, body mass and $\dot{V}o_{2max}$ for boys and girls aged 13 years in the Growth and Fitness Study in Sydney 1972–1973. From Russo *et al.* (1975).

Characteristics	Range of scores at the age of 13 years	
	Boys	Girls
Height (m)	1.34–1.81 ($R = 0.47$)	1.41–1.70 ($R = 0.29$)
Body mass (kg)	29–84 ($R = 55$)	28–79 ($R = 51$)
$\dot{V}o_{2max}$ (ml·kg^{-1}·min^{-1})	31–77 ($R = 46$)	18–74 ($R = 56$)

tal reports of intense, successful coaching in high-jumping or basketball with prepubertal girls and boys. If the height gain after PHV age stops at 1.6 and 1.7 m, respectively, then the wrong sports were chosen for these children. Again, these individuals perhaps had talents for sports where body height was not a basic prerequisite for success. Therefore, children and teenagers should be stimulated to be physically active and to try many different sports — a 'smörgåsbord'. It is a special challenge for parents, teachers, coaches and administrators to promote activities that maintain the late maturer's interest in and adherence to an active lifestyle.

A study of Swedish élite tennis players reported that five male players who were ranked among the 15 top tennis players in the world had participated in all-round sports activities up to the age of about 14 years. They then discovered that they were most successful in tennis, and so specialized 100% in tennis. They were compared with another group of players who were as good or better when 11–13 years old. Those players specialized much earlier in tennis, they trained more and matured earlier. However, they were apparently not gifted enough to reach world-class competition (Carlson 1988). Perhaps they should have tried and been successful in another sport? One conclusion from the study of tennis players mentioned above is that the performance at age 11–13 is not a good predictor of future élite achievements. Malina (1994) points out that, with few exceptions, interage correlations for indicators of growth, fitness and cardiovascular status are generally moderate to low and thus have limited predictive utility.

Another example of a sport with early selection based on chronological age is soccer. Junior players are often selected during phases of rapid growth and development. One of the problems faced by those responsible for the identification of élite players at junior level is to identify those who possess talent, but who are still at a relatively low level of physical maturity. It may be difficult for the talented but less physically mature individuals to be selected for junior representative squads (Brewer *et al.* 1995). These authors reported that English professional clubs employ a limited number of junior players aged between 17 and 19 years, with the intent that they will become future senior professional players. In England, the selection year is consistent with the academic year, starting in September and ending in August. They noted that between 1992 and 1994, 53% of these players were born between September and December, and only 16% between May and August! In view of the tendency to select physically mature individuals at a given chronological age, and the consequent large-scale omission of equally talented but less mature individuals, it would seem sensible to review procedures for selecting junior squads.

It is still debatable whether a high intensity and volume of training may affect PHV age and the time of menarche. After a review of the literature, Malina (1994) concluded that in the vast majority of athletes, intensive training for sport had no effect on growth and maturation. Menarche is to a large extent determined by biological selection and social factors.

Training can improve muscular strength and aerobic and anaerobic power in children (Armstrong & Welsman 1997). However, athletic training should be under the guidance and supervision of experienced coaches. Parents, teachers and coaches must have a good knowledge of the distinction between chronological and biological age.

Maffulli (1990) points out that 'during the growth spurt a dissociation between bone matrix formation and bone mineralization occurs, thus leaving the child with the risks of chronic moderate-to-high overloading, sudden great overload, and diminished bone strength'. Also, epiphyseal plate ('growth plate') injuries can have disastrous consequences. An early specialization with frequent, repetitive, monotonous activities may induce an overloading of the young athlete's musculoskeletal system. (Certainly the adult athlete also takes risks: see Chapters 35 and 52.) Endurance running is a typical stress factor, and each step can contribute to cumulative microtrauma. The marathon should be prohibited for children and young teenagers. In Sweden the minimum age for participation is 17 years, which is quite logical because, according to Fig. 27.2, all individuals have by then passed their PHV age.

Talent identification and development

At the 1988 Seoul Olympic Scientific Congress, two sessions were devoted to this theme. No doubt it is the ambition of sports associations and coaches to find young presumptive champions and keep them in a 'nursery' with efficient training facilities. In my opinion this is a doubtful strategy. As pointed out, children and teenagers should be stimulated and helped to try a wide variety of sports. Sports for young people should not be too serious: they should be fun and games. During growth it is hard to decide who will develop the best physical structure for a particular sport discipline. At one stage it was believed that muscle biopsy might reveal whether a person had a fibre type that was optimal for a specific type of sport. However, with the exception of long-distance runners and skiers, top athletes in other types of sport, e.g. players in ball games, exhibit a wide variety of fibre types. Success in a sport is highly genotype dependent. The person who wants to become a champion must be very careful when selecting her or his parents! Figure 27.3

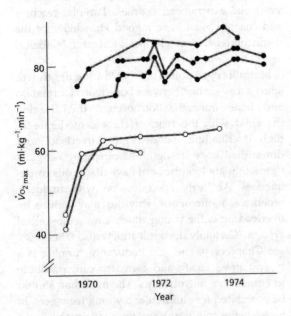

Fig. 27.3 Maximal oxygen intake in three internationally successful cross-country skiers (●) and in two 'normal' subjects (○) who started intensive training of aerobic power in 1969. Courtesy of U. Bergh and B. Ekblom.

Table 27.2 Number of medals won by the East German national swimming team in the European Championship (EC) and the World Championship (WC) out of the possible totals.

	Women		Men	
	Gold	Silver	Gold	Silver
EC in Rome 1983	15/15	12/12	1/15	6/15
EC in Sofia 1985	14/15	10/12	2/15	6/15
WC in Madrid 1986	13/16	8/13	1/16	4/15

gives an example of two sedentary males who started an intensive training programme comparable to those of top athletes. They made impressive progress, with an increase in maximal oxygen intake from $40–45\,ml\cdot kg^{-1}\cdot min^{-1}$ to about $60\,ml\cdot kg^{-1}\cdot min^{-1}$, but that was their definite ceiling: it is far from the 80 $ml\cdot kg^{-1}\cdot min^{-1}$ that characterizes élite cross-country skiers and middle-distance runners. Bouchard *et al.* (1988) reported that 77% of the variance in maximal aerobic power training response seemed to be genotype dependent. The subjects were monozygotic twins. About 5% of a sedentary population were estimated to have improved by less than 5% with a given training programme. Another 5% of the population were reported to have improved their maximal aerobic power by 60% or more. The authors pointed out that at present there are no genetic markers that can be used to type an individual for sensitivity to training (Chapter 15).

At the Seoul Congress there was a discussion of East German successes in talent identification and development. East German female swimmers have been extremely successful in European and World Championships (Table 27.2). However, the male swimmers were not so outstanding. In the 1988 Olympic Games in Seoul the East German women won 10 out of 15 gold medals, but the men only one out of 16. In the 1992 Olympic Games in Barcelona, with a joint Germany, the female team only won one gold medal. Trials are taking place in Germany in which the 1988 team physicians and coaches have been accused of 'manipulating' the athletes with various drugs listed as doping agents.

References

Armstrong N. & Welsman J. (1997) *Young People and Physical Activity*. Oxford University Press, Oxford.

Bouchard, C., Boulay, M.R., Simoneau, J.-A., Lortie, G. & Pérusse, L. (1988) Heredity and trainability of aerobic and anaerobic performances. *Sports Medicine* 5, 69–73.

Brewer, R.M., Balsom, P. & Davis, J. (1995) Seasonal birth distribution amongst European soccer players. *Sports Exercise and Injury* 1, 154–157.

Carlson, R. (1988) The socialization of élite tennis players in Sweden: an analysis of the players' backgrounds and development. *Sociology of Sport Journal* 5, 241–256.

Lindgren, G. (1978) Growth of schoolchildren with early, average and late ages of peak height velocity. *Annals of Human Biology* 5, 253–267.

Maffulli, N. (1990) Intensive training in young athletes: the orthopaedic surgeon's viewpoint. *Sports Medicine* 9, 229–243.

Malina, R.M. (1994) Physical growth and biological maturation of young athletes. *Exercise and Sport Sciences Reviews* 22, 389–434.

Tanner, J.M. (1962) *Growth of Adolescence*, 2nd edn. Blackwell Scientific Publications, Oxford.

Tanner, J.M. (1980) *Foetus into Man. Physical Growth from Conception to Maturity*, 2nd edn. Castlemead Publications, Ware.

Chapter 28

Endurance Conditioning

JAN SVEDENHAG

Introduction

Some of the basic training principles and physiological changes of endurance conditioning have been known for half a century or more. However, the increased interest in endurance training and especially long-distance running during the last decades has created unique opportunities for more thorough studies on the physiology of endurance conditioning and racing performance. This has led to a better understanding of the factors determining endurance capacity.

In this chapter, general training considerations and specific training factors will be discussed. Firstly, the basic physiological factors determining success in endurance events will be reviewed. Since most of the applied research carried out by the present author has dealt with male middle- and long-distance runners (of various abilities), and since running is one of the oldest and most widespread sports around the globe, the runner will also form the basis of these discussions.

Physiological factors related to endurance performance and their interrelationships

Maximal oxygen intake

Since the 1930s it has been known that the maximal oxygen intake ($\dot{V}_{O_{2max}}$) is exceptionally high in élite endurance-event athletes. These high values are thought to be due to a combination of training and natural endowment. Early studies of élite runners

(Robinson *et al.* 1937; Åstrand 1955) measured values of up to $81.5 \, \text{ml·kg}^{-1}\text{·min}^{-1}$ in champion athletes. This is comparable to the $\dot{V}_{O_{2max}}$ found in élite runners of today (the highest value ever obtained by us in a runner: $87.1 \, \text{ml·kg}^{-1}\text{·min}^{-1}$; the mean for a 5000–10 000-m group: $78.7 \, \text{ml·kg}^{-1}\text{·min}^{-1}$). Thus, the last 50 years of improvements in competitive results in middle and long distance events cannot be ascribed to a higher $\dot{V}_{O_{2max}}$ of the present cohort of élite runners. Although evidently important, the maximal oxygen intake is only one of the factors that determine success in long-distance events. This is illustrated by the large differences in performance between marathon runners of equal $\dot{V}_{O_{2max}}$ (Sjödin & Svedenhag 1985).

Running economy

Since the early 1970s, there has been growing interest in how best to utilize the maximal aerobic capacity in endurance events. During running, the submaximal oxygen intake of an individual is directly and linearly related to his or her running velocity. However, at a given running speed, the submaximal oxygen requirement (in $\text{ml·kg}^{-1}\text{·min}^{-1}$) may vary considerably between subjects (Costill *et al.* 1973; Svedenhag & Sjödin 1984). The lower the $\dot{V}_{O_{2submax}}$ at a given running speed, the better the individual's running economy. In contrast, the differences may be small or non-existent when groups of élite runners from different distances are compared (Svedenhag & Sjödin 1984). In élite distance runners with a relatively narrow range of $\dot{V}_{O_{2max}}$, the running economy at different speeds is significantly correlated ($r = 0.79$–0.83) with performance in a 10-km race (Conley & Krahenbuhl 1980). A low $\dot{V}O_{2submax}$ (i.e. a good running economy) is thus truly beneficial. There is also a surprisingly wide (about 20%) variation in running economy ($ml \cdot kg^{-1} \cdot min^{-1}$) at a speed of 15 km·h^{-1} between marathon runners at the good or élite level (Sjödin & Svedenhag 1985). However, in a heterogeneous sample, there may be a relatively poor correlation between the $\dot{V}O_{2submax}$ during running and endurance performance (e.g. $r = -0.55$ in a marathon with a large variation in performance; Sjödin & Svedenhag 1985).

Because running economy has been thoroughly studied for only three decades, any long-term trend for élite runners cannot be assessed. Leaving aside improvements in long-distance racing shoes, and in track and spikes, the last 50 years of enhanced results (especially in long-distance running) are still probably explained by improvements in running economy and/or the ability to exercise at a high percentage of $\dot{V}O_{2max}$ for long periods.

Total aerobic running capacity

A given performance in an endurance event like distance running can be attained in different ways. We can distinguish two kinds of élite runner with different physiological characteristics. One category has a high $\dot{V}O_{2max}$ but a relatively poorer running economy. The second category has an excellent running economy but a relatively smaller $\dot{V}O_{2max}$. In many cases the overall result of these differences is a fairly even level of performance. Only the outstanding runner has excellent values in both aspects (thus creating a third category). Both the training accomplished and varying natural abilities may explain differences in running economy and $\dot{V}O_{2max}$. In addition, the body mass may incorrectly influence the $\dot{V}O_2$ values that are obtained if results are expressed as $ml \cdot kg^{-1} \cdot min^{-1}$ (see below).

To account better for individual differences in relation to performance, the fractional utilization of $\dot{V}O_{2max}$ when running at a specific speed (e.g. 15 km·h^{-1}, 20 km·h^{-1}) can be calculated. This $\%\dot{V}O_{2max}$ value is significantly correlated with performance over various long distances. It can be regarded as the total aerobic running capacity of a runner. For instance, the relationship between fractional utilization of $\dot{V}O_{2max}$ at a submaximal speed of 15 km·h^{-1} and performance was as good as $r = -0.94$ ($n = 35$) in a heterogeneous sample of marathon competitors (Sjödin & Svedenhag 1985). The good correlation between $\%\dot{V}O_{2max}$ at a specific submaximal speed and performance is attributable to the fact that the $\%\dot{V}O_{2max}$ value expresses the effects of both $\dot{V}O_{2max}$ and running economy, each of which may be independently related to performance. Furthermore, the mode of expressing $\dot{V}O_2$ (see below) does not influence $\%\dot{V}O_{2max}$ values.

In more recent years, another way of expressing the combined effect of running economy and $\dot{V}O_{2max}$ has won some popularity. This is to extrapolate the running economy line of an individual up to her or his $\dot{V}O_{2max}$ and to report the running velocity at which this occurs (Morgan *et al.* 1989). If the running economy extrapolation can be accepted, this may be the preferred way of presenting test results, particularly for middle-distance runners with high racing velocities.

Training advice can be given depending on the treadmill test results. A runner with poor running economy should, thus, place more emphasis on training to improve running economy (such as interval techniques with relatively long rest periods, hill training and general strength work). On the other hand, a runner who needs an increase in $\dot{V}O_{2max}$ (and is judged to have the capacity to achieve it) may adjust his or her training programme accordingly (e.g. more '*fartlek*' work in hilly terrain, long intense intervals and lactate threshold training). However, when such comparisons are made, the $\dot{V}O_{2max}$ and running economy should be expressed as $ml \cdot kg^{-0.75} \cdot min^{-1}$ (see below).

Lactate threshold

The 'anaerobic threshold' concept is reviewed elsewhere (Chapter 22). We have used the 4 mmol·l^{-1} blood lactate concentration as the highest steady-state level of lactate that can be tolerated during running (expressed as the corresponding running velocity of each subject, V_{La4}). Leaving aside theoretical considerations, we have found that from a practical and experimental viewpoint the V_{La4} is an excellent marker of training status and form. Several studies (e.g. Farrell *et al.* 1979) have shown a good relationship between lactate threshold and performance over long distances. For a marathon sample (with marathon times ranging from 2 h 12 min to 3 h 52 min) a correlation of $r = 0.97$ was found between V_{La4} and competitive marathon speed (Sjödin & Svedenhag 1985). The lactate threshold is also the best single predictor of performance in long-distance running over distances from 5 km to the marathon.

The high correlations found between the lactate threshold and long-distance running speed reflect dependency of the lactate threshold on several variables that are all related to performance. The 4 $mmol \cdot l^{-1}$ lactate threshold (expressed as a running velocity) is thus a function of both $\dot{V}O_{2max}$ and running economy, together with $\%\dot{V}O_{2max}$ at V_{La4} (Fig. 28.1). An improvement in one of these factors (e.g. in running economy, with the other factors unchanged) will therefore improve the lactate threshold to an analogous degree. However, an unbalanced training programme, overemphasizing one or a few training elements, may lead to an opposing change in some other factor with, at best, an unchanged lactate threshold as the overall result.

With physical endurance training, the lactate curve is shifted to the right relative to $\dot{V}O_{2max}$. This reduces lactate levels at the same $\%\dot{V}O_{2max}$ and increases $\%\dot{V}O_{2max}$ at the lactate threshold (as V_{La4}). In our marathon sample, the $\%\dot{V}O_{2max}$ at V_{La4} was similar (88%) in two sub 3-h groups but was slightly, although significantly, lower (85%) in the slow

runners. However, the $\%\dot{V}O_{2max}$ at V_{La4} did not differ significantly between élite marathon runners and élite runners in the 400- and 800-m events (88, 84 and 83%, respectively) (Svedenhag & Sjödin 1984). Furthermore, if trained long-distance runners have their individual lactate thresholds at a slightly lower blood lactate concentration than untrained or less well endurance-trained subjects (as suggested by Stegmann *et al.* 1981), the $\%\dot{V}O_{2max}$ value at the individual lactate threshold in the above comparisons could be very similar. In all, this may indicate that the rightward shift of the lactate threshold relative to $\dot{V}O_{2max}$ occurs largely as an early response to training. The excessive amounts of training that some endurance athletes undertake appear to have relatively little or no effect in shifting the lactate curve further to the right.

Training at the speed corresponding to the 'anaerobic threshold' is widely used as a means of improving performance in marathon running. As for the early rightward shift of the lactate curve (above), such a training plan seems rather fruitless for a previously trained individual. However, an improvement in the anaerobic threshold velocity after threshold training in a previously well-trained runner may be due mainly to effects on the running economy and the $\dot{V}O_{2max}$ (Sjödin *et al.* 1982; see below). Evidently, there may be an intricate interplay between training and the different physiological variables determining running performance.

The endurance factor

Another aspect of performance is the question of how close to $\dot{V}O_{2max}$ an athlete can run during competition. This depends on the distance to be covered as well as on environmental factors. During a marathon race, the $\%\dot{V}O_{2max}$ at the race pace ($\%\dot{V}O_{2Ma}$) has ranged from 60% in slow to 86% in élite marathon runners. In our marathon material, the $\%\dot{V}O_{2Ma}$ was the same, on average 80%, in both élite runners (mean time 2 h 21 min) and good runners (2 h 37 min), but it was significantly lower (71%) in the slow runners (3 h 24 min) (Sjödin & Svedenhag 1985). Likewise, the percentage of lactate threshold velocity ($\%V_{La4}$) reached during a marathon event was significantly less in slow

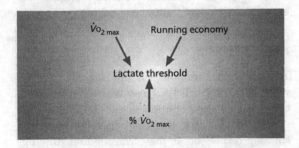

Fig. 28.1 Interrelationships between different physiological variables of importance for performance in middle- and long-distance running.

runners (85%) than in good or élite runners (92–93%). These findings suggest that the $\%\dot{V}O_{2max}$ that can be maintained during a marathon race differs between runners showing large differences in performance. These differences would be even greater if account were taken of the effect of wind resistance (proportional to the third power of velocity). In experienced runners prepared for the event with adequate endurance training (such as our sub 3-h marathon runners) the $\%\dot{V}O_{2max}$ may be similar. The lower $\%\dot{V}O_{2max}$ in the slowest runners may be due not only to a lack of adequate endurance training (with a lower capacity to metabolize fat and save glycogen) but also to the longer period of exertion and/or to inadequate running and racing experience.

Expressing oxygen intake

Theoretically, and from a strictly dimensional point of view, maximal oxygen intake ($\dot{V}O_{2max}$, l·min^{-1}) should be proportional to body mass raised to the 2/3 power (see Åstrand & Rodahl 1986). Based on calculated limitations imposed by the elastic components of biological material, aerobic power has been suggested to be proportional to the 3/4 power of body mass. This is in conformity with relationships between resting and maximal oxygen intake and body mass raised to the power 0.73–0.79 as reported in comparative animal studies (for references, see Svedenhag 1995). From calculations based on a large series of tests on adult humans, Bergh *et al.* (1991) suggested that the submaximal and maximal $\dot{V}O_2$ attained during running are better related to kg$^{2/3}$ or kg$^{3/4}$ than to kg^1. Furthermore, Sjödin and Svedenhag (1992) suggested that changes in running economy and $\dot{V}O_{2max}$ (ml·kg^{-1}·min^{-1}) during the growth of adolescent boys may be largely due to an overestimation of the dependence of $\dot{V}O_2$ on body mass during running; calculations have favoured oxygen intake expressed as kg$^{0.75}$. Thus, in recent years, several lines of evidence have suggested that oxygen intake determined during submaximal or maximal running should be related to kg$^{0.75}$ rather than to kg^1 (Svedenhag 1995). For the above-mentioned 5000–10 000-m group of runners, the corresponding

mean $\dot{V}O_{2max}$ value would be 221 ml·kg$^{-0.75}$·min^{-1} (the largest value obtained in a runner would be 243 ml·kg$^{-0.75}$·min^{-1}). For the running economy at 15 km·h^{-1} the mean would be 125 ml·kg$^{-0.75}$·min^{-1}. Such a mode of expressing $\dot{V}O_2$ should increase our understanding of differences and changes in $\dot{V}O_{2max}$ and running economy, particularly at the individual level. However, this mode of expressing $\dot{V}O_2$ should also be used when comparing groups with differences (or changes) in body masses.

General training considerations

Even though there may be several ways of getting to the goal, there ought to be an optimal training programme for each individual that provides the easiest, fastest and/or least hazardous way of achieving a given performance level. Today, a complete adjustment of the training programme for an individual athlete is rather Utopian. With a good training log, recurrent physiological and medical tests and *'Fingerspitzgefühl'* (i.e. fingertip sense), the athlete and the coach, together with their physiological and medical advisers, may be well on their way. To get even further, however, more knowledge regarding the normal responses to different types of training is needed.

The more you train, the less the added training effect. However, relatively little is known about the physiological changes that accompany the smaller but important improvements in performance in already well-trained athletes. For the completely untrained individual, the exact training elements do not seem as important; he or she will probably improve in condition anyway. For example, several studies of previously untrained subjects have not found any difference in physiological effects or performance improvements between continuous and interval running training programmes (although training intensity is positively related to $\dot{V}O_{2max}$ increases when a meta-analysis of different study populations is performed; Wenger & Bell 1986). For the well trained, on the other hand, the composition and variations in the different training elements (with quantity and quality clearly specified) together with the timing and length of the recovery periods, may (to say the least) be decisive.

Less training may be needed to preserve a raised physiological capacity/performance level than to attain it in the first place (which is quite reassuring for the athlete who has put much effort into her or his training). However, this seems mostly applicable to rather 'slowly responding' variables such as $\dot{V}_{O_{2max}}$, whereas endurance or skeletal muscle mitochondrial capacity need an almost continuous or more or less unaltered stimulation (i.e. training) to maintain their capacity, especially during the earlier years of training.

Physiological effects of specified training

Effects on $\dot{V}_{O_{2max}}$

Ten well-trained élite runners from the Swedish National Team, with judged capacity for improvement, were followed by regular treadmill tests throughout 1 year (January to the following January) (Svedenhag & Sjödin 1985). Five of these individuals were middle-distance runners (mean age 21.2 years) and five were long-distance runners (22.6 years). From the competitive season preceding to the one following the test year, the 1500-m time improved from 3 min 45.0 s to 3 min 40.8 s, but the 800-m time remained essentially unchanged (1 min 50 s) (middle-distance runners), and the 5000-m time improved from 14 min 11 s to 13 min 43 s (long-distance runners).

The $\dot{V}_{O_{2max}}$ (ml·kg^{-1}·min^{-1}) rose significantly from winter to the competitive summer season (from 74.2 to 77.4; +4.5%) (Fig. 28.2). In some part (+1.3%), this was due to a slight reduction in body mass during the competitive season. The following winter, the $\dot{V}_{O_{2max}}$ was almost back to the starting level. The summer increase in $\dot{V}_{O_{2max}}$ may seem small, but is likely to be of great importance in a race with runners at a similar level of performance. The increase in $\dot{V}_{O_{2max}}$ from winter to summer is probably related to an increase in the number of weekly high intensity workouts. These tripled from January to May and the competitive summer season in these runners (Svedenhag & Sjödin 1985). Changes are also illustrated by the blood lactate concentration 30 s after the $\dot{V}_{O_{2max}}$ test, which rose significantly

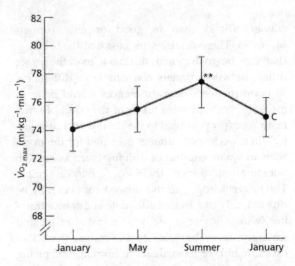

Fig. 28.2 Maximal oxygen intake ($\dot{V}_{O_{2max}}$, ml·kg^{-1}·min^{-1}) of 10 élite runners on four occasions during the course of a year. Analysis of variance (ANOVA) was applied with subsequent calculation of least significant differences. The symbol ** denotes a significant ($p < 0.01$) difference from the initial January value. The letter C denotes a significant ($p < 0.05$) difference from the summer value. Values are means ± standard errors. From Svedenhag and Sjödin (1985), with permission.

during the same period. The relationship between training intensity and $\dot{V}_{O_{2max}}$ is compatible with the findings of Wenger and Bell (1986) (see above).

Effects on running economy

In the above follow-up study on 10 élite middle- and long-distance runners (Svedenhag & Sjödin 1985) running economy at 15 km·h^{-1} and 20 km·h^{-1} was also determined. The training response differed from that for $\dot{V}_{O_{2max}}$. The $\dot{V}_{O_{2submax}}$ (ml·kg^{-1}·min^{-1}) decreased progressively during the test year and was between 3 and 4% lower at the last compared to the first test occasion. For $\dot{V}_{O_2}$ at 20 km·h^{-1} ($\dot{V}_{O_{2\,20}}$), the improvement in running economy was statistically significant (Fig. 28.3). There was no change in body mass on a year-to-year basis. Furthermore, successive and significant improvements in both $\dot{V}_{O_{2\,15}}$ and $\dot{V}_{O_{2\,20}}$ were found in a larger group of élite runners who were followed for 22 months (Svedenhag & Sjödin 1985). All runners had been familiarized with and tested on the treadmill at least once

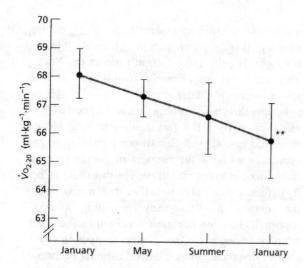

Fig. 28.3 Running economy at $20\,km\cdot h^{-1}$ ($\dot{V}_{O_{2}\,20}$). Data for 10 élite runners on four occasions during the course of a year. Analysis of variance (ANOVA) was applied with a subsequent calculation of least significant difference. The symbol ** denotes a significant ($p < 0.01$) difference from the initial January value. Values are means ± standard errors. From Svedenhag and Sjödin (1985), with permission.

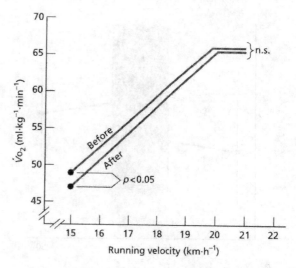

Fig. 28.4 Running economy in 11 marathon runners before and after 12 weeks of added hill training. At $15\,km\cdot h^{-1}$ there was a significant improvement in running economy ($p < 0.05$). $\dot{V}_{O_{2}max}$ was unchanged. B. Sjödin and J. Svedenhag (unpublished observations).

before commencing the study. Thus, our data suggest a slow but progressive improvement in running economy in these élite runners. At the same time, the $\dot{V}_{O_{2}max}$ remained unchanged from year to year (comparisons for the same month). This indicates that it may take a longer time to improve the running economy than it takes to reach an individual's maximal obtainable level of $\dot{V}_{O_{2}max}$ (which in itself may take several years of hard and rational training). This could at least partly explain continuing improvements in performance levels in runners who have already been training for many years.

The effect of hill training on different physiological characteristics was investigated in 11 marathon runners (B. Sjödin & J. Svedenhag, unpublished observations). Their normal training routine was supplemented by a programme of hill training, with 'bounce' running over an almost 400-m long, firm and even uphill slope. The hill training was performed with periodic variations in intensity during a 12-week period. After this training, the submaximal oxygen intake during running was significantly lower (Fig. 28.4). Improvement was greatest at rela-

tively low running velocities (3% at $15\,km\cdot h^{-1}$). This effect may, theoretically, be related to development of the elastic components in the musculature engaged in running.

Effects on the lactate threshold

The effect of specific training at the lactate threshold was studied in a group of middle- and long-distance runners (two 800-m and six 1500–5000-m runners). In addition to their normal training, the subjects ran a fast 20-min distance workout on a treadmill once a week for 14 weeks. The speed was set at each individual's $4\,mmol\cdot l^{-1}$ lactate threshold. Blood lactate concentrations were determined at each workout. As a result of this threshold training, the speed at the lactate threshold (V_{La4}) increased significantly (Sjödin *et al.* 1982) (Fig. 28.5). Normal training before and after the lactate threshold training period did not affect the threshold velocity (Fig. 28.5). The runners who were closest to their individual lactate threshold (i.e. had the smallest accumulation of blood lactate during the fast distance training) showed the greatest improvements. The enhancement of the lactate threshold velocity was related to

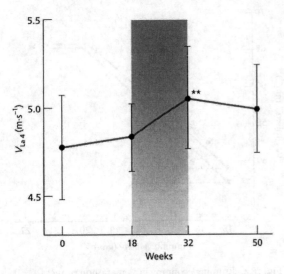

Fig. 28.5 The running velocity corresponding to a blood lactate concentration of $4\,mmol\cdot l^{-1}$ (V_{La4}). Data for seven well-trained runners measured twice before and twice after 14 weeks of added 'V_{La4}' training. The symbol ** denotes a significant difference ($p < 0.01$) from the previously measured value. Values are means ± standard deviations. From Sjödin *et al.* (1982), with permission.

a decrease (i.e. improvement) in $\dot{V}O_{2submax}$ during running ($\dot{V}O_{2\,15}$: from 50.6 to 49.2 ml·kg^{-1}·min^{-1}, $p < 0.05$). For the 1500–5000-m runners the $\dot{V}O_{2max}$ also increased significantly (from 68.7 to 71.0 ml·kg^{-1}·min^{-1}, $p < 0.01$).

Lactate threshold training thus had a good overall effect on two of the factors determining lactate threshold (see above). Fast distance training seems especially suitable for runners in events ranging from 10000 m to the marathon. The threshold velocity in these cases is at or near the actual racing velocity, thereby simultaneously providing a good (optimal?) training of running technique. For other running categories (i.e. those competing over shorter distances) more planned running economy training is also needed and indeed recommended (e.g. technique intervals at racing speed).

In conclusion, this chapter has discussed some basic physiological variables, training principles and specific factors influencing performance in endurance events. The findings that have been reviewed should improve the understanding of endurance and how best to achieve outstanding performances.

References

Åstrand, P.-O. (1955) New records in human power. *Nature* **176**, 922–923.

Åstrand, P.-O. & Rodahl, K. (1986) *Textbook of Work Physiology*. McGraw-Hill, New York.

Bergh, U., Sjödin, B., Forsberg, A. & Svedenhag, J. (1991) The relationship between body mass and oxygen intake during running in humans. *Medicine and Science in Sports and Exercise* **23**, 205–211.

Conley, D.L. & Krahenbuhl, G.S. (1980) Running economy and distance running performance of highly trained athletes. *Medicine and Science in Sports and Exercise* **12**, 357–360.

Costill, D.L., Thomason, H. & Roberts, E. (1973) Fractional utilization of the aerobic capacity during distance running. *Medicine and Science in Sports and Exercise* **5**, 248–252.

Farrell, P.A., Wilmore, J.H., Coyle, E.F., Billing, J.E. & Costill, D.L. (1979) Plasma lactate accumulation and distance running performance. *Medicine and Science in Sports and Exercise* **11**, 338–344.

Morgan, D.W., Baldini, F.D., Martin, P.E. & Kohrt, W.M. (1989) Ten kilometer performance and predicted velocity at $\dot{V}O_{2max}$ among well-trained male runners. *Medicine and Science in Sports and Exercise* **21**, 78–83.

Robinson, S., Edwards, H.T. & Dill, D.B. (1937) New records in human power. *Science* **83**, 409–410.

Sjödin, B. & Svedenhag, J. (1985) Applied physiology of marathon running. *Sports Medicine* **2**, 83–99.

Sjödin, B. & Svedenhag, J. (1992) Oxygen uptake during running as related to body mass in circumpubertal boys: a longitudinal study. *European Journal of Applied Physiology and Occupational Physiology* **65**, 150–157.

Sjödin, B., Jacobs, I. & Svedenhag, J. (1982) Changes in onset of blood lactate accumulation (OBLA) and muscle enzymes after training at OBLA. *European Journal of Applied Physiology* **49**, 45–57.

Stegmann, H., Kindermann, W. & Schnabel, A. (1981) Lactate kinetics and individual anaerobic threshold. *International Journal of Sports Medicine* **2**, 160–165.

Svedenhag, J. (1995) Maximal and submaximal oxygen uptake during running: how should body mass be accounted for? *Scandinavian Journal of Medicine and Science in Sports* **5**, 175–180.

Svedenhag, J. & Sjödin, B. (1984) Maximal and submaximal oxygen uptakes and blood lactate levels in elite male middle- and long-distance runners. *International Journal of Sports Medicine* **5**, 255–261.

Svedenhag, J. & Sjödin, B. (1985) Physiological characteristics of élite male runners in and off-season. *Canadian Journal of Applied Sport Sciences* **10**, 127–133.

Wenger, H.A. & Bell, G.J. (1986) The interactions of intensity, frequency and duration of exercise training in altering cardiorespiratory fitness. *Sports Medicine* **3**, 346–356.

Chapter 29

Food and Fluids Before, During and After Prolonged Exercise

RONALD J. MAUGHAN

Introduction

When athletes seek to perform at the highest level, training schedules, injury and diet are their main concerns. The last of these factors, the foods that are eaten in training and competition, cannot turn a club athlete into an Olympic champion, but poor food choices will prevent the athlete's potential from being realized. When other factors, including talent, training, skill and motivation, are equal, diet can make the difference between winning and losing, or even between first and last place in an Olympic final. Good food choices can further improve performance by enhancing the quality of training and may help to reduce the risk of illness and injury.

In planning a nutritional strategy for the athlete, there are several issues that require careful attention. The diet should be consistent with current recommendations for maintaining good health, but must meet the additional demands of the training programme. Special nutritional strategies before and during competition may be necessary to optimize performance, and recovery after training sessions or competition may also require a change from the normal eating pattern. Although the basic principles are well established, there are still many areas where some uncertainty remains, and within the broad nutritional goal, there is considerable scope for different food choices to provide the necessary nutrients. Food is an important part of the athlete's daily life, and eating should provide pleasure as well as sustenance.

Two aspects of the athlete's diet must be considered: the first is the diet in training, and the second is the diet in the period around competitions. Although most athletes and coaches focus on nutritional strategies for competition, diet may play a bigger role in allowing the athlete to sustain a high training load for prolonged periods.

The training diet

The athlete engaged in hard regular training must consume a diet that will cover the requirements of daily living and will also meet any additional nutrient requirements imposed by the training load. The most obvious effect of the intensive training involved in preparation for élite-level sport is an increase in daily energy expenditure. The metabolic rate during running or cycling, for example, may be 15–20 times the resting rate, and such levels of activity may be sustained by trained athletes for several hours. Professional cyclists may compete for up to 200 days per year, and training becomes almost indistinguishable from competition. Mean daily energy expenditure in a laboratory simulation of the Tour de France was measured at 32 MJ (8000 calories), with individual values much higher than this (Westerterp et al. 1986). Even the sprinter or weightlifter, whose events last only a few seconds, may spend several hours per day in training. There is evidence that the metabolic rate may remain elevated for at least 12 and possibly up to 24 h after exercise if the exercise is prolonged and close to the maximum intensity that can be sustained (Bahr 1992). For the athlete training two or even three times per day, the metabolic rate is therefore likely to be chronically elevated even at rest, further increasing the total daily energy expenditure.

If body mass and performance levels are to be maintained, the high rate of energy expenditure in training must be matched by a high energy intake. When athletes engaged in simple locomotor sports such as running are studied, a good relationship is seen between the daily energy intake and the distance run in training each week (Fig. 29.1). Available data for most athletes suggest that they are in energy balance within the limits of the techniques used for measuring intake and expenditure. This is to be expected, as a chronic deficit in energy intake would lead to a progressive loss of body mass. However, data for women engaged in sports where a low body mass, and especially a low body fat content, are important, including events such as gymnastics, distance running and ballet, consistently show a lower than expected energy intake (Maughan & Piehl Aulin 1997). There is no obvious physiological explanation for this finding other than methodological errors inherent in the estimation of energy intake and expenditure. It may seem odd that such errors should apply specifically to this group of athletes, but in these sports, body mass and body fat content are crucial factors. Many of these women have a very low body fat content; a value of less than 10% is not uncommon in female long-distance runners (see Chapter 24). Secondary amenorrhoea, possibly related more to the training regimen than to the low body fat content, is common in these women, but is usually reversed when training stops (Drinkwater et al. 1986).

The effects of exercise in stimulating an increased energy intake are important from a nutritional perspective. The increased amount of food that must be eaten to meet the energy requirement means that the intake of most nutrients will be increased if a varied diet is consumed. Where the increase in intake of any individual nutrient exceeds any increase in requirement resulting from the exercise, the possibility of an inadequate intake is reduced.

Energy substrates

The energy requirements of training are largely met by oxidation of fat and carbohydrate, although a number of factors will influence the relative contributions of these two fuels. The higher the intensity of exercise, the greater the reliance on carbohydrate as a fuel in both absolute terms and as a fraction of total energy metabolism (Fig. 29.2). During low-intensity exercise at a level corresponding to about 50% of maximum oxygen intake ($\dot{V}O_{2max}$), approximately two-thirds of the total energy requirement is met by fat oxidation, with oxidation of carbohydrate (blood glucose and muscle glycogen) supplying about one-third. If the exercise intensity is increased to about 75% of $\dot{V}O_{2max}$, the total energy expenditure is increased, and carbohydrate (mostly muscle glycogen) is now the major fuel. Endurance training, restriction of dietary carbohydrate intake and an increased dietary fat intake will all shift fuel selection in the direction of an increased fat oxidation and a sparing of carbohydrate. At very high intensity, conversion of carbohydrate to lactic acid

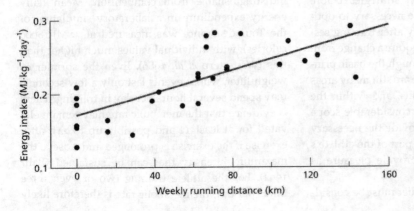

Fig. 29.1 Measured energy intake of runners in steady state with regard to training and body mass shows a good relationship between the weekly training distance and the daily energy intake.

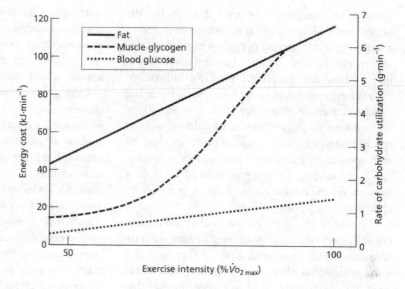

Fig. 29.2 The total energy demand increases as the exercise intensity increases, and the relative contributions of the different energy substrates also change. Fat oxidation can meet most of the energy demand at low exercise intensities, but carbohydrate (especially muscle glycogen) is the main fuel used when the exercise intensity is high.

can provide energy at high rates, but this anaerobic metabolism places great demands on the limited carbohydrate stores. If carbohydrate is not available, or is available in only a limited amount, the intensity of the exercise must be reduced to a level where the energy requirement can be met by fat oxidation.

The total carbohydrate store in the body is small. In the average 70-kg adult male, it amounts to about 350 g in the muscles and about 90 g in the liver in the fed state (Newsholme & Leech 1983). Even at rest, there is a relatively high rate of carbohydrate use, primarily by the nervous tissues and the red blood cells. In the absence of dietary carbohydrate intake, the liver will release glucose into the bloodstream by breaking down its glycogen store. During exercise, the muscles will use carbohydrate from their own glycogen store and from blood glucose, causing both liver and muscle glycogen concentrations to fall. The rate of muscle glycogen breakdown is directly related to the exercise intensity, and in continuous cycling exercise that causes exhaustion within about 1–2 h, the point of fatigue coincides closely with a critically low level of glycogen in the working muscles (Saltin & Karlsson 1971).

Because of this reliance on carbohydrate as an energy source for the athlete who must follow an intensive training schedule, it is essential that the carbohydrate intake be sufficient to enable training to be sustained at a level that will produce the optimum response. During each strenuous training session, substantial depletion of glycogen stores takes place in the exercising muscles (Bergstrom & Hultman 1967) and in the liver (Hultman & Nilsson 1971). If this carbohydrate reserve is not replenished before the next training session, training intensity must be reduced, leading to corresponding decrements in the training response. Even when large fat stores are present, these cannot be converted to carbohydrate, so glycogen resynthesis can only occur if sufficient carbohydrate is provided by the diet.

Recognition of the need for dietary carbohydrate has led to the recommendation that athletes should obtain a large fraction of their total energy needs from carbohydrate. However, several studies have looked at the carbohydrate needs of athletes engaged in hard training, and the results of these surveys do not entirely support the idea that a diet with a very high carbohydrate content must be consumed if an intensive training schedule is carried out (see Sherman & Wimer 1991 for a review). It may be better to think of the dietary carbohydrate intake in absolute amounts (grams per kg body mass per day) in relation to the amount used in training, rather than as a percentage of the total energy intake. Well-trained athletes with a body mass of about 70 kg exercising at a level that can be sustained for 1–2 h can use carbohydrate at a rate of about 3–5 g·min⁻¹. During periods of intensive training, where the total exercise duration can be more than 2–3 h per day, this would result in a daily carbohydrate requirement of about 8–12 g·kg⁻¹. When the energy demand is extremely high, it seems likely that the exercise intensity must be reduced and the contribution of fat to energy metabolism must be correspondingly increased. In this situation, the diet can accommodate a greater amount of fat than is possible for the athlete whose training is relatively short and at very high intensity.

The rate of glycogen synthesis after exercise is crucially dependent on the amount of carbohydrate consumed in the postexercise period (Fig. 29.3). If a low carbohydrate diet, providing less than about 200 g of carbohydrate per day, is consumed at this time, little or no resynthesis of muscle glycogen will take place (Bergstrom *et al.* 1967). At least 50–100 g of carbohydrate foods should be consumed within the first 1–2 h after exercise in order to maximize the rate of glycogen resynthesis (Ivy *et al.* 1988). Although some studies have shown little effect of varying the type of carbohydrate consumed, there may be advantages in consuming high glycaemic index foods at this time if the speed of recovery is crucial (Coyle 1991). Such foods will cause a rapid elevation

of the blood glucose concentration, making glucose readily available to the muscle at a time when it is most required. Some examples of foods with different effects on blood glucose concentration are shown in Table 29.1.

During very heavy training, a dietary carbohydrate intake of 500–800 g per day may be necessary to ensure adequate glycogen resynthesis, and these high levels of intake are difficult to achieve without consuming large amounts of simple sugars. Many athletes find that they can only satisfy the requirement for carbohydrate by eating confectionery and sweet snacks between, or even instead of, meals (Coyle 1991). Athletes may find that sugar, jam, honey, confectionery and other high sugar foods as well as carbohydrate-containing drinks are a convenient, low-bulk way of achieving a high carbohydrate intake at this time (Clark 1994). For the athlete training two or more times per day, there are special problems with recovery of muscle glycogen stores. Most athletes do not like to train hard for a few hours after eating, and appetite is usually suppressed for some time after hard exercise. Such athletes usually adopt a 'grazing' pattern of eating, with many small meals throughout the day (Burke 1995).

It is well recognized that feeding a high fat, low carbohydrate diet for prolonged periods can

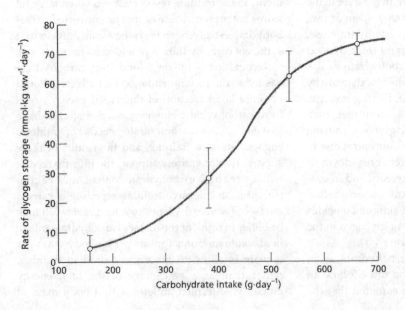

Fig. 29.3 The rate of glycogen resynthesis in the muscle after exercise is closely related to the carbohydrate content of the diet. For complete and effective recovery of the muscle glycogen stores, a high carbohydrate diet should be eaten.

Table 29.1 Some examples of high carbohydrate foods with different effects on the blood glucose concentration. Also shown for each food is the amount that must be eaten to provide 50 g of carbohydrate (CHO).

Food	Amount (in g) to give 50 g of CHO
High glycaemic index foods	
White bread	200
Breakfast cereal	60–80
Potato (boiled)	250
Banana	260
Sugar (glucose or sucrose)	50
Moderate glycaemic index foods	
Pasta	200
Sponge cake	90
Potato chips (crisps)	100
Orange	500
Grapes	300
Low glycaemic index foods	
Apple	400
Baked beans	480
Lentils	300
Fructose	50
Milk	1100

Table 29.2 Hard exercise increases the requirement for dietary protein intake above that of the sedentary individual. These values are recommended daily intakes expressed per unit of body mass, except for the cycle tour value which is an estimated requirement (Lemon, 1991).

Individual	Recommended dietary protein intake ($g \cdot kg^{-1} \cdot day^{-1}$)
Sedentary individual	0.8–1.2
Endurance athlete	1.2–1.4
Strength athlete	1.2–1.7
Very hard training (cycle tour)	1.6

increase the capacity of muscle to oxidize fat and hence improve endurance capacity in the rat, but this strategy may not be effective in humans. Similarly, short-term fasting increases endurance capacity in the rat, but results in a decreased exercise tolerance in humans. There have been suggestions that the athlete should consume a high fat diet in training in order to increase the capacity of the muscles to oxidize fat, switching to a high carbohydrate diet shortly before competition to ensure adequate carbohydrate availability (Hawley *et al.* 1998). However, the limited capacity of humans to adapt to a high fat diet suggests that the training diet should be high in carbohydrate (Coyle 1997). A large proportion of the dietary carbohydrate should be in the form of complex carbohydrates rather than simple sugars, to meet the need for the micronutrients associated with these foods (Coyle 1991). This suggestion conforms to the recommendations of various governmental expert committees that carbohydrates should provide at least 50% of total dietary energy intake in a healthy diet.

Protein intake

Athletes engaged in strength and power events have traditionally been concerned with achieving a high dietary protein intake, in the belief that this is necessary for muscle hypertrophy. In a survey of American college athletes, 98% believed that a high protein diet would improve performance. Although it is undoubtedly true that a diet deficient in protein will lead to loss of muscle, slowed tissue repair and wound healing and other symptoms, there is no evidence to support the idea that protein synthesis can be stimulated simply by increasing dietary protein intake. If the protein intake exceeds the requirement, the carbon skeletons of the unwanted amino acids will be used as a substrate for oxidative metabolism, either directly or as a precursor of glucose, and the excess nitrogen will be lost in the urine.

There is good evidence, though, that exercise, whether it is long-distance running, aerobics or weight training, will cause an increased protein oxidation compared with the resting state (Table 29.2), and this leads to an increase in the intake necessary to ensure nitrogen balance. It is important to distinguish between the actual requirement of an individual and the intake recommended by various expert committees. The recommended intake is a population value designed to ensure that 98% of the general population achieves an adequate intake: this amount is not necessary for everyone, and there may occasionally be an outlier who needs more. A recent survey of the published data on élite-level athletes during training led Tarnopolsky (1999) to conclude that the protein requirement of these athletes is about $1.5–1.8\,g\cdot kg^{-1}\cdot day^{-1}$.

Although the contribution of protein oxidation to energy production during exercise may decrease to about 3–6% of the total energy demand, compared with about 10–15% (i.e. the normal fraction of protein in the diet) at rest, the absolute rate of protein degradation is increased during exercise (Dohm 1986). This leads to an increase in the minimum daily protein requirement, but the additional requirement should easily be met if a normal mixed diet adequate to meet the increased energy expenditure is consumed. In spite of this, many athletes ingest large quantities of foods with a high protein content and many also use expensive protein supplements; daily protein intakes of up to 400 g are not unknown in some sports. Disposal of the excess nitrogen is theoretically a problem if renal function is compromised, but there is no good evidence that excessive protein intake among athletes is in any way damaging to health (Lemon 1991). The recommended diet for athletes may even contain a lower than normal proportion of protein, on account of the increased total energy intake. The effect of increasing energy intake on protein intake is shown in Table 29.3. There is not at present good evidence of major differences between men and women in terms of protein requirements or the effects of exercise on protein metabolism.

It should be stressed that the effects of exercise on protein metabolism cannot be seen in isolation from the effects on other nutrients. If the energy intake, and more especially the carbohydrate intake, is inadequate, protein synthesis will be depressed and protein breakdown enhanced (Krempf et al. 1993). These observations have important implications for

athletes on energy-restricted diets, and there may be a need for such athletes to increase the total protein intake to allow adaptation to the training stimulus. There are also some recent data suggesting that feeding carbohydrate in the first hour after a strength training session can result in a more positive nitrogen balance (Roy et al. 1997). Although further experimental support is needed before guidelines can be established, this suggests that there may be benefits, in addition to the stimulation of glycogen synthesis, from encouraging athletes to consume carbohydrate as soon as possible after exercise.

Micronutrients

With regular strenuous training, there must be an increased total food intake to balance the increased energy expenditure, as pointed out above. Provided that a varied diet containing items from all the major food groups is consumed, this will supply more than adequate amounts of protein, minerals, vitamins and other dietary requirements. With a very limited number of possible exceptions detailed below, there is no good evidence to suggest that specific supplementation with any of these dietary components is necessary. Nor will it improve performance, unless a specific deficiency exists. It may be worth pointing out that the majority of studies that purport to show nutritional deficiencies or inadequate nutrient intakes in athletes are worthless. Most of these studies are based on comparisons of estimated intake with one or other value for the recommended intake. The methodology for estimating intake is rather imprecise, and depends on compliance of the athlete for recall or recording of food consumption. The tables of nutrient contents of foods are incomplete, and are at best approximations, adding to the problem of obtaining reliable estimates. The recommended intakes are intended for use with populations rather than individuals, and failure to meet the recommended standards is not an indication of an inadequate intake. Indeed, the recommended intake is calculated in such a way that all but 4% of those whose actual intake is less than the recommended value will meet their requirement.

Table 29.3 Energy intake and protein intake for a diet containing 12–15% protein.

70-kg athlete (typical male)
12 MJ (3000 cal) = 90–112 g protein = $1.3–1.6\,g\cdot kg^{-1}$
20 MJ (5000 cal) = 150–188 g protein = $2.1–2.7\,g\cdot kg^{-1}$
60-kg athlete (typical female)
8 MJ (2000 cal) = 60–75 g protein = $1–1.3\,g\cdot kg^{-1}$
12 MJ (3000 cal) = 90–112 g protein = $1.5–1.9\,g\cdot kg^{-1}$

The nutrient density of the diet becomes vitally important when energy intake is low. A selection of foods that may be considered inadequate for a sedentary individual consuming 4 MJ per day may meet the requirements of an athlete taking 12–15 MJ per day. Indeed without resorting to sweets (candies), snacks and convenience foods, which provide energy but may not contain large amounts of micronutrients, such a high intake may be difficult to achieve. There is no evidence that this pattern of eating is harmful; for the athlete who has to fit an exercise programme into a busy day, it is inevitable that changes to eating patterns must be made, but these need not compromise the quality of the diet. When the energy expenditure is very high, as in cycle stage races, carbohydrate-rich drinks and snacks become an essential part of the diet (Brouns et al. 1989).

Two significant exceptions to the generalization about dietary supplements may be iron (Eichner 1986) and, particularly in the case of very active women, calcium (Clarkson 1991). Highly trained endurance athletes commonly have low circulating haemoglobin levels relative to population norms, although total red cell mass may be elevated due to an increased blood volume. This may be considered an adaptation to the trained state, but hard training may result in an increased iron requirement and exercise tolerance is impaired in the presence of anaemia. A reduced level of iron stores as indicated by low serum folate and serum ferritin levels, but without anaemia, is not associated with impaired performance, and correction of these deficiencies does not appear to influence performance in trained athletes. The prevalence of anaemia in athletes seems to be similar to that in the general population and, although therefore rare, it should always be considered as a possibility when an athlete performs below expectation. Iron supplements may be necessary if there is severe iron deficiency, but both prevention and treatment are possible by attention to diet. This should certainly be the long-term solution. Iron is present in many foods, and it is not difficult to achieve an adequate dietary intake. The aims should be to identify foods high in iron that are acceptable to the athlete, and to maximize the availability of the iron in the diet (Deakin 1994).

The haem iron found in red meat, liver and some other meats is more easily absorbed in the intestine than other forms of iron, but such foods are avoided by many athletes. Vegetarians should have no difficulty in achieving an iron intake that will be well in excess of their needs, but they may need special advice to ensure an adequate intake of available iron. Eating large amounts of dietary fibre can reduce the absorption of iron, and added fibre is generally not necessary. Iron supplements are used by many athletes as a form of insurance against iron deficiency, but these are of limited value, since they fail to address overall dietary adequacy. In general, iron supplements should be taken only on the advice of a qualified sports doctor or dietitian, and only when clinical and haematological testing indicates a true iron deficiency caused by a low intake. If iron deficiency has not been established by a blood test, there is no justification for recommending supplementation.

Moderate exercise has been reported to increase bone mineral density in women, and for most women this may be a significant benefit of participation in a recreational exercise programme. Hard training, however, may reduce circulating oestrogen levels and hence accelerate bone loss. There is evidence of low bone mineral density and increased risk of fracture in some groups of female athletes. For these athletes, an adequate calcium intake should be ensured, although calcium supplements themselves will not reverse bone loss while oestrogen levels remain low. Restoration of normal menstrual function is normally associated with a gain of bone mass (Drinkwater et al. 1986). Reduced fat dairy produce is a good source of dietary calcium, but many women restrict their intake of dairy products because of concerns about fat intake.

Supplements

Many different food supplements are on sale to the athlete, and the manufacture and sale of sports nutrition products is a lucrative business. Most of the substances categorized as ergogenic aids are completely ineffective, neither improving performance nor having any detrimental effect. Some, indeed most, of the compounds that are effective in improving exercise performance contravene the doping regulations and have no place in sport. Many supplements are widely used, in spite of the absence of any proven benefit. Carnitine, for example, is sold widely, but a comprehensive review of the published literature led Heinonen (1996) to conclude that 'although there are some theoretical points favouring potential ergogenic effects of carnitine supplementation, there is currently no scientific basis for healthy individuals or athletes to use carnitine supplementation to improve exercise performance.' There are, however, a small number of food components that are not against the rules of sport, are not harmful to health, and yet may confer benefits.

Creatine is now widely used by athletes, and its effects on performance have been reviewed by Greenhaff (1995) and Maughan (1995). A few days of supplementation of the diet with large (20–30 g per day) amounts of creatine increase the creatine content of the muscles and a part of this creatine is in the form of the high-energy compound creatine phosphate. Creatine and creatine phosphate play a number of important roles in muscle metabolism during, and during recovery from, high-intensity exercise. These include provision for rapid resynthesis of ATP during periods of intense activity, buffering of the acidity associated with anaerobic glycolysis in intense exercise, and transport of ATP equivalents across the mitochondrial membrane, although there is no evidence that this last process is normally limiting in endurance exercise. The normal dietary source of creatine is from meat. The daily requirement is about 2 g, with about half that amount normally coming from the diet and the remainder synthesized by the body. Vegetarians, who have no dietary source of creatine, must synthesize all their requirement.

The creatine stores in the muscles seem to be maximized if about 5 g of creatine is taken four times per day for about 2–4 days. The effectiveness is increased if this is taken together with a high carbohydrate snack to increase circulating insulin levels, as the transport of creatine into muscle seems to be stimulated by insulin. Each individual may respond differently, and the biggest increases in muscle creatine content are seen in those individuals with the lowest starting levels. If this loading phase is followed by a daily supplement of about 2 g per day, the muscle creatine stores will remain high for several weeks.

A large number of controlled scientific studies have now been performed, and a large amount of practical experience in the use of creatine has been gained by the many thousands of athletes who have used it. The available evidence supports a beneficial effect of creatine supplementation on muscle strength and on high-intensity exercise, especially performance involving repeated bouts of high-intensity exercise with only short recovery periods. There are no reports of beneficial effects on performance of endurance exercise, but it appears that creatine supplementation may particularly benefit athletes who undertake interval-type training sessions; the biggest benefit may be to improve performance by allowing more intensive training. The application of creatine supplementation to multiple sprint sports (e.g. team games, racquet sports) has not been well studied, although it appears that this pattern of exercise should be one where supplementation would be beneficial.

In the case of creatine, use among athletes is now widespread, and each athlete who decides to use creatine should monitor their own response to supplementation, as they would evaluate any new training method, or a new pair of shoes. This accumulated experience will ultimately decide whether creatine is effective or not. There is no evidence of any adverse side-effects associated with the use of creatine, even after long-term use of amounts in excess of those that are recommended for the improvement of performance. An acute weight gain of about 1–2 kg normally accompanies creatine loading, but this is mostly in the form of water (muscle tissue is 75% water).

Creatine is a good example of a nutritional ergogenic aid which has the potential to improve athletic performance. There is still much to be learned, though, about optimum doses, supplementation protocols and the types of sport situations where supplementation may be beneficial. Some of the evidence will come from scientific laboratories where carefully controlled studies can be carried out, but such experimentation can involve only a few individuals, and these are seldom highly trained athletes. Athletes are usually (and rightly) unwilling to disrupt training routines to accommodate participation in controlled scientific investigations. Usually, the laboratory evidence therefore comes from recreationally active, but not well-trained, subjects.

Recovery during periods of intensive training is vital if the training load is to be sustained. The recovery period is a time for tissue repair and adaptation. There is good evidence for a role of free radicals in the mediation of the muscle damage and inflammation that occurs in the hours and days after a bout of prolonged intense exercise (Ebbeling & Clarkson 1989). There is also growing support for the suggestion that dietary antioxidants can neutralize these free radicals and reduce the extent of muscle damage that occurs (Dekkers et al. 1996). Interest has focused particularly on the effects of supplementation with vitamins C and E. Again, it would be premature to advise athletes to supplement their diet with large amounts of these nutrients, especially as excessive supplementation with single components of the antioxidant defence system may disturb the balance of the various factors which are involved (Halliwell 1996). None the less, it seems a sensible precaution to encourage athletes to ensure that their diet contains a plentiful amount of fruits, vegetables and nuts, which contain complex mixtures of essential micronutrients and phytochemicals that can act as antioxidants themselves or can participate in endogenous enzymatic defence systems.

There is some evidence that athletes may be at increased risk of minor illness and infection during periods of intensive training or immediately after a strenuous competition (Nieman 1996) (Chapter 50). A fall in the circulating concentration of glutamine, which acts as an essential fuel for cells of the immune system, is commonly observed after prolonged intense exercise. This in turn has led to suggestions that supplementation of the diet with glutamine may be beneficial for athletes at these times. Once again, though, in spite of the sound theoretical basis, there is not at present sufficient experimental evidence to support the sale of this supplement to athletes.

Diet for competition

There is no doubt that the ability to perform prolonged exercise can be substantially modified by dietary intake in the pre-exercise period, and this becomes important for the individual aiming to produce peak performance on a specific day. The pre-exercise period can conveniently be divided into two phases—the few days prior to the competition, and the day of competition itself.

Dietary manipulation to increase muscle glycogen content in the few days prior to exercise has been extensively recommended for endurance athletes, following observations that these procedures were effective in increasing endurance capacity in cycle ergometer exercise lasting about $1\frac{1}{2}$–2 h (Fig. 29.4). Hawley et al. (1997) concluded that when the exercise duration exceeds about 90 min, an increase in the muscle glycogen content prior to exercise can postpone fatigue by about 20% of the total exercise time. Where a set distance is covered as quickly as possible, performance can be improved by 2–3%. The suggested procedure, based on a comprehensive series of studies carried out in Scandinavia in the 1960s, was to deplete muscle glycogen by prolonged exercise about 1 week prior to competition and to prevent resynthesis by consuming a low carbohydrate diet for 2–3 days before changing to a high carbohydrate diet for the last 3 days during

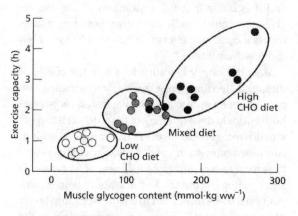

Fig. 29.4 Effects of variations in the carbohydrate content of the diet on muscle glycogen content and on exercise time to exhaustion at an exercise intensity of about 75% of maximal oxygen intake. Data of Bergstrom et al. (1967).

which little or no exercise was performed. This procedure can double the muscle glycogen content and is effective in increasing cycling or running performance, measured as the time for which a given work load can be sustained (Coyle 1991).

There is now a considerable amount of evidence that it is not necessary to include the low carbohydrate glycogen depletion phase of the diet for well-trained endurance athletes (O'Connor 1994; Coyle 1997). All that is necessary is to reduce the training load over the last few days before competition and to simultaneously increase the dietary carbohydrate intake. This avoids many of the problems associated with the more extreme forms of the diet. Although an increased precompetition muscle glycogen content is undoubtedly beneficial, there is a faster rate of muscle glycogen utilization when the glycogen content itself is increased, thus nullifying some of the advantage gained.

Consumption of a high carbohydrate diet in the days prior to competition may also benefit competitors in games such as rugby, soccer or hockey, although it appears unusual for these players to pay attention to this aspect of their diet. Saltin and Karlsson (1973) showed that players starting a soccer game with low muscle glycogen content did less running, and much less running at high speed, than players who began the game with a normal muscle glycogen content. It is common for players to have one game midweek as well as one at the weekend, and it is likely that full restoration of the muscle glycogen content will not occur between games unless a conscious effort is made to achieve a high carbohydrate intake.

Most laboratory investigations into the effects of diet and feeding on exercise performance are carried out on subjects who have fasted for several hours prior to the beginning of the study. It is important to recognize, however, that athletes seldom compete under such conditions. Especially where time for recovery and replenishment of fuel stores is short, eating during the last few hours before competition may be important to ensure optimum levels of liver and muscle glycogen. Preparation in the days beforehand should have resulted in muscle glycogen stores being optimal. On the day of competition, a high carbohydrate meal 3–4 h before competition will ensure that the liver glycogen stores are also full. This final meal should have a low fat content so that gastric emptying and the processes of digestion and absorption are not delayed. Although some athletes may prefer not to eat before competition, it is clear that ingestion of carbohydrate 3–4 h before exercise is effective in improving performance.

Some experiments carried out in the 1970s suggested that feeding a high carbohydrate meal within the last hour before exercise was best avoided because of the possibility of a reactive hypoglycaemia. The logic is persuasive: the carbohydrate causes a sharp rise in the circulating insulin level which inhibits fat mobilization and promotes carbohydrate storage. When exercise begins, there is a reduced availability of fat as a fuel and also a limited availability of carbohydrate from the body's stores. The blood glucose concentration is therefore likely to fall rapidly, and this can lead to the early onset of fatigue. On the basis of this result, it was recommended that high carbohydrate meals should be avoided for at least 2 h before exercise. More recent studies do not support this advice, and have shown that most individuals benefit from ingesting carbohydrate at this time, especially if they have fasted overnight (see Coyle 1997 for a review of these studies). The important point is that sufficient carbohydrate must be consumed to offset the inhibition of fat mobilization and utilization caused by the elevated insulin level after eating carbohydrate (Wright et al. 1991). It is also apparent that the glycaemic index of foods ingested in the pre-exercise period is not a good predictor of subsequent metabolic and performance responses (Horowitz & Coyle 1993). Again, athletes should practise with different meals before training or minor competitions to find out what best suits them. For many individuals, the last meal may be most easily taken in liquid form: this reduces the risk of gastrointestinal upset during exercise, as well as providing extra fluid to meet the needs during exercise.

Nutrition and central fatigue

Fatigue in prolonged exercise is normally ascribed to failure of thermoregulatory or cardiovascular control, or to depletion of substrate (glycogen) in the working muscles. It is, however, difficult to account for fatigue due to glycogen depletion in metabolic terms, as the ATP concentration of the muscles is well maintained even at the point of subjective exhaustion (Tsintzas *et al.* 1996). It is also difficult to identify the mechanisms by which an elevated body temperature causes fatigue. Nielsen believes that fatigue in prolonged exercise in a warm environment is limited by core temperature rather than by circulatory failure, and has suggested that this is mediated by an inhibitory effect of the high internal temperature on motivation (Nielsen *et al.* 1993).

One possible mechanism by which prolonged exercise may reduce the neural drive to the muscles has been termed 'central fatigue'. This proposes a mechanism mediated by the action of the brain neurotransmitters 5-hydroxytryptamine (5-HT, also known as serotonin) and dopamine (Newsholme & Castell 1996; Davis & Bailey 1997). The role of 5-HT in pain, sleep and other physiological events is well established. It is possible that it also plays a role in the fatigue process, but the evidence is largely circumstantial. The rate of synthesis of 5-HT in nerve cells and, by extrapolation, its rate of release, is influenced by the plasma concentrations of the 5-HT precursor tryptophan and of other amino acids (particularly the branched-chain amino acids) that compete for the transporter protein that conveys them across the cell membrane. According to this hypothesis, nutritional factors that influence the plasma amino acid profile would be expected to affect exercise performance. The experimental evidence (including studies involving feeding of tryptophan or of branched-chain amino acids) is not conclusive, but on the whole it does not support the hypothesis. Other lines of evidence involving drugs that affect 5-HT or dopamine do, however, give reason to believe that such a mechanism may be operational (Wilson & Maughan 1992). There is also a recent report that feeding branched-chain amino acids may be effective in improving endurance performance in the heat (Mittleman *et al.* 1998). It would be wrong to place too much emphasis on the results of a single study and, notwithstanding the fact that drinks containing branched-chain amino acids are on sale to athletes, further evidence is required

before nutritional strategies can be devised to manipulate this aspect of central fatigue.

Fluid requirements

High rates of sweat secretion are necessary during hard exercise in order to limit the rise in body temperature which would otherwise occur. When the ambient temperature is higher than the skin temperature, evaporation of sweat from the skin surface is the only means available for the body to lose heat (Chapters 17 and 20). The rates of sweat loss vary greatly between individuals as well as being influenced by exercise intensity and the ambient conditions: information on sweat losses in different sports has recently been collated by Rehrer and Burke (1996). Sweating rates of 1–2 l per hour are not unusual during hard work in hot environments, and if the exercise is prolonged, this leads to progressive dehydration and loss of electrolytes. During hard training in the heat, the daily water requirement may be in excess of 10–12 l. The major electrolytes lost will be sodium, which is typically present in sweat at a concentration of about 40–60 mmol·l^{-1}, chloride and potassium (Maughan & Shirreffs 1998).

Fatigue towards the end of a prolonged event may result as much from the effects of dehydration as from substrate depletion. It is often reported that exercise performance is impaired when an individual is dehydrated by as little as 2% of body mass, and that losses in excess of 5% of body mass can decrease the capacity for work by about 30%. Although there is little opportunity for sweat loss during short-duration events, athletes who travel to hot climates are likely to experience chronic dehydration because of the increased fluid needs of daily living and training in the heat. Beginning exercise in a hypohydrated condition will seriously impair performance. Armstrong *et al.* (1985) showed that athletes who ran a 10-km track race after diuretic-induced dehydration of 2% of body mass ran about 6.3% slower than when they were fully hydrated.

It has been proposed that hyperhydration induced prior to exercise by the addition of glycerol (or possibly also other osmotically active but relatively metabolically inert agents) may improve

the thermoregulatory capacity and lead to enhanced exercise performance. The evidence from
well-controlled studies, however, is not altogether
supportive of this idea, and the ingestion of
glycerol-containing drinks cannot be recommended
at this time (Sawka *et al*. 1998). It is clear that any
athlete who is not fully hydrated at the beginning of
exercise will not achieve an optimum performance:
furthermore, dehydration negates the beneficial
effects of heat acclimatization on thermoregulation
and exercise capacity (Sawka *et al*. 1998). Athletes
should therefore ensure that fluid intake in the hours
before exercise is sufficient to ensure full hydration.

The composition of drinks to be taken during
exercise should be chosen to suit individual circumstances, but the primary aims are to supply water
and energy substrate in the form of carbohydrate
(Maughan & Shirreffs 1998). During exercise in the
cold, the need for fluid replacement will be reduced
because of the lower sweat rates, but there is still a
need to supply additional glucose to the exercising
muscles. Even in the cold, ingestion of dilute carbohydrate–electrolyte drinks is effective in improving
performance, and athletes should not assume that
rehydration is not important in these conditions.
Consumption of a high carbohydrate diet in the
days prior to exercise should reduce the need for
carbohydrate ingestion during exercise in events
lasting less than about 2 h, but it is not always possible to boost carbohydrate stores. Competition on
successive days, for example, may prevent adequate
glycogen replacement between exercise periods.
This situation often arises in tournaments, where
more than one competition may even take place on
the same day, and carbohydrate-containing drinks
are then effective in improving performance. In
cycle stage races which are held over many consecutive days, concentrated glucose drinks, and even
solid food, may be necessary during the event to
ensure an adequate intake of energy and carbohydrates. These will supply more glucose, thus
sparing the limited glycogen stores in the muscles
and liver without overloading the body with fluid.
In many sports there is little provision for fluid
replacement: participants in games such as football
or hockey can lose large amounts of fluid, but
opportunities for replacement are limited to brief
stoppages in play and to the half-time interval. Until
very recently, opportunities for drinking during
long road races were severely restricted, but the
rules have now been relaxed to allow a more frequent intake. In spite of this, few athletes practise
drinking in training, so the occurrence of gastrointestinal problems when drinks are consumed
during competition is not surprising.

The effects on performance of replacing water
and carbohydrate are independent and additive
(Below *et al*. 1995), and a variety of carbohydrate
types, including glucose, sucrose and maltodextrin,
may be used. Even when substantial sweat losses
are incurred, there is little evidence that there is a
need to replace the electrolytes lost in sweat. The
addition of sodium to carbohydrate-containing
drinks, however, in concentrations of 20–50
mmol·l^{-1} may promote water absorption in the
small intestine, and will help to maintain plasma
volume. In hot weather, there are benefits in cooling
drinks to improve palatability: although fluid availability may be limited by the rates of gastric emptying and intestinal absorption (Maughan & Shirreffs
1998), few athletes reach this physiological limit
to replacement. Anything that encourages an
increased consumption should be exploited, and
athletes should experiment in training with different types and flavours of drinks.

In the postexercise period, it is essential that the
carbohydrate stores are replenished and that hydration status is returned to normal. Replacement of
fluid and electrolytes can usually be achieved
through the normal dietary intake, but will require
special attention when sweat losses are high. Fluid
loss can be assessed by weight loss during exercise:
a weight loss of 1 kg represents a sweat loss of
approximately 1 l. The volume consumed after exercise must be sufficient to replace this loss as well as
providing for the ongoing water loss by all routes.
An intake of 1.5 times the sweat loss is recommended for effective restoration of fluid balance
(Shirreffs *et al*. 1996). If large volumes of electrolyte-
free fluid are ingested, a marked diuresis will be
stimulated, even though the individual is still hypohydrated, and electrolyte (especially sodium) losses
must be replaced if fluid balance is to be restored
and maintained (Fig. 29.5). If there is a need to

Fig. 29.5 Fluid balance in the post-exercise recovery period when drinks with different sodium concentrations were consumed. The experiments began with subjects in fluid balance: they then exercised in the heat to lose 2% of body mass before drinking a volume of fluid equal to 1.5 times the sweat loss. Over the next 6 h, fluid balance was assessed. The drinks with a low sodium content promoted large losses in the urine, leading to a rapid return to a dehydrated state. Only when a high sodium drink was consumed did subjects remain in positive fluid balance. From Maughan and Leiper (1995).

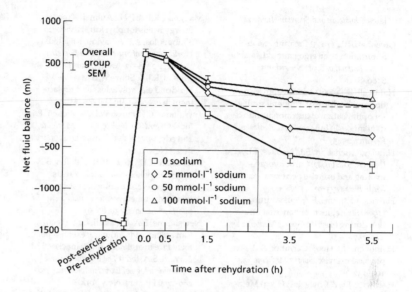

ensure adequate replacement before exercise is repeated, extra fluids should be taken and additional salt (sodium chloride) might usefully be added to food. If no solid food is taken in the recovery period, drinks should contain sufficient sodium to replace the amount lost in sweat. The requirement for the other major electrolytes, particularly potassium and magnesium, can normally be met from the diet. Mineral supplements are not normally necessary, even when sweat losses are exceptionally high, provided that a variety of foods are eaten in amounts sufficient to meet the energy demand.

References

Armstrong, L.E., Costill, D.L. & Fink, W.J. (1985) Influence of diuretic-induced dehydration on competitive running performance. *Medicine and Science in Sports and Exercise* **17**, 456–461.

Bahr, R. (1992) Excess postexercise oxygen consumption—magnitude, mechanisms and practical implications. *Acta Physiologica Scandinavica* **144** (Suppl. 605), 1–70.

Below, P., Mora-Rodriguez, R., Gonzalez-Alonso, J. & Coyle, E.F. (1995) Fluid and carbohydrate ingestion independently improve performance during 1 h of intense cycling. *Medicine and Science in Sports and Exercise* **27**, 200–210.

Bergstrom, L. & Hultman, E. (1967) A study of the glycogen metabolism during exercise in man. *Scandinavian Journal of Clinical and Laboratory Investigation* **19**, 218–228.

Bergstrom, J., Hermansen, L., Hultman, E. & Saltin, B. (1967) Diet, muscle glycogen and physical performance. *Acta Physiologica Scandinavica* **71**, 140–150.

Brouns, F., Saris, W.H.M., Stroecken, J. *et al.* (1989) Eating, drinking and cycling. A controlled Tour de France simulation study. *International Journal of Sports Medicine* **10**, S41–S48.

Burke, L. (1995) *The Complete Guide to Food for Sports Performance*, 2nd edn. Allen & Unwin, St Leonards, Sussex.

Clark, K. (1994) Nutritional guidance to soccer players for training and competition. *Journal of Sports Sciences* **12** (Special Issue), S43–S50.

Clarkson, P.M. (1991) Minerals: exercise performance and supplementation. *Journal of Sports Sciences* **9** (Special Issue), 91–116.

Coyle, E.F. (1991) Timing and method of increased carbohydrate intake to cope with heavy training, competition and recovery. *Journal of Sports Sciences* **9** (Special Issue), 29–52.

Coyle, E.F. (1997) Fuels for sport performance. In: Lamb, D.R. & Murray, R. (eds) *Optimising Sport Performance*, pp. 95–139. Cooper Publishing Group, Carmel.

Davis, M. & Bailey, S.P. (1997) Possible mechanisms of central nervous system fatigue during exercise. *Medicine and Science in Sports and Exercise* **29**, 45–57.

Deakin, V. (1994) Iron deficiency in athletes: identification, prevention and dietary treatment. In: Burke, L. & Deakin, V. (eds) *Clinical Sports Nutrition*, pp. 174–199. McGraw-Hill, Sydney.

Dekkers, J.C., van Doornen, L.J.P. & Kemper, H.C.G. (1996) The role of antioxidant vitamins and enzymes in the prevention of exercise-induced muscle damage. *Sports Medicine* **21**, 213–238.

Dohm, G.L. (1986) Protein as a fuel for endurance exercise. *Exercise and Sport Science Reviews* **14**, 143–173.

Drinkwater, B.L., Nilson, K., Ott, S. & Chestnet, C.H. (1986) Bone mineral density after resumption of menses in amenorrheic athletes. *Journal of the American Medical Association* **256**, 380–382.

Ebbeling, C.B. & Clarkson, P.M. (1989) Exercise-induced muscle damage and adaptation. *Sports Medicine* **7**, 207–234.

Eichner, E.R. (1986) The anemias of athletes. *Physician and Sportsmedicine* **14**, 122–130.

Greenhaff, P.L. (1995) Creatine and its application as an ergogenic aid. *International Journal of Sport Nutrition* **5**, S100–S110.

Halliwell, B. (1996) Oxidative stress, nutrition and health. Experimental strategies for optimisation of nutritional antioxidant intake in humans. *Free Radical Research* **25**, 57–74.

Hawley, J., Schabort, E.J., Noakes, T.D. & Dennis, S.C. (1997) Carbohydrate-loading and exercise performance. *Sports Medicine* **24**, 73–81.

Hawley, J., Brouns, F. & Jeukendrup, A. (1998) Strategies to enhance fat utilisation during exercise. *Sports Medicine* **25**, 241–257.

Heinonen, O.J. (1996) Carnitine and physical exercise. *Sports Medicine* **22**, 109–132.

Horowitz, J.F. & Coyle, E.F. (1993) Metabolic responses to preexercise meals containing various carbohydrates and fat. *American Journal of Clinical Nutrition* **58**, 235–241.

Hultman, E. & Nilsson, L.H. (1971) Liver glycogen in man. *Advances in Experimental Medicine and Biology* **11**, 143–151.

Ivy, J.L., Katz, A.L., Cutler, C.L., Sherman, W.M. & Coyle, E.F. (1988) Muscle glycogen synthesis after exercise: effects of time of carbohydrate ingestion. *Journal of Applied Physiology* **65**, 1480–1485.

Krempf, M., Hoerr, R.A., Pelletier, V.A., Marks, L.M., Gleason, R. & Young, V.R. (1993) An isotopic study of the effect of dietary carbohydrate on the metabolic fate of dietary leucine and phenylalanine. *American Journal of Clinical Nutrition* **57**, 161–169.

Lemon, P.W.R. (1991) Effect of exercise on protein requirements. *Journal of Sports Sciences* **9** (Special Issue), 53–70.

Maughan, R.J. (1995) Creatine supplementation and exercise performance. *International Journal of Sport Nutrition* **5**, 94–101.

Maughan, R.J. & Leiper, J.B. (1995) Effects of sodium content of ingested fluids on postexercise rehydration in man. *European Journal of Applied Physiology* **71**, 311–319.

Maughan, R.J. & Piehl Aulin, K. (1997) Energy needs for physical activity. In: Simopoulos, A.P. & Pavlou, K.N. (eds) *World Review of Nutrition and Dietetics*, Vol. 82, pp. 18–32. Karger, Basel.

Maughan, R.J. & Shirreffs, S.M. (1998) Fluid and electrolyte loss and replacement in exercise. In: Harries, M., Williams, C., Stanish W.D. & Micheli, L.J. (eds) *Oxford Textbook of Sports Medicine*, 2nd edn, pp. 97–113. Oxford University Press, New York.

Mittleman, K.D., Ricci, M.R. & Bailey, S.P. (1998) Branched-chain amino acids prolong exercise during heat stress in men and women. *Medicine and Science in Sports and Exercise* **30**, 83–91.

Newsholme, E.A. & Castell, L.M. (1996) Can amino acids influence exercise performance in athletes?. In: Steinacker, J.M. & Ward, S.A. (eds) *The Physiology and Pathophysiology of Exercise Tolerance*, pp. 269–274. Plenum, New York.

Newsholme, E.A. & Leech, A.R. (1983) *Biochemistry for the Medical Sciences*. John Wiley & Sons, Chichester.

Nielsen, B., Hales, J.R.S., Strange, S., Christensen, N.J., Warberg, J. & Saltin, B. (1993) Human circulatory and thermoregulatory adaptations with heat acclimation and exercise in a hot, dry environment. *Journal of Physiology (London)* **460**, 467–485.

Nieman, D.C. (1996) Prolonged aerobic exercise, immune response, and risk of infection. In: Hoffman-Goetz, L. (ed.) *Exercise and Immune Function*, pp. 143–162. CRC Press, Boca Raton.

O'Connor, H. (1994) Competition nutrition issues: preparation and recovery. In: Burke, L. & Deakin, V. (eds) *Clinical Sports Nutrition*, pp. 307–332. McGraw-Hill, New York.

Rehrer, N.J. & Burke, L.M. (1996) Sweat losses during various sports. *Australian Journal of Nutrition and Dietetics* **53**, S13–S16.

Roy, B.D., Tarnopolsky, M.A., MacDougall, J.D., Fowles, J. & Yarasheski, K.E. (1997) Effect of glucose supplement timing on protein metabolism after resistance training. *Journal of Applied Physiology* **82**, 1822–1888.

Saltin, B. & Karlsson, J. (1971) Muscle glycogen utilization during work of different intensities. In: Pernow, B. & Saltin, B. (eds) *Muscle Metabolism During Exercise*, pp. 289–300. Plenum, New York.

Saltin, B. & Karlsson, J. (1973) Die Ernahrung Des Sportlers. In: Hollmann, W. (ed.) *Zentrale Themen der Sport-Medizin*, pp. 245–260. Springer, Berlin.

Sawka, M.N., Latzka, W.A., Matott, R.P. & Montain, S.P. (1998) Hydration effects on temperature regulation. *International Journal of Sports Medicine* **19**, S108–S110.

Sherman, M. & Wimer, G.S. (1991) Insufficient dietary carbohydrate during training: does it impair athletic performance? *International Journal of Sport Nutrition* **1**, 28–44.

Shirreffs, S.M., Taylor, A.J., Leiper, J.B. & Maughan, R.J. (1996) Post-exercise rehydration in man: effects of volume consumed and sodium content of ingested fluids. *Medicine and Science in Sports and Exercise* **28**, 1260–1271.

Tarnopolsky, M. (1999) Protein metabolism in strength and endurance activities. In: Spriet, L.L. & Hargreaves, M.A. (eds) *The Metabolic Bases of Exercise and Sport Performance*, pp. 125–163. Cooper, Carmel.

Tsintzas, O.K., Williams, C., Boobis, L. & Greenhaff, P. (1996) Carbohydrate ingestion and single muscle fibre glycogen metabolism during prolonged running in men. *Journal of Applied Physiology* **81**, 801–809.

Westerterp, K.R., Saris, W.H.M., Van Es, M. et al. (1986) Use of doubly-labelled water technique in humans during heavy sustained exercise. *Journal of Applied Physiology* **61**, 2162–2167.

Wilson, W.M. & Maughan, R.J. (1992) A role for serotonin in the genesis of fatigue in man: administration of a 5-hydroxytryptamine reuptake inhibitor (Paroxetine) reduces the capacity to perform prolonged exercise. *Experimental Physiology* **77**, 921–924.

Wright, D.A., Sherman, W.M. & Dernbach, A.R. (1991) Carbohydrate feedings before, during, or in combination improve cycling endurance performance. *Journal of Applied Physiology* **71**, 1082–1088.

Chapter 30

Haemoglobin, Blood Volume and Endurance

NORMAN GLEDHILL AND DARREN WARBURTON

Determinants of endurance performance

Endurance performance is influenced by several factors, in particular maximal oxygen intake ($\dot{V}_{O_{2max}}$), anaerobic threshold and running efficiency (see Chapters 16, 21 and 22). However, since $\dot{V}_{O_{2max}}$ can vary among individuals by as much as 300% (from $< 30\,ml\cdot kg^{-1}\cdot min^{-1}$ to $> 80\,ml\cdot kg^{-1}\cdot min^{-1}$), this factor must be regarded as the major determinant of endurance performance. By comparison, anaerobic threshold and running efficiency influence to only a modest degree the portion of an individual's $\dot{V}_{O_{2max}}$ that is utilized during endurance performance (up to 20% and 5% of $\dot{V}_{O_{2max}}$, respectively). $\dot{V}_{O_{2max}}$, in turn, is determined by oxygen transport—the product of cardiac output ($\dot{Q}$) and arterial oxygen content (C_aO_2). Further, $\dot{Q}$ is influenced by blood volume (BV), and the sea-level C_aO_2 is determined almost entirely by the blood haemoglobin concentration ([Hb]). Manipulation of BV and [Hb] thus can markedly affect the provision of oxygen to the working muscles, thereby having a significant influence on $\dot{V}_{O_{2max}}$ and endurance performance.

Role of haemoglobin in oxygen transport

Oxygen is carried by the blood both in physical solution and in combination with haemoglobin. According to Henry's law, the amount of dissolved oxygen is proportional to the partial pressure of oxygen (P_{O_2}, torr) in blood as follows: $P_{O_2} \times 0.03\,ml$ oxygen per litre of blood. Hence, under normal sea-level atmospheric conditions, dissolved oxygen

contributes no more than $3\,ml\cdot l^{-1}$ to the overall blood transport of oxygen. In addition, oxygen undergoes an easily reversible chemical combination with haemoglobin, and this accounts for most of the blood's capacity to transport oxygen.

Normal adult haemoglobin (haemoglobin A) is a complex molecule containing four polypeptide chains (globins), two α chains and two β chains (Hsia 1998). Each polypeptide chain contains one haem group, which is capable of binding to one oxygen molecule. Thus, each haemoglobin molecule is capable of binding to four oxygen molecules, with the formation of oxyhaemoglobin. Each gram of haemoglobin can combine with up to 1.39 ml of oxygen when it is fully saturated with oxygen. Therefore, the oxygen-carrying capacity of haemoglobin can be calculated as follows: ($1.39\,ml\ O_2\cdot g^{-1}$ Hb) $\times$ (Hb concentration (g Hb$\cdot l^{-1}$ blood)). The percentage oxygen saturation of haemoglobin in blood is calculated as follows: (O_2 content of Hb)/(O_2 capacity of Hb) $\times$ 100. Hence, the C_aO_2 depends on the arterial P_{O_2}, the oxygen-carrying capacity of haemoglobin and the percentage oxyhaemoglobin saturation. It is calculated as ($1.39 \times$ [Hb] $\times$ % saturation) + ($0.003\,P_{O_2}$).

The binding of one molecule of oxygen to haemoglobin changes the conformational structure of the haemoglobin complex (Hsia 1998), such that the remaining haemoglobin binding sites have a greater affinity for oxygen. Therefore, as more haemoglobin binding sites are coupled with oxygen, the affinity for oxygen increases, resulting in the characteristic sigmoidal shape of the oxygen dissociation curve (ODC) (Hsia 1998). Most observers argue that the shape of the ODC is beneficial during exercise and during hypoxia. Variations in [Hb] and resultant changes in the ODC can markedly affect oxygen transport.

Given the substantial influence of the oxygen-carrying capacity of blood upon endurance performance, a consideration of the relevant measurements is informative. Since haemoglobin is contained in red blood cells (RBC), the total number of RBC can have a considerable influence on oxygen carriage. The RBC count is generally determined via automated counters, although measurements are possible using the older and simpler technology of a standard light microscope and counting chambers. In normal healthy males, the mean RBC count is 5.2 × 10^{12}.l^{-1} (range 4.5–6.0 × 10^{12}.l^{-1}). Red blood cells make up approximately 45% of the BV of a normal healthy male; this measurement is called the haematocrit. In normal healthy females, the mean red cell count is 4.8 × 10^{12}.l^{-1} (range 4.0–5.5 × 10^{12}.l^{-1}) and the mean haematocrit is 41% (range 37–47%). The haematocrit can be determined via automated counters, or more simply by centrifugation to a packed cell volume. Except when it is used in the determination of BV, the reported haematocrit is not usually corrected for the effect of trapped plasma (factor = 0.96), or for the venous to whole body ratio (factor = 0.91). The concentration of haemoglobin in blood is generally determined using automated counters or a spectrophotometric cyanmethaemoglobin assay. The mean [Hb] in normal healthy males is 155 g·l^{-1} (range 140–180 g·l^{-1}), and in normal healthy females it is 138 g·l^{-1} (range 120–160 g·l^{-1}).

Anaemia and endurance performance

Severe clinical anaemia ([Hb] < 70–80 g·l^{-1}) is associated with both a reduction in $\dot{V}_{O_{2max}}$ and an impairment of endurance performance (Sproule *et al.* 1960). However, the impact of more modest reductions in haemoglobin is more controversial (Beutler *et al.* 1960; Cotes *et al.* 1972; Davies *et al.* 1973). Of greater relevance to the topic of endurance performance is the condition of 'sports anaemia' — when the [Hb] of an athlete is below normal in the absence of any medical explanation (Clement & Sawchuk 1984). Although the incidence of clinical anaemia is very low in well-nourished athletes, a suboptimal (low normal) [Hb] is frequently reported (Pate 1983). In fact, [Hb] decreases as a function of the intensity of endurance training (Frederickson *et al.* 1983), and small reductions in [Hb] have been associated with reductions in $\dot{V}_{O_{2max}}$ and endurance performance (Ekblom *et al.* 1972; Kanstrup & Ekblom 1982). As an approximation of the relationship between [Hb] and $\dot{V}_{O_{2max}}$, a reduction in [Hb] of 3 g·l^{-1} corresponds to a fall in $\dot{V}_{O_{2max}}$ of 1% (Gledhill 1982) over the [Hb] range from 120 to 170 g·l^{-1}. Thus, if the [Hb] of an endurance athlete falls from 155 g·l^{-1} to 140 g·l^{-1}, it may be accompanied by a 5% decrease in $\dot{V}_{O_{2max}}$ and a parallel impairment of endurance performance.

'Sports anaemia' has been related to a series of mechanisms, including: (i) footstrike destruction of RBC (haemolytic anaemia); (ii) blunted erythropoietic drive due to improved tissue oxygenation; (iii) expanded plasma volume (PV) leading to a dilutional anaemia; and (iv) low iron storage (iron-deficiency anaemia) due to (a) inadequate dietary iron intake; (b) loss of iron through sweat and/or urine; and (c) low iron absorption in the digestive tract (Pate 1983; Hallberg & Magnusson 1984; Magnusson *et al.* 1984a,b; Ricci *et al.* 1988; Weight *et al.* 1992). The impact of footstrike destruction of RBC on 'sports anaemia' is negligible (Ricci *et al.* 1988) and is easily offset by an increased RBC production (Hallberg & Magnusson 1984). However, the role the other factors play in the so-called 'sports anaemia' is equivocal.

Given the performance implications of haematological status, it is important to monitor this variable in athletes. Haemoglobin is an iron-containing protein, and its synthesis thus depends on the presence of adequate amounts of iron in the bone marrow. Iron deficiency in athletes may result in 'sports anaemia.' Therefore, in addition to customary measurements of [Hb], haematocrit and RBC count, current monitoring includes measurements of iron-related variables that can detect impending haematological problems before they become overtly manifested. Such indices include serum ferritin, serum iron, total iron-binding capacity and iron saturation of transferrin. Individually, these indicators do not monitor iron deficiency very accurately, but when several indicators are measured concurrently, abnormalities are more easily and promptly detected. If only one index of iron status is to be monitored, serum ferritin is recommended. However, care must be taken in comparing values for the same athlete if samples have been measured using different assay kits or tested in different laboratories. In addition, the use of a single value to distinguish 'normal' from 'iron-deficient' serum ferritin (or other iron status indicator) values should be avoided in favour of kit-specific and laboratory-specific normative values (Ondracka & Gledhill 1988).

Men and women normally lose approximately 1 mg of iron each day in sweat and stool, and women lose additional iron during menstruation. This loss must be balanced by the dietary intake of iron. The recommended daily intake is 10 mg for males and 14 mg for females. Because only 10% of the ingested iron is absorbed, the daily intake normally matches the daily loss. Computer-processed analyses of nutritional intake can be employed to monitor the adequacy of dietary iron intake.

Deficiencies should be offset by increased dietary intake of iron and other nutrients involved in the absorption of iron and the synthesis of haemoglobin. In situations in which excessive iron levels are needed (i.e. high-intensity training) deficiencies can be corrected using a variety of tablet or liquid supplements (Clement & Sawchuk 1984).

The contribution of iron deficiency to the development of 'sports anaemia' and the potential decrease in endurance performance of athletes is debatable. It is clear that iron deficiency may result in reduced erythropoiesis and perhaps decreased endurance performance. However, it is not clear whether the athlete's iron stores are reduced to the point at which endurance performance is adversely affected. Many endurance athletes, especially females (Rowland 1990; Weight et al. 1991), are iron depleted without having a 'true' clinical iron deficiency (Hallberg & Magnusson 1984; Magnusson et al. 1984a,b). That is, iron depletion does not limit erythropoiesis (Hallberg & Magnusson 1984; Magnusson et al. 1984a,b) and/or lead to a reduction in endurance performance unless an iron-deficiency anaemia exists. Iron supplementation will only improve performance in those athletes with iron-deficiency anaemia.

Erythrocythaemia and endurance performance

Blood doping, blood boosting and blood packing are terms used to describe the procedure of inducing erythrocythaemia—an above normal [Hb]. Early investigators of blood doping employed a blood storage technique which resulted in considerable RBC loss, and they were therefore unable to achieve a significant increase in [Hb]. Consequently, it was commonly concluded that blood doping had no effect on $\dot{V}_{O_{2max}}$ or endurance performance. However, given this major methodological shortcoming, the findings from such studies must be largely ignored. More recent investigators of blood doping avoided this methodological problem and induced a significant increase in [Hb]; they reported consequent increases in $\dot{V}_{O_{2max}}$ and endurance performance (Buick et al. 1980; Williams et al. 1981; Robertson et al. 1982; Spriet et al. 1986; Brien & Simon 1987; Celsing et al. 1987). The $\dot{V}_{O_{2max}}$ increases by approximately 1% for each 3 g·l^{-1} increase in [Hb] (Gledhill 1982; Celsing et al. 1987) over the [Hb] range from 120 to 170 g·l^{-1}.

Improvements in endurance performance have been observed not only in laboratory experiments, but also in competitive cross-country skiing (Berglund & Hemmingson 1987) and 10-km running (Brien & Simon 1987). Moreover, the results on those members of the US cycling team who engaged in blood doping at the Los Angeles Olympics appear to substantiate the improvement of competitive performance (Pavelka 1985). Inducing erythrocythaemia before exercising at altitude very effectively erases the adverse effect of aerohypoxia on $\dot{V}_{O_{2max}}$ and endurance performance (Robertson et al. 1982). It was long accepted that oxygen transport and haematocrit had an 'inverted U' relationship, such that increases in [Hb] above the optimal haematocrit (postulated to be 45%) would cause a decrease in oxygen transport. This was thought to result from a decrease in $\dot{Q}$, due to increased blood viscosity and a concomitant increase in peripheral resistance. However, the relationship was based on in vitro observations which do not simulate *in vivo* conditions accurately, especially during exercise. The effective *in vivo* viscosity, both at and above the optimal haematocrit, is considerably less than the corresponding *in vitro* value, due to exercise-induced increases in temperature and blood vessel dimensions (Celsing *et al.* 1987). Therefore, $\dot{Q}_{max}$, and hence oxygen transport, is not impaired up to a haematocrit of at least 52% (Thomson *et al.* 1982; Spriet *et al.* 1986).

METHODOLOGY OF INDUCING ERYTHROCYTHAEMIA

Erythrocythaemia can be induced by transfusing fresh blood from a matched donor (homologous transfusion), as was undertaken by some members of the US cycling team during the 1984 Los Angeles Olympics (Pavelka 1985). Homologous transfusions are utilized routinely during the treatment of life-threatening medical conditions. However, even when strict clinical precautions are taken, such transfusions are associated with significant risks. For example, despite appropriate typing and matching of blood, there is a 3–4% incidence of minor transfusion reactions, consisting of fever, chills or malaise, and such reactions can result in the destruction of transfused RBC. Homologous transfusions also pose a risk of acquiring potentially fatal infections such as hepatitis B and acquired immune deficiency syndrome.

Inducing erythrocythaemia via the removal, storage and subsequent reinfusion of a person's own blood (autologous infusion) avoids these dangers. The conventional clinical method of storing blood for autologous transfusion is to preserve the cells by refrigeration at 4°C. During refrigeration and storage, the erythrocytes continue to age, and since the average lifespan of an RBC is 120 days, approximately 1% of any RBC population is lost each day. In the body, the by-products of RBC degradation are recycled, and the destruction of RBC is matched by RBC synthesis through erythropoiesis. However, when blood is refrigeration stored, there is a progressive build-up of cellular aggregates, and health authorities in North America impose a 3-week maximum refrigeration storage

time on blood banks. (In some countries the allowable storage time is extended to 4–5 weeks.) At the end of a 3-week period of refrigeration, the number of stored RBC has declined by approximately 15–20% (Valeri 1976). Additional erythrocytes are lost during processing because they adhere to the storage containers and transfer tubing. Additionally, some erythrocytes become so fragile during storage that they rupture shortly after they are infused (Valeri 1976). The net result is that when blood is refrigeration stored for the maximum allowable 3-week period, only approximately 60% of the RBC that were removed are viable after infusion.

The glycerol cell-freezing technique of blood storage is utilized by blood banks to maintain a supply of rare blood types. Freeze preservation requires laboratory personnel with considerable expertise and the use of sophisticated equipment. Unlike normal refrigeration, when blood is stored as frozen cells, the ageing process of the RBC is interrupted, and the fragility of the stored cells is unchanged after reinfusion. Loss due to RBC handling is similar to that in normal refrigeration, amounting to approximately 15% whether the storage time is 2 days or 2 years. Freeze-preserved cells can be stored safely for an indefinite period (Valeri 1976). Therefore, by employing freeze preservation it is possible not only to maximize recovery of the stored RBC (approximately 85%), but also to delay reinfusion of the cells as long as is necessary to ensure that the normal RBC count has been re-established in the donor.

Before blood is freeze preserved, it is centrifuged, and the separated RBC are combined with glycerol at a haematocrit of approximately 90%. At the conclusion of storage, the RBC are carefully thawed, deglycerolysed via a series of washings, and reconstituted with physiological saline to a haematocrit of approximately 50%. Since this reconstituted 'blood' has essentially the same haematocrit as normal blood, the BV of the recipient is transiently increased, and there is no immediate increase in haematocrit. The acute hypervolaemia disappears over the next 24 h, as excess fluid is lost, and this produces the elevated haematocrit and [Hb] that is termed erythrocythaemia.

TIME COURSE OF CHANGES IN HAEMOGLOBIN CONCENTRATION FOLLOWING BLOOD REMOVAL AND INFUSION

Following blood removal, the donor's [Hb] drops by approximately 1–1.5% (1–1.5 g·l^{-1}) for each 100 ml of blood that has been removed. Thereafter, the [Hb] remains low for 1–2 weeks before increasing rapidly towards the control level (Gledhill 1982). The time required to re-establish the control [Hb] following phlebotomy depends on: (i) the volume of blood removed (450 ml requires 3–4 weeks' recovery and 900 ml requires 4–5 weeks' recovery); and (ii) the activity level of the donor (after a 900-ml phlebotomy, up to 10 weeks' recovery is required for donors who continue endurance training). Consequently, 3 weeks after a 900-ml phlebotomy, the blood has regained only half of its 10–12% reduction in [Hb]. After refrigeration storage, infusion of the 60% of the removed RBC that are still viable cannot achieve a significant increase in [Hb]. Not surprisingly, therefore, studies of blood doping in which the refrigeration storage technique was employed did not achieve a significant increase in [Hb], and hence the authors should not have expected to observe any increase in $\dot{V}O_{2max}$ or endurance performance. However, when RBC are freeze preserved, it is possible to wait until the control [Hb] has been re-established before infusing the 85% of the removed RBC that are still viable, thereby achieving a significant increase in [Hb].

After reinfusion of 900 ml freeze-preserved blood, the [Hb] increases to approximately 10% above control, then progressively declines toward the control level over the next 120 days; a condition of erythrocythaemia is present for an extended period while the RBC count gradually decreases to the control level (Gledhill 1982).

DETECTION OF BLOOD DOPING

The practice of blood doping to improve athletic performance was banned by the International Olympic Committee in 1987, but there exists no reliable method for detecting its use. Currently, athletes selected for doping control must provide a urine sample. However, the provision of a blood sample may also be required, so that the presence of a high [Hb], haematocrit and RBC count can easily be determined. The International Skiing Federation used blood sampling as part of their doping control in the 1989 World Cross-Country Ski Championship and withdrew blood samples from their athletes during the XVII Olympic Winter Games at Lillehammer in 1994 (Souillard et al. 1996). The International Amateur Athletic Federation also decided to include blood sampling as part of their doping control for World Cup events in 1993 and 1994 (Birkeland et al. 1997). An *abnormally* high [Hb] (i.e. greater than 50%) is generally the criterion used to detect potential blood doping in athletes. The problem in detecting the use of blood doping is that of determining unequivocally that there is an *abnormally* high [Hb]. In all of the studies of induced erythrocythaemia to date, the [Hb] was within the range found in the general population, and a high normal [Hb] could be due to genetic endowment or altitude acclimatization. In fact, some athletes (who were not suspected of blood doping) competed in the 1976 Montreal Olympics with a [Hb] as high as 18 g·100 ml^{-1} (Clement et al. 1977).

Investigators have attempted to develop an effective technique to detect blood doping. Berglund et al. (1987, 1989) proposed that it might be possible to detect blood doping from analysis of a blood sample and an algorithm incorporating [Hb], erythropoietin, serum iron and bilirubin. As an indication of the effectiveness of this potential detection technique, if 20 athletes were tested for blood doping, and 10 had actually employed this manipulation, the detection technique would catch five of the 10 guilty athletes and would not falsely detect any of the 10 who had not employed blood doping. However, five guilty athletes would still not be detected, and because the technique is equivocal it is not commonly employed.

Birkeland and coworkers (Birkeland et al. 1997) recently reported the results of blood sampling on 99 athletes tested during a series of International Amateur Athletic Federation World Cup meetings in 1993 and 1994. With regard to homologous blood doping, the authors postulated that the transfusion of 450 ml of whole blood would add approximately

10% allogenic erythrocytes to the circulation. To detect such levels of blood doping, the authors utilized a gel technique capable of detecting less than 10% of allogenic cells. Thus, their doping control methodology for homologous blood transfusion was based on the detection of blood group differences between the athlete's own blood and the transfused RBC. The authors found no evidence of non-autologous blood doping and concluded that either no athletes used homologous blood doping, or the blood groups they chose to examine (which were based on the European population) may not be the best for the detection of homologous blood transfusions in athletes from around the world.

With further investigation into appropriate combinations of antisera, this technique may hold promise for future detection of homologous blood transfusions. However, it does not address the problem of autologous blood transfusions. Interestingly, the athletes who were examined also had [Hb] values that were generally lower than in controls. The authors postulated that this may have been the result of dilutional anaemia (as the result of excessive drinking following competition but before doping control) and/or it may have indicated that there is no widespread use of homologous blood doping in athletics. The findings suggest that an excessively high [Hb] is rare and may not be an effective doping control. Therefore, at present the only deterrents to the use of blood doping are concern over associated health risks and the integrity of the athletes and coaches involved.

Erythropoietin: a new form of blood doping

Erythropoietin is a glycoprotein hormone produced mainly by the kidneys (90%), with up to 10% being produced in the liver (Macdougall *et al.* 1991). Erythropoietin is synthesized in the tubular epithelial cells of the renal cortex and/or peritubular interstitial cells in response to low oxygen delivery to the tissues (hypoxia) (Eckardt *et al.* 1989; Macdougall *et al.* 1991; Fisher 1997). Tissue hypoxia can be the result of a series of factors, including a reduced arterial Po_2 (as seen at altitude ('hypobaric hypoxia') or in patients with pulmonary disease ('hypoxic hypoxia')); low levels of circulating haemoglobin (anaemia); reduced oxygen affinity by the preferential binding of toxins, such as carbon monoxide to haemoglobin; increased metabolic rate (as seen during exercise); reduced tissue blood flow (ischaemia); and interference with the tissue utilization of oxygen by toxins (for example, cyanide inhibition of cytochrome oxidase) (Macdougall *et al.* 1991; West 1995).

Erythropoietin binds specifically to the cell surface of erythroid progenitor cells in the bone marrow (Macdougall *et al.* 1991; Wide *et al.* 1995; Fisher 1997) and it is the primary regulator of erythrocyte differentiation (Egrie *et al.* 1986). Tissue hypoxia controls the synthesis of erythropoietin via a negative feedback mechanism (De Paoli Vitali *et al.* 1988; Macdougall *et al.* 1991). Thus, tissue hypoxia increases synthesis of erythropoietin, which results in the stimulation of marrow erythropoiesis, an increased production of RBC and an improved oxygen transport. This improvement corrects the tissue hypoxia and decreases the stimulus for erythropoietin production (Macdougall *et al.* 1991).

Recombinant DNA technology has allowed a cloning of the gene for erythropoietin (Jacobs *et al.* 1985; Lin *et al.* 1985). The use of recombinant human erythropoietin (rHuEPO) was approved for the treatment of anaemia in North America (Cowart 1989). It is an effective treatment of anaemia in patients with chronic renal failure (Winearls *et al.* 1986; Eschbach *et al.* 1987). Unfortunately, erythropoietin could also be employed to improve endurance performance in the same manner as blood doping—by enhancing [Hb] and thereby oxygen transport (Adamson & Vapnek 1991). Therefore, the use of rHuEPO has the potential to be a 'pharmacological alternative to blood doping' (Wagner 1991). In this case, though, the increase would be accomplished by a series of injections.

Recent investigations have revealed that rHuEPO administration results in an improved aerobic power (Rosenlof *et al.* 1989; Ekblom 1996) and endurance performance (Ekblom 1996). Both haematocrit and haemoglobin are increased as a result of erythropoiesis (Casoni *et al.* 1993; Ekblom 1996), causing an increased oxygen content. Hence, the use of rHuEPO as a doping substance represents a major threat for endurance sports.

DANGERS OF ERYTHROPOIETIN USE

The use of rHuEPO has been associated with a series of problems, including hypertension, seizures and thrombotic events. For instance, the use of rHuEPO is associated with an increase in blood pressure in patients with end-stage renal disease (Berglund & Ekblom 1991; Fisher 1997). Fisher (1997) outlined a series of mechanisms for the observed increase in blood pressure after the administration of rHuEPO. Increased blood viscosity and possibly direct vascular effects are major reasons (Berglund & Ekblom 1991; Fisher 1997). During exercise, when a 5–10% haemoconcentration occurs (owing to a loss of PV), it would be reasonable to assume that these problems may be worsened.

Some investigators have reported that rHuEPO does not result in hypertensive, convulsive or thrombotic episodes in healthy individuals (McMahon et al. 1990; Souillard et al. 1996). McMahon et al. (1990) postulated that the absence of these events in healthy volunteers after rHuEPO usage indicates that the associated problems may be a result of the patients' underlying disease or the effects of increasing haematocrit, and not of a direct pressor effect of erythropoietin. However, others have reported that after the administration of rHuEPO, healthy volunteers show an elevated blood pressure during submaximal exercise (Berglund & Ekblom 1991).

In both anaemic and normal subjects, haematocrit levels increase in direct relation to the dosage of rHuEPO (McMahon et al. 1990; Adamson & Vapnek 1991). Treatment is generally acceptable and safe for persons with renal anaemia during resting conditions (Adamson & Vapnek 1991). However, in athletes the administration of rHuEPO may cause serious complications, since haematocrit levels may rise to dangerous levels (Adamson & Vapnek 1991). It is quite possible that erythropoietin injections could increase a normal haematocrit to the point that viscosity impairs $\dot{Q}_{max}$ and thereby $\dot{V}_{O_{2max}}$ and endurance performance. Further, the considerable accompanying increase in viscosity could lead to heart failure and death. A series of mysterious deaths in élite cyclists from the Netherlands and Swedish orienteers may have been associated with the misuse of erythropoietin (although this speculation has yet to be substantiated). However, at the present time it is a formidable task to identify those who have used this pharmacological advantage, since detection of rHuEPO is difficult and training itself may modify endogenous levels of erythropoietin.

EFFECT OF TRAINING ON SERUM ERYTHROPOIETIN LEVELS

Investigators have examined the influence of various exercise regimes on serum erythropoietin levels (De Paoli Vitali et al. 1988; Schwandt et al. 1991; Weight et al. 1992; Klausen et al. 1993a). Haemoglobin concentration is partially controlled by erythropoietin levels (Ekblom 1996) and therefore serum erythropoietin levels are related to changes in the ODC (Weight et al. 1992). A rightward shift of the ODC is beneficial for the unloading of oxygen within the muscle capillaries during exercise (West 1995). Strenuous exercise results in metabolic acidosis and an increased body temperature, which serve to enhance the unloading of oxygen from haemoglobin and may reduce the stimulus for erythropoietin production. Combined with the elevated PV as a result of training, this could result in a reduced [Hb] and may give a further explanation for sports anaemia (Hallberg & Magnusson 1984; Weight et al. 1992). On the other hand, an increased haemoglobin oxygen affinity, which may also be observed during endurance exercise, may stimulate the production of erythropoietin (Klausen et al. 1993a).

There is considerable debate as to whether serum erythropoietin levels are decreased, increased or unchanged as a result of short- and long-term exercise. Some investigators have found that erythropoietin is increased both immediately after exercise (De Paoli Vitali et al. 1988; Ricci et al. 1988) and 3–31 h after a marathon run (Schwandt et al. 1991). In contrast, unchanged serum erythropoietin levels after strenuous exercise were found by other investigators (Berglund et al. 1988; Weight et al. 1992; Klausen et al. 1993a). Weight and coworkers (Weight et al. 1992) reported that a 42-km marathon did not result in a significant reduction in serum erythropoietin levels, despite a significant rightward shift in the ODC. Thus, this level of exercise was not sufficient to cause a decrease in the stimulus for erythropoietin production.

Cross-sectional comparisons of athletes and sedentary controls are also unclear with regard to the effects of long-term endurance training on serum erythropoietin levels. For instance, Ricci and coworkers (Ricci et al. 1988) revealed that 18 male long-distance runners had significantly greater serum erythropoietin levels than their untrained counterparts. Other investigators (Berglund et al. 1988; Weight et al. 1992) found no significant difference between endurance athletes and untrained individuals. In a recent investigation, Klausen et al. (1993a) reported that both short- and long-term exercise had no significant impact on serum erythropoietin concentrations in healthy male athletes. The authors concluded that the duration of endurance exercise has no direct effect on serum levels of erythropoietin. Therefore, findings are conflicting with regard to the effects of endurance training and/or exercise on endogenous erythropoietin levels. However, it appears that endurance-trained athletes possess similar levels of erythropoietin to their untrained counterparts.

DETECTION OF RECOMBINANT HUMAN ERYTHROPOIETIN

The Medical Commission of the International Olympic Committee has classified rHuEPO as a 'banned doping' substance (International Olympic Committee 1990). Unfortunately, rHuEPO has a short half-life (5–13 h) (Birkeland et al. 1997) and, since it is virtually indistinguishable from its endogenous counterpart (Egrie et al. 1986), there is presently no effective technique for detecting unequivocally the use of synthetic erythropoietin (Berglund & Ekblom 1991). The use of rHuEPO results in characteristic improvements in haematological properties (i.e. increased haematocrit, haemoglobin and RBC), which can be monitored via blood samples. High levels of serum erythropoietin can also be determined within the early hours after its administration (Birkeland et al. 1997). However, detection of rHuEPO becomes increasingly difficult as the time postinfusion increases.

Several investigators have examined methods of detecting rHuEPO in blood or urine (Casoni et al. 1993; Wide et al. 1995; Souillard et al. 1996). Casoni et al. (1993) revealed that there is a significant increase in large erythrocytes with low haemoglobin content (hypochromic macrocytes). They postulated that the use of a cut-off value for hypochromic macrocytes would detect approximately 50% of rHuEPO-treated athletes, without yielding any false positives. Despite this relatively low detection rate, the authors postulated that such a cut-off value could be a deterrent for rHuEPO misuse in athletes. However, the technique still needs to be conducted on a wide variety of athletes differing in sex, race and type of sport before it can be implemented as a doping control measure. The effects of other factors, such as altitude training, on the prevalence of hypochromic macrocytes also need to be examined.

Klausen et al. (1993a) wrote that serum erythropoietin levels can be determined within low, normal and high ranges using radioimmunoassays and enzyme-linked immunoassays. Therefore, a standard criterion for serum erythropoietin levels could potentially be created, allowing abnormally high or low levels of erythropoietin to be detected. However, an inherent problem with this approach would be the variability of endogenous erythropoietin levels as a result of training, training at altitude and circadian variations. Therefore, more direct techniques are needed to determine the use of rHuEPO.

Recently, investigators revealed that serum and urine samples can be analysed using an immunoradiometric assay to determine misuse of rHuEPO (Souillard et al. 1996). Souillard et al. (1996) also used an exponential model of the change in reticulocytes as an index of the effects of rHuEPO. However, they noted that serum and urine concentrations of rHuEPO can only detect such doping during or within 4–7 days after injection. Thus, detection of rHuEPO misuse using blood and urine samples may be more suited to 'out-of-competition' situations.

A recent technique of Wide et al. (1995) appears promising. This method is based on the fact that rHuEPO consists of a wide range of isoforms that have a differing median charge from endogenous erythropoietin. Thus, these authors have postulated that an electrophoretic method may be useful for the detection of rHuEPO in both blood and urine samples. The authors found that rHuEPO is less negatively charged and has a lower electrophoretic mobility than its endogenous counterpart. Wide and coworkers (Wide *et al.* 1995) were therefore able to detect rHuEPO in both serum and urine samples up to 48 h after injection. However, they were unable to detect rHuEPO in serum or urine 1–3 weeks after injection. The probability of detecting rHuEPO more than 3 days after injection was less than 50%. This is important, since the effects of rHuEPO may be maintained for a longer period (Ekblom 1996) than the detection capabilities of the method. This technique may be more useful for 'out-of-competition' tests, since athletes using rHuEPO would need 6–8 weeks of rHuEPO injections to gain its full benefits. This method presently holds the greatest potential for the detection of rHuEPO, but it is a very labour-intensive and costly procedure (Birkeland *et al.* 1997).

The lack of a definitive method for measuring exogenous erythropoietin, combined with uncertainties regarding the effects of training, altitude, diurnal variations and stress on basal erythropoietin levels, make it difficult to set standard criteria for erythropoietin levels (Klausen *et al.* 1993b; Ekblom 1996). Until an analytical technique is made available that detects rHuEPO during competition, we must once again rely on the integrity of the athletes and coaches to refrain from utilizing this unfair advantage. However, the recent controversy surrounding the 1998 Tour de France, during which several athletes and teams admitted to the use of rHuEPO for performance enhancement, reveals that this may not be possible. Therefore, a suitable doping control technique for erythropoietin is very much needed.

Role of blood volume in oxygen transport and endurance performance

Changes in BV affect oxygen transport by altering stroke volume (SV) and thereby $\dot{Q}$ through changes in ventricular preload and the Frank–Starling mechanism. Resultant changes in $\dot{Q}_{max}$ in turn affect oxygen transport capacity and consequently

$\dot{V}_{O_{2max}}$. Hence, alterations in BV can influence endurance performance capacity.

Blood volume can be estimated from body mass (77.5 ml blood per kg body mass), or it can be measured by dilution techniques, using radioactive labelled RBC or Evan's blue dye (current supplier: New World Trading Corporation, Longwood, Florida, USA). In addition, changes in BV subsequent to the infusion of blood can be determined from a knowledge of both the [Hb] and the volume of infused blood (generally by weighing it, then converting it to a volume, using an assumed density of 1.037). The BV following infusion can then be calculated, based on the principle of mass balance, assuming 100% erythrocyte survival *in vivo*. (With freeze-preserved cells, it is reasonable to assume 100% *in vivo* survival following infusion, but with refrigeration storage some erythrocytes become fragile and break up shortly after they are infused.) The BV following infusion is determined via the equation:

$$(BV\ post \times [Hb]\ post) = (BV\ pre \times [Hb]\ pre) + (BV\ infused \times [Hb]\ infused)$$

Because alterations in BV are interrelated to changes in [Hb], when examining the effect of changes in BV on $\dot{V}_{O_{2max}}$ and endurance performance, it is necessary to specify the [Hb] that accompanies the hypervolaemia or hypovolaemia. For example, in the hours immediately following the infusion of RBC for blood doping, there exists a transient hypervolaemia, with no change in [Hb]. Within 1 day, or at the most 2 days, the excess fluid is excreted to re-establish normovolaemia, with an elevated [Hb] (although a very slight hypervolaemia may persist due to the increase in oncotic pressure) (Spriet *et al.* 1986).

Original investigators of the effects of BV manipulations generally concluded that [Hb] (through alterations in total body haemoglobin) plays the dominant role in the influence of BV and [Hb] on $\dot{V}_{O_{2max}}$ and endurance performance. For instance, a series of investigations by Kanstrup and coworkers revealed that the effects of hypervolaemia are dependent on the resultant [Hb] of blood. Hypervolaemia, accompanied by an above-normal [Hb], increased both $\dot{V}_{O_{2max}}$ and endurance performance (Kanstrup & Ekblom 1984), but when hypervolaemia was accompanied by a mildly subnormal [Hb], there was no change in $\dot{V}_{O_{2max}}$ and possibly a decrease in endurance performance (Kanstrup & Ekblom 1982, 1984). When a greater reduction in [Hb] accompanied hypervolaemia, both $\dot{V}_{O_{2max}}$ and endurance performance were impaired (Kanstrup & Ekblom 1984). Therefore, an increase in $\dot{V}_{O_{2max}}$ and endurance performance can be achieved after BV expansion through an increase in oxygen-carrying capacity of the blood (brought about by an increase in total body haemoglobin). However, if hypervolaemia is associated with a significantly reduced [Hb], it tends to be associated with a decreased $\dot{V}_{O_{2max}}$ and endurance performance.

Acute decreases in PV and a consequent elevation in [Hb] are compensated within several hours by an expansion of the PV back to normovolaemia. However, the acute hypovolaemia and increased [Hb] are accompanied by a decrease in both $\dot{V}_{O_{2max}}$ (Danzinger & Cumming 1964) and endurance performance (Saltin 1964). When a subnormal [Hb] is accompanied by hypovolaemia, both $\dot{V}_{O_{2max}}$ and endurance performance are considerably impaired (Kanstrup & Ekblom 1982).

Volume loading independent of changes in red blood cells

Recent investigations have shown that $\dot{V}_{O_{2max}}$ and perhaps endurance performance can be improved as a result of training or acute PV expansion, independently of changes in RBC. Increases in PV can take place without concomitant increases in RBC volume, resulting in a decreased [Hb] (Green et al. 1987; Shoemaker et al. 1996). Thus, PV expansion presents an opportunity to examine the effects of BV on $\dot{V}_{O_{2max}}$ and endurance performance independently of changes in RBC.

Volume expansion can take place through training, acute expansion and/or the use of volume-regulating hormones. Training results in a significantly larger BV (hypervolaemia), which reaches a plateau after 1 week of training (Convertino 1991); the upper limit may be set by heredity. Short-term exercise-induced increases in BV are almost entirely due to increases in PV and not RBC volume

(Kanstrup & Ekblom 1982, 1984; Green et al. 1987; Shoemaker et al. 1996). However, as the training duration increases, an increase of RBC accounts for approximately half of the BV expansion (Convertino 1991). Acute PV expansion is generally brought about by the intravenous infusion of 400–700 ml of 6% dextran in saline (Coyle et al. 1986, 1990; Kanstrup et al. 1992; Krip et al. 1997; Warburton et al. 1999). Dextran (Macrodex™, Kabi Pharmacia Inc.) has an average molecular weight of 70 000 (similar to the plasma protein albumin). This, combined with the inclusion of isotonic saline in the mixture, means that an elevated PV equivalent to the amount infused can occur without a significant escape of the infusate. There is relatively low risk to patients' health in using Macrodex™. However, a few cases of marked hypotension and/or cardiac and respiratory arrest have been reported. These reactions usually take place early during infusion (Krogh (1994): Compendium of Pharmaceutical and Specialties). To minimize the possibility of anaphylactic reactions, 20 ml of Promiten™ (Pharmacia, Hillerod, Denmark) is injected either immediately before (Warburton et al. 1999) or after (Kanstrup et al. 1992) the infusion of Macrodex™. The plasma expander is generally infused over a 30–40-min period (Kanstrup et al. 1992). Exercise tests are generally conducted 30–60 min after infusion (Krip et al. 1997; Warburton et al. 1999).

The amount of PV expansion sustained over an exercise programme will have a direct effect on the magnitude of enhancements in $\dot{V}_{O_{2max}}$ and endurance performance. This is because substantial losses in water and electrolytes can occur during exercise (especially in the heat) (Convertino 1991). To offset losses in PV as a result of exercise, two mechanisms must be stimulated: (i) an increased thirst mechanism; and/or (ii) a reduced urine output (Convertino 1991). Renal manipulation for the maintenance of PV levels can be achieved by the release of a series of hormones. For instance, several investigators have reported that the plasma levels of renin, angiotensin, aldosterone and the antidiuretic hormone (i.e. vasopressin) increase during exercise (Convertino et al. 1980, 1981, 1983; Convertino & Kirby 1985). These hormones serve to enhance the retention of water and electrolytes, and contribute to the regulation of PV during exercise. Therefore, it is possible that acute supplementation of these hormones may lead to a further expansion of PV during exercise, such that the volume benefits (i.e. increased SV and $\dot{Q}$) are maintained throughout exercise. This may be particularly important for ultra-endurance events in the heat. It is also possible that the combination of acute PV expansion and acute supplementation of volume-regulating hormones may enhance the benefits seen as a result of acute PV expansion. This is because acute PV expansion may be associated with decreased circulating levels of renin–angiotensin, vasopressin and aldosterone (Share & Claybaugh 1972; Grant et al. 1996), which promote diuresis and bring BV back to normal levels. The extra volume provided by acute volume expansion may be maintained to a greater extent with simultaneous manipulation of the volume-regulating hormones.

To our knowledge, no investigators have examined the effects of acute supplementation of the volume-regulating hormones on endurance performance and $\dot{V}_{O_{2max}}$. However, numerous investigators have examined the effects of PV expansion, due to endurance training or acute PV expansion. A great deal of controversy (Kanstrup 1998; Warburton 1998) exists as to whether PV expansion results in an improved $\dot{V}_{O_{2max}}$ and endurance performance. It holds that if an increased $\dot{V}_{O_{2max}}$ is found after PV expansion, independent of changes in RBC, BV plays a greater role in the determination of $\dot{V}_{O_{2max}}$ and endurance performance than was previously thought.

Several investigators have reported that a PV expansion of 500–700 ml has little effect on $\dot{V}_{O_{2max}}$ despite a significant reduction (8–11%) in the oxygen content of blood (Kanstrup & Ekblom 1982, 1984; Green et al. 1987; Coyle et al. 1990; Mier et al. 1996; Warburton et al. 1999). Plasma volume expansion is thought to result in an increased central venous pressure (i.e. cardiac preload), which results in increased ventricular filling (via the Frank–Starling effect) (Kanstrup & Ekblom 1982, 1984; Green et al. 1987; Coyle et al. 1990; Kanstrup et al. 1992; Warburton et al. 1999). The resultant increases in SV and $\dot{Q}$ compensate for the haemodilution effects of PV expansion, allowing $\dot{V}_{O_{2max}}$ to remain

unchanged (Kanstrup & Ekblom 1982, 1984; Green et al. 1987; Coyle et al. 1990; Mier et al. 1996; Warburton et al. 1999).

However, other investigators have reported that PV expansion in untrained subjects may result in a significant improvement in $\dot{V}_{O_{2max}}$ (Convertino 1983; Coyle et al. 1986; Krip et al. 1997). These authors postulate that if the haemodilution effects of PV expansion are sufficiently offset by increases in SV and $\dot{Q}$, $\dot{V}_{O_{2max}}$ may be increased. This provides support for the contention that BV plays a greater role in the determination of $\dot{V}_{O_{2max}}$ than was previously thought. In fact, we have shown that a large portion of the difference in cardiovascular function between untrained and trained individuals is due to differences in BV. It is believed that endurance-trained athletes may be at an optimum BV for exercise performance (Krip et al. 1997; Warburton et al. 1999). This is supported by research in which the effects of acute PV on endurance athletes were examined, and minimal changes in their cardiovascular function were found (Coyle et al. 1986; Hopper et al. 1988; Warburton et al. 1999).

Comparison of investigations in which the effects of acute PV expansion on endurance performance have been examined reveals that endurance performance tends to be reduced, in both trained and untrained individuals, despite a maintained or increased $\dot{V}_{O_{2max}}$ (Kanstrup & Ekblom 1982, 1984; Coyle et al. 1986). That is, acute PV expansion may affect endurance performance differently from $\dot{V}_{O_{2max}}$. Therefore, endurance performance is dependent on more factors than $\dot{V}_{O_{2max}}$ alone (Coyle et al. 1986).

In the majority of these investigations, participants complained of an enhanced local fatigue of the legs during submaximal exercise. Hence, it is possible that the extra weight of the volume expander may have inhibited the participant's performance (Kanstrup & Ekblom 1982). It is also possible that an increased local lactate production (Kanstrup & Ekblom 1982) resulted in the increased feeling of leg fatigue. Another hypothesis is that the excessive haemodilution of the PV expander resulted in a decreased buffering capacity of blood, thereby impairing performance (Gledhill 1982; Coyle et al. 1990).

Other investigators have reported that if the amount of haemodilution is minimal as a result of acute PV expansion, endurance performance may be maintained (Coyle *et al.* 1990; Warburton *et al.* 1997) or improved (Coyle *et al.* 1990; Luetkemeimer & Thomas 1994). In the investigations in which endurance performance was increased, it is likely that the increase in PV resulted in an enhanced SV and $\dot{Q}$, allowing an increased aerobic power. As Coyle and coworkers (Coyle *et al.* 1990) wrote, these data indicate that there may be an 'optimal' PV for increases in $\dot{V}O_{2max}$ and endurance performance in untrained people. Given the findings of Warburton and coworkers (Warburton *et al.* 1999), it is also possible that endurance-trained athletes may be at an optimum BV for both endurance performance and $\dot{V}O_{2max}$, such that any further increases in BV without concomitant changes in RBC volume do not improve endurance performance or $\dot{V}O_{2max}$.

DETECTION OF ARTIFICIAL VOLUME LOADING: IS IT NECESSARY?

Several researchers have reported that basal levels of circulating hormones involved with fluid volume regulation (i.e. renin–angiotensin, vasopressin and aldosterone) are unchanged as a result of endurance training (Convertino *et al.* 1980, 1991; Carroll *et al.* 1995). Therefore, it may be possible that artificially elevated levels of these circulating hormones could be detected using standard radioimmunoassay procedures (Carroll *et al.* 1995). However, the difficulty in this procedure, as with all other doping controls, would be the development of a criterion level for each of the hormones.

The effects of Macrodex™ infusion on vascular volume remain relatively constant for up to 4 h, even with exercise participation, after which time substantial quantities of Macrodex™ are eliminated through normal renal excretion (Krip *et al.* 1997). It is generally reported that within 24 h 40% of the Macrodex™ solution is eliminated through normal renal excretion (Kabi Pharmacia Inc., Quebec). The remaining Macrodex™ is broken down enzymatically at a rate of approximately 70–90 mg·kg^{-1}·day^{-1} (Krogh (1994): Compendium of Pharmaceutical and Specialties) and it is fully dissipated within 1 week

(Convertino *et al.* 1980). Therefore, the benefits of Macrodex™ are short term, such that prerace infusions are required. Thus, postrace urine analysis would be suitable for the detection of this potential ergogenic aid.

It is likely that there has not been much interest in the potential ergogenic effects of volume loading because training results in significant increases in PV, and acute PV expansion results in minimal improvements in the cardiovascular function of endurance athletes. However, there may be situations in which volume loading and/or renal manipulation of the volume-regulating hormones give an athlete an unfair advantage. For instance, it may be advantageous during ultra-endurance events in the heat. No researchers have examined the effects of acute PV expansion and/or acute supplementation of volume-regulating hormones on the endurance performance of élite athletes during ultra-endurance events. If PV is maintained at a higher level, cardiovascular and thermoregulatory stability will not be as compromised, possibly allowing an improved performance. However, it is foreseeable that the same benefits could be achieved by proper hydration before and during a competition (Noakes 1993; Convertino *et al.* 1996). Therefore, testing athletes for the presence of dextran or abnormal levels of volume-regulating hormones may not be warranted.

In summary, if [Hb] remains unchanged, an accompanying decrease in BV will generally lead to decreases in $\dot{V}O_{2max}$ and endurance performance. However, an increase in BV with a reduction in [Hb] will either have no effect on or reduce $\dot{V}O_{2max}$ or endurance performance in endurance-trained athletes. An increased BV with a reduced [Hb] may result in an improved $\dot{V}O_{2max}$ and endurance performance in moderately active and/or untrained individuals. Also, if BV remains unchanged, accompanying decreases in [Hb] will lead to decreases in $\dot{V}O_{2max}$ and endurance performance, while an increase in [Hb] with no change in BV will produce increases in $\dot{V}O_{2max}$ and endurance performance. It can be concluded that [Hb] (through alterations in total body haemoglobin) and BV both play important roles in the determination of $\dot{V}O_{2max}$ and endurance performance. However, blood doping techniques which increase [Hb] are the most effective form of abuse for highly trained endurance athletes. Nevertheless, BV expansion, independent of changes in [Hb], may represent a possible ergogenic aid in untrained individuals. Also, given the potential ergogenic effects of acute PV expansion, preevent hydration is extremely important for optimal performance.

References

Adamson, J.W. & Vapnek, D. (1991) Recombinant erythropoietin to improve athletic performance. *New England Journal of Medicine* **324**, 698–699.

Berglund, B. & Ekblom, B. (1991) Effect of recombinant human erythropoietin treatment on blood pressure and some haematological parameters in healthy men. *Journal of Internal Medicine* **229**, 125–130.

Berglund, B. & Hemmingson, P. (1987) Effect of reinfusion of autologous blood on exercise performance in cross-country skiers. *International Journal of Sports Medicine* **8**, 231–233.

Berglund, B., Hemmingson, P. & Birgegard, G. (1987) Detection of autologous blood transfusions in cross-country skiers. *International Journal of Sports Medicine* **8**, 66–70.

Berglund, B., Birgegard, G. & Hemmingsson, P. (1988) Serum erythropoietin in cross-country skiers. *Medicine and Science in Sports and Exercise* **20**, 208–209.

Berglund, B., Birgegard, G., Wide, L. & Pihlstedt, P. (1989) Effects of blood transfusions on some hematological variables in endurance athletes. *Medicine and Science in Sports and Exercise* **21**, 637–642.

Beutler, E., Larsh, S. & Tanzi, F. (1960) Iron enzymes in iron deficiency. VII. Oxygen consumption measurements in iron-deficient subjects. *American Journal of the Medical Sciences* **239**, 759–765.

Birkeland, K.I., Donike, M., Ljungqvist, A. *et al.* (1997) Blood sampling in doping control. First experiences from regular testing in athletics. *International Journal of Sports Medicine* **18**, 8–12.

Brien, A.J. & Simon, T.L. (1987) The effects of red blood cell infusion on 10-km race time. *Journal of the American Medical Association* **257**, 2761–2765.

Buick, F., Gledhill, N., Froese, A.B., Spriet, L. & Meyers, E.C. (1980) Effect of induced erythrocythemia on aerobic work capacity. *Journal of Applied Physiology* **48**, 636–642.

Carroll, J.F., Convertino, V.A., Wood, C.E., Graves, J.E., Lowenthal, D.T. & Pollock, M.L. (1995) Effect of training on blood volume and plasma hormone concentrations in the elderly. *Medicine and Science in Sports and Exercise* **27**, 79–84.

Casoni, I., Ricci, G., Ballarin, E. *et al.* (1993) Hematological indices of erythropoietin administration in athletes. *International Journal of Sports Medicine* **14**, 307–311.

Celsing, F., Svedenhag, J., Pihlstedt, P. & Ekblom, B. (1987) Effects of anaemia and stepwise-induced polycythaemia on maximal aerobic power in individuals with high and low haemoglobin concentrations. *Acta Physiologica Scandinavica* **129**, 47–54.

Clement, D.B. & Sawchuk, L.L. (1984) Iron status and sports performance. *Sports Medicine* **1**, 65–74.

Clement, D.B., Asmundson, R.C. & Medhurst, C.W. (1977) Hemoglobin values: comparative survey of the 1976 Canadian Olympic team. *Canadian Medical Association Journal* **117**, 614–616.

Convertino, V.A. (1983) Heart rate and sweat rate response associated with exercise-induced hypervolemia. *Medicine and Science in Sports and Exercise* **15**, 77–82.

Convertino, V.A. (1991) Blood volume: its adaptation to endurance training. *Medicine and Science in Sports and Exercise* **23**, 1338–1348.

Convertino, V.A. & Kirby, C.R. (1985) Plasma aldosterone and renal sodium conservation during exercise following heat acclimation. *Federation Proceedings* **44**, 1562.

Convertino, V.A., Brock, P.J., Keil, L.C., Bernauer, E.M. & Greenleaf, J.E. (1980) Exercise training-induced hypervolemia: role of plasma albumin, renin, and vasopressin. *Journal of Applied Physiology* **48**, 665–669.

Convertino, V.A., Keil, L.C., Bernauer, E.M. & Greenleaf, J.E. (1981) Plasma volume, osmolality, vasopressin, and renin activity during graded exercise in man. *Journal of Applied Physiology* **50**, 123–128.

Convertino, V.A., Keil, L.C. & Greenleaf, J.E. (1983) Plasma volume, renin, and vasopressin responses to graded exercise after training. *Journal of Applied Physiology* **54**, 508–514.

Convertino, V.A., Mack, G.W. & Nadel, E.R. (1991) Elevated central venous pressure: a consequence of exercise training-induced hypervolemia. *American Journal of Physiology* **29**, R273–R277.

Convertino, V.A., Armstrong, L.E., Coyle, E.F. *et al.* (1996) American College of Sports Medicine. Position stand on exercise and fluid replacement. *Medicine and Science in Sports and Exercise* **28**, i–vii.

Cotes, J.E., Dobbs, J.M., Elwood, P.C., Hall, A.M., McDonald, A. & Saunders, M.J. (1972) Iron deficiency anaemia: its effect on transfer factor for the lung (diffusing capacity) and ventilation and cardiac frequency during submaximal exercise. *Clinical Science* **42**, 325–335.

Cowart, V.S. (1989) Erythropoietin: a dangerous new form of blood doping? *Physician and Sportsmedicine* **17** (8), 115–118.

Coyle, E.F., Hemmert, M.K. & Coggan, A.R. (1986) Effect of detraining on cardiovascular responses to exercise: role of blood volume. *Journal of Applied Physiology* **60**, 95–99.

Coyle, E.F., Hopper, M.K. & Coggan, A.R. (1990) Maximal oxygen uptake relative to plasma volume expansion. *International Journal of Sports Medicine* **11**, 116–119.

Danzinger, R.G. & Cumming, G.R. (1964) Effects of chlorothiazide on working capacity of normal subjects. *Journal of Applied Physiology* **33**, 636–638.

Davies, C.T.M., Chukweumeka, A.C. & Van Haaren, J.P.M. (1973) Iron-deficiency anaemia: its effect on maximum aerobic power and responses to exercise in African males aged 17–40 years. *Clinical Science* **44**, 555–562.

De Paoli Vitali, E., Guglielmini, C., Casoni, I. *et al.* (1988) Serum erythropoietin in cross-country skiers. *International Journal of Sports Medicine* **9**, 99–101.

Eckardt, K.U., Kurtz, A. & Bauer, C. (1989) Regulation of erythropoietin production is related to proximal tubular function. *American Journal of Physiology* **256**, F942–F947.

Egrie, J.C., Strickland, T.W., Lane, J. *et al.* (1986) Characterization and biological effects of recombinant human erythropoietin. *Immunobiology* **172**, 213–224.

Ekblom, B. (1996) Blood doping and ery-thropoietin. The effects of variation in hemoglobin concentration and other related factors on physical performance. *American Journal of Sports Medicine* 24, S40–S42.

Ekblom, B., Goldbarg, A.N. & Gullberg, B. (1972) Response to exercise after blood loss and reinfusion. *Journal of Applied Physiology* 33, 175–180.

Eschbach, J.W., Egrie, J.C., Downing, M.R., Browne, J.K. & Adamson, J.M. (1987) Correction of anemia of end-stage renal disease with recombinant human ery-thropoietin: results of combined phase I and phase II clinical trial. *New England Journal of Medicine* 316, 73–78.

Fisher, J.W. (1997) Erythropoietin: physio-logic and pharmacologic aspects. *Pro-ceedings of the Society for Experimental Biology and Medicine* 216, 358–369.

Frederickson, L.A., Puhl, J.L. & Runyan, W.S. (1983) Effects of training on indices of iron status of young female cross-country runners. *Medicine and Science in Sports and Exercise* 15, 271–276.

Gledhill, N. (1982) Blood doping and related issues: a brief review. *Medicine and Science in Sports and Exercise* 14, 183–189.

Grant, S.M.H.J.G., Phillips, S.M., Enns, D.L. & Sutton, J.R. (1996) Fluid and elec-trolyte hormonal responses to exercise and acute plasma volume expansion. *Journal of Applied Physiology* 81, 2386–2392.

Green, H.J., Jones, L.L., Hughson, R.L., Painter, D.C. & Farrance, B.W. (1987) Training-induced hypervolemia: lack of an effect on oxygen utilization during exercise. *Medicine and Science in Sports and Exercise* 19, 202–206.

Hallberg, L. & Magnusson, B. (1984) The etiology of 'sports anemia'. A physiolog-ical adaptation of the oxygen-dissociation curve of hemoglobin to an unphysiological exercise load. *Acta Medica Scandinavica* 216, 147–148.

Hopper, M.K., Coggan, A.R. & Coyle, E.F. (1988) Exercise stroke volume relative to plasma-volume expansion. *Journal of Applied Physiology* 64, 404–408.

Hsia, C.C.W. (1998) Respiratory function of hemoglobin. *New England Journal of Medicine* 338, 239–247.

International Olympic Committee (1990) Preliminary minutes from the meeting of the IOC Medical Commission. Lau-sanne.

Jacobs, K., Shoemaker, C., Rudersdorf, R. *et al.* (1985) Isolation and characterization of genomic and cDNA clones of human erythropoietin. *Nature* 313, 806–810.

Kanstrup, I. (1998) Effect of alterations in blood volume on cardiac functioning during maximal exercise [letter]. *Medi-cine and Science in Sports and Exercise* 30, 1339.

Kanstrup, I. & Ekblom, B. (1982) Acute hypervolemia, cardiac performance and aerobic power during exercise. *Journal of Applied Physiology* 52, 1186–1191.

Kanstrup, I. & Ekblom, B. (1984) Blood volume and hemoglobin concentration as determinants of maximal aerobic power. *Medicine and Science in Sports and Exercise* 16, 256–262.

Kanstrup, I.L., Marving, J. & Hoilund-Carlsen, P.F. (1992) Acute plasma expan-sion: left ventricular hemodynamics and endocrine function during exercise. *Journal of Applied Physiology* 73, 1791–1796.

Klausen, T., Breum, L., Fogh-Andersen, N., Bennett, P. & Hippe, E. (1993a) The effect of short and long duration exercise on serum erythropoietin concentrations. *European Journal of Applied Physiology* 67, 213–217.

Klausen, T., Dela, F., Hippe, E. & Galbo, H. (1993b) Diurnal variations of serum ery-thropoietin in trained and untrained subjects. *European Journal of Applied Phys-iology* 67, 545–548.

Krip, B., Gledhill, N., Jamnik, V. & Warburton, D. (1997) Effect of alterations in blood volume on cardiac function during maximal exercise. *Medicine and Science in Sports and Exercise* 29, 1469–1476.

Krogh, C.E. (ed.) (1994) *Compendium of Pharmaceuticals and Specialties*, 29th edn. Canadian Pharmaceutical Association, Ottawa.

Lin, F.K., Suggs, S., Lin, C.H. *et al.* (1985) Cloning and expression of the human erythropoietin gene. *Proceedings of the National Academy of Sciences of the USA* 82, 7580–7585.

Luetkemeimer, M.J. & Thomas, E.L. (1994) Hypervolemia and cycling time trial performance. *Medicine and Science in Sports and Exercise* 26, 503–509.

Macdougall, I.C., Roberts, D.E., Coles, G.A. & Williams, J.D. (1991) Clinical pharma-cokinetics of epoetin (recombinant human erythropoietin) *Clinical Pharma-cokinetics* 20, 99–113.

McMahon, F.G., Vargas, R., Ryan, M. *et al.* (1990) Pharmacokinetics and effects of recombinant human erythropoietin after intravenous and subcutaneous injec-tions in healthy volunteers. *Blood* 76, 1718–1722.

Magnusson, B., Hallberg, L., Rossander, L. & Swolin, B. (1984a) Iron metabolism and 'sports anemia'. I. A study of several iron parameters in elite runners with dif-ferences in iron status. *Acta Medica Scan-dinavica* 216, 149–155.

Magnusson, B., Hallberg, L., Rossander, L. & Swolin, B. (1984b) Iron metabolism and 'sports anemia'. II. A hematological comparison of elite runners and control subjects. *Acta Medica Scandinavica* 216, 157–164.

Mier, C.M., Domenick, M.A., Turner, N.S. & Wilmore, J.H. (1996) Changes in stroke volume and maximal aerobic capacity with increased blood, in men and women. *Journal of Applied Physiology* 80, 1180–1186.

Noakes, T.D. (1993) Fluid replacement during exercise. *Exercise and Sport Science Reviews* 21, 297–330.

Ondracka, S. & Gledhill, N. (1988) Evalua-tion of serum ferritin analysis tech-niques. *Canadian Journal of Sport Sciences* 13, 73–74.

Pate, R.R. (1983) Sports anemia: a review of the current research literature. *Physician and Sportsmedicine* 11 (2), 115–127.

Pavelka, E. (1985) Olympic blood boosting. *Bicycling* April, 32–39.

Ricci, G., Masotti, M., De Paoli Vitali, E., Vedovato, M. & Zanotti, G. (1988) Effects of exercise on haematologic parameters, serum iron, serum ferritin, red cell 2,3-diphosphoglycerate and creatine con-tents, and serum erythropoietin in long-distance runners during basal training. *Acta Haematologica* 80, 95–98.

Robertson, R.J., Gilcher, R., Metz, K.F. *et al.* (1982) Effect of induced erythrocythemia on hypoxia tolerance during physical exercise. *Journal of Applied Physiology* 53, 490–495.

Rosenlof, K., Gronhagen-Riska, C., Sovi-jarvi, A. *et al.* (1989) Beneficial effects of erythropoietin on haematological para-meters, aerobic capacity, and body fluid composition in patients on haemodialy-sis. *Journal of Internal Medicine* 226, 311–317.

Rowland, T.W. (1990) Iron deficiency in the young athlete. *Pediatric Clinics of North America* 37, 1153–1163.

Saltin, B. (1964) Circulatory response to submaximal and maximal exercise after thermal dehydration. *Journal of Applied Physiology* 19, 1125–1132.

Schwandt, H.J., Heyduck, B., Gunga, H.C. & Rocker, L. (1991) Influence of pro-longed physical exercise on the erythro-poietin concentration in blood. *European Journal of Applied Physiology* 63, 463–466.

Share, L. & Claybaugh, J.R. (1972) Regula-tion of body fluids. *Annual Review of Physiology* 34, 235–260.

Shoemaker, J.K., Green, H.J., Coates, J., Ali, M. & Grant, S. (1996) Failure of prolonged exercise training to increase red cell mass in humans. *American Journal of Physiology* **270**, H121–H126.

Souillard, A., Audran, M., Bressolle, F., Gareau, R., Duvallet, A. & Chanal, J.L. (1996) Pharmacokinetics and pharmacodynamics of recombinant human erythropoietin in athletes. Blood sampling and doping control. *British Journal of Clinical Pharmacology* **42**, 355–364.

Spriet, L., Gledhill, N., Froese, A.B. & Wilkes, D.L. (1986) Effect of graded erythrocythemia on cardiovascular and metabolic responses to exercise. *Journal of Applied Physiology* **61**, 1942–1948.

Sproule, B.J., Mitchell, J.H. & Miller, W.F. (1960) Cardiopulmonary physiological responses to heavy exercise in patients with anemia. *Journal of Clinical Investigation* **39**, 378–388.

Thomson, J.M., Stone, J.A., Ginsburg, A.D. & Hamilton, P. (1982) O₂ transport during exercise following blood reinfusion. *Journal of Applied Physiology* **53**, 1213–1219.

Valeri, C.R. (1976) *Blood Banking and the Use of Frozen Blood Products.* CRC Press, Cleveland.

Wagner, J.C. (1991) Enhancement of athletic performance with drugs. An overview. *Sports Medicine* **12**, 250–265.

Warburton, D.E.R. (1998) Effect of alterations in blood volume on cardiac functioning during maximal exercise [letter]. *Medicine and Science in Sports and Exercise* **30**, 1339–1341.

Warburton, D.E.R., Gledhill, N., Jamnik, V., Krip, B. & Card, N. (1999) Induced hypervolemia, cardiac function, $\dot{V}O_{2max}$ and performance of élite cyclists. *Medicine and Science in Sports and Exercise* **31**, 800–808.

Weight, L.M., Darge, B.L. & Jacobs, P. (1991) Athletes' pseudoanaemia. *European Journal of Applied Physiology* **62**, 358–362.

Weight, L.M., Alexander, D., Elliot, T. &

Jacobs, P. (1992) Erythropoietic adaptations to endurance training. *European Journal of Applied Physiology* **64**, 444–448.

West, J.B. (1995) *Respiratory Physiology— the Essentials*, 5th edn. Williams & Wilkins, Baltimore.

Wide, L., Bengtsson, C., Berglund, B. & Ekblom, B. (1995) Detection in blood and urine of recombinant erythropoietin administered to healthy men. *Medicine and Science in Sports and Exercise* **27**, 1569–1576.

Williams, M.H., Wesseldine, S., Somma, T. & Schuster, R. (1981) The effect of induced erythrocythemia upon 5-mile treadmill run time. *Medicine and Science in Sports and Exercise* **13**, 169–175.

Winearls, C.G., Oliver, D.O., Pippard, M.J., Reid, C., Downing, M.R. & Cotes, P.M. (1986) Effect of human erythropoietin derived from recombinant DNA on the anemia of patients maintained by chronic haemodialysis. *Lancet* **2**, 1175–1178.

Chapter 31

Smoking, Alcohol, Ergogenic Aids, Doping and the Endurance Performer

MELVIN H. WILLIAMS

Introduction

As documented elsewhere in this monograph, highly successful endurance performers are genetically endowed (Chapter 15) with specific physiological (Chapters 5–11, 21–23), psychological (Chapters 14, 25, 26) and biomechanical (Chapters 4, 16, 24) characteristics, associated with optimal energy production, control and efficiency for the various aerobic endurance sport events described in Chapters 54–64.

In order to optimize genetic potential, the endurance performer must receive state-of-the-art physiological, psychological and biomechanical training (Chapters 28, 32). Physiologically, the athlete trains the cardiovascular–respiratory oxygen transport system and intramuscular oxidative metabolic pathways to increase aerobic energy production. Psychologically, the athlete trains the mind to adapt to stressful physiological circumstances encountered during prolonged exercise tasks, improving control of energy production in attempts to prevent mental fatigue. Biomechanically, the athlete masters skills and attains the desirable body composition appropriate for his or her sport in order to increase energy efficiency. To achieve these ends, many national Olympic training centres employ sports physiologists, psychologists and biomechanists to optimize training (Chapter 28) and prevent sport injuries (Chapters 33, 53) or overtraining (Chapters 34, 52) that may impair effective endurance training.

Factors other than genetics and state-of-the-art training, such as environmental temperature (Chap-

ters 17, 40), altitude (Chapter 48), air pollution (Chapter 42), diet and nutrition (Chapter 29), and use of tactics such as blood doping (Chapter 30), may also influence endurance performance. Another factor that may affect performance is the athlete's general lifestyle, including such behaviours as sleeping habits, interpersonal relationships and, in particular, drug use.

Endurance athletes may use drugs for medical, social or ergogenic reasons. Medicinal drugs may be used to treat acute health problems, such as inflammation, or chronic health problems, such as asthma. Social drugs are used for mind-altering experiences. Ergogenic drugs may be used in attempts to enhance endurance performance beyond that attributable to genetics and training. Although athletes may use drugs specifically for one of these three reasons, various interactions may occur. For example, drugs taken for medicinal or social purposes may influence endurance performance. Conversely, drugs used for their ergogenic potential may affect health and social behaviour.

This chapter focuses primarily on the effect of purported ergogenic drugs used to enhance endurance performance. Also highlighted are several social drugs that may influence endurance performance, most often in an adverse, or ergolytic, manner. Given the plethora of individual studies evaluating the effect of ergogenic aids on performance and the limited space allocated for this presentation, most references cited are expertly detailed reviews that may provide in-depth information for the interested professional. Other ergogenic strategies for endurance athletes, particularly use of blood doping and the hormone recombinant erythropoietin (rEPO), are covered in Chapter 30.

Ergogenic drugs

In order to provide equal opportunities for success, the International Olympic Committee (IOC) has prohibited the use by athletes of numerous substances or methods (see Table 31.1). The practice known as doping may artificially enhance performance. Most prohibited substances are drugs.

Sport scientists (Smith & Perry 1992) indicate that athletes depend on ergogenic aids to compete. Indeed, allegations of drug use plagued the 1998 Tour de France, the definitive endurance sport. Literally scores of drugs are banned by the IOC. Unfortunately, although research should be the basis to determine whether or not a particular drug will improve sport performance, there are few well-designed studies evaluating the efficacy of most purported ergogenic drugs, especially studies involving élite athletes. Williams (1989a) indicated that an ideal study would use:

1 highly trained subjects in the sport performance theorized to be improved by an ergogenic drug;

Table 31.1 International Olympic Committee prohibited substances and methods. Adapted from United States Olympic Committee (1996).

1 Doping classes
  A Stimulants
  B Narcotic analgesics
  C Anabolic agents
  D Diuretics
  E Peptide and glycoprotein hormones and analogues
2 Doping methods
  A Blood doping
  B Pharmacological, chemical and physical manipulation
3 Classes of drugs subject to certain restrictions
  A Alcohol
  B Marijuana
  C Local anaesthetics
  D Corticosteroids
  E β-blockers
  F Specified β_2-agonists

2 a drug dosage comparable to that used by athletes;
3 a performance test that mimics the actual performance as closely as possible, but minimizes extraneous factors;
4 a double-blind, placebo protocol;
5 a repeated-measures, crossover design, if possible; and
6 graded dosage levels to evaluate a trend effect.

Ergogenic drugs are used to improve aerobic endurance performance via several mechanisms. Some drugs are used to increase physiological energy production, either by boosting oxygen delivery/utilization or by optimizing fuel supply/utilization. Other drugs may be used to stimulate psychological functions, improving energy control to help prevent mental fatigue. Drugs may also be used to reduce body fat in attempts to improve biomechanical efficiency. Several drugs may be purported ergogenics for multiple reasons. For example, some stimulants, as discussed below, may increase cardiovascular function, influence fuel utilization, elicit psychological arousal and suppress appetite.

Amphetamine

Amphetamine and its derivatives are sympathomimetic amines, chemical analogues to the natural endogenous catecholamine hormones epinephrine, norepinephrine and dopamine. Several derivatives such as methamphetamine (speed) and methylenedioxymethamphetamine (ecstasy) are used as social drugs, but amphetamine (Benzedrine) and dextroamphetamine (Dexedrine) have been used by athletes for their ergogenic potential. Amphetamine use was widespread in sports during the 1950s–1970s, and the amphetamine-related death of a Danish cyclist in the 1960 Olympics was a catalyst for IOC doping legislation (Williams 1974).

Conlee (1991) indicated that although the underlying pharmacological mechanism of action is unclear, amphetamine appears to potentiate the activity of the natural catecholamines. Amphetamine may elicit both central and peripheral nervous system responses, inducing both physiological and psychological effects at rest that theoretically might enhance exercise endurance performance. Physiologically, at rest, amphetamines will increase heart rate, cardiac output, blood pressure, glycogenolysis, serum glucose and free fatty acids (FFA), vasodilatation in the musculature, vasoconstriction in the cutaneous circulation and muscle cell irritability. Amphetamines may also invoke a subjective psychological state of excitability, arousal, motivation, self-confidence and mental and physical stimulation, factors that may elicit a decreased sense of fatigue (Martin 1971).

However, strenuous exercise induces a strong catecholamine effect that may negate the effects attributable to amphetamine use during rest. Indeed, the vast majority of physiological responses to exercise, particularly maximal exercise, do not appear to be influenced significantly by amphetamines in dosages ranging from 7 to 21 mg·kg^{-1} body mass, although Chandler and Blair (1980) reported a significantly higher maximal heart rate. Of importance to the endurance athlete, most research reveals that amphetamines have no effect on aerobic power ($\dot{V}_{O_{2max}}$) (Chandler & Blair 1980; Williams 1989a).

Although amphetamines do not appear to influence physiological responses to maximal exercise favourably in humans, numerous reviews (Cooter 1980; Ivy 1983; Lombardo 1986; Williams 1989a; Conlee 1991) indicate that their effect on various exercise tasks is equivocal. This equivocality may be attributed to the fact that amphetamines have neither consistent effects for all people, nor consistent effects when administered to the same individual on separate occasions (Chandler & Blair 1980). Nevertheless, several reviewers have indicated that amphetamines may decrease the rate of fatigue and enhance endurance performance (Ivy 1983), particularly in fatigued subjects (Williams 1989a; Conlee 1991). Several individual studies support this viewpoint.

Smith and Beecher (1959) conducted the most extensive field study with athletes. Although beset with numerous extraneous variables that could have affected the outcome, they concluded that amphetamines could enhance performance in a wide variety of athletic endeavours, including long-distance running. In one phase of their overall experiment, nine marathon runners timed themselves over their normal daily running courses, ranging in distance from 6.7 to 20.5 km (4.5–12.7 miles). Amphetamine dosages ranged from 7 to 21 mg·kg^{-1} body mass. Overall, amphetamines improved performance by over 24 s, significant at $P < 0.10$. Although this study was justifiably criticized for some methodological shortcomings, subjects were highly trained athletes.

The last well-controlled laboratory study was conducted by Chandler and Blair (1980) nearly 20 years ago. Although the six subjects were former high-school athletes, they were not participating in a regular programme of endurance activities. The investigators used a double-blind, placebo protocol, and tested subjects three times under both amphetamine and placebo conditions. Although amphetamines did not increase $\dot{V}_{O_{2max}}$ significantly, the subjects significantly improved their time to exhaustion in the treadmill $\dot{V}_{O_{2max}}$ test, and this increased time was associated with a significantly higher maximal heart rate and serum lactate concentration.

Chandler and Blair (1980) indicated that amphetamines do not prevent fatigue, but they may mask the effects of fatigue as documented by the increased serum lactate concentration. Theoretically, amphetamines may enhance performance via psychological mechanisms, removing normal inhibitions that might otherwise limit endurance performance. However, by interfering with the body's natural fatigue alarm system, amphetamine use could have serious health consequences, particularly heat illnesses under extreme environmental conditions.

Because amphetamines may increase serum FFA, Ivy (1983) hypothesized that endurance performance could be improved via a muscle glycogen-sparing effect. Although there are no experimental data with humans to evaluate this hypothesis, considerable research has investigated such an effect with another, more common stimulant—caffeine.

Caffeine

Caffeine, chemically 1,3,7-trimethylxanthine, is an alkaloid derived from dried seeds of *Coffea arabica* or dried leaves of *Thea sinensis*. Caffeine may be classified as a food drug, appearing naturally in coffee, tea, chocolate and guarana, but it is also found in other commercial products (see Table 31.2).

Caffeine is a stimulant that, comparable to amphetamine, exerts widespread effects on human physiological and psychological functions. Several recent reviews (Tarnopolsky 1994; Spriet 1995; Graham & Spriet 1996; Graham 1997) have detailed the possible mechanisms whereby caffeine supplementation may improve endurance performance. Although all reviewers acknowledge that the mechanisms have not been clearly established, caffeine appears to cross the membranes of all tissues in the body, including both the central nervous system (CNS) and skeletal muscle, and it may directly or indirectly affect neural, metabolic or hormonal factors that may enhance endurance performance. Some of these effects may also be mediated by caffeine metabolites, particularly the dimethylxanthine paraxanthine. Reviewers (Spriet 1995; Graham 1997) indicate that, because of its role as a competitive antagonist for adenosine receptors, caffeine may possibly influence endurance performance via the following mechanisms.

1 Caffeine may exert a direct stimulant effect on some portion of the CNS, which in turn may influence the cardiovascular system, endocrine secretion and activity of the sympathetic nervous system (Graham 1997). In particular, caffeine may increase epinephrine secretion. The CNS stimulant effect could prevent mental fatigue, whereas the resultant physiological effects, such as arterial dilatation, increased heart function and bronchodilatation, could benefit oxygen transport.

2 Caffeine may exert a direct effect on excitation–contraction coupling in the skeletal muscle by potentiating calcium release from the sarcoplasmic reticulum, which could increase the force of muscle contraction at lower frequencies of stimulation (Tarnopolsky 1994), increasing energy efficiency.

3 Caffeine may affect metabolic processes, increasing fat oxidation and decreasing carbohydrate oxidation. Caffeine may increase FFA mobilization from adipose or intramuscular stores indirectly by increasing epinephrine or directly by antagonizing adenosine receptors that normally inhibit FFA mobilization (Spriet 1995; Graham & Spriet 1996). This metabolic effect could spare muscle glycogen for use during the latter portions of prolonged endurance events.

Individually, each of these factors may enhance endurance performance, but they also may be operating collectively.

Numerous studies have evaluated the effect of caffeine supplementation on exercise performance. Conlee (1991) noted that equivocal findings could be attributed to experimental design problems, including exercise modality, exercise power output and caffeine dose. Spriet (1995) identified other problems, including nutritional status, training status, previous caffeine use and individual variation.

Nevertheless, most reviewers (Nehlig & Debry 1994; Tarnopolsky 1994; Spriet 1995; Graham & Spriet 1996; Graham 1997) concluded that caffeine appears to improve endurance performance. For example, caffeine dosages ranging from 3 to 13 mg·kg^{-1} increase endurance time by over 20% in exercise tasks carried to exhaustion at 80–85% $\dot{V}O_{2max}$ (Graham & Spriet 1995; Pasman et al. 1995). However, the underlying ergogenic mechanism has not been unequivocally identified. Although some research has demonstrated that caffeine ingestion is frequently associated with increases in plasma epinephrine and FFA, as well as muscle glycogen sparing, Graham (1997) indicates that this hypothesis is far from complete. For example, studies have

Table 31.2 Approximate caffeine content in selected drinks and other products.

Item	Caffeine (mg)
Coffee, regular, brewed, 175 ml	100
Espresso, 60 ml	120
Coffee, decaffeinated, 175 ml	5
Tea, black, 175 ml	50
Iced tea, 355 ml	70
Cola soda, 355 ml	50
Java juice, 355 ml	90
Hershey Special Dark Chocolate Bar	30
Excedrin tablet	65
No Doz tablet	100
Vivarin tablet	200

reported improved endurance without significant elevation of plasma epinephrine (Graham & Spriet 1995) and, as discussed below, caffeine has improved endurance performance in events not dependent upon muscle glycogen sparing.

Several studies have shown that caffeine may enhance endurance performance in events of shorter duration, such as a 5 min test of cycling to exhaustion at $\dot{V}O_{2max}$ (Jackman *et al.* 1996) and in a 20 min, 1500-m swim (MacIntosh & Wright 1995). In such events, glycogen is not limiting and fat metabolism is not important (Graham 1997). Either a stimulation of the CNS or a skeletal muscle effect could be operative. For example, in a recent study (Cole *et al.* 1996) subjects were asked on six separate occasions to generate as much total work as possible in 10 min. Three different ratings of perceived exertion (RPE of 9, 12 and 15) were set, once each with caffeine or placebo. Compared to the placebo, caffeine significantly increased total work output by approximately 12%, suggesting a beneficial neuromuscular effect.

Caffeine is also a diuretic and could compromise endurance performance in the heat by impairing temperature regulation. However, when consumed in a carbohydrate–electrolyte drink before and after a prolonged cycling task, caffeine (8.7 mg·kg^{-1}) had no effect on urine production and apparently did not compromise body hydration status (Wemple *et al.* 1997). Moreover, caffeine (5 mg·kg^{-1}) administered to highly trained subjects who ran for 2 h had no significant effect on sweat loss, water deficit, percentage change in plasma volume, serum electrolyte losses or final rectal temperature (Gordon *et al.* 1982). Although caffeine (5 or 9 mg·kg^{-1}) had no ergogenic effect on 21-km race performance under hot and humid conditions, it did not have any ergolytic effect either (Cohen *et al.* 1996). It appears that caffeine use will not impair endurance performance under warm environmental conditions.

Overall, research data suggest that caffeine may play an ergogenic role in endurance exercise performance of varying durations by altering neuromuscular or metabolic factors. However, Spriet (1995) notes that although group studies suggest that caffeine use may produce significant endurance performance improvements in recreational and élite

athletes, because of individual variability, we do not know how caffeine will affect any given individual is not known.

In general, although caffeine use may pose some health risks for certain individuals, such as those with hypertension or abnormal heart rhythms, research suggests relatively low or non-existent levels of risk associated with moderate caffeine consumption (Lamarine 1994; Consumers Union 1997). This would appear to be particularly so with healthy athletes.

Because caffeine is a common ingredient of beverages normally consumed by athletes, the IOC lists caffeine as a controlled or restricted substance. The maximal permitted level is 12 μg·ml^{-1} in urine; in a 70-kg individual, this level could be achieved by drinking about six 150-ml cups of coffee. A caffeine dose of 5–6 mg·kg^{-1} is ergogenic, but would result in urinary caffeine concentrations lower than the current IOC restricted level (Tarnopolsky 1994; Pasman *et al.* 1995). Spriet (1995) recommends that the IOC reconsider its policy on caffeine use.

Ephedrine and related sympathomimetics

The stimulant ephedrine, like amphetamine, is a synthetic sympathomimetic drug, a non-selective agent that elicits a general sympathetic response. Ephedrine may be useful in the treatment of asthma, and many over-the-counter products containing ephedrine are marketed for treating cold symptoms (Bronkotabs; Vicks Inhaler) or promoting weight loss (Herbal Phen-Fen). Ephedrine is also found in herbal teas and herbal ephedrine (Chinese Ephedra or Ma huang).

Theoretically, ephedrine and related stimulants, such as pseudoephedrine, could elicit physiological and psychological effects comparable to amphetamines and caffeine that could prove ergogenic for endurance performance.

The effect of ephedrine or pseudoephedrine supplementation on exercise performance has received little research attention, and recent studies do not support any ergogenic benefits. Swain *et al.* (1997) studied the effect of varying dosages of pseudoephedrine (1 or 2 mg·kg^{-1}) and phenylpropanolamine (0.33 or 0.66 mg·kg^{-1}) on well-trained cyclists during a maximal cycling test. The drugs had no significant effect on physiological responses, including $\dot{V}o_{2max}$, or maximal and sub-maximal heart rate and blood pressure, perception of effort as evaluated by the Borg RPE, or perfor-mance as measured by cycling time to exhaustion. Similar findings were reported in a double-blind, placebo-controlled, crossover study with female athletes undertaking a graded treadmill test (Bruce protocol); pseudoephedrine (60 mg) exerted no effect on submaximal or maximal $\dot{V}o_2$, ventilation, respiration rate, tidal volume, systolic and diastolic blood pressure, core temperature, RPE or total exer-cise time. However, submaximal heart rate was higher during the first four stages of the treadmill test and during recovery, a finding not considered to be ergogenic (Clemons & Crosby 1993). In a double-blind, placebo-controlled, crossover design involv-ing a simulated sport event, Gillies *et al.* (1996) found that a single dose of pseudoephedrine (120 mg) exerted no significant effect on the perfor-mance of 10 male cyclists in a 40-km trial (time to completion: placebo, 58.7 min; pseudoephedrine, 58.1 min).

These recent well-controlled studies, as well as previous studies and reviews (Sidney & Lefcoe 1977; Fitch 1986), indicate that ephedrine or related compounds do not exert an ergogenic effect on endurance performance as observed with ampheta-mine and caffeine.

Epidemiological data indicate that use of ephedrine or other sympathomimetics may elicit various side-effects, including nervous tension, headache, gastrointestinal distress, irregularities of heart rhythm and, in some cases, death. In one 2-year period over 500 reports of adverse health effects associated with use of dietary supplements containing ephedrine and associated alkaloids (pseudoephedrine, norephedrine and *N*-methyl ephedrine) were reported in the state of Texas, including eight deaths. Most of the deaths were attributed to myocardial infarction or cerebrovascu-lar accident (United States Department of Health and Human Services 1996).

The IOC prohibits the use of ephedrine and other sympathomimetics. Athletes should know that all cold medications with decongestants are likely to contain prohibited sympathomimetics. Intranasal administration of an over-the-counter ephedrine-containing cold medicine can lead to a urinary ephedrine concentration above $5 \mu g \cdot ml^{-1}$, a positive drug test (Lefebvre *et al.* 1992). In the 1996 Olympics, at least six athletes tested positive for drug use, mostly because of stimulants obtained from over-the-counter products. However, not all athletics-governing organizations prohibit ephedrine-like substances, so athletes should check with their spe-cific organization regarding legality.

Anabolic–androgenic steroids (AAS)

Anabolic–androgenic steroids (AAS) are synthetic drugs designed to mimic testosterone, the male sex hormone that elicits both anabolic and androgenic effects. Both oral (17-carbon alkyl group) and injectable (17-carbon ester) AAS are used by ath-letes; some commonly used products are high-lighted in Table 31.3.

Strength/power athletes use AAS as an ergogenic aid to alter body composition by increasing lean mass and decreasing body fat, primarily with the intent of increasing muscular strength and endurance. Surveys reveal that athletes such as weightlifters, bodybuilders, throwers (javelin, discus, hammer and shot-put), American football players and sprinters are predominant users of AAS (Lombardo *et al.* 1991). Although results from indi-vidual studies evaluating the ergogenicity of AAS are equivocal, most recent reviews and well-controlled studies (American College of Sports Medicine 1987; Elashoff *et al.* 1991; Lombardo *et al.*

Table 31.3 Commonly used oral and injectable anabolic–androgenic steroids (AAS). Trade (and generic) names. Adapted from Friedl (1993).

Oral
Dianabol (methandrostenolone)
Anavar (oxandrolone)
Winstrol (stanozolol)
Anadrol (oxymetholone)

Injectable
Delatestryl (testosterone enanthate)
Deca-durabolin (nandrolone decanoate)

1991; Lombardo 1993; Bhasin *et al.* 1996; Cable 1997) indicate that AAS use may modify body composition favourably by increasing muscle mass and decreasing body fat. They may also increase muscular strength and endurance.

AAS may be used by endurance athletes for several reasons. Firstly, AAS have been shown to stimulate erythropoiesis and increase red cell production (Alen 1985). They may also potentiate the effect of recombinant erythropoietin (Ballal *et al.* 1991). Such an effect could increase $\dot{V}O_{2max}$. Several studies reported that AAS increased indirect measures of $\dot{V}O_{2max}$ as predicted from submaximal exercise heart rate responses (Lombardo 1993), but studies using direct measurements of $\dot{V}O_{2max}$ reported no significant effect of AAS (Williams 1974, 1989a).

Secondly, AAS may facilitate recovery from intense exercise. Endurance athletes reportedly use AAS to perform more frequent, longer, high-intensity training sessions. Available surveys reveal very limited AAS use by endurance athletes, but anecdotal reports suggest some use by Tour de France cyclists, presumably for more rapid daily recovery during the 3-week race. Unfortunately, research investigating the effect of AAS on actual aerobic endurance performance is virtually non-existent. Lombardo (1993) noted that until such investigations are conducted, the question as to the effect of AAS on performance in endurance events will remain unanswered.

AAS use has been associated with a variety of relatively minor adverse health effects, including cosmetic effects (development of acne, alopecia and facial hair in females), psychological effects (increased aggressiveness) and reproductive effects (decreased libido, testicular shrinkage). It may also be associated with more chronic health problems (Williams 1998). Friedl (1993) indicates that although it is not readily apparent that we can attribute significant adverse health effects to AAS as a general class, oral AAS clearly affect liver function, one effect being a substantial reduction in high density lipoprotein cholesterol, a risk factor for coronary heart disease. In addition to altering lipoprotein metabolism, other reviewers (Melchert & Welder 1995; Cable 1997) indicate that AAS may increase the risk of coronary heart disease by increasing clot formation, by changing the reactivity of the endothelium to vasoactive substances or by modulating cardiac dimensions. Friedl (1993) notes that injectable steroids appear to produce fewer adverse effects, although there are several case reports suggesting increased susceptibility to thrombotic stroke, possibly associated with administration of high doses. Additionally, prostate carcinoma is linked to androgen excess.

Summarizing, Friedl (1993) states that an athlete would be foolish to conclude that there is a safe way to use anabolic steroids, noting that the long-term consequences of AAS use have not been investigated and are simply unknown. Case reports subsequent to Friedl's review indicate involvement of AAS in major mood disturbances (Pope & Katz 1994), peliosis hepatitis, or blood-filled liver cysts (Cabasso 1994), and fatal cardiac arrests (Kennedy & Lawrence 1993).

The IOC and most other athletics-governing organizations prohibit the use of AAS.

Social drugs

Many athletes use social or 'recreational' drugs for their mind-altering effects, but not usually in conjunction with sports performance. Nevertheless, some illegal social drugs have been theorized to be ergogenic, such as cocaine (Conlee 1991) and marijuana (Williams 1991), as have two commonly used social drugs, nicotine (in tobacco products) and alcohol.

Nicotine and cigarette smoking

Nicotine, a stimulant derived from tobacco leaves, is readily available in commercial products such as cigarettes, smokeless tobacco, nicotine gum and nicotine patches. In laboratory experimentation, nicotine has been infused intravenously. Depending on the form (cigarette; plug tobacco; moist snuff), 1 g of tobacco contains about 10–20 mg of nicotine, enough to provide a stimulant effect. Nicotine reaches the brain in fewer than 10 s via cigarette smoking, but may take 30 min with other delivery methods (Christen *et al.* 1990; Williams 1998).

Small doses of nicotine, as delivered by one cigarette, may imitate the effects of acetylcholine, stimulating the CNS and sympathetic nervous system. Nicotinic receptors in the adrenal medulla may release norepinephrine and epinephrine, responsible for some of the stimulating effects of nicotine analogous to amphetamine (Williams 1974; Krogh 1991).

As a stimulant, nicotine is theorized to improve neural functions such as reaction time, visual acuity and vigilance, possibly one of the reasons why smokeless tobacco is widely used by baseball players (Krogh 1991). In this regard, some consider nicotine as a doping agent (Williams 1974).

Research data relative to the effects of nicotine, cigarette smoking and smokeless tobacco on aerobic endurance performance are limited (Williams 1998). Nicotine infusion in miniswine increased heart rate and vascular resistance at rest, but these detrimental haemodynamic effects were minimized during exercise, possibly being counteracted by local vasodilators (Symons & Stebbins 1996). In humans, most laboratory studies have investigated the acute effect of smoking or smoking cessation on physiological or performance responses of habituated smokers, whereas epidemiological data compare responses of smokers with non-smokers.

Most research has been stimulated by the possible adverse effects of cigarette smoking (Williams 1974). Cigarette smoke contains compounds other than nicotine that may influence exercise performance, particularly carbon monoxide (CO). CO forms carboxyhaemoglobin (COHb), blocking oxygen binding to haemoglobin. It is thus ergolytic to aerobic endurance (Krogh 1991; Williams 1998).

Several studies have provided data suggesting that acute smoking may impair physiological functions important to aerobic endurance. For example, Rode and Shephard (1971), testing habitual smokers immediately after smoking two cigarettes, reported an increased oxygen cost of breathing when running on a treadmill at approximately 80% of $\dot{V}O_{2max}$. The increased oxygen cost of breathing decreased substantially when the subjects abstained from smoking for 24 h. Other studies indicate that acute smoking may decrease airway conductance (attributed to factors in cigarette smoke other than

nicotine) and may elicit a higher heart rate and lower stroke volume during submaximal exercise, decreasing heart efficiency (Williams 1974). However, other investigators reported no adverse effect of acute smoking on heart rate, oxygen consumption, oxygen debt in submaximal exercise or endurance performance. Based on these early findings, Williams (1974) concluded that the acute effects of smoking on endurance performance in habitual smokers were neither ergogenic nor ergolytic, but noted also that this did not infer that chronic smoking patterns had no effect on endurance performance.

Several epidemiological studies indicate that chronic smoking may impair aerobic endurance performance by affecting cardiovascular–respiratory functions negatively. Although Cooper et al. (1968) reported no significant effect of chronic cigarette smoking on $\dot{V}O_{2max}$ in young military recruits, smoking was associated with impaired minute ventilation, a lower oxygen consumption at equivalent heart rates and decreased aerobic endurance capacity as evaluated by a 12-min field running test. Sidney et al. (1993), using a graded exercise treadmill test with nearly 5000 subjects, reported that the mean maximum heart rate was lower (ranging from 6.7 to 11.2 beats lower) and the mean exercise test duration was shorter for smokers compared to non-smokers. Any deleterious effects of cigarette smoking may be attributed to factors in cigarette smoke other than nicotine. Bolinder et al. (1997) reported no adverse effects of 20-year smokeless tobacco use on exercise capacity, as evaluated by $\dot{V}O_{2max}$, in healthy, physically well-trained subjects.

Nicotine is considered an addictive drug, and cigarette smoke contains over 4000 chemicals, many possibly carcinogenic. Chronic cigarette smoking has been associated with numerous health problems, including heart disease, chronic obstructive lung disease and lung cancer; smokeless tobacco use is associated with oral cancer (Williams 1994).

Alcohol

Ethyl alcohol (C_2H_5OH) is classified as a drug, and it may also be regarded as a nutrient because it provides 43 kJ (7 kcal)·g^{-1}. One average drink of alcohol

(344 ml beer; 126 ml wine; 36 ml 80° proof liquor) contains about 14 g of pure ethanol (Williams 1991).

Ingested alcohol is absorbed rapidly from the stomach and small intestine, and the distribution in the body is related to the water content of the tissue. Organs with a high water content and rich blood supply, such as the brain, receive the highest initial concentration (Williams 1991). Alcohol is catabolized in the liver by alcohol dehydrogenase, being converted to acetylaldehyde and eventually metabolized to carbon dioxide and water. In a 70-kg individual, the liver oxidizes approximately $7 g \cdot h^{-1}$, but a small amount is also eliminated by the breath (Reilly 1997).

Alcohol may affect almost all tissues in the body, but its most prevalent effects are upon the CNS. Alcohol has differential effects on central neurotransmitters, including acetylcholine, serotonin, norepinephrine and dopamine. Alcohol may increase activity in central noradrenergic pathways and may increase plasma norepinephrine, eliciting a paradoxical stimulant effect; however, this response is inconsistent and transient. Alcohol acts primarily as a depressant, disrupting acetylcholine synthesis and release with a resultant slowing of nerve conduction. The overall depressant effects of alcohol are dependent primarily upon the blood alcohol concentration, ranging from mild relaxation to coma (Williams 1991; Reilly 1997).

Reilly (1997) has noted that sports competition, particularly important contests, may induce stress that disrupts optimal performance. Because alcohol may be an anxiolytic and antitremor agent for some individuals, its most prevalent use in athletic competition appears to be in target sports such as archery, darts and riflery (Williams 1991; Reilly 1997). However, the acute ingestion of alcohol may impair performance in sports that require fast reactions, complex decision making and highly skilled actions (American College of Sports Medicine 1982; Williams 1991; Reilly 1997).

Although the primary ergogenic application of alcohol to sport performance is psychological in nature, it may also affect physiological responses important to aerobic exercise. In this regard, Jokl (1968) reported evidence that alcohol was in wide use on the European sport scene at the turn of the century, citing cases of endurance athletes imbibing rum, champagne, cognac or beer during competition. However, as noted below, alcohol is likely to be ergolytic to aerobic endurance performance, rather than ergogenic.

The physiological effects of alcohol on cardiovascular–respiratory and metabolic responses to mild or moderate aerobic endurance exercise appear to be inconsistent. Although various investigators have reported neither beneficial nor detrimental effects of small to moderate amounts of alcohol (a blood alcohol concentration ranging from 0.5 to $1.0 mg \cdot l^{-1}$) on heart rate, myocardial efficiency, arteriovenous oxygen difference, respiratory dynamics or oxygen consumption during mild to moderate aerobic exercise tasks, other investigators using similar alcohol dosages and exercise protocols have reported significant increases in heart rate, oxygen consumption and blood lactate, an indication of impaired physiological efficiency that could be caused by decreased neuromuscular efficiency (American College of Sports Medicine 1982; Williams 1992; Reilly 1997). With higher alcohol dosages (a blood alcohol concentration greater than $2.0 mg \cdot l^{-1}$) heart function may be impaired, as suggested by a reported 6% reduction in left ventricular ejection fraction (Williams 1992).

During maximal exercise, the reported effects of alcohol on cardiovascular–respiratory and metabolic responses are more consistent; alcohol appears to exert no significant effect on maximal levels of oxygen intake, heart rate, stroke volume, cardiac output, arteriovenous oxygen difference, blood pressure, peripheral vascular resistance or peak blood lactate concentrations (Williams 1985; Reilly 1997).

Alcohol contains chemical energy, but several studies (Schurch et al. 1982; Massicotte et al. 1993) have reported that alcohol does not appear to be utilized as a major energy source during prolonged aerobic exercise. Massicotte et al. (1993) found that during aerobic exercise ethanol oxidation represented 5.2% of the total energy expenditure, much less than that previously reported for exogenous carbohydrates (8–18%) or medium-chain FFA (7–14%). Additionally, the small contribution of ethanol to energy metabolism did not modify endogenous carbohydrate or fat oxidation significantly during moderately prolonged exercise tasks (40–60 min) at low to moderate exercise intensities (30–60% $\dot{V}O_{2max}$) (Schurch et al. 1982).

Alcohol ingestion may theoretically impair aerobic endurance performance in more prolonged events, such as a marathon run, by interfering with optimal carbohydrate metabolism. Although alcohol does not impair lipolysis or FFA utilization during exercise, it may interfere with liver function, decreasing gluconeogenesis and glucose output from the liver, increasing the likelihood of hypoglycaemia developing during prolonged exercise (Williams 1992; Reilly 1997).

In an earlier review, Williams (1985) concluded that small to moderate doses of alcohol exerted no significant beneficial or detrimental effect on tests of aerobic endurance. Subsequent to that review, some research supported this conclusion, but other investigators reported that alcohol impaired performance. Despite an apparent trend towards a deterioration in performance with increased alcohol intake (0.0, 0.22 and 0.44 ml·kg^{-1}), Houmard et al. (1987) reported no significant effects of these alcohol doses on 8-km (5-mile) treadmill run time. Conversely, McNaughton and Preece (1986), using trained middle-distance athletes as subjects, observed a detrimental effect of alcohol in both an 800-m and a 1500-m run, the effect being dose related over blood alcohol concentrations ranging from 0.1 to 1.0 mg·l^{-1}. One study provides some support for adverse effects of a hypoglycaemic response, discussed above. Kendrick et al. (1993) reported that 25 ml of alcohol consumed by trained runners before and during a 60-min treadmill run at 80–85% $\dot{V}O_{2max}$ elicited a hypoglycaemic response (a 24% decrease in blood glucose) during the latter half of the test; 75% of the subjects could not complete the run during the alcohol trial.

Alcohol ingestion may decrease the release of antidiuretic hormone, possibly impairing temperature regulation during exercise under warm/hot environmental conditions. As a rehydration fluid after dehydration, drinks containing 4% alcohol or more, such as beer, tend to delay the recovery process as measured by restoration of blood and plasma volume (Shirreffs & Maughan 1997). Start-

ing a prolonged endurance event under warm/hot conditions in a dehydrated state could certainly impair performance. In a related vein, beer appears to have no advantage as a fluid replacement during exercise. Compared to water, beer had no significant effect on skin or rectal temperature while exercising for 45 min at 50% $\dot{V}O_{2max}$ (Mangum et al. 1986).

Alcohol ingestion may elicit cutaneous vasodilatation, possibly increasing heat loss from the body. Reilly (1997) has indicated that consuming alcohol while undertaking endurance exercise in the cold, e.g. during mountaineering, may not be a good idea because of heat loss from the skin surface, possibly predisposing to hypothermia.

Most athletes who drink alcohol do so for social, not ergogenic, reasons, so there is some concern that social drinking may affect endurance performance negatively. Limited available data suggest that social alcohol consumption, in moderation, has no beneficial or detrimental effect upon physical performance. For example, light drinking (one drink) the previous evening had no effect on physiological responses to aerobic exercise the following morning (Williams 1991). However, Reilly (1997) indicates that alcohol ingestion may lower muscle glycogen at rest. He advises against alcohol ingestion in the 24 h before an event, because prestart glycogen levels are important for sustained exercise at an intensity of 70–90% $\dot{V}O_{2max}$.

Heavy social alcohol consumption, leading to a hangover the following day, may significantly impair aerobic endurance, as noted by significant impairments in $\dot{V}O_{2max}$ and cycle performance time at 250 W (Karvinin et al. 1962; O'Brien 1993).

Alcohol is a popular social drug, and a major international drug problem. Health problems associated with alcohol misuse are numerous and varied, contributing substantially to health-care costs. Excessive use has been associated with alcoholic liver disease, the aetiology of some human cancers (oral, pharyngeal, oesophageal and breast cancer), high blood pressure, cardiomyopathy and heart failure, and fetal alcohol syndrome. Moderate drinking (1–2 glasses of wine·day^{-1}), however, has been associated with reduced mortality from coronary heart disease (Williams 1994).

Although alcohol consumption is not prohibited

for aerobic endurance athletes, there are no data supporting an ergogenic effect, and some data to suggest an ergolytic effect. Athletes who drink should do so in moderation, and possibly abstain 24 h prior to a prolonged contest.

Conclusions

Aerobic endurance athletes have used drugs and other ergogenic aids in attempts to enhance performance for centuries. Use continues, even if now illegal, as attested by recent administration of rEPO in the Tour de France. Stimulant drugs have long been popular, and are usually effective ergogenics. Although the use of amphetamine and ephedrine has been prohibited by the IOC, a limited amount of caffeine is permitted, and the legal amount may be a very effective ergogenic for some athletes. Other prohibited agents, such as AAS, have not been

shown to increase physiological or metabolic functions important to aerobic endurance, but they may enable more intense training, possibly improving competitive performance.

Athletes may use numerous medicinal drugs to cope with acute and chronic illnesses. Some of these drugs, such as diuretics and β-blockers (Williams 1989b, 1991), may impair aerobic endurance performance, but others, particularly stimulants and β-agonists found in cold/asthmatic medications, may be ergogenic and are prohibited by the IOC.

Authorities advising athletes should be aware of the drugs that are currently prohibited by their respective athletics-governing organizations, who normally provide detailed lists of proscribed substances. The IOC has developed a standard model for use by most organizations, and the current list of proscribed substances may be obtained from respective national Olympic committees.

References

Alen, M. (1985) Androgenic steroid effects on liver and red cells. *British Journal of Sports Medicine* **19**, 15–20.

American College of Sports Medicine (1982) Position statement on the use of alcohol in sports. *Medicine and Science in Sports and Exercise* **14** (6), ix–x.

American College of Sports Medicine (1987) American College of Sports Medicine position stand on use of anabolic–androgenic steroids in sports. *Medicine and Science in Sports and Exercise* **19**, 534–539.

Ballal, S.H., Domoto, D.T., Polack, D.C., Marciulonis, P. & Martin, K.J. (1991) Androgens potentiate the effects of erythropoietin in the treatment of anemia of end-stage renal disease. *American Journal of Kidney Disease* **17**, 29–33.

Bhasin, S., Storer, T.W., Berman, N. *et al.* (1996) The effects of supraphysiologic doses of testosterone on muscle size and strength in normal men. *New England Journal of Medicine* **335**, 1–7.

Bolinder, G., Noren, A., Wahren, J. & DeFaire, U. (1997) Long-term use of smokeless tobacco and physical performance in middle-aged men. *European Journal of Clinical Investigation* **27**, 427–433.

Cabasso, A. (1994) Peliosis hepatitis in a young adult bodybuilder. *Medicine and Science in Sports and Exercise* **26**, 2–4.

Cable, N.T. (1997) Anabolic–androgenic steroids, ergogenic and cardiovascular effects. In: Reilly, T. & Orme, M. (eds) *The Clinical Pharmacology of Sport and Exercise*, pp. 135–144. Excerpta Medica, Amsterdam.

Chandler, J.V. & Blair, S.N. (1980) The effect of amphetamines on selected physiological components related to athletic success. *Medicine and Science in Sports and Exercise* **12**, 65–69.

Christen, A.G., McDaniel, R.K. & McDonald, J.L. (1990) The smokeless tobacco 'time bomb'. *Postgraduate Medicine* **87** (7), 69–74.

Clemons, J.M. & Crosby, S.L. (1993) Cardiopulmonary and subjective effects of a 60-mg dose of pseudoephedrine on graded treadmill exercise. *Journal of Sports Medicine and Physical Fitness* **33**, 405–412.

Cohen, B.S., Nelson, A.G., Prevost, M.C., Thompson, G.D., Marx, B.D. & Morris, G.S. (1996) Effects of caffeine ingestion on endurance racing in heat and humidity. *European Journal of Applied Physiology* **73**, 358–363.

Cole, K.J., Costill, D.L., Starling, R.D., Goodpaster, B.H., Trappe, S.W. & Fink, W.J. (1996) Effect of caffeine on perception of effort and subsequent work production. *International Journal of Sport Nutrition* **6**, 14–23.

Conlee, R.K. (1991) Amphetamine, caffeine, and cocaine. In: Lamb, D.R. & Williams, M.H. (eds) *Ergogenics: Enhancement of Performance in Exercise and Sport*, pp. 285–330. WCB/Brown & Benchmark, Dubuque, IA.

Consumers Union (1997) What caffeine can do for you—and to you. *Consumer Reports on Health* **9**, 97–101.

Cooper, K.H., Gey, G.O. & Bottenberg, R.A. (1968) Effects of cigarette smoking on endurance performance. *Journal of the American Medical Association* **203**, 189–192.

Cooter, G.R. (1980) Amphetamine use, physical activity and sport. *Journal of Drug Issues* **10**, 323–330.

Elashoff, J.D., Jacknow, A.D., Shain, S.G. & Braunstein, G.D. (1991) Effects of anabolic–androgenic steroids on muscular strength. *Annals of Internal Medicine* **115**, 387–393.

Fitch, K. (1986) The use of anti-asthmatic drugs. Do they affect sports performance. *Sports Medicine* **3**, 136–150.

Friedl, K.E. (1993) Effects of anabolic steroids on physical health. In: Yesalis, C.E. (ed.) *Anabolic Steroids in Sport and Exercise*, pp. 107–150. Human Kinetics, Champaign, IL.

Gillies, H., Derman, W.E., Noakes, T.D., Smith, P., Evans, A. & Gabriels, G. (1996) Pseudoephedrine is without ergogenic effects during prolonged exercise. *Journal of Applied Physiology* **81**, 2611–2617.

Gordon, N., Myburgh, J.L., Kruger, P.E. et al. (1982) Effect of caffeine ingestion on thermoregulatory and myocardial function during endurance performance. *South African Medical Journal* **62**, 644–647.

Graham, T.E. (1997) The possible actions of methylxanthines on various tissues. In: Reilly, T. & Orme, M. (eds) *The Clinical Pharmacology of Sport and Exercise*, pp. 257–267. Excerpta Medica, Amsterdam.

Graham, T.E. & Spriet, L.L. (1995) Metabolic, catecholamine, and exercise performance responses to various doses of caffeine. *Journal of Applied Physiology* **78**, 867–874.

Graham, T.E. & Spriet, L.L. (1996) Caffeine and exercise performance. *Sport Sciences Exchange* **9** (1), 1–6.

Houmard, J.A., Langenfeld, M.E., Wiley, R.L. & Siefert, J. (1987) Effects of the acute ingestion of small amounts of alcohol upon 5-mile run times. *Journal of Sports Medicine and Physical Fitness* **27**, 253–257.

Ivy, J.L. (1983) Amphetamines. In: Williams, M.H. (ed.) *Ergogenic Aids in Sport*, pp. 101–127. Human Kinetics, Champaign, IL.

Jackman, M., Wendling, P., Friars, D. & Graham, T.E. (1996) Metabolic, catecholamine, and endurance responses to caffeine during intense exercise. *Journal of Applied Physiology* **81**, 1658–1663.

Jokl, E. (1968) Notes on doping. In: Jokl, E. & Jokl, P. (eds) *Exercise and Altitude*, pp. 55–57. S. Karger, Basel.

Karvinin, E., Miettinen, A. & Ahlman, K. (1962) Physical performance during hangover. *Quarterly Journal of Studies on Alcohol* **23**, 208–215.

Kendrick, Z.V., Affrime, M.B. & Lowenthal, D.T. (1993) Effect of ethanol on metabolic responses to treadmill running in well-trained men. *Journal of Clinical Pharmacology* **33**, 136–139.

Kennedy, M.C. & Lawrence, C. (1993) Anabolic steroid abuse and cardiac death. *Medical Journal of Australia* **158**, 346–348.

Krogh, J. (1991) *Smoking: The Artificial Passion*. W. H. Freeman, New York.

Lamarine, R.J. (1994) Selected health and behavioral effects related to the use of caffeine. *Journal of Community Health* **19**, 449–466.

Lefebvre, R.A., Surmont, F., Bouckaert, J. & Moerman, E. (1992) Urinary excretion of ephedrine after nasal application in healthy volunteers. *Journal of Pharmacy and Pharmacology* **44**, 672–675.

Lombardo, J.A. (1986) Stimulants and athletic performance (part 1 of 2): amphetamines and caffeine. *Physician and Sportsmedicine* **14** (11), 128–141.

Lombardo, J.A. (1993) The efficacy and mechanisms of action of anabolic steroids. In: Yesalis, C.E. (ed.) *Anabolic Steroids in Sport and Exercise*, pp. 89–106. Human Kinetics, Champaign, IL.

Lombardo, J.A., Hickson, R.C. & Lamb, D.R. (1991) Anabolic/androgenic steroids and growth hormone. In: Lamb, D.R. & Williams, M.H. (eds) *Ergogenics: Enhancement of Performance in Exercise and Sport*, pp. 249–284. WCB/Brown & Benchmark, Dubuque, IA.

MacIntosh, B.R. & Wright, B.M. (1995) Caffeine ingestion and performance of a 1500-metre swim. *Canadian Journal of Applied Physiology* **20**, 168–177.

Mangum, M., Gatch, W., Cooke, T. & Brooks, E. (1986) The effects of beer consumption on the physiological responses to submaximal exercise. *Journal of Sports Medicine and Physical Fitness* **26**, 301–305.

Martin, W. (1971) Physiologic, subjective and behavioral effects of amphetamine. *Clinical Pharmacology and Therapeutics* **12**, 245–258.

Massicotte, D., Provencher, S., Adopo, E. et al. (1993) Oxidation of ethanol at rest and during prolonged exercise in men. *Journal of Applied Physiology* **75**, 329–333.

McNaughton, L. & Preece, D. (1986) Alcohol and its effects on sprint and middle distance running. *British Journal of Sports Medicine* **20**, 56–59.

Melchert, R.B. & Welder, A.A. (1995) Cardiovascular effects of androgenic-anabolic steroids. *Medicine and Science in Sports and Exercise* **27**, 1252–1262.

Nehlig, A. & Debry, G. (1994) Caffeine and sports activity: a review. *International Journal of Sports Medicine* **15**, 215–223.

O'Brien, C.P. (1993) Alcohol and sport. *Sports Medicine* **15**, 71–77.

Pasman, W.J., van Baak, M.A., Jeukendrup, A.E. & de Haan, A. (1995) The effect of different dosages of caffeine on endurance performance time. *International Journal of Sports Medicine* **16**, 225–230.

Pope, H.G. & Katz, D.L. (1994) Psychiatric and medical effects of anabolic–androgenic steroid use. A controlled study of 160 athletes. *Archives of General Psychiatry* **51**, 375–382.

Reilly, T. (1997) Alcohol: its influence in sport and exercise. In: Reilly, T. & Orme, M. (eds) *The Clinical Pharmacology of Sport and Exercise*, pp. 281–292. Excerpta Medica, Amsterdam.

Rode, A. & Shephard, R.J. (1971) The influence of cigarette smoking upon the oxygen cost of breathing in near-maximal exercise. *Medicine and Science in Sports and Exercise* **3**, 51–55.

Schurch, P., Radinsky, J., Iffland, R. & Hollmann, W. (1982) The influence of moderate prolonged exercise and a low carbohydrate diet on ethanol elimination and on metabolism. *European Journal of Applied Physiology* **48**, 407–414.

Shirreffs, S.M. & Maughan, R.J. (1997) Restoration of fluid balance after exercise-induced dehydration: Effects of alcohol consumption. *Journal of Applied Physiology* **83**, 1152–1158.

Sidney, K.H. & Lefcoe, N.M. (1977) The effects of ephedrine on the physiological and psychological responses to submaximal and maximal exercise in man. *Medicine and Science in Sports* **9**, 95–99.

Sidney, S., Sternfeld, B., Gidding, S.S. et al. (1993) Cigarette smoking and submaximal exercise test duration in a biracial population of young adults: the CARDIA study. *Medicine and Science in Sports and Exercise* **25**, 911–916.

Smith, D.A. & Perry, P.G. (1992) The efficacy of ergogenic agents in athletic competition. *Annals of Pharmacotherapy* **26**, 653–659.

Smith, G.M. & Beecher, H.K. (1959) Amphetamine sulfate and athletic performance. *Journal of the American Medical Association* **170**, 542–557.

Spriet, L.L. (1995) Caffeine and performance. *International Journal of Sport Nutrition* **5**, S84–S99.

Swain, R.A., Harsha, D.M., Baenziger, J. & Saywell, R.M. (1997) Do pseudoephedrine or phenylpropanolamine improve maximum oxygen uptake and time to exhaustion. *Clinical Journal of Sports Medicine* **7**, 168–173.

Symons, J.D. & Stebbins, C.L. (1996) Hemodynamic and regional blood flow responses to nicotine at rest and during exercise. *Medicine and Science in Exercise and Sport* **28**, 457–467.

Tarnopolsky, M.A. (1994) Caffeine and endurance performance. *Sports Medicine* **18**, 109–125.

United States Department of Health and Human Services (1996) Adverse events associated with ephedrine-containing products. *Morbidity and Mortality Weekly Report* **45** (32), 689–693.

United States Olympic Committee (1996) *US Olympic Committee Drug Education Handbook*. USOC, Colorado Springs, CO.

Wemple, R.D., Lamb, D.R. & McKeever, K.H. (1997) Caffeine vs caffeine-free sports drinks: Effects on urine production at rest and during prolonged exercise. *International Journal of Sports Medicine* 18, 40–46.

Williams, M.H. (1974) *Drugs and Athletic Performance*. C. C. Thomas, Springfield, IL.

Williams, M.H. (1985) *Nutritional Aspects of Human Physical and Athletic Performance*. C.C. Thomas, Springfield, IL.

Williams, M.H. (1989a) Drugs and sports performance. In: Ryan, A.J. & Allman,
F.L. (eds) *Sports Medicine*, pp. 183–210. Academic Press, San Diego.

Williams, M.H. (1989b) *Beyond Training: How Athletes Enhance Performance Legally and Illegally*. Human Kinetics, Champaign, IL.

Williams, M.H. (1991) Alcohol, marijuana and beta blockers. In: Lamb, D.R. & Williams, M.H. (eds) *Ergogenics: Enhancement of Performance in Exercise and Sport*, pp. 331–372. WCB/Brown & Benchmark, Dubuque, IA.

Williams, M.H. (1992) Alcohol and sport performance. *Sport Sciences Exchange* 4 (40), 1–4.

Williams, M.H. (1994) Physical activity, fitness, and substance misuse and abuse. In: Bouchard, C., Shephard, R. & Stevens, T. (eds) *Physical Activity, Fitness, and Health*, pp. 898–915. Human Kinetics, Champaign, IL.

Williams, M.H. (1998) *The Ergogenics Edge: Pushing the Limits of Sports Performance*. Human Kinetics, Champaign, IL.

Chapter 32

Psychological Preparation of Endurance Performers

SUZANNE TUFFEY

If you have any negative doubts about anything during the race, I don't think it's going to go right. I mean if you think one bad incident that happened during warm-up or something, I think it's really going to affect you. I think everything that you think has to be positive. I mean I go into a race and I think of everything that I have done and what I have done to prepare for this race—I've worked hard for this. (Distance swimmer from 1998 US World Championship Team.)

Mental preparation started, you know, as soon as I made it. As soon as I made the team I was thinking about how I'm going to swim this race. So it started a long time before [the event]. I guess it gets more and more intense as it gets closer and closer to the meet. You know, you start thinking about exactly what you want to do, but for me it is a long process. (Open Water swimmer from the 1998 US World Championship Team.)

Sport performance is influenced by numerous variables. Analysis suggests that the factors impacting on performance can, for the most part, be grouped into three primary categories—physical, technical and psychological—with the quotations above illustrating the role of psychological factors in endurance performance.

Physical factors that influence athletic performance include factors such as strength, endurance, speed, flexibility and power. For the most part, athletes practise and develop these skills on a daily

basis through a structured, regimented physical training programme.

Technical factors involve executing a given skill with correct technique or biomechanics. For example, staying streamlined off the wall in swimming, rotating one's hips in a golf swing and applying force throughout the pedal rotation in cycling are technical factors that impact on performance. A portion of weekly training is often focused on developing and perfecting technique-related skills.

Psychological factors involve mental or attitudinal skills and characteristics of the athlete, for instance confidence, goal setting, use of self-talk and anxiety. Although physical and technical skills are often practised regularly, in a systematic and purposeful manner, this is less often the case for psychological skills. Nevertheless, athletes could benefit from training this mental aspect by:

• identifying psychological skills that could enhance their individual performance;
• working to develop and practise these skills; and
• implementing these skills and strategies as needed in practice and competition.

This chapter will focus on understanding how psychological factors impact on performance and exploring how endurance athletes can use this information to enhance their performance. Specific areas that are discussed include published literature on the psychological characteristics or skills of élite performers; the unique demands and challenges faced by participants in endurance sports such as distance running, cycling and distance swimming; and how endurance performers can use specific mental skills to deal with the unique challenges they face and to enhance their competitive performance.

Psychological characteristics related to successful performance

Anecdotal accounts from athletes and coaches suggest that mental skills influence performance. For example, Jack Nicklaus has often been quoted as saying that golf is 90% mental, and Vince Lombardi, coach of a well-known football team, the Green Bay Packers, believes that 'mental toughness is essential to success. You've got to be mentally tough' (Ferguson 1991, pp. 6–16).

What does research tell us about psychological skills/preparation and performance? Past research with élite-level athletes indicates that the mind (i.e. thoughts, focus, attitude, cognitive tactics and confidence) plays a role in performance. For example, Orlick and Partington (1988) investigated the mental control and mental readiness of Canadian Olympic athletes. They used both survey and interview techniques to understand the influence of psychological skills and characteristics on athletic performance. Their data indicated that mental readiness was a significant factor influencing performance across sports. The authors also identified what they termed common elements of success, including:

• a total commitment to pursuing excellence;
• quality training that included setting daily goals, competition simulation and imagery training; and
• quality mental preparation for competition.

Orlick and Partington concluded that the mental aspect of performance was an essential determinant of high achievement in important events.

Similarly, Gould et al. (1990) studied various psychological attributes of the 1988 US Olympic wrestling teams. Their qualitative investigation identified four dimensions of psychological skills that were discussed most often by this class of athletes:

• use of imagery;
• emotional control skills;
• thought control techniques; and
• skills used as part of a routine of mental preparation for competition.

Williams and Krane (1998) reviewed the literature to identify psychological characteristics related to successful performance. Specifically, they explored three sources of information: research related to athletes' recall of peak performance experiences; research comparing psychological characteristics of less versus more successful athletes; and athletes', coaches' and sport psychologists' perceptions of characteristics that were related to success. Williams and Krane (1998) concluded that certain mental skills and attributes were associated with superior athletic performance, including:

• self-regulation of arousal such that the athlete is energized yet relaxed;
• a high level of self-confidence;
• an ability to concentrate appropriately and effectively;
• a feeling of control over the performance;
• a positive preoccupation with sport; and
• determination and commitment.

Williams and Krane also identified the mental skills used most often by élite performers. These included a use of imagery, goal setting, tactics of thought control, techniques of arousal control, well-developed competition plans and coping strategies, and precompetition mental readying plans.

More recently, Gould et al. (1998) attempted to identify the positive and negative factors influencing US Olympic athletes' performances at the 1996 Olympic Games in Atlanta. Using both surveys and interviews, the investigators were able to identify factors that discriminated between athletes who performed well and those who failed to meet performance expectations. The following factors were deemed worthy of consideration in future preparation plans:

• distraction preparation;
• development of preparation plans and adherence to those plans;
• an optimization of physical training;
• mental preparation for unexpected events and stressors; and
• team cohesion and harmony.

Many of these factors are tied to the mental aspect of performance, suggesting that mental factors played an influential role in the performance of US 1996 Olympians.

These and other empirical investigations of élite-level athletes have reached similar conclusions to Williams and Krane, namely that enhanced performance is related to mental preparation using specific mental skills and strategies. The research cited to this point has been based on participants in numerous types of sports. Our interest, however, is strictly with endurance sport. What does research tell us about psychological skills and strategies that can enhance *endurance* performance? And why should we look at endurance performers separately from those engaged in other disciplines?

Psychological demands and challenges in endurance sports

Before reviewing research on the mental aspect of endurance performance, it seems important to identify how endurance athletes differ from other categories of athletes, to identify the unique physical and psychological challenges and demands faced by endurance competitors. The nature of these unique demands and challenges necessitates a separate examination of the mental skills and techniques that can help the endurance performer. Many of the skills that enhance performance across sports would also facilitate the performance of endurance athletes, but by understanding the nature of specific challenges, we can adapt such skills to the particular needs of the endurance competitor.

Among the numerous challenges endurance performers must overcome or learn how to manage, a few are especially pervasive, including:

Maintaining motivation on a daily basis despite long, repetitive training sessions. In sports such as distance running, distance or open water swimming and road cycling, athletes spend an inordinate amount of time in repetitive training. Hour after hour and day after day is spent performing a similar activity and pattern of movement. It is a major challenge for these athletes to maintain motivation and intensity on a daily (and often twice-daily) basis. Nevertheless it is crucial to do so, as practice of the required performance impacts directly on competitive outcome. An athlete will therefore want to maximize what he/she is doing in practice. In a later section, we discuss goal setting as a psychological skill that can be used by endurance athletes to deal with this challenge.

Enduring, and persevering through, the pain, discomfort and fatigue that are expected in endurance events—in both training and competition.

A lot of people run a race to see who is fastest. I run to see who has the most guts, who can punish himself into an exhausting pace and then at the end, punish himself even more. Nobody is going to win a 5000 meter race after running an easy two miles. Not with me. If I lose forcing the pace all the way, well, at least I can live with myself. (Steve Prefontaine, Ferguson 1991, pp. 6–14.)

As any endurance athlete knows, the physiological stress placed on the body—working at a high intensity level for an extended period of time—is extremely uncomfortable, and at times painful. This taxes and stresses the athlete mentally. Letting up mentally can have a profoundly adverse impact on performance, as noted by a distance swimmer who said: 'I got physically beat down from the conditions and that hurt me mentally. Once I started slipping back, it kind of went downhill from there'.

Athletes must strive to ensure that their internal thoughts are productive in spite of how they are feeling physically. We will discuss the use of cognitive control strategies to help manage this challenge/demand.

Mentally preparing for competition. The endurance athlete faces several unique competition-related challenges, in addition to the inherent stresses and pressures of competition. Firstly, as mentioned above, endurance athletes must be mentally prepared to manage the physical discomfort and pain that they know will occur in their competitive event. Secondly, endurance athletes must manage their physical and mental energy to optimize their performance. Prior to the event, this probably means conserving physical energy, yet maintaining a sharp mental focus. During the event, athletes must manage their energies and stay in control of themselves. Lastly, because of the importance of managing physical and mental energy, athletes would benefit from a well-developed race plan and a commitment to this plan. In a later section, we will discuss the use of mental preparation strategies to optimize preparation for competition.

Psychological aspects of endurance performance

As discussed above, research has identified specific psychological characteristics and mental skills that are related to successful performance across a variety of sports. What do we know about the psychological aspects of endurance performances?

The most frequently studied psychological characteristic of endurance performers is the cognitive tactic of associative versus dissociative thinking. Associative strategies are thought processes whereby the performer focuses on internal sensations such as muscular tension, breathing and race tactics. Dissociative strategies, such as listening to music, talking or singing to oneself, or imaging other more pleasant situations, are thought processes where the athlete focuses on external sensations. Dissociative strategies serve to distract the athlete from the discomfort or pain they are experiencing while training or competing.

Early research by Morgan and Pollock (1977) on the coping thought processes of distance runners found that non-élite runners tended to use dissociative coping tactics, whereas élite runners tended to use associative coping. They concluded that élite-level endurance runners used associative coping and attended to bodily sensation in order to endure distance runs. Conversely, non-élite endurance runners dissociated from pain and discomfort to endure distance runs. A second study of experienced versus non-experienced runners (Underleider et al. 1989) noted similar findings in terms of the use of dissociative versus associative coping. Schomer (1986) found a relationship between associative tactics and the perceived intensity, a greater perceived effort being related to a greater use of associative cognitive tactics. Tammen (1996) considered intensity to be the critical variable in determining the mental coping tactics of endurance performers. Although his sample size was small, he suggested that as running

intensity increased, élite distance runners adopted more associative cognitive tactics and their use of dissociative tactics decreased. Gill (1986) suggested that no one strategy was best, but rather both tactics were effective in specific situations. She noted that associative tactics might be more effective when attempting to attain a specific time or placing, and that dissociative tactics were beneficial when trying to maintain performance. Taken together, this research suggests that cognitive control tactics, both associative and dissociative, exert an influence on the performance of endurance athletes.

The notion that both associative and dissociative cognitive tactics are used by endurance athletes seems to contradict our understanding of effective concentration, which suggests that an athlete should focus on task-relevant cues. Although élite performers use associative tactics, where they are focused on task-relevant cues during specific parts of the event, they also adopt dissociative attentional tactics. Hardy et al. (1996) explained this seeming discrepancy by suggesting that the demands of endurance events present a unique situation. 'Clearly, the application of this form of attentional control [dissociation] is at best limited to those sports which are relatively low in terms of skill complexity and which involve intense physical pain and fatigue' (p. 197). The implication is that endurance athletes may need to be trained in the use of both dissociative and associative tactics in order to manage pain and discomfort, while at the same time enhancing their performance.

In addition to research on cognitive control tactics, empirical studies have assessed psychological skills and characteristics as they relate to endurance performers. For example, Bull (1989) developed an individualized mental training programme for an ultradistance runner that included imagery, relaxation and self-talk; success was reported with this mental training intervention. Burhans et al. (1988) reported performance benefits when athletes used mental imagery prior to running. Patrick and Hrycaiko (1998) used a single-subject multiple baseline design to measure the effects of a mental training regimen on performance. Their results indicated that the mental training, which consisted of relaxation, imagery rehearsal, self-talk and goal setting, was effective in improving the endurance running performance of participants. Although much research exists to demonstrate the relationship between psychological skills/characteristics and enhanced sport performance, these findings support the efficacy of using psychological skills training to enhance *endurance* performance. In the last section, we discuss the application of specific mental skills and techniques to address the challenges that we have noted and to enhance endurance performance.

Development of specific mental skills to enhance endurance performance

Systematic goal setting by endurance athletes to maintain daily motivation

Goal setting has been shown to facilitate performance. In a review of over 100 studies on goal setting, Locke *et al.* (1981) found that over 90% of the research demonstrated positive or partially positive effects, making it one of the most robust findings in the psychological literature. The effectiveness of goal setting in sport has not received such strong empirical support, but several methodological issues have been advanced to explain the equivocal findings (for a review, see Locke 1991). Despite inconsistent findings, the use of goal setting to enhance athletic performance has received both anecdotal and empirical support, and is a skill that can benefit endurance performers.

Several suggestions have been put forth to explain how goal setting facilitates performance. In his comprehensive review, Burton (1992) noted that 'goals motivate individuals to take direct action by focusing attention, increasing effort and intensity, prompting development of new problem-solving strategies, and/or encouraging persistence in the face of failure' (p. 269). Given this explanation, it is suggested that systematic goal setting be used by endurance athletes to help them overcome the challenge of maintaining motivation on a daily basis. By developing a structured goal-setting system, these athletes could enhance the focus, intensity and persistence with which they train, and

thereby help to maintain their motivation for practice despite the long and repetitive hours of training.

Although the empirical literature supports the use of goal setting to enhance performance, not all types of goals are equally effective. Research and experiential work with athletes has helped identify specific principles of goal setting (for a review, see Gould 1998); three of these principles are discussed below and may be applied to endurance performers.

Guidelines for effective goal setting

SET LONG-TERM AND SHORT-TERM GOALS

While long-term goals often have a motivational effect on the athlete, short-term goals can help in skill acquisition and can provide feedback regarding progress towards long-term goals. Identifying a daily or weekly goal may assist the athlete in training with a focused intensity. For example, a road cyclist may have a long-term goal of competing in the World Championships. Recalling this goal may provide motivation to train, but by setting shorter-term goals of maintaining a specific cadence and staying aerodynamic, the athlete has more specific objectives that, when accomplished, will bring him or her closer to the long-term goal. Short-term goals provide a purpose to training, enhance daily focus and increase training intensity.

SET PROCESS AND PERFORMANCE GOALS AS OPPOSED TO ONLY OUTCOME GOALS

Hardy *et al.* (1996) have distinguished between these three types of goals and discussed the benefits of each. All types of goals probably exert some positive influence but they argue that outcome goals are less effective for several reasons: they are not completely under the athlete's control, they increase anxiety and, unlike outcome goals, process goals direct attention to task-relevant cues. For the endurance athlete, the setting of process goals that tell the athlete what he or she needs to do may enhance daily motivation to train with an appropriate intensity and purpose.

If goals are to aid in practice motivation, they must be specific as opposed to general admonitions to 'work hard' or 'do your best'. They must also be measurable, so the athlete will know if the goal has been achieved. Such an approach keeps the athletes accountable for their daily training.

Cognitive control strategies to help manage physical pain and discomfort

As discussed above, the endurance performer uses both associative and dissociative tactics to aid performance during practice and competition. Some research has examined when each strategy may be most beneficial, but further study is needed. Nevertheless, we can begin to educate endurance athletes concerning specific dissociative and associative tactics that can be implemented to help manage discomfort while enhancing performance, taking into account individual goals and preferences. Often-suggested associative tactics, which should be taught and practised by the athlete to manage discomfort, include: concentration/focusing; use of mental imagery; and engaging in self-talk. Dissociative cognitive tactics that are used by endurance athletes to facilitate performance vary extensively. As with the associative tactics, the approach that is most beneficial depends on the goals, preferences and personality of the individual athlete; the tactic must be one that serves the athlete's purpose of distraction from bodily discomfort. Some commonly discussed dissociative approaches include: singing a specific song to oneself; engaging in distracting self-talk; and the use of imagery of task-irrelevant people, places or events.

Mental preparation to optimize preparation for competition

Research suggests that athletes need to develop and adhere to competition preparation plans which include both physical and mental preparation (Orlick & Partington 1988; Gould *et al.* 1990, 1998). Investigators have begun to assess what is 'optimal' preparation for athletes, but much more empirical

research is needed. One hypothesis receiving initial support is Hanin's individual zone of optimal functioning (IZOF) hypothesis (see Gould & Tuffey 1996 for a review). This hypothesis attempts to explain the anxiety–performance relationship by suggesting that each athlete has a zone or state in which he or she tends to perform best. If athletes are 'in their individual zone' prior to competition, they tend to have better performances than when they are out of their zone. The majority of research on the IZOF hypothesis has looked at state anxiety, but Hanin (1995) has extended his hypothesis to other arousal-related emotions. This hypothesis, in combination with research on élite-level athletes, suggests that individual athletes may have a unique combination of emotions that are related to better performances. In a more applied vein, Orlick (1986) has developed a form for athletes to complete, called 'Competitive Reflections'; this device helps to enhance the athlete's awareness of optimal mental preparation. Through a series of questions, the competitor is asked to compare thoughts, feelings, focus, nervousness and activation prior to a best performance versus prior to a worst performance. Such reflection helps the individual to identify what must go on internally to achieve better performances. The challenge for the athlete, then, is not only to identify how he or she tends to perform best, but to develop a routine that will help to attain this state/zone; to develop a mental preparation plan to enhance performance. Individual precompetition routines include a variety of psychological skills such as mental rehearsal, positive self-talk, confidence-building, goal setting and concentration, all serving to help the athlete manage his/her internal environment.

Conclusions

In order to enhance their performance, athletes need to train and control a variety of factors that have an impact on performance. Primary areas that need to be addressed include the physical, technical and mental aspects of performance. This chapter has focused specifically on the mental aspect of performance of endurance performers, presenting research to illustrate the contribution of psychological skills and characteristics to élite-level endurance performance. Endurance performers can use specific psychological skills to aid in dealing with the unique challenges and demands of their discipline and to enhance both their practice and their competitive performance.

References

Bull, S.J. (1989) The role of the sport psychology consultant: a case study of ultra distance running. *Sport Psychologist* 3 (3), 254–264.

Burhans, R., Richman, C. & Bergey, D. (1988) Mental imagery training: Effects on running speed performance. *International Journal of Sport Psychology* 19 (1), 26–37.

Burton, D. (1992) The Jekyll/Hyde nature of goals: Reconceptualizing goal setting in sport. In: Horn, T. (ed.) *Advances in Sport Psychology*, pp. 267–298. Human Kinetics, Champaign, IL.

Ferguson, H. (1991) *The Edge*. Getting the Edge Co., Cleveland, OH.

Gill, D. (1986) *Psychological Dynamics of Sport*. Human Kinetics, Champaign, IL.

Gould, D. (1998) Goal setting for peak performance. In: Williams, J. (ed.) *Applied Sport Psychology: Personal Growth to Peak Performance*, pp. 182–196. Mayfield, Mountain View, CA.

Gould, D. & Tuffey, S. (1996) Zones of optimal functioning research: a review and critique. *Anxiety, Stress, and Coping* 9, 53–68.

Gould, D., Eklund, R. & Jackson, S. (1990) *An indepth examination of mental factors and preparation techniques associated with 1988 U.S. Olympic team wrestling excel-lence*. Unpublished final project report to USA Wrestling.

Gould, D., Guinan, D., Greenleaf, C. *et al.* (1998) *Positive and negative factors influencing U.S. Olympic athletes and coaches: Atlanta games assessment*. Unpublished final report to USOC Sport Science and Technology.

Hanin, Y. (1995) Individual Zones of Optimal Functioning (I.Z.O.F.) model, idiographic approach to performance anxiety. In: Henschen, K. & Straub, W. (eds) *Sport Psychology: An Analysis of Athlete Behavior*, 3rd edn, pp. 103–119. Mouvement, Ithaca, NY.

Hardy, L., Jones, G. & Gould, D. (1996) *Understanding Psychological Preparation for Sport: Theory and Practice of Élite Performers*. John Wiley & Sons, Chichester.

Locke, E.A. (1991) Problems with goal-setting to sports — and their solutions. *Journal of Sport and Exercise Psychology* 13, 311–316.

Locke, E., Shaw, K., Saari, L. & Latham, G. (1981) Goal setting and task performance. *Psychological Bulletin* 90, 125–152.

Morgan, W. & Pollock, M. (1977) Psychological characterization of the élite distance runner. *Annals of the New York Academy of Science* 301, 382–403.

Orlick, T. (1986) *Psyching for Sport: Mental Training for Athletes*. Leisure Press, Champaign, IL.

Orlick, T. & Partington, J. (1988) Mental links to excellence. *Sport Psychologist* 2, 105–130.

Patrick, T. & Hrycaiko, D. (1998) Effects of a mental training package on an endurance performance. *Sport Psychologist* 12 (3), 283–299.

Schomer, H.H. (1986) Mental strategies and the perceptions of effort: implications for the training of marathon runners. *International Journal of Sport Psychology* 16, 41–59.

Tammen, V. (1996) Élite middle and long distance runners associative/dissociative coping. *Journal of Applied Sport Psychology* 8, 1–8.

Underleider, S., Golding, J., Porter, K. & Foster, J. (1989) An exploratory examination of cognitive strategies used by Masters track and field athletes. *Sport Psychologist* 3, 245–253.

Williams, J. & Krane, V. (1998) Psychological characteristics of peak performance. In: Williams, J.M. (ed.) *Applied Sport Psychology: Personal Growth to Peak Performance*, pp. 137–147. Mayfield, Mountain View, CA.

Chapter 33

Prevention of Injuries in Endurance Athletes

PER A.F.H. RENSTRÖM AND PEKKA KANNUS

Introduction

Interest in sports participation has increased tremendously during recent decades. There is a great interest among the general population in improving both their health and their body composition. Regular aerobic exercise has been linked to a decreased risk of cardiovascular disease (Paffenbarger *et al.* 1986; Chapters 47 & 51), and regular exercise and resultant fitness have been shown to decrease the morbidity of ageing and mortality (Bortz 1982; Blair *et al.* 1992; Chapters 38 & 51). Furthermore, inactivity and immobilization are detrimental to and regular physical activity is beneficial to all musculoskeletal tissues in the body (Kannus *et al.* 1992a) Sporting activities in general are therefore beneficial for the individual as well as for society, and a certain amount of physical activity is an important element in health promotion (Blair *et al.* 1992).

With increased mass media attention, top-level competitive participation has become more common, thus demanding more intensive and longer-duration training. Training has also become more specialized. Serious and specialized training starts at an ever younger age and continues until an older age; in consequence, an increased exposure time increases the likelihood of sustaining an injury. Sport was previously confined mainly to amateurs, but the attention of the mass media and commercial interests has resulted in a growing participation by professionals.

The increased interest in sport participation at all levels has resulted in an increased frequency and severity of sports injuries, both from acute trauma and from overuse. An acute injury may be defined as a single impact macrotrauma (for example, a blow to a leg resulting in a fracture, a rotational injury of a joint resulting in a ligament sprain or a direct blow to a muscle resulting in muscle strain). An overuse injury may be defined as a long-standing or recurring orthopaedic problem, starting during training or performance and due to repetitive overloading of the tissue.

Despite adequate treatment based on advanced knowledge, modern technology and improved skills in sports medicine, some athletes fail to regain their preinjury level and intensity of physical activity. Injuries are usually considered as a disaster by the athletes concerned. Moreover, most injuries are unnecessary. The prevention of injuries should therefore be a major goal for every physician, physiotherapist, trainer, nurse, coach, parent, athlete and others who are active in sports and sports medicine.

Tactics for the prevention of sports injuries

Efforts at individual, group and societal levels

Direct or indirect prevention of sports injury may be at an individual level. Medical preseason examination, an adequate warm-up before competition and the use of appropriate protective equipment (helmets, face masks, knee, shoulder and elbow pads, safety-release ski bindings, braces, tape, etc.) are typical examples of individual preventive tactics (Table 33.1).

The most common tactic is the provision of information and education at the group level. Lectures to athletes and coaches may stress the importance of proper warming up and cooling down, careful following of the rules (fair play), the disadvantages of illicit drugs, alcohol and tobacco, and known risk factors for injuries. Any decision taken within an individual sporting event which makes that particular sport safer can also be considered as a form of group prevention.

Efforts undertaken at the societal level will not normally yield benefit until many years after the tactics have been planned and made effective. One example might be a political decision to build new,

safe cycling routes and to separate them completely from motor vehicle traffic. A legislative decision to forbid all blows to the head in boxing would also be a form of societal prevention. Table 33.1 summarizes the three different sorts of injury prevention.

The concept of three levels of prevention can also apply to a given individual (Hlobil *et al.* 1987). Using this scheme of classification, prevention of an injury before its occurrence may be termed primary prevention. Efforts to prevent reinjury, or to prevent existing injuries from becoming chronic, may be termed secondary prevention. Finally, tertiary prevention limits the progression of irreversible loss of function from a chronic injury.

Sequence of prevention

Measures to prevent sports injuries do not stand by themselves, but rather form part of what may be termed 'a sequence of prevention' (Fig. 33.1) (Van Mechelen *et al.* 1987). Firstly, the problem needs to be identified and described in terms of the incidence and severity of sports injuries. Secondly, risk factors and exact mechanisms of injury must be identified. The third step includes the introduction of measures likely to reduce the risk and/or severity of injuries. Finally, the effects of these measures must be evaluated by repeating the first step.

Success in evaluating the incidence of sports injuries depends upon valid and reliable definitions of the severity of injury and the extent of sports participation. Incidence data are important for several reasons: they guide sports injury prevention and

Table 33.1 Tactics for the prevention of sports injuries. From Renström and Kannus (1991).

Prevention at individual level
Medical screening
Use of protective equipment
Flexibility and strength training
Nutrition

Prevention at group level
Enforcement and amendment of rules
Agreements
Information
Education

Prevention at societal level
Societal planning
Legislation
Budgetary measures
Investment

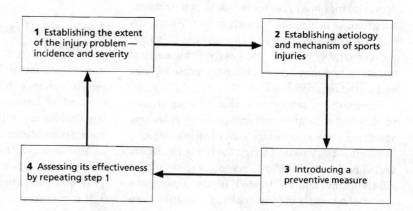

Fig. 33.1 Sequence of prevention. Adapted from van Mechelen *et al.* (1987).

1 Establishing the extent of the injury problem — incidence and severity

2 Establishing aetiology and mechanism of sports injuries

4 Assessing its effectiveness by repeating step 1

3 Introducing a preventive measure

research into improving sports safety; they assist in identifying priority areas for injury prevention and research in terms of particular sports activities and levels of participation. Attention must be directed towards the definition of both risk and exposure, since the validity and usefulness of research activities, data collection and surveillance systems depend on this.

Injury epidemiology

Numerous epidemiological studies of sports injuries are available (Sandelin *et al.* 1987; Sandelin 1988). It is estimated that about 1.5 million acute medically treated injuries occurred in the adult population of Finland in 1980. Work-related injuries made up 17% of this total, sports injuries 14% and traffic injuries 12%.

In the Netherlands, the overall incidence has been calculated at 3.3 injuries per 1000 h spent on sports (van Galen & Diederiks 1990). In the study cited, 2.2 million sports injuries were identified, of which 1.7 million were treated medically. In West Germany, Steinbrück and Kotta (1983) estimated that sports injuries accounted for 10–15% of accidents. In a Swedish community with 31620 inhabitants, Loes (1990) registered all emergency visits to the public health-care unit over a 1-year period: 571 acute sports injuries were recorded. They comprised 17% of all acute visits, with acute home injuries, acute work injuries and acute traffic accidents making up 26, 19 and 7% of the total, respectively.

Despite such figures, the population at risk is extremely difficult to identify, and the incidence of sports injuries in a given society or in some specific subgroup is, in general, not well known. An important drawback to figures of this kind is that they reflect relatively serious accidents requiring medical attention, and they ignore chronic overuse injuries and less serious accidents.

The number of acute sports injuries treated in hospital, however, is fairly well known. Forty years ago, sports injuries accounted for 1.4% of all injuries seen in the emergency room. During the 1970s, this figure varied between 5% and 7%, but today some 10% of all traumatic injuries treated in the emergency rooms of hospitals in industrialized countries have

been sustained in sports (van Galen & Diederiks 1990; Renström & Kannus 1991).

The incidence of overuse injuries is difficult to calculate. The absolute number of overuse injuries has probably increased dramatically during recent decades, due to the general increase in sport participation. However, claims that the incidence has increased remain without scientific evidence.

Both acute and overuse sports injuries are generally considered relatively benign. Up to 75% of all sports injuries can be classified as mild to moderate, requiring only a short absence from sport and a short period of sick-leave. The proportion of patients requiring further inpatient treatment because of a sports injury is around 10%. The proportion of patients requiring operative treatment for an acute or overuse injury varies from 5% to 10% (Kannus *et al.* 1989).

Sports injuries have a large societal cost. In the Netherlands, the total costs of treatment and sick-leave have been estimated at $350 million per year (Toom & Schuurman 1988). Athletes in Ireland and the UK suffer from the effects of sports injury for 52 days in the year (Watson 1993). The cost of sports injuries in the UK has been estimated at half a billion pounds annually (Nicholl 1991).

Step two in the sequence of prevention focuses on the aetiology and mechanisms of sports injuries; it is described later in this chapter.

The third and fourth steps (measures to reduce the future risk of sports injury and/or the severity of sports injuries) are also discussed later on. Such measures should be based on the aetiological factors identified in the second step.

Aetiological factors and injury mechanisms

Aetiological factors can be extrinsic or intrinsic; they lead to a change in the incidence, prevalence, duration and/or seriousness of sports injuries if manipulated under controlled circumstances (Backus *et al.* 1988, *Sports Medicine* Sept 1997, p. 175).

Aetiological factors should be studied in a sports injury surveillance system, based on the following principles (van Mechelen 1997).

1 It is necessary to begin with a hypothesis about

the factors that are causing sports injuries. Ideally, the effect of eliminating the hypothesized factor can then be studied in a randomized clinical trial.

2 A prospective observational study is a routine approach. There are several problems with this tactic. One issue is how to obtain a valid measurement of potential risk factors for sports injuries. Secondly, one must deal with the specificity of the sports injury. A third problem concerns the nature of the risk factors. Prospective observational studies can only be performed if a surveillance system is tailored to the specific sport and the research question to be investigated.

3 An alternative approach is to use a retrospective case-controlled study. Cases can be matched to a control group of uninjured individuals.

Extrinsic factors predisposing to injury

Injury mechanisms

It is important to identify risk factors and injury mechanisms that play an important role in the aetiology of injuries. Acute injuries are common in many sports, especially contact sports. Large impact traumas, such as collision against another player, a fall against the ground, a tackling against the boards of a rink or a blow by the club or puck in ice hockey, are common. An acute impact injury deforms tissues beyond their recoverable limit, thus damaging the anatomical structures or altering normal function. The risk of injury depends on both the energy delivered to the body by the impacting object, and the shape of the object (Viano et al. 1989). The individual's capacity to withstand the trauma is of importance. For example, an osteoporotic bone fractures more readily than a normal bone that is subjected to the same trauma. It is important to identify and define the mechanism of impact injury, to quantify the biomechanical response to such impact, to determine the impact tolerance level and to develop injury assessment devices and techniques for evaluating injury prevention. It would also be of value if the resulting forces from the impact could be decreased and/or dispersed, thus avoiding deformation and severe tissue damage.

Repeated overload in running and jumping activ-

ities is often associated with overuse injuries. In running, a force in the range of three to five times the body mass ascends the lower extremity at each heel-strike. This force has a short duration (20–40 ms) and rapid dissipation. Even if the impact force were only 250% of body mass, a runner would absorb a force of 68.5 Mg (68.5 tons) on each foot per km (Mann et al. 1981). The cumulative effect can be imagined in a long-distance runner, who runs 160 km per week and plants each foot about three million times a year. The cumulative forces are so large, it is not surprising that they contribute to injuries. Equally, it seems likely that a reduction in these forces may reduce the frequency and extent of injury.

One possible way of decreasing the load on the body is to change the type of motion. For example, one can run by landing on the heel or landing on the forefoot. When landing on the heel, the point of application of the ground reaction force and the line of action of that force both lie behind the ankle joint. Therefore, structures in the anterior part of the leg are loaded on first contact and the Achilles tendon is unloaded. Heel landing can be used to unload the Achilles tendon, for example when recovering from an Achilles tendinitis or peritendinitis.

Another possibility is to decrease the speed of motion; if the speed of heel–toe running is decreased from $6\,m\cdot s^{-1}$ to $3\,m\cdot s^{-1}$, the vertical impact and active forces are decreased by 40% and 20%, respectively (Nigg 1988). A change in the speed of motion also changes the speed of the limbs that are involved, and it can therefore influence the forces acting on the athlete's body.

Little is known about the number of repetitions and their effects during loading of the human body. Biological materials can show a positive response to an applied stress, provided that the rate of stress increase is sufficiently slow. If the adaptive response is stronger than the effects of mechanical fatigue, then the tissue becomes stronger. Generally, bones and muscles have large and rapid responses, whereas cartilage and tendons show a smaller and slower response, because they have a lower nutritional blood flow and metabolism. Fatigue injuries such as stress fractures occur frequently. It is thus important to increase the number of repetitions slowly.

Training errors

Overuse injuries are associated with extrinsic and/or intrinsic factors. The most common extrinsic factors are application of excessive loads on the body, training errors, bad environmental conditions, poor equipment and ineffective rules (Table 33.2). Training errors are probably present in 60–80% of reported injuries of runners (James et al. 1978). The most common errors are too long a distance, too high an intensity, too fast a progression and too much hill work. Monotony, asymmetry and specialization are major risk factors in training in most sports. For instance, running on the edge of the road implies running with one leg shortened and one leg extended; this results in overuse injuries such as trochanteric bursitis and iliotibial band friction syndrome. By varying the exercise method (cycling, swimming and cross-country skiing in addition to running), a much larger total amount of work can be carried out, with a lesser risk of injury.

Poor technique and fatigue also play a role. Even minor technical faults, continuously repeated, can cause overuse injuries. Fatigued muscles have a decreased ability to absorb repetitive shock or stress, leading to injuries such as stress fractures, tennis elbow and medial tibial stress syndrome.

Few studies have explored how important different risk factors are in terms of the injuries sustained. van Mechelen (1994) found that in non-contact sports such as running, previous injuries, lack of running experience, running to compete and excessive weekly running distances were all significantly associated with injuries. The association between running injuries and other risk factors, such as running frequency, performing, warming up and stretching exercises, body height, malalignment, muscle imbalance, restricted range of motion, level of performance, stability of running patterns, types of shoes and inshoes, orthoses and running on one side of the road, was less clear and sometimes contradicted by other research findings. Factors not associated with running injuries included age, gender, body mass index, type of running heels, running on hard surfaces, participation in other sports, time of year and time of day.

Table 33.2 Extrinsic factors related to injuries in sports. From Renström and Kannus (1991).

Excessive load on the body
Type of movement
Speed of movement
Number of repetitions
Footwear
Surface

Training errors
Excessive distances
Fast progression
High intensity
Hill work
Poor technique
Monotonous or asymmetrical training
Fatigue

Poor environmental conditions
Inadequate illumination
Heat/cold
Humidity
High altitude
Wind chill

Poor equipment

Ineffective rules

Sports surface adjustment

As each foot makes contact with the ground, a ground reaction force is applied, and the foot acts on the ground with a force of the same magnitude but in the opposite direction. The forces encountered during landing and take-off are quite different on different surfaces. The impact force is much higher when running on asphalt than when running on grass or sand (Nigg 1988). However, the active part of the ground reaction force remains about the same for grass and asphalt. High impact forces are a major cause of injuries in running and other sports. Adolescents often sustain overuse injuries such as medial tibial stress syndrome and Achilles tendinitis when playing tennis on surfaces with a high friction. These problems are rarely seen on clay courts (Renström 1988). It is therefore very important that people who are responsible for the development of sports facilities appreciate the possibilities of reducing impact forces through an appropriate selection of playing surfaces. Additional shock absorption can be achieved by the use of proper orthotics and shoes (see below).

Poor equipment

Equipment can be divided into instrumental and protective. Poor instrumental equipment can cause overuse injuries, especially if it is used in combination with poor technique. One of the few areas where research has been carried out is in tennis, where the size of the racquet is important. Oversized racquets absorb vibrations well from tennis balls that are hit off-centre along the vertical axis (Elliott *et al.* 1980). The frequency of tennis elbow is thus lower in players who use oversized racquets. Tennis elbow is generally thought to be more likely to occur in players who use a heavy racquet than in those who use a light one (Kulund *et al.* 1979), but there are some studies suggesting that the mass of the racquet does not influence the incidence of tennis elbow (Carroll 1986). The material from which the racquet is made may be an important determinant of the incidence of tennis elbow: tennis elbow may result from using oversized aluminium racquets. Studies of the muscle activity generated in the forearm and shoulder muscles of players using racquets with different grip sizes have shown that force changes were not sufficient to warrant a change of grip size (Adelsberg 1986).

In tennis, gut stringing provides better control, higher ball velocities, lower levels of vibration transmission to the hand and improved player characteristics (Groppel 1984). Gut stringing should thus be used when a player has tennis elbow. String tension is also a factor in the occurrence of tennis elbow. The looser the strings, the higher the positive impact velocity. In general, tightly strung racquets give better control, whereas loosely strung racquets generate more force. The racquet should be strung at a tension of around 220–250N (50–55 lb) in order to reduce the risk of tennis elbow. Heavy balls should be avoided, as well as 'dead', wet or pressureless balls, because such balls increase the impact against the tennis racquet, thereby increasing the risk of tennis elbow. The use of slow courts is also suggested for athletes with tennis elbow problems.

An extensive prospective study of downhill skiing injuries has been carried out by the Department of Orthopedics and Rehabilitation at the University of Vermont, USA under the leadership of Robert J. Johnson. Between 1972 and 1994, the overall injury rate decreased by 50%, to about 2.5 injuries per 1000 skier visits. Injuries below the knee declined by approximately 85%, and tibial fractures and ankle sprains and fractures decreased by 90%; most of these gains were attributed to improved equipment and slopes. However, the rate of severe knee sprains involving a tear or rupture of one or more ligaments rose from 3% of all injuries in 1972 to almost 20% in 1994. Better-designed and functioning ski binding release systems have been a major factor in the improvement in below-knee injury rates. However, no statistically significant relationship has been observed between the quality or the description of the release system and the increased incidence of severe knee sprains. Releasable ski bindings of the 19th century were designed to help reduce the risk of tibial fractures, but no product has yet been introduced that can sense and respond appropriately to potentially injurious loads on the knee (Ettlinger *et al.* 1995). The provision of information concerning the importance of setting ski bindings at a proper release level is effective in reducing the incidence of ski injuries (Eriksson & Johnson 1980).

These examples indicate the importance of proper, good quality equipment in various sports. Equipment should also be used in a prescribed and tested fashion. Moreover, the efficacy of equipment can be increased significantly by community and societal approaches such as provision of information, education, legislation and planning.

Arena equipment

Recreational organized softball league play is a very common team sport in the US, attracting over 40 million individuals every year. A retrospective review revealed that this sport was responsible for the majority of sports injuries seen in emergency room visits. Between 1983 and 1989, the consumer product safety division documented more than 2.5 million injuries that were referred to emergency rooms. This figure does not include non-hospital physician visits. Sliding into the base was the cause of 71% of all softball-related injuries sustained in recreational leagues. Several efforts, including abolishing the act of sliding and providing instructional courses on how to slide proved unsuccessful. It was then discovered that break-away bases as opposed to standard stationary bases were an effective remedy, preventing impact loading on a stationary object. Half of the fields at the University of Michigan were therefore switched to break-away bases (Janda 1997). Injury surveillance showed a 96% reduction in sliding-related injuries and a 99% reduction in associated health-care costs. The Centers for Disease Control in the US concluded that if all fields across the US switched from stationary to break-away bases, this would prevent approximately 1.7 million injuries per year and would save $2 billion in associated health-care costs per year. This is a remarkable example of how preventive thinking can reduce both injuries and health-care costs.

Ineffective rules

One less well-known extrinsic predisposing factor is the inefficacy of many rules. Improvement of the rules to make sports safer is a key factor in reducing injuries. Interest in improving rules, however, is a fairly recent development. Rules are now becoming more concerned with facilities, environmental circumstances such as weather, use of personal equipment and tactics or practices demonstrated to be unsafe (Ryan & Stoner 1989). Coaches and athletes have shown considerable resistance to changing the rules, because frequently these place restrictions on a style of play that is popular, even though it may be quite dangerous.

Rules that prevent contact likely to produce injuries have been instituted in American football. The clipping injury and down-field blocking below the waist are now forbidden (Peterson 1970). Other rule changes have resulted in a dramatic decrease in both the total number of cervical spine injuries and the number of lesions resulting in quadriplegia (Torg et al. 1990).

Rules for safety have been developed gradually;

for example, in American football a helmet is now compulsory. In ice hockey, it has long been compulsory to wear a helmet, and in university and junior hockey face masks are required as well. These rule changes have reduced the number of facial and eye injuries dramatically. Despite research showing the benefits of face masks, many professional ice hockey players still refuse to use them, and therefore facial and dental injuries continue to be a great problem in professional ice hockey. It is strange that these players do not realize how such potentially serious injuries can be avoided. In most countries, amateur boxers must use a protective head cover.

In junior baseball, there is a restriction on the number of pitches that may be thrown per season, to avoid little leaguer's elbow. In volleyball, stepping on the net line is prohibited, in order to avoid ankle sprains. Bahr et al. (1997) found a two-fold reduction in the incidence of acute ankle sprains in Norwegian volleyball players after the introduction of an injury prevention programme that included injury awareness instruction, technical training with an emphasis on proper take-off and landing techniques for blocking and attacking, and a balance-board training programme for players with recurrent sprains.

Jörgensen (1993) showed that allowing free substitution in soccer decreased the number of injuries. In badminton, treatment of an injury during a match is not allowed. This seems an old-fashioned rule, out of keeping with the development of sports medical treatment. Application of this rule often forces a player to continue a game, with the risk of incurring a more serious injury. The rule should be changed to allow an adequate examination and any necessary minor short treatment. This has happened in tennis, where a trainer has 3 min to examine and treat a player he feels has been injured. Common sense makes these rules important, but on the other hand, they must not be misused by the athletes.

Sports techniques are developing rapidly and will force further changes to existing rules; so will improved technology. It is necessary to review and to revise the rules continuously. Rule changes may be a very important way of reducing the future number of sports injuries, since new sports, often with a high risk of injury, and the number of participants both seem to be increasing exponentially.

Poor environmental conditions

Weather may affect the frequency of injury during sports. The rules provide that a baseball game should be cancelled in the event of rain, because wet fields increase the risk of injury. Poor illumination, too high or low a temperature or humidity, high altitude and a strong wind may also play a key role in the pathogenesis of injury. The time of nightfall has to be taken into account when planning orienteering competitions. High temperature and humidity without wind restrict the cooling of marathon runners, with potentially serious consequences (see Chapter 40). Low temperatures with a strong wind may produce frostbite, hypothermia and other cold injuries in sports such as downhill or cross-country skiing, ski jumping, bandy (floor hockey on ice) and mountain climbing.

It is always essential to have clear rules about when training or competition must be cancelled because of poor environmental conditions. Cross-country skiing competitions are cancelled if the temperature falls below −20°C (−4°F), in order to avoid cold injuries. Other weather factors should also be taken into consideration. For example, the wind chill factor is critical in many winter sports, since the wind velocity has a marked effect on body heat loss. If the thermometer reads −7°C (20°F) and the wind velocity is 32 km·h^{-1} (20 miles·h^{-1}), the rate of cooling is equivalent to −23°C (−10°F) in still air (Boswick *et al.* 1983).

Intrinsic factors predisposing to injury

Intrinsic factors predisposing to injury can be divided into basic, primary and secondary. Basic intrinsic factors include gender, age, growth, body mass and height. Important primary intrinsic factors are different malalignments, leg length discrepancies, muscle imbalance, inadequate strength, poor flexibility and poor neuromuscular coordination. Secondary, acquired factors can include kinetic chain dysfunctions and previous injuries (Table 33.3). Intrinsic predisposing factors were present in 40% of cases of running injury, but in only 10% were they the only demonstrable factor (Lysholm & Wiklander 1987).

Table 33.3 Intrinsic factors related to overuse injuries in sports.

Basic
Gender
Age
Growth
Body mass
Height

Primary
Bone and joint alignments
    Foot, tibia, knee, hip, pelvis, leg length
Structural variations
Muscular condition
    Strength
    Flexibility
    Neuromuscular coordination
    Ligamentous laxity

Secondary or acquired dysfunction
Mechanical
    Foot, ankle, knee, hip, spine, sacroiliac joints
Muscular asymmetries
    Imbalance
    Localized weakness
    Localized inflexibility
Previous and recurrent injuries

Basic intrinsic factors

WOMEN IN SPORT

Women are participating increasingly in sport and other forms of physical activity. There is also an increased female interest in sporting events with a high risk of injury, such as gymnastics, soccer and team handball. Injuries are therefore becoming increasingly common in women. A prospective study showed that 31% of injured athletes were female (Kannus *et al.* 1987b).

Anterior cruciate ligament injuries of the knee among contact sport participants are three to four times more common in women than in men. One reason for this may be that women are more dependent on their quadriceps muscles, and their hamstring function is not as good as in men. Women also have a longer electromechanical delay (the time interval between the change in electrical activity of the muscle and movement) (presentation by E. Wojtys,

American Academy of Orthopedic Surgeons, Anaheim 1999).

There is a high incidence of overuse injuries among women. The reason for this may be that the repetitive impact of the body mass must be absorbed by a weaker musculoskeletal system in women compared with men of equal body mass (Lloyd *et al.* 1986). Women have less muscle mass per kg of body mass (20–25%) than equally trained men (40%), and their overall muscle strength averages only about two-thirds that of men (Drinkwater 1988). Men also have greater bone mass than women. These factors, together with other known female risk factors such as wider hips and more mobile joints, predispose women to overuse injuries.

Menstrual irregularities, which are much more common among female athletes than among non-athletes, constitute a risk factor for certain overuse injuries. There is an increased incidence of stress fractures among amenorrhoeic athletes compared with eumenorrhoeic athletes who are participating in the same sport (Marcus *et al.* 1985) (Fig. 33.2). A prolonged hypoestrogenic state may result in a loss of bone mass (especially in trabecular bone areas) and, therefore, an increased risk of osteoporotic acute fractures. In strenuous endurance sports, continuous recording of menstrual cycles and follow-up of dietary habits (to ensure an adequate intake of protein, calcium and vitamin D) should be compulsory.

YOUNG AGE

The regular training of children and young adults is becoming ever more common in sports. Competitive sports are carried out at increasing intensity and at ever younger ages. In some sports such as figure-skating, swimming and gymnastics, children start regular training at 4–5 years of age; 2–4 h of training for 5–6 days a week is not unusual. As a result, the risks of acute and overuse injuries are increasing.

Before puberty, a child's body seems to withstand repeated voluntary stress amazingly well. During the growth spurt, which occurs in most girls at about 12 years of age and in boys at about 14 years, there is a gross imbalance between muscle strength,

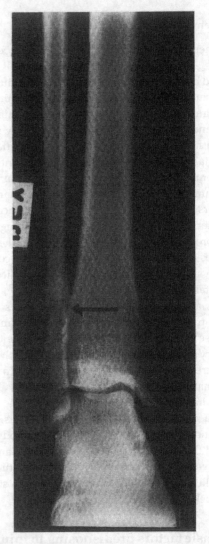

Fig. 33.2 Stress fractures can occur in females with amenorrhoea or osteoporosis. The figure shows a 26-year-old female who had worked for 1 year as an aerobic dance teacher. She sustained simultaneous bilateral stress fractures of the fibulae. When the stress fractures occurred, her menstrual cycle was very irregular due to hard training.

tightness, joint mobility and coordination. In addition, the growth plates are extremely vulnerable to external forces during that phase of development, with an associated increase in the risk of acute and overuse injuries (Micheli 1983). Well-known examples of injuries during the pubertal growth spurt include traumatic epiphysiolyses of the hip joints, and traction epiphysitis of the tibial tubercle in jumpers (Osgood–Schlatter disease) or of the humeral medial epicondyle in young pitchers (little leaguer's elbow). The incidence of little leaguer's elbow has decreased with restriction of the number of pitches allowed for the growing athlete.

Prolonged one-sided training in childhood can cause permanent asymmetrical adaptive changes. One example of this is the so-called tennis shoulder; the end results are an increased laxity in the joint capsule, ligaments and tendons, and an increased bone growth, resulting in a dropping of the shoulder and a relative lengthening of the racquet arm (Fig. 33.3). Intensive and prolonged training of gymnasts may produce hypermobility of the vertebral column and other joints, and the end result may be spondylosis and spondylolisthesis or early osteoarthritis (Sward 1990). Hyperextension (Fig. 33.4) in competitive gymnastics is stimulated by the award of high scores. These rules should be analysed by sports medicine specialists, with a view to their modification.

It is essential that regular hard training during adolescence be carried out under supervision.

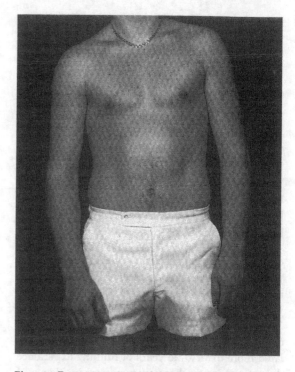

Fig. 33.3 Repetitive one-sided isometric tennis training can cause laxity in the joint capsule, ligament and tendons with a resultant dropping of the shoulder — 'tennis shoulder'.

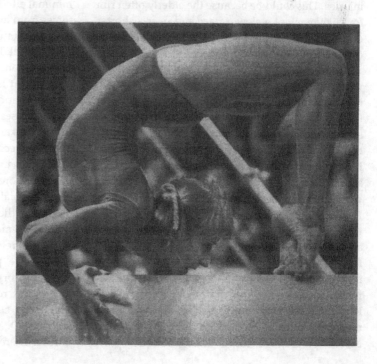

Fig. 33.4 Hyperextension is a risk factor for injury to the spinal vertebrae in gymnasts, especially in very young competitors (Olga Korbut, winner of many gold medals in the 1972 Olympic Games; photograph courtesy of Pressens Bild).

Group and societal preventive measures such as protective rules, information and education are also of great importance at this age.

OLD AGE

Various functions of the body including the musculoskeletal system gradually deteriorate with ageing (Chapter 38). Musculoskeletal function deteriorates more slowly in long-distance runners aged 50–72 years than in non-running control groups (Lane *et al.* 1987). Runners show less physical disability, maintain a better functional capacity and have fewer physician visits per year.

In elderly athletes, sports injuries are more frequently overuse related than acute. Compared with young adults, the injuries of elderly athletes more commonly have a degenerative basis (Kannus *et al.* 1989). Degenerative changes decrease the capacity for shock absorption and thereby augment the risk of injury. Nevertheless, people who have accumulated more than 30–40 years of running experience do not appear to show an increased incidence of osteoarthritis of the hip. Age also does not seem a primary factor increasing the incidence of running injuries. This could be because the elderly often run for enjoyment, at a slower pace and over a shorter distance, and because they are in general more careful than are younger adults.

Among veteran élite athletes competing in the world master championships, the most common injuries were muscle and tendon strains of the lower leg (Peterson & Renström 1980). Prevention of sports injuries in master athletes should therefore concentrate on these areas. Maintenance of flexibility and neuromuscular coordination through daily stretching and calisthenics is recommended. Long warm-up and cool-down periods should be the rule. A slow progression of training is especially important for elderly people. Participation in sports such as swimming, cycling or rowing is recommended for most elderly individuals, since the lower extremities do not then support the entire body mass. Postmenopausal women, on the other hand, need to load their skeletons to prevent osteoporosis. Common sense must be used when planning long-term exercise programmes for the elderly. Racquet sports

such as tennis have a low risk of injury, and are therefore suitable for elderly people. Regular medical checkups are recommended.

EXCESS WEIGHT

Excess weight may be a problem in weight-bearing recreational physical activities; the development of knee and hip symptoms and osteoarthritis is associated with an excess body mass (Hartz *et al.* 1986; Felson *et al.* 1988). Physical activity may accelerate the osteoarthritic process. A prospective study has shown that, in several obese individuals, weight reduction significantly relieves musculoskeletal symptoms (McGoey *et al.* 1990). The recommended regimen for overweight people includes a reduced energy intake and participation in activities where the entire body mass does not stress the lower extremities.

Primary intrinsic factors

MALALIGNMENTS

Forces associated with initiated ground impact have minimal effects on typical chronic injuries. The high forces from increased muscle activity are associated with midstance and push-off phases and result in greater peak loads on the tissue. A maximum point of pronation is usually reached at around 40% of stance (that is, at midstance). The foot levels over into supination at around 60% of stance. As pronation increases, there is an excessively weighted rear foot valgus and a compensatory internal rotation of the tibia secondary to movement of the subtalar joint (Fig. 33.5). The degree of this subtalar eversion and therefore pronation determines the degree of internal tibial rotation. This rotation of the tibia can also affect the femur and the pelvis, with increased internal femoral rotation. The lower extremity should therefore be considered a functional unit.

Excessive pronation can be physiological, but compensatory hyperpronation may also occur for anatomical reasons (tibia vara of more than 10°, functional equinus, talar varus and/or forefoot supination). Many good runners have a mild genu varum. There seems to be a low likelihood of injury

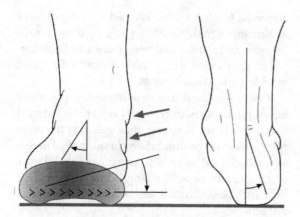

Fig. 33.5 Hyperpronation causes secondary effects such as an increased tension on the medial aspect of the ankle and foot, valgus deviation of the calcaneus, oblique traction on the calcaneus tendon and increased internal rotation of the tibia. The hyperpronation can be prevented by use of orthotics. From Renström (1988).

if the total varus is less than 8°, but the risk increases if the varus is greater than 18° (Ross & Schuster 1983).

Different malalignments may be combined. The so-called 'miserable malalignment syndrome' is seen in some runners. This syndrome combines femoral neck anteversion with internal rotation of the hip, genu valgum, squinting patella, excessive q-angle, tibia varum, functional equinus and compensatory foot pronation. A miserable malalignment syndrome can cause such problems that some of the affected individuals simply should not be running long distances.

James *et al.* (1978) noticed that increased pronation was present in 60% of a group of injured runners. Excessive pronation may predispose to injuries on the medial aspect of the lower extremities, such as medial tibial stress syndrome, posterior tibial tendinitis, pes anserinus tendinitis and bursitis, fibular and tibial stress fractures, chronic Achilles problems and plantar fasciitis. However, excessive pronation has not been shown to be the direct cause of these injuries; specific anatomical abnormalities and abnormal biomechanics of the extremity have not been correlated with specific injuries on a predictable basis.

Cavus feet are also associated with running

injuries. Cavus feet are present in about 20% of injured runners. Cavus feet have decreased motion of the subtalar joints, with a resulting decrease in flexibility of the midfoot and an excessive rear foot varus. At footstrike, the heel remains in varus, the longitudinal arch is maintained and the foot does not unlock. The tibia remains in external rotation, and the net result is a decreased stress, because the arch remains rigid throughout the midstance phase of running. With a reduction in internal tibial rotation, stress is passed through the lateral foot and knee, resulting in injuries such as iliotibial band friction syndrome, trochanteric bursitis, stress fractures, Achilles tendinosis, perioneal muscle strain, plantar fasciitis and metatarsalgia (Lorentzon 1988; James 1991).

If excessive or prolonged pronation occurs, with associated pain in the lower extremities, shoe orthotics may be indicated. In hyperpronation, the medial side of the sole and forefoot is elevated. If hyperpronation is found in an asymptomatic person, shoe corrections are seldom necessary. The same principles can be followed in the prevention and treatment of other injuries associated with malalignments.

In the patellofemoral pain syndrome, some additional risk factors may be present, such as patella alta and an excessive lateral displacement or tilting of the patella. Patellar bracing or taping may be beneficial in preventing reinjury. Activity modification and quadriceps muscle training are, however, the most common routes to successful treatment (Kannus *et al.* 1999).

LEG LENGTH DISCREPANCY

Leg length discrepancy is a commonly discussed factor in orthopaedics and sports medicine. The traditional orthopaedic view has been that discrepancies of less than 20 mm are largely cosmetic (Friberg *et al.* 1985). In élite athletes, however, a discrepancy of more than 5–6 mm may be symptomatic, and a built-up shoe or insert type of orthotic may be indicated for a discrepancy of 10 mm or more (Lysholm & Wiklander 1987).

A functional leg length discrepancy can be created if a runner runs consistently on the side of the road. Functional leg shortening can also result from sacroiliac joint dysfunction, unilateral excessive pronation, lumbar muscular pain and contractions or imbalance.

Many biomechanical alterations have been proposed to result from leg length discrepancy: pelvic tilt to the shorter side, followed by a compensatory lumbar scoliosis and compression of the intervertebral disc on the concave (inner) side of the curve, increased abduction of the hip (longer leg), excessive pronation of the foot (on the longer or shorter side), secondary increased knee valgus, and outward rotation of the leg. As a result, leg length discrepancy has been suggested as a causal factor in the development of lower back pain, hip osteoarthritis, trochanteric bursitis, patellar tendinitis, iliotibial band friction syndrome and stress fractures.

STRUCTURAL VARIATIONS

Structural variations can predispose to injuries. A prominent posterior aspect of the calcaneus can cause Achilles tendon and/or bursa problems (the so-called Haglund's deformity). A large os trigonum or a prominent posterior talar break can cause posterolateral ankle pain. Tarsal coalition of various kinds can cause abnormal and painful foot motion. An accessory navicular bone can cause medial foot pain.

MUSCLE STRENGTH AND IMBALANCE

The contributions of muscle weakness and imbalance to injury are also a matter for discussion. Muscle imbalance implies an asymmetry between the agonist and antagonist muscles in one extremity, asymmetry between the extremities, or a differential with an anticipated normal value (Grace et al. 1984; Grace 1985). An athlete with a greater than 10% difference in quadriceps or hamstring strength between the right and left sides is thought to be at increased risk of musculotendinous injury. An athlete who has a hamstring to quadriceps strength ratio of 60% or less in one leg is believed to have propensity for muscle injury (Safran et al. 1989). Heiser et al. (1984) showed that the University of

Nebraska football team sustained a 7.7% incidence of hamstring injury with a 31.7% recurrence rate, but after imbalances had been recognized and corrected, the incidence of hamstring strains decreased to 1.1%, with no recurrences.

Muscle weakness due to scarring from previous injury predisposes to recurrent injury, because the scar tissue is not as strong or as elastic as the other components of the musculotendinous unit. There is an increased risk of muscle injury, not only because of inadequate muscle strength but also because there may be inadequate corelaxation of the antagonist muscle.

Athletes with previous joint injury have long-lasting muscular strength, power and endurance deficits in their affected extremity, and these joints are at greater danger of reinjury than uninjured joints (Kannus et al. 1987a). Many such athletes feel fully rehabilitated and return to their sport too early. There is a persistent 20% loss of muscle strength in the affected leg 5–10 years after knee surgery, although the athletes who have been treated resume full activity, believing themselves to be completely rehabilitated (Grimby et al. 1980). The same persistent functional loss is observed after conservatively treated anterior cruciate ligament injuries of the knee. It is not clear how important muscle imbalance per se is as a causative factor for reinjury, since persistent joint instability, pain, swelling and impairment of neuromuscular coordination are also involved.

There is some evidence that multifactorial conditioning programmes can reduce injury rates (Hlobil et al. 1987), although other studies have found no direct relationship between muscle weakness or imbalance and injury (Grace 1985). Nevertheless, rehabilitation after injury is a tool not only for increasing muscle strength, but also for improving dynamic stability of the joint and coordination of the whole extremity. Therefore, it should always be a most important step in preparing an athlete for return to sport.

FLEXIBILITY

Good flexibility is often considered to be one of the most important measures for the prevention of sports injuries. It is logical to anticipate that an improvement of flexibility through stretching will result in a lengthening of the muscle–tendon unit, which in turn should reduce the likelihood of muscle strains during physical activities. Increasing flexibility will, however, alter the dynamics of the stretch–shortening cycle, which is likely to have unpredictable effects on the athlete and his or her susceptibility to injury (Watson 1995).

Knapic (1992) reviewed studies on the relationship between flexibility and injury and found insufficient information to reach any major conclusions. A few studies linking the risk of injury to an imbalance of left–right flexibility were more convincing. Walter *et al.* (1989) found that runners who sometimes stretched were at greater risk of injury than those who never stretched. Jakobs (1986) found that injured runners stretched before running as opposed to those who did not stretch. Van Mechelen *et al.* (1993) carried out a randomized controlled trial of the effects of 16 weeks of education in warm-up and stretching on the incidence of injuries in runners. The programme increased the knowledge of warm-up and cooling down in the experimental group, but the number of injuries remained unchanged. More prospective follow-up studies are clearly needed. In the meantime, flexibility training should be regarded as an important tool in preventing muscle and tendon injuries.

NEUROMUSCULAR CONDITIONS

A breakdown in balance and motor control can predispose to injury. Any deficit in proprioceptive capacity may lead to a functional instability that makes the athlete more prone to injury. This is especially true of chronic ankle instability, but is probably also true in chronic knee ligament instability.

Caraffa *et al.* (1996) studied 600 Italian soccer players in 40 soccer teams; 300 players were induced to train 20 min per day, including balance training, both with and without balance-boards. A control group underwent the same soccer training, but without balance training. The incidence of anterior cruciate ligament injuries was 1.15 per team per year in the control group, compared to 0.15 injuries per team per year in the proprioceptively trained group.

These results need to be verified, as they are almost too good to be true! They indicate that proprioceptive training can significantly reduce the incidence of anterior cruciate ligament injuries in soccer players.

JOINT LAXITY AND INSTABILITY

In some people, especially women, joints can be hypermobile. The range of movement may be excessive in normal, physiological directions of movement, in abnormal directions, or in both (Fig. 33.6). Joint hypermobility is often genetic (Grahame 1990). As a rule, this does not require special attention in injury prevention, but more research is needed.

A ligamentous injury may lead to joint instability and residual problems, especially in the knee, ankle and shoulder joints. Athletes with post-traumatic instability often complain of fear of 'giving way', recurrent sprains and pain of swelling during activity. Serious long-term consequences, such as post-traumatic osteoarthritis, may follow complete ligament tears where the joint has become unstable (Fig. 33.7) (Kannus 1988; Kannus & Järvinen 1989).

Specific muscle-strengthening exercises are of great value in preventing reinjury of these unstable joints. Good muscle function can to some extent compensate for ligamentous instability. Joint braces and taping may be of value in preventing abnormal movements and reinjuries (American Academy of Orthopedic Surgeons 1984).

Secondary intrinsic factors

The kinetic chain is a series of mobile segments and linkages that allows forward propulsion during gait. Anything that interferes with the normal progression and mechanics of force transfer can lead to alterations in gait, and compensatory changes in motion at another site in the chain. In athletes with recurrent and previous injuries, it is especially important to focus on dysfunction of the kinetic chain. As the kinetic chain is very complicated in nature, it is frequently overlooked in the aetiology of sports injuries. Secondary dysfunction can result from hyper- or hypomobility of a segment of the

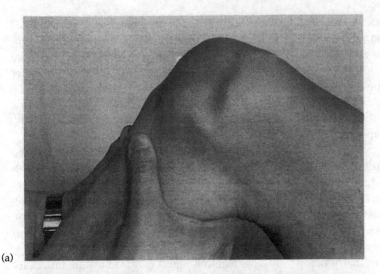

(a)

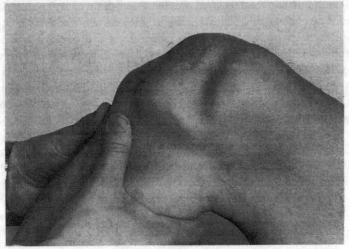

(b)

Fig. 33.6 Unstable joints resulting from untreated or maltreated ligamentous injury may result in osteoarthritis, for example of the knee. Correct initial treatment is important in preventing future complications. The figure shows the knee of a 27-year-old male athlete who had been conservatively treated for rupture of the anterior cruciate ligament; 10 years after injury, the knee shows a major anterior laxity, with a soft endpoint indicating insufficiency of the ligament. (a) Shows the starting position of the drawer test and (b) shows the end position of the test.

kinetic chain after an injury. Any dysfunction in the kinetic chain can lead to compensatory alterations in stand and gait, and in turn can lead to tissue microtrauma and other injuries.

Changes in the position and motion of the sacroiliac joint are fairly common. Although this joint is usually stable, it has been claimed that motion may occur and can lead to asymmetry of the pelvic ring structure. The main symptom is pain, localized to the sacroiliac joint, but it can also radiate to the buttocks and groin region. In order to identify sacroiliac joint dysfunction, one must be aware of its existence and understand the biomechanics involved.

PREVIOUS INJURIES AND PREDISPOSING DISEASES

Most injuries heal sooner or later, but they can leave a residual scar. This scar may have an elastic component that differs from that of normal tissue, thereby creating a weak area with increased risk of injury. Multiple, recurrent injuries may be indicative of kinetic chain dysfunction. Previous injuries can lead to fibrosis, with adhesions and limited joint motion and function. Long-standing joint injury may result in chronic instability, and even the slightest effusion can result in reflex inhibition of the muscles and sec-

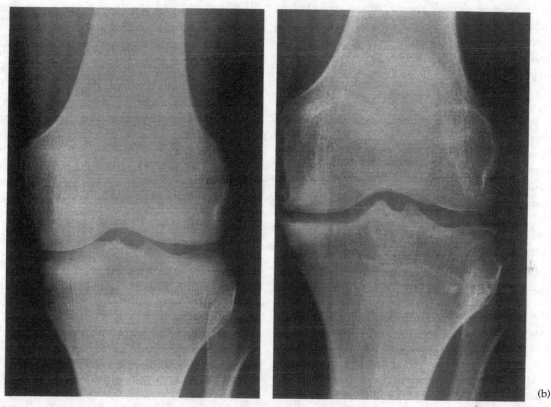

(a)

(b)

Fig. 33.7 Good muscle function developed through proper muscle exercises can, to some extent, compensate for ligamentous instability and prevent future problems. (a) Radiographs of a normal knee in a 34-year-old male who sustained complete anterior cruciate and medial–collateral ligament injuries in 1973. These injuries were treated conservatively. (b) Fifteen years later osteoarthritis has developed in the injured knee, which is now unstable.

ondary alterations of gait. Restricted motion of subtalar ankle, knee, shoulder and elbow joints increases stresses on other areas. Joint instability often results in muscle hypotrophy and a compensatory increase of stress on other structures.

An athlete may have a predisposing disease, making him or her prone to injury. A diabetic patient who is involved in long-distance running competition needs special care, since a low blood sugar level may cause a loss of concentration and coordination. Children who have had Perthes' disease may have a major loss of rotatory function in the hip, and they may develop secondary hip or knee swelling and irritation as a result of strenuous physical activities. Children with Osgood–Schlatter disease of their knees have an increased risk of patella alta in adulthood, and of patellofemoral subluxation or chondromalacia problems during physical activity.

General preventive methods

The general prevention of sports injuries includes activities that concern everyone involved in physical activity.

Basic physical fitness

A good level of physical fitness is of the utmost importance in avoiding injury. Athletes whose basic fitness level is below normal are more prone to injury, both from acute trauma and from overuse (Peterson & Renström 1986).

An appropriate basic physical fitness level can be achieved by regular exercise and general physical activity throughout the year. General conditioning and training of the large muscle groups are of great importance in most sports. Training should progress gradually, especially in those who are no longer young.

Physical inactivity and immobilization have deleterious effects on the musculoskeletal tissues. Bones become decalcified, tendons and ligaments lose their tensile strength, muscle tissue atrophies, and cartilage loses its elasticity (Kannus *et al.* 1992a,b). Following illness or injury, or after a break in training, it is important that a reasonable level of basic physical fitness be reached before competition is resumed.

Warm-up

Warm-up exercises are designed to prepare the body for the ensuing sporting activity. They have two functions: to prevent injury and to enhance performance.

The resting blood flow to the skeletal muscles is relatively low, and most of the small blood vessels (capillaries) supplying them are closed. When activity begins, the blood flow to the muscles increases. At rest, 15–20% of the blood flow is directed to the skeletal muscles, but the corresponding figure after 10–12 min of all-round exercise is 70–75%. A muscle can achieve maximal aerobic performance only when all its blood vessels are functional and maximally dilated.

The elastic components of muscle are more susceptible to injury when the tissue is cold (Zarins & Ciullo 1983). An increase in muscle temperature speeds the metabolic processes, allowing faster and more forceful contractions (Safran *et al.* 1989), and it also increases the elasticity of intramuscular connective tissue, making the contractions smoother. The thermally dependent increase in connective tissue elasticity may be the reason why warmed-up muscles stretch to a greater length before tearing, and withstand application of a greater force before failure. Rosenbaum *et al.* (1995) investigated the influence of stretching and warm-up on force development in the human triceps surae muscle.

Stretching reduced the peak force, suggesting a change in muscle compliance. After warm-up, the peak force remained unchanged, but the rate of rise in force was increased. The increase in compliance might be expected to reduce the risk of muscle strains, but the increase in rise rate would have the opposite effect. Common and important injuries to be prevented by warm-up include not only muscle strains, but also tendon, ligament and other soft tissue injuries.

A warm-up is also a way of preparing an athlete's mind for physical activity. A proper warm-up may relax the athlete, and aid concentration. Brain–muscle coordination and cooperation are improved, with less likelihood of uncontrolled muscle activity and strain.

Warm-up can be passive or active. A passive warm-up may involve a sauna, a warm shower, warm clothes or massage. The circulation is somewhat increased thereby, but the response is smaller than that achieved with an active warm-up. An active warm-up should be both general and sport specific. The general part includes jogging or stationary cycling in order to involve large muscle groups. After the general warm-up, more sport-specific exercises can begin. Runners, for example, should concentrate the further warm-up on the muscles, tendons, joints and ligaments of the lower extremities.

The final stage of warm-up concentrates on technique, and practice of sport-specific movements. The pace of exercise can be gradually increased, with the whole warm-up session lasting for at least 15–20 min, depending on the sport involved. The effect of the warm-up wears off rapidly, and mild exercise should therefore be continued. Ideally, the delay before competition should be no longer than 10 min. During this time the athlete also prepares psychologically.

Cooling down

Cooling down exercises are desirable after training or competition. They enhance clearance of the products of muscle metabolism, such as lactic acid, shortening the recovery time. They also offer a unique possibility for stretching exercises, since the muscle temperature is still high and stretching can be performed safely and easily.

Cooling down is normally performed in two phases. The first phase includes aerobic sport-specific movements at 50–70% of maximal aerobic power. For example, after a cross-country skiing competition, the athlete should ski for an additional 1–3 km at mild or moderate speed. The second phase consists of general large muscle exercise, such as gentle jogging, performed at 30–50% of maximal aerobic power. Stretching for 5–15 min, depending on the sport, is included in this phase.

Slow progression

The musculoskeletal system must be allowed to adapt gradually to increasing loads. At least 50% of all overuse injuries are caused by training errors, usually a breaking of this principle of slow progression.

After 10 years, a male competitive runner who has increased his weekly training distance slowly but steadily every year is able to run more than 200 km per week without musculoskeletal problems. However, a colleague who has increased the distance faster is much more prone to overuse troubles while running the same distance per week.

Musculoskeletal adaptation to stress is a slow but very reliable process. Athletes and their coaches must understand the importance of slow progression in order to avoid injury to muscle (e.g. pain, soreness, strain and compartment syndromes), tendons (tendinitis, peritendinitis, insertionitis, partial or complete ruptures), joints (cartilage softening or avulsion, meniscal ruptures, ligament sprains, synovitis and osteoarthritis) and bones (stress fractures, osteoporotic fractures and apophysitis). This is of particular concern to children and adolescents.

Preventive training

Training of the musculoskeletal system is the key to both prevention of injury and successful recovery after an injury. Repeated, slowly progressive exercises improve the mechanical and structural properties of the muscles, tendons, joints, ligaments and bones by increasing their mass and tensile strength. Preventive training includes muscle training, flexibility training, coordination and proprioceptive training and sport-specific training.

Muscle training

Muscle training can be isometric, concentric or eccentric. Isometric exercise is an effective method of increasing strength, but the response is greatest around the angle at which training is carried out. Isokinetic training is a form of concentric or eccentric training, performed at a constant angular velocity throughout the range of motion; it is very effective in increasing muscle strength, power and endurance. However, this type of motion is not used in sport.

In many types of exercise, for example in running, there is a stretch–shortening cycle where the stretch (eccentric action) precedes shortening (concentric action) (Komi 1984). Eccentric exercises combined with stretching can be used in the preventive as well as rehabilitative phases of overuse injuries (Curwin & Stanish 1984; Alfredsson 1998). It is, however, important to realize that eccentric contractions may sometimes contribute to both acute and chronic overuse tendon and muscle problems (e.g. muscle soreness). Therefore, eccentric exercises are not recommended as a part of regular training for elderly athletes.

Flexibility training

Strength training has a negative effect on joint flexibility (Moller 1984). This can be counteracted by flexibility training. The flexibility of a particular joint is limited primarily by tightness of the connective tissue. Flexibility exercises should be started after the growth spurt, when there is a rapid increase in muscle volume and power. Flexibility decreases with age, and flexibility training should therefore be emphasized more and more with increasing age.

Flexibility training aims to maintain and/or improve joint mobility, to reduce the risk of overloading at extreme joint angles, to increase muscle and tendon strength, to enhance coordination between various parts of the musculoskeletal system, and to adapt the musculoskeletal system to the specific demands of a particular sport.

Stretching is one of the most important methods of flexibility training. It should be preceded by a 3–5-min warm-up. Dynamic (or ballistic, spring, bounce or rebound) stretching implies repeated muscle extension to its limit, followed by immediate relaxation. This type of stretching is not effective, as it activates protective reflexes, and it is seldom used nowadays.

Static stretching involves slowly stretching the muscle as far as possible and then holding that position for 20–60 s. This technique is commonly used. Static contract–relax–hold stretching includes first a slow stretch to the limit of motion, and then a maximum isometric contraction in that position, held for 4–6 s. This is followed by a relaxation for 2–3 s. Thereafter, a passive stretch is made to the extreme position, and that position is held for 10–60 s. This technique is a modification of the proprioceptive neuromuscular facilitation technique frequently used by physical therapists.

The 3S system (scientific stretching for sport) is a fourth type of stretching. The muscle is stretched passively and then exposed to an isometric contraction. This technique is effective, but a partner is required to hold and stretch the leg.

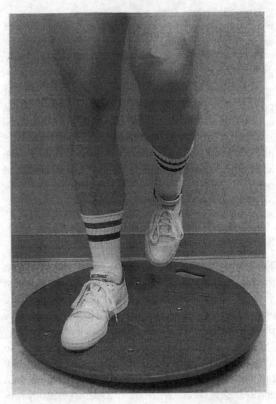

Fig. 33.8 Tilt board exercises can improve proprioceptive capacity and strength in ankle joints with functional instability, thereby preventing recurrence of ankle sprains.

Coordination and proprioceptive training

This involves training the interaction between the nervous system, muscles, tendons, joints and ligaments. In many sports, good technique and coordination are essential to prevent acute and overuse injuries.

An ankle injury often damages the nerves in the joint capsule, along with the ankle ligaments, and 10–20% of patients show a residual functional instability. Proprioceptive training is then one of the major treatments. Such training can be carried out on a tilt-board (Fig. 33.8). Gauffin (1988) has shown that a steady state is reached after 10 weeks with this type of training.

As mentioned earlier, this type of proprioceptive training is also very effective in preventing anterior cruciate ligament injuries (Caraffa *et al.* 1996).

Sport-specific training

Sport-specific conditioning can usually be achieved by training within the sport itself. For example, many soccer and tennis coaches prefer training carried out on the soccer field or tennis court, respectively. However, if the sports event is dangerous by nature (such as boxing, motor sports or aerial freestyle skiing), or if it carries a high risk of injury (for instance, gymnastics or American football), simulation exercises should be performed before taking part in the sport itself. In the case of freestyle skiing, this involves training and jumping into a pool.

Sport-specific training often includes all other aspects of preventive training, and it is therefore one of the most effective approaches to the primary prevention of sports injuries. After injury, a sport-specific exercise programme should be the final step in rehabilitation before return to the sports arena.

Education

Health education can be an effective way of preventing sports injuries. Nevertheless, its effectiveness depends on the quality of planning and the extent of cooperation with sports injury specialists. Planning requires a careful analysis of the problem, the behaviour, the determinants, the intervention, the implementation, and the strength of interrelationships between these five aspects (Renström 1994). The optimal stage at which particular advice on prevention should be given has yet to be determined. Epidemiological studies on the aetiology of sports injuries, followed by research on behavioural determinants, are necessary to fill gaps in our current knowledge.

Information on injury mechanisms is effective in preventing anterior cruciate ligament injuries among skiers. Videotapes of the occurrence of anterior cruciate ligament sprains in alpine skiers and data associated with more than 1400 anterior cruciate ligament injuries observed over 22 years allowed Ettlinger *et al.* (1995) to identify two common mechanisms underlying such injuries. A study based on this information showed that serious knee sprains declined by 62% among trained patrollers and instructors who were given information on how to fall, compared with the experience of the two previous seasons, but there was no decline in a control group who were given no information.

Medical examination

Some sports require a medical examination immediately before competition (for example, boxing or ultramarathon running) in order to prevent injury or general medical complications. A medical screening examination is also recommended for middle-aged and older people (35 years and over) who have decided to start a regular exercise programme (International Federation of Sports Medicine 1989a). Such screening should include a complete orthopaedic evaluation to discover possible risk factors for musculo-skeletal injury.

Nutrition and diet

Nutrition becomes important in injury prevention during training and competition that is sufficiently prolonged to deplete the body's carbohydrate stores. At this stage, performance, reactions and coordination become impaired, and the athlete is at increased risk of injury.

Other nutritional elements of food (fat, proteins, vitamins and minerals) are of secondary value in injury prevention, although they have a tremendous effect on general well-being. A well-balanced diet is therefore recommended for every active individual (Chapters 13 and 29).

Drugs, medication and doping

Athletes who are taking part in competitions should not normally be receiving medication of any kind. If medication is essential (for example, in asthma or diabetes), is prescribed by the athlete's own physician and is not a banned substance, it will enhance general well-being and allow the athlete to take an enjoyable part in sports. Stimulants, narcotics, anabolic steroids, diuretics, alcohol, local anaesthetics and corticosteroids are dangerous from the viewpoint of injury prevention.

Pain is a guide to correct diagnosis and treatment and is also a warning signal. Pain inhibition is dangerous in combination with sports injuries. If pain has been reduced by use of local anaesthetics or corticosteroids, the athlete should not be allowed to participate in competition. Corticosteroid injections may cause hypoxic degenerative alterations in tendons, weakening their tensile strength and inducing muscle necrosis.

Overall hygiene

The skin secretes sweat and grease. Dust and dirt may adhere to this, forming a breeding ground for bacteria, and producing unpleasant odours, rashes, irritation and pimples. Inadequate foot care allows dirt to collect between the toes, again providing a breeding ground for bacteria and fungi.

General preparation for sports

An athlete who is preparing for regular hard training and competition should lead a well-regulated daily life, with regular dietary habits, enough sleep and avoidance of drug abuse. The importance of a regular, healthy lifestyle cannot be overemphasized for an athlete who wishes to reach or to stay at the top. The competitor must be well prepared, not only physically, but also mentally. The degree of mental tension varies from sport to sport. Excessive mental tension can cause reactions such as lack of appetite, headaches and, occasionally, defective coordination with an increased risk of injury. If mental tension is excessive, the coach must find a way to restore an optimal level. Discussion with the athlete and a gradual increase in the competitive element of training are often used to prepare the athlete. A competitor usually learns quickly what is her or his optimal level of mental tension for competitive performance.

Preventive equipment

Preventive equipment is of the utmost importance. Appropriate measures include the use of protective equipment, braces, tapes, shoes and orthotics.

Protective equipment

Protective equipment plays an important safety role, especially in contact sports such as American football, ice hockey, lacrosse, team handball, volleyball and soccer. This is also true in some popular racquet sports such as squash. The equipment must be chosen carefully and fitted by a knowledgeable individual. The player's cooperation is also necessary. Modification of the equipment to increase its comfort may sacrifice its protective effect, thereby increasing the risk of injury.

Protective head equipment is used in many sports, especially ice hockey and American football. No helmet is designed well enough to prevent a head injury completely, but such equipment can

reduce the magnitude of a blow, dispersing its force over as large an area as possible (Gieck 1990). The American football helmet and the ice hockey helmet have been well tested. Chin straps and face masks may be added; face masks are now compulsory in junior and university ice hockey (Fig. 33.9), and the number of facial and eye injuries has decreased dramatically since adoption of this rule.

There are other sports with a substantial risk of eye injury where eye-protecting devices are not worn, for example professional ice hockey, racquet sports (such as racquetball and badminton), lacrosse and baseball. Adequate protective eye devices are now available (International Federation of Sports Medicine 1989b). In low risk sports, protective eye wear can consist of normal eye glass frames

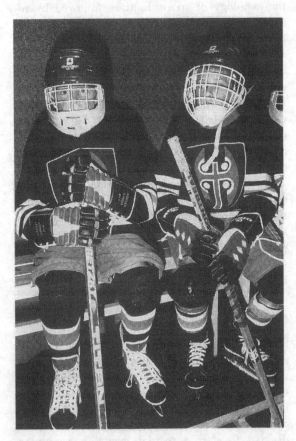

Fig. 33.9 Helmets with face masks are now compulsory in junior ice hockey. This protective device prevents many injuries.

with polycarbonate lenses. Moulded polycarbonate frames and lenses are also suggested for athletes who ordinarily do not wear glasses, but who participate in moderate to high risk non-contact sports. Face masks or helmets with face protection are required in sports with a high risk of contact or collision. Some basketball players have begun wearing protective eye guards as well.

Ear guards are often worn by water polo players and wrestlers; they should be well fitted to the head, and should not come off during competition. Such protective devices have partially eliminated the cauliflower ear that was previously common among wrestlers.

Mouthpieces have been mandatory in boxing and in American football since the 1960s. Participants in other sports, for example lacrosse, field hockey and ice hockey, have also begun to wear mouthpieces. Well-designed shoulder and elbow pads as well as other protective pads over the thorax are used in ice hockey and in American football (Fig. 33.10).

Protective equipment for the lower extremities is worn in American football. Ice hockey goalkeepers wear special padding to protect themselves against the puck. Shin padding is compulsory in soccer.

Protective equipment should be designed to absorb and distribute impact forces. The equipment is continuously being developed and improved to meet the increasing requirements of sports.

Role of braces in injury prevention

Braces are commonly used to prevent injuries, to protect against reinjury and to aid in rehabilitation following injury. Braces are specially designed for use on ankle, knee, elbow and wrist joints. The most commonly used are knee stabilizing braces; the American Academy of Orthopedic Surgeons (1984)

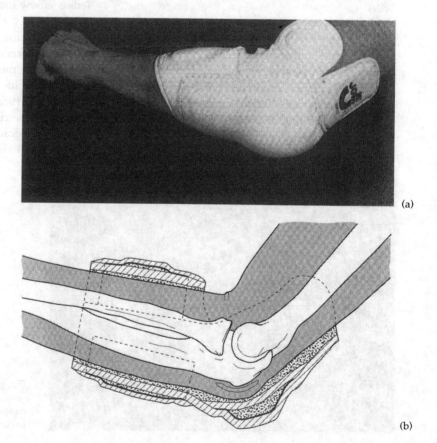

(a)

(b)

Fig. 33.10 Protective padding should take up and distribute impact forces correctly. (a) An elbow protective device used in ice hockey. (b) The principles of distribution of shock absorption. From Peterson and Renström (1986), with permission.

has classified these into three types: prophylactic, rehabilitative and functional.

Prophylactic knee braces are designed to prevent or reduce the severity of damage to the knee joint caused by an injury. Such braces are not common in Europe, because they cannot be used in soccer, but they are appropriate for American football. They usually have one lateral hinge. Prophylactic braces have a limited capacity to protect the medial collateral ligament from direct lateral stress when the knee is in full extension. The efficacy of these braces is probably small, and their future role in sports medicine is unclear.

Rehabilitative knee braces are designed to immobilize the knee, or to allow limited and controlled flexion after injury or operative procedures. They provide accurate control over motion, and avoid excessive loading of the healing tissue. They may provide some stability, but cannot duplicate the function of the undamaged ligaments (Hofman *et al.* 1984).

Functional knee braces are designed to assist the functional stability of unstable knee joints. There are many varieties, but they are limited in their direct control of the rotation of the tibia and femur by the soft tissues covering the limbs; these provide the principal mechanical interface for the brace. Functional braces attempt to control secondary rotation by blocking the principal components of instability, which are translations in multiple planes. Many patients are satisfied with this type of brace, and feel it is of some value (Colville *et al.* 1986). Biomechanically, the braces decrease anterior translation, but only at low loads and slow speeds (Beynnon *et al.* 1997).

Braces for patellofemoral pain syndromes have been developed with the aim of preventing lateral subluxation of the patella. These braces have limited value, but are still used, as some patients experience a reduction in pain.

Ankle stabilizing braces are becoming more popular than tape (Fig. 33.11). Ankle braces decrease the recurrence of sprains and also the severity of injury (Schwellnus 1994). The most effective support of the ankle, producing the lowest incidence of ligament injuries, is a combination of high-top shoes and laced ankle stabilizers (Rovere *et al.* 1988). Different types of ankle brace are available, and can be used in shoes.

Tennis elbow braces are also receiving growing popularity. They are applied to relaxed muscles, thereby preventing the lower arm extensor muscles from full contraction and protecting the insertion of the extensor muscles at the lateral epicondyle. Electromyographic studies have verified the effectiveness of these braces (Groppel & Nischl 1983).

The role of braces in injury prevention remains controversial, because of the lack of scientific data.

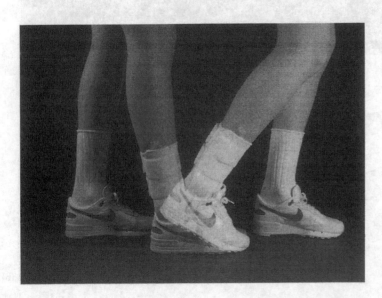

Fig. 33.11 Ankle braces help to prevent recurrence of ankle injuries. Their support is increased when they are used in combination with a sport shoe.

Biomechanically, braces seem to have a limited effect, but injured athletes often experience some symptomatic relief while wearing them.

Heat retainers or neoprene sleeves have been applied in the treatment of overuse injuries and in rehabilitation from most injuries for many years. They have also been used by many alpine skiers to prevent injury in cold weather. The idea behind such braces is that heat enhances circulation around the injured area, facilitating the healing process. Heat also enhances elasticity, potentially preventing and rehabilitating muscle tendon injuries (Fig. 33.12).

Role of tape in injury prevention

Medical tape is used extensively to support different

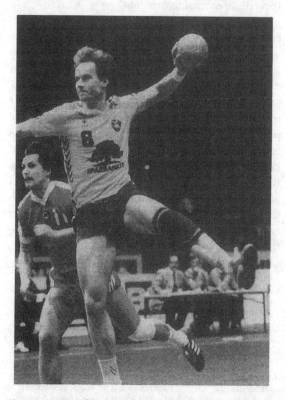

Fig. 33.12 Heat plays an important role in the prevention of sports injuries, as it increases the circulation and improves the elasticity of the collagen in tendons, muscles and ligaments. Heat-retaining braces are therefore used increasingly in both prevention and rehabilitation after injury.

joints, especially the ankle, where it is claimed to prevent ankle injuries. Ekstrand (1982) showed that the number of ankle sprains in soccer was reduced by 75% by a preventive programme that included prophylactic taping, stretching and player education. Likewise, a combination of prophylactic taping and the use of high-top shoes in basketball reduced the number of ankle sprains (Garrick 1977). Tape also had a significant prophylactic effect against injuries of the lateral ligaments of the ankle in a 2-year prospective randomized study of team handball players (Londenberger *et al.* 1990).

The role of taping is probably decreasing; there are associated skin problems, the effect of taping is not long lasting, and tape is expensive. It often requires trained application and use of a sharp instrument to remove it.

Role of shoes in injury prevention

Shoes have great importance in the reduction of impact forces. The design of shoes has been revolutionized during the last 15 years. Most modern shoes are designed to provide both stability and shock absorption. Good running shoes should absorb and/or reduce impact forces, and provide medial–lateral stability, avoiding excessive pronation and oversupination of the foot. It is a question of cushioning, support and friction. Appropriate shoes are now available for almost every sport event.

The ideal shoe should hold the foot so that it functions much as when barefoot. Shock-absorbing characteristics are important, and shoe design has a great influence on the extent of shock absorption at heelstrike (Jörgensen & Ekstrand 1988). Shoes also have a stabilizing function, and hyperpronation can be prevented by stable shoes with a firm and high heel counter. Running shoes should control the rolling movement at push-off (Pforringer & Segesser 1986). Shoes should be very flexible in the forefoot, or they can cause forefoot overuse problems during push-off. An ideal shoe should not wear out within the first few months of use. It is more important to buy good shoes than expensive clothing.

The importance of purchasing the correct shoe

for different sports activities cannot be overemphasized. Correct shoe wear is very important in the prevention of injuries, particularly overuse injuries.

Role of shoe orthotics in injury prevention

During the past 20 years, custom-made orthotic devices have been used increasingly, as sports physicians have come to understand the role of malalignments in the genesis of overuse injuries.

The biomechanical goals of orthotic devices have been summarized by Doxey (1985) as follows.
1 To prevent abnormal movements of the subtalar and metatarsal joints.
2 To rebalance the malaligned foot to a more neutral position.
3 To resist or normalize the foot's abduction to the ground at heelstrike.
4 To resist or normalize the foot's propulsive function as a rigid lever at push-off.
5 To maximize hallux function.
6 To maximize toe function in propulsion.
7 To allow normal foot movements and muscle activity at the proper time.

The failure of orthotic treatment experienced by some people may reflect failure to adjust the orthotics as needed. Support diminishes owing to the person's progressive pronation or compression of the orthotic appliance material. The orthotic control of pronation is satisfactory for daily activities, but may not be adequate for the increased pronation in running, which can be resumed gradually when the athlete is asymptomatic.

There is a lack of scientific support for the use of orthotics. However, a success rate of 70% has been reported in typical running injuries (Smith *et al.* 1986). Some clinical reports also imply that orthotics are effective in the treatment of stress injuries and pain syndromes of the lower limbs (Darrigan & Ganley 1985). Orthotics have mostly been prescribed to control excessive pronation. Both maximum pronation and the initial maximal velocity of pronation can be reduced in this way (Clarke *et al.* 1983), while the total movement is maintained. Orthotics for pronation can significantly decrease abduction of the foot during walking and running, and can also correct leg length discrepancies. No prospective randomized studies are available, but a vast experience in sports medicine suggests the value of orthotics in compensating for and neutralizing different malalignments.

Custom-made orthotics allow the sports physician to treat the cause of injuries and not merely the symptoms. The use of orthotics should be encouraged if there are clear biomechanical indications for such treatment.

When prescribing orthotics, some caution is recommended. Biomechanical factors are only one potential aetiological factor in any injury. It is wise to view biomechanical factors as contributory to and not causative of injury (Craton & McKenzie 1994; Renström 1994). They represent only one of a host of intrinsic and extrinsic causes of injury, although they can be a very significant factor. The use of orthotics should be part of a comprehensive preventive programme.

References

Adelsberg, S. (1986) The tennis stroke. An EMG analysis of selected muscles with rackets in increasing grip size. *American Journal of Sports Medicine* 14, 139–142.

Alfredson, H., Pietilä, T., Jonsson, P. & Lorentzon, R. (1998) Heavy-load eccentric calf muscle training for the treatment of chronic achilles tendinosis. *American Journal of Sports Medicine* 26, 360–366.

American Academy of Orthopedic Surgeons (1984) *Knee braces.* Seminar report, Annual Meeting, 18–19 August, Chicago, IL.

Backous, D.D., Friedl, K.E., Smith, N.J. *et al.* (1988) Soccer injuries and their relation to physical maturity. *Am J Dis Child* 142, 839–842.

Bahr, R., Lian, O. & Bahr, I.A. (1997) A two-fold reduction in the incidence of acute ankle sprains in volleyball after the introduction of an injury prevention program: a prospective cohort study. *Scandinavian Journal of Medicine and Science in Sports* 7, 172–177.

Beynnon, B.D., Johnson, R.J., Fleming, B.C. *et al.* (1997) The effect of functional knee

bracing on the anterior cruciate ligament in the weight-bearing and non-weight-bearing knee. *American Journal of Sports Medicine* 25, 353–359.

Blair, S.N., Kohl, H.W., Gordon, N.F. & Paffenberger, R.S.J. (1992) How much physical activity is good for health. *Annual Reviews of Public Health* 13, 99–126.

Bortz, W.M. (1982) Disuse and aging. *Journal of the American Medical Association* 248, 1203.

Boswick, J.A. Jr, Danzl, D.F., Hamlet, M.P.

& Schultz, A.L. (1983) Helping the frost-bitten patient. *Patient Care* **17**, 90–115.

Caraffa, A., Cerulli, G., Projetti, M., Aisa, G. & Rizzo, A. (1996) Prevention of anterior cruciate ligament injuries in soccer. A prospective controlled study of proprioceptive training. *Knee Surgery, Sports Traumatology, Arthroscopy* **4**, 19–21.

Carroll, R. (1986) Tennis elbow and tennis rackets: case studies of club tennis players. In: MacGregor & Moncur (eds) *Sports and Medicine*, pp. 281–288. E. & F.N. Spon, London.

Clarke, T.E., Freerick, E.C. & Hlavac, H.F. (1983) Effects of a soft orthotic device on rear foot movement in running. *Pediatric Sports Medicine* **1**, 20–23.

Colville, M.R., Lee, C.L. & Ciullo, J.V. (1986) The Lennox Hill brace. An evaluation of effectiveness in treating knee instability. *American Journal of Sports Medicine* **14**, 257–261.

Craton, N. & McKenzie, D.C. (1994) Orthotics in injury prevention. In: Renström P.A.F.H. (ed.) *Sports Injuries: Basic Principles of Prevention and Care*, pp. 417–423. Blackwell Scientific Publications, Oxford.

Curwin, S. & Stanish, W.D. (1984) *Tendinitis: its Etiology and Treatment*. The Collamore Press, Lexington, Massachusetts.

Darrigan, R.D. & Ganley, J.V. (1985) Functional orthoses with intrinsic rear foot post. *Journal of the American Podiatric Medical Association* **75**, 619–624.

Doxey, G.E. (1985) Clinical use and fabrication of molded thermoplastic foot orthotic devices. Suggestion from the field. *Physical Therapy* **11**, 1679–1682.

Drinkwater, B. (1988) Training of female athletes. In: Dirix, A., Knuttgen, H.G. & Tittel, K. (eds) *The Olympic Book of Sports Medicine*, pp. 309–327. Blackwell Scientific Publications, Oxford.

Ekstrand, J. (1982) *Soccer injuries and their prevention*. Doctoral Dissertation. Linköping University, Linköping, Sweden.

Elliott, B.C., Blanksby, B.A. & Ellis, R. (1980) Vibration and rebound velocity characteristics of conventional and over-sized tennis rackets. *Research Quarterly* **51**, 608–615.

Eriksson, E. & Johnson, R. (1980) The etiology of downhill ski injuries. *Exercise and Sport Sciences Reviews* **8**, 1–17.

Ettlinger, C.F., Johnson, R.J. & Shealy, J.E. (1995) A method to help reduce the risk of serious knee sprains incurred in alpine skiing. *American Journal of Sports Medicine* **23**, 531–537.

Felson, D.T., Andersson, J.J., Neimvk, A.,

Walker, A.M. & Meenan, R.F. (1988) Obesity and knee osteoarthritis. The Framingham Study. *Annals of Internal Medicine* **109**, 18–24.

Friberg. O., Kvist, M., Aalto, T. & Kujula, V. (1985) Leg length inequality in the etiology of low back pain and low limb overuse injuries in young athletes. *Idrottsmedicin (Stockholm)* **3**, 5–7.

van Galen, W.Ch.C. & Diederiks, J.P.M. (1990) *Sportblessures breed uitgementen* (English summary). Publishers Comp. De Vrieseborvh, Haarlem, The Netherlands.

Garrick, J.G. (1977) The frequency of injury, mechanism of injury and epidemiology of ankle sprains. *American Journal of Sports Medicine* **5**, 241–242.

Gauffin, H., Tropp, H., Odenrick, P. (1988) Effect of ankle disk training on postural control in patients with functional instability of the ankle joint. *International Journal of Sports Medicine* **9**, 141–144.

Gieck, I. (1990) Protective equipment for sports. In: Ryan, A. & Allman, F. (eds) *Sports Medicine*, pp. 211–242. Academic Press, San Diego, CA.

Grace, T.G. (1985) Muscle imbalance and extremity injury. A perplexing relationship. *Sports Medicine* **2**, 77–82.

Grace, T.G., Sweetser, E.R. & Nelson, M.A. (1984) Isokinetic muscle imbalance and knee-joint injuries. *Journal of Bone and Joint Surgery* **66A**, 734–740.

Grahame, R. (1990) The hypermobility syndrome. *Annals of the Rheumatic Diseases* **49**, 199–200.

Grimby, G., Gustafsson, E., Peterson, L. & Renström, P. (1980) Quadriceps function and training after knee ligament surgery. *Medicine and Science in Sports and Exercise* **12**, 70–75.

Groppel, J.L. (1984) *Tennis for Advanced Players and Those Who Would Like to Be*. Human Kinetics, Champaign, IL.

Groppel, J.L. & Nischl, R.P. (1983) A mechanical and electromyographical analysis of the effects of various joint counterforce braces on the tennis player. *American Journal of Sports Medicine* **14**, 195–200.

Hartz, A.J., Fischer, M.E., Bril, G. *et al.* (1986) The association of obesity with joint pain and osteoarthritis in the HANES data. *Journal of Chronic Diseases* **39**, 311–319.

Heiser, T.M., Weber, J., Sullivan, G., Clare, P. & Jacobs, R.R. (1984) Prophylaxis and management of hamstring muscle injuries in intercollegiate football players. *American Journal of Sports Medicine* **12**, 368–370.

Hlobil, H., van Mechelen, W. & Kemper, H.C.G. (1987) *How can Sports Injuries be Prevented?*, pp. 1–236. NISGZ Publication 25E, Oosterbeek, Netherlands.

Hofman, A.A., Wyatt, R.W., Bourne, M. & Daniels, A.U. (1984) Knee stability in orthotic knee braces. *American Journal of Sports Medicine* **12**, 371–374.

International Federation of Sports Medicine (1989a) Physical exercise—an important factor for health. A position statement. *International Journal of Sports Medicine* **10**, 460–461.

International Federation of Sports Medicine (1989b) Eye injuries and eye protection in sports. *Australian Sports Medicine Federation* **7** (2), 19–20.

Jacobs, S.L. & Berson, B.L. (1986) Injuries to runners: a study of entrants to a 10000 metre race. *American Journal of Sports Medicine* **14**, 151–155.

James, S.L., Bates, B.T. & Osternig, L.R. (1978) Injuries to runners. *American Journal of Sports Medicine* **6**, 40–50.

Janda, D.H. (1997) Sports surveillance has everything to do with sports medicine. *Sports Medicine* **24**, 169–171.

Jörgensen, U. (1993) Regulations and officiating in injury prevention. In: Renström P.A.F.H. (ed.) *Sports Injuries: Basic Principles of Prevention and Care*, pp. 213–219. Blackwell Scientific Publications, Oxford.

Jörgensen, U. & Ekstrand, J. (1988) Significance of heel pad confinement for the shock absorption at heel strike. *International Journal of Sports Medicine* **9**, 468–473.

Kannus, P. (1988) *Conservative treatment of acute knee distortions—long-term results and their evaluation methods*. Doctoral Dissertation, University of Tampere, Tampere, Finland.

Kannus, P. & Järvinen, M. (1989) Posttraumatic anterior cruciate ligament insufficiency as a cause of osteoarthritis in a knee joint. *Clinical Rheumatology* **8**, 251–260.

Kannus, P., Latvala, K. & Järvinen, M. (1987a) Thigh muscle strengths in the anterior cruciate ligament deficient knee: isokinetic and isometric long-term results. *Journal of Orthopedic and Sports Physical Therapy* **9**, 223–227.

Kannus, P., Niittymaki, S. & Jarvinen, M. (1987b) Sports injuries in women: a one-year prospective follow up study at an outpatient sports clinic. *British Journal of Sports Medicine* **21**, 37–39.

Kannus, P., Niittymaki, S., Jarvinen, M. & Lehto, M. (1989) Sports injuries in elderly athletes: a three-year prospective, controlled study. *Age and Ageing* 18, 263–270.

Kannus, P., Josza, L., Renström, P. *et al.* (1992a) The effects of training immobilization and remobilization on musculoskeletal tissues. *Scandinavian Journal of Medicine and Science in Sports* 2, 100–118.

Kannus, P., Jozsa, L., Renström, P. *et al.* (1992b) The effects of training immobilization and remobilization on musculoskeletal tissues. Remobilization and prevention of immobilization atrophy. *Scandinavian Journal of Medicine and Science in Sports* 2, 164–176.

Kannus, P., Natri, A., Paakkala, T. & Järvinen, M. (1999) An outcome study of chronic patellofemoral pain syndrome. *Journal of Bone and Joint Surgery (America)* 81, 355–363.

Knapikk, J.J., Jones, B.H., Bauman, C.L., Harris, J.M. (1992) Strength, flexibility and athletic injuries. *Sports Medicine* 14, 277–288.

Komi, P.V. (1984) Physiological and biomechanical correlates of muscle function: effects of muscle structure and stretch–shortening cycle on force and speed. *Exercise and Sport Sciences Reviews* 12, 81–121.

Kulund, D.N., McCue, F.C. III, Rockwell, D.A. & Gieck, J.H. (1979) Tennis injuries: prevention and treatment, a review. *American Journal of Sports Medicine* 7, 249–253.

Lane, N.E., Bloch, D.A. & Wood, P.D. (1987) Aging, long-distance running, and the development of musculoskeletal disability: a controlled study. *American Journal of Medicine* 82, 772–780.

Lloyd, T., Traintafyllou, S.J., Baker, E.R. *et al.* (1986) Women athletes with menstrual irregularity have increased musculoskeletal injuries. *Medicine and Science in Sports and Exercise* 18, 374–379.

de Loës, M. (1990) Medical treatment and costs of sports-related injuries in a total population. *International Journal of Sports Medicine* 11, 66–72.

Londenberger, U., Reese, D., Renström, P., Andreasson, G. & Peterson, L. (1990) A prospective study of the effect of ankle taping. *FIMS Proceedings of the XXIV World Congress of Sports Medicine.* Amsterdam.

Lorentzon, R. (1988) Causes of injuries: intrinsic factors. In: Dirix, A., Knuttgen, H.G. & Tittel, K. (eds) *The Olympic Book of Sports Medicine*, pp. 376–390. Blackwell Science, Oxford.

Lysholm, J. & Wiklander, J. (1987) Injuries in runners. *American Journal of Sports Medicine* 15, 168–171.

van Mechelen, W. (1997) Sports injury surveillance system: 'One size fits all?' *Sports Medicine* 24, 164–168.

van Mechelen, W., Hlobil, H. & Kemper, H.C.G. (1987) How can sports injuries be prevented? NISGZ, Papendahl, The Netherlands.

van Mechelen, W., Hlobil, H., Kemper, H.C.G., Voom, W.J., Jongh, H.R. (1993) Prevention of running injuries by warmup, cool-down and stretching exercises. *American Journal of Sports Medicine* 21, 711–719.

Mann, R.A., Baxter, D.E. & Lutter, L.D. (1981) Symposium. *Foot and Ankle* 1, 190–224.

Marcus, R., Cann, C., Madvig, P. *et al.* (1985) Menstrual function and bone mass in elite women distance runners. *Annals of Internal Medicine* 102, 158–163.

McGoey, B.V., Deitel, M., Saplys, R.J.F. & Kliman, M.E. (1990) Effect of weight loss on musculoskeletal pain in the morbidly obese. *Journal of Bone and Joint Surgery* 72B, 322–323.

Micheli, L.J. (1983) Overuse injuries in children's sports: the growth factor. *Orthopedic Clinics of North America* 14, 337–360.

Moller, M. (1984) *Athletic training and flexibility. A study on range of motion in the lower extremity.* Medical Dissertation, Linköping University, Linköping, Sweden.

Nicholl, J.P., Coleman, P., Williams, B.T. (1991) *Injuries in Sport and Exercise.* Sports Council, London.

Nigg, B. (1988) Causes of injuries: extrinsic factors. In: Dirix, A., Knuttgen, H.G. & Tittel, K. (eds) *The Olympic Book of Sports Medicine*, pp. 363–375. Blackwell Science, Oxford.

Paffenbarger, R.S., Hyde, R.T., Wing, A.L. & Hsieh, C. (1986) Physical activity, allcause mortality, and longevity of college alumni. *New England Journal of Medicine* 314, 605–613.

Peterson, L. (1970) The cross body block, the major cause of knee injuries. *Journal of the American Medical Association* 211, 449–452.

Peterson, L. & Renström, P. (1980) Världsmästerskapen för veteraner — en medicinsk utmaning. (Championships for veterans — a medical challenge.) *Läkartidningen (Stockholm)* 77, 3618.

Peterson, L. & Renström, P. (1986) *Sports Injuries. Their Prevention and Treatment.* Martin Dunitz, London.

Pforringer, W. & Segesser, B. (1986) The sports shoe. *Orthopade* 15, 260–263.

Renström, P. (1988) Diagnosis and management of overuse injuries. In: Dirix, A.,

Knuttgen, H.G. & Tittel, K. (eds) *The Olympic Book of Sports Medicine*, pp. 446–468. Blackwell Science, Oxford.

Renström, P. (1994) *Clinical Practice of Sports Injury Prevention and Care.* Blackwell Science, Oxford.

Renström, P. & Kannus, P. (1991) Chapter 21. In: Strauss, R.H. (ed.) *Sports Medicine.* W.B. Saunders, Philadelphia.

Rosenbaum *et al.* (1995)

Ross, C.F. & Schuster, R.O. (1983) A preliminary report on predicting injuries in distance runners. *Journal of the American Podiatric Association* 73, 275–277.

Rovere, G.D., Clarke, T.J., Yates, C.S. & Burley, K. (1988) Retrospective comparison of taping on ankle stabilizers in preventing ankle injuries. *American Journal of Sports Medicine* 16, 228–233.

Ryan, A.J. & Stoner, C.J. (1989) Role of skills and rules in the prevention of sports injuries. In: Ryan, A.J. & Allman, F.L. Jr (eds) *Sports Medicine*, 2nd edn, pp. 263–278, Academic Press, San Diego, CA.

Safran, M., Seaber, A. & Garnett, W. (1989) Warm-up and muscular injury prevention. An update. *Sports Medicine* 8, 239–249.

Sandelin, J. (1988) *Acute sports injuries: a clinical and epidemiological study.* Doctoral Dissertation, Yliopistopaino, Helsinki.

Sandelin, J., Santavirta, S., Lattila, R. *et al.* (1988) Sports injuries in a large urban population: occurrence and epidemiology aspects. *International Journal of Sports Medicine* 9, 61–66.

Schwellnus (1994)

Smith, L.S., Clarke, T.E., Hamill, C.L. & Santopietro, F. (1986) The effects of soft and semi-rigid orthoses upon rear foot movement in running. *Journal of the American Podiatric Medical Association* 76, 227–233.

van Steinbrück, K. & Cotta, H. (1983) Epidemiologie von Sportverlezungen. *Dtsch Z Sportmed* 6, 173–186.

Sward, L. (1990) *The back of the young top athlete; symptoms, muscle strength, mobility, anthropometric and radiological findings.* Doctoral Thesis, University of Göteborg, Göteborg, Sweden.

den Toom, P.J. & Schuurman, M.I.M. (1988) Een model voor berekening van kosten van ongevallen in de privé-sfer. St Cons en Veiligheid, Amsterdam.

Torg, J.S., Vegso, J.J., O'Neill, M.J. & Sennett, B. (1990) The epidemiologic pathologic, biomechanical, and cinematographic analysis of football induced cervical spine trauma. *American Journal of Sports Medicine* 18, 50–57.

Viano, D., King, A., Melvin, J. & Weber, K.

(1989) Injury biomechanics research; an essential element in the prevention of trauma. *Journal of Biomechanics* **22**, 403–417.

Walter, S.D., Hart, L.E., McIntosh, J.M. & Sutton, J.R. (1989) The Ontario cohort study of running-related injuries.

Archives of Internal Medicine **146**, 2561–2564.

Watson, A.W.S. (1993) Sports injuries in Ireland, an analysis of four different types of sport. *American Journal of Sports Medicine* **21**, 137–143.

Watson, A.W.S. (1997) Sports injuries: incidence, causes, prevention. *Physical Therapy Review* **2**, 135–151.

Zarins, B. & Ciullo, J. (1983) Acute muscle and tendon injuries in athletes. *Clinical Sports Medicine* **2**, 167–182.

Chapter 34

Monitoring for Overtraining in the Endurance Performer

DAVID G. ROWBOTTOM, ALAN R. MORTON AND DAVID KEAST

Initial considerations

Identifying the optimal balance of training and recovery required to improve athletic performance is a question that continues to challenge athletes, coaches and sports scientists alike. An imbalance between training and recovery may result in impaired, rather than improved, performance and has become known as overtraining. The number of athletes who continue to suffer the consequences of overtraining is testimony to the fact that an optimal training balance remains elusive, and that the distinction between training and overtraining is a fine one indeed. Consequently, the main emphasis of research in the field of overtraining in recent years has been an attempt to develop strategies for the monitoring of athletes in order to identify the onset of overtraining at an early stage. This chapter outlines the current status of research in this area, highlights topics in which knowledge is deficient, and provides practical recommendations and direction for future research.

Definitions and terminology

A review of the literature reveals that a variety of terms and definitions have been used in this field of research, including overreaching (Kreider *et al.* 1998), overload training (Fry *et al.* 1992a), staleness (Hooper *et al.* 1995), burnout, overfatigue, overstrain (Czajkowski 1982), short-term overtraining (Fry *et al.* 1991), overtraining syndrome (Rowbottom *et al.* 1995b) and simply overtraining (Urhausen *et al.* 1998a). Often, the terms have been used some-

what interchangeably, but some authors have drawn clear distinctions between them. This has hindered the comparison of published studies from different research groups. A number of authors have lamented the lack of a standard, worldwide terminology to define the condition, and have attempted to establish discrete definitions (Kuipers & Keizer 1988; Fry *et al.* 1991). Most recently, the following definitions were adopted by the International Conference on Overtraining in Sport held at The University of Memphis in 1996 (Kreider *et al.* 1998); they will be used in this review.

Overtraining was defined as 'an accumulation of training and non-training stress resulting in a long-term decrement in performance capacity with or without related physiological and psychological signs and symptoms of overtraining in which restoration of performance capacity may take several weeks or months'. *Overreaching* was defined as 'an accumulation of training and non-training stress resulting in a short-term decrement in performance capacity with or without related physiological and psychological signs and symptoms of overtraining in which restoration of performance capacity may take from several days to several weeks' (Kreider *et al.* 1998). The implication from these two definitions is that a period of training, especially of an intensive or extensive nature, may result in a reduction of performance capacity. The length of time for which the impairment persists defines the description of the condition, regardless of the degree of impairment, or the amount of training required to reach that state. In reviewing the available literature, it is not always possible to

486

determine clearly the terminology which is most appropriate in a given case, since details of the restoration of performance are not always provided.

Incidence of overtraining

Coaches and athletes have been rightly concerned about the apparently high incidence of overtraining among athletes—both élite and sub-élite. However, only a limited number of studies have attempted to quantify the incidence of overtraining in specific population groups. In college swimmers training up to 14 000 m·day^{-1}, the annual incidence of overtraining was reported to be about 10% (Morgan *et al.* 1987a). Other authors have reported higher incidence rates, albeit in smaller samples. Based on coaches' observations during a 6-month training period leading up to a national championship, O'Connor *et al.* (1989) classified three of 11 (27%) swimmers as 'stale'. Hooper *et al.* (1995) classified three of 14 (21%) swimmers as 'stale' based on performance decrements during a similar training period. Raglin and Morgan (1994) used a two-tiered classification system and reported that over a 4-year period 32% of college swimmers showed signs of training 'distress' each season, but only 6.8% of athletes met the authors' criterion of overtraining—a performance decrement of 5% or greater. Longer-term estimates have suggested that the career prevalence of overtraining in élite female distance runners may be as high as 60% (Morgan *et al.* 1987b).

The most comprehensive study to date was completed on 257 élite athletes from a variety of different sports during a 12-month training season (Koutedakis & Sharp 1998). The authors reported 38 cases of overtraining during the training year (15% of the cohort); the incidence was slightly higher in male (17%) than in female athletes (11%). Perhaps more importantly, 50% of the cases of overtraining that were diagnosed through the year occurred during the 3-month period of competition from June to August (Table 34.1). Despite anecdotal reports that overtraining is more prevalent in endurance sports, Koutedakis and Sharp (1998) found no difference in the incidence of overtraining between predominantly endurance athletes (rowers, middle- to long-distance runners, cyclists and endurance swimmers) and competitors in events involving a larger anaerobic component (wrestlers, fencers, canoeists and field hockey players). Although studies of the incidence of overtraining have been confined mainly to élite-level competitors, the problem is not restricted to this small subgroup of competitive athletes. Therefore, any strategies for the effective monitoring of overtraining must be equally applicable through all levels of competitive sport.

Overtraining research

Three approaches have traditionally been used in the study of overtraining, all of which have limitations. The simplest research design has been to make observations on athletes diagnosed with symptoms of overtraining (Parry-Billings *et al.* 1992; Rowbottom *et al.* 1995b). There are two significant problems with this approach. Firstly, any measurements have to be compared to an appropriate control group of healthy athletes or their equivalent. Therefore, it is not always apparent whether the observed differences are indeed due to the overtrained state, or simply reflect individual variation. There is also no indication of the degree of performance impairment in such studies, since it is very rare that an athlete for whom healthy training data are available will present with symptoms of

Table 34.1 The percentage of male and female élite athletes presenting with symptoms of overtraining during three phases of their 12-month training season. Data recalculated from Koutedakis and Sharp (1998).

	Preparation (Oct–Feb)	Precompetition (March–May)	Competition (June–Aug)
Male athletes ($n = 163$)	3.5%	5.6%	8.2%
Female athletes ($n = 94$)	1.6%	2.8%	6.1%

overtraining in this fashion (Rowbottom *et al.* 1998a). Secondly, early markers which may be useful for identifying the onset of overtraining may no longer be apparent in individuals who have been suffering performance impairment for a number of weeks or months.

A number of longitudinal studies have conducted serial measurements on athletes over a 6–12-month period during their normal training programme. This is probably the most realistic setting in which to observe the onset of overreaching or overtraining. Although some studies have reported cases of athletes whose performance decreased during the season (Vervoorn *et al.* 1991; Hooper *et al.* 1993; Flynn *et al.* 1994), others have only been able to report a healthy progression of performance measures, with no indications of overreaching or overtraining (Baj *et al.* 1994; Baum *et al.* 1994; Rowbottom *et al.* 1997). Despite the need for comparative information with regard to the normal training process, the return of pertinent information on the onset of overtraining has been minimal in comparison to the time-consuming nature of such investigations. Even in the few studies which have identified overtrained athletes successfully during a competitive season, the numbers of athletes involved have been limited, providing only limited statistical power.

The final approach, and seemingly the one of choice for many researchers, has been to use a 10–28-day period of intensified training to induce an overreached state artificially in a group of athletes (Lehmann *et al.* 1991; Fry *et al.* 1992a; Jeukendrup *et al.* 1992; Snyder *et al.* 1995; Urhausen *et al.* 1998a). There are a number of problems associated with this method, not the least of which is the ethical concern of deliberately inducing an overreached or overtrained state in competitive athletes. From a coaching perspective, the validity of an unrealistic imposition of excessive training volumes and/or intensities has been questioned. From a scientific perspective, it could be argued that a time-constrained period of intensified training does not allow individual variations in training response to be taken into account. The practice of pooling subjects into a single group following a predefined training period assumes that the degree of performance impairment experienced during that time is homogeneous. Given our current understanding of individual variability in susceptibility to overtraining, a heterogeneous performance decrement would be more likely. It should be questioned whether reported changes in associated parameters would be expected to be homogeneous and useful as markers of overtraining, given a heterogeneous training response. Although these methodological restrictions have tended to limit the usefulness of much of the data in a prospective setting, researchers have striven, and continue to strive, to identify indicators of the onset of overtraining.

Potential markers of overtraining

The consensus among researchers seems to be that no single parameter will ultimately stand alone as a means of screening athletes to prevent overtraining. Many studies have combined indicators in an effort to improve diagnostic power (Hooper *et al.* 1995). However, for the purposes of this review, the literature is summarized under discrete headings of potential performance, biochemical, hormonal, immunological, psychological and central fatigue markers, in order to evaluate their relative merits. We have previously attempted to establish criteria for an effective marker of the onset of overtraining (Rowbottom *et al.* 1998b). It is our belief that any potential indicator should fulfil three basic criteria (Fig. 34.1). Briefly, an indicator must: (i) demonstrate a consistent, predictable change in response to overreaching and overtraining which precedes, or at least coincides, with performance impairment; (ii) be able to delineate an abnormal training response from a normal response; and (iii) be distinguishable from the normal changes associated with intensive training (Rowbottom *et al.* 1998b). The first two criteria are reflections of the appropriateness of the marker itself, while the third may be more a result of appropriate administration. Markers and tactics for monitoring overtraining are discussed in relation to these criteria.

Performance

Overtraining is often considered as a process whereby exercise training and recovery become

	Increase in potential overtraining marker	No change in potential overtraining marker	Decrease in potential overtraining marker
Well-trained athletes		✓	✓
Overtrained athletes	✓		

(a)

	Increase in potential overtraining marker	No change in potential overtraining marker	Decrease in potential overtraining marker
Well-trained athletes		✓	✓
Overtrained athletes	✓	✓	✓

(b)

Fig. 34.1 A schematic diagram of the essential criteria for a potential marker of overtraining. A marker should be consistent in response to overtraining (a) rather than inconsistent (b); and be able to delineate well-trained from overtrained athletes (a) rather than demonstrating similar changes in both groups (b).

imbalanced, resulting in decrements rather than enhancements in performance (Snyder 1998). It is therefore remarkable how rarely athletic performance data have been reported in research studies involving intensive training, overtraining and associated changes. Although overtraining is as much the process as the result, it is important to distinguish studies inducing a performance decrement or stagnation which would indicate overtraining or overreaching (Fry *et al.* 1992a; Jeukendrup *et al.* 1992; Hooper *et al.* 1993; Flynn *et al.* 1994; Snyder *et al.* 1995; Lehmann *et al.* 1996; Urhausen *et al.* 1998a), from those which found no performance impairment despite intensified training (Costill *et al.* 1988; O'Connor *et al.* 1991; Verde *et al.* 1992; Baj *et al.* 1994; Tanaka *et al.* 1997).

A distinction also needs to be drawn between those studies which have reported the results of a sport- or event-specific performance test, such as a time trial, and those which have reported physiological variables related to performance, such as maximal oxygen intake ($\dot{V}O_{2max}$). In the first category, race performances at the Australian National Swimming Trials were reported to be 2.4% slower than previous best times in overtrained athletes compared to the 1.1% faster times that were recorded by well-trained swimmers (Hooper *et al.* 1993). Jeukendrup *et al.* (1992) reported 5% slower time trial performances in road cyclists (871 s versus

830 s) following 14 days of intensified training, and Fry *et al.* (1992a) reported a 29% decrease in running time to exhaustion at $18 \, \text{km·h}^{-1}$ (261 s versus 369 s) in élite soldiers following 10 days of twice-daily interval training. Urhausen *et al.* (1998a) allowed athletes to self-impose a period of intensified training, and used a cycle ergometer test at 110% of individual anaerobic threshold as a criterion measure of performance. The authors reported a decrease in endurance time (996 s versus 1362 s; –27%) of similar magnitude to Fry *et al.* (1992a) following the intensified training. In each case, the decrement in performance was clear, although the magnitude varied depending on the choice of performance assessment. Many authors have contrasted the substantial magnitudes of performance impairments during overtraining with the small changes in performance (< 1%) required to make the difference between a world or Olympic champion and a runner-up (Fry *et al.* 1991; Levin 1991; Kuipers 1998). Table 34.2 highlights a similar analysis of the 1998 World Half-Marathon Championships.

Other studies have chosen to report a number of physiological variables related to performance, but without a specific performance test. These data need to be reviewed critically to establish the extent to which the measured variables would contribute to a competitive performance. Jeukendrup *et al.* (1992) reported an 8% decrease in peak oxygen intake

Table 34.2 The potential effects of small reductions in performance on the finishing time and position of the winner of the 1998 IAAF World Half-Marathon Championship.

Potential reduction in performance (%)	New finishing time (h:min:s)	New finishing position
0	1:00:01	1st
1	1:00:37	5th
2	1:01:13	8th
3	1:01:49	16th
4	1:02:25	26th
5	1:03:01	39th

(4.41 versus 4.80 l·min^{-1}) following 14 days of intensified training; this change was associated with a reduced peak heart rate (178 versus 185 beats·min^{-1}) and peak blood lactate concentration (5.9 versus 11.8 mmol·l^{-1}). Similarly, Snyder et al. (1995) used 15 days of intensified training in cyclists; they reported a decrease in peak oxygen intake (4.65 versus 4.94 l·min^{-1}), associated with a reduced peak respiratory exchange ratio (1.07 versus 1.11), peak blood lactate concentration (11.3 versus 13.1 mmol·l^{-1}) and peak heart rate. Lehmann et al. (1991) reported that following 28 days of increased training a decreased distance was run during an incremental treadmill test (4361 versus 4732 m). Although they did not report peak oxygen uptake, the endpoint of the test was associated with a reduced maximal heart rate (178 versus 184 beats·min^{-1}) and a reduced blood lactate concentration (8.7 versus 11.3 mmol·l^{-1}). Taken together, these data would suggest that a period of intensified training is associated with reduced peak oxygen consumption and reduced peak exercise capacity. However, these data present a picture of a submaximal effort by comparison to normal training in relation to peak respiratory exchange ratio, blood lactate concentrations and heart rate responses. It could be argued that these observations are the result of an athlete's inability to achieve a 'maximal' effort during incremental tests, possibly due to centrally mediated fatigue mechanisms, rather than peripherally mediated. Irrespective of the reason for the impairment, peak oxygen intake is only one of the determinants of endurance performance. Maximal exercise data need to be viewed in conjunction with other physiological indicators of performance before conclusions can be drawn about the performance capacity of an athlete.

Since the anaerobic threshold (Chapter 22) has been recognized as the best single indicator of endurance performance (Tanaka et al. 1986; Maffulli et al. 1991), a number of studies have documented changes in this parameter following a period of intensified training. Despite significant decreases in maximal exercise capacity, Lehmann et al. (1991) reported no change in the running speed at the anaerobic threshold (4.50 versus 4.44 m·s^{-1}) following 28 days of increased training. A number of other studies have highlighted decreases in submaximal and maximal blood lactate concentrations following intensified training (Jeukendrup et al. 1992; Snyder et al. 1993; Jeukendrup & Hesselink 1994); consequently, both running speed and cycling power output at a specified blood lactate concentration may actually increase during overreaching and overtraining. Lehmann et al. (1996) found no change in running speed at 4 mmol·l^{-1} lactate (4.91 versus 4.88 m·s^{-1}) and an increase in running speed at 2 mmol·l^{-1} lactate (4.31 versus 4.16 m·s^{-1}) following a 28-day period when the volume of training was increased, despite a significant decrease in maximal exercise capacity. Jeukendrup et al. (1992) reported an increase in power output at 4 mmol·l^{-1} lactate (267 versus 234 W) following 14 days of intensified training, despite a reduced peak oxygen intake and an impaired time-trial performance. Urhausen et al. (1998a) reported a trend for the anaerobic threshold to be slightly, but not significantly, higher in athletes who were overtrained compared to their own results in a normal trained state. Importantly, they found no significant difference in the blood lactate concentration following 10 min of a cycling test at 110% of anaerobic threshold (5.58 versus 5.19 mmol·l^{-1}), even though the time to volitional exhaustion was reduced by 27% in the overtrained condition. Conversely, decreased power outputs at 4 mmol·l^{-1} lactate were observed in members of the German Junior National Rowing Team following a period of intensive training, despite maximal exercise performance being maintained (Steinacker et al. 1998).

These data underline the necessity to select appropriate performance tests for the endurance athlete as a means of detecting overreaching and overtraining. An increase in the anaerobic threshold would normally be indicative of improved endurance performance. These observations of increased anaerobic threshold in overtrained athletes, despite decreased endurance performance, bring into question the usefulness of this measure as an indicator of overtraining. It is suggested that event-specific performance measures, such as time trials or competitive race performances, offer the clearest indication that performance capacity is impaired and they should thus be used to recognize overtraining and overreaching.

Biochemical markers

It is probable that once an athlete presents with a recognizable decrease in performance capacity, it is too late to initiate training changes that would avoid a period of enforced recovery. Therefore, there has been a sustained search for early biochemical indicators of an overreached or overtrained state. Unfortunately, the one consistent finding of the overtraining literature has been the stability of many biochemical variables in the face of fatigue and decreased performance. Resting plasma levels of urea, glucose, uric acid, creatinine, iron and ferritin have all been suggested as potential indicators of overtraining, but prospective research studies have been unsuccessful in sustaining these hypotheses (Lehmann *et al.* 1991; Fry *et al.* 1992a; Urhausen *et al.* 1998a). Other potential indicators, although apparently sensitive to intensive training, have failed to meet the criteria laid out (Rowbottom *et al.* 1998b). For example, elevated plasma levels of creatine kinase (CK), considered a marker of muscle damage, were at one time thought to indicate an overtrained state. More recent studies have reported that elevated CK levels may occur in the absence of any performance impairment (Kirwan *et al.* 1988), and indeed they are found in asymptomatic long-distance runners on routine blood tests (Apple 1992). Conversely, overtraining and overreaching have been identified in the absence of elevated CK levels (Lehmann *et al.* 1991; Rowbottom *et al.*

1995b; Urhausen *et al.* 1998a). In non-impact sports, such as swimming and cycling, serum CK may not rise in spite of severe fatigue (Kuipers & Keizer 1988).

Similarly, the role of muscle glycogen depletion in the aetiology of overtraining has been investigated with disappointing results. It had been proposed that observations of reduced blood lactate concentrations during both submaximal and maximal exercise were indicative of glycogen depletion in overreached athletes (Costill *et al.* 1988; Jeukendrup *et al.* 1992; Snyder *et al.* 1993; Jeukendrup & Hesselink 1994). Unfortunately, 10 days of intensified training in collegiate swimmers was sufficient to reduce muscle glycogen content (110.2 ± 7.7 versus $130.5 \pm 9.8 \, \text{mmol·kg}^{-1}$ wet weight) without reducing submaximal or maximal swimming performance (Costill *et al.* 1988). In a study of competitive cyclists, Snyder *et al.* (1995) were able to maintain muscle glycogen content (571.2 ± 27.5 versus $530.9 \pm 42.5 \, \mu\text{mol·g}^{-1}$ dry weight) during 15 days of intensive training and yet they induced an overreached state in all eight athletes. There is clearly a need to maintain muscle glycogen in endurance athletes, but the contribution of glycogen depletion to the onset of overreaching and overtraining is uncertain and its use as a marker of overreaching and overtraining appears limited.

One of the most promising biochemical indicators of overreaching and overtraining has been the plasma concentration of the amino acid glutamine (Rowbottom *et al.* 1996). Cross-sectional studies have observed significantly lower levels of plasma glutamine in overtrained athletes compared to well-trained controls (Parry-Billings *et al.* 1992; Rowbottom *et al.* 1995b). In longitudinal studies, 10 days of intensive training resulted in a significant decrease in both endurance performance and plasma glutamine in élite soldiers (Table 34.3); both variables returned to pretraining levels after 5 days of recovery (Keast *et al.* 1995). MacKinnon and Hooper (1996) reported that overtrained swimmers had 26% and 23% lower plasma glutamine levels than their well-trained counterparts after 2 and 4 weeks of intensive training, respectively, although the difference was only significant at the 2-week

Table 34.3 Changes in running performance (time to exhaustion at $18 \, km \cdot h^{-1}$) and plasma glutamine concentration following 10 days of intensive training and 5 days of recovery. Data combined from Fry *et al.* (1992a) and Keast *et al.* (1995).

	Pretraining (day 1)	Post-training (day 11)	Postrecovery (day 16)
Plasma glutamine ($\mu mol \cdot l^{-1}$)	630 ± 83	328 ± 49	755 ± 157
Time to exhaustion (s)	369 ± 33	261 ± 27	359 ± 34

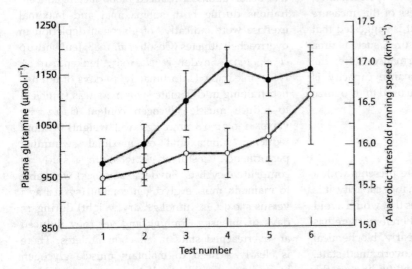

Fig. 34.2 The increase in anaerobic threshold running speed (○) and plasma glutamine concentration (●) during a 9-month training season in well-trained male triathletes. Redrawn from data in Rowbottom *et al.* (1997).

assessment. In this study, the well-trained swimmers demonstrated an 18.4% increase in plasma glutamine relative to pretraining levels. This important observation has been reported elsewhere, with well-trained triathletes showing an increase in plasma glutamine concentration (Fig. 34.2) during a 9-month training season (Rowbottom *et al.* 1997). Lehmann *et al.* (1996) observed a variety of changes in plasma amino acid levels following separate periods of increased-intensity and increased-volume training. An average 6.5% decrease of amino acid concentrations was reported with decreased performance and an 8.8% increase with improved performance. Such observations suggest that glutamine may not be the only amino acid which is susceptible to overtraining and overreaching. The divergence of plasma glutamine responses to training and overtraining may allow an overtrained athlete to be distinguished effectively from a well-trained athlete, although further work is needed in this area.

Hormonal markers

Since overtraining has often been considered an imbalance between training and recovery, it has been seen as an imbalance between catabolic and anabolic processes. The primary hormones that modulate these processes, notably cortisol and testosterone, have been investigated as potential indicators of an overtrained or overreached state. Although considered at one time useful indicators of overtraining, more recent data suggest that the behaviour of testosterone and cortisol may be more indicative of the current training load than of overtraining *per se* (Urhausen *et al.* 1995; Rowbottom *et al.* 1998b). This change in emphasis has predominantly been the result of contradictory observations in a number of overtraining and overreaching studies.

Significant decreases in serum concentrations of both total and free testosterone have been observed in both male and female athletes following intensive training (Urhausen *et al.* 1987; Vervoorn *et al.* 1991; Flynn *et al.* 1994). This has been accompanied by a decrease in performance in some studies (Flynn *et al.* 1994), but not in others (Vervoorn *et al.* 1991); other studies have not reported performance measures that would enable a comparison to be made (Urhausen *et al.* 1987). Conversely, Urhausen *et al.* (1998a) did not observe any change in either total testosterone (17.2 ± 1.5 versus 18.4 ± 2.2 nmol·l^{-1}) or the testosterone/sex hormone-binding globulin ratio (0.56 ± 0.06 versus 0.57 ± 0.07) following a self-imposed period of intensified training which resulted in a decrease in endurance performance.

Serum cortisol concentrations following over-reaching or overtraining are equally contradictory. Some authors have reported an increased concentration in overtrained athletes (Barron *et al.* 1985; Stray-Gundersen *et al.* 1986) and others have reported a significant decrease (381.8 ± 52.0 versus 541.8 ± 56.8 nmol·l^{-1}) following overreaching (Snyder *et al.* 1995), but the majority have found no change in serum cortisol despite significant performance impairments (Fry *et al.* 1992a; Hooper *et al.* 1993; Flynn *et al.* 1994; Urhausen *et al.* 1998a). We have suggested that free rather than total cortisol should be measured (Rowbottom *et al.* 1995a), since only the unbound component is biologically active (Garrell 1996). Free testosterone has been measured for many years, but free serum or salivary cortisol measurements, quantitatively representative of the free serum concentration, are rare. O'Connor *et al.* (1989) reported significantly higher salivary cortisol levels (4.8 ± 1.1 versus 2.9 ± 1.1 μg·l^{-1}) when three swimmers diagnosed as 'stale' were compared to 11 well-trained swimmers following a 6-month training programme. Rowbottom *et al.* (1997) found no change in serum free cortisol levels during a 9-month season of training and competition in well-trained triathletes. Potentially, free cortisol concentrations may be more sensitive to overreaching and overtraining than total cortisol concentrations, although further work is required.

The suggestion that an unfavourable testosterone/cortisol ratio may be indicative of an overtrained state led Adlercreutz *et al.* (1986) to define discrete criteria for the use of this ratio. Following the authors' observations in runners, they proposed

that an athlete could be diagnosed as overtrained if the free testosterone/cortisol ratio fell below 0.35 × 10^{-3}, or decreased by 30%. This suggestion has not been supported by further research. Other reports have shown no change in the ratio in overtrained athletes (Urhausen *et al.* 1998a), and decreased ratios without performance decrements following intensive training (Vervoorn *et al.* 1991). During a 9-month training season, élite rowers showed decreased ratios predominantly following a 2-week training camp. Although no athlete reached the criterion ratio of 0.35 × 10^{-3}, many showed a 30% decrease from baseline. Physiological measures taken at corresponding times showed an improved maximal exercise capacity and an increased power output at 4 mmol·l^{-1} lactate; this suggested that the athletes were not overtrained (Vervoorn *et al.* 1991), although specific performance data were not reported. Consequently, neither of the criteria proposed by Adlercreutz *et al.* (1986) are widely accepted as sensitive indicators of an overreached or overtrained state.

The primary action of adrenocorticotrophic hormone (ACTH) is to increase the secretion of cortisol from the adrenal cortex. It has been suggested that hormonal imbalances in overtrained athletes may be attributable, at least in part, to higher levels of regulation of hormone secretion (Urhausen *et al.* 1995). Barron *et al.* (1985) investigated the hypothalamic–pituitary axis in overtrained athletes, using a challenge of insulin-induced hypoglycaemia. They reported a decreased ACTH, and hence cortisol, response which was significantly improved following 4 weeks of rest. Urhausen *et al.* (1998a) observed a tendency towards a lower resting ACTH level (2.10 ± 0.26 versus 2.65 ± 0.27 pmol·l^{-1}) following a self-imposed period of overtraining, and a significantly lower exercise-induced ACTH production after a cycling test to exhaustion. Since performance was impaired in the overtrained condition, the cycling test had a 27% shorter duration (996 s versus 1356 s) than during normal training. Thus, it cannot be discounted that the shorter test duration may account for the lower hormone production. Taken together, these data may indicate a hypothalamic dysfunction in overtrained athletes, although routine hypothalamic monitoring is problematic due to considerable individual variability, the need to standardize conditions, particularly diet, and the high cost involved in measuring pituitary hormones.

An alternative area of investigation has been the role of catecholamines, particularly adrenaline (epinephrine) and noradrenaline (norepinephrine), in overreaching and overtraining. Plasma catecholamine levels are elevated during exercise in proportion to the intensity of training (Urhausen et al. 1994), and they may be further elevated with the psychological stress of competition. Hooper et al. (1993) reported significantly higher plasma noradrenaline levels (457.7 ± 67.5 versus $236.5 \pm 15.8\,pg\cdot ml^{-1}$) in 'stale' compared to well-trained swimmers during a taper period at the end of a 6-month training season. Both adrenaline and noradrenaline concentrations were positively correlated with training volume. Lehmann et al. (1991) found no significant change in resting plasma adrenaline or noradrenaline levels after a 28-day period of increased training volume, but there was an increase in resting adrenaline levels after a similar period of increased training intensity (Lehmann et al. 1992).

Lehmann et al. (1992) also reported that at a given submaximal exercise intensity, plasma noradrenaline levels were increased after 28 days of increased training volume if this was associated with decreased performance, but they were decreased following 28 days of increased training intensity associated with increased performance. The authors suggested that the latter may be a positive adaptive response, whereas the former may be the result of a counter-regulatory decrease in adrenoreceptor sensitivity. In contrast, following a period of self-imposed overtraining, Urhausen et al. (1998a) found no significant difference in either submaximal or maximal plasma catecholamine concentrations during a cycle test to exhaustion at 110% of the anaerobic threshold. In addition to these somewhat contradictory results, there are a number of other problems in using plasma catecholamines as indicators of an overreached or overtrained state. Inter- and intraindividual variability are relatively high, and since the half-life of plasma catecholamines may be as short as 2 min, careful sample handling and rapid freezing are required (Urhausen et al. 1995). An alternative has been the measurement of either 24-h or overnight urinary excretion of catecholamines (Lehmann et al. 1992).

Immunological markers

Many authors have drawn attention to an association between overtraining and an increased incidence of infections (Fitzgerald 1991; Fry et al. 1991; Nieman 1994; Keast 1996), particularly upper respiratory tract infections (URTI) (Chapter 50). Although there are a number of reports of higher infection rates in athletes who have completed extensive training schedules (Nieman et al. 1990; Heath et al. 1991), and following particularly intensive endurance events (Peters & Bateman 1985; Nieman et al. 1990), few studies have quantified the rates of infection in overtrained, compared to well-trained athletes. In a 19-month study of competitive cyclists and triathletes, Gabriel et al. (1998) reported that on 70 occasions when athletes did not exhibit overtraining, symptoms of URTI were evident on 17 occasions (24%). By comparison, on 15 occasions when overtraining was diagnosed, URTI symptoms were reported on five occasions (33%). Mackinnon and Hooper (1996) reported an infection rate of 42% during a 4-week period of intensified training in swimmers. When the athletes were classified as either well trained or stale on the basis of swimming performance, only one of eight stale swimmers (12.5%) exhibited URTI, compared to nine of 16 well-trained swimmers (56%). Although further research is required, these data suggest that increased infection rates may be more a consequence of intensive training than overtraining per se.

It is still open to debate whether the observed changes in immune cell distribution and function following both acute and chronic exercise carry any clinical significance for an athlete. Despite this uncertainty, researchers have investigated a number of immunological measures as potential markers of overreaching and overtraining. Numerical changes in circulating cells have been reported by a number of authors. Lehmann et al. (1996) reported a decrease in leucocyte counts (4288 ± 892 versus 5428 ± 1669

cells·μl^{-1}) following 28 days of increased-volume training that was associated with a decreased maximal exercise capacity. However, a similar 28-day period of increased-intensity training, which resulted in increased maximal exercise capacity, was not accompanied by a change in circulating leucocyte numbers (5150 ± 1030 versus 5300 ± 820 cells·μl^{-1}). Baj et al. (1994) also reported decreases in leucocyte and lymphocyte counts in trained cyclists following a 6-month season of training and competition, although the athletes' performances improved significantly ($\dot{V}O_{2max}$ 81.0 $\pm$ 1.7 versus 74.1 $\pm$ 1.4 ml·kg^{-1}·min^{-1}) during this time. On the other hand, neither Gabriel et al. (1998) nor Fry et al. (1992a) found any differences in leucocyte, neutrophil, eosinophil, monocyte or lymphocyte counts in athletes following a period of overreaching or overtraining. These data suggest that changes in circulating immune cell numbers in response to overtraining are not consistent, and cannot be used to distinguish overtrained from well-trained athletes.

In terms of lymphocyte subsets, the majority of studies of overtrained athletes have failed to detect any significant changes in circulating numbers of T cells, B cells or natural killer (NK) cells (Fry et al. 1992a; Hooper et al. 1993; Rowbottom et al. 1995b; Gabriel et al. 1998). A particular exception was the observation of decreased NK cell counts (0.36 ± 0.05 versus $0.60 \pm 0.06 \times 10^9$ cells·l^{-1}) following 10 days of intensive training; these changes persisted through 5 days of recovery (Fry et al. 1992a). Decreased NK cell counts have also been reported in élite swimmers over a 7-month intensive training programme without performance decrements (Gleeson et al. 1995). An area which has attracted recent attention has been the increased expression of lymphocyte activation markers following intensified training and overtraining. Fry et al. (1994) reported that the interleukin-2 receptor (CD25) was expressed on 10% of T cells before overreaching, increasing to 33% of T cells following 10 days of intensive training and remaining at 31% even when endurance performance was restored following 5 days of recovery. Baum et al. (1994) reported a similar increase in CD25 expression on T-helper cells (34 ± 7 versus $26 \pm 10\%$) in track and field athletes following a train-

ing and competition season. Unfortunately, no performance measures were reported, and it is not possible to determine whether these changes were the result of intensive training, or specific to overtraining. Gabriel et al. (1998) recently reported that the expression of the activation marker CD45RO on T cells was able to predict overtraining correctly in 67% of cases, with a test specificity of 84%.

As well as circulating numbers, researchers have assessed the function of immune cells following intensive training, overreaching and overtraining, as a means of assessing immunocompetence. Parry-Billings et al. (1992) reported that lymphocyte proliferation in response to the mitogen concanavalin-A was unimpaired in athletes suffering from the overtraining syndrome, when they were compared to a control group of athletes matched for training volume and intensity. Verde et al. (1992) observed an increase in proliferative response to both phytohaemagglutinin and concanavalin-A following 3 weeks of increased training in élite male runners. This would appear to be in response to the intensive training alone, since physiological measures of exercise capacity and efficiency were not impaired during this time. Similarly, Baj et al. (1994) reported an increased proliferative response to phytohaemagglutinin following a competitive track and field season, although performance measures were not reported. Unfortunately, traditional proliferation assays have the potential to produce artefactual increases or decreases in response as a result of shifts in the proportion of T lymphocytes in the peripheral circulation. Hinton et al. (1997) reported that after acute exercise observed changes in T-lymphocyte function can be accounted for if a purified sample of T lymphocytes is used instead of a mixed lymphocyte culture (Fig. 34.3). The data suggest that T-lymphocyte function may not be affected adversely by either intensive training or overtraining, and may not offer a useful indicator of the early onset of overreaching and overtraining.

Secretion of immunoglobulins, particularly salivary IgA, has been reported to be 18–32% lower in swimmers diagnosed as overtrained compared to well-trained athletes observed over the same 6-month training period (Mackinnon & Hooper 1994). Neutrophil function has also been observed to

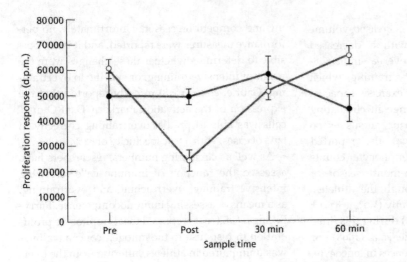

Fig. 34.3 Changes in mitogen-induced T-lymphocyte blastogenesis of peripheral blood mononuclear leucocytes (○) and purified T lymphocytes (●) following intensive interval training (15 × 1-min intervals at 95% $\dot{V}_{O_{2max}}$). Reprinted from Hinton *et al.* (1997), with permission.

decrease during a 12-week intensive training period (Pyne *et al.* 1995), although it remains unclear whether these changes are specific to overtraining, or simply a result of intensive training. In general, a number of indicators of immune function are affected by periods of intensive training. It is presently uncertain to what degree these changes have clinical significance in terms of the susceptibility of athletes to infection, or indeed whether overtrained athletes are at any greater risk of infection than well-trained athletes undergoing intensive training. In terms of being potential indicators of overtraining, many of the immune function tests do not fulfil the criteria set out, and in many cases the data are simply insufficient to decide on their value.

The amino acid glutamine has been recognized as a key substrate for cells of the immune system. During periods of immunological challenge, glutamine metabolism is increased to support the processes of rapid cell division, protein synthesis and the production of antibodies and cytokines. Cells of the immune system rely on the plasma supply of glutamine to meet their metabolic needs; ultimately, this glutamine is thought to be released from skeletal muscle (Newsholme 1994). Decreased plasma concentrations of glutamine during periods of intensive training, overreaching and overtraining have been suggested to cause impairment of immune function, a compromised ability to respond to immune challenge and an increased risk of infec-

tion (Parry-Billings *et al.* 1992; Keast *et al.* 1995). Unfortunately, the results of studies investigating the association between plasma glutamine level and infection rates in athletes have been contradictory (Castell *et al.* 1996; MacKinnon & Hooper 1996).

Psychological markers

Anecdotal evidence has suggested that an overreached or overtrained athlete may suffer psychological disturbances coincident with performance decrements. Following a self-imposed period of overtraining, athletes complained of intense daily fatigue, lack of mental concentration, sleep disorders and diminished appetite (Urhausen *et al.* 1998b). Fry *et al.* (1994) reported lethargy, lack of interest in everyday tasks, quick temperedness, concentration difficulties, sleep problems and loss of appetite in élite soldiers after 10 days of intensive training. Jeukendrup *et al.* (1992) asked athletes to respond to specific questions following a 2-week period of intensified training. Athletes complained of incomplete recovery, increased difficulty in completing training and problems falling asleep. Decreases in other factors such as motivation, satisfaction and sociability have also been reported (Urhausen *et al.* 1998b).

A more quantifiable approach taken by many researchers has been to use the profile of mood states (POMS) questionnaire. Results have been expressed either as a global POMS score, or as individual scores for the six subscales of tension, depression, anger, vigour, fatigue and confusion. Fry *et al.* (1994) reported that following intensified training associated with impaired performance, élite soldiers showed significant increases in global POMS scores (100.0 ± 5.5 versus 75.8 ± 3.4) as well as an increased score on the fatigue subscale and a decreased score on the vigour subscale. Flynn *et al.* (1994) reported an elevated global POMS score in collegiate swimmers (189 ± 14 versus 159 ± 12) following a 2-week winter training camp, compared to normal training. This was associated with a significant reduction in the swimming velocity during a 365.8-m time trial. Berglund and Safstrom (1994) reported an increase in global POMS score in canoeists from 130 ± 15.7 preseason to 160 ± 27.2 following a period of heavy training; scores returned to 120 ± 22.1 after a taper to the Olympic games. Although the increase in score was associated with an increased subjective rating of training load, no performance data were reported to confirm that these changes were associated with overtraining and not simply intensive training.

Increases in POMS scores may not be sufficiently sensitive to distinguish intensive training from overtraining. Morgan *et al.* (1988) reported POMS scores for a group of 12 swimmers following a 10-day period of increased training distance (9000 versus 4000 m·day^{-1}). Although neither maximal nor submaximal swimming performances were decreased in 365.8-m time trials (Costill *et al.* 1988), significant increases in global POMS scores were reported (153 ± 42 versus 133 ± 32) as well as increases in scores on the depression, anger and fatigue subscales (Morgan *et al.* 1988). Furthermore, changes in global scores were evident following only 3–4 days of training, and remained at elevated levels for the remainder of the trial. Similarly, O'Connor *et al.* (1991) reported elevations in global POMS scores in both male (132 ± 22 versus 115 ± 16) and female (137 ± 33 versus 119 ± 24) swimmers after only 3 days of increased training volume. Swimmers were able to maintain an established training pace (90% of best performance) throughout the period of intensified training, but no measure of maximal performance was recorded. These obser-

vations raise the question of whether POMS scores or subscales are truly sensitive to overtraining, or whether changes are more a reflection of intensive training. The fact that changes can occur within only a few days of intensified training raises concerns about a lack of temporal relationship between performance decrements and elevated POMS scores.

In contrast, a number of studies have reported an ability to distinguish overtrained athletes from their well-trained counterparts during longitudinal observations. Hooper *et al.* (1995) classified three swimmers from a cohort of 14 athletes as 'stale' on the basis of performance decrements during a 6-month training season. The stale swimmers reported higher scores for fatigue and muscle soreness than the 11 well-trained swimmers, and also complained of poor sleep quality. Raglin and Morgan (1994) reported that over a 4-year period the global POMS scale could identify 'distressed' athletes successfully on 73.7% of occasions for male collegiate swimmers and 89.2% of occasions for female collegiate swimmers. Unfortunately, the identification of a 'distressed' athlete was based on the subjective and objective criteria of the team coach, and no performance data were reported. Following a 4-month period of intensified training, O'Connor *et al.* (1989) reported a significant increase in global POMS score in collegiate swimmers; this was associated with elevated subscale scores for fatigue, tension, depression and anger, and a decreased subscale score for vigour. Three of the 11 athletes were identified as 'stale' based on a 5–10% decrease in performance, although the selected performance measure was not identified. The three 'stale' swimmers had significantly higher global POMS scores than the other eight athletes (190 ± 19 versus 168 ± 20) following intensive training. These data suggest that both intensive training and overtraining may increase global POMS scores, irrespective of a performance decrement. To be an objective indicator of overtraining, it is critical that a criterion score be determined to distinguish a normal training response from any further increase in response due to overtraining. Whether this is expressed as a percentile increase from baseline or an absolute cutoff, an appropriate score has yet to be determined.

The use of global POMS scores or subscale scores to identify an overtrained or overreached athlete may be further confounded. The characteristic of 'hardiness' may enable some athletes to cope better with the stress of intensive training. Goss (1994) reported that athletes with higher scores for hardiness had significantly fewer POMS disturbances during intensive training. Since no performance data were reported, it is difficult to draw conclusions on its implications for monitoring overtraining. It could be concluded that athletes with high hardiness scores will be less likely to suffer performance decrements, but equally it could be concluded that these athletes will display fewer POMS disturbances in the face of a performance impairment. If the latter is correct, the use of POMS to monitor overtraining or overreaching may be confounded in athletes who have particularly high scores for the hardiness trait.

One simple variable which has been reported as sensitive to overreaching and overtraining is an athlete's rating of perceived exertion (RPE) during exercise. Immediately after a 2-week winter training camp, Flynn *et al.* (1994) reported that RPE scores for collegiate swimmers were significantly elevated (14.2 ± 0.6 versus 11.2 ± 1.1) during a submaximal 365.8-m swim at 90% $\dot{V}O_{2max}$. This was associated with a reduced swimming velocity during a maximal time trial. Following 10 min of a cycle ergometer test at 110% of anaerobic threshold, RPE scores were significantly higher (16.3 ± 0.4 versus 14.6 ± 0.3) after self-imposed overtraining than during normal training (Urhausen *et al.* 1998a).

Other authors have reported that RPE does not change significantly following intensified training, even when there is an associated decrease in maximal exercise capacity (Snyder *et al.* 1993, 1995). However, these authors have proposed a ratio between blood lactate concentration (BLa) and RPE as a potential marker of overtraining. Using BLa in $mmol \cdot l^{-1}$ with the modified 10-point RPE scale (Borg *et al.* 1987), and expressing the ratio as a percentage (BLa/RPE × 100), they concluded that during normal training the ratio should be greater than 100 for work rates above the anaerobic threshold. A decrease below 100 was associated with overreaching in all seven subjects (Fig. 34.4), although this was predominantly the result of decreased BLa rather than increased RPE scores (Snyder *et al.* 1993). Since all athletes in this study were classified as overreached, it was not possible to determine whether a BLa/RPE ratio of less than 100 could distinguish between overtraining or overreaching *per se* and intensive training without performance impairment.

Some researchers have observed a temporal relationship between POMS scores and RPE during intensive training (Morgan *et al.* 1988; Berglund & Safstrom 1994). Furthermore, strong associations between submaximal RPE scores and subscales of

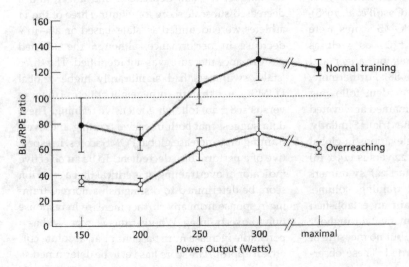

Fig. 34.4 The blood lactate/rating of perceived exertion (BLa/RPE) ratio at five exercise intensities during normal training and overreaching in male road cyclists. Redrawn from data in Snyder *et al.* (1993).

depression, anxiety and fatigue have been reported previously (Morgan 1992; Rowbottom *et al.* 1998c). Since changes in RPE scores may be related to changes in mood states, the problems outlined with using POMS scores to monitor overtraining may be applicable, by association, to the use of RPE scores.

Central fatigue mechanisms

A variety of theories have been advanced to explain the phenomena of fatigue and performance decrements in the overtrained athlete. One hypothesis has been a centrally mediated fatigue mechanism, giving rise to premature sensations of fatigue, independent of peripheral indicators of fatigue such as lactic acid accumulation or muscle glycogen depletion. Prolonged and intensive exercise gives rise to an increased rate of oxidation of branched-chain amino acids (BCAA), potentially as a result of muscle glycogen depletion, and thus leads to a decrease in circulating BCAA (Bloomstrand *et al.* 1988, 1991). At the same time, an increase in plasma levels of free fatty acids means that these compete with tryptophan (TRP) for their mutual carrier of albumin, resulting in increased levels of circulating free TRP during prolonged exercise (Bloomstrand *et al.* 1988, 1991). Since both BCAA and free TRP cross the blood–brain barrier on the same neutral amino acid carrier, it has been suggested that prolonged exercise will favour the entry of free TRP into the brain (Newsholme *et al.* 1991). The TRP is then converted to 5-hydroxytryptamine (5-HT). Elevated 5-HT in the brain is associated with increased tiredness and fatigue, sleep disturbances, suppression of appetite and modulation of perceptions of exertion, as well as disturbances of temperature regulation and control of hypothalamic function (Young 1986). Administration of selective agonists of the 5-HT receptor significantly heightens RPE scores and reduces the time to exhaustion (16 versus 26 min) during exercise at 80% $\dot{V}O_{2max}$ in healthy individuals (Marvin *et al.* 1997).

To date, only two studies have reported the effects of intensified training on the ratio between plasma levels of free TRP and BCAA. Tanaka *et al.* (1997) increased the training volume in highly trained distance runners by 40% for 2 weeks. This training regime did not induce any decrements in physiological measures which would indicate overtraining or overreaching, and the well-trained athletes showed no significant change in free TRP/BCAA ratio (0.027 versus 0.025) following intensified training. Lehmann *et al.* (1996) reported an increase in free TRP/BCAA ratio (0.019 versus 0.014) following 28 days of increased training volume, coincident with a decrease in maximal exercise capacity. Unfortunately, following a 28-day period of increased training intensity, associated with improved maximal exercise capacity, a similar increase in free TRP/BCAA ratio (0.021 versus 0.014) was observed. These data suggest that the free TRP/BCAA ratio does not show a consistent change in response to intensified training, and is thus unable to distinguish between overtrained and well-trained athletes.

An alternative hypothesis is that 5-HT receptors in the hypothalamus may be up- and down-regulated in different situations, giving rise to the possibility that receptor sensitivity may be more important than availability of 5-HT *per se*. Cross-sectional studies have revealed that 5-HT receptor response to a standard serotoninergic challenge is decreased in endurance-trained athletes (Jakeman *et al.* 1994), but it is increased in individuals diagnosed with chronic fatigue syndrome (Sharpe *et al.* 1996) and postviral fatigue syndrome (Bakheit *et al.* 1992). It remains to be shown whether overreaching or overtraining results in a modulation of 5-HT receptor sensitivity. However, from our current understanding of the function of the 5-HT receptor, it could be hypothesized that an up-regulation of 5-HT receptor sensitivity during overtraining or overreaching leads to elevated fatigue, an increased RPE, a reduced time to exhaustion in endurance performance tests, mood state changes, sleep disturbances and suppressed appetite. Although 5-HT receptor function provides an interesting theory about overtraining aetiology and its onset, it does not as yet provide a marker which would be useful for athletes and coaches to detect its early onset.

Providing a framework

At the outset of this review, a number of criteria

were laid out (Rowbottom *et al.* 1998b). In many cases potential indicators do not demonstrate a consistent change in response to overreaching and overtraining, nor do they delineate a training response from an overtraining response. Many new areas are starting to produce fruitful insight into possible mechanisms for the onset of overtraining, but they are perhaps still some way short of enabling diagnostic tests to be devised. Ultimately, a criterion for a positive diagnosis will need to be established for any test, including an appropriate threshold value and sensitivity and specificity scores, as well as both positive and negative predictive values (Zweig & Campbell 1993). To date, only one study has attempted to provide sensitivity and specificity data for a proposed indicator of overreaching and overtraining (Gabriel *et al.* 1998), although unpublished data have attempted to establish similar criteria for plasma glutamine as an indicator of the related chronic fatigue syndrome (Fig. 34.5). Gabriel *et al.* (1998) were careful to point out that a 'gold standard' to diagnose overtraining

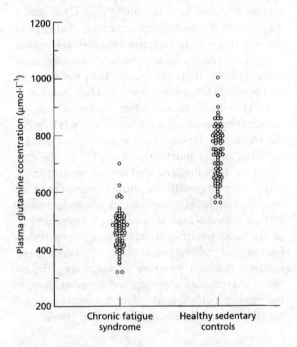

Fig. 34.5 Plasma glutamine concentrations in 85 chronic fatigue syndrome subjects and age- and gender-matched healthy, sedentary controls.

and overreaching does not exist and therefore the clinical diagnosis with which to compare any diagnostic test is at best open to question. There is at present no simple 'golden bullet' in terms of a fail-safe monitoring tool for recognizing overreaching and overtraining. This may remain the case for some time to come. It may even be unrealistic to rely solely on a monitoring tool to detect when things start to go wrong, rather than structuring an athlete's training in such a way as to prevent excessive fatigue developing in the first place.

The discussion of potential markers of overtraining has so far only dealt with the appropriateness of particular markers. Another consideration must be the practical administration of any routine tests. Any discussion of monitoring an athlete must inevitably raise the question of how frequently testing should be carried out. Given that overreaching has been achieved effectively with only 10–15 days of intensive training (Fry *et al.* 1992a; Jeukendrup *et al.* 1992; Snyder *et al.* 1995), the answer would seem to be more often than is practically achievable, unless the test is simple to administer. Secondly, concerns have been raised that changes associated with overreaching and overtraining need to be separated from the acute effects of exercise (Fry *et al.* 1991; Rowbottom *et al.* 1998b). The most effective approach would be to enforce a period of recovery over a number of days following a training period before any tests were conducted. This would allow the acute changes associated with training stress to diminish, and long-term changes associated with overtraining to be highlighted. The use of a periodized training programme has been proposed as a means of achieving this end (Fry *et al.* 1991, 1992b; Rowbottom *et al.* 1998b), as well as providing the necessary structure to enable training adaptation without placing an athlete at risk of overtraining (Rowbottom 2000).

However, we may need to redefine our thinking about what we describe as overreaching and overtraining if effective strategies for monitoring athletes are to be put in place. There is a tendency to refer to training programmes in very black and white terms, as either 'training' or 'overtraining', and then attempt to identify the boundary which is supposed to exist between the two states. Perhaps it would be helpful to recognize that a grey scale is more likely to exist. Any training session will displace the homeostasis of the body, resulting in a number of catabolic events. These may include the breakdown of structural and functional proteins and the utilization of endogenous energy stores. Consequently, a single training session will result in a certain level of fatigue, changes in biochemical, hormonal and immunological measures and a temporary reduction of an athlete's performance. A recovery period is then required, during which time the body works to re-establish homeostasis, replenish endogenous energy stores, synthesize new protein and restore performance capacity. The length of time required for recovery will depend on the intensity and duration of training, but will also be influenced by any further training that is imposed during the recovery period.

An athlete's performance at any given time will be determined by the combination and distribution of previous training sessions and recovery periods. Mathematical models have even been developed and tested to predict these effects (Banister et al. 1992; Morton 1997). Any imbalance between training and recovery, whether over a number of months, a few weeks or even a couple of days, will produce the characteristic impairment in physical performance which we refer to as overtraining. Distinguishing between each situation may not be possible on the basis of performance capacity, or biochemical, hormonal or other variables, but only in terms of the time required to regain peak performance. It may therefore be helpful to view training as a continuum (Fry et al. 1991) or grey scale extending from the acute fatigue of a single training session through the cumulative fatigue of a number of days of training (overreaching) to the fatigue of long-term training imbalance or overtraining (Fig. 34.6). The degree of training adaptation achieved by an athlete depends on the magnitude of the overload imposed (Fry et al. 1992b). Consequently, a series of training sessions undertaken by an athlete without sufficient recovery time may produce a more powerful stimulus for subsequent adaptation during a prolonged recovery phase, from which the practice of periodization has developed (Rowbottom 2000). Is it therefore possible to define a boundary between

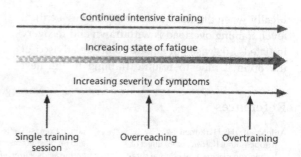

Fig. 34.6 A continuum of training and overtraining. Adapted from Fry et al. (1991).

what is a normal training process and what we would consider overtraining? Perhaps it should be regarded more as a task of optimization not only of training load but also of training distribution.

As a framework for structuring an athlete's training, the practice of periodization has much to offer. Although performance is allowed to decrease temporarily (overreaching), complete recovery is ensured between each period of training and long-term performance decrement (overtraining) is not allowed to develop. The way forward for overtraining research may indeed be in terms of trying to optimize overreaching. As a means of trying to help athletes avoid overtraining, it may be beneficial to help them to achieve a predefined degree of overreaching as an optimal stimulus for training adaptation during an enforced recovery period. Questions remain as to where lies the point of overreaching when the training stimulus should be withdrawn and recovery initiated. At present, this is a very subjective decision. In this context, a performance test has often been promoted as the criterion measure of choice in both experimental and coaching settings (Fry et al. 1991; 1992b; Jeukendrup et al. 1992; Urhausen et al. 1998a). It has been assumed that performance measures will give a valid and reliable indication of the degree of overreaching and the extent of recovery during a training programme. Although periodic performance assessment is essential for monitoring athletic development, it may not be the most suitable measure in all situations. As an alternative it may be possible to exploit some of the newly suggested potential markers as a means of identifying the point of optimal overload.

Ideally, when the chosen indicator reaches a critical level, training overload is withdrawn and recovery initiated. Likewise, an athlete could be advised of the optimal time to resume training in the next 'period' of training when recovery has reached a critical level. However, research is still some way from this utopia of guiding the coach and athlete to optimal performance tactics.

References

Adlercreutz, H., Härkönen, M., Kuoppasalmi, K. *et al.* (1986) Effect of training on plasma anabolic and catabolic steroid hormones and their response during physical exercise. *International Journal of Sports Medicine* 7, S27–S28.

Apple, F.S. (1992) The creatine kinase system in the serum of runners following a doubling of training mileage. *Clinical Physiology* 12, 419–424.

Baj, Z., Kantorski, J., Majewska, E. *et al.* (1994) Immunological status of competitive cyclists before and after the training season. *International Journal of Sports Medicine* 15, 319–324.

Bakheit, A.M.O., Behan, P.O., Dinan, T.G., Gray, C.E. & O'Keane, V. (1992) Possible upregulation of hypothalamic 5-hydroxytryptamine receptors in patients with postviral fatigue syndrome. *British Medical Journal* 304, 1010–1012.

Banister, E.W., Morton, R.H. & Fitz-Clarke, J. (1992) Dose/response effects of exercise modeled from training: physical and biochemical measures. *Annals of Physiology and Anthropology* 11, 345–356.

Barron, J.L., Noakes, T.D., Levy, W., Smith, C. & Millar, R.P. (1985) Hypothalamic dysfunction in overtrained athletes. *Journal of Clinical Endocrinology and Metabolism* 60, 803–806.

Baum, M., Liesen, H. & Enneper, J. (1994) Leucocytes, lymphocytes, activation parameters and cell adhesion molecules in middle-distance runners under different training conditions. *International Journal of Sports Medicine* 15, S122–S126.

Berglund, B. & Safstrom, H. (1994) Psychological monitoring and modulation of training load of world-class canoeists. *Medicine and Science in Sports and Exercise* 26, 1036–1040.

Bloomstrand, E., Celsing, F. & Newsholme, E.A. (1988) Changes in plasma concentrations of aromatic and branch-chain amino acids during sustained exercise in man and their possible role in fatigue. *Acta Physiologica Scandinavica* 133, 115–121.

Bloomstrand, E., Hassmen, P. & Newsholme, E. (1991) Administration of branch-chain amino acids during sustained exercise—effects on performance and on plasma concentration of some amino acids. *European Journal of Applied Physiology* 63, 83–88.

Borg, G., Hassmen, P. & Langerstrom, M. (1987) Perceived exertion related to heart rate and blood lactate during arm and leg exercise. *European Journal of Applied Physiology* 65, 679–685.

Castell, L.M., Poortmans, J.R. & Newsholme, E.A. (1996) Does glutamine have a role in reducing infections in athletes? *European Journal of Applied Physiology* 73, 488–490.

Costill, D.L., Flynn, M.G., Kirwan, J.P. *et al.* (1988) Effects of repeated days of intensified training on muscle glycogen and swimming performance. *Medicine and Science in Sports and Exercise* 20, 249–254.

Czajkowski, W. (1982) A simple method to control fatigue in endurance training. In: Komi, P.V. (ed.) *Exercise and Sport Biology.* International Series on Sport Sciences 12, pp. 207–212. Human Kinetics, Champaign, IL.

Fitzgerald, L. (1991) Overtraining increases the susceptibility to infection. *International Journal of Sports Medicine* 12, S5–S8.

Flynn, M.G., Pizza, F.X., Boone, J.B., Andres, F.F., Michaud, T.A. & Rodriguez-Zayas, J.R. (1994) Indices of training stress during competitive running and swimming seasons. *International Journal of Sports Medicine* 15, 21–26.

Fry, R.W., Morton, A.R. & Keast, D. (1991) Overtraining in athletes—an update. *Sports Medicine* 12, 32–65.

Fry, R.W., Morton, A.R., Garcia-Webb, P., Crawford, G.P.M. & Keast, D. (1992a) Biological responses to overload training in endurance sports. *European Journal of Applied Physiology* 64, 335–344.

Fry, R.W., Morton, A.R. & Keast, D. (1992b) Periodisation and the prevention of overtraining. *Canadian Journal of Sport Sciences* 17, 241–248.

Fry, R.W., Grove, J.R., Morton, A.R., Zeroni, P.M., Gaudieri, S. & Keast, D. (1994) Psychological and immunological correlates of acute overtraining. *British Journal of Sports Medicine* 28, 241–246.

Gabriel, H.H.W., Urhausen, A., Valet, G., Heidelbach, U. & Kindermann, W. (1998) Overtraining and immune system: a prospective longitudinal study in endurance athletes. *Medicine and Science in Sports and Exercise* 30, 1151–1157.

Garrell, D.R. (1996) Corticosteroid-binding globulin during inflammation and burn injury: nutritional modulation and clinical implications. *Hormone Research* 45, 245–251.

Gleeson, M., McDonald, W.A., Cripps, A.W., Pyne, D.B., Clancy, R.L. & Fricker, P.A. (1995) The effect on immunity of long-term intensive training in élite swimmers. *Clinical and Experimental Immunology* 102, 210–216.

Goss, J.D. (1994) Hardiness and mood disturbances in swimmers while overtraining. *Journal of Sport and Exercise Psychology* 16, 135–149.

Heath, G.W., Ford, E.S., Craven, T.E., Macrea, C.A., Jackson, K.L. & Pate, R.E. (1991) Exercise and the incidence of upper respiratory tract infection. *Medicine and Science in Sports and Exercise* 23, 152–157.

Hinton, J.R., Rowbottom, D.G., Keast, D. & Morton, A.R. (1997) Acute intensive interval training and *in vitro* T-lymphocyte function. *International Journal of Sports Medicine* 18, 130–135.

Hooper, S.L., MacKinnon, L.T., Gordon, R.D. & Bachmann, A.W. (1993) Hormonal responses of élite swimmers to overtraining. *Medicine and Science in Sports and Exercise* 25, 741–747.

Hooper, S.L., MacKinnon, L.T., Howard, A., Gordon, R.D. & Bachmann, A.W. (1995) Markers for monitoring overtraining and recovery. *Medicine and Science in Sports and Exercise* 27, 106–112.

Jakeman, P.M., Hawthorne, J.E., Maxwell, S.R., Kendall, M.J. & Holder, G. (1994) Evidence for downregulation of hypothalamic 5-hydroxytryptamine receptor function in endurance-trained athletes. *Experimental Physiology* 79, 461–464.

Jeukendrup, A.E. & Hesselink, M.K.C. (1994) Overtraining: what do lactate curves tell us? *British Journal of Sports Medicine* 28, 239–240.

Jeukendrup, A.E., Hesselink, M.K.C., Snyder, A.C., Kuipers, H. & Keizer, H.A. (1992) Physiological changes in male competitive cyclists after two weeks of intensified training. *International Journal of Sports Medicine* **13**, 534–541.

Keast, D. (1996) Immune responses to overtraining and fatigue. In: Hoffman-Goetz, L. (ed.) *Exercise and Immune Function*, pp. 121–141. CRC Publishers, Boca Raton, FL.

Keast, D., Arstein, D., Harper, W., Fry, R.W. & Morton, A.R. (1995) Depression of plasma glutamine following exercise stress and its possible influence on the immune system. *Medical Journal of Australia* **162**, 15–18.

Kirwan, J.P., Costill, D.L., Flynn, M.G. *et al.* (1988) Physiological responses to successive days of intense training in competitive swimmers. *Medicine and Science in Sports and Exercise* **20**, 255–259.

Koutedakis, Y. & Sharp, N.C.C. (1998) Seasonal variations of injury and overtraining in élite athletes. *Clinical Journal of Sports Medicine* **8**, 18–21.

Kreider, R.B., Fry, A.C. & O'Toole, M.L. (1998) Overtraining in sport: terms, definitions, and prevalence. In: Kreider, R.B., Fry, A.C. & O'Toole, M.L. (eds). *Overtraining in Sport*, vii–ix. Human Kinetics, Champaign, IL.

Kuipers, H. (1998) Training and overtraining: an introduction. *Medicine and Science in Sports and Exercise* **30**, 1137–1139.

Kuipers, H. & Keizer, H.A. (1988) Overtraining in élite athletes; review and directions for the future. *Sports Medicine* **6**, 79–92.

Lehmann, M., Dickhuth, H.H., Gendrisch, G. *et al.* (1991) Training–overtraining: a prospective, experimental study with experienced middle- and long-distance runners. *International Journal of Sports Medicine* **12**, 444–452.

Lehmann, M., Gastmann, U., Petersen, K.G. *et al.* (1992) Training–overtraining: performance, and hormone levels, after a defined increase in training volume versus intensity in experienced middle- and long-distance runners. *British Journal of Sports Medicine* **26**, 233–242.

Lehmann, M., Mann, H., Gastmann, U. *et al.* (1996) Unaccustomed high-mileage vs intensity training-related changes in performance and serum amino acid levels. *International Journal of Sports Medicine* **17**, 187–192.

Levin, S. (1991) Overtraining causes Olympic-sized problems. *Physician and Sportsmedicine* **19** (5), 112–118.

Mackinnon, L.T. & Hooper, S. (1994) Mucosal (secretory) immune system responses to exercise of varying intensity and during overtraining. *International Journal of Sports Medicine* **15**, S179–S183.

Mackinnon, L.T. & Hooper, S.L. (1996) Plasma glutamine and upper respiratory tract infection during intensified training in swimmers. *Medicine and Science in Sports and Exercise* **28**, 285–290.

Maffulli, N., Capasso, G. & Lancia, A. (1991) Anaerobic threshold and performance in middle and long distance running. *Journal of Sports Medicine and Physical Fitness* **31**, 332–338.

Marvin, G., Sharma, A., Aston, W., Field, C., Kendall, M.J. & Jones, D.A. (1997) The effects of buspirone on perceived exertion and time to fatigue in man. *Experimental Physiology* **82**, 1057–1060.

Morgan, W.P. (1992) Psychological components of effort sense. *Medicine and Science in Sports and Exercise* **26**, 1071–1077.

Morgan, W.P., Brown, D.R., Raglin, J.S. & O'Connor, P.J. (1987a) Psychological monitoring of overtraining and staleness. *British Journal of Sports Medicine* **21**, 107–114.

Morgan, W.P., O'Connor, P.J., Sparling, P.B. & Pate, R.R. (1987b) Psychologic characterization of the élite female distance runner. *International Journal of Sports Medicine* **8**, 124–131.

Morgan, W.P., Costill, D.L., Flynn, M.G., Raglin, J.S. & O'Connor, P.J. (1988) Mood disturbance following increased training in swimmers. *Medicine and Science in Sports and Exercise* **20**, 408–414.

Morton, R.H. (1997) Modelling training and overtraining. *Journal of Sports Sciences* **15**, 335–340.

Newsholme, E.A. (1994) Biochemical mechanisms to explain immunosuppression in well-trained and overtrained athletes. *International Journal of Sports Medicine* **15**, S142–S147.

Newsholme, E.A., Parry-Billings, M., McAndrew, M. & Budgett, R. (1991) Biochemical mechanisms to explain some characteristics of overtraining. In: Brouns, F. (ed.) *Medical Sports Science*, Vol. 32. *Advances in Nutrition and Top Sport*, pp. 79–93. Karger, Basel.

Nieman, D.C. (1994) Exercise, infection and immunity. *International Journal of Sports Medicine* **15**, S131–S141.

Nieman, D.C., Johanssen, L.M., Lee, J.W. & Arabatzis, K. (1990) Infectious episodes in runners before and after the Los Angeles marathon. *Journal of Sports Medicine and Physical Fitness* **30**, 316–328.

O'Connor, P.J., Morgan, W.P., Raglin, J.S., Barksdale, C.M. & Kalin, N.H. (1989) Mood state and salivary cortisol levels following overtraining in female swimmers. *Psychoneuroendocrinology* **14**, 303–310.

O'Connor, P.J., Morgan, W.P. & Raglin, J.S. (1991) Psychobiologic effects of 3 days of increased training in female and male swimmers. *Medicine and Science in Sports and Exercise* **23**, 1055–1061.

Parry-Billings, M., Budgett, R., Koutedakis, Y. *et al.* (1992) Plasma amino acid concentrations in the overtraining syndrome: possible effects on the immune system. *Medicine and Science in Sports and Exercise* **24**, 1353–1358.

Peters, E.M. & Bateman, E.D. (1985) Ultramarathon running and upper respiratory tract infection. *South African Medical Journal* **64**, 582–584.

Pyne, D.B., Baker, M.S., Fricker, P.A., McDonald, W.A., Telford, R.D. & Weidemann, M.J. (1995) Effects of an intensive 12-week training program by élite swimmers on neutrophil oxidative activity. *Medicine and Science in Sports and Exercise* **27**, 536–542.

Raglin, J.S. & Morgan, W.P. (1994) Development of a scale for use in monitoring training-induced distress in athletes. *International Journal of Sports Medicine* **15**, 84–88.

Rowbottom, D.G. (2000) Periodisation of training. In: Garrett, W.E. & Kirkendall, D.T. (eds). *Exercise: Basic and Applied Science*, pp. 499–512. Williams & Wilkins, Baltimore.

Rowbottom, D.G., Keast, D., Garcia-Webb, P. & Morton, A.R. (1995a) Serum free cortisol responses to a standard exercise test among élite triathletes. *Australian Journal of Science and Medicine in Sport* **27**, 103–107.

Rowbottom, D.G., Keast, D., Goodman, C. & Morton, A.R. (1995b) The haematological, biochemical and immunological profile of athletes suffering from the overtraining syndrome. *European Journal of Applied Physiology* **70**, 502–509.

Rowbottom, D.G., Keast, D. & Morton, A.R. (1996) The emerging role of glutamine as an indicator of exercise-stress and overtraining. *Sports Medicine* **21**, 80–97.

Rowbottom, D.G., Keast, D., Garcia-Webb, P. & Morton, A.R. (1997) Training adaptation and biological changes among well-trained male triathletes. *Medicine and Science in Sports and Exercise* **29**, 1233–1239.

Rowbottom, D.G., Keast, D., Green, S., Kakulas, B. & Morton, A.R. (1998a) The case study of an élite ultra-endurance cyclist who developed the Chronic

Fatigue Syndrome. *Medicine and Science in Sports and Exercise* **30**, 1345–1349.

Rowbottom, D.G., Keast, D. & Morton, A.R. (1998b) Monitoring and preventing of overreaching and overtraining in endurance athletes. In: Kreider, R.B., Fry, A.C. & O'Toole, M.L. (eds) *Overtraining in Sport*, pp. 47–66. Human Kinetics, Champaign, IL.

Rowbottom, D.G., Keast, D., Pervan, Z. & Morton, A.R. (1998c) The physiological response to exercise in chronic fatigue syndrome. *Journal of Chronic Fatigue Syndrome* **4**, 33–49.

Sharpe, M., Clements, A., Hawton, K., Young, A.H., Sargent, P. & Cowen, P.J. (1996) Increased prolactin response to buspirone in chronic fatigue syndrome. *Journal of Affective Disorders* **41**, 71–76.

Snyder, A.C. (1998) Overtraining and glycogen depletion hypothesis. *Medicine and Science in Sports and Exercise* **30**, 1146–1150.

Snyder, A.C., Jeukendrup, A.E., Hesselink, M.K., Kuipers, H. & Foster, C. (1993) A physiological/psychological indicator of over-reaching during intensive training. *International Journal of Sports Medicine* **14**, 29–32.

Snyder, A.C., Kuipers, H., Cheng, B., Servais, R. & Fransen, E. (1995) Overtraining following intensified training with normal muscle glycogen. *Medicine and Science in Sports and Exercise* **27**, 1063–1070.

Steinacker, J.M., Lormes, W., Lehmann, M. & Altenburg, D. (1998) Training of rowers before world championships. *Medicine and Science in Sports and Exercise* **30**, 1158–1163.

Stray-Gundersen, J., Videman, T. & Snell, P.G. (1986) Changes in selected objective parameters during overtraining. *Medicine and Science in Sports and Exercise* **18** (Suppl.), 54–55.

Tanaka, K., Watanabe, H. & Konishi, Y. (1986) Longitudinal association between anaerobic threshold and distance running performance. *European Journal of Applied Physiology* **55**, 248–252.

Tanaka, H., West, K.A., Duncan, G.E. & Bassett, D.R. (1997) Changes in plasma tryptophan/branched chain amino acid ratio in response to training volume variation. *International Journal of Sports Medicine* **18**, 270–275.

Urhausen, A., Kullmer, T. & Kindermann, W. (1987) A 7-week follow-up study of the behaviour of testosterone and cortisol during the competition period in rowers. *European Journal of Applied Physiology* **56**, 528–533.

Urhausen, A., Weiler, B., Coen, B. & Kindermann, W. (1994) Plasma catecholamines during endurance exercise of different intensities as related to the individual anaerobic threshold. *European Journal of Applied Physiology* **69**, 16–20.

Urhausen, A., Gabriel, H. & Kindermann, W. (1995) Blood hormones as markers of training stress and overtraining. *Sports Medicine* **40**, 251–276.

Urhausen, A., Gabriel, H.H.W. & Kindermann, W. (1998a) Impaired pituitary hormonal response to exhaustive exercise in overtrained endurance athletes. *Medicine and Science in Sports and Exercise* **30**, 407–414.

Urhausen, A., Gabriel, H.H.W., Weiler, B. & Kindermann, W. (1998b) Ergometric and psychological findings during overtraining: a long term follow-up study in endurance athletes. *International Journal of Sports Medicine* **19**, 114–120.

Verde, T., Thomas, S.G., Moore, R.W., Shek, P. & Shephard, R.J. (1992) Immune responses and increased training of the élite athlete. *Journal of Applied Physiology* **73**, 1494–1499.

Vervoorn, C., Quist, A.M., Vermulst, L.J.M. et al. (1991) The behaviour of the plasma free testosterone/cortisol ratio during a season of élite rowing training. *International Journal of Sports Medicine* **12**, 257–263.

Young, S.N. (1986) The clinical pharmacology of tryptophan. In: Wurtman, R.J. & Wurtman, J.J. (eds) *Nutrition and the Brain*, pp. 49–88. Raven Press, New York.

Zweig, M.H. & Campbell, G. (1993) Receiver-operating curve (ROC) plots: A fundamental evaluation tool in clinical medicine. *Clinical Chemistry* **39**, 561–577.

PART 5

SPECIFIC POPULATION GROUPS AND ENDURANCE TRAINING

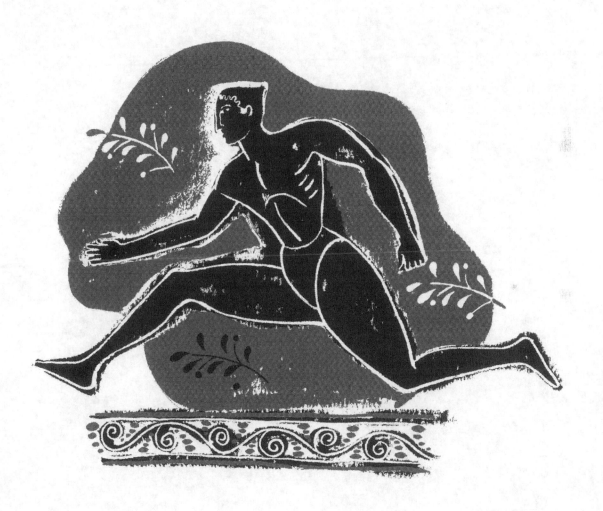

PART

SKELETAL POPULATION GROUPS AND
ENDURANCE TRAINING

Chapter 35

Endurance Training and Children

THOMAS W. ROWLAND

Introduction

The burgeoning involvement of child athletes in endurance sports has prompted an examination of responses to training and risks of early intense athletic play in the prepubertal age group. Do children demonstrate unique physiological responses to endurance training that differ from those of adults? Are there physical and emotional risks to intensive sports training and competition that are unique to the growing athlete? If so, what are the limits of safe sports participation for the child?

The research information available to address these critical issues is limited. Indeed, the increasing popularity of endurance events in child athletes has clearly exceeded the scientific data upon which guidelines for safe involvement can be based. This chapter will review our current understanding of the responses of children to endurance training and the potential risks that might be incurred by early sports participation, particularly in endurance sports such as distance running, cycling and swimming. It will be apparent to the reader that considerable additional information is necessary to close the gap between the need to guide the growing number of young athletes into safe participation and the scientific data available to create such recommendations.

Participation by children in organized sports has generally been considered in a positive light, given the enjoyment and physical benefits provided by athletic play. Still, the potential for adverse mental and physical outcomes for children has been identified at the extreme of intense sports involvement. In addition, research evidence indicates that improvements in physiological aerobic fitness following a period of endurance training may be less in children compared to adults. Such findings may have an important bearing on appropriate endurance training regimens in the paediatric age group.

Issues surrounding élite-level sports play by children as well as aerobic trainability have been addressed comprehensively elsewhere (Cahill & Pearl 1993; Bompa 1995; Armstrong & Welsman 1997; Chan & Micheli 1998). The reader is referred to these sources for additional information.

Aerobic trainability of children

Maximal oxygen intake ($\dot{V}_{O_{2max}}$) serves as the physiological hallmark of aerobic fitness (Chapter 21). A previously sedentary adult placed in an endurance programme of sufficient intensity (60–90% maximal heart rate), frequency (three to five sessions per week) and duration (30 min per session) will typically demonstrate a rise in $\dot{V}_{O_{2max}}$ of 15–30%. While such responses may be largely controlled by hereditary factors (Chapter 15), several non-genetic variables influence the magnitude of rise in $\dot{V}_{O_{2max}}$ with training, particularly the level of pretraining aerobic fitness.

Data from training studies in adults reviewed by Saltin et al. (1969) indicate that normal young men with an initial $\dot{V}_{O_{2max}}$ of 40 ml·kg^{-1}·min^{-1} can be expected to demonstrate a 30% rise with training. However, those with a pretraining value of 50 ml·kg^{-1}·min^{-1} typically show only a 15% increase in $\dot{V}_{O_{2max}}$.

Cardiovascular responses to acute bouts of exercise are similar in children and adults (Rowland et al. 1997b). There is no reason to expect a priori, then, that prepubertal subjects should demonstrate differences in improvements in $\dot{V}O_{2max}$ with endurance training. None the less, two initial observations suggested that this is the case. First, highly trained male child distance runners typically demonstrate a $\dot{V}O_{2max}$ of 60–65 ml·kg^{-1}·min^{-1}, while values of 70–75 ml·kg^{-1}·min^{-1} are usually seen in mature endurance runners. While this could reflect duration and/or intensity of training, this observation has led some authors to suggest that prior to the age of puberty there is a 'ceiling' for increase of $\dot{V}O_{2max}$ with endurance training.

Second, Bar-Or (1989) reviewed a series of nine exercise training studies in children performed between 1969 and 1985 which demonstrated little (less than 10%) or no improvement in $\dot{V}O_{2max}$. Although these increases were far less than those in adult training studies, most involved training regimes that did not satisfy recognized criteria for improving $\dot{V}O_{2max}$ (at least in adults). Several, for instance, utilized short-burst interval runs one or two times per week as the training stimulus.

Rowland (1985) examined $\dot{V}O_{2max}$ responses in only those paediatric training studies which appeared to meet such adult-based criteria. Of eight studies, six demonstrated a significant rise in $\dot{V}O_{2max}$, ranging from 7 to 26% (average 14%). A subsequent review of 12 training studies in children (Pate and Ward 1990) reached similar conclusions

(mean increase 10.4%). It was recognized by these authors that the studies exhibited a number of important methodological weaknesses, including small subject numbers, lack of controls, no documentation of training intensity and non-representative subject populations (for instance, swimming clubs). The importance of these issues as confounding factors in assessing the aerobic trainability of children has been reviewed by Shephard (1997).

When Payne and Morrow (1993) performed a meta-analysis of all 23 paediatric training studies reported to that time, however, the average increase in $\dot{V}O_{2max}$ was only approximately 5%. They failed to find any differences in change of $\dot{V}O_{2max}$ in training studies which did and did not conform to traditional training criteria for eliciting improvements in aerobic fitness.

A number of paediatric endurance training studies since that time have avoided the methodological pitfalls of earlier reports (Table 35.1). These reports have included adequate training intensity (target heart rate 160–170 beats·min^{-1}), frequency and duration; use of larger numbers of subjects, who have not been involved in sports training; and inclusion of appropriate non-training controls. Improvements in $\dot{V}O_{2max}$ in these more recent reports have ranged from 0 to 10%, with an average rise of 4.6%. This corresponds closely to that determined in the earlier meta-analysis of paediatric training studies by Payne and Morrow (1993).

Several of these studies have provided particular insights into the aerobic trainability of children.

Table 35.1 Recent aerobic training studies evaluating $\dot{V}O_{2max}$ response in children.

Study	n	Age (years)	Sex	Duration (weeks)	% change $\dot{V}O_{2max}$
McManus et al. (1997)	12	9.6	F	8	7.8
Rowland & Boyajian (1995)	37	10.9–12.8	M, F	12	6.7
Welsman et al. (1997)	17	10.2	F	8	1.5
	18	10.1	F	8	1.0
Williford et al. (1996)	12	12	M	15	10.3
Rowland et al. (1996)	31	10.9–12.9	M, F	13	5.4
Shore & Shephard (1998)	15	10.3	M, F	12	0
Tolfrey et al. (1998)	12	10.5	M	12	1
	14	10.5	F	12	7.9

Rowland and Boyajian (1995) examined variability and gender influences as well as the magnitude of $\dot{V}_{O_{2max}}$ increase in 35 children (24 girls, 13 boys, ages 10.9–12.8 years) who were trained for 12 weeks, 20–30 min three times per week. The average heart rate during the training sessions, as recorded by monitors, was 166 beats·min^{-1}. No difference in change in $\dot{V}_{O_{2max}}$ was observed between boys and girls, with an overall mean increase of 6.7%.

One-third of the children demonstrated a rise of less than 3%, while the greatest single increase was 19.7%. This observation suggests that the interindividual variability of $\dot{V}_{O_2}$ response to training in children might be smaller than in adults. In the 20-week training study of Lortie et al. (1984) involving sedentary adults, for instance, $\dot{V}_{O_{2max}}$ rose from 5 to 88% (Chapter 15). Rowland and Boyajian (1995) observed no relationship between pretraining $\dot{V}_{O_{2max}}$ and the magnitude of its increase after 12 weeks of training, a finding also observed in the review of studies by Pate and Ward (1990).

Some studies continue to show no overall effect of endurance training on $\dot{V}_{O_{2max}}$ in children. Ignico and Mahon (1995) reported responses to 10 weeks of aerobic training in 18 low-fitness children aged 8–11 years who had failed to meet at least three out of four fitness criteria in a standardized testing protocol. The mean pretraining $\dot{V}_{O_{2max}}$ was 45.6 ml·kg^{-1}·min^{-1}. Following training, the mean time required for a 1.6-km (1-mile) walk/run improved significantly, from 13.33 to 12.06 min. However, no increase was observed in maximal aerobic power (average post-training $\dot{V}_{O_{2max}}$ 44.5 ml·kg^{-1}·min^{-1}). A control group demonstrated no significant changes in either field performance or $\dot{V}_{O_{2max}}$. Similarly, Welsman et al. (1997) showed no significant changes in $\dot{V}_{O_{2max}}$ when 10-year-old girls completed either an 8-week aerobic training programme or one involving cycle ergometer training.

Taken collectively, the available research data appear to indicate the following.
1 Given an endurance training programme of appropriate frequency, duration and intensity (that is, consistent with adult criteria), most prepubertal children will demonstrate an improvement in $\dot{V}_{O_{2max}}$.
2 The magnitude of increase in $\dot{V}_{O_{2max}}$ from 8 to 12 weeks of aerobic training in children is typically 5–10%, substantially less than that observed in training studies of adult subjects.
3 The aerobic trainability of children is independent of gender.
4 Increases in $\dot{V}_{O_{2max}}$ response to endurance training appear to occur in the teen years coincident with the timing of puberty.

It would appear logical to test these conclusions by performing studies that compare $\dot{V}_{O_2}$ responses to endurance training directly in pre- and postpubertal groups, or by conducting training studies in subjects across the pubertal years. The results of such investigations, however, have proven inconclusive and sometimes conflicting. Small numbers of subjects and difficulties in equating training intensity in different age groups may contribute to the variable findings.

Eisenman and Golding (1975) compared aerobic responses to a 14-week programme of distance running and bench stepping by 12–13-year-old girls (presumably not entirely prepubertal) and 18–21-year-old women. Average increases in $\dot{V}_{O_{2max}}$ for the two groups were 17.6% and 16.1%, respectively.

Savage et al. (1986) trained 12 boys (mean age 8 years) and 12 men (mean age 37 years) at a running intensity of 75% $\dot{V}_{O_{2max}}$ for 10 weeks. The average improvement in $\dot{V}_{O_{2max}}$ was 4.6% for the boys and 7.9% for the men, a difference that was not statistically significant. Kobayashi et al. (1978) reported that postpubertal subjects demonstrated a greater improvement in $\dot{V}_{O_{2max}}$ with endurance training compared to when they were prepubertal. Seven boys were tested annually with endurance activities from the ages of 9–10 to 15–16 years. Mean $\dot{V}_{O_{2max}}$·kg^{-1} did not begin to rise until the age of 13 years (the age of peak height velocity). However, Weber et al. (1976) could find no difference in aerobic trainability when comparing the effects of exercise programmes in 10- and 16-year-olds.

Mechanisms

If children truly have a dampened physiological response to endurance training compared to adults, what is the reason? Efforts to answer this question might pay dividends in understanding not only maturational effects on aerobic trainability but also the basic mechanisms responsible for the improvement in $\dot{V}O_{2max}$ with training.

It appeared logical to earlier investigators that the inherent greater level of daily physical activity in children might be responsible for their lack of ability to improve aerobic fitness with training. That is, through their higher habitual activities, children were essentially training themselves in their daily lives, leaving less scope for increased fitness with training. This concept was supported by the observation that prepubertal children exhibit higher levels of $\dot{V}O_{2max}$ (expressed per kg body mass) than at any other time in life. A typical 10-year-old boy has a $\dot{V}O_{2max}$ of approximately $52\,\mathrm{ml\cdot kg^{-1}\cdot min^{-1}}$. Once the mid-teen years are reached, this value begins to decline, with cross-sectional studies showing average values of about $45\,\mathrm{ml\cdot kg^{-1}\cdot min^{-1}}$ at the age of 30 years and $40\,\mathrm{ml\cdot kg^{-1}\cdot min^{-1}}$ at 40 years (Robinson 1938).

Although this concept is intuitively attractive, several lines of evidence fail to support it. First, little association has been observed between $\dot{V}O_{2max}$ and the amount of habitual physical activity in the paediatric years. Recognizing that the ability to measure the level of daily physical activity accurately is limited, Morrow and Freedson (1994) comprehensively reviewed 13 studies which examined the relationship between habitual physical activity and $\dot{V}O_{2max}$ in children. Of these, nine showed no significant association. Of those indicating a relationship between physical activity and aerobic fitness, correlation coefficients ranged from $r = 0.12$ to $r = 0.59$. The authors concluded that typical daily physical activity 'probably has a weak association with $\dot{V}O_{2max}$' in children.

Although children are, in fact, physically more active than adults, such activity is typically very short burst in nature. The pattern of activity in children does not include the types of sustained exercise that are necessary to improve $\dot{V}O_{2max}$ (at least in adults). In addition, during the course of childhood and early adolescence, levels of daily energy expenditure (relative to body size) decline progressively. Over the same age span, values of $\dot{V}O_{2max}\cdot kg^{-1}$ remain stable, at least in males.

Most of the training studies in adults have been performed with subjects who had a pretraining $\dot{V}O_{2max}$ value of $30–45\,\mathrm{ml\cdot kg^{-1}\cdot min^{-1}}$. As initial $\dot{V}O_{2max}$ levels in paediatric studies have been higher, it could be that the greater pretraining levels in children are responsible for the smaller increases in $\dot{V}O_{2max}$ with training. In fact, training of adults who have an initial $\dot{V}O_{2max}$ of $50–60\,\mathrm{ml\cdot kg^{-1}\cdot min^{-1}}$ typically results in a rise of only a few percentage points (Saltin et al. 1969). This explanation for the dampened $\dot{V}O_{2max}$ rise in children is weakened by the observation that endurance training of prepubertal subjects with low fitness has resulted in little change in $\dot{V}O_{2max}$ (Ignico & Mahon 1995). Also, Rowland and Boyajian (1995) could find no relationship between initial $\dot{V}O_{2max}$ and the change in aerobic power with training in a group of children who entered their study with a wide range of fitness.

It is possible that true biological differences between pre- and postpubertal subjects are responsible for their differences in responsiveness of $\dot{V}O_{2max}$ to endurance training. This concept was, in fact, set forth early by Katch (1983) as the 'trigger hypothesis': there exists a critical age in the growing years before which the effects of endurance training will be minimal. That time is puberty, and the enhancement of the training effect that occurs during the pubertal years results from hormones which stimulate adaptations to physical conditioning.

It is difficult to assess the truth of this hypothesis, given our minimal understanding of the triggers and mechanisms for physiological adaptations to endurance training at any age. Still, there are enough pieces of this puzzle that fit together to suggest that it has at least some validity.

The Fick equation dictates that improvements in maximal oxygen intake must reflect increases in maximal heart rate, stroke volume and/or arteriovenous oxygen difference. Heart rate has been shown clearly to be unaltered by endurance training, and most studies in adults indicate that a combination of increases in stroke volume and arteriovenous oxygen difference are responsible for training adaptations in aerobic fitness. Adult–child differences in the magnitude of such adaptations should then be expected to involve these factors. Unfortunately, due largely to methodological and ethical constraints, little information is available on the responses of these components to endurance training in children.

Eriksson and Koch (1973) trained nine boys aged 11–13 years for 16 weeks and reported a 16% increase in $\dot{V}O_{2max}$ (although they had no non-trained control subjects). Maximal stroke volume rose by 20%, but no significant changes were seen in maximal arteriovenous oxygen difference. Mobert et al. (1997) reported changes in resting stroke volume in a group of 12–14-year-old boys after 7 months of aerobic training. The six boys who trained most consistently demonstrated an average increase in $\dot{V}O_{2max}$ from 49 to 55 ml·kg^{-1}·min^{-1} (12%). In this group resting upright stroke volume rose from 55 to 66 ml.

It is interesting to speculate on how possible hormonal changes developing at the time of puberty might influence responses of stroke volume and arteriovenous oxygen difference to endurance training. Serum testosterone levels rise dramatically in males at puberty and demonstrate a significant but smaller rise in females. Testosterone acts to increase cardiac muscle mass and function, as well as increasing peripheral skeletal muscle strength. The latter effect may improve function of the 'skeletal muscle pump', partly responsible for augmenting systemic venous return during exercise.

Testosterone also stimulates red blood cell production, resulting in a 20 g·l^{-1} increase in haemoglobin concentration in the postpubertal compared to prepubertal male. This appears to explain the greater maximal arteriovenous oxygen difference values in men compared to boys (Rowland et al. 1997b).

Growth hormone also has prominent anabolic effects, on both peripheral and cardiac muscle. Resting and exercise-induced levels of growth hormone increase approximately three-fold at the time of puberty. How the influences of these anabolic hormones might affect responses to training is unclear. However, there is some evidence that they can. Testosterone administered to adult men in a 10-week weight-training programme caused greater improvements in strength and muscle size than in a control training group (Bhasin et al. 1996).

An increase in plasma volume is a well-documented response to endurance training in adults and contributes significantly to improvements in maximal stroke volume. The mechanism for this response is unknown, but it may be influenced by a number of hormones, including aldosterone, vasopressin and atrial natriuretic peptide. Plasma volume responses to endurance training have not been studied in children. Similarly, the effects of biological maturation on the levels of hormones influencing plasma volume are not well understood. These factors deserve future research attention in efforts to understand the potential mechanisms behind the lower aerobic responses of children to endurance training.

Implications

As Shephard (1997) has pointed out, evidence indicating a limited aerobic response to training in children has significant implications for public health initiatives and physical education curricula. Specifically, the rationale behind instituting exercise training for children with low endurance fitness to promote health is weakened. Shephard concluded that 'rather than focusing upon the development of maximal oxygen intake, it seems important to emphasize attitudes and behaviour, allowing the child to try a wide range of active pursuits. . . . Such programmes should increase the likelihood that physical activity will be maintained into adult life . . .'.

The implications of the diminished aerobic trainability in children for the child endurance athlete are not clear. From one perspective, changes in $\dot{V}O_{2max}$ are typically manifested by parallel changes in endurance performance. If a prepubertal athlete cannot be expected to improve endurance performance substantially with training (in the same way that he or she cannot increase $\dot{V}O_{2max}$), intensive training regimens in sports such as distance running prior to the age of puberty may not be justified.

On the other hand, improvements in $\dot{V}O_{2max}$ are not typical of highly trained adult endurance athletes. The training regimen of an adult marathon runner is more geared to improving performance through changes in substrate utilization and maximizing such submaximal factors as a higher anaerobic threshold or improving ability to run at a greater fractional percentage of $\dot{V}_{O_{2max}}$. It is not known if the prepubertal athlete can improve performance through these mechanisms.

Studies examining $\dot{V}_{O_{2max}}$ changes in training child athletes have produced mixed findings. Van Huss *et al.* (1988) could find no changes in $\dot{V}_{O_{2max}}$ in serial measurements of $\dot{V}_{O_{2max}}$ over 3 years in élite male and female distance runners aged 10–11 and 12–13 years. Daniels and Oldridge (1971) described no improvement in $\dot{V}_{O_{2max}}$ in 14 boys who trained with distance running over 22 months. However, significant improvements in $\dot{V}_{O_{2max}}$ have been described in child swimmers (Zauner & Benson 1981) and hockey players (Paterson *et al.* 1987).

In the late teen, postpubertal years, improvements in $\dot{V}_{O_{2max}}$ in athletes have been more impressive. Finnish cross-country skiers increased their $\dot{V}_{O_{2max}}$ from 55 to 80 ml·kg^{-1}·min^{-1} from the age of 14 to 20 years (Rusko 1992). Kobayashi *et al.* (1978) described four élite distance runners who improved their mean $\dot{V}_{O_{2max}}$ from 63.8 to 73.9 ml·kg^{-1}·min^{-1} between the ages of 14 and 17 years. Murase *et al.* (1981) described an average increase in $\dot{V}_{O_{2max}}$ from 65.1 to 72.8 ml·kg^{-1}·min^{-1} in highly trained Japanese males over 5–7 years, beginning at the age of 14.

Little research has addressed the performance trainability of the prepubertal athlete. A study of the responses to 22 months of running training by 10–15-year-old boys (Daniels & Oldridge 1971) has been cited as evidence that performance improvements can occur, even without increases in $\dot{V}_{O_{2max}}$. During the training period, there were no significant changes in $\dot{V}_{O_{2max}}$ (per kg), which averaged approximately 59.5 ml·kg^{-1}·min^{-1}. During the study period of 1 year, average 1.6-km (1-mile) race time fell from 6 min 10 s to 5 min 38 s (8.6% decrease). Such improvement might, however, reflect normal maturational change rather than a training effect. Average 1.6-km (1-mile) run times in school fitness testing of boys between 11 and 12 years of age have been reported to decrease from 9 min 6 s to 8 min 20 s (an 8.4% improvement) (American Alliance for Health Physical Education, Recreation, and Dance 1980).

Based on these data, it is difficult to draw clear-cut conclusions as to whether the apparently diminished $\dot{V}_{O_2}$ response to endurance training in children has particular implications for young athletes. Further research efforts will be important in determining whether this phenomenon signals the need for unique approaches to training for children.

Risks and benefits of endurance training

Participation in regular endurance exercise provides health benefits, both physical and psychological. While these effects have been documented principally in adults, there is evidence for a similar salutary influence of endurance training in child athletes. Cross-sectional studies indicate that highly trained child endurance athletes have a favourable serum lipid profile in respect to risk for future coronary artery disease (especially an elevated high density lipoprotein (HDL)-cholesterol). These athletes typically demonstrate a lower percentage of body fat than the general paediatric population, and the augmented bone density observed in weight-bearing sports may be protective against future osteoporosis (Rowland 1990).

Child athletes may demonstrate superior academic achievement, decreased high risk health behaviours (smoking, alcohol consumption) and a lower incidence of juvenile delinquency. A cause and effect relationship, however, has not yet been proven. Athletic participation may improve social competence and self-esteem as well as serving to reduce anxiety.

More attention has been focused on the potential physical and emotional risks of sports training by children, particularly when such involvement reaches highly intensive, élite levels. Some authors have suggested that such participation is tantamount to 'child abuse'. The reality of such risks and the extent to which they are present among training child athletes are not yet clear. Several factors have clouded a true picture of the hazards that might be faced by young competitors. Child athletes are involved in many different forms of sport at varying levels of intensity. The number of such athletes is not large. In addition, there has been insufficient time to determine if early intense sports training has long-term side-effects.

The attention focused on the risks of intensive sports play by children reflects a concern that certain risks are unique to growing athletes. By its nature, endurance training is designed to stress body systems—heart, lungs, skeletal muscle—and adaptations to such stress are expected to improve performance. Children are different from adults in that their tissues are growing in size and developing in function. The key question is: Can the recurrent stresses imposed by intensive training interfere with normal growth and development in young competitors? The following sections examine the current information that addresses this important issue.

The heart

Both child and adult endurance athletes exhibit a superior cardiac functional reserve (i.e. a higher maximal cardiac output) than non-athletes. Still, there is evidence from animal studies and clinically in adult ultramarathoners that extended bouts of exercise can depress myocardial function transiently (Maher *et al.* 1972; Niemela *et al.* 1984). Monitoring child athletes for any adverse effects of such stress is therefore important.

Limited research information fails to suggest any adverse effect of intensive endurance training on the heart of the child athlete. Rowland *et al.* (1997a) found no evidence of changes in cardiac function in highly trained child distance runners following a 4-km road race. The heart sizes in young swimmers followed longitudinally by Rost (1987) were greater than in non-athletes, but no evidence of cardiac damage was evident.

Child endurance athletes and non-athletes demonstrate no differences in resting electrocardiograms (Rowland *et al.* 1984). Cardiac changes during prolonged submaximal exercise are similar in children and adults, with increases in heart rate, decreases in stroke volume and small rises in cardiac output (Asano & Hirakoba 1984). Thus, although research data are far from complete, there is currently no evidence for untoward influences of endurance training on the heart of the prepubertal child.

The musculoskeletal system

Physical activity is an important stimulus to bone development, but excessive stress can lead to fractures and/or diminished development, particularly if there is an associated negative energy balance.

Concern has been raised that intensive endurance training, particularly in weight-bearing sports such as running, might damage growth centres (epiphyseal plates) and lead to degenerative arthritis and/or stunted linear growth.

In groups of child athletes, however, epiphyseal overuse injuries have been primarily limited to gymnasts. Highly competitive gymnasts have been described as exhibiting stress fractures of the distal radial epiphysis, shortening of the radius and rarefaction of the wrist bones (Caine 1990). Such epiphyseal injuries have not been encountered in the lower extremities of prepubertal distance runners.

Cross-sectional and longitudinal studies of young endurance athletes have not found any disturbance in linear growth (Malina 1994). The one possible exception among child athletes is in gymnasts. Heights for both male and female gymnasts tend to cluster at about the 10th percentile for age, and skeletal age tends to lag behind chronological age during the adolescent years. Similar patterns are observed in ballet dancers. In reviewing these data, Malina (1998) concluded that 'the short stature and later maturation of female gymnasts and average stature and later maturation of female ballet dancers are to a major extent familial and not the result of intensive training. They also likely reflect the extreme selectivity of participants in both activities, especially at élite levels'.

Current information indicates, then, that intensive endurance sports training by children, even in weight-bearing endurance events, does not interfere with normal growth in stature.

Nutrition

Proper nutrition is critically important for young athletes, not only for good health and optimizing performance, but also for meeting the needs of normal growth and development. An inadequate diet therefore places the child athlete at jeopardy in these three separate areas. Little is known regarding the dietary practices of young competitors, but the available research insights have proven disturbing. Child athletes tend to consume inadequate total amounts of food, often fail to ingest a well-rounded diet, and commonly exhibit deficiencies of particular nutrients, especially iron and calcium. Moreover, young athletes appear to have little understanding of the proper components of a diet for training and competition and are subject to fads and misinformation from team-mates and coaches.

Improper diets, especially a low energy intake, may be manifestations of a more serious eating disorder (i.e. anorexia nervosa). More commonly, the young endurance athlete may be limiting food intake with the mistaken perception that 'thinner is better', and that a lower body mass will be reflected in improved performance. Monitoring of weights of training child athletes is important in correcting such improper tactics. Energy intake for these athletes must exceed the needs of training if growth is not to be compromised.

Many young athletes focus on carbohydrate intake, assuming that this 'fuel' is all they need for sports performance. It is essential to educate the athlete that protein and fat, plus a well-rounded diet that will provide essential vitamins and minerals, is critical for endurance performance as well as health. Many athletes are averse to consuming red meat, either on aesthetic grounds or from fear of eating fat. This practice places the athlete at risk for depletion of body iron, a mineral which is essential for athletic performance (oxygen transport, cellular aerobic metabolism) as well as growth and health. The needs for iron are greater during the growing years than at any other time in life. Similarly, calcium intake is often low in young athletes, partly from their aversion to dairy products. Adequate dietary calcium needs to be assured to diminish risks of future osteoporosis and perhaps to decrease the likelihood of stress fractures with training.

Sexual maturation

Female child endurance athletes typically demonstrate a later age of menarche compared to non-athletes. The usual age of menarche in North American females is 12.3–12.8 years, while that of the athlete is often 1–2 years later. It is reasonable to assume that intense training is at least partially responsible for this phenomenon. Vigorous training is associated with loss of monthly menstrual cycles once menarche has been achieved (secondary amenorrhoea), a consequence principally of energy

imbalance (inadequate food intake relative to energy expended). In addition, the later age of menarche in endurance athletes may reflect a preselection phenomenon: girls with narrow hips, slender physiques, long legs and low body fat are typically successful in sports, and these characteristics are also associated with a later age of menarche.

The concern regarding absence of menses — either primary or secondary — surrounds lack of circulating oestrogen. This hormone is important in the development of bone mass. A prolonged hypoestrogenaemia may pose a risk of skeletal fractures and, in the long run, osteoporosis in the adult years. Most authorities now feel that amenorrhoea associated with sports training should not be considered 'normal'. Following an investigation to rule out other causes, athletic amenorrhoea should be managed with a reduction in training and/or an improvement of diet. Oestrogen supplementation should be considered in those with prolonged amenorrhoea who are over the age of 16 years.

Thermoregulation

The responses of children to exercise in the heat differ from those of the adult. Children sweat less, relying more on thermal convection from the skin for cooling. They have a larger surface area/mass ratio than the adult, a disadvantage for heat exchange when environmental temperatures become high. Children also acclimatize to heat more slowly than mature athletes.

These unique thermoregulatory characteristics of child athletes may place them at increased risk of heat injury during extended endurance training and competition. The usual concerns of adequate fluid intake, avoiding excessive ambient temperature and humidity and recognizing early signs of heat injury are thus particularly critical in the child endurance athlete.

Psychosocial factors

Perhaps the greatest concern regarding risks to the intensively training child athlete involves possible negative influences on social development and emotional health. Childhood is a time of psychosocial as well as physical growth. There is concern that long hours of daily training, particularly in endurance sports where training is performed alone, might interfere with the development of social competence. Failure of normal interaction with peers, interference with schooling and the identification of success in sports with self-image may also result from excessive commitment to sport training at an early age.

At the élite level this commitment may become sufficiently intense to disrupt family life, increase competitive anxiety and stress and result in a 'disappearance of childhood'. Reports of sexual and physical abuse, deaths from anorexia nervosa and adverse behaviours (drinking and drug abuse) have fuelled these concerns.

Little research has addressed the reality or extent of these issues. Most élite child athletes, in fact, have reported that their participation in high-level sports was a positive experience (Donnelly 1993). While adverse psychosocial effects do occur in this group, these occurrences may be less common than has been assumed.

One preventable risk from early intense endurance training, however, deserves particular consideration. It is not uncommon that child athletes involved in intensive training regimens 'burn out' at an early age and drop out of athletic participation altogether. The young star athlete will demonstrate a rapid peaking of performance, but injury risk, athletic longevity and consistency of performance are likely to suffer. The young athlete who remains involved in multiple sports at an early age and then specializes in the teen years typically peaks later, but has a more effective overall athletic career, with fewer injuries and more consistent performance (Bompa 1995). For this reason, specialization in sports should be avoided until the child reaches the pubertal years.

Summary

The physiological response of the prepubertal child to endurance training differs from those of the adult. Children typically demonstrate a blunted response of $\dot{V}_{O_{2max}}$ to such training programmes, a characteristic which may have a biological basis. Whether this decreased aerobic trainability can be translated into a dampened response in performance gains with training in child endurance athletes is not known.

The child endurance athlete may face certain unique risks from intensive training. Particularly pertinent is the need for adequate nutrition to provide not only for performance but for normal growth. The female athlete with extended amenorrhoea deserves attention to reduce risks of hypoestrogenaemia. Young athletes should avoid sports specialization before the pubertal years, and situations of unwarranted psychosocial stress need to be identified. Given proper supervision, the potential risks of early endurance training should be avoidable, allowing the young competitor to gain the full benefits of sports participation.

References

American Alliance for Health, Physical Education, Recreation, and Dance (1980) *Youth Fitness Testing Manual.* Washington, D.C.

Armstrong, N. & Welsman, J. (1997) *Young People & Physical Activity.* Oxford University Press, Oxford.

Asano, K. & Hirakoba, K. (1984) Respiratory and circulatory adaptations during prolonged exercise in 10- to 12-year-old children and adults. In: Ilmarinen, J. & Valimaki, I. (eds) *Children and Sport,* pp. 119–128. Springer-Verlag, Berlin.

Bar-Or, O. (1989) Trainability of the prepubescent child. *Physician and Sportsmedicine* **17** (3), 65–81.

Bhasin, S., Storer, T.W., Berman, N. *et al.* (1996) The effects of supraphysiologic doses of testosterone on muscle size and strength in normal men. *New England Journal of Medicine* **335**, 1–7.

Bompa, T. (1995) *From Childhood to Champion Athlete.* Veritas Publishing, Toronto.

Cahill, B.R. & Pearl, A.J. (1993) *Intensive Participation in Children's Sports.* Human Kinetics, Champaign, IL.

Caine, D.J. (1990) Growth plate injury and bone growth: an update. *Pediatric Exercise Science* **2**, 209–229.

Chan, K.-M. & Micheli, L.J. (1998) *Sports and Children.* Williams & Wilkins, Hong Kong.

Daniels, J. & Oldridge, N. (1971) Changes in oxygen consumption of young boys during growth and running training. *Medicine and Science in Sports* **3**, 161–165.

Donnelly, P. (1993) Problems associated with youth involvement in high-performance sport. In: Cahil, B.R. & Pearl, A.J. (eds) *Intensive Participation in Children's Sports,* pp. 95–126. Human Kinetics, Champaign, IL.

Eisenman, P.A. & Golding, L.A. (1975) Comparison of effects of training on $\dot{V}_{O_{2max}}$ in girls and young women. *Medicine and Science in Sports* **7**, 136–138.

Eriksson, B.O. & Koch, G. (1973) Effect of physical training on hemodynamic response during submaximal and maximal exercise in 12–13-year-old boys. *Acta Physiologica Scandinavica* **87**, 27–39.

Ignico, A.A. & Mahon, A.D. (1995) The effects of a physical fitness program on low-fit children. *Research Quarterly for Exercise and Sport* **66**, 85–90.

Katch, V.L. (1983) Physical conditioning of children. *Journal of Adolescent Health Care* **3**, 241–246.

Kobayashi, K., Kitamura, K., Miura, M. *et al.* (1978) Aerobic power as related to body growth and training in Japanese boys: a longitudinal study. *Journal of Applied Physiology* **44**, 666–672.

Lortie, G., Simoneau, J.A., Hamel, P., Boulay, M.R., Landry, F. & Bouchard, C. (1984) Responses of maximal aerobic power and capacity to aerobic training. *International Journal of Sports Medicine* **5**, 232–236.

McManus, A.M., Armstrong, N. & Williams, C.A. (1997) Effect of training on the aerobic power and anaerobic performance of prepubertal girls. *Acta Paediatrica* **86**, 456–459.

Maher, J.T., Goodman, A.L. & Francesconi, R. (1972) Responses of rat myocardium to exhaustive exercise. *American Journal of Physiology* **222**, 207–212.

Malina, R.M. (1994) Physical growth and biological maturation of young athletes. *Exercise and Sport Sciences Reviews* **22**, 389–434.

Malina, R.M. (1998) Growth and maturation of young athletes—is training for sport a factor? In: Chan, K.-M. & Micheli, L.J. (eds) *Sports and Children*, pp. 133–161. Williams & Wilkins, Hong Kong.

Mobert, J., Koch, G., Humplik, O. & Oyen, E.-M. (1997) Cardiovascular adjustment to supine and seated postures: Effect of physical training. In: Armstrong, N., Kirby, B. & Welsman, J. (eds) *Children and Exercise XIX*, pp. 429–433. E & FN Spon, London.

Morrow, J.R. & Freedson, P.S. (1994) Relationship between habitual physical activity and aerobic fitness in adolescents. *Pediatric Exercise Science* **6**, 315–329.

Murase, Y., Kobayashi, K., Kamei, S. & Matsui, H. (1981) Longitudinal study of aerobic power in superior junior athletes. *Medicine and Science in Sports and Exercise* **13**, 180–184.

Niemela, K.O., Palatski, I.J. & Ikaheimo, M.J. (1984) Evidence of impaired left ventricular performance after an uninterrupted 24-hour run. *Circulation* **70**, 350–356.

Pate, R.R. & Ward, D.S. (1990) Endurance exercise trainability in children and youth. In: Grana, W.A., Lombardo, J.A., Sharkey B.J. & Stone, J.A. (eds) *Advances in Sports Medicine and Fitness*, Vol. 3, pp. 37–55. Year Book Medical Publishers, Chicago.

Paterson, D.H., McLellan, T.M., Stella, R.S. & Cunningham, D.A. (1987) Longitudinal study of ventilation threshold and maximal O_2 uptake in athletic boys. *Journal of Applied Physiology* **62**, 2051–2057.

Payne, V.G. & Morrow, J.R. (1993) The effect of physical training on prepubescent $\dot{V}O_{2max}$: a meta-analysis. *Research Quarterly* **64**, 305–313.

Robinson, S. (1938) Experimental studies of physical fitness in relation to age. *Arbeitsphysiologie* **10**, 251–323.

Rost, R. (1987) *Athletics and the Heart.* Year Book Medical Publishers, Chicago.

Rowland, T.W. (1985) Aerobic response to endurance training in prepubescent children: a critical analysis. *Medicine and Science in Sports and Exercise* **17**, 493–497.

Rowland, T.W. (1990) *Exercise and Children's Health.* Human Kinetics, Champaign, IL.

Rowland, T.W. & Boyajian, A. (1995) Aerobic response to endurance training in children. *Pediatrics* **96**, 654–658.

Rowland, T.W., Unnithan, V.B., McFarlane, N.G. & Paton, J. (1994) Clinical manifestations of the 'athlete's heart' in prepubertal male runners. *International Journal of Sports Medicine* **15**, 515–519.

Rowland, T.W., Martel, L., Vanderburgh, P., Manos, T. & Charkoudian, N. (1996) The influence of short-term aerobic training on blood lipids in healthy 10–12-year-old children. *International Journal of Sports Medicine* **17**, 487–492.

Rowland, T.W., Goff, D., DeLuca, P. & Popowski, B. (1997a) Cardiac effects of a competitive road race in trained child runners. *Pediatrics* electronic pages **100** (3).

Rowland, T., Popowski, B. & Ferrone, L. (1997b) Cardiac responses to maximal upright cycle exercise in healthy boys and men. *Medicine and Science in Sports and Exercise* **29**, 1146–1151.

Rusko, H.K. (1992) Development of aerobic power in relation to age and training in cross-country skiers. *Medicine and Science in Sports and Exercise* **24**, 1040–1047.

Saltin, B., Hartely, L.H., Kilbom, A. & Astrand, I. (1969) Physical training in sedentary middle-aged and older men. II. Oxygen uptake, heart rate and blood lactate concentrations at submaximal and maximal exercise. *Scandinavian Journal of Clinical and Laboratory Investigation* **24**, 323–334.

Savage, M.P., Petratis, M.M., Thomsen, W.H., Berg, K., Smith, J.L. & Sady, S.P. (1986) Exercise training effects on serum lipids of prepubescent boys and adult men. *Medicine and Science in Sports and Exercise* **18**, 197–204.

Shephard, R.J. (1997) Assessing physiological responses to training in young children. *British Journal of Sports Medicine* **31**, 415–418.

Shore, S. & Shephard, R.J. (1998) Immune responses to exercise and training: a comparison of children and young adults. *Pediatric Exercise Science* **10**, 210–226.

Tolfrey, K., Campbell, I.G. & Batterham, A.M. (1998) Aerobic trainability of prepubertal boys and girls. *Pediatric Exercise Science* **10**, 248–263.

Van Huss, W., Evans, S.A., Kurowski, T., Anderson, D.J., Allen, R. & Stephens, K. (1988) Physiologic characteristics of male and female age-group runners. In: Brown, E.W. & Branta, C.F. (eds) *Competitive Sports for Children and Youth*, pp. 148–153. Human Kinetics, Champaign, IL.

Weber, G., Kartodihardjo, W. & Klissouras, V. (1976) Growth and physical training with reference to heredity. *Journal of Applied Physiology* **40**, 211–215.

Welsman, J.R., Armstrong, N. & Withers, S. (1997) Responses of young girls to two modes of aerobic training. *British Journal of Sports Medicine* **31**, 139–142.

Williford, H.N., Blessing, D.L., Duey, W.J. *et al.* (1996) Exercise training in black adolescents: changes in blood lipids and $\dot{V}O_{2max}$. *Ethnicity and Disease* **6**, 279–285.

Zauner, C.W. & Benson, N.Y. (1981) Physiological alteration in young swimmers during three years of intensive training. *Journal of Sports Medicine and Physical Fitness* **21**, 179–185.

Chapter 36

Endurance Training for Women

MARY L. O'TOOLE

Introduction

Women as endurance athletes

Women athletes have been competing in Olympic events since the IInd Olympiad (1900) of the modern games. At that time, only a few women contestants participated in just three sports—tennis, golf and croquet. Although tennis has an endurance component, none of these sports are truly endurance sports and serious endurance training was not part of a woman athlete's routine. In the 1996 summer Olympic Games, 36% of competing athletes were women. These women athletes were contestants in a broad range of sporting events, including endurance contests as well as sports with a large endurance component. Most of these endurance events were identical to those in which men competed. For example, the women's marathon was a 42.2-km road race; a basketball game consisted of two 20-min halves; and a soccer game two 45-min halves. Serious endurance training, thus, is currently as important for women as for men.

Endurance sport needs

ENERGY REQUIREMENTS

Endurance sport races require that an athlete expend a certain amount of energy to get from the starting line to the finish line. Examples from two of the more common endurance sports (running and cycling) serve to illustrate this point. In running,

because the relationship between aerobic energy expenditure (kJ) and movement velocity is linear (approximately $4 \, kJ \cdot kg^{-1}$ body mass $\cdot km^{-1}$), the overall energy cost for running a given distance is relatively independent of speed and can be estimated in accordance with race distance. For example, it is generally accepted that running 1 km on flat terrain requires an average energy expenditure of approximately 260 kJ (± 39 kJ to allow for variations in body size and running economy) (Margaria *et al.* 1963). So, for a 10-km race, the energy requirement would be approximately 2.6 MJ. Factors such as topography of the race course and environmental variables such as temperature or wind may alter this estimate. Similar, albeit less precise, estimates of energy requirements can also be made for cycling (Sherman & Lamb 1988). The energy costs of cycling are less consistent, in part, because they vary with movement velocity (Chapter 58). Air resistance increases with cycling speed. External factors, such as the design of the bicycle and the nature of the road surface, also affect the energy cost of cycling. So, although the energy costs of various endurance contests can be estimated, actual costs for an individual athlete may differ from those of a fellow competitor as a result of both intrinsic and extrinsic factors.

Despite an energy requirement that is sometimes large, energy stores in both men and women athletes are more than adequate to provide energy needed for endurance contests. However, the athlete with the fastest rate of energy transfer (the one who expends the required amount of energy in the shortest time) is likely to be the winner if other factors are equal. Thus, the primary physiological determinant of success in an endurance race is the ability to sustain a high rate of energy expenditure for a prolonged period of time.

TRAINING REQUIREMENTS

The ultimate goal of endurance training is to improve performance. The general assumption is that training will affect physiological variables related to the rate of energy turnover and improvements in these physiological variables will, in turn, improve performance. A core set of techniques forms the basis for endurance training. These techniques have been adopted by women athletes, so that prolonged and intense daily training regimens have become as common for women as for men. The stimulus is the training overload; the response, a physiological adaptation that allows the athlete to go faster for a longer period of time. The physiological adaptations are manifested as changes in those variables usually cited as determinants of endurance performance: i.e. maximal oxygen intake ($\dot{V}_{O_{2max}}$), lactate threshold and economy of movement. Although evidence for the adaptive responses of women is not as voluminous as that for male athletes, existing evidence suggests that men and women respond to the same training with the same adaptations (Wells 1991; Plowman & Smith 1997).

Basic endurance training techniques

Endurance training techniques target both aerobic and anaerobic energy systems (Chapter 28). Sustained distance training and aerobic interval training are methods commonly used for training the aerobic energy transformation systems. Sustained distance training has the greatest effect on $\dot{V}_{O_{2max}}$, whereas aerobic interval training also affects movement economy and lactate thresholds (Wells & Pate 1988). Pace or tempo training, although providing some stress to the oxidative energy systems, is performed at a high enough intensity to have its greatest effects on movement economy and lactate thresholds.

Sustained distance training

During sustained distance (long slow distance) training, workouts are bouts of continuous, rhythmic and comfortably paced activity lasting for relatively long periods of time. The specific distance is somewhat arbitrary and may vary considerably depending on the length and type of competitive event. Eight km of running or at least 30 min of continuous swimming are typical distances for rowers and swimmers, respectively (Kearney 1996), whereas marathon runners use 2–3-h runs and cyclists ride 130–250 km for sustained distance training (Wells & Pate 1988). The pace should be one that is easily performed for the specified time. Exercise intensity can be monitored by the athlete, using the rating of perceived exertion (RPE) or heart rates. RPE (Chapter 26) should be 'fairly light to light' (RPE = 10–12). If information is available from an incremental exercise test, heart rates representing a pace well below the lactate threshold (see below) can be used to guide pace. Heart rate monitors (on which lower and upper limits can be set) are useful in guiding the athlete to maintain an appropriate pace. During sustained distance running, transport (cardiovascular) and utilization (metabolic) systems are stressed. Additional stresses on the athlete include elevation of body temperature, loss of fluid and electrolytes in sweat, repeated microtrauma to joints and muscles and the need to maintain energy balance.

Aerobic interval training

During aerobic interval training, workouts consist of repeated intervals of exercise (usually between 5 and 15 min each in duration) interspersed with short rest periods (5–15 s each). This type of training allows more absolute work to be performed during a workout session than would be possible with sustained distance training. Neither circulation nor oxygen intake has time to recover appreciably during the short recovery intervals, but the musculoskeletal system gets brief periods of respite. As with sustained distance training, the duration of the exercise interval depends on the exercise mode and the length of the competitive event. For example, a

10-km runner might incorporate 800–1600-m repeats into her workout plan. Repetitions may be as few as five per session or as many as 20. The longer the exercise interval in relation to the total length of the event, the fewer the number of repetitions (Costill 1986). The pace should be slightly below the lactate threshold, but faster than for sustained distance training (above). Intensity can be guided by keeping RPE in the 'somewhat hard to hard' range (RPE = 13–15), with heart rates kept in a range slightly below those corresponding to the lactate threshold. It is commonly recommended that such intervals be undertaken no more than 1–3 days per week, because of the risk of injury (Costill 1986). Transport and utilization systems are enhanced as with sustained distance training, but additional benefits accrue as well. The movement patterns are more similar to those encountered in competitive events, thus potentially improving the economy of movement (see below). A greater use of fat as substrate also results from this type of training. Additionally, some lactate may accumulate during the workout, stressing systems involved in tolerating higher lactate levels and those involved in removing lactate.

Pace training

Pace training involves exercise performed at a pace slightly faster than that corresponding to the lactate threshold (Wells & Pate 1988). Intervals of 3–10 min are interspersed with 30–90-s periods of slower-paced activity. The number of intervals performed during any exercise session depends on the exercise mode and on the length of competition. During the exercise intervals, RPE should represent subjective feelings of 'hard to very hard' exercise (RPE = 15–17). Heart rates that represent an exercise intensity approximately 5% greater than the lactate threshold can be used to monitor training (Dwyer & Bybee 1983; Gilman & Wells 1993). Since lactate thresholds vary according to exercise mode, heart rates that have been measured in an appropriate training mode should be used. For example, in both men and women triathletes, lactate thresholds $(4 mmol \cdot l^{-1})$ are 72–88% $\dot{V}O_{2max}$ for cycling, but 80–85% $\dot{V}O_{2max}$ for running (Kohrt et al. 1989;

O'Toole et al. 1989). Because the training pace is above the threshold, lactate accumulates in the muscle during the exercise intervals. During the recovery intervals, adenosine triphosphate (ATP) and phosphocreatine (PCr) stores are replenished, allowing the athlete to maintain a high intensity at the beginning of the next exercise interval. However, only some of the lactate is removed and metabolized, so that the athlete must try to maintain pace in the face of a more acidic local muscle environment (Plowman & Smith 1997). Pace training, thus, stimulates and causes adaptive responses in both aerobic and anaerobic energy systems. Since many endurance sports require intermittent anaerobic activity over a long period of time, this type of training can be particularly useful to a competitor. Following a training session, approximately 50% of the lactate is removed with 15–20 min of rest and near-resting levels are regained within an hour. Lactate removal can be accelerated by approximately 20 min of continuous jogging at a comfortable pace just below the lactate threshold. However, continuous jogging may delay muscle glycogen resynthesis and may therefore be disadvantageous for some athletes, e.g. one who faces repeated heats in a middle-distance event.

Training-induced physiological adaptations

$\dot{V}O_{2max}$

Improvements in $\dot{V}O_{2max}$ augment the ability to circulate oxygen and substrate (Chapter 21). The key adaptation is an increase in stroke volume and therefore cardiac output. The increased stroke volume results from a variety of cardiac adaptations that allow greater efficiency in performance of the heart's primary function, that of a muscular pump (Harrison 1985). Until recently, traditional wisdom has been that stroke volumes of women as well as men plateau at exercise intensities of 40–50% maximal aerobic power and that training increases the height of this plateau. Endurance athletes were thought to have larger stroke volumes at each exercise intensity, and higher plateaus than untrained or less well-trained individuals (Saltin 1969). Recently, however, Gledhill *et al.* (1994) confirmed earlier reports (Ekblom & Hermanson 1968; Vanfraechem 1979; Crawford *et al.* 1986) of continued increases in stroke volume as exercise intensities were increased to maximal effort in highly trained male cyclists. The resultant slowing of heart rates at any given submaximal exercise intensity reduces myocardial oxygen demand for that level of exercise. Parallel information is lacking for female athletes, but they exhibit many of the physiological changes that could potentially contribute to increased stroke volumes.

Increased left ventricular cavity size and left ventricular mass are common findings in female as well as in male endurance-trained athletes over a wide age range and from a variety of sports (Pollack *et al.* 1987; Douglas *et al.* 1988; Douglas & O'Toole 1992; Pelliccia *et al.* 1996). The increased wall thickness allows a reduction in the tension applied to each individual fibre as wall stress is distributed across a greater mass of myocardium (Douglas 1989). Additionally, preload is increased, in part because of an increase in total blood volume (particularly plasma volume) (Oscai *et al.* 1968); this results in an increase of stroke volume via the Frank–Starling mechanism. The increased left and right ventricular end-diastolic volumes allow a similar volume of blood to be ejected with less fibre shortening and with less friction, but with increased tension. Endurance training appears to result also in an increased left ventricular compliance, enhancing preload at maximal exercise (Levine *et al.* 1991). Studies of male and female Ironman triathletes have shown an enhanced diastolic function at rest (greater ratio of early to late left ventricular inflow velocities), which would presumably result in increased preload during strenuous exercise (Douglas 1989). Others, also, have reported enhanced diastolic function, with peak filling rates of male athletes being up to 71% greater than in controls at matched heart rates (Gledhill *et al.* 1994). In longitudinal studies, training has improved cardiac filling in both younger and older subjects, both at rest and during exercise (Levy *et al.* 1993). Others have reported resting diastolic performance to be an independent determinant of $\dot{V}O_{2max}$ in both sedentary individuals and

athletes (Vanoverschelde *et al.* 1991), although our studies in triathletes have not confirmed this relationship (P. S. Douglas & M. L. O'Toole, unpublished observations).

The effects of endurance training on contractile function are less clear, since contractile function is increased during maximal exercise in untrained as well as highly trained athletes. Gledhill *et al.* (1994) demonstrated a progressive training-related increase in peak left ventricular emptying rates with maximal exercise testing in cyclists, but not in controls. They also reported a longer left ventricular ejection time, suggesting that augmentation of systolic function during exercise is a mechanism by which male athletes can enhance performance. It has been postulated that the athlete's ability to enhance systolic function leads to a smaller end-systolic volume which, by reducing intraventricular pressure, enhances early diastolic filling. Similar information on female athletes is lacking.

Peripheral cardiovascular adaptations may contribute to the training-induced increases in $\dot{V}O_{2max}$. Aerobic training increases capillary density; a close correlation has been shown between $\dot{V}O_{2max}$ and the number of capillaries per muscle fibre in both women and men athletes (Saltin *et al.* 1977). Endurance training also reduces systolic and diastolic blood pressures and total peripheral resistance, thereby enabling the endurance athlete to achieve high cardiac outputs during hard exercise with an afterload similar to that of sedentary subjects who are developing much smaller cardiac outputs. Additionally, a close relationship between submaximal exercise blood pressures and left ventricular mass has been reported for male and female Ironman triathletes (Douglas *et al.* 1986).

All of these findings suggest that the cardiovascular system is functioning more efficiently in highly trained athletes. Some of this information, including the work of Gledhill *et al.* (1994), has been derived from studies of male athletes, but Douglas and colleagues and Pelliccia and colleagues both included women athletes in their samples, and they found no gender-related differences in responses. The time course of adaptations and the limits to adaptation in any single athlete remain unknown.

Economy of movement

Adaptive changes in the muscular system in response to sustained distance or aerobic interval training improve the efficiency of substrate utilization (Saltin & Rowell 1980; Klausen *et al.* 1981). Metabolic adaptations, including increases in myoglobin, in the size and number of mitochondria and in the levels of various enzymes and transfer agents that enhance aerobic metabolism, can contribute as much as 50% to the initial improvement in ability to extract and use oxygen during the aerobic re-synthesis of ATP (Holloszy 1975; Clausen 1977). Gollnick *et al.* (1972) demonstrated in males that adaptations were specific to the mode of exercise stimulus (e.g. the patterns of enzyme activities in the arm and leg muscles of swimmers differed from those of cyclists). Both fat and carbohydrate metabolism are enhanced by training (Gollnick *et al.* 1972; Holloszy & Coyle 1984). All of these factors have the potential to improve movement economy. The time course of adaptations is somewhat variable, but Hamel *et al.* (1986) reported that skeletal muscle enzyme adaptations peaked after 15 weeks.

Interindividual differences in movement economy occur in highly trained élite athletes (Daniels 1985). As in male runners, élite female runners have a lower $\dot{V}O_2$ (better movement economy) than non-élite runners at two different submaximal running speeds (230 and 248 m·min⁻¹) (Pate *et al.* 1987). Morgan and Craib (1992) have suggested that these differences reflect muscle fibre type. However, Williams and Cavanagh (1987) found no difference in fibre type among trained runners with good, medium and poor running economy. Similarly, Costill *et al.* (1987) confirmed that muscle fibre characteristics and enzyme activities in female runners were directly related to the length of the competitive event, but not to skill level. Women marathoners had a greater percentage of type I fibres than middle-distance runners, but muscle enzyme activities were similar between élite and non-élite runners over matched distances (Costill *et al.* 1987).

Both muscle and liver glycogen reserves are increased with this pattern of training. Studies have shown an increased relative contribution of fat as compared with carbohydrate as substrate with training (Gollnick 1985). So, at the same absolute work rate (for example, the same running speed), muscle and liver glycogen are metabolized at a slower rate after than before training (Holloszy & Coyle 1984; Gollnick *et al.* 1986; Abernathy *et al.* 1990). The main advantage to this is a delay in glycogen depletion. This not only allows physical activity to continue at a particular pace for a longer time, but also allows brief spurts of high-intensity activity that rely on glycolytic energy sources (a common practice in most sports events). However, the oxygen cost of burning fat is greater than that of burning carbohydrate, thus adversely affecting movement economy. Therefore, one could hypothesize that it would be to the advantage of the successful athlete not only to conserve muscle glycogen, but also to oxidize exogenous carbohydrate. No studies have specifically addressed this issue in female athletes.

Lactate thresholds

Lactate thresholds (Chapter 22) are altered by both sustained distance training and aerobic interval training. Lactate production is decreased and/or clearance rates are increased at submaximal exercise intensities (i.e. specific movement speeds). The benefits of pace training include many of the adaptations described above for sustained distance and aerobic interval training. Additionally, pace training effectively stimulates an increase in the lactate threshold by increasing the capacity to remove lactate, increasing tolerance of high lactate concentrations, enhancing the capacity for glycolytic energy transfer (by increasing the activity of glycolytic enzymes) and increasing the capacity to store muscle glycogen. Pace-training benefits include a muscle fibre recruitment pattern that is similar to that encountered in competition, thus contributing to an improved economy of movement. Male and female athletes have similar resting lactate levels, and reach similar lactate concentrations at matched relative intensities of effort (Plowman & Smith 1997). As with aerobic training, the time course and upper limits of trainability for female athletes remain unknown.

Relationship to performance

The effectiveness of training is ultimately judged by performance. However, it is difficult to assign a causal relationship between the specifics of training and performance or between training-induced physiological adaptations and performance. For example, the relative importance of training distance versus training intensity is not well understood, but probably varies with race distance. Likewise, the relative contributions of $\dot{V}_{O_{2max}}$, movement economy and lactate thresholds to performance are not well defined and may vary with race distance.

Training and performance

Although women endurance athletes follow similar training patterns to men, women frequently have lower absolute training volumes (distance × pace) than men. For example, the weekly training distances for élite women middle- and long-distance runners have been reported to average 104 km per week compared with an average 137 km per week for élite male runners (Sparling et al. 1987). However, performance times in similar events are only 10% slower for women (Sparling et al. 1987; Noakes 1991).

In an attempt to clarify the relationship of training practices to performance, O'Toole et al. (1989) compared swim, cycle and run training practices of men and women Ironman triathletes who finished the event (a combination of a 3.9-km swim, a 180.1-km cycle and a 42.2-km run) with similar performances (i.e. a time < 10.5 h). Men and women did not differ in weekly swim training distance or pace. During cycle training, the women rode 11% less distance at a 5% slower pace. Run distances were similar, but the pace of the women was again 5–7% slower than that of the men. The reasons for the ability to perform similarly with less training are unexplained, but suggest that there may be a training ceiling above which increased training does little to augment performance. The complexity of training

and/or physiological influences on performance is further illustrated by Speechly et al. (1995) who matched men and women endurance athletes according to training practices and performance in a standard marathon (42.2-km run). Although the $\dot{V}_{O_{2max}}$ of the women runners was significantly less than that of their male counterparts (48.3 versus 51.3 ml·kg^{-1}·min^{-1}), running economies and lactate thresholds did not differ between groups. Male and female performance times were similar not only for the marathon, but also for 10- and 21.1-km races. The performance times of the women, however, were significantly better than those of the men during a 90-km race (Comrades Marathon). Both of these examples point out how difficult it is to define precisely how much and how hard one should train in order to optimize endurance performance.

$\dot{V}_{O_{2max}}$ and performance

Several gender-related physiological differences may limit the effects of endurance training on $\dot{V}_{O_{2max}}$ and could also limit a woman's performance (Table 36.1). For example, women typically have smaller hearts, smaller blood volumes and lower haemoglobin concentrations, thus limiting peak oxygen transport. These factors, in combination with a woman's greater percentage of body fat, may limit $\dot{V}_{O_{2max}}$ (ml·kg^{-1}·min^{-1}) in women athletes regardless of how hard they train. None the less, there is some evidence that $\dot{V}_{O_{2max}}$ is related to performance in some groups of women athletes. For example, $\dot{V}_{O_{2max}}$ appears to be a fairly good predictor of performance in heterogeneous groups of athletes (variable training and racing backgrounds). Butts et al. (1991) reported a relatively close correlation between event-specific $\dot{V}_{O_{2max}}$ values and performance ($r = -0.49, -0.78, -0.84$; swimming, cycling and running, respectively) for recreational women triathletes. However, in part because of a smaller variance in the data, the relationship between event-specific $\dot{V}_{O_{2max}}$ and performance appears to be less strong for homogeneously trained groups of triathletes and competitors in long or ultradistance races. A dissociation between $\dot{V}_{O_{2max}}$ and race performance was noted by Kohrt et al. (1989) for experienced, short-course triathletes; they improved

Table 36.1 Summary of gender differences potentially important for endurance performance.

Factor	Gender difference (%)	Supporting evidence*	Type of athlete	References
$\dot{V}O_{2max}$	14	75.4 versus 66.2 ml·kg⁻¹·min⁻¹	Élite runners	Daniels & Daniels (1992)
Lactate threshold	None documented	85.5% versus 87.1%	Élite runners	Daniels & Daniels (1992)
Economy of movement	7	48.3 versus 51.7 ml·kg⁻¹·min⁻¹ @ 268 m·min⁻¹	Élite runners	Daniels & Daniels (1992)
	6	53.6 versus 56.6 ml·kg⁻¹·min⁻¹ @ 290 m·min⁻¹		
	4	58.4 versus 61 ml·kg⁻¹·min⁻¹ @ 310 m·min⁻¹		
Physiological contributors				
Cardiac dimensions				
LVIDd†	11	54.2 versus 48.9 mm	Athletes from multiple sports	Pelliccia et al. (1996)
LV wall thickness	25	10.1 versus 8.1 mm	Athletes from multiple sports	Pelliccia et al. (1996)
LV mass	32	249 versus 189 g	Ultradistance triathletes	Douglas et al. (1997)
Blood volume	Approximately 20	5–6 l in men; 4–5 l in women	Untrained men versus women	Åstrand & Rodahl (1986)
Haemoglobin concentration	11	15.5 ± 0.9 versus 14.0 ± 1.1	Élite runners	Martin et al. (1977) Durstine et al. (1987)
Body composition (sum of six skinfolds)	34	35.4 mm versus 47.3 mm	Élite runners	Daniels & Daniels (1992)

* Male versus female values, respectively.

† Left ventricular internal diameter in diastole.

performance over the course of 1 year of competition without any change in $\dot{V}O_{2max}$. Similarly, in ultradistance (Hawaii Ironman) triathletes we found virtually no relationship between any event-specific $\dot{V}O_{2max}$ (arm crank ergometry, leg cycle ergometry and treadmill running) and overall race performance ($r = 0.19$, 0.04 and 0.09, respectively) (O'Toole *et al.* 1987). Several factors probably contribute to the weak relationship between $\dot{V}O_{2max}$ and triathlon performance in experienced triathletes, but the time course for training-induced improvement in $\dot{V}O_{2max}$ may be the greatest factor. Training-induced improvements in $\dot{V}O_{2max}$ are essentially complete in most individuals after 3 months of serious training. So, although endurance athletes have high $\dot{V}O_{2max}$ values, other physiological variables are also closely related to race performance. There is no evidence of a gender difference in the relationship between $\dot{V}O_{2max}$ and performance.

Economy of movement and performance

The average mechanical efficiency of human locomotion has been estimated at between 20 and 30% during running or cycling, but it is only 5–9.5% during swimming (McArdle *et al.* 1992; Toussaint & Beck 1992). Even in well-trained competitors, there is marked interindividual variation within these average ranges, particularly in swimming. For a given energy output (submaximal $\dot{V}O_2$), the athlete with the greatest mechanical efficiency can move at the fastest pace. From the opposite perspective, the energy requirement to go at a given pace is lowest in the most efficient athletes, thus delaying the depletion of their substrate stores, particularly glycogen.

Studies of runners have consistently shown a close relationship between running economy and running performance. In distance runners with similar $\dot{V}O_{2max}$ values, running economy correlates well with performance (Conley & Krahenbuhl 1980). Also, élite distance runners have better running economies than same-gender runners of lesser ability (Conley & Krahenbuhl 1980). Although some élite women distance runners have similar running economies to those of élite men

runners (e.g. Grete Waitz, a world record holder in the marathon for a number of years, had a running economy virtually identical to that of Derek Clayton, an élite male marathoner), Daniels and Daniels (1992) reported a 4–7% better economy for élite male compared to élite female runners (Table 36.1). Technical skill may account for much of interindividual differences in movement economy among cyclists, but specific reasons for differences in cycling are unclear (Dengel *et al.* 1989; Miura *et al.* 1997). Factors such as seat position, crank length, wheel size, body position, aerobars and shoe/pedal interfaces have all been investigated (Cullen *et al.* 1992; Berry *et al.* 1994; Gregor & Wheeler 1994; Sheel *et al.* 1996). None of these factors entirely explain differences in cycling economy among athletes, but all probably contribute in varying amounts, with different factors being more important to the performance of individual athletes.

Lactate threshold and performance

It has long been thought that distance running performance is directly related to the ability of an athlete to use a large fraction of $\dot{V}O_{2max}$ (Costill *et al.* 1973). The ability to use a large percentage of $\dot{V}O_{2max}$ depends in large part on the athlete's lactate threshold. Lactate thresholds, expressed as a percentage of $\dot{V}O_{2max}$, are similar for equally well-trained men and women (Table 36.1), and are equally important to successful endurance performance (e.g. O'Toole *et al.* 1989; Daniels & Daniels 1992; Laurenson *et al.* 1993; O'Toole & Douglas 1995). Élite marathon runners run their races at an average pace equivalent to 86% of $\dot{V}O_{2max}$ or 93% of their $4 \, mmol \cdot l^{-1}$ lactate threshold (Sjodin & Svedenhag 1985). Slower marathon runners reportedly run at only 65% $\dot{V}O_{2max}$. There is some evidence that highly trained athletes (both men and women), who have reached their genetic ceiling for $\dot{V}O_{2max}$ through hard training, can still improve performance by augmenting their lactate threshold. Kohrt *et al.* (1989) reported increased thresholds for cycling (6%) and running (10%) during the course of a season where performance improved. Neither the time course nor the optimal training stimulus for improvement of lactate thresholds is known.

Better performance times are associated with use of a lower percentage of $\dot{V}_{O_{2max}}$ at a specific pace. For example, runners show a highly significant correlation ($r = 0.94$) between marathon performance and the percentage of $\dot{V}_{O_{2max}}$ used during a treadmill run at $15\,km\cdot h^{-1}$ (Sjodin & Svedenhag 1985). Similarly, élite women triathletes require a significantly ($P < 0.01$) lower percentage of $\dot{V}_{O_{2max}}$ than club triathletes when running at $15\,km\cdot h^{-1}$ (Laurenson et al. 1993). In a comprehensive study of triathletes, event-specific percentage $\dot{V}_{O_{2max}}$ was calculated for swimming at $1\,m\cdot s^{-1}$, cycling at $200\,W$ and running at $12\,km\cdot h^{-1}$. These were significantly related to swimming ($r = 0.91$), cycling ($r = 0.78$) and running ($r = 0.86$) performance times in a half-Ironman distance triathlon (Dengel et al. 1989). As with other physiological measures, the relationship between $\%\dot{V}_{O_{2max}}$ and performance becomes weaker as the length of the triathlon increases. However, we have previously reported a moderately good correlation ($r = 0.61$) between $\%\dot{V}_{O_{2max}}$ during cycling at $160\,W$ and cycle finish times for both men and women competing in an Ironman triathlon (O'Toole et al. 1989). There is no evidence that men and women differ in this aspect of performance.

Other practices to enhance endurance training

Although winning performances require optimization of the above-mentioned training adaptations, additional factors also contribute to competitive outcome. Other practices that are used to enhance the effects of endurance training include altitude training, nutritional modification and resistance training. Periodization of training schedules is employed to minimize the chance of injury and/or overtraining.

Nutritional modification

To derive optimal training benefits from sustained distance and aerobic interval training, energy balance as well as fluid and electrolyte balance must be maintained on a daily basis. During sustained distance and aerobic interval training, the athlete metabolizes a combination of fat and carbohydrate.

Since fat stores are essentially unlimited, the focus should be on the overall energy balance and consumption of sufficient carbohydrate to maintain glycogen stores. It is generally accepted that $8–10\,g$ carbohydrate$\cdot kg^{-1}\cdot day^{-1}$ ($600–650\,g$ carbohydrate) are necessary to maintain maximal glycogen storage (Sherman & Lamb 1988). How well female athletes comply with these recommendations depends on the specific sport for which they are training. For example, triathletes have an energy intake appropriate to the amount and type of training, and carbohydrate intake ($6.7–8.8\,g$ carbohydrate$\cdot kg^{-1}\cdot day^{-1}$) is also quite close to recommended amounts (Burke & Read 1987; Khoo et al. 1987; Applegate 1989). Conversely, female cross-country runners (for whom thinness may be perceived as more important) fall short of both energy and carbohydrate requirements (Tanaka et al. 1995). The effects on performance of failing to follow these recommendations are not clear, since women athletes demonstrate greater lipid and less carbohydrate or protein metabolism during moderate-intensity exercise than equally trained male athletes (Tarnopolsky et al. 1990).

In addition to daily energy/carbohydrate balance, many endurance athletes follow carbohydrate loading regimens before important competitions. During typical carbohydrate loading, dietary carbohydrate is increased to 75% of energy intake for 4 days before competition (Chapter 29). Recent research, however, has cast doubt on the usefulness of this practice for female athletes. Tarnopolsky et al. (1995) reported that although men increased muscle glycogen concentration by 41% following such a routine, no change in glycogen concentration was seen in women athletes. This resulted in a 45% improvement in cycling performance at 85% $\dot{V}_{O_{2max}}$ for men, but no significant change (5%) in women. Confirmation of these apparent gender differences is needed in larger groups of women athletes and in different exercise modes.

Another major consideration is the maintenance of fluid and electrolyte balance (Chapter 29). To maintain body temperature within tolerable limits, the high rate of heat production that occurs with aerobic exercise training and competition must be balanced by a high rate of heat loss. This requires a high sweat rate and, therefore, loss of both fluids and electrolytes (Nadel 1988). Particularly in a hot environment, sustained distance training and aerobic interval training place large thermoregulatory demands on the female athlete. Tolerance of fluid consumption during endurance exercise appears to be a trainable phenomenon and should be incorporated into sustained distance and aerobic interval training (Sparling *et al.* 1993).

Resistance training

Many male and female athletes augment their endurance training with resistance training. Resistance training manipulates the load, velocity of movement, number of repetitions, number of sets and length of rest periods (Fleck & Kramer 1987; Perrin 1993). Of these variables, load seems the most important for the development of strength. No single combination of these components has been documented to produce the best results. Resistance must be at least 60% of maximum in order to make strength gains. However, most commonly, 80–90% maximal capacity (one repetition maximum, 1RM) is lifted for three to six repetitions per set and for three to five sets (Fleck & Kramer 1987). Many athletes quantify and manipulate the volume of training (the number of repetitions × sets × load) per session to optimize improvement in strength without undue fatigue (Tesch 1992). If muscular endurance (for instance, the ability to repeat submaximal efforts continually, as in tennis swings) is the desired outcome, a lower resistance can be used. Muscular endurance gains have been reported with resistance as low as 30% of maximal capacity if repetitions are continued until the muscle group is fatigued (Cureton *et al.* 1988). In addition to the resistance that is applied, the velocity of movement seems important in training for power (Perrin 1993). Slow-velocity training increases torque only at the training velocity. Fast-velocity training seems to have the added advantage of increasing torque not only at the training velocity, but also at movement speeds slower than the training velocity. Since angular velocities for most sport movements are greater than commonly used isokinetic training velocities, it makes intuitive sense that the athlete

should train at the highest velocity possible for a given power requirement. The length of the rest periods is also important. Relatively long (several minutes) rest periods between sets are used when the goal is to increase strength. Conversely, shorter rest periods (<1 min) are used between sets when training muscular endurance (Fleck & Kramer 1987). Training 2–4 days a week is thought by weightlifters to be the most effective schedule. However, they frequently emphasize only one muscle group during a workout. This muscle group is then rested for 48–72 h before carrying out another strength training session. Whether this is an appropriate way to train strength in other than competitive resistance athletes remains unknown. Once the athlete has achieved the desired level of strength (usually within 1 year of serious training), this level can be maintained by as little as one training session per week, or by multiple sessions with reduced volume as long as the resistance load is maintained. The male athlete is typically stronger than the female competitor, but both respond to resistance training by similar patterns of strength gains and similar changes in muscle cross-sectional area (Wilmore 1974; Weltman *et al.* 1978; Cureton *et al.* 1988; Tesch 1992). Some controversy continues regarding concurrent strength and endurance training (Dudley & Djamil 1985; Callister *et al.* 1990; Chromiak & Mulvaney 1990), although most studies suggest that concurrent training has little effect on aerobic power or capacity. The optimal combination of endurance and resistance training for endurance athletes is unknown.

Altitude training

Athletes attempt to increase their haematocrits in a number of ways in order to increase oxygen transport in the blood. The most common approach is altitude training (Chapter 41). Acclimatization to an altitude of more than 2200 m is likely to increase the haematocrit within 8–10 days. Unfortunately for the athlete, the initial increase in haematocrit results from a decrease in plasma volume, rather than from a large increase in red cell mass (Selby & Eichner 1994). With continued altitude exposure, hypoxia-induced increases in erythropoiesis cause haematocrits to rise, while the plasma volume returns to pre-exposure levels. Berglund (1992) suggested that a much longer altitude acclimatization period than is commonly used (10–12 weeks rather than 2–3 weeks) would be necessary for athletes to achieve the desired increments in haematocrit and plasma volume levels. More recently, Levine and Stray-Gundersen (1997) suggested a 'living high, training low' regimen, whereby red cell mass could be increased without change in blood volume. These physiological increases in haematocrit are anecdotally perceived by athletes to be beneficial to endurance performance. Scientific evidence of the benefits of altitude training for sea-level perfor-mance is less clear in either men or women athletes (Chapter 41).

Periodization

Periodization is the purposeful variation of a train-ing programme over time, so that the athlete will approach her optimal adaptive potential just before an important competition. A systematic, sequential approach is used, organizing training into blocks of time. In its simplest form, athletes use a hard/easy pattern for daily workouts. In its more complete form, the training year is divided into time blocks ranging from days to weeks to months. During each of these blocks, a particular aspect of training is emphasized.

The longest blocks of time are called macrocycles; these usually last for 2–4 months. There may be three or four macrocycles per year. Smaller blocks, mesocycles, are organized within each macrocycle. A mesocycle typically lasts 8–10 weeks. In turn, microcycles, usually of 1 week's duration, make up the mesocycles. Training volumes and intensities are varied by cycle. Volume and intensity of effort are typically varied inversely. The exact make-up of each cycle, however, depends on the specific demands of the competitive event, including one primary and several secondary foci. For example, during the first macrocycle of a training period (fre-quently referred to as the preparatory phase), high-volume/low-intensity workouts are emphasized. For an endurance athlete, sustained distance and aerobic interval training make up the bulk of train-ing, perhaps supplemented by some low-resistance and medium- to high-volume weight training. As the athlete progresses toward competition, training volumes are decreased and intensities increased. The last mesocycle before an important event is typically divided into two parts. During the first part, the emphasis is on maximal intensity, very short-duration specific training (based on the strength, power and endurance requirements for that particular sport). The second part of the last mesocycle is the taper. Some tapering is universally accepted. It is a means of optimizing performance by allowing adequate recovery from hard training before an important competition (Wells & Pate 1988). During a taper, some combination of training frequency, intensity and volume is altered to reduce the training stimulus. Most evidence indicates that a rather drastic reduction in volume (dropping to 10–15% of usual training volume) in combination with short intense workouts gives an optimal result (Shepley et al. 1992; Houmard & Johns 1994). This type of taper improves performance by approxi-mately 3% in swimmers and distance runners. Nev-ertheless, athletes find the taper a difficult part of training to accept. Typically, athletes reduce their training volume by at least two-thirds for about a week. This may not be a long enough change for an optimal response. Costill et al. (1985) reported a 3–4% improvement in swim times following a 15-day taper where training distance was reduced by two-thirds. This work, as well as that of Hickson and Rosenkoetter (1981), shows that training adap-tations can be maintained and perhaps even poten-tiated by appropriate use of tapering. Although evaluation of individual periodization routines is difficult, shorter mesocycles can be evaluated to determine the efficacy of specific aspects of training. There is no evidence that periodization schedules should be different for men and women athletes.

Avoidance of overtraining

Overtraining, a long-term (weeks to months) decre-ment in performance with or without related physiological and psychological signs or symptoms, can be a serious problem for the competitive athlete (Chapter 34; Kreider et al. 1997). To achieve optimal athletic performance, serious athletes devote many years to rigorous training. An athlete who does not train hard enough may never reach her potential, so that many athletes adopt a 'more is better' philosophy. Unfortunately, training too often and/or too intensely may lead to physiological maladaptations and a decrease in performance. It can be difficult to determine the optimal amount of training to optimize the performance of individual athletes. Amounts of training that are optimal for one athlete may undertrain or overtrain others. To complicate the issue further, both undertraining and overtraining may result in performance plateaus. The usual response to a performance plateau is to increase the amount and intensity of training. If the reason for the plateau is undertraining, additional training may be of benefit. If, on the other hand, the reason for the plateau is overtraining, further training will exacerbate the problem and, in all likelihood, it will lead to further decrements in performance.

The maladaptations of overtraining are essentially an imbalance between stimulus and recovery. Multiple signs and symptoms have been associated with overtraining (Fry *et al.* 1991), ranging from generalized fatigue to more specific physiological symptoms. Alternatively, a specific physiological system may break down (for example, an overuse injury such as a stress fracture). Reports are sometimes contradictory, e.g. both increased and decreased resting heart rates have been described in overtrained runners. Single or multiple symptoms in any combination or the absence of physiological symptoms may be found in an overtrained athlete. The one universal finding is a decrease in performance. Not all aspects of performance, however, are affected simultaneously or to the same degree. Identification of physiological markers prodromal to the overtraining syndrome in women endurance athletes is currently difficult and should be addressed in future research.

Summary

The physiological demands of most sporting events are similar for men and women athletes. Likewise, training methods seem to be similar. Although men athletes may be swifter and stronger than women athletes in absolute terms, women athletes respond to training with many of the same physiological adaptations. Much is known about the initial responses of women to training and about the physiological adaptations (e.g. changes in cardiac structure and function) attributed to multiyear training. Much less is known about the small adaptations that occur throughout an athlete's career, allowing her to reach her full potential. This gap in knowledge should be addressed in future studies of women athletes.

References

Abernathy, P.J., Thayer, R. & Taylor, A.W. (1990) Acute and chronic responses of skeletal muscle to endurance and spring exercise: a review. *Sports Medicine* 10, 365–389.

Applegate, E. (1989) Nutritional concerns of the ultraendurance athlete. *Medicine and Science in Sports and Exercise* 21 (Suppl.), S205–S208.

Åstrand, P.-O. & Rodahl, K., (1986) *Textbook of Work Physiology*, 3rd edn. McGraw-Hill Book Company, New York.

Berglund, B. (1992) High-altitude training: aspects of haematological adaptation. *Sports Medicine* 14, 289–303.

Berry, M.J., Pollock, W.E., van Nieuwenhuizen, K. & Brubaker, P.H. (1994) A comparison between aero and standard racing handlebars during prolonged exercise. *International Journal of Sports Medicine* 15, 16–20.

Burke, L.M. & Read, R.S.D. (1987) Diet patterns of élite Australian male triathletes. *Physician and Sportsmedicine* 15, 140–155.

Butts, N.K., Henry, B.A. & Mclean, D. (1991) Correlations between $\dot{V}_{O_2max}$ and performance times of recreational triathletes. *Journal of Sports Medicine and Physical Fitness* 31, 339–344.

Callister, R., Callister, R.J., Fleck, S.J. & Dudley, G.A. (1990) Physiological and performance responses to overtraining in élite judo athletes. *Medicine and Science in Sports and Exercise* 22, 816–824.

Chromiak, J.A. & Mulvaney, D.R. (1990) A review: the effects of combined strength and endurance training on strength development. *Journal of Applied Sport Science Research* 4, 55–60.

Clausen, J.P. (1977) Effect of physical training on cardiovascular adjustments to exercise in man. *Physiological Reviews* 57, 779–815.

Conley, D.L. & Krahenbuhl, G.S. (1980) Running economy and distance running performance of highly trained athletes. *Medicine and Science in Sports and Exercise* 12, 357–360.

Costill, D.L. (1986) *Inside Running: Basics of Sport Physiology*. Benchmark Press, Indianapolis.

Costill, D.L., Thomason, H. & Roberts, E. (1973) Fractional utilization of aerobic capacity during distance running. *Medicine and Science in Sports and Exercise* 5, 248–252.

Costill, D.L., King, D.S., Thomas, R. & Hargreaves, M. (1985) Effects of reduced training on muscular power in swimmers. *Physician and Sportsmedicine* **13** (2), 94–101.

Costill, D.L., Fink, W.J., Flynn, M. & Kirwan, J. (1987) Muscle fiber composition and enzyme activities in élite female distance runners. *International Journal of Sports Medicine* **8**, 1031–1036.

Crawford, M.H., Petru, M.A. & Rabinowitz, C. (1986) Effect of isotonic exercise training on left ventricular volume during upright exercise. *Circulation* **72**, 1237–1243.

Cullen, L.K., Andrew, K., Lair, K.R., Widger, M.J. & Timson, B.F. (1992) Efficiency of trained cyclists using circular and noncircular chainrings. *International Journal of Sports Medicine* **13**, 264–269.

Cureton, K.J., Collins, M.A., Hill, D.W. & Mcelhannon, F.M. (1988) Muscle hypertrophy in men and women. *Medicine and Science in Sports and Exercise* **20**, 338–344.

Daniels, J.T. (1985) A physiologist's view of running economy. *Medicine and Science in Sports and Exercise* **17**, 332–338.

Daniels, J. & Daniels, N. (1992) Running economy of élite male and élite female runners. *Medicine and Science in Sports and Exercise* **24**, 483–489.

Dengel, D.R., Flynn, M.G., Costill, D.L. & Kirwan, J.P. (1989) Determinants of success during triathlon competition. *Research Quarterly for Exercise and Sport* **60**, 234–238.

Douglas, P.S. (1989) Cardiac considerations in the triathlete. *Medicine and Science in Sports and Exercise* **21** (Suppl.), S214–S218.

Douglas, P.S. & O'Toole, M.L. (1992) Aging and physical activity determine cardiac structure and function in the older athlete. *Journal of Applied Physiology* **72**, 1969–1973.

Douglas, P.S., O'Toole, M.L., Hiller, W.D.B. & Reichek, N. (1986) Left ventricular structure and function by echocardiography in ultraendurance athletes. *American Journal of Cardiology* **58**, 805–809.

Douglas, P.S., O'Toole, M.L., Hiller, W.D.B., Hackney, K. & Reichek, N. (1988) Electrocardiographic diagnosis of exercise-induced left ventricular hypertrophy. *American Heart Journal* **116**, 786–790.

Douglas, P.S., O'Toole, M.L., Katz, S.E., Ginsburg, G.S., Hiller, W.D.B. & Laird, R.H. (1997) Left ventricular hypertrophy in athletes. *American Journal of Cardiology* **80**, 1384–1388.

Dudley, G.A. & Djamil, R. (1985) Incompat- ibility of endurance and strength training modes of exercise. *Journal of Applied Physiology* **59**, 1446–1451.

Durstine, J.L., Pate, R.R., Sparling, P.B., Wilson, G.E., Senn, M.D. & Bartoli, W.P. (1987) Lipid, lipoprotein, and iron status of élite women distance runners. *International Journal of Sports Medicine* (Suppl. 2) **8**, 119–123.

Dwyer, J. & Bybee, R. (1983) Heart rate indices of the anaerobic threshold. *Medicine and Science in Sports and Exercise* **15**, 72–76.

Ekblom, B. & Hermanson, L. (1968) Cardiac output in athletes. *Journal of Applied Physiology* **25**, 619–625.

Fleck, S.J. & Kramer, W.J. (1987) *Designing Resistance Training Programs.* Human Kinetics, Champaign, IL.

Fry, R.W., Morton, A.R. & Keast, D. (1991) Overtraining in athletes. *Sports Medicine* **12**, 32–65.

Gilman, M.B. & Wells, C.L. (1993) The use of heart rates to monitor exercise intensity in relation to metabolic variables. *International Journal of Sports Medicine* **14**, 3334–3339.

Gledhill, N., Cox, D. & Jamink, R. (1994) Endurance athletes' stroke volume does not plateau: major advantage is diastolic function. *Medicine and Science in Sports and Exercise* **26**, 1116–1121.

Gollnick, P.D. (1985) Metabolism of substrates during exercise and as modified by training. *Federation Proceedings* **44**, 353–357.

Gollnick, P.D., Armstrong, R.B., Saubert, C.W., Piehl, K. & Saltin, B. (1972) Enzyme activity and fiber composition in skeletal muscle of untrained and trained men. *Journal of Applied Physiology* **33**, 312–319.

Gollnick, P.D., Bayly, W.M. & Hodgson, D.R. (1986) Exercise intensity, training, diet, and lactate concentration in muscle and blood. *Medicine and Science in Sports and Exercise* **18**, 334–340.

Gregor, R.J. & Wheeler, J.B. (1994) Biomechanical factors associated with shoe/pedal interfaces. Implications for injury. *Sports Medicine* **17**, 117–131.

Hamel, P., Simoneau, J.-A., Lortie, G., Boulay, M.R. & Bouchard, C. (1986) Heredity and muscle adaptation to endurance training. *Medicine and Science in Sports and Exercise* **18**, 690–699.

Harrison, M.H. (1985) Effects of thermal stress and exercise on blood volume in humans. *Physiological Reviews* **65**, 149–199.

Hickson, R.C. & Rosenkoetter, M.A. (1981) Reduced training frequencies and main- tenance of increased aerobic power. *Medicine and Science in Sports and Exercise* **13**, 13–16.

Holloszy, J.O. (1975) Adaptation of skeletal muscle to endurance exercise. *Medicine and Science in Sports and Exercise* **7**, 155–164.

Holloszy, J.O. & Coyle, E.F. (1984) Adaptations of skeletal muscle to endurance exercise and their metabolic consequences. *Journal of Applied Physiology* **56**, 831–838.

Houmard, J.A. & Johns, R.A. (1994) Effects of taper on swim performance. Practical implications. *Sports Medicine* **17**, 224–232.

Kearney, J.T. (1996) Training the Olympic athlete. *Scientific American* **274**, 52–63.

Khoo, C.S., Rawson, N.E. & Robinson, M.L. (1987) Nutrient intake and eating habits of triathletes. *Annals of Sports Medicine* **3**, 144–150.

Klausen, K., Andersen, L.B. & Pelle, I. (1981) Adaptive changes in work capacity, skeletal muscle capilliarization, and enzyme levels during training and detraining. *Acta Physiologica Scandinavica* **113**, 9–16.

Kohrt, W.M., O'Connor, J.S. & Skinner, J.S. (1989) Longitudinal assessment of responses by triathletes to swimming, cycling, and running. *Medicine and Science in Sports and Exercise* **21**, 569–575.

Kreider, R.B., Fry, A.C. & O'Toole, M.L. (eds) (1997) *Overtraining in Sport.* Human Kinetics, Champaign, IL.

Laurenson, N.M., Fulcher, K.Y. & Korkia, P. (1993) Physiological characteristics of élite and club level female triathletes during running. *International Journal of Sports Medicine* **14**, 455–459.

Levine, B.D. & Stray-Gundersen, J. (1997) 'Living high–training low': effect of moderate-altitude acclimatization with low-altitude training on performance. *Journal of Applied Physiology* **83**, 102–112.

Levine, B.D., Lane, L.D., Buckey, J.C., Friedman, D.B. & Blomqvist, C.G. (1991) Left ventricular pressure–volume and Frank–Starling relations in endurance athletes: Implications for orthostatic tolerance and exercise performance. *Circulation* **84**, 1016–1023.

Levy, W.C., Cerqueira, M.D.S., Abrass, I.B., Schwartz, R.S. & Stratton, J.R. (1993) Endurance exercise training augments diastolic filling at rest and during exercise in healthy young and older men. *Circulation* **88**, 116–126.

McArdle, W.D., Katch, F.I. & Katch, V.L. (1992) *Exercise Physiology. Energy, Nutri-

tion and Performance, 3rd edn, p. 177. Lea & Febiger, Philadelphia.

Margaria, R., Cerretelli, P. & Aghens, P. (1963) Energy cost of running. *Journal of Applied Physiology* 18, 367–370.

Martin, R.P., Haskell, W.L. & Wood, P.D. (1977) Blood chemistry and lipid profiles of élite distance runners. In: Milvy, P. (ed.) *The Marathon: Physiological, Medical, Epidemiological, and Psychological Studies* 301, pp. 346–360. Annals of the New York Academy of Sciences, New York.

Miura, H., Kitagawa, K. & Ishiko, R. (1997) Economy during a simulated laboratory test triathlon is highly related to Olympic distance triathlon. *International Journal of Sports Medicine* 18, 276–280.

Morgan, D.W. & Craib, M. (1992) Physiological aspects of running economy. *Medicine and Science in Sports and Exercise* 24, 456–461.

Nadel, E.R. (1988) Temperature regulation and prolonged exercise. In: Lamb, D.R. & Murray, R. (eds) *Prospectives in Exercise Science and Sports Medicine*, Vol. 1. *Prolonged Exercise*, pp. 25–47. Benchmark Press Inc, Indianapolis.

Noakes, T.D. (1991) *Lore of Running*, pp. 60–61. Oxford University Press, Cape Town.

O'Toole, M.L. & Douglas, P.S. (1995) Applied physiology of triathlon. *Sports Medicine* 19, 251–267.

O'Toole, M.L., Hiller, W.D.B., Crosby, L.O. & Douglas, P.S. (1987) The ultra-endurance triathlete: a physiologic profile. *Medicine and Science in Sports and Exercise* 19, 45–50.

O'Toole, M.L., Douglas, P.S. & Hiller, W.D.B. (1989) Lactate, oxygen uptake, and cycling performance in triathletes. *International Journal of Sports Medicine* 10, 413–418.

Oscai, L.B., Williams, B.T. & Hertig, B.A. (1968) Effect of exercise on blood volume. *Journal of Applied Physiology* 26, 622–624.

Pate, R.R., Sparling, P.B., Wilson, G.E., Cureton, K.J. & Miller, B.J. (1987) Cardiorespiratory and metabolic responses to submaximal and maximal exercise in élite women distance runners. *International Journal of Sports Medicine* 8 (Suppl.), 91–95.

Pelliccia, A., Maron, B.J., Culasso, F., Spataro, A. & Caselli, G. (1996) Athlete's heart in women. Echocardiographic characterization of highly trained élite female athletes. *Journal of the American Medical Association* 276, 211–215.

Perrin, D.H. (1993) *Isokinetic Exercise and Assessment*. Human Kinetics, Champaign, IL.

Plowman, S.A. & Smith, D.L. (1997) *Exercise Physiology for Health, Fitness and Performance*. Allyn & Bacon, Boston.

Pollack, S.J., McMillan, S.T., Mumpower, E. *et al.* (1987) Echocardiographic analysis of élite women distance runners. *International Journal of Sports Medicine* 8 (Suppl.), 81–83.

Saltin, B. (1969) Physiological effects of physical conditioning. *Medicine and Science in Sports* 1, 50.

Saltin, B. & Rowell, L.B. (1980) Functional adaptations to physical activity and inactivity. *Federation Proceedings* 39, 1506–1513.

Saltin, B., Henriksson, J., Nygaard, E. & Andersen, P. (1977) Fiber types and metabolic potentials of skeletal muscles in sedentary man and endurance runners. In: Milvy, P. (ed.) *The Marathon: Physiological, Medical, Epidemiological, and Psychological Studies* 301, pp. 3–29. Annals of the New York Academy of Sciences, New York.

Selby, G.B. & Eichner, E.R. (1994) Hematocrit and performance: the effect of endurance training on blood volume. *Seminars in Hematology* 31, 122–127.

Sheel, A.W., Lama, I., Potvin, P., Coutts, K.D. & McKenzie, D.C. (1996) Comparison of aerobars versus traditional cycling postures on physiological parameters during submaximal cycling. *Canadian Journal of Applied Physiology* 21, 16–22.

Shepley, B., MacDougall, J.D., Cipriano, N. & Sutton, J.R. (1992) Physiological effects of tapering in highly trained athletes. *Journal of Applied Physiology* 72, 706–711.

Sherman, W.M. & Lamb, D.R. (1988) Nutrition and prolonged exercise. In: Lamb, D.R. & Murray, R. (eds) *Perspectives in Exercise Science and Sports Medicine*, Vol. 1. *Prolonged Exercise*, pp. 213–276. Benchmark Press Inc, Indianapolis.

Sjodin, B. & Svedenhag, J. (1985) Applied physiology of marathon running. *Sports Medicine* 2, 83–99.

Sparling, P.B., Wilson, G.E. & Pate, R.R. (1987) Project overview and description of performance, training, and physical characteristics in élite women distance runners. *International Journal of Sports Medicine* 8 (Suppl.), 73–76.

Sparling, P.B., Nieman, D.C. & O'Connor, P.J. (1993) Selected scientific aspects of marathon racing. An update on fluid replacement, immune function, psychological factors and the gender difference. *Sports Medicine* 15, 116–132.

Speechly, D.P., Taylor, S.R. & Rogers, G.G. (1995) Differences in ultra-endurance exercise performance-matched male and female runners. *Medicine and Science in Sports and Exercise* 28, 359–365.

Tanaka, J.A., Tanaka, H. & Landis, W. (1995) An assessment of carbohydrate intake in collegiate distance runners. *International Journal of Sport Nutrition* 5, 206–214.

Tarnopolsky, L.J., MacDougall, J.D., Atkinson, S.A., Tarnopolsky, M.A. & Sutton, J.R. (1990) Gender differences in substrate for endurance exercise. *Journal of Applied Physiology* 68, 302–308.

Tarnopolsky, M.A., Atkinson, S.A., Phillips, S.M. & MacDougall, J.D. (1995) Carbohydrate loading and metabolism during exercise in men and women. *Journal of Applied Physiology* 78, 1360–1368.

Tesch, P.A. (1992) Training for body building. In: Komi, P.V. (ed.) *Strength and Power in Sport*, pp. 357–369. Blackwell Scientific Publications, Oxford.

Toussaint, H.M. & Beck, P.J. (1992) Biomechanics of competitive front crawl swimming. *Sports Medicine* 13, 8–24.

Vanfraechem, J.H.P. (1979) Stroke volume and systolic time interval adjustments during bicycle exercise. *Journal of Applied Physiology* 46, 588–592.

Vanoverschelde, J.L.J., Younis, L.T., Melin, J.A. *et al.* (1991) Prolonged exercise induces left ventricular dysfunction in healthy subjects. *Journal of Applied Physiology* 70, 1356–1363.

Wells, C.L. (1991) *Women, Sport and Performance: a Physiological Perspective*, 2nd edn. Human Kinetics, Champaign, IL.

Wells, C.L. & Pate, R.R. (1988) Training for performance of prolonged exercise. In: Lamb, D.R. & Murray, R. (eds) *Perspectives in Exercise Science and Sports Medicine*, Vol. 1. *Prolonged Exercise*, pp. 357–391. Benchmark Press, Indianapolis.

Weltman, A.R., Moffatt, R.J. & Stamford, B.A. (1978) Supramaximal training in females: effects on anaerobic power output, anaerobic capacity, and aerobic power. *Journal of Sports Medicine and Physical Fitness* 18, 237–244.

Williams, K. & Cavanagh, P. (1987) Relationship between distance running mechanics, running economy and performance. *Journal of Applied Physiology* 63, 1236–1245.

Wilmore, J.H. (1974) Alterations in strength, body composition, and anthropometric measurements consequent to a 10 week weight training program. *Medicine and Science in Sports* 6, 133–138.

Chapter 37

Pregnant Women and Endurance Exercise

LARRY A. WOLFE

Introduction

There is a substantial overlap between a woman's childbearing years and those that comprise the competitive years of female endurance athletes. Since regular intensive endurance exercise may compromise fetal growth and development, many female athletes choose to interrupt their athletic careers temporarily in order to have children (Hale & Milne 1996). This usually includes a reduction in training intensity and avoidance of competition during pregnancy, followed by a gradual return to intensive conditioning and competition postpartum. There are many known examples of women who have recorded personal best performances following childbirth (Zaharieva 1972), and there is reason to believe that pregnancy may enhance cardiovascular capacities (Wolfe *et al.* 1999).

The purpose of this chapter is to summarize current information on the interactive effects of pregnancy and endurance exercise, providing advice for maintenance of basic fitness during pregnancy and for return to strenuous training and competition after delivery.

Physiological effects of pregnancy

The physiological and anatomical changes of pregnancy are initiated and maintained by ovarian and placental hormones. Functions of virtually all of the systems of the body are altered in order to accommodate the various needs of the growing fetus (Table 37.1). The most important of these for endurance performance include carbohydrate metabolism, heart and circulatory function and circulation, respiration and acid–base balance, and thermoregulation.

Carbohydrate metabolism

During the first trimester of pregnancy (known as the 'anabolic' phase) insulin secretion by the pancreas increases, causing an increase in maternal adiposity (Hollingsworth 1985). During the latter half of pregnancy, there is an increase in peripheral insulin sensitivity caused by circulating placental hormones. This in turn causes an increase in maternal fat metabolism and carbohydrate sparing, protecting fetal access to the maternal blood glucose pool (Hollingsworth 1985). This is especially important for fetal growth, since glucose is its main source of energy.

Heart and circulation

Gestational hormones cause substantial remodelling of the maternal cardiovascular system (Morton *et al.* 1985; Capeless & Clapp 1989). Changes include dilatation of all four chambers of the heart, widening of the aortic diameter (Wolfe *et al.* 1999), enlargement of the venous capacitance vessels and dilatation of arteriolar resistance vessels (Duvekot *et al.* 1993). These changes are accompanied by a gradual 40–50% increase in blood volume (Lund & Donovan 1967), and a 10–15 beat·min^{-1} increase in resting heart rate (HR) (Clapp 1985), as well as increases in stroke volume (SV) and cardiac output ($\dot{Q}$) in the resting state and during standard

Table 37.1 Pregnancy-induced changes that may alter endurance performance in late gestation.

Change	Postulated mechanism	Effect on endurance performance
Increased resting metabolic rate	Fetal energy requirements	Less energy available for muscle contraction
Increased diaphragmatic work of breathing	Reduced expiratory reserve volume	Maximum breathing capacity may be reduced
Reduced maximal heart rate	Blunted sympathoadrenal response to strenuous exercise	Reduced maximal heart rate reserve
Increased resting heart rate	Reduced parasympathetic cardiac modulation at rest	
Increased maternal body mass	Fetal growth increases maternal adiposity	Increased energy cost of weight-supported work
Reduced peak blood lactate levels after strenuous exercise	Insulin resistance, dilution of lactate in expanded maternal blood volume; fetal/placental lactate utilization	Possible reduction in ability to use carbohydrate and produce lactate during strenuous exercise

submaximal exercise (Guzman & Caplan 1970; Sady *et al.* 1989, 1990; Pivarnik *et al.* 1990).

Respiration and acid–base balance

The anatomical changes of pregnancy tend to raise the midposition of the diaphragm, reducing expiratory reserve volume, residual lung volume and total lung volume (Ratigan 1983). However, there is an increase in inspiratory capacity and no appreciable change in vital capacity despite the fact that the total lung capacity is moderately reduced (Ratigan 1983).

Owing to the effects of augmented circulating progesterone (and perhaps other factors), pregnant women exhibit a marked increase in respiratory sensitivity (Wolfe *et al.* 1998). In the resting state (Lyons & Antonio 1959; Moore *et al.* 1987), this results in an increase in minute ventilation ($\dot{V}_E$) from approximately $6 \, l \cdot min^{-1}$ to approximately $9 \, l \cdot min^{-1}$, primarily as a result of an increase in tidal volume (Knuttgen & Emerson 1974; Pernoll *et al.* 1975). This in turn causes an increase in arterial oxygen tension and a reduction in carbon dioxide tension. To compensate for the decrease in carbon dioxide tension, the kidneys excrete bicarbonate, resulting in a partly compensated state of respiratory alkalosis (pH $\approx$ 7.46) (Hytten 1968; Blechner 1993). These changes

help to facilitate maternal–fetal gas exchange before the fetal cardiovascular system becomes functional (Liberatore *et al.* 1984). Dyspnoea (a feeling of breathlessness) is a commonly reported subjective symptom during pregnancy and may be related to the increase in ventilatory drive described above (Gilbert *et al.* 1962; Field *et al.* 1991).

Thermoregulation

By late gestation, maternal body core temperature increases by approximately 0.5°C compared to the non-pregnant state (i.e. to 37.5°C). Fetal temperature is approximately 39°C, and thus it is theoretically possible to gain heat from rather than lose heat to the maternal system if the maternal core temperature rises too high (Lotgering *et al.* 1983b). Maternal heat loss is made more difficult by the progressive increase in the woman's body mass/body surface area ratio with advancing gestational age. However, this is compensated via augmented peripheral vasodilatation and a reduced threshold for sweating (Clapp *et al.* 1987; Clapp 1991).

Effects of pregnancy on endurance performance

The effects of pregnancy on endurance performance

depend greatly on whether the exercise modality is weight-bearing (e.g. walking, running) or non-weight-bearing (e.g. stationary cycling). Whenever exercise involves significant weight-bearing, there is a progressive reduction in performance measures, because of the additional energy required to move an increased body mass (Artal *et al.* 1989). Values for aerobic power ($\dot{V}_{O_{2max}}$) expressed per kg body mass fall progressively with advancing gestational age.

Values for $\dot{V}_{O_{2max}}$ expressed in absolute terms ($l \cdot min^{-1}$) have variously been reported to be decreased, unchanged or increased compared to the non-pregnant state (Sady *et al.* 1990; Clapp & Capeless 1991; Lotgering *et al.* 1991; Wolfe & Mottola 1993). These contradictory findings may be related to differences in aerobic fitness prior to pregnancy and subsequent changes in activity during the puerperium. Very fit women are likely to reduce their activity levels during pregnancy to maintain comfort and preserve fetal safety (Clapp & Capeless 1991). Conversely, women who have very low fitness levels before pregnancy may actually become better conditioned as a result of carrying a greater body mass during the activities of daily living (Webb *et al.* 1994).

Physiological responses to strenuous exercise

Because of concerns for maternal and fetal safety, studies of maternal responses to maximal or near-maximal exercise are few in number. As noted above, reported effects on $\dot{V}_{O_{2max}}$ ($l \cdot min^{-1}$) have been variable. There appears to be little or no effect on the mechanical efficiency (i.e. $\dot{V}_{O_2}$ or energy expended per unit of external work). However, resting O_2 consumption increases with advancing gestational age and therefore the energy available to perform external work is slightly reduced in late pregnancy.

Depending on posture, HR and SV are increased in pregnancy both at rest and during standard submaximal steady-state exercise. However, several studies have reported a moderate reduction in maximal HR during graded exercise testing (Lotgering *et al.* 1992). This effect is observed in association with a blunted sympathetic nervous system response to strenuous exercise (Bonen *et al.* 1992), and along with a higher resting HR (Clapp 1985), it

results in a substantially reduced maximal HR reserve (Fig. 37.1).

Recent research supports the concept that the ventilatory anaerobic threshold (T_{vent}) is not altered by pregnancy or advancing gestational age (Wolfe *et al.* 1994b; Lotgering *et al.* 1995). However, several studies in late gestation have reported reductions in the respiratory exchange ratio (RER) at peak exercise and/or peak postexercise lactate concentration during graded exercise testing (Clapp *et al.* 1987; McMurray *et al.* 1988; Lotgering *et al.* 1991; Wolfe *et al.* 1994b). Such findings can be explained by the reduced ability to metabolize carbohydrate and produce lactate, reduced glucose availability caused by blunted liver glycogenolysis, dilution of lactate in an expanded maternal blood volume, fetal/placental utilization of lactate as a metabolic fuel, or a combination of these factors (Wolfe *et al.* 1994a,b).

Healthy, active pregnant women maintain lower plasma hydrogen ion concentrations than non-pregnant women, both at rest and during and following strenuous exercise testing (Kemp *et al.* 1997). Exercise-induced changes are similar in magnitude to the non-pregnant state and the highest values achieved with maximal exercise testing are probably not high enough to reverse the maternal–fetal hydrogen ion gradient (Blechner *et al.* 1967; Kemp *et al.* 1997).

Effects of pregnancy on responses to aerobic conditioning

Pregnancy and aerobic conditioning are both powerful processes that result in substantial structural and functional changes. As described in detail elsewhere (Wolfe *et al.* 1989), these changes can be in the same direction or in opposite directions, depending on the specific variable that is being considered.

The effects of training on HR appear to be masked in the resting state (Wolfe *et al.* 1999). Presumably, the powerful endocrine effects of pregnancy reduce parasympathetic modulation and override the usual conditioning-induced enhancement of resting parasympathetic tone. Training-induced reductions of HR are seen during standard submaximal exercise, and they become more evident with increasing exercise intensity (Wolfe *et al.* 1999).

Pregnancy and regular exercise tend to increase

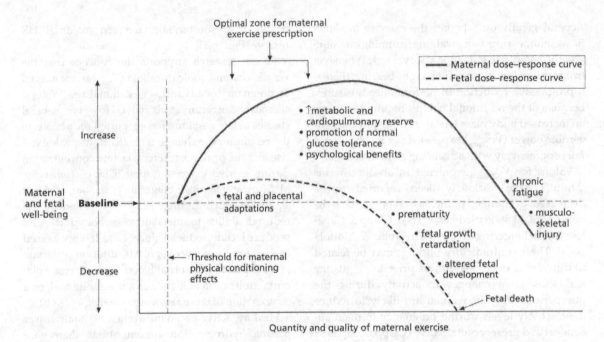

Fig. 37.1 Possible dose–response association between the quantity and quality of prenatal exercise and maternal/fetal well-being. From Wolfe *et al.* (1994a), with permission.

the blood volume and left ventricular mass. However, the effects of pregnancy are greater quantitatively, and they may obscure the effects of training on these variables, since training-induced changes in resting and exercise SV depend on an enhancement of blood volume and venous return. Therefore, the effects of aerobic conditioning on SV may also be masked in pregnant women (Morton *et al.* 1985; Wolfe *et al.* 1990).

Physical conditioning usually reduces subcutaneous adiposity, whereas pregnancy causes increases during the first and second trimesters (Taggart *et al.* 1967). In our experience, moderate conditioning does not prevent increases in adiposity in early pregnancy and it may help to conserve maternal energy stores in late gestation (Greer & Wolfe 1994). Presumably, this is because conditioning tends to attenuate the pregnancy-induced insulin resistance which occurs in late gestation (López-Luna *et al.* 1998). This effect may also help to prevent or treat gestational diabetes (Bung & Artal 1996).

From a metabolic viewpoint, the usual effects of

conditioning (to enhance fat versus carbohydrate utilization, and reduce carbon dioxide output and the RER during standard submaximal exercise) have been documented in healthy pregnant women (Ohtake & Wolfe 1998). The reduced carbon dioxide output may reduce the drive to ventilate and tends to offset pregnancy-induced increases in respiratory sensitivity. Since respiratory perception of effort is reduced, this effect may help to prevent or treat dyspnoea in pregnancy (Ohtake & Wolfe 1998).

Fetal responses to strenuous maternal exercise

Due to the inaccessibility of the human fetus, information on fetal responses to strenuous maternal exercise must be obtained using safe non-invasive methodologies (usually involving diagnostic ultrasound technology). The most important variables have included fetal heart rate (FHR) characteristics, fetal movements, FHR reactivity and fetal breathing movements (Wolfe *et al.* 1994a).

The most important concern with strenuous

maternal exercise is that maternal blood flow may be redistributed away from the uterus and toward contracting maternal skeletal muscle. Studies involving laboratory animals have shown that this effect is proportional to both the intensity and duration of exercise (Lotgering *et al.* 1983a). However, several protective mechanisms are available to preserve fetal oxygenation. These include exercise-induced haemoconcentration, redistribution of uterine blood flow favouring the uterine cotyledons over the myometrium, and enhanced fetal arteriovenous oxygen extraction (Wolfe *et al.* 1994b).

Fetal bradycardia (FHR ≤ 120 beats·min^{-1}) is a protective reflex that helps to conserve oxygen. It is associated with a fetal blood flow distribution that favours vital organs during fetal hypoxia. Reductions in fetal limb and breathing movements are also consistent with fetal conservation of oxygen. Fetal tachycardia (FHR > 160 beats·min^{-1}) may be observed during recovery from fetal hypoxia and as a reaction to mild hypoxia (Clapp *et al.* 1993), increases in fetal temperature (Lotgering *et al.* 1992) or leakage across the placenta of catecholamines from the maternal system (Sodha *et al.* 1984).

The most common fetal reaction to maternal exercise is an increase in FHR baseline (Watson *et al.* 1991; Clapp *et al.* 1993) which is often accompanied by a transient reduction in FHR reactivity (i.e. FHR acceleration, in association with fetal movement). Instances of transient fetal bradycardia in association with light to moderate exercise are rare in healthy, normally active women. Studies involving strenuous maximal or near-maximal exercise testing protocols have reported a significantly higher incidence of fetal bradycardia (overall incidence approximately 10–15%) during or following such exercise (Wolfe *et al.* 1994a) than during light to moderate exertion.

In healthy women undergoing a normal pregnancy, fetal bradycardia is usually transient and is most often observed immediately postexercise (Carpenter *et al.* 1988; Webb *et al.* 1994). The most likely cause is a temporary reduction in uterine blood flow, caused by a reduction in maternal venous return when skeletal muscle vascular beds are still vasodilated. Factors which may determine the incidence of exercise-induced fetal bradycardia include maternal characteristics (age, physical fitness, etc.), gestational age, the exercise modality, the muscle mass involved and the interactive effects of exercise intensity and duration (Lotgering *et al.* 1983a,b). Fetal bradycardia may be accompanied by reductions in fetal reactivity and breathing movements (Manders *et al.* 1997). Significant reductions in FHR variability (a measure of fetal central nervous system function) are rare and we are unaware of any reports of fetal decompensation or injury in association with maternal exercise testing.

Effects of endurance exercise on pregnancy outcome

The bulk of the available literature has focused on the interactive effects of endurance exercise and fetal growth (Wolfe *et al.* 1994a; Pivarnik 1998). Early investigations reported that continued participation in strenuous exercise by recreational athletes resulted in significant reductions in birthweight (Clapp & Dickstein 1984). Parallel studies of neonatal morphometrics further suggested that this was the result of reduced fetal adiposity (Clapp & Capeless 1990). Subsequent studies reported varying effects of regular endurance exercise, depending on the intensity and volume of maternal physical conditioning.

Data from our laboratory (Brenner *et al.* 1991; Webb *et al.* 1994; Wolfe *et al.* 1994a), including a recent prospective randomized trial (Wolfe *et al.* 1999), have shown no significant effect if moderate aerobic conditioning is conducted in conformity with guidelines published by the Canadian Society for Exercise Physiology (CSEP 1996). Other investigations, involving more strenuous exercise, have reported higher birthweights than in sedentary control subjects (Hatch *et al.* 1993), possibly because of augmented placental growth (Clapp & Rizk 1992). Finally, some investigations involving pregnant women who exercised very strenuously have reported significant growth retardation (Bell *et al.* 1995). Thus, existing information suggests a complicated dose–response relationship (Fig. 37.1).

Only a few studies have examined birth outcome in female athletes. A number of case reports indicate favourable pregnancy outcomes among active women who continued to run or jog throughout pregnancy (Hutchinson *et al.* 1981; Lutter *et al.* 1984; Cohen *et al.* 1989). However, owing to small sample sizes, these reports do not provide a sound basis on which to advise pregnant endurance athletes in general.

Other reports have included retrospective surveys of obstetric outcomes in athletic populations. For example, Erdelyi (1962) compared the pregnancy outcomes of 172 Hungarian athletes to those of 150 non-athlete controls. Two-thirds of the athletes continued to train during the first 3–4 months of pregnancy, but the proportion who exercised in late gestation was not reported. The athletes had a lower incidence of Caesarean sections, threatened abortions and toxaemia, as well as shorter mean labour durations than controls.

Zaharieva (1972) reported obstetric outcomes for 150 Bulgarian athletes, including 27 women who participated in the Olympic games between 1952 and 1972, 59 female 'masters of sport' and 64 female 'first-grade athletes'. The majority (63, 76 and 77%, respectively) continued to train during pregnancy. Most of the Olympic athletes (70.4%) reported completely normal pregnancy outcomes and the others had only 'mild' complications. However, masters of sport had somewhat higher occurrences of 'disturbances of the perineum' (42.3%), and of the need for episiotomy, perineotomy and Caesarean section.

Safe limits for physical conditioning in pregnancy

Although pregnancy is clearly not a time for intensive training or serious competition in endurance sports, it is advantageous to maintain reasonable levels of aerobic and muscular fitness. This facilitates a faster subsequent return to normal sports participation and may help to prevent and/or treat serious maternal–fetal disease including gestational diabetes mellitus (Jones *et al.* 1990; Bung & Artal 1996; López-Luna *et al.* 1998) and pre-eclampsia/toxaemia (Zaharieva 1972; Marcoux *et al.* 1989), as well as other conditions such as dyspnoea (Ohtake & Wolfe 1998), gestational low back pain

(American College of Obstetricians & Gynecologists (ACOG) 1994), diastasis recti and varicose veins. Whether or not regular activity facilitates or shortens labour remains an open question (Wolfe *et al.* 1994a), but it is reasonable to suggest that fit women may have a greater physiological reserve to cope with the labour process, regardless of its difficulty and energy requirements.

The Physical Activity Readiness Medical Examination for Pregnancy (PARmed-X for Pregnancy) was developed in our laboratory in cooperation with the Ontario Fitness Safety Standards Committee (1990) and the Canadian Society for Exercise Physiology (Appendix). Its contents are based on a current review of available literature, as well as more than a decade of research. Guidelines in the PARmed-X for Pregnancy were aimed originally at providing advice to previously inactive pregnant women who wanted to start new exercise programmes. However, methods for medical screening, identification of safe exercise limits, exercise prescription and monitoring and safety guidelines are directly applicable to active women who wish to maintain fitness during pregnancy.

Medical screening

To ensure that the physiological demands of the fetus are met and to ensure safety, all pregnant women (regardless of their physical fitness) should be screened medically by a qualified physician or midwife before initiating or continuing an exercise regimen during pregnancy. In the absence of infectious diseases or serious metabolic or cardiopulmonary disease states, the most important contraindications to exercise are: premature labour (e.g. ruptured membranes); placental injury or dysfunction; an incompetent cervix; presence of pregnancy-induced hypertension, pre-eclampsia or toxaemia; and intrauterine growth retardation (ACOG 1994; CSEP 1996).

Women with a history of spontaneous abortion or premature labour should exercise with caution and in compliance with advice from the physician or midwife who is monitoring their pregnancy. Similarly, women with twin pregnancies should exercise moderately in accordance with individual medical advice after the 28th week of gestation. It is accepted practice for pregnant women to take specific prenatal vitamin supplements and have regular haemoglobin measurements to ensure that they are not anaemic. Since fetal growth can be adversely affected by low maternal energy stores, women with little body fat should pay strict attention to nutritional guidelines for pregnant women (ACOG 1994; CSEP 1996) and avoid participation in strenuous exercise regimens that may contribute to inadequate substrate availability.

Aerobic exercise prescription — general advice

The PARmed-X for Pregnancy states that pregnant women should not begin a new aerobic exercise programme or increase the quantity and quality of aerobic exercise prior to the 14th week or after the 28th week of pregnancy. The best time to increase exercise participation is during the second trimester, when the discomforts and theoretical risks are lowest. However, this advice is directed primarily towards women who were inactive prior to pregnancy, and it needs to be modified for women who were involved in strenuous competitive or recreational aerobic exercise prior to pregnancy. Pregnancy is not a time for intensive aerobic conditioning or involvement in competition. In particular, strenuous exercise is not recommended during the time surrounding closure of the fetal neural tube (at approximately the 4th week of gestation), since overheating due to intensive exercise and/or heat exposure could, in theory, cause neural tube defects, facial defects or other fetal malformations. Such adverse effects have been reported as a result of chronic heating in animal studies (Edwards 1986), and following sauna or hot tub exposure (Milunski *et al.* 1991), but we are unaware of any reports which attribute fetal malformations directly to participation in strenuous exercise.

Since the safety of strenuous exercise in early pregnancy cannot be confirmed, it is prudent for women who have just learned that they are pregnant (or women who are trying to become pregnant) to exercise moderately. The occurrence of discomforts such as morning sickness also suggests that exercise should be limited to moderate intensities and durations early in pregnancy. The potential competition between the developing fetus and contracting maternal skeletal muscle for blood flow, substrate availability and heat dissipation is greatest during the period of rapid fetal growth (i.e. the third trimester). Therefore, involvement in strenuous exercise is not recommended at this time and, in most cases, exercise intensity and duration should be reduced relative to the second trimester.

Modality

In general, it is appropriate to continue with the types of endurance exercise normally used in training, but within the limits discussed above for intensity, duration and frequency. However, it is also important to apply common sense in making exercise choices and adjustments. For example, a competitive cyclist may choose to use an upright cycle ergometer rather than cycling on the road, to avoid the possibility of injury by falling. A runner may substitute inclined treadmill walking to circumvent the discomfort and potential trauma to the fetus encountered during running in late gestation. Swimming is a particularly good form of exercise for endurance athletes from other sports, since the body mass is supported by the buoyant effects of water and heat dissipation is facilitated (provided that the water temperature is below skin temperature during exercise). Thus, swimming may be used in conjunction with other exercise modalities to maintain fitness.

Intensity

As discussed above, resting HR is increased by approximately 10–15 beats·min^{-1} compared to the non-pregnant state, and there is also evidence for a moderate reduction in maximal HR (Fig. 37.2). Since the maximal HR reserve is reduced, conventional HR target zones for exercise prescription have been modified in the PARmed-X for Pregnancy. The recommended target HR range has been reduced by 10–15 beats·min^{-1} and the upper limit has been

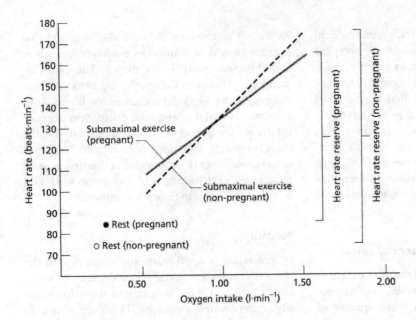

Fig. 37.2 Maximal heart rate reserve in human pregnancy. From Wolfe and Mottola (1993), with permission.

reduced by 5 beats·min⁻¹. These changes are supported by recent studies of cardiac autonomic function at rest and during exercise (Avery *et al.* 1998a,b).

Since the maximal HR reserve is reduced, the use of the HR as an indicator of exercise intensity is less accurate than in the non-pregnant state. However, the perception of effort is not significantly altered by pregnancy or advancing gestational age (Ohtake *et al.* 1988; Pivarnik *et al.* 1991). Thus, use of Borg's 15-point (6–20) rating of perceived exertion (RPE) scale along with HR is recommended for monitoring exercise intensity in the PARmed-X for Pregnancy. A target RPE of 12–14 ('somewhat hard') is appropriate for most pregnant women. It corresponds to the same intensity range as the recommended target HR. Use of the 'talk test' provides a final check to prevent overexertion. If the pregnant woman cannot maintain a verbal conversation while exercising, then the exercise intensity is considered to be too high.

Duration

The degree of fetal thermal and hypoxic stress (Lotgering *et al.* 1983a,b), as well as the magnitude of exercise-induced FHR baseline elevation (Clapp *et*

al. 1993), depend on the interaction between maternal exercise intensity and duration. In conjunction with the exercise intensity guidelines cited above, aerobic exercise durations of up to 30 min per session (performed 3–4 days per week) are safe for healthy pregnant women and their unborn fetuses (Brenner *et al.* 1991; Webb *et al.* 1994; Wolfe *et al.* 1994b; Ohtake & Wolfe 1998).

Given that endurance athletes normally participate in much greater volumes of aerobic conditioning, it is not unreasonable to suggest that such women may safely exceed the exercise limits recommended for previously inactive non-athletes. In the absence of scientific information to support this idea, it is strongly recommended that pregnant athletes participate in more strenuous exercise only with the approval and continuing advice of the physician or midwife monitoring their pregnancies. In such cases, particular attention should be paid to optimal prenatal nutrition and to replacement of the energy expended during exercise, to ongoing monitoring of maternal–fetal weight gain, and to avoidance of warm/humid exercise environments. If the individual experiences feelings of fatigue or lack of energy following exercise or on the day following an exercise session, then the exercise intensity and duration of exercise should be reduced.

Reasons to contact a physician

The most important contraindications to exercise in pregnancy are premature labour (as reflected by persistent uterine contractions and/or a loss of fluid from the vagina due to ruptured membranes), placental injury or dysfunction (as reflected by persistent second or third trimester bleeding), an incompetent cervix (which usually results in preterm delivery), intrauterine growth retardation (as reflected by failure to gain weight), and pre-eclampsia (involving swelling of the extremities, headaches, dizziness or disturbances of vision). It is essential that all pregnant women become familiar with the signs and symptoms of these problems and seek medical attention if they occur.

Return to strenuous training and competition after childbirth

Pregnancy-induced changes in anatomical and physiological variables return to preconceptual levels at different rates, depending on the variables in question. After delivery of the fetus, placenta and body fluids, there is an immediate loss of 5–7 kg of body mass. Blood volume also returns quickly to preconceptual levels although some women may remain anaemic. Respiration returns to normal because of withdrawal of the stimulatory effects of progesterone. HR normalizes quickly after child-birth, but systemic vascular resistance, end-diastolic volume and SV remain elevated compared to pre-conceptual values for up to 12 weeks postpartum (Capeless & Clapp 1991). Body mass and adiposity return toward preconceptual values over several weeks or months postpartum (South-Paul et al. 1992).

Soon after a normal, uncomplicated delivery, activities such as walking, and recumbent bed exercises such as abdominal tightening, Kegel (pelvic floor) exercises and pelvic tilts can be initiated, along with deep breathing and static muscular contractions for a variety of muscle groups (Fitness Ontario 1983). Women with diastasis recti during pregnancy should avoid intensive abdominal exercises until abdominal muscle separation is corrected. The rate of recovery from Caesarean section varies greatly; resumption of normal activities and initiation of physical conditioning should be decided on an individual basis, in accordance with medical advice.

In the absence of complications, and following initial recovery from labour and delivery, the quantity and quality of physical conditioning can be increased gradually in accordance with individual tolerance. Both metabolic rate and endocrine factors are normally increased during lactation, and this may increase susceptibility to fatigue. Lactating women should keep in mind that lactic acid may be found in breast milk following strenuous maternal exercise and concern has been expressed that it may affect infant acceptance of breast milk (Wallace et al. 1992).

Conclusions

Human pregnancy involves a wide range of metabolic, circulatory and respiratory changes that can alter a woman's responses to endurance exercise and aerobic conditioning. These effects are driven by gestational hormones. Current information supports the concept of a dose–response relationship between the quantity and quality of regular maternal exercise. Moderate exercise, as outlined in the PARmed-X for Pregnancy, has been shown to be safe for healthy women with uncomplicated pregnancies, is useful to maintain aerobic fitness, and may be helpful in preventing serious maternal–fetal diseases (gestational diabetes, pre-eclampsia). However, more strenuous exercise may adversely affect fetal growth and development. Thus, it is recommended that pregnant endurance athletes exercise within limits recommended in the PARmed-X for Pregnancy. More strenuous programmes should be attempted only with close medical supervision and monitoring. All pregnant women should be screened medically before involvement in a prenatal exercise regimen and they should know the reasons to stop exercise and consult a physician.

The time required for safe return to intensive endurance training and competition varies, depending on whether or not complications were encountered during labour and delivery. Women with uncomplicated deliveries can gradually increase the quantity and quality of exercise after cessation of postpartum bleeding, in accordance with energy levels. Women with Caesarean sections, persistent bleeding or fatigue should resume activity more slowly, in accordance with medical advice. Lactation tends to reduce maternal energy levels. Involvement in strenuous exercise may result in the presence of lactate in breast milk, and may affect infant acceptance of breast milk.

Acknowledgements

The Exercise/Pregnancy Research Program at Queen's University has received financial support from the US Army Medical Research and Materiel Command (Contract #DAMD17-96-C-6112), the Ontario Thoracic Society, Canadian Fitness and Lifestyle Research Institute, Health Canada (NHRDP) and N.S.E.R.C. (Canada).

References

American College of Obstetricians & Gynecologists (1994) Exercise during pregnancy and the post partum period. *American College of Obstetricians and Gynecologists Technical Bulletin* **189**, 2–7.

Artal, R., Masaki, D.L., Khodiguian, N., Romem, Y., Rutherford, S.E. & Wiswell, R.A. (1989) Exercise prescription in pregnancy: weight-bearing versus non-weight-bearing exercise. *American Journal of Obstetrics and Gynecology* **161**, 1464–1469.

Avery, N.D., Wolfe, L.A. & McGrath, M.J. (1998a) Effects of human pregnancy on heart rate variability (HRV) above and below the ventilatory anaerobic threshold (abstract). *Canadian Journal of Applied Physiology* **23**, 462.

Avery, N.D., Wolfe, L.A. & McGrath, M.J. (1998b) Effects of human pregnancy on spontaneous baroreflex (SBR) function above and below the ventilatory anaerobic threshold (abstract). *Canadian Journal of Applied Physiology* **23**, 463.

Bell, R.J., Palma, S.M. & Lumley, J.M. (1995) The effect of vigorous exercise during pregnancy on birth-weight. *Australian and New Zealand Journal of Obstetrics and Gynaecology* **35**, 46–51.

Blechner, J.H. (1993) Maternal–fetal acid–base physiology. *Clinical Obstetrics and Gynecology* **36**, 3–12.

Blechner, J.N., Stenger, V.G., Eitzman, D.V. & Prystowsky, H. (1967) Effects of maternal metabolic acidosis on the human fetus and newborn infant. *American Journal of Obstetrics and Gynecology* **99**, 46–54.

Bonen, A., Campagna, P., Gilchrist, L., Young, D.C. & Beresford, P. (1992) Substrate and endocrine responses during exercise at selected stages of pregnancy. *Journal of Applied Physiology* **73**, 134–142.

Brenner, I.K.M., Monga, M., Webb, K., McGrath, M.J. & Wolfe, L.A. (1991) Controlled prospective study of aerobic conditioning effects on pregnancy outcome (abstract). *Medicine and Science in Sports and Exercise* **23**, S169.

Bung, P. & Artal, R. (1996) Gestational diabetes and exercise: a survey. *Seminars in Perinatology* **20**, 328–333.

Canadian Society for Exercise Physiology (1996) *Physical Activity Readiness Medical Examination for Pregnancy (Parmed-X for Pregnancy)*. Available from CSEP, 185 Somerset St. West, Suite 202, Ottawa, ON, K2P 0J2, Canada.

Capeless, E.L. & Clapp, J.F. (1989) Cardiovascular changes in early phase of pregnancy. *American Journal of Obstetrics and Gynecology* **161**, 1449–1453.

Capeless, E.L. & Clapp, J.F. III (1991) When do cardiovascular parameters return to their preconception values? *American Journal of Obstetrics and Gynecology* **165**, 883–886.

Carpenter, M.W., Sady, S.P., Hoegsborg, B. *et al.* (1988) Fetal heart rate response to maternal exertion. *Journal of the American Medical Association* **259**, 3006–3009.

Clapp, J.F. (1985) Maternal heart rate in pregnancy. *American Journal of Obstetrics and Gynecology* **132**, 659–660.

Clapp, J.F. III (1991) The changing thermal response to endurance exercise in pregnancy. *American Journal of Obstetrics and Gynecology* **165**, 1684–1689.

Clapp, J.F. III & Capeless, E. (1990) Neonatal morphometrics following endurance exercise during pregnancy. *American Journal of Obstetrics and Gynecology* **163**, 1803–1811.

Clapp, J.F. III & Capeless, E. (1991) The $\dot{V}o_{2max}$ of recreational athletes before and after pregnancy. *Medicine and Science in Sports and Exercise* **23**, 1128–1133.

Clapp, J.F. III & Dickstein, S. (1984) Endurance exercise and pregnancy outcome. *Medicine and Science in Sports and Exercise* **16**, 556–562.

Clapp, J.F. III & Rizk, K.D. (1992) Effect of recreational exercise on midtrimester placental growth. *American Journal of Obstetrics and Gynecology* **167**, 1518–1521.

Clapp, J.F. III, Wesley, M. & Sleamaker, R.H. (1987) Thermoregulatory and metabolic responses prior to and during pregnancy. *Medicine and Science in Sports and Exercise* **19**, 124–180.

Clapp, J.F. III, Little, C.D. & Capeless, E.L. (1993) Fetal heart rate response to sustained recreational exercise. *American Journal of Obstetrics and Gynecology* **168**, 198–206.

Cohen, G.C., Prior, J.C., Vigna, Y. & Pride, S.M. (1989) Intense exercise during the first two trimesters of unapparent pregnancy. *Physician and Sportsmedicine* **17** (1), 87, 88, 91–94.

Duvekot, J.J., Cleriex, E.C., Pieters, F.A.A., Menheere, P.P.C.A. & Peeters, L.L.H. (1993) Early pregnancy changes in hemodynamics and homeostasis as consecutive adjustments triggered by a primary fall in systemic vascular tone. *American Journal of Obstetrics and Gynecology* **169**, 1382–1392.

Edwards, M.J. (1986) Hyperthermia and a teratogen: a review of experimental studies and their clinical significance. *Teratogenesis, Carcinogenesis and Mutagenesis* **6**, 563–572.

Erdelyi, G.J. (1962) Gynecological survey of female athletes. *Journal of Sports Medicine and Physical Fitness* **2**, 174–179.

Field, S.K., Bell, G., Cenaiko, D.T. & Whitelaw, W.A. (1991) Relationship between inspiratory effort and breathlessness in pregnancy. *Journal of Applied Physiology* **71**, 1897–1902.

Fitness Ontario (1983) *Pre/Post Natal Fitness*. Ontario Ministry of Tourism and Recreation, Sports and Fitness Branch, Toronto.

Fitness Safety Standards Committee (February, 1990) *Final Report to the Minister of Tourism and Recreation on the Development* of Fitness Safety Standards in Ontario (Canada). Ministry of Tourism and Recreation, Toronto.

Gilbert, R., Epifano, L. & Auchincloss, J.H. (1962) Dyspnea of pregnancy. *Journal of the American Medical Association* **182** (11), 1073–1077.

Greer, F.A. & Wolfe, L.A. (1994) Chronic exercise effects on subcutaneous adiposity in pregnancy (abstract). *Medicine and Science in Sports and Exercise* **26**, S119.

Guzman, C.A. & Caplan, R. (1970) Cardiorespiratory responses to exercise during pregnancy. *American Journal of Obstetrics and Gynecology* **108**, 600–605.

Hale, R.W. & Milne, L. (1996) The elite athlete and exercise in pregnancy. *Seminars in Perinatology* **20**, 277–284.

Hatch, M.C., Shu, X., McLean, D.E. et al. (1993) Maternal exercise during pregnancy, physical fitness and fetal growth. *American Journal of Epidemiology* **137**, 1105–1114.

Hollingsworth, D.R. (1985) Maternal metabolism in normal pregnancy and pregnancy complicated with diabetes mellitus. *Clinics in Obstetrics and Gynecology* **28**, 457–472.

Hutchinson, P.L., Careson, K.J. & Sparling, P.B. (1981) Metabolic and circulatory responses to running during pregnancy. *Physician and Sportsmedicine* **9** (8), 35–38, 61.

Hytten, F.E. (1968) Physiological changes in early pregnancy. *Journal of Obstetrics and Gynaecology of the British Commonwealth* **75**, 1193–1197.

Jones, M.T., Norton, K.I., Dengel, D.R. & Armstrong, R.B. (1990) Effects of training on reproductive tissue blood flow in exercising pregnant rats. *Journal of Applied Physiology* **69**, 2097–2103.

Kemp, J.G., Greer, F.A. & Wolfe, L.A. (1997) Acid–base balance following maximal exercise testing in pregnancy. *Journal of Applied Physiology* **83**, 644–651.

Knuttgen, H.G. & Emerson, K. (1974) Physiological response to pregnancy at rest and during exercise. *Journal of Applied Physiology* **36**, 549–553.

Liberatore, S.M., Pistelli, R., Patolano, F., Moncto, E., Incolzi, R.A. & Gappi, G. (1984) Respiratory function during pregnancy. *Respiration* **46**, 145–150.

López-Luna, P., Iglesias, M.A., Muñoz, C. & Herrera, E. (1998) Aerobic exercise during pregnancy reveals maternal insulin resistance in rats. *Medicine and Science in Sports and Exercise* **30**, 1510–1514.

Lotgering, F.K., Gilbert, R.D. & Longo, L.D. (1983a) Exercise responses in pregnant

sheep: oxygen consumption, uterine blood flow and blood. *Journal of Applied Physiology* **55**, 834–841.

Lotgering, F.K., Gilbert, R.D. & Longo, L.D. (1983b) Exercise responses in pregnant sheep: blood gases, temperatures and fetal cardiovascular system. *Journal of Applied Physiology* **55**, 842–850.

Lotgering, F.K., Van Doorn, M.K., Struijk, P.C., Pool, J. & Wallenberg, H.C.S. (1991) Maximal aerobic exercise in pregnant women: heart rate, O_2 consumption, CO_2 production, and ventilation. *Journal of Applied Physiology* **70**, 1016–1023.

Lotgering, F.K., Struijk, P.C., Van Doorn, M.B. & Wallenberg, H.C.S. (1992) Errors in predicting maximal oxygen consumption in pregnant women. *Journal of Applied Physiology* **72**, 562–567.

Lotgering, F.K., Struijk, P.C., Van Doorn, M.B., Spinnewijn, W.E.M. & Wallenberg, H.C.S. (1995) Anaerobic threshold and respiratory compensation in pregnant women. *Journal of Applied Physiology* **78**, 1772–1777.

Lund, C.J. & Donovan, J.C. (1967) Blood volume during pregnancy. Significance of plasma and red cell volumes. *American Journal of Obstetrics and Gynecology* **98**, 393–403.

Lutter, J.M., Lee, V. & Cushman, S. (1984) Fetal outcomes of women who ran while pregnant. *Melpomene Report* **3**, 6–8.

Lyons, H.A. & Antonio, R. (1959) The sensitivity of the respiratory center in pregnancy and after the administration of progesterone. *Transactions of the American Association of Physicians* **72**, 173–180.

McMurray, R.G., Katz, V.L., Berry, M.J. & Cefalo, R.C. (1988) The effect of pregnancy on metabolic responses during rest, immersion and aerobic exercise in the water. *American Journal of Obstetrics and Gynecology* **158**, 481–486.

Manders, M.A., Sonder, G.J., Mulder, E.J. & Visser, G.H. (1997) The effects of maternal exercise on fetal heart rate and movement patterns. *Early Human Development* **48**, 237–247.

Marcoux, S., Brisson, J. & Fabra, J. (1989) The effect of leisure time physical activity on the risk of pre-eclampsia and gestational hypertension. *Journal of Epidemiology and Community Health* **73**, 147–152.

Milunski, A., Uleickas, M., Rothman, K.J., Willest, S.S. & Jick, H. (1991) Maternal heat exposure and neural tube defects. *Journal of the American Medical Association* **268**, 882–885.

Moore, L.G., McCullough, R.E. & Weil, J.V. (1987) Increased HVR in pregnancy:

relationship to hormonal and metabolic changes. *Journal of Applied Physiology* **62**, 158–163.

Morton, M.J., Paul, M.S. & Metcalfe, J. (1985) Exercise during pregnancy. *Medical Clinics of North America* **69**, 97–108.

Ohtake, P.J. & Wolfe, L.A. (1998) Physical conditioning attenuates respiratory responses to exercise in late gestation. *Medicine and Science in Sports and Exercise* **30**, 17–27.

Ohtake, P.J., Wolfe, L.A., Hall, P. & McGrath, M.J. (1988) Physical conditioning effects on heart rate and perception of exertion in pregnancy (abstract). *Candian Journal of Sport Sciences* **13**, 71P (Abstract).

Pernoll, M.L., Metcalfe, J., Kovack, P.A., Wachtel, R. & Durham, M.J. (1975) Ventilation at rest and exercise in pregnancy and postpartum. *Respiration Physiology* **25**, 295–310.

Pivarnik, J.M. (1998) Potential effects of maternal physical activity on birth weight: a brief review. *Medicine and Science in Sports and Exercise* **30**, 400–406.

Pivarnik, J.M., Lee, W., Clark, S.L., Cotton, D.B., Spillman, H.T. & Miller, J.F. (1990) Cardiac output responses in primigravid women during exercise determined by the direct Fick technique. *Obstetrics and Gynecology* **75**, 954–959.

Pivarnik, J.M., Lee, W. & Miller, J.F. (1991) Physiological and perceptual responses to cycle and treadmill exercise during pregnancy. *Medicine and Science in Sports and Exercise* **23**, 470–475.

Ratigan, T.R. (1983) Anatomic and physiologic changes of pregnancy: anesthetic considerations. *Journal of the American Association of Nurse Anesthesiologists* **31**, 38–42.

Sady, S.P., Carpenter, M.W., Thompson, P.D., Sady, M.A., Haydon, B. & Coustan, D.R. (1989) Cardiovascular response to cycle exercise during and after pregnancy. *Journal of Applied Physiology* **66**, 336–341.

Sady, M.A., Haydon, B.B., Sady, S.P., Carpenter, M.W., Thompson, P.D. & Coustan, D.R. (1990) Cardiovascular response to maximal cycle exercise during pregnancy and at two and seven months postpartum. *American Journal of Obstetrics and Gynecology* **162**, 1181–1185.

Sodha, R.J., Proegler, M. & Schneider, H. (1984) Transfer and metabolism of norepinephrine studied from maternal-to-fetal and fetal-to-maternal sides of the *in vitro* profused human placental lobe.

American Journal of Obstetrics and Gynecology **148**, 474–481.

South-Paul, J.E., Rajogopal, K.R. & Tenholder, M.F. (1992) Exercise responses prior to pregnancy and the postpartum state. *Medicine and Science in Sports and Exercise* **24**, 410–414.

Taggart, N.R., Halliday, R.M., Billewitz, W.Z., Hytten, F.E. & Thomson, A.M. (1967) Changes in skinfolds during pregnancy. *British Journal of Nutrition* **21**, 439–451.

Wallace, J.P., Inbar, G. & Ernsthausen, K. (1992) Infant acceptance of postexercise breast milk. *Pediatrics* **89**, 1245–1247.

Watson, W.J., Katz, V.L., Hackney, A.C., Gall, M.M. & McMurray, R.G. (1991) Fetal responses to maximal swimming and cycling exercise during pregnancy. *Obstetrics and Gynecology* **77**, 382–386.

Webb, K.A., Wolfe, L.A. & McGrath, M.J. (1994) Effects of acute and chronic maternal exercise on fetal heart rate.

Journal of Applied Physiology **97**, 2207–2213.

Wolfe, L.A. & Mottola, M.F. (1993) Aerobic exercise in pregnancy: an update. *Canadian Journal of Applied Physiology* **18**, 119–147.

Wolfe, L.A., Ohtake, P.J., Mottola, M.F. & McGrath, M.J. (1989) Physiological interactions between pregnancy and aerobic exercise. *Exercise and Sport Sciences Reviews* **17**, 295–351.

Wolfe, L.A., Ohtake, P.J., George, K.A. & McGrath, M.J. (1990) Aerobic training effects on exercise hemodynamics during pregnancy (abstract). *Medicine and Science in Sports and Exercise* **22**, S28.

Wolfe, L.A., Brenner, I.K.M. & Mottola, M.F. (1994a) Maternal exercise, fetal well-being and pregnancy outcome. *Exercise and Sport Sciences Reviews* **22**, 145–194.

Wolfe, L.A., Walker, R.M.C., Bonen, A. & McGrath, M.J. (1994b) Effects of pregnancy and chronic exercise on respira-

tory responses to graded exercise. *Journal of Applied Physiology* **76**, 1928–1934.

Wolfe, L.A., Kemp, J.G., Heenan, A.P., Preston, R.J. & Ohtake, P. (1998) Acid–base regulation and respiratory control in human pregnancy. *Canadian Journal of Physiology and Pharmacology* **76**, 815–827.

Wolfe, L.A., Preston, R.J., Burggraf, G.W. & McGrath, M.J. (Submitted December, 1998) Effects of pregnancy and chronic exercise on maternal cardiac structure and function. *Canadian Journal of Physiology and Pharmacology* **77**, 909–917.

Wolfe, L.A., Mottola, M.F., Bonen, A. *et al.* (1999) Controlled, randomized study of aerobic conditioning effects on neonatal morphometrics. *Medicine and Science in Sports and Exercise* **31**, S138.

Zaharieva, E. (1972) Olympic participation by women. Effects on pregnancy and child birth. *Journal of the American Medical Association* **221**, 992–995.

Appendix: Physical activity readiness medical examination for pregnancy (PARmed-X for pregnancy)

PARmed-X for PREGNANCY PHYSICAL ACTIVITY READINESS MEDICAL EXAMINATION

PARmed-X for PREGNANCY is a guideline for health screening prior to participation in a prenatal fitness class or other exercise.

Healthy women with uncomplicated pregnancies can integrate physical activity into their daily living and can participate without significant risks either to themselves or to their unborn child. Postulated benefits of such programs include improved aerobic and muscular fitness, promotion of appropriate weight gain, and facilitation of labour. Regular exercise may also help to prevent gestational glucose intolerance and pregnancy-induced hypertension.

The safety of prenatal exercise programs depends on an adequate level of maternal-fetal physiological reserve. PARmed-X for PREGNANCY is a convenient checklist and prescription for use by physicians to evaluate pregnant patients who want to enter a prenatal fitness program and for ongoing medical surveillance of exercising pregnant patients.

Instructions for use of the 4-page PARmed-X for PREGNANCY are the following:

1. The patient should fill out the section on PATIENT INFORMATION and the PRE-EXERCISE HEALTH CHECKLIST (PART 1, 2, 3, and 4 on p. 1) and give the form to the physician monitoring her pregnancy.

2. The physician should check the information provided by the patient for accuracy and fill out SECTION C on CONTRAINDICATIONS (p. 2) based on current medical information.

3. If no exercise contraindications exist, the HEALTH EVALUATION FORM (p. 3) should be completed, signed by the physician, and given by the patient to her prenatal fitness professional.

In addition to prudent medical care, participation in appropriate types, intensities and amounts of exercise is recommended to increase the likelihood of a beneficial pregnancy outcome. PARmed-X for PREGNANCY provides recommendations for individualized exercise prescription (p. 3) and program safety (p. 4).

NOTE: Sections A and B should be completed by the patient before the appointment with the physician.

A PATIENT INFORMATION

NAME _____

ADDRESS _____

TELEPHONE _____ BIRTHDATE _____ HEALTH INSURANCE No. _____

NAME OF
PRENATAL FITNESS PROFESSIONAL _____

PRENATAL FITNESS
PROFESSIONAL'S PHONE NUMBER _____

B PRE-EXERCISE HEALTH CHECKLIST

PART 1: GENERAL HEALTH STATUS

In the past, have you experienced (check YES or NO):

	YES	NO
1. Miscarriage in an earlier pregnancy?	❑	❑
2. Other pregnancy complications?	❑	❑
3. I have completed a PAR-Q within the last 30 days.	❑	❑

If you answered YES to question 1 or 2, please explain:

_____

Number of previous pregnancies? _____

PART 2: STATUS OF CURRENT PREGNANCY

Due Date: _____

During this pregnancy, have you experienced:

	YES	NO
1. Marked fatigue?	❑	❑
2. Bloody discharge from the vagina ("spotting")?	❑	❑
3. Unexplained faintness or dizziness?	❑	❑
4. Unexplained abdominal pain?	❑	❑
5. Sudden swelling of ankles, hands or face?	❑	❑
6. Persistent headaches or problems with headaches?	❑	❑
7. Swelling, pain or redness in the calf of one leg?	❑	❑
8. Absence of fetal movement after 4th month?	❑	❑
9. Failure to gain weight after fourth month?	❑	❑

If you answered YES to any of the above questions, please explain:

PART 3: ACTIVITY HABITS DURING THE PAST MONTH

1. List only regular fitness/recreational activities:

_____

INTENSITY	FREQUENCY (times/week)			TIME (minutes/day)		
	1-2	2-4	4+	<20	20-40	40+
Heavy	—	—	—	—	—	—
Medium	—	—	—	—	—	—
Light	—	—	—	—	—	—

2. Does your regular occupation (job/home) activity involve:

	YES	NO
Heavy Lifting?	❑	❑
Frequent walking/stair climbing?	❑	❑
Occasional walking (>once/hr)?	❑	❑
Prolonged standing?	❑	❑
Mainly sitting?	❑	❑
Normal daily activity	❑	❑
3. Do you currently smoke tobacco?*	❑	❑
4. Do you consume alcohol?*	❑	❑

PART 4: PHYSICAL ACTIVITY INTENTIONS

What physical activity do you intend to do?

_____

Is this a change from what you currently do? ❑ YES ❑ NO

*NOTE: PREGNANT WOMEN ARE STRONGLY ADVISED NOT TO SMOKE OR CONSUME ALCOHOL DURING PREGNANCY AND DURING LACTATION.

C CONTRAINDICATIONS TO EXERCISE: to be completed by physician

Absolute Contraindications		
Does the patient have:	YES	NO
1. Ruptured membranes, premature labour?	❏	❏
2. Persistent second or third trimester bleeding/placenta previa?	❏	❏
3. Pregnancy-induced hypertension pre-eclampsia or toxemia?	❏	❏
4. Incompetent cervix?	❏	❏
5. Evidence of intrauterine growth retardation?	❏	❏
6. Multiple pregnancy (e.g., triplets)?	❏	❏
7. Uncontrolled Type I diabetes, hypertension or thyroid disease, other serious cardiovascular, respiratory or systemic disorder?	❏	❏

Relative Contraindications		
Does the patient have:	YES	NO
1. History of spontaneous abortion or premature labour in previous pregnancies?	❏	❏
2. Mild/moderate cardiovascular or respiratory disease (e.g., chronic hypertension, asthma?)	❏	❏
3. Anemia or iron deficiency? (Hb < 10 g/dl)?	❏	❏
4. Very low body fatness, eating disorder (anorexia, bulimia)?	❏	❏
5. Twin pregnancy after 28th week?	❏	❏
6. Other significant medical condition?	❏	❏
Please specify: _____		

NOTE: Risk may exceed benefits of regular physical activity. The decision to be physically active or not should be made with qualified medical advice.

PHYSICAL ACTIVITY RECOMMENDATION: ❏ Recommended/Approved   ❏ Contraindicated

Prescription for Aerobic Activity

RATE OF PROGRESSION: The best time to progress is during the second trimester since risks and discomfort of exercise are lowest at that time. It is not advisable to begin a new exercise program or increase the amount of exercise prior to the 14th week of pregnancy or after the 28th week. Aerobic exercise should be gradually and progressively increased during the second trimester from a minimum of 15 minutes per session to a maximum of approximately 30 minutes per session.

WARM-UP/COOL-DOWN: Aerobic activity should be preceded by a brief (10-15 min.) warm-up and followed by a short (10-15 min.) cool-down. Low intensity calesthenics, stretching and relaxation exercises should be included in the warm-up/cool-down.

PRESCRIPTION/MONITORING OF INTENSITY: The best way to prescribe and monitor exercise is by combining the heart rate and rating of perceived exertion (RPE) methods.

F I T T

FREQUENCY	INTENSITY	TIME	TYPE
Begin at 3 times per week and progress to four or five times per week	Exercise within an appropriate RPE range and/or target heart rate zone	Attempt 15 minutes, even if it means reducing the intensity. Rest intervals may be helpful	Non weight-bearing or low-impact endurance exercise using large muscle groups (e.g., walking, stationary cycling, swimming, aquatic exercises, low impact aerobics)

TARGET HEART RATE ZONES

The heart rate zones shown below are appropriate for most pregnant women. Work during the lower end of the HR range at the start of a new exercise program and in late pregnancy.

Age	Heart Rate Range
< 20	140-155
20-29	135-150
30-39	130-145
≥ 40	125-140

RATING OF PERCEIVED EXERTION (RPE)

Check the accuracy of your heart rate target zone by comparing it to the scale below. A range of about 12-14 (somewhat hard) is appropriate for most pregnant women.

6	
7	Very, very light
8	
9	Somewhat light
10	
11	Fairly light
12	
13	Somewhat hard
14	
15	Hard
16	
17	Very hard
18	
19	Very, very hard
20	

"TALK TEST" - A final check to avoid overexertion is to use the "talk test". The exercise intensity is excessive if you cannot carry on a verbal conversation while exercising.

The original PARmed-X for PREGNANCY was developed by L.A. Wolfe, Ph.D. of Queen's University, Kingston, Ontario. The muscular conditioning component was developed by M.F. Mottola, Ph.D. of The University of Western Ontario, London, Ontario. It has been revised by an Expert Advisory Committee assembled by the Canadian Society for Exercise Physiology and the Fitness Program-Health Canada (1996).

Translation and reproduction in its entirety is encouraged

Disponible en français sous le titre «Examination medicale sur l'aptitude à l'activité physique pour les femmes enceintes (X-AAP pour les femmes enceintes)»

To order additional printed copies of the PARmed-X for PREGNANCY, the PARmed-X and/or the PAR-Q, (for a nominal charge) contact the:

Canadian Society for Exercise Physiology
185 Somerset St. West, Suite 202
Ottawa, Ontario CANADA K2P 0J2
tel. (613) 234-3755   FAX (613) 234-3565

Prescription for Muscular Conditioning

It is important to condition all major muscle groups during both prenatal and postnatal periods.

WARM-UPS & COOL DOWN:
Range of Motion: neck, shoulder girdle, back, arms, hips, knees, ankles, etc.
Static Stretching: all major muscle groups
(DO NOT OVER STRETCH!)

EXAMPLES OF MUSCULAR STRENGTHENING EXERCISES

CATEGORY	PURPOSE	EXAMPLE
Upper back	Promotion of good posture	Shoulder shrugs, shoulder blade pinch
Lower back	Promotion of good posture	Modified standing opposite leg & arm lifts
Abdomen	Promotion of good posture, prevent low-back pain, prevent diastasis recti, strengthen muscles of labour	Abdominal tightening, abdominal curl-ups, head raises lying on side or standing position
Pelvic floor ("Kegels")	Promotion of good bladder control, prevention of urinary incontinence	"Wave", "elevator"
Upper body	Improve muscular support for breasts	Shoulder rotations, modified push-ups against a wall
Buttocks, lower limbs	Facilitation of weight-bearing, prevention of varicose veins	Buttocks squeeze, standing leg lifts, heel raises

Precautions for Muscular Conditioning During Pregnancy

VARIABLE	EFFECTS OF PREGNANCY	EXERCISE MODIFICATIONS
Body Position	• in the supine position (lying on the back), the enlarged uterus may decrease the flow of blood returning from the lower half of the body as it presses on a major vein (inferior fena cava)	• past 4 months of gestation, exercises normally done in the supine position should be altered • such exercises should be done side lying or standing
Joint Laxity	• ligaments become relaxed due to increasing hormone levels • joints may be prone to injury	• avoid rapid changes in direction and bouncing during exercises • stretching should be performed with controlled movements
Abdominal Muscles	• presence of a rippling (bulging) of connective tissue along the midline of the pregnant abdomen (diastasis recti) may be seen during abdominal exercise	• abdominal exercises are not recommended if diastasis recti develops
Posture	• increasing weight of enlarged breasts and uterus may cause a forward shift in the centre of gravity and may increase the arch in the lower back • this may also cause shoulders to slump forward	• emphasis on correct posture
Precautions for Resistance Exercise	• emphasis must be placed on continuous breathing throughout exercise • exhale on exertion, inhale on relaxation • Valsalva Manoevre (holding breath while working against a resistance) causes a decrease in blood pressure and therefore should be avoided • avoid exercise in supine position past 4 months gestation	

Health Evaluation Form

(to be completed by patient and given to the prenatal fitness professional after obtaining medical clearance to exercise)

I, _____ PLEASE PRINT (patient's name), have discussed my plans to participate in physical activity during my current pregnancy with my physician and I have obtained his/her approval to begin participation.

Signed: _____
(patient's signature)

Date: _____

Name of Physician: _____ M.D.

Address: _____

_____

Telephone: _____

PHYSICIAN'S COMMENTS:

_____

_____

_____

_____ M.D.
(physician's signature)

Advice for Active Living During Pregnancy

Pregnacy is a time when women make beneficial changes in their health habits to protect and promote the healthy development of their unborn babies. These changes include adopting improved eating habits, abstinence from smoking and alcohol intake, and participating in regular moderate physical activity. All of these changes can be carried over into the postnatal period and many health experts believe that pregnancy is a very good time to adopt healthy lifestyle habits that are permanent by integrating physical activity with enjoyable healthy eating and a positive self and body image.

Active Living:

➤ see your doctor before increasing your activity level during pregnancy

➤ exercise regularly but don't overexert

➤ exercise with a pregnant friend or join a prenatal exercise program

➤ follow FITT principles modified for pregnant women

➤ know safetey considerations for exercise in pregnancy

Healthy Eating:

➤ the need for calories is higher (about 300 more per day) than before pregnancy

➤ follow Canada's Food Guide to Healthy Eating and choose healthy foods from the following groups: whole grain or enriched bread or cereal, fruits and vegetables, milk and milk products, meat, fish, poultry and alternatives

➤ drink 6-8 glasses of fluid, including water, each day

➤ salt intake should not be restricted

➤ limit caffeine intake i.e., coffee, tea, chocolate, and cola drinks

➤ dieting to lose weight may be harmful

Positive Self and Body Image:

➤ remember that it is normal to gain weight during pregnanoy

➤ accept that your body shape will change during pregnancy

➤ enjoy your pregnancy as a unique and meaningful experience

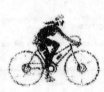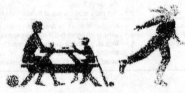

Enjoy eating well, being active and feeling good about yourself. That's VITALIT

SAFETY CONSIDERATIONS

◆ Avoid prolonged or strenuous exertion during the 1st trimester

◆ Avoid isometric exercise or straining while holding your breath

◆ Maintain adequate nutrition and hydration - drink liquids before and after exercise

◆ Avoid exercising in warm/humid environments

◆ Avoid exercise while lying on your back past the 4th month of pregnancy

◆ Avoid activities which involve physical contact or danger of falling

◆ Periodic rest periods may help to minimize possible low oxygen or temperature stress to the fetus

◆ Know the reasons to stop exercise and consult a qualified physician immediately if they occur

** CAUTION **   It is important to monitor the temperature of heated pools. Maternal body temperature during exercise may be increased more by exercising in a warm environment.

REASONS TO CONSULT A PHYSICIAN

◆ Persistent uterine contractions (more than 6-8 per hour)

◆ Bloody discharge from vagina

◆ Any "gush" of fluid from vagina (suggesting premature rupture of the membranes)

◆ Unexplained pain in abdomen

◆ Sudden swelling of extremities (ankles, hands, face)

◆ Swelling, pain and redness in the calf of one leg (suggesting phlebitis)

◆ Persistent headaches or disturbances of vision

◆ Unexplained dizziness or faintness

◆ Marked fatigue, heart palpitations or chest pain

◆ Failure to gain weight (less than 1 kg per month during last two trimesters)

◆ Absence of usual fetal movement

Chapter 38

The Elderly and Endurance Training

MICHAEL L. POLLOCK, DAVID T. LOWENTHAL, JOAN F. CARROLL
AND JAMES E. GRAVES

Introduction

The population in North America and most industrialized countries is living longer. US Census
Bureau data (1996) show that from 1980 to 1990 the
US population increased by 15.8% in the age range
of 65–74 years, 29.5% for those aged 75–84 years and
34.9% for those above 85 years. In 1990, the number
of persons in the US over 65 years of age was 31.1
million, but it is projected to reach over 40 million by
the year 2010, and over 70 million by 2030. With
increased life expectancy, Americans who reach 65
years of age can expect to live an average of 17 additional years (Beck 1989).

Stephens (1987) reported that the activity level of
elderly persons had increased over the preceding
two decades. Even so, it was estimated that at most
10–20% of elderly North Americans participated
in regular vigorous physical activity (defined as
activity that involved an energy expenditure of
$12.5\,kJ\cdot kg^{-1}$ body mass, three times per week for a
minimum of 20 min per session) (Haskell *et al.* 1985).
Further, approximately 37% of North Americans
over 65 years of age rated themselves as having a
sedentary lifestyle (US Department of Health and
Human Services, 1996).

Ageing is associated with a dramatic increase
in health problems and physical limitations. The
physical and physiological limitations to be discussed here are related to changes in aerobic
power/maximal oxygen intake ($\dot{V}O_{2max}$), body composition, muscular strength and the ability to
perform the activities of daily living. We will also
discuss how these limitations are related to a variety
of chronic diseases. Many health problems and
physical limitations are related to the individual's
lifestyle. Thus, sedentary living has a significant
adverse effect on health and physical well-being.
With the elderly population living longer, the
importance of leisure-time activity and regular
exercise training is apparent. The purposes of this
chapter are to discuss the various health problems
and physical/physiological limitations associated
with ageing, to review studies dealing with
endurance training in the elderly, and to give recommendations for exercise prescription in older individuals. Special concerns of and contraindications
to exercise in the elderly will also be addressed.

Physiological and pathological changes related to ageing and exercise science

Physical capacity and physiological function
decline with age (Dehn & Bruce 1972; Raven &
Mitchell 1980; Shephard 1993). The loss of physical
capacity has been attributed to age, reduced physical activity, chronic disease and the medications that
are used to treat chronic disease. The majority of the
elderly do not exercise, and until recently they have
not been encouraged to participate in regular exercise. It is unclear therefore whether the reduced state
of physical conditioning associated with ageing is
a result of deconditioning (a sedentary lifestyle),
ageing, or both. Several reports have suggested that
the age-associated decline in physical performance
and increased incidence of disease can be minimized by regular endurance training (Ordway &
Wekstein 1979; Buskirk & Hodgson 1987; Pollock &

Wilmore 1990; US Department of Health and Human Services 1996). Indeed, participation in regular physical activity results in many favourable responses that contribute to healthy ageing (Huang et al. 1998; Mazzeo et al. 1998). Age-associated changes such as a decline in fat-free mass, total body water and intracellular water, and an increase in fat mass (Sidney et al. 1977; Suominen et al. 1977a), may alter the physiological responses to exercise and influence drug dynamics and kinetics (Richey & Bender 1975; Epstein 1979).

Changes in cardiac function

Cardiac performance undergoes direct and indirect age-associated changes. With increasing age, there is a small reduction in the contractility of the myocardium (Becklake et al. 1965; Dock 1966; Gerstenblith et al. 1976) which may be due to a decrease in myocardial responses to catecholamines (Gerstenblith et al. 1976). Plasma norepinephrine concentrations are increased in the elderly, but the cardiovascular responses are diminished (Palmer et al. 1978; Eisdorfer 1980). The myocardium increases in stiffness, which impairs ventricular diastolic filling (Templeton et al. 1979; Weisfeldt 1981). This suggests that exercised-induced increases in heart rate would be less well tolerated in older individuals than in younger populations.

The age-associated decline in maximal heart rate (Åstrand & Rodahl 1986) is probably less than the 10 beat per decade value commonly reported (Londeree & Moeschberger 1982; Graves et al. 1993). There are multiple causes of this decline, but the most important seems to be a decrement in sympathetic nervous system (adrenergic) reactivity. Reductions in maximal values for cardiac output, stroke volume and stroke index have all been observed with increasing age (Brandfonbrenner et al. 1955; Raven & Mitchell 1980), especially in those individuals with heart disease. The healthy elderly human heart tends to maintain its cardiac output by increasing stroke volume through the Starling effect (Weisfeldt 1981). Nevertheless, cardiac output at the same relative exercise load is lower and arteriovenous O_2 difference is greater than in younger persons (Ogawa et al. 1992).

In a young adult, acute exercise results in a redistribution of the cardiac output from inactive to active tissues (Clausen 1977); in particular, there is a reduction in resting splanchnic flow in order to increase perfusion of the exercising muscle. In the elderly, the resting splanchnic blood flow is reduced to a greater extent than cardiac output, thereby allowing other tissues to be perfused adequately (Bender 1965). The reduction in resting splanchnic blood flow limits the availability of blood flow for redirection to skeletal muscle and the skin during exercise.

Older persons do not tolerate high ambient temperatures as well as younger persons (Shock 1977), because decreases in cardiovascular and hypothalamic function compromise heat-dissipating mechanisms (Irion et al. 1984). The dissipation of heat is further compromised by the decrease in fat-free mass and intracellular and total body water, and the increase in body fat.

Regular endurance exercise favourably alters coronary artery disease (CAD) risk factors, including hypertension, serum concentrations of triglycerides and high density lipoprotein (HDL) cholesterol, glucose tolerance and obesity (US Department of Health and Human Services 1996). In addition, regular exercise raises the angina threshold (Pollock & Wilmore 1990) by improving coronary circulation to the affected myocardium (Laughlin 1994).

Coronary artery disease and graded exercise testing

In spite of a downward trend in CAD mortality rates over the past two decades, cardiovascular disease is still the leading cause of death among older North Americans; CAD accounts for 80% of all cardiovascular deaths. Fifty per cent of US citizens aged 70 years or more show coronary artery stenoses of 75% or more at autopsy (Gersh et al. 1983).

Disease has many atypical manifestations in the elderly. Silent ischaemia may present as confusion, a disturbance of mobility or dizziness. However, angina pectoris remains the most common presenting symptom of CAD. Dyspnoea is also a common presenting symptom in elderly people who have either a myocardial infarction or transient ischaemia (Gottlieb *et al.* 1988).

As many as 50% of North Americans over the age of 65 years have a diagnostically abnormal resting electrocardiogram (ECG). This may reflect age-related changes in the heart, such as mild thickening of the ventricular wall and fibrosis of the conduction system. Electrocardiographic observation of deep Q waves, 1–2 mm of ST segment depression, and T-wave changes associated with symptoms of ischaemia, remain classical features of clinically significant disease (Gottlieb *et al.* 1988).

The aforementioned ECG changes may be interpreted as a false-negative graded exercise test, especially if no further ischaemic changes are noted because the exercise test is terminated after an inadequate peak effort. However, further ST segmental depression to 3–4 mm, if superimposed on a baseline resting ECG of 1–2 mm depression, may connote ischaemia (Bruce 1985). The baseline resting ECG and the patterns observed during graded exercise testing must be interpreted with knowledge of the confounding effects of ageing and underlying conditions, including CAD, hypokalaemia, hypomagnesaemia, hypercalcaemia and hypoxaemia.

Peripheral vascular disease and musculoskeletal disorders may also compromise exercise test performance. Individualization of the graded exercise test (treadmill or cycle ergometer) is important, and protocol selection must depend on the individual's capabilities (Wasserman *et al.* 1994).

The use of radionuclide scintigraphy and thallium in graded exercise testing may improve test sensitivity relative to the ECG alone, particularly at lower levels of intensity. However, some decrease in specificity is found, since other concomitant illnesses may cause abnormalities of coronary perfusion and myocardial function. The gold standard for the diagnosis of CAD remains coronary arteriography.

Changes in blood pressure

Systolic blood pressure usually rises with advancing age (Kannel 1976; Amery *et al.* 1978). Longitudinal data from the Framingham study (Kannel 1976;

Kannel *et al.* 1987) showed a mean increase of 20–25 mmHg between the ages of 36 and 74 years in both men and women. In the same study, the diastolic blood pressure tended to fall in both men and women who were older than 60 years of age.

Ageing is associated with a progressive increase in the rigidity of the aorta and peripheral arteries (Dustan 1974; Hollander 1976), due to a loss of elastic fibres, increases in the collagenous materials and calcium deposition in the media. As aortic rigidity develops, the pulse generated during systole is transmitted to the arterial tree relatively unchanged. Therefore, systolic hypertension predominates in elderly hypertensive patients.

Because of the rise in diastolic blood pressure with isometric or dynamic resistance exercise (Lewis *et al.* 1985; McCartney 1998), elderly individuals with poorly controlled hypertension and/or left ventricular dysfunction should limit their strength training and concentrate more on moderate endurance exercise (Sheldahl *et al.* 1983; MacDougall *et al.* 1985). Hagberg and Seals (1986) noted that aerobic training resulted in an 8-mmHg reduction in both systolic and diastolic blood pressure in elderly hypertensive subjects.

Baroreceptor reflex function

Baroreceptor sensitivity decreases with age (Gribbin *et al.* 1971; Pickering *et al.* 1972). Therefore, rapid adjustment of the cerebral circulation to changes in posture may be impaired in the elderly. Adrenergic blocking agents should be carefully titrated, and blood pressure should be checked in the supine, sitting and standing positions. Regular endurance training does not seem to rectify the gradual deterioration in orthostatic blood pressure regulation with age. Carroll *et al.* (1995), however, found an improved tolerance of postural changes in elderly men and women who had experienced presyncopal symptoms during head-up tilt prior to endurance training.

Renal function

Glomerular filtration rate (GFR) and renal plasma flow are well maintained through the fifth decade of life. Even so, a linear decrease in GFR and renal plasma flow after the age of 20 years leads to a loss of GFR amounting to $4\,ml\cdot min^{-1}$ per decade of GFR, and a loss of renal plasma flow of $35\,ml\cdot min^{-1}$ per decade of renal plasma flow (Slack & Wilson 1976).

Redistribution of cardiac output during exercise results in an acute yet reversible reduction in GFR and renal plasma flow. There is a need to investigate whether these changes become superimposed on the alterations associated with ageing, adversely affecting renal function.

A defect in renal concentrating ability and sluggish renal conservation of sodium intake make elderly patients more liable to dehydration (Papper 1973; Epstein & Hollenberg 1976). Therefore, diuretic agents should be used cautiously, and elderly participants in endurance events should be encouraged to drink plenty of fluids. Hyponatraemia and an oversecretion of antidiuretic hormone further compromise normal salt, water and electrolyte homeostasis in the elderly, a problem that can be compounded by overzealous administration of diuretics.

Renin–angiotensin–aldosterone system

Plasma renin activity and plasma aldosterone concentrations decrease with age in normotensive subjects, and values are even lower in elderly individuals with hypertension (Hayduck et al. 1973; Amery et al. 1978; Ogihara et al. 1979). Sympathetic nervous system deterioration with ageing is due, in part, to a decrease in β-receptor reactivity; on the other hand, plasma catecholamine levels are elevated. This is reflected in a gradual decrease of renin–angiotensin–aldosterone activity. As a result, patients have high normal or slightly elevated resting serum potassium concentrations. This tendency is clinically augmented by the administration of potassium-sparing diuretics, β-adrenergic blocking drugs, angiotensin-converting enzyme inhibitors and non-steroidal anti-inflammatory drugs. The hyperkalaemia may be further exacerbated if the patient is an insulin-dependent diabetic with a degree of renal insufficiency.

Serum potassium increases as a result of vigorous endurance exercise. The elderly have some protection against a lethal hyperkalaemia because skeletal muscle mass, the major source of intracellular potassium, is reduced. After endurance training, exercise-induced increases in potassium are not as large as in the untrained (Braith et al. 1990). Carroll et al. (1994) found that increases in plasma volume and total blood volume following endurance training in men and women 60–82 years old were not associated with changes in resting levels of adrenocorticotrophic hormone, vasopressin, aldosterone, norepinephrine, epinephrine, sodium, potassium or protein.

Hepatic function

Senescence affects hepatic function, with a decrease in the production of albumin, alteration in its molecular structure or changes in receptor affinity. This affects many drugs that are bound to albumin and it also decreases phase I (oxidation, methylation, hydroxylation) pathways of drug biotransformation (Lowenthal 1990). Exercise, acutely and reversibly, decreases hepatic blood flow, and it is therefore possible that changes in liver function with age and exercise exaggerate certain pharmacodynamic effects. Panton et al. (1995), however, found no effect of aerobic training on propranolol pharmacokinetics in healthy men and women 60–80 years of age.

Musculoskeletal changes

Manifestations of disease are at times difficult to distinguish from age-related physiological changes (Cummings et al. 1985; Lane et al. 1986). A decrease in muscle mass relative to total body mass starts in the fifth decade of life, and it becomes marked in the seventh decade. This change leads to decreases in muscle strength, muscular endurance, muscle mass and the number of muscle fibres. There is also a selective reduction in type II (fast-twitch) skeletal muscle relative to type I (slow-twitch) muscle. Enzymes that regulate glycolytic energy metabolism are reduced more than those enzymes involved in oxidative metabolism. The diaphragm and cardiac muscle do not seem to incur metabolic changes with age.

Hyaline cartilage on the articular surface of various joints generally shows degenerative changes with age. Clinically, this is the fundamental alteration in degenerative osteoarthritis (Lane *et al.* 1986).

Bone loss is also a hallmark of ageing (Cummings *et al.* 1985; Heidrich & Thompson 1987). The rate of bone loss is highly individual, and is greatly augmented in postmenopausal women. A decrease in bone mass (osteoporosis) can reduce body stature as well as predispose an individual to spontaneous fractures. Dynamic weight-bearing exercise slows the decrement in bone mass. Older women are more prone to osteoporosis than older men; this may reflect hormonal differences affecting bone (Lane *et al.* 1986).

Exercise in preventive geriatrics

Health in older people is best measured in terms of function, mental status, mobility, continence and a range of activities of daily living. Primary preventive strategies, including proper nutrition (Wheeler *et al.* 1993), can forestall the onset of disease. Whether exercise can prevent the development of atherosclerosis, delay the occurrence of clinical CAD or prevent the evolution of hypertension is at present debatable. But moderate endurance exercise (leisure-time activity or physical training) significantly decreases cardiovascular mortality (Paffenbarger *et al.* 1986; Leon *et al.* 1987; Blair *et al.* 1989; US Department of Health and Human Services 1996). Risk factors associated with CAD are still relevant for the elderly, and should be taken into consideration when planning a preventive regimen (Kannel *et al.* 1987; Mazzeo *et al.* 1998). Secondary prevention is aimed at the early diagnosis and treatment of subclinical disease. Endurance exercise can alter the contributions of stress, a sedentary lifestyle, obesity and diabetes to the development of CAD (Kannel *et al.* 1987; US Department of Health and Human Services 1996). Tertiary prevention focuses on maintaining or improving functional status after the onset of symptomatic disease; the latter con-

tribution is particularly useful in the elderly (Williams 1984).

Special concerns related to medical clearance for exercise

Exercise for the healthy elderly person needs to be addressed in the same manner as that for a younger individual. The US position is that a physician should perform a comprehensive history, physical and mental status examination, basic laboratory studies and a dynamic graded exercise test. Clearance for graded exercise testing and the absolute and relative contraindications to exercise are generally similar for elderly and younger participants (Table 38.1). However, there are some special concerns for the elderly individual (Table 38.2).

The graded exercise test must include careful attention to changes in cardiac rhythm and changes in blood pressure indicative of ischaemia. Abnormalities in patient response and/or symptomatology are not necessarily signs of disease. Careful

Table 38.1 Contraindications to exercise testing in 35–64-year-olds.

Recent acute myocardial infarction
Unstable angina pectoris
Uncontrolled hypertension
Uncontrolled arrhythmia
Symptomatic left ventricular dysfunction
Acute myocarditis
Acute pericarditis
Thrombophlebitis and/or recent pulmonary embolus
Tertiary heart block
Psychotic mental illness

Table 38.2 Contraindications to exercise testing or training unique to the elderly population.

Dementia
Frailty
Global cerebrovascular accident with no evidence of reversibility
Multiple pressure sores
Idiopathic gait disturbances and falls
Urinary incontinence

observation during recovery from the graded exercise test is critical, since dysrhythmias and sudden changes of blood pressure may occur during this phase. Older patients may need a short, active, walking recovery period after both testing and training sessions in order to decrease venous pooling and to attenuate abrupt increases in intravascular volume that would occur if they were placed promptly supine. Once the formal test recovery period has been completed, the patient should be observed while upright for at least an additional 5 min, and the blood pressure should be checked before normal activity is resumed.

Effects of endurance training in the elderly

Even though endurance training has a favourable effect on blood pressure (Hagberg 1990; Fagard & Tipton 1994), glucose tolerance (Holloszy et al. 1986; Durstine & Haskell 1994), concentrations of HDL cholesterol (Wood et al. 1983; Haskell 1986), cardiovascular mortality (Paffenbarger et al. 1986; Leon et al. 1987; Blair et al. 1989; Sherman et al. 1994; LaCroix et al. 1996), bone density (Smith et al. 1981; Chow et al. 1987; Drinkwater 1993) and other physical and health-related factors, this section focuses on the effects of endurance training on aerobic power and body composition (body mass, percentage fat and fat-free mass). The importance of resistance training and its effect on strength and fat-free mass are also discussed. The important question is no longer whether elderly participants can improve function with exercise, but to what extent training-induced adaptations can improve their fitness and well-being. Also, how do their training results compare with the responses of middle-aged and younger participants?

Aerobic power ($\dot{V}O_{2max}$)

$\dot{V}O_{2max}$ decreases with age (Robinson 1938; Dehn & Bruce 1972; Buskirk & Hodgson 1987; Rowell & Tipton 1993). This decline can be attributed to a decrease in maximal cardiac output and arteriovenous O_2 difference (Ogawa et al. 1992; Stratton et al. 1994; Fleg et al. 1995). Heath et al. (1981) reported a

5–15% reduction in $\dot{V}O_{2max}$ for each decade after the age of 30 years. Longitudinal studies on average participants (Kasch & Wallace 1976; Kasch et al. 1985; Åstrand & Rodahl 1986) and athletes (Pollock et al. 1987, 1997; Kohrt et al. 1991) have shown that an active lifestyle (chronic endurance training) significantly attenuates this decline. When such training is maintained, there may be little or no decline in $\dot{V}O_{2max}$ over 10–20 years of follow-up evaluations. Thus, it has been concluded that the decline in $\dot{V}O_{2max}$ is less than 5% per decade for active individuals (Buskirk & Hodgson 1987).

Early studies showed moderate to no improvement in $\dot{V}O_{2max}$ with endurance training in persons over 60 years of age (Benestad 1965; deVries 1970) (Table 38.3). This led many to suggest that elderly participants did not adapt to endurance training to the same extent as middle-aged and younger subjects. However, the short duration of the Benestad (1965) study and the relatively low intensity of training used by deVries (1970) may have limited the potential for improvements. More recent studies confirm that changes in aerobic power are minimal following light-intensity training (Seals et al. 1984; Hagberg et al. 1989).

Recent reviews (Pollock & Wilmore 1990; American College of Sports Medicine (ACSM) 1998; Mazzeo et al. 1998) have shown that aerobic power is increased by 15–30% in most populations following 3–12 months of endurance training. The ACSM's position stand (1998) on *The recommended quantity and quality of exercise for developing and maintaining cardiorespiratory and muscular fitness and flexibility in healthy adults* is shown in Table 38.4.

Intensity and duration of training are interrelated. Lower-intensity exercise must be pursued for a longer duration in order to elicit results that are comparable to those found with higher-intensity training. Within this framework, the total amount of energy expended appears to be the important factor (ACSM recommends 1050–1260 kJ (250–300 kcal) per exercise session for a 70-kg person). Thus, activities with an intensity similar to moderate walking require a training duration of 40–50 min and jogging/running requires 20–30 min.

Table 38.3 shows the effects of endurance training on $\dot{V}O_{2max}$ in the elderly. Even though several

Table 38.3 Effect of exercise training on improvement of $\dot{V}O_{2max}$ in the elderly.

Study	n	Mean age (years)	Training (weeks)	Type	Intensity (% HRR_{max})	Frequency (days·week^{-1})	Duration (min)	$\dot{V}O_{2max}$ (%)
Sidney &	14	62	14	W	60	>2	30	14*
Shephard	8	64	14	W	80	>2	30	29*
(1978)	8	65	14	W	80	<2	30	19*
	12	71	14	W	60	<2	30	−1
Cunningham et al. (1987)	100	63	52	W/J	60 + max MET‡	3	30	11*
Seals et al. (1984)	11	63	26	W	40–50	3	20–30	12*
			26	W/J, B, WG	85	3	30–45	17*
Schwartz (1988)	10	65	12	W/J	80–85	3	40	10*
Meredith et al. (1989)	10	65	12	B	70	3	45	20*
Niinimaa &	10	65	11	W/J, C	HR 125–145	3	10–15	0.5
Shephard (1978)	9	65	11	W/J, C	HR 145–155	3	10–15	10
Chow et al. (1987)	19	66	54	W, D, C	80% HR_{max}	3	30	72*
Adams & deVries (1973)	17	66	12	W/J, C	60	3	15–20	20*†
Badenhop et al.	14	66	9	B	30–45	3	25	16*
(1983)	14	68	9	B	60–75	3	25	15*
deVries (1970)	68	69	6	W/J, C	n.r.	3	30–45	5*†
deVries (1970)	8	69	42	W/J, C	n.r.	3	30–45	8†
Suominen et al. (1977b)	26	69	8	W/J, S, BG, G	n.r.	3	60	11*†
Barry et al. (1996)	8	70	12	B-INT	n.r.	3	40	38*
Hagberg et al. (1989)	16	72	26	W/J	75–85	3	35–45	20*
Benestad (1965)	13	75	5–6	WG-INT	n.r.	3	10–22	0
Kohrt et al. (1991)	110	60–71	39–52	W/J	80%	4	45	18–21*
Satchenfeld et al. (1998)	9	71	24	W	75% HR_{max}	3–4	40–50	14.2*
Kirwan et al. (1993)	12	65	39	W/J	80% HR_{max}	4	45	23.0*
Schwartz et al. (1991)	15	68	26	W/J	85% HRR	5	45	22*

* Significantly different from baseline measurement at $p \leq 0.05$ or less.

† $\dot{V}O_2$ predicted by Åstrand–Ryhming submaximal cycle test.

‡ 1 Met = resting metabolic equivalent, usually 3.5 ml oxygen·kg^{-1}·min^{-1}.

B, bicycling; BG, ball game; C, calisthenics; D, dance; G, gymnastics; HR, heart rate: HRR_{max}, maximal heart rate reserve; INT, intervals; n.r., not reported; S, swimming; W, walk; WG, walking on an uphill grade; W/J, walk/jog.

Table 38.4 The American College of Sports Medicine's position stand on 'The recommended quantity and quality of exercise for developing and maintaining cardiorespiratory and muscular fitness and flexibility in healthy adults' (ACSM 1998).

Factor	Recommendation
Cardiorespiratory fitness and body composition	
Frequency of training	3–5 days·week^{-1}
Intensity of training	55/65–90% of maximum heart rate (HR_{max}), or 40/50–85% of maximum oxygen uptake reserve ($\dot{V}o_{2R}$) or HR_{max} reserve (HRR)*. The lower-intensity values, i.e. 40–49% of $\dot{V}o_{2R}$ or HRR and 55–64% of HR_{max}, are most applicable to individuals who are quite unfit.
Duration of training	20–60 min of continuous or intermittent (minimum of 10-min bouts accumulated throughout the day) aerobic activity. Duration is dependent on the intensity of the activity; thus, lower-intensity activity should be conducted over a longer period of time (30 min or more), and conversely, individuals training at higher levels of intensity should train at least 20 min or longer. Because of the importance of 'total fitness' and the fact that it is more readily attained with exercise sessions of longer duration, and because of the potential hazards and adherence problems associated with high-intensity activity, moderate-intensity activity of longer duration is recommended for adults not training for athletic competition.
Mode of activity	Any activity that uses large muscle groups, which can be maintained continuously, and is rhythmic and aerobic in nature, e.g. walking–hiking, running–jogging, cycling–bicycling, cross-country skiing, aerobic dance/group exercise† (213), rope skipping, rowing, stair climbing, swimming, skating and various endurance game activities or some combination thereof.
Muscular strength and endurance, body composition and flexibility	
Resistance training	Resistance training should be an integral part of an adult fitness programme and of a sufficient intensity to enhance strength and muscular endurance, and maintain fat-free mass (FFM). Resistance training should be progressive in nature, individualized and provide a stimulus to all the major muscle groups. One set of 8–10 exercises that conditions the major muscle groups 2–3 days·week^{-1} is recommended. Multiple-set regimens may provide greater benefits if time allows. Most persons should complete 8–12 repetitions of each exercise; however, for older and more frail persons (approximately 50–60 years of age and above), 10–15 repetitions at a lower intensity may be more appropriate.
Flexibility training	Flexibility exercises should be incorporated into the overall fitness programme sufficiently to develop and maintain range of motion (ROM). These exercises should stretch the major muscle groups and be performed a minimum of 2–3 days·week^{-1}. Stretching should include appropriate static and/or dynamic techniques.

* Maximum heart rate reserve (HRR) and maximum $\dot{V}o_2$ reserve ($\dot{V}o_{2R}$) are calculated from the difference between resting and maximum heart rate and resting and maximum $\dot{V}o_2$, respectively. To estimate training intensity, a percentage of this value is added to the resting heart rate and/or resting $\dot{V}o_2$ and is expressed as a percentage of HRR or $\dot{V}o_{2R}$.
† Aerobic dance refers to a variety of activities such as high- and low-impact aerobics and jazz dancing. The term 'group exercise' has been coined to encompass the broad spectrum of these activities, such as step aerobics, slide-board exercise, strength aerobics and spinning, which are usually performed to music.

investigations did not report precise information on training intensity, it appears that elderly participants who meet the guidelines for fitness recommended by the ACSM increase their $\dot{V}O_{2max}$ to a similar magnitude as younger participants. For example, Sidney and Shephard (1978) showed that subjects who trained at 60% or 80% of maximal heart rate reserve (HRR_{max}) for 30 min more than 2 days per week had a 14% and a 29% increase in $\dot{V}O_{2max}$, respectively, whereas a group who trained at 60% of HRR_{max} for less than 2 days per week showed no change. Hagberg et al. (1989) found a 20% improvement in $\dot{V}O_{2max}$ following 6 months of aerobic training in men and women 70–79 years of age, and Kohrt et al. (1991) found an 18–21% increase in $\dot{V}O_{2max}$ following 9–12 months of training in men and women 60–71 years of age.

Muscular strength

Resistance training does little to promote aerobic fitness, although it is an effective means of developing and maintaining fat-free mass (Hagberg et al. 1989). Likewise, endurance training does little to promote the development and maintenance of muscular strength and muscle mass (Pollock et al. 1987). As mentioned earlier, muscular strength and fat-free mass decrease with age, with more dramatic changes developing after 50–60 years of age (Forbes 1976, 1987). Thus, some type of strength training can benefit most elderly people. Recent research has shown that resistance training is effective in elderly persons up to and exceeding 90 years of age (Fiatarone et al. 1994; Evans 1999).

Body composition

Changes in body composition (body mass, percentage fat and fat-free mass) associated with aerobic training are shown in Table 38.5. Although body mass is reported in most studies, body fat and fat-free mass are mentioned infrequently. Many of the aerobic training programmes that met the aerobic fitness guidelines of the ACSM (see Table 38.4) showed a modest, but significant decrease of body mass (from 0.0 to –2.8 kg, $\bar{x} = -1.1$ kg) (note, one study showed no loss of mass). The average loss

(Table 38.5) was less than the average of 1.5 kg found in 32 studies on young and middle-aged subjects (Wilmore 1983; ACSM 1998). The change in percentage fat in the elderly ranged from –0.9 to –2.6% ($\bar{x} = -1.4$%), again less than the –2.2% loss of fat reported in Wilmore's review (1983). However, one study (Schwartz et al. 1991) noted that intra-abdominal fat decreased by 25% in older men who had lost just 2.5 kg of body mass following 26 weeks of aerobic training. This finding is especially relevant, due to the relationship between abdominal fat and cardiovascular disease. A valid comparison of reductions in body mass and fat with aerobic training between elderly and younger participants is not yet possible, but it appears that elderly exercisers make similar modest changes.

Most studies have not reported fat-free mass data in regard to aerobic training.

Exercise prescription in the elderly

Most elderly men and women can benefit from a regular and appropriately designed exercise programme. Like middle-aged and younger participants, exercise prescription for the elderly is dependent on their needs, goals, physical and health status, available time, equipment and facilities, and personal preference (Larson & Bruce 1987; Pollock & Wilmore 1990). Shephard (1990) adds that when prescribing exercise for the elderly, safety of the programme, compliance and potential effectiveness should be considered. Lower-intensity programmes aid participants in avoiding injury and a potential cardiovascular event, both of which are associated with higher-intensity exercise (Waller 1987; Pollock & Wilmore 1990). Because elderly subjects vary more in health status and level of fitness than middle-aged participants, the art of prescribing safe and adequate training regimens becomes more challenging.

Guidelines for exercise in the elderly

In general, guidelines for the prescription needed to develop and maintain cardiorespiratory fitness in the elderly do not differ much in principle from the guidelines used for middle-aged or younger

Table 38.5 Effect of aerobic training on body composition in the elderly.

Study	n	Mean age (years)	Weeks	Type	Intensity (%HRR$_{max}$)	Frequency (days·week^{-1})	Duration (min)	Criterion	BM (kg)	BF (%)	SF (mm)	FFM (kg)
Cunningham et al. (1987)	102	63	52	W/J	60 + max MET‡	3	30	Σ8 SF[1]	−0.4			+1.1
Seals et al. (1984)†	11	63	20	W	40	3	20–30	Σ6 SF[2]	−0.5		−5.0	
Schwartz (1988)	10	65	12	W/J	80–85	3	40	HW	−2.8*	−2.6*		+0.08
Meredith et al. (1989)	10	65	12	B	70	3	45	HW	+0.1	−1.3		
Niinimaa & Shephard (1978)	10	65	52	W/J,C	HR$_{125-145}$	3	10–15		−1.1			
	9	65	52	W/J,C	HR$_{145-155}$	3	10–15		+0.4			
Adams & deVries (1973)	17	66	12	W/J,C	60	3	15–20 W/J 20–25 C	Σ2 SF[3]	−0.5$^{n.a.}$		−1.8$^{n.a.}$	
deVries (1970)	68	69	6	W/J,C	n.a.	3	30–45	Σ3 SF[4]	−0.9*	−0.9*		
	8	69	42	W/J,C	n.a.	3	30–45		−1.0	−0.9		
Suominen et al. (1977b)	26	69	8	W/J,S, BG,G	n.a.		60		−0.3			
Hagberg et al. (1989)	17	72	26	W/J	85	3	35–45	Σ7 SF[5]	−1.0*	−1.5*	12.5*	
Schwartz et al. (1991)	15	68	26	W/J	85% HRR	5	45	HW	−0.8	−2.3		−0.01

* Significantly different from baseline measurement at $P \leq 0.05$ or less.
† Complete study was 52 consecutive weeks of training, same subjects throughout.
‡ See Table 38.3.
B, bicycling; BF, body fat; BG, ball games; BM, body mass; C, calisthenics; FFM, fat-free mass; G, gymnastics; HR, heart rate; HRR$_{max}$, maximal heart rate reserve; HW, hydrostatic weighting; n.a., no statistics available; S, swimming; SF, skinfolds; W, walk; WG, walking on an uphill grade; W/J, walk/jog.
[1] Chest, triceps, biceps, subscapular, umbilical, suprailiac, anterior thigh and medial calf.
[2] Triceps, subscapular pectoral, umbilical, suprailiac, anterior thigh and medial calf.
[3] Triceps and suprailiac.
[4] Triceps, subscapular and chest.
[5] Chest, axilla, triceps, subscapular, abdominal, suprailiac and anterior thigh.

participants (see Table 38.4). The major difference is in how these guidelines are applied to the elderly. A position stand on *Exercise and physical activity for older adults* has been published by the American College of Sports Medicine (Mazzeo *et al*. 1998) and guidelines for prescribing exercise training for the elderly have also been published (Evans 1999). Programmes most often recommended are similar to those prescribed for unfit, obese, cardiac or fragile participants. Thus, it is suggested typically that relative to younger individuals, old people should exercise at a lower intensity for a longer duration, use activities that avoid stress on the joints and progress in training at a slower rate (deVries 1979; Lampman 1987; Pollock & Wilmore 1990; Shephard 1990; ACSM 1998).

The programme should include an adequate warm-up, some muscular conditioning, a substantial aerobic phase and a cool-down period. The total programme for an average individual should not last longer than 1 h (Pollock & Wilmore 1990). Long-duration programmes usually have high dropout rates.

The elderly participant should place more emphasis on the warm-up and cool-down periods than a younger person. The warm-up should include stretching, low-level calisthenics, and low-level aerobic activities such as slow walking, cycling or swimming. The muscular conditioning period could come either before or after the main aerobic period, depending on personal preference. However, it is recommended that aerobic conditioning follow strength training in the frail elderly (Mazzeo *et al*. 1998). The muscular conditioning period should include moderate-intensity calisthenics and/or weight training. The aerobic period would normally be specific to the participant's needs and sport, but could include any of a variety of endurance activities such as fast walking, swimming, cycling, stair climbing or rowing.

The biggest difference between endurance training programmes for the elderly and those prescribed for younger participants is the intensity/duration component (Pollock & Wilmore 1990; ACSM 1998). For the average elderly person, the intensity of training would be more moderate (50–70% HRR_{max}) and the duration would be longer

(40–50 min). Current guidelines for exercise point out that health benefits may be obtained from quite low-intensity exercise (40–49% HRR_{max}) if this is performed for long periods. Younger participants may benefit from high-intensity interval training (short-duration sprints and rest periods), but this is not usually recommended for the elderly, due to an increased risk of injury and the potential for precipitating a cardiac event. If the subject has not recently been active in sport, a training intensity of 30–40% of HRR_{max} is often appropriate during the first few weeks. The starting programme is usually conducted for 15–20 min. It is important to increase intensity and duration gradually, in order to minimize the risk of injury or untoward event. Thus, several weeks or months may be needed to achieve the appropriate maintenance level of training. Our experience suggests that the duration of training should be increased by 5 min and the intensity by increments of 5% of HRR_{max} approximately every 2 weeks. Unfit subjects should progress first by increasing the duration and then by increasing the intensity of their exercise programmes (Pollock & Wilmore 1990).

The training intensity for each workout can be monitored easily by determining the heart rate at the midpoint and the end of each training session, and making an appropriate calculation of the percentage of HRR_{max}. More recently, the rating of perceived exertion (RPE) scale (Borg 1982) has also been used to help monitor exercise intensity (Birk & Birk 1987; Pollock & Wilmore 1990; ACSM 1998). The RPE scale relates well to heart rate, $\dot{V}O_2$, pulmonary ventilation and blood lactate (Borg 1982). Thus, knowledge of the RPE allows the participant to regulate the training programme perceptually. Exercising at an intensity that produces a training effect is important and, at the same time, regulating the programme at a perceptually acceptable level ('moderate to somewhat hard') helps long-term adherence (Table 38.6).

Is the intensity of an exercise prescription calculated and interpreted in the same manner for elderly participants as for young and middle-aged adults? In our experience with healthy elderly subjects and cardiac patients, it is acceptable to establish exercise intensity as a percentage of HRR_{max} and to use the

Table 38.6 Classification of intensity of exercise based on 30–60 min of endurance training. Adapted from Pollock and Wilmore (1990).

Relative intensity ($\dot{V}o_{2max}$ or HRR_{max})	Rating of perceived exertion	Classification of intensity
<30%	<10	Very light
30–49%	10–11	Light
50–74%	12–13	Moderate (somewhat hard)
75–84%	14–16	Heavy
>85%	>16	Very heavy

HRR_{max}, maximal heart rate reserve.

Table 38.7 Comparison of injuries by age*.

Study	n	Age range (years)	Mode	Injuries (%)
Pollock *et al.* (1977)	50	20–35	W	18
Pollock *et al.* (1971)	19	40–56	W	12
Pollock *et al.* (1976)	22	49–65	W/J	41
Pollock *et al.* (1991)	14	70–79	W, W/J	57

*All programmes were conducted with healthy, previously sedentary individuals. Except for Pollock *et al.* (1971), all programmes had a walk/jog (W/J) component; the 1971 study included only walking (W) as the mode of training. Injuries occurred mainly in the foot, ankle, leg or knee and led to withdrawal from training for at least 1 week. From Pollock (1988).

RPE scale (Pollock *et al.* 1986; Pollock 1988). Table 38.6 shows the recommended classification of exercise programmes lasting 30–60 min (Pollock & Wilmore 1990). The table lists the relationship between the percentage of HRR_{max} and RPE. Based on individualized exercise test results, these markers of intensity have similar values and meaning in the training and progression of training in elderly as in younger participants.

Flexibility is perhaps the most overlooked component of physical fitness. The 1998 ACSM position stand on *The recommended quantity and quality of exercise for developing and maintaining cardiorespiratory and muscular fitness and flexibility in healthy adults* included for the first time recommendations for flexibility exercise. Flexibility exercise assumes an even greater importance in the elderly, because flexibility and mobility are lost with ageing (Greey 1955) and there are potential relationships among flexibility, ambulation, proprioception and balance (Mazzeo *et al.* 1998). Unfortunately flexibility data

from carefully controlled scientific studies are still lacking.

Because of the strong relationship between high-impact activities (such as jogging, running and aerobic dance) and musculoskeletal injuries, low-impact activities are most appropriate for the elderly (Kilbom *et al.* 1969; Mann *et al.* 1969; Oja *et al.* 1974; Pollock *et al.* 1977, 1991; Richie *et al.* 1985). The incidence of orthopaedic injury during participation in jogging programmes is related to the age of the participant (Table 38.7; Pollock 1988). The programmes listed in Table 38.7 were conducted with healthy, previously sedentary volunteers; they trained for 5–6 months by walking (W) and walk/jogging (W/J) for 30–40 min, 3 days (W/J) or 4 days (W) per week (Pollock *et al.* 1971, 1976, 1977, 1991). In the experiments conducted by Pollock *et al.* in 1976 and 1977, training began with equal amounts of W/J and progressed to more continuous jogging as adaptation to training occurred. In our 1991 investigation (Pollock *et al.* 1991), jogging was not introduced until after 3 months of moderately paced walking (40–60% of HRR_{max}, RPE 11–12) and fast walking (60–70% of HRR_{max}, RPE 12–13).

It was surprising that even after 3 months of preliminary training (W), the injury rate was high when the 70–79-year-old subjects began to walk fast or jog. Injuries occurred within the first 2 weeks of W/J; in all cases but one, they were resolved within 3 weeks, while subjects continued to train on a stationary cycle ergometer or to walk slowly on a treadmill. One woman had a stress fracture of the tibia and could not continue in the study. Eventually, all subjects could develop a training heart rate of 70–85% of HRR_{max} (RPE 14–15). The injured subjects continued to walk on the treadmill at an elevation that elicited the desired heart rate response. All of the six women who began to W/J were injured, but only two of eight men were affected. Although the sample was small, this suggests that elderly females are more susceptible to injury than their male peers.

In the above-mentioned W/J study on 70–79-year-old participants (Pollock et al. 1991), the average increases in $\dot{V}O_{2max}$ were 16% and 22%, after 3 and 6 months' training, respectively (Hagberg et al. 1989). The W/J programme that was prescribed was limited not by the cardiorespiratory system, but by the musculoskeletal system (orthopaedic limitations). Further, since a 16% increase in $\dot{V}O_{2max}$ was attained by moderate walking during the first 3 months of the programme, the additional 6% increase in $\dot{V}O_{2max}$ found with W/J was probably not worth the additional risk of injury.

In a follow-up to the Pollock et al. (1991) study, Carroll et al. (1992) compared the incidence of injury from aerobic activity in elderly men and women who trained at either moderate (60–65% HRR_{max}) or high (80–85% HRR_{max}) intensity. In both groups, orthopaedic stress was minimized by walking uphill instead of jogging as exercise intensity was increased. Using this approach, high-intensity training was not associated with an increased incidence of orthopaedic injury. Thus, the high prevalence of injuries in older exercisers is probably due to their inability to tolerate orthopaedic stress.

The fast walking study reported in Table 38.7 (Pollock et al. 1971) produced a 30% increase in $\dot{V}O_{2max}$ and had the lowest injury (12%) and dropout rate of any of the 25 endurance training studies conducted by Pollock and colleagues since 1968. These data and others have shown clearly that walking offers a safe and effective programme both for developing a moderate level of aerobic fitness and for improving body composition (Sharkey & Holleman 1967; Pollock et al. 1975; Leon et al. 1979; Rippe et al. 1988). Walking is also simple to carry out and requires little in terms of skill, special facilities or equipment. Its lower intensity and impact forces make it safe and easily adaptable for elderly participants.

If exercise training cannot be sustained for the required time, low-level interval training may be necessary. This would include periods of slow to moderate walking interspersed with periods of very slow walking or sitting. As adaptation develops, longer periods of moderate to fast walking can be used. The RPE scale is useful in rating peripheral discomfort/pain. Our experience has shown that when discomfort reaches a score of 13 ('moderate to somewhat hard') on the RPE scale, a rest period should begin. Stopka et al. (1998) reported significant improvements of performance in patients with intermittent claudication who were trained below the claudicant threshold for 12 weeks. Shephard (1990) recommended circuit training, whereby 1–2-min bouts of light activity are interspersed with short bouts of exercise using different tasks/exercise stations.

Strength training

A well-rounded stretching and muscle conditioning programme is particularly useful in the elderly, because of a loss of muscle mass and functional capacity in various body segments (Forbes 1976, 1987; Åstrand & Rodahl 1986; Pollock & Wilmore 1990; Evans 1999). For example, Pollock et al. (1987) completed a 10-year follow-up study on master runners whose ages ranged from 50 to 82 years. The study was designed to assess the runners' ability to maintain their aerobic power. Eleven of the 25 subjects evaluated continued to train at the same level throughout the 10-year period, and their $\dot{V}O_{2max}$ did not change (54.2 versus 53.3 ml·kg^{-1}·min^{-1}), whereas the group who reduced their training showed a significant decrease (52.5 versus 45.9 ml·kg^{-1}·min^{-1}). The striking finding in this investigation was a significant loss of fat-free mass in both groups. As a whole, they showed a slight loss of body mass, an increase in body fat and a 2.0-kg decline in fat-free mass over the 10-year timespan. Considering their low body fat (13.2%) and continued training, the change in fat-free mass was a surprising finding. Short-term studies with younger individuals have shown that fat-free mass is usually maintained with endurance training (Pollock & Wilmore 1990), whereas weight/resistance-training activities generally increase muscle mass (Gettman & Pollock 1981; Fleck & Kraemer 1997).

Although ageing is an important consideration, the manner in which the runners trained (just by running) probably contributed to their inability to maintain fat-free mass. The training mode shows significant specificity (Åstrand & Rodahl 1986). Specificity of training was illustrated by circumference measurements on the upper arm and thigh. The upper arm girth showed a significant reduction, whereas the thigh remained constant. An interview with each athlete revealed that most of them had trained aerobically and had undertaken little strength training. Three of the 25 athletes included upper body training as a part of their regular regimen; two weight trained and one was an avid cross-country skier. These three athletes were the only ones who maintained their fat-free mass over the 10-year follow-up period. Age did not seem to be a factor, because there was one athlete representing each decade of age from 50 to 80 years. These data illustrate the need for a well-rounded exercise programme to develop and maintain both aerobic power and muscle mass. It is also one of the reasons why the ACSM added a strength component to their 1990 position stand and continue to emphasize the importance of resistance training (ACSM 1998) (see Table 38.4).

Although calisthenics can provide enough overload to increase strength in the elderly, moderate weight training is safe and can produce better results (Fleck & Kraemer 1997; Mazzeo et al. 1998; Evans 1999). The eight to ten exercises recommended by the ACSM (see Table 38.4) should be adequate to train the major muscles of the body (arms, shoulders, trunk, hips and legs). The development of new equipment such as variable resistance exercise devices makes this type of training particularly suitable and safe for the elderly population (Pollock 1988; Pollock & Wilmore 1990).

Conclusions

Aerobic power, muscular strength, muscle mass and flexibility decline after maturation. Declines in physiological function are associated with a reduction in muscle mass, a concomitant increase in relative body fat and an increase in the incidence of chronic disease. Although they were traditionally considered a direct consequence of the ageing process, recent studies indicate that many age-related declines in functional capacity and health status can be reduced by regular physical activity. This suggests that reduced physiological function is related to a sedentary lifestyle, and that elderly men and women would benefit from exercise training. Indeed, individuals of all ages derive benefits in physical function and health status from participation in regular physical activity.

Exercise programmes for elderly persons should emphasize fitness development, but the maintenance of functional capacity and quality of life are equally important. The basic guidelines of frequency, intensity and duration of training and mode of activity recommended by the ACSM are appropriate for the elderly, but the manner in which they are applied is important. Given that many elderly people are more fragile and have more physical–medical limitations than middle-aged exercisers, the intensity of the programme should be lower, and the frequency and duration of training should be increased. High-impact activities should be avoided and progression of training should be more gradual. The training heart rate, 50–85% of HRR$_{max}$, and its relationships to relative metabolic work and RPE are similar to those found in younger participants. Health benefits may result from aerobic activities as low as 40–49% of HRR$_{max}$. Because of the importance of maintaining muscle mass and bone density in middle and old age, a well-rounded endurance training programme should include strength/resistance exercise for the major muscle groups. Exercises for the development and maintenance of flexibility are also a critical component of a well-rounded exercise programme for older adults. Such exercises may be easily incorporated into the warm-up and/or cool-down. Finally, exercise prescription for most elderly persons should emphasize moderate-intensity, low-impact activities; it should avoid heavy static–dynamic lifting, and allow a slow, gradual period of adaptation.

References

Adams, G. & deVries, H. (1973) Physiological effects of an exercise training regimen upon women aged 52–79. *Journal of Gerontology* **28**, 50–55.

American College of Sports Medicine (ACSM) (1998) The recommended quantity and quality of exercise for developing and maintaining cardiorespiratory and muscular fitness and flexibility in healthy adults. *Medicine and Science in Sports and Exercise* **30**, 975–991.

Amery, A., Wasir, H., Bulpitt, C. *et al.* (1978) Aging and the cardiovascular system. *Acta Cardiologica (Bruxelles)* **6**, 443.

Åstrand, P. & Rodahl, K. (1986) *Textbook of Work Physiology*, 3rd edn. McGraw-Hill, New York.

Badenhop, D., Cleary, P., Schall, S., Fox, E. & Bartels, R. (1983) Physiological adjustments to higher or lower-intensity exercise in elders. *Medicine and Science in Sports and Exercise* **15**, 496–502.

Barry, A., Daly, J., Pruett, E. *et al.* (1996) The effects of physical conditioning on older individuals. I. Work capacity, circulatory–respiratory function and work electrocardiogram. *Journal of Gerontology* **21**, 182–191.

Beck, J. (1989) General principles of aging: demography of aging. In: Beck, J. (ed.) *Geriatrics Review Syllabus: a Core Curriculum in Geriatric Medicine*, pp. 1–5. American Geriatrics Society, New York.

Becklake, M., Frank, H., Dagenais, G., Ostiguy, G. & Guzman, C. (1965) Age changes in myocardial function and exercise response. *Progress in Cardiovascular Diseases* **19**, 1–21.

Bender, A. (1965) The effect of increasing age on the distribution of peripheral blood flow in man. *Journal of the American Geriatric Society* **13**, 192–198.

Benestad, A. (1965) Trainability of old men. *Acta Medica Scandinavica* **178**, 321–327.

Birk, T. & Birk, C. (1987) Use of ratings of perceived exertion for exercise prescription. *Journal of Sports Medicine and Physical Fitness* **4**, 1–8.

Blair, S., Kohl, H., Paffenberger, R., Clark, D., Cooper, K. & Gibbons, L. (1989) Physical fitness and all-cause mortality: a prospective study of healthy men and women. *Journal of the American Medical Association* **262**, 2395–2401.

Borg, G. (1982) Psychophysical bases of perceived exertion. *Medicine and Science in Sports and Exercise* **14**, 377–381.

Braith, R., Lowenthal, D., Graves, J., Leggett, S., Wilcox, C. & Pollock, M. (1990) The influence of exercise training on the renin–aldosterone system of the elderly. *Medicine and Science in Sports and Exercise* (abstract) **22**, S33.

Brandfonbrenner, M., Landowne, M. & Shock, N. (1955) Changes in cardiac output with age. *Circulation* **12**, 557–566.

Bruce, R. (1985) Functional aerobic capacity, exercise and aging. In: Andres, R., Bierman, E. & Hazzard, W. (eds) *Principles of Geriatric Medicine*, pp. 87–103. McGraw-Hill, New York.

Buskirk, E. & Hodgson, J. (1987) Age and aerobic power: the rate of change in men and women. *Federation Proceedings* **46**, 1824–1829.

Carroll, J., Pollock, M.L., Graves, J.E. *et al.* (1992) Incidence of injury during moderate- and high-intensity walking training in the elderly. *Journals of Gerontology* **47**, 61–66.

Carroll, J.F., Convertino, V.A., Wood, C.E., Graves, J.E., Lowenthal, D.T. & Pollock, M.L. (1994) Effect of training on blood volume and plasma hormone concentrations in the elderly. *Medicine and Science in Sports and Exercise* **27**, 79–84.

Carroll, J.F., Wood, C.E., Pollock, M.L., Graves, J.E., Convertino, V.A. & Lowenthal, D.T. (1995) Hormonal responses in elders experiencing presyncopal symptoms during head-up tilt before and after exercise training. *Journals of Gerontology* **50**, 324–329.

Centers for Disease Control and Prevention (1992) National Center for Chronic Disease Prevention and Health Promotion, Behavioural Risk Factor Social Survey, Atlanta, GA.

Chow, R., Harrison, J., Sturtridge, W. *et al.* (1987) The effect of exercise on bone mass of osteoporotic patients on fluoride treatments. *Clinical and Investigative Medicine* **10**, 59–63.

Clausen, J. (1977) Effect of physical training on cardiovascular adjustments to exercise in man. *Physiological Reviews* **57**, 779–815.

Cummings, S., Kelsey, J., Nevitt, M. *et al.* (1985) Epidemiology of osteoporosis and osteoporotic fractures. *Epidemiological Reviews* **7**, 178–208.

Cunningham, D., Rechnitzer, P., Howard, J. & Donner, A. (1987) Exercise training of men at retirement: a clinical trial. *Journals of Gerontology* **42**, 17–23.

Dehn, M. & Bruce, R. (1972) Longitudinal variations in maximal oxygen intake with age and activity. *Journal of Applied Physiology* **33**, 805–807.

Dock, W. (1966) How some hearts age. *Journal of the American Medical Association* **195**, 442–444.

Drinkwater, B.L. (1993) Exercise in the prevention of osteoporosis. *Osteoporosis International* **1**, S169–S171.

Durstine, J.L. & Haskell, W.L. (1994) Effects of exercise training on plasma lipids and lipoproteins. *Exercise and Sport Sciences Reviews* **22**, 477–521.

Dustan, H. (1974) Atherosclerosis complicating chronic hypertension. *Circulation* **50**, 871.

Eisdorfer, C. (1980) Neurotransmitters and aging: clinical correlates. In: Adelman, R. *et al.* (eds) *Neural Regulatory Mechanisms During Aging*, pp. 53–69. Alan R. Liss, New York.

Epstein, M. (1979) Effects of aging of the kidney. *Federation Proceedings* **38**, 168–173.

Epstein, M. & Hollenberg, N. (1976) Age as a determinant of renal sodium conservation in normal man. *Journal of Laboratory and Clinical Medicine* **87**, 411.

Evans, W. (1999) Exercise training guidelines for the elderly. *Medicine and Science in Sports and Exercise* **31**, 12–17.

Fagard, R.H. & Tipton, C.M. (1994) Physical activity, fitness, and hypertension. In: Bouchard, C., Shephard, R.J. & Stephans, T. (eds) *Physical Activity, Fitness, and Health: International Proceedings and Consensus Statement*, pp. 633–655. Human Kinetics, Champaign, IL.

Fiatarone, M.A., O'Neill, E.F., Ryan, N.D. *et al.* (1994) Exercise training and nutritional supplementation for physical frailty in very elderly people. *New England Journal of Medicine* **330**, 1769–1775.

Fleck, S. & Kraemer, W. (1997) *Designing Resistance Training Programs*, 2nd edn. Human Kinetics, Champaign, IL.

Fleg, J.L., O'Connor, F., Gerstenblith, G., Becker, L., Clulow, J., Schulman, S. & Lakatta, E. (1995) Impact of age on the cardiovascular response to dynamic upright exercise in healthy men and women. *Journal of Applied Physiology* **78**, 890–900.

Forbes, G. (1976) The adult decline in lean body mass. *Human Biology* **48**, 161–173.

Forbes, G. (1987) *Human Body Composition Growth, Aging, Nutrition and Activity*. Springer-Verlag, New York.

Gersh, B., Kronmal, R., Frye, R. *et al.* (1983) Coronary arteriography and coronary artery bypass surgery: morbidity and mortality in patients age 65 years or older: a report from the coronary artery surgery study. *Circulation* **67**, 483.

Gerstenblith, G., Lakatta, E. & Weinsfeldt, M. (1976) Age changes in myocardial function and exercise response. *Progress in Cardiovascular Diseases* **19**, 1–21.

Gettman, L. & Pollock, M. (1981) Circuit weight training: a critical review of its physiological benefits. *Physician and Sportsmedicine* **9** (1), 44–60.

Gottlieb, S.O., Gottlieb, S.H., Achuff S.C., Baumgardner R., Mellits E.D., Weisfeldt M.L. & Gerstenblith G. (1988) Silent ischemia on Holter monitoring predicts mortality in high risk post infarction patients. *Journal of the American Medical Association* **259**, 1030–1035.

Graves, J.E., Pollock, M., Swart, D., Panton, L.B., Garzarella, L., Lowenthal, D.T., Limacher, M. & Menglekoch, L. (1993) Does 220 – age accurately predict maximal heart rate in the elderly? *Medicine and Science in Sports and Exercise* **25** (5), 186.

Greey, C.W. (1955) *A Study of Flexibility in Selected Joints of Adult Males Ages 18–72*. Doctoral Dissertation, University of Michigan.

Gribbin, B., Pickering, T., Sleight, P. & Peto, R. (1971) Effect of age and high blood pressure on baroflex sensitivity in man. *Circulation Research* **29**, 424.

Hagberg, J. (1990) Exercise, fitness, and hypertension. In: *Exercise Fitness, and Health: a Consensus of Current Knowledge*, pp. 455–466. Human Kinetics, Champaign, IL.

Hagberg, J. & Seals, D. (1986) Exercise training and hypertension. *Acta Medica Scandinavica* **711** (Suppl.), 131–136.

Hagberg, J., Graves, J., Limbacher, M. *et al.* (1989) Cardiovascular responses of 70–79 year old men and women to exercise training. *Journal of Applied Physiology* **66**, 2589–2594.

Haskell, W. (1986) The influence of exercise training on plasma lipids and lipoproteins in health and disease. *Acta Medica Scandinavica* (**Suppl.** 711), 25–37.

Haskell, W., Montoye, H. & Orenstein, D. (1985) Physical activity and exercise to achieve health-related physical fitness components. *Public Health Reports* **100**, 202–212.

Hayduck, K., Krause, D., Kaufmann, W., Huenges, R., Schillmoeller, U. & Unbehaun, V. (1973) Age dependent changes of plasma renin concentration in humans. *Clinical Science and Molecular Medicine* **45** (Suppl. 1), 273.

Heath, G., Hagberg, J., Ehsani, A. & Holloszy, J. (1981) A physiological comparison of young and older endurance athletes. *Journal of Applied Physiology* **51**, 634–640.

Heidrich, F. & Thompson, R.S. (1987) Osteoporosis prevention: strategies applicable for general population groups. *Journal of Family Practice* **25**, 33–39.

Hollander, W. (1976) Role of hypertension in atherosclerosis and cardiovascular disease. *American Journal of Cardiology* **38**, 786.

Holloszy, J., Schultz, J., Kusnierkiewicz, J., Hagberg, J. & Ehsani, A. (1986) Effect of exercise on glucose tolerance and insulin resistance. *Acta Medica Scandinavica* **711** (Suppl.), 55–65.

Huang, Y., Macera, S., Blair, S., Brill, P., Kohl, H. & Kronenfeld, J. (1998) Physical fitness, physical activity, and functional limitation in adults aged 40 and older. *Medicine and Science in Sports and Exercise* **30**, 1430–1435.

Irion, G., Wailgum, T., Stevens, C., Kendrick, Z. & Paolone, A. (1984) The effect of age on the hemodynamic response to thermal stress during exercise. In: Cristfalo, V., Baker, G., Adelman, R. & Roberts, I. (eds) *Altered Endocrine States During Aging*, pp. 187–195. H.A. Liss, New York.

Kannel, W. (1976) Blood pressure and the development of cardiovascular disease in the aged. In: Caird, F., Dahl, J. & Kennedy, R. (eds) *Cardiology in Old Age*, pp. 143–175. Plenum Press, New York.

Kannel, W., Doyle, J., Shepard, R., Stamler, J. & Vokonas, P. (1987) Prevention of cardiovascular disease in the elderly. *Journal of the American College of Cardiology* **10**, 25A–28A.

Kasch, F. & Wallace, J. (1976) Physiological variables during 10 years of endurance exercise. *Medicine and Science in Sports* **8**, 5–8.

Kasch, F., Wallace, J. & vanCamp, S. (1985) Effects of 18 years of endurance exercise on physical work capacity of older men. *Journal of Cardiopulmonary Rehabilitation* **15**, 308–312.

Kilbom, A., Hartley, L., Saltin, B., Bijure, J., Grimby, G. & Åstrand, I. (1969) Physical training in sedentary middle-aged and older men. *Scandinavian Journal of Laboratory and Clinical Investigation* **24**, 315–322.

Kirwan, J.P., Kohrt, W.M., Wojta, D.M., Bourey, R.E. & Holloszy, J.O. (1993) Endurance exercise training reduces glucose-stimulated insulin levels in 60- to 70-year-old men and women. *Journals of Gerontology* **48**, 84–90.

Kohrt, W., Malley, M., Coggan, A. *et al.* (1991) Effects of gender, age, and fitness level on response of $\dot{V}O_{2max}$ to training in 60–71 year olds. *Journal of Applied Physiology* **71**, 2004–2011.

LaCroix, A.Z., Leveille, S.G., Hecht, J.A., Grothaus, L.C. & Wagner, E.H. (1996) Does walking decrease the risk of cardiovascular disease hospitalizations and death in older adults? *Journal of the American Geriatric Society* **44**, 113–120.

Lampman, R. (1987) Evaluating and prescribing exercise for elderly patients. *Geriatrics* **42**, 63–76.

Lane, C., Bloch, D., Jones, S. *et al.* (1986) Long distance running, bone density, and osteoarthritis. *Journal of the American Medical Association* **255**, 1147–1151.

Larson, E. & Bruce, R. (1987) Health benefits of exercise in an aging society. *Archives of Internal Medicine* **147**, 353–356.

Laughlin, M.H. (1994) Effects of exercise training on coronary circulation: introduction. *Medicine and Science in Sports and Exercise* **26**, 1226–1229.

Leon, A., Conrad, J., Hunninghake, D. & Serfass, R. (1979) Effects of a vigorous walking program on body composition, and carbohydrate and lipid metabolism of obese young men. *American Journal of Clinical Nutrition* **32**, 1776–1787.

Leon, A., Connett, J., Jacobs, D. & Rauramaa, R. (1987) Leisure-time physical activity levels and risk of coronary heart disease and death: the multiple risk factor intervention trial. *Journal of the American Medical Association* **258**, 2388–2395.

Lewis, S., Snell, P., Taylor, W. *et al.* (1985) Role of muscle mass and mode of contraction in circulatory responses to exercise. *Journal of Applied Physiology* **58**, 146–151.

Londeree, B.R. & Moeschberger, M.L. (1982) Effect of age and other factors on maximal heart rate. *Research Quarterly* **53**, 29.

Lowenthal, D. (1990) Geriatric clinical pharmacology. In: Abrams, W. & Berkow, R. (eds) *Merck Manual of Geriatrics*, pp. 181–193. Merck, Rahway, New Jersey.

MacDougall, J., Tuxen, D., Sale, D., Moroz, J. & Sutton, J. (1985) Arterial blood pressure responses to heavy resistance exercise. *Journal of Applied Physiology* **58**, 785–790.

McCartney, N. (1998) Acute responses to resistance training and safety. *Medicine and Science in Sports and Exercise* **31**, 31–37.

Mann, G., Garrett, L., Farhi, A. *et al.* (1969) Exercise to prevent coronary heart disease. *American Journal of Medicine* **46**, 785–790.

Mazzeo, R.S., Cavanagh, P., Evans, W. *et al.* (1998) ACSM position stand: exercise and physical activity for older adults. *Medicine and Science in Sports and Exercise* **30**, 992–1008.

Meredith, C., Frontera, W., Fisher, E. *et al.* (1989) Peripheral effects of endurance training in young and old subjects. *Journal of Applied Physiology* **66**, 2844–2849.

Niinimaa, V. & Shephard, R. (1978) Training and oxygen conductance in the elderly. *Journal of Gerontology* **33**, 354–361.

Ogawa, T., Spina, R., Martin, W. III *et al.* (1992) Effects of aging, sex and physical training on cardiovascular responses to exercise. *Circulation* **86**, 494–503.

Ogihara, T., Hata, T., Maruyama, A. *et al.* (1979) Studies on the renin–angiotensin aldosterone system in elderly hypertensive patients with an angiotensin II antagonist. *Clinical Science* **57**, 461–463.

Oja, P., Terslinna, P., Partanen, T. & Karava, R. (1974) Feasibility of an 18 months' physical training program for middle-aged men and its effect on physical fitness. *American Journal of Public Health* **64**, 459–465.

Ordway, G. & Wekstein, D. (1979) The effect of age on selected cardiovascular responses to static (isometric) exercise. *Proceedings of the Society for Experimental Biology and Medicine* **161**, 189–192.

Paffenbarger, R., Hyde, R., Wing, A. & Hsieh, C. (1986) Physical activity and all-cause mortality, and longevity of college alumni. *New England Journal of Medicine* **314**, 605–613.

Palmer, G., Ziegler, M. & Lake, C. (1978) Response of norepinephrine and blood pressure to stress increases with age. *Journal of Gerontology* **33**, 482–487.

Panton, L.B., Guillen, G.J., Williams, L. *et al.* (1995) The lack of effect of aerobic exercise training on propranolol pharmacokinetics in young and elderly adults. *Journal of Clinical Pharmacology* **35**, 885–894.

Papper, S. (1973) The effects of age in reducing renal function. *Geriatrics* **28**, 83–87.

Pickering, T., Gribbin, B. & Oliver, D. (1972) Baroflex sensitivity in patients on long term hemodialysis. *Clinical Science* **43**, 645–657.

Pollock, M. (1988) Exercise prescriptions for the elderly. In: Spirduso, W. & Eckert, H. (eds) *Physical Activity and Aging*, pp. 163–174. Human Kinetics, Champaign, IL.

Pollock, M. & Wilmore, J. (1990) *Exercise in Health and Disease: Evaluation and Prescription for Prevention and Rehabilitation*, 2nd edn. W.B. Saunders, Philadelphia.

Pollock, M., Miller, H., Janeway, R., Linnerud, A., Robertson, B. & Valentino, R. (1971) Effects of walking on body composition and cardiovascular function of middle aged men. *Journal of Applied Physiology* **30**, 126–130.

Pollock, M., Dimmick, J., Miller, H., Kendrick, Z. & Linnerud, A. (1975) Effects of mode of training on cardiovascular function and body composition of middle-aged men. *Medicine and Science in Sports* **7**, 139–145.

Pollock, M., Dawson, G., Miller, H. *et al.* (1976) Physiologic responses of men 49–65 years of age to endurance training. *Journal of the American Geriatric Society* **24**, 97–104.

Pollock, M., Gettman, L., Milesis, C., Bah, M., Durstine, L. & Johnson, R. (1977) Effects of frequency and duration of training on attrition and incidence of injury. *Medicine and Science in Sports and Exercise* **19**, 31–36.

Pollock, M., Jackson, A. & Foster, C. (1986) The use of the perception scale for exercise prescription. In: Borg, G. & Ottoson, D. (eds) *The Perception of Exertion in Physical Work*, pp. 161–176. MacMillan, London.

Pollock, M., Foster, C., Knapp, D., Rod, J. & Schmidt, D. (1987) Effect of age and training on aerobic capacity and body composition of master athletes. *Journal of Applied Physiology* **62**, 725–731.

Pollock, M., Carrol, J., Graves, J., Leggett, S., Braith, R. & Hagberg, J. (1991) Injuries and adherence to walk/jog and resistance training programs in the elderly.

Medicine and Science in Sports and Exercise **23**, 1194–1200.

Pollock, M., Mengelkoch, L., Graves, J. *et al.* (1997) Twenty-year follow-up of aerobic power and body composition of older track athletes. *Journal of Applied Physiology* **82**, 1508–1516.

Raven, P. & Mitchell, J. (1980) The effect of aging on the cardiovascular response to dynamic and static exercise. In: Wisfelt, M. (ed.) *The Aging Heart*, pp. 269–296. Raven Press, New York.

Richey, D. & Bender, A. (1975) Effects of human aging on drug absorption and metabolism. In: Goldman, R. & Rockstein, M. (eds) *Physiology and Pathology of Human Aging*, pp. 59–71. Academic Press, New York.

Richie, D., Kelso, S. & Bellucci, P. (1985) Aerobic dance injuries: a retrospective study of instructors and participants. *Physician and Sportsmedicine* **13** (2), 114–120.

Rippe, J., Ward, A., Porcari, J. & Freedson, P. (1988) Walking for health and fitness. *Journal of the American Medical Association* **259**, 2720–2724.

Robinson, S. (1938) Experimental studies of physical fitness in relation to age. *Arbeitsphysiologie* **10**, 251–323.

Rowell, L.B. & Tipton, C.M. (1993) Cardiovascular adjustments to exercise and physical conditioning in midlife. *American Academy of Orthopedic Surgeons* **5**, 61–76.

Satchenfeld, N.S., Mack, G.W., DiPietro, L., Morocco, T.S., Jozsi, A.C. & Nadel, E.R. (1998) Regulation of blood volume during training in post-menopausal women. *Medicine and Science in Sports and Exercise* **30**, 92–98.

Schwartz, R. (1988) Effects of exercise training on high-density lipoproteins and apolipoprotein A-I in old and young men. *Metabolism* **37**, 1128–1133.

Schwartz, R.S., Shuman, W.P., Larson, V. *et al.* (1991) The effect of intensive endurance exercise training on body fat distribution in young and older men. *Metabolism: Clinical and Experimental* **40**, 545–551.

Seals, D., Hagberg, J., Hurley, B., Ehsani, A. & Holloszy, J. (1984) Endurance training in older men and women. I. Cardiovascular responses to exercise. *Journal of Applied Physiology* **57**, 1024–1029.

Sharkey, B. & Holleman, J. (1967) Cardiorespiratory adaptations to training at specified intensities. *Research Quarterly* **38**, 698–704.

Sheldahl, L., Wilkie, N., Tristani, F. & Kalbfleisch, J. (1983) Responses of patients after myocardial infarction to carrying a graded series of weight loads. *American Journal of Cardiology* **52**, 698–703.

Shephard, R. (1990) The scientific basis of exercise prescribing for the very old. *Journal of the American Geriatric Society* **38**, 62–70.

Shephard, R. (1993) Physiologic changes over the years. In: American College of Sports Medicine. *ACSM's Resource Manual for Guidelines for Exercise Testing and Prescription* (2nd edn), pp. 397–408. Lea & Febiger, Philadelphia, PA.

Sherman, S.E., D'Agostino, R.B., Cobb, J.L. & Kannel, W.B. (1994) Physical activity and mortality in women in the Framingham Heart Study. *American Heart Journal* **128**, 879–884.

Shock, N. (1977) Systems integration. In: Finch, C. & Hayflick, L. (eds) *Handbook of the Biology of Aging*, pp. 639–665. Van Nostrand Reinhold, New York.

Sidney, K. & Shephard, R. (1978) Frequency and intensity of exercise training for elderly subjects. *Medicine and Science in Sports and Exercise* **10**, 125–131.

Sidney, K., Shephard, R. & Harrison, J. (1977) Endurance training and body composition in the elderly. *American Journal of Clinical Nutrition* **30**, 326–333.

Slack, T. & Wilson, D. (1976) Normal renal function: C_{in} and C_{pah} in healthy donors before and after nephrectomy. *Mayo Clinic Proceedings* **51**, 296–300.

Smith, E., Reddan, W. & Smith, P. (1981) Physical activity and calcium modalities for bone mineral increase in aged women. *Medicine and Science in Sports and Exercise* **13**, 60–64.

Stephens, T. (1987) Secular trends in adult physical activity: exercise boom or bust? *Research Quarterly* **58**, 94–105.

Stopka, C., Wolper, R., Scott, K., Seegar, J., Ballinger, R., Graves, J. (1998) Pain-free exercise training for people with peripheral vascular disease? *Palaestra* **14**, 20–23.

Stratton, J., Levy, W., Cerqueira, M., Schwartz, R. & Abrass, I. (1994) Cardiovascular responses to exercise effects of aging and exercise training in healthy men. *Circulation* **89**, 1648–1655.

Suominen, H., Heikkinen, E., Leisen, H., Michael, D. & Hollman, W. (1977a) Effects of 8 weeks' endurance training on skeletal muscle metabolism in 56–70 year old sedentary men. *European Journal of Applied Physiology* **37**, 173–180.

Suominen, H., Heikkinen, E. & Parkatti, T. (1977b) Effect of eight weeks' physical training on muscle and connective tissue of the m. vastus lateralis in 69-year-old men and women. *Journal of Gerontology* **32**, 33–37.

Templeton, G., Platt, M., Willerson, J. & Weisfeldt, M. (1979) Influence of aging on left ventricular hemodynamics and stiffness in beagles. *Circulation Research* **44**, 189–194.

US Bureau of the Census (1996) *Current Population Reports, Special Studies, 65+ in the United States*, pp. 23–190. US Government Printing Office, Washington, DC.

US Department of Health and Human Services (1996) *Physical Activity and Health: a Report of the Surgeon General*. US Department of Health and Human Services,

Centers for Disease Control and Prevention, National Center for Chronic Disease Prevention and Health Promotion, Atlanta, GA.

deVries, H. (1970) Physiological effects of an exercise training program upon men aged 52–88. *Journal of Gerontology* **24**, 325–336.

deVries, H. (1979) Tips on prescribing exercise regimens for your older patient. *Geriatrics* **34** (4), 75–77, 80–81.

Waller, B. (1987) Sudden death in middle-aged conditioned subjects: Coronary atherosclerosis is the culprit. *Mayo Clinic Proceedings* **62**, 634–636.

Wasserman, K., Hansen, J.E., Sue, D.Y., Whipp, B.J. & Casaburi, R. (1994) *Principles of Exercise Testing and Interpretation*. Lea & Febiger, Philadelphia.

Weisfeldt, M. (1981) Left ventricular function. In: Weisfeldt, M.L. (ed.) *The Aging Heart*, pp. 297–316. Raven Press, New York.

Wheeler, D.L., Graves, J.E. & Lowenthal, D.T. (1993) Exercise and nutrition at midlife. *American Academy of Orthopedic Surgeons* **22**, 375–411.

Williams, T. (1984) *Rehabilitation in the Aging*. Raven Press, New York.

Wilmore, J. (1983) Body composition in sport and exercise: directions for future research. *Medicine and Science in Sports and Exercise* **15**, 21–31.

Wood, P., Haskell, W., Blair, S. *et al.* (1983) Increased exercise level and plasma lipoprotein concentrations: a one-year, randomized, controlled study in sedentary, middle-aged men. *Metabolism* **32**, 31–39.

Chapter 39

Endurance Training for Persons with Disabilities

KENNETH H. PITETTI AND J. LARRY DURSTINE

Introduction

According to the Americans with Disability Act (ADA), a disability is defined as 'a physical or mental impairment that substantially limits one or more of the major life activities' (McNeil 1993). Using this definition, it has been reported that there are 48.9 million persons (19.4% of the population) with disabilities in the United States (McNeil 1993). This includes persons who use wheelchairs or are long-term users of crutches, canes or walkers. Other examples would be persons with limited or no vision, and persons with mental retardation, arthritis, obesity or asthma. All of these conditions limit the individual's ability to interact successfully with society or the environment. As major life activities become limited, the need for physical exercise or endurance training increases.

The principles of endurance training for non-disabled persons have been well documented and are equally applicable to persons with disabilities. The essential components of an endurance exercise programme are mode(s), intensity, duration, frequency and progression of physical activity (American College of Sports Medicine 1995). The mode of exercise involves the use of large muscle groups over prolonged periods (e.g. 15–60 min) and is rhythmic in nature (e.g. walking, jogging, cycling, rowing, combined arm and leg ergometry or swimming). Intensity is determined by the level of heart rate during exercise and/or the use of rating of perceived exertion (RPE) scales. Exercise duration is the length of the exercise session, and exercise frequency is the number of exercise sessions per day

and per week. Rate of progression involves three stages: initial conditioning, improvement and maintenance. Methods and criteria for determining the mode, intensity, duration, frequency and rate of progression are specified by the American College of Sports Medicine (1995).

In order to prescribe the proper endurance exercise regimen for each person, a graded exercise test (GXT) of functional capacity should be conducted prior to the onset of the exercise programme. This test is usually performed on a treadmill or cycle ergometer while heart rate, blood pressure, RPE and subjective response to exercise (e.g. feelings of breathlessness, extreme muscle fatigue) are monitored (American College of Sports Medicine 1995). The results of the functional capacity test help to identify any cardiopulmonary anomalies and provide the necessary information for prescribing a safe and effective exercise regimen. However, many persons with disabilities, because of the uniqueness of each disability (e.g. spinal cord injury, cerebral palsy, multiple sclerosis, cystic fibrosis), have distinctive limitations and therefore special consideration must be given when evaluating their functional capacity. For the chronically diseased and disabled, recommendations for exercise testing have also been provided by the American College of Sports Medicine (1997).

The benefits of endurance training and regular physical activity for the general population have been well established (Blair 1993; Paffenbarger et al. 1993; Chapters 47 & 51). Epidemiological and laboratory data demonstrate that regular exercise protects against the development and progression of many chronic diseases and is an important ingredient of a healthy lifestyle. Additionally, increases in the physical activity of sedentary adults have reduced mortality, thus supporting the hypothesis that regular exercise increases longevity. Indeed, Hahn *et al.* (1990) reported that enormous public health benefits within the general population would result from an increase in their physical activity. For the disabled, however, the rewards of regular exercise far surpass the benefits of reducing the risk of developing a secondary chronic disease or of extending longevity. Regular exercise improves the *quality* of life for the disabled.

To clarify why endurance training or regular exercise is *more* important for persons with disabilities than for able-bodied individuals, one must consider how a person's physical capacity to perform the activities of daily living (ADL) is determined. As in able-bodied people, the physical capacity of persons with disabilities is expressed as peak aerobic power, or $\dot{V}_{O_{2peak}}$ (Wasserman *et al.* 1994), reported in millilitres of oxygen consumed per kilogram of body mass per minute ($ml \cdot kg^{-1} \cdot min^{-1}$). The $\dot{V}_{O_{2peak}}$ is measured by a GXT, as discussed above. Data for both adults and young people, with a wide range of physical and mental disabilities, have indicated physical fitness profiles that reflect a very inactive and sedentary group of persons (American College of Sports Medicine 1997). The $\dot{V}_{O_{2peak}}$ for most participants in these studies was less than $25\,ml \cdot kg^{-1} \cdot min^{-1}$ and often it was less than $20\,ml \cdot kg^{-1} \cdot min^{-1}$. Many common ADL that are taken for granted by healthy and able-bodied persons require a $\dot{V}_{O_{2peak}}$ in the range of 12–$30\,ml \cdot kg^{-1} \cdot min^{-1}$. Therefore, many of those with disabilities have a $\dot{V}_{O_{2peak}}$ which is *below* that required for ADL, employment and independent living. The fact that endurance training or regular exercise can improve the peak aerobic power of those who are disabled relates directly to their quality of life and the maximizing of their potential for independence.

This chapter is divided into five sections covering various types of disabilities/diseases: cardiovascular and pulmonary; metabolic; orthopaedic; neuromuscular; and cognitive and sensory (Table 39.1). Each disability or disorder is addressed in the following manner: a brief description of the pathophysiology; the known effects of exercise training; medications; and recommendations for prescribing an endurance training programme.

Cardiovascular and pulmonary diseases/disabilities

Myocardial infarction

PATHOPHYSIOLOGY

Myocardial infarction (MI) is one reflection of the ongoing process of atherosclerosis. There is a gradual occlusion of the coronary artery lumen, due to growing lipid plaques and infiltration of the smooth muscle cells lining the inner arterial wall. Partial or complete occlusion of one or more coronary arteries or their branches results in decreased perfusion in areas of the myocardium served by those vessels. When perfusion is insufficient to meet metabolic demands, myocardial ischaemia develops. Prolonged myocardial ischaemia results in MI, with death of myocardial muscle tissue distal to the occlusion. The extent of left ventricular damage and dysfunction plays a major role in determining subsequent exercise capacity as well as the risk of future cardiovascular morbidity and mortality.

EFFECTS OF EXERCISE TRAINING

The rationale of exercise training for persons with previous MI is to increase aerobic power ($\dot{V}_{O_{2peak}}$). This, in turn, increases functional capacity and usually relieves any residual anginal symptoms. Aerobic training lowers heart rate and/or blood pressure at any given submaximal work rate and therefore reduces myocardial oxygen demand (Franklin 1997). Modest decreases in body mass and body fat should occur and if the activity is sufficiently prolonged there are increases in the 'antiatherogenic' high density lipoprotein (HDL) cholesterol.

MEDICATIONS

Several cardiovascular medications can influence responses to exercise and endurance training.

Table 39.1 Classification of diseases and disabilities.

Section	Disease/disability
Cardiovascular and pulmonary	Myocardial infarction
	Peripheral arterial disease
	Aneurysms and Marfan's syndrome
	Chronic obstructive pulmonary disease
	Cystic fibrosis
Metabolic	Renal failure
	Diabetes mellitus
	Obesity
Orthopaedic	Arthritis
	Osteoporosis
	Lower extremity amputees
Neuromuscular	Stroke and head injury
	Spinal cord injury
	Muscular dystrophy
	Epilepsy
	Multiple sclerosis
	Anterior poliomyelitis and post-polio syndrome
	Amyotrophic lateral sclerosis
	Cerebral palsy
	Parkinson's disease
Cognitive and sensory	Mental retardation
	Deafness and hardness of hearing
	Visual impairment and blindness

Diuretics do not usually alter the heart rate response to exercise or aerobic power, although they may do so if plasma volume is greatly reduced.

α-Receptor blockers significantly lower systolic and diastolic blood pressures; thus, they can induce episodes of hypotension following exercise, warranting a prolonged cool-down period. α-Receptor blockers have minimal effects on heart rate and on metabolic responses when exercising.

β-Blockers decrease submaximal and maximal heart rates, but do not compromise exercise trainability. If a patient is receiving β-blockers, the intensity of exercise can best be determined by an RPE.

Calcium channel blockers do not generally affect exercise trainability, but some may alter the heart rate response to exercise (e.g. verapamil).

Vasodilators and angiotensin-converting enzyme inhibitors do not suppress the normal heart rate response to exercise. Thus, the exercise training intensity can to be prescribed in the usual manner. However, hypotensive episodes can occur immediately postexercise when using such medication and the cool-down period must therefore be prolonged.

RECOMMENDATIONS FOR ENDURANCE TRAINING

Intermittent sitting or standing is recommended during Phase I of treatment (while the patient is in hospital), in order to prevent much of the physiological deterioration that would otherwise follow an acute MI. Progressive, rhythmic, large muscle group exercise (walking, cycle ergometry, rowing, stair climbing, etc.), together with briefly held isometric contractions of the main muscle groups, is recommended during the outpatient phases of treatment (Phases II–IV). The recommended intensity of effort corresponds to an RPE of 11–16 (Borg 6–20 scale); the frequency should be at least 3 days per week, and the duration 20–40min. A warm-up and cool-down, each of 10-min duration, should be adequate.

Peripheral arterial disease

PATHOPHYSIOLOGY

Peripheral arterial disease (PAD) results in atherosclerotic stenosis and occlusion of the arteries serving the lower extremities. Blood flow is reduced below the point of obstruction. The severity of disease is generally classified into four categories: (i) Grade 0, asymptomatic; (ii) Grade 1, intermittent claudication (lameness or limping, associated with cramping pains in the calf muscles when walking); (iii) Grade 2, ischaemic pain in the leg(s) at rest; and (iv) Grade 3, minor or major tissue loss from the foot, progressing to gangrene and amputation of the limb.

EFFECTS OF EXERCISE TRAINING

Exercise tolerance can be improved through physical conditioning (Gardner 1997). The improvement in clinical status is due to the following adaptations: (i) an improved distribution of available blood flow to the limb; (ii) a reduced blood viscosity; (iii) a higher concentration of oxidative enzymes and less reliance upon anaerobic metabolism in the limb muscles; and (iv) an improved efficiency of walking.

MEDICATIONS

Common medications provided for patients with intermittent claudication include anticoagulants (Dipyridamole, warfarin, aspirin) and agents that lower blood viscosity (Pentoxifylline). Little information is available on interactions between exercise training and medications for the treatment of intermittent claudication.

RECOMMENDATIONS FOR ENDURANCE TRAINING

Initially, the intensity of exercise training is limited by claudicant symptoms. Training is recommended to begin with interval walking or stair climbing; such activity is performed three times a week at an intensity that causes mild to moderate discomfort in the lower extremities. The programme starts with 15–20min per session at an RPE between 9 and 12 (a rating of the overall effects of exercise, not local claudicant pain) and the prescription progresses to 40min per session at an RPE of 12–16. Non-weight-bearing tasks such as cycle ergometry may be used for warm-up and cool-down. Exercise training for this population should not be initiated until completion of medical clearance, including a physical examination and a GXT.

Aneurysms and Marfan's syndrome

PATHOPHYSIOLOGY

An aneurysmic dilatation of an artery could lead to the serious and even deadly sequelae of dissection and rupture of the vessel. Common sites for aneurysms include the cerebral arteries and the aorta. The regions of the aorta most frequently affected are the aortic root and the abdominal aorta near the kidneys.

Marfan's syndrome is a genetic disorder of connective tissue causing, among other things, weakness in the aortic wall leading to an aortic aneurysm. Other conditions that can cause an aortic aneurysm include hypertension, atherosclerosis and syphilitic infection. Enlargement of the aorta is usually painless and progressive, so that substantial dilatation can develop before the diagnosis is discovered. The larger the diameter of the aneurysm, the greater the risk of dissection and rupture, both of which can cause death, even if treated promptly.

EFFECTS OF EXERCISE TRAINING

Exercise increases blood pressure, which in turn increases tension within the wall of an aneurysm and, most probably, promotes its enlargement and progression. Therefore, aneurysmal disease is a relative contraindication for exercise training (Pyeritz 1997).

MEDICATIONS

The usual medication prescribed for this group of patients is a β-adrenergic blocking drug (atenolol or propranolol) to limit increases of blood pressure.

RECOMMENDATIONS FOR ENDURANCE TRAINING

The permissible extent of exercise depends on the degree of aneurysmal dilatation. The larger the aneurysm, the less exercise a person should undertake. But many people with aneurysms *want* to exercise and such individuals should not be totally denied the physiological, medical, and psychological benefits that exercise has to offer. Pyeritz (1997) has suggested the following guidelines: (i) contact and competitive sports should be avoided; (ii) the mode of choice is aerobic exercise, and this should be performed at a low to moderate intensity (i.e. for adults, the exercise intensity should be such that the pulse rate does not increase above 100 beats·min^{-1}). Special consideration must be given to those with Marfan's syndrome, who may seem suited to sports such as basketball or volleyball because of their stature and flexibility; these sports are contact, competitive activities whose nature will elevate blood pressure significantly. The serious consequences of possible rupture of an aneurysm should be weighed against the possible psychological benefits of athletic success and an informed decision may warrant the guidance and expertise of a medical sport psychologist (Graham et al. 1994).

Chronic pulmonary disease

PATHOPHYSIOLOGY

Chronic pulmonary disease (CPD) leads to many exercise-related physiological limitations other than impairments of ventilation and gas exchange. The pathophysiology can be divided into various pulmonary, cardiovascular and muscular categories (Cooper 1997). Chronic obstructive pulmonary disease due to bronchitis, bronchiolitis, emphysema and/or asthma, and restrictive pulmonary disease due to such conditions as pulmonary fibrosis or kyphoscoliosis can pose single or multiple pathophysiological problems: (i) ventilatory impairments such as increased airway resistance and reduced compliance augment the work of breathing, leading to ventilatory muscle fatigue; ventilation also becomes inefficient, due to increased dead space and/or ventilation–perfusion inequality; (ii) cardiovascular function is impaired because of deconditioning due to reduced physical activity and/or the development of cor pulmonale; (iii) muscular deconditioning, weakness and wasting may arise from physical inactivity; (iv) symptomatic limitation of effort may be caused by breathlessness (dyspnoea); and (v) psychological disturbances may arise, for example chronic anxiety because of experiencing dyspnoea, or depression due to social isolation (i.e. a limited ability to perform the normal ADL).

EFFECTS OF EXERCISE TRAINING

When a person with CPD participates in regular physical activity, beneficial changes include: (i) improved ventilatory efficiency due to a strengthening of the ventilatory muscles; (ii) cardiovascular reconditioning, reversing the downward spiral of physical inactivity, increased dyspnoea and greater cardiovascular deconditioning; (iii) improved skeletal muscle strength, reversing the process of peripheral muscle deconditioning and muscle wasting; (iv) habituation to the frightening symptoms of breathlessness; and (v) a reversal of psychological disturbances due to an improved physical appearance and an enhanced body image (Cooper 1997).

MEDICATIONS

The medications prescribed for persons with CPD are intended to optimize respiratory function, thus enabling these individuals to increase their physical work capacity. Several of these medications have implications for exercise training.

Sympathomimetic agents (e.g. albuterol, metaproterenol, salmeterol) are selective β_2-adrenoceptor agonists, and are intended to induce bronchodilatation, but they can also stimulate α-adrenoceptors in the peripheral vasculature, causing vasoconstriction and an increase in systemic blood pressure. They may stimulate β_1-adrenoceptors, leading to tachycardia and/or dysrhythmias.

Methylxanthines (e.g. theophylline and aminophylline) are potent vasodilators but, like the sympathomimetic drugs, they can also cause tachycardia and/or dysrhythmias.

Diuretics (e.g. thiazide diuretics such as hydrochlorothiazide or loop diuretics such as frusemide (furosemide)) help to prevent fluid retention in cases where cor pulmonale is coexistent with CPD, but potential side-effects include hypotension during exercise, and potassium depletion predisposing to cardiac dysrhythmias and muscle weakness.

Glucocorticoids such as prednisone reduce the inflammatory process of bronchitis/bronchiolitis, but chronic use of these drugs can result in atrophy and fragility of the skin, osteoporosis, muscle atrophy and a myopathy of both skeletal and ventilatory muscles.

Antidepressants such as tricyclic compounds may cause tachycardia both at rest and during exercise.

RECOMMENDATIONS FOR ENDURANCE TRAINING

Endurance training begins as *exercise rehabilitation*, often under the supervision of several health professionals. Respiratory therapists teach the proper use of bronchodilators and oxygen; exercise professionals adjust the exercise prescription; and occupational therapists improve the efficiency of movement for the ADL. During the rehabilitation phase, a typical person with chronic respiratory disease cannot sustain a single bout of exercise for as long as 20–30 min and therefore a sequence of 5–10-min sessions is necessary until some adaptation has occured. When formal rehabilitation has been completed, walking, cycling, swimming or any other aerobic mode of exercise is recommended for the continuing phase of exercise training. Exercise specific to energy centring and balance, such as Tai Chi, is also helpful. Individuals with CPD are at particular risk of relapsing into a state of physical inactivity and progressive deconditioning. Therefore, it is important to develop tactics to encourage maintenance of a regular physical activity regimen. Membership of a health and fitness facility will increase motivation for some individuals.

Cystic fibrosis

PATHOPHYSIOLOGY

Cystic fibrosis (CF) is a genetic defect that affects the regulation of chloride transport in sweat glands, the mucus and serous glands in the airways and the pancreatic ducts. The defect causes: (i) an increased concentration of sodium chloride in sweat; (ii) the formation of mucus 'plugs' in the airways, leading to infection, chronic inflammation, fibrosis and, eventually, an irreversible loss of pulmonary function; and (iii) blockage of the pancreatic ducts, preventing digestive enzymes from reaching the small intestine and thus resulting in malnutrition and poor growth. Pulmonary involvement accounts for over 90% of the mortality, with most deaths occurring between the ages of 15 and 30 years.

EFFECTS OF EXERCISE TRAINING

There has not yet been a well-controlled randomized study to establish the effects of long-term endurance training on persons with CF (Nixon 1997). Current research suggests that persons with CF *may*, like their non-disabled peers, increase physical work capacity and peak oxygen consumption with endurance training. Training may also: (i) increase ventilatory muscle endurance; (ii) improve mucus clearance; and (iii) temporarily delay deterioration in certain indices of pulmonary function (Cerny *et al.* 1982; Nixon 1997).

MEDICATIONS

Persons with CF are prescribed many of the same medications as persons with CPD. For example, they take inhaled (e.g. albuterol) and oral (theophylline) bronchodilators, corticosteroids (inhaled or oral) to diminish bronchial hyperreactivity and anti-inflammatory agents to reduce airway inflammation. Specific medications for CF are: (i) *pancreatic enzyme supplements,* which improve exercise capacity indirectly by improving nutritional status; (ii) *sodium cromolyn and nedocromil* (inhaled), which improve exercise tolerance by preventing or reversing exercise-induced bronchoconstriction; and (iii) *mucolytic therapy,* which reduces the viscosity of bronchial mucus, improving its clearance.

RECOMMENDATIONS FOR ENDURANCE TRAINING

The physical work capacity of a person with CF depends on the glands that are affected and the severity of their involvement. In some individuals, the disease is quite mild and does not seriously disturb growth or development; such patients readily survive into young adulthood. In other cases, pancreatic and pulmonary involvement are severe and cause death in childhood. Given that most persons with CF now live through their adolescent years, participation in school or community-supported competitive sports (soccer, baseball, basketball, volleyball, etc.) and/or recreational activities (swimming, cycling and hiking) is an important consideration. Youths with CF are encouraged to engage in as active a lifestyle as possible. Young adults with CF who wish to participate in endurance training can do so in moderate intensity sessions of 20–30-min duration. Persons with severe lung involvement should limit bouts to 5–10 min, interspersed with rest periods, and they should also consider use of supplemental oxygen, particularly in the early stages of training. The intensity of training needs to be reduced during acute exacerbations of pulmonary infections.

Other special considerations in CF are as follows: (i) loss of excessive amounts of salt when exercising on hot days requires an increased fluid and dietary intake of salt; (ii) the risk of developing diabetes mellitus increases with age; exercise training for individuals with this complication follows the guidelines outlined in the next section; and (iii) those who have developed end-stage lung disease may develop right heart failure, so they should exercise at a low intensity in order to conserve their functional capacity for the ADL.

Metabolic diseases

Renal failure

PATHOPHYSIOLOGY

Renal failure (RF) or end-stage renal disease results in a failure to clear waste products from the blood. The common consequences of RF are metabolic acidosis, hypertension, left ventricular hypertrophy, anaemia, secondary hyperparathyroidism, peripheral neuropathy, muscle weakness, autonomic dysfunction, elevated serum triglycerides and reduced concentrations of HDL cholesterol. Thirty per cent of persons with RF are diabetic. Additionally, persons with RF are usually inactive and possess low functional capacities.

EFFECTS OF EXERCISE TRAINING

Skeletal muscle dysfunction is considered the major factor limiting work capacity for persons with RF (Painter 1997). Aerobic power ($\dot{V}O_{2peak}$) correlates with skeletal muscle strength; therefore, restoration of muscle strength and resultant increases in work capacity are the major objective of exercise therapy for persons with RF. Since limitation of the ADL is related to muscle weakness, both resistance and aerobic training programmes should be considered. In addition, exercise training improves blood pressure control, lipid profiles and psychological profiles.

MEDICATIONS

The main component of maintenance therapy is haemodialysis. Other options are peritoneal dialysis and renal transplantation. Medical management includes: (i) blood pressure control by a variety of antihypertensive agents, as addressed in a previous section; (ii) the control of anaemia, using recombinant human erythropoietin (EPO); (iii) the control of secondary hyperparathyroidism by phosphate-binding agents; and (iv) the provision of insulin for diabetic patients. Persons with RF may develop the following problems before initiation of dialysis, with inadequate dialysis or with an indiscretion of fluid intake: (i) congestive heart failure due to fluid overload; (ii) pericardial effusion; (iii) an abnormal electrocardiogram and dysrhythmias due to abnormal serum electrolyte concentrations; or (iv) cardiomegaly. Other complications are accelerated atherosclerosis, due to an abnormal blood lipid profile, renal osteodystrophy from secondary hyperparathyroidism, persistent anaemia due to non-response to EPO, and in patients treated with peritoneal dialysis, peritonitis due to catheter infection.

RECOMMENDATIONS FOR ENDURANCE TRAINING

Because the medical schedule is already complex and intensive, an exercise programme is not part of routine patient care. However, exercise training provides the only possible chance to increase functional capacity for these individuals. Studies have reported the feasibility of exercise programming immediately before or following dialysis treatment, using either treadmill walking or cycle ergometry at low to moderate intensities. Attachment of a portable cycle ergometer to the treatment chair *during* dialysis is also a feasible form of endurance training.

Diabetes mellitus

PATHOPHYSIOLOGY

This disease is characterized by an absolute or relative deficiency in insulin, resulting in hyperglycaemia. Chronic hyperglycaemia increases the risk of developing microvascular complications (e.g. retinopathy and nephropathy), macrovascular diseases (e.g. atherosclerosis) and various neuropathies, both autonomic and peripheral. There are three main forms of diabetes mellitus.

Diabetes mellitus: type I (insulin dependent or juvenile onset)

Type I diabetes involves an autoimmune response directed at the insulin-secreting β cells of the pancreas, and ultimately leading to their destruction. Consequently, insulin must be supplied by injection or an insulin pump. The marked hyperglycaemia caused by insulin deficiency potentiates the life-threatening condition of ketoacidosis. This form of diabetes usually develops before the age of 30. Of the 16 million people with diabetes in the US, 10–15% have type I diabetes.

Diabetes mellitus: type II (non-insulin dependent or adult onset)

In this form of diabetes, peripheral tissue insulin resistance and defective insulin secretion are common features. The aetiology involves the following sequence of events: (i) glucose does not readily enter the insulin-sensitive tissues (primarily muscle and adipose tissue) because they have developed an insulin resistance; (ii) the rise in blood glucose causes the β cells to secrete more insulin to maintain normal blood glucose concentrations; (iii) the increase in endogenous insulin is often ineffective in lowering blood glucose, due to insulin resistance; and (iv) over time the β cells become exhausted and insulin secretion decreases. Eighty per cent of people with type II diabetes are obese at the onset of the condition. Unlike patients with type I diabetes, those with type II diabetes usually do not develop ketoacidosis. Of the 16 million diabetic persons in the US, 85–90% have type II diabetes.

Gestational diabetes

Gestational diabetes develops during pregnancy. This category of disorder does not include those women who had diabetes prior to pregnancy or those with type II diabetes who were undiagnosed until pregnancy. Risk factors include a family history of gestational diabetes, previous delivery of a large birthweight baby and obesity. The classic characteristic of gestational diabetes is that it resolves postpartum. However, 50% of those who develop gestational diabetes develop type II diabetes later in life.

EFFECTS OF EXERCISE TRAINING

It is important to distinguish between type I and type II diabetes when considering the benefits that an exercise training programme can provide (Albright 1997).

Improvement in blood glucose control. For type II diabetes, exercise should be part of standard therapy, along with diet and medication to improve blood glucose control. For type I diabetics, insulin therapy, not exercise, is the main component of treatment. However, those with type I diabetes are encouraged to exercise to gain other benefits (see below).

Improved insulin sensitivity/lower medication requirement. This translates into reduction in dosage of insulin (type I) or oral hypoglycaemic agents (type II).

Reduction in body fat. The majority of type II diabetics are obese, and exercise coupled with a reduced energy intake is considered the most effective way to lose weight. A decrease in body mass increases insulin sensitivity and reduces the amounts of insulin or oral hypoglycaemic agents that are needed.

Prevention of type II diabetes. Epidemiological studies strongly suggest that exercise may play a role in preventing type II diabetes.

Stress reduction. Stress can exacerbate diabetes by increasing the secretion of counter-regulatory hormones (e.g. glucocorticoids, growth hormone) and augmenting plasma concentrations of free fatty acids.

MEDICATIONS

The goal of diabetes management is to keep blood glucose under control ($<250\,mg\cdot dl^{-1}$; no ketones).

Insulin allows glucose to enter insulin-sensitive tissue. It is important to know what type of insulin the patient has been prescribed, as different types vary in onset, peak and duration of action.

Oral hypoglycaemic agents are medications that help the pancreas secrete more insulin (first- and second-generation sulphonylureas) or increase insulin sensitivity (biguanides). The most significant effect of both insulin and oral hypoglycaemic agents on exercise training is their ability to cause hypoglycaemia. Attention must be paid to the onset, peak and duration of action of medications, food intake and blood glucose level before and after exercise. Medications may also include antihypertensives and lipid-lowering agents.

RECOMMENDATIONS FOR ENDURANCE TRAINING

The most beneficial modes of aerobic exercise involve the large muscles (e.g. cycle ergometry, rowing ergometry, use of a Stair-Master, etc.). The timing of activity is individualized to fit the medication schedule and the presence and severity of diabetic complications. Food intake must also be considered. For example, it is recommended that 15 g of carbohydrate be consumed either before or after 1 h of exercise and, if the exercise is vigorous and of longer duration, an additional 15–20 g of carbohydrate is recommended (Albright 1997). Exercise is contraindicated if: (i) there is active retinal haemorrhage or a history of recent therapy for retinopathy (e.g. laser treatment); (ii) infection is present; (iii) the blood glucose concentration is $>250–300\,mg\cdot dl^{-1}$ and/or ketones are present; or (iv) if the blood glucose is $80–100\,mg\cdot dl^{-1}$. As carbohydrates are eaten and time is allowed for absorption, an increase in blood sugar will help to prevent exercise-induced hypoglycaemia. Precautions against hypoglycaemia include: (i) availability of a quick source of rapidly active carbohydrate (e.g. sweets) during exercise; (ii) an adequate fluid intake before, during and after exercise; (iii) the wearing of proper exercise shoes and cotton socks; and (iv) carrying medical identification.

Obesity

PATHOPHYSIOLOGY

Although the cause of obesity includes factors such as endocrine and genetic disorders, an excessive intake of food and physical inactivity are the primary causes. Many physiological and metabolic functions influence fat storage and release, but an excessive intake of dietary fat and sugar and physical inactivity are important lifestyle factors that contribute to this condition. Obesity is commonly defined in terms of body mass index (BMI = body mass in kilograms divided by height (m)^2) or percentage body fat. The risk of obesity is increased in men if the BMI is greater than $27.8\,kg\cdot m^{-2}$ or the percentage body fat is > 25%. For women the criteria are a BMI greater than $27.3\,kg\cdot m^{-2}$ or a percentage body fat > 32% (Wallace 1997). Body fat distribution also plays a major role when considering the contribution of obesity to the risk of other diseases. Truncal or upper body fat distribution is associated with an increased risk of coronary artery disease, hypertension, hyperlipidaemia and diabetes, whereas an abdominal distribution increases the risk of coronary artery disease specific to an increase in very low density lipoprotein (VLDL).

EFFECTS OF EXERCISE TRAINING

Exercise training is very effective in reducing body mass in individuals with moderate obesity (BMI = $30.1-40.0\,kg\cdot m^{-2}$), although it is not as effective in morbid obesity (BMI > $40.0\,kg\cdot m^{-2}$). Moreover, physical activity and diet are the most important factors in *maintenance* of weight loss. The *maintenance* of weight loss is influenced directly by an increase in energy expenditure and indirectly by a decrease in energy intake. As stated previously, 80% of persons with type II diabetes are obese at the onset of this condition. Exercise training has a pro-

found effect in reducing the risk of type II diabetes for both moderately and morbidly obese individuals, decreasing the fasting blood glucose and fasting insulin concentrations and decreasing insulin resistance. These changes have been found, even *without changes in body mass or body fat content*.

MEDICATIONS/MANAGEMENT

Management, rather than medication, is the primary approach to the reduction and control of body weight/fat. Behavioural change focuses on improving diet (reduction in total energy and fat intake) and increasing physical activity (exercise training programmes along with an increase in habitual activity). Medications for weight control act by suppressing appetite. FDA-approved medications include sympathomimetic drugs that stimulate the sympathetic nervous system (e.g. certain amphetamines, isoindoles and caffeine). Serotonin uptake inhibitors have also been tried as appetite suppressants, but these drugs do not have FDA approval and are of questionable clinical value. Thyroid hormone *should not* be considered, because of its dangerous cardiovascular side-effects and potential contribution to osteoporosis.

RECOMMENDATIONS FOR ENDURANCE TRAINING

There is a debate concerning whether two short exercise sessions per day rather than one long exercise session will enable obese individuals to reach a higher total energy expenditure. The total energy expenditure associated with exercise includes not only the energy expended during exercise, but also the recovery period, when there is an *excess post-exercise oxygen consumption (EPOC)*. The use of two shorter sessions has been recommended because the elevated energy expenditure due to EPOC may be sustained for a longer time than with a long single session. On the other hand, long single sessions are easier to incorporate into most individuals' lifestyles. To guard against injury, the best mode of exercise is low-impact (e.g. walking rather than jogging) or non-weight-bearing (e.g. cycle ergometry) aerobic exercise. It is just as important to increase daily living activities (e.g. using the stairs rather than the lift or escalator). The frequency of exercise should be five to seven sessions per week, using one long session (40–60 min) or two short sessions (20–30 min) per day, beginning at a low intensity and progressing to a moderate intensity. Thermoregulatory considerations include exercising in a thermally neutral environment or during cool times of the day, drinking plenty of water and wearing loose-fitting clothes.

Orthopaedic conditions

Arthritis

PATHOPHYSIOLOGY

The two most common arthritic conditions are osteoarthritis and rheumatoid arthritis. Osteoarthritis is a degenerative joint disease commonly affecting the hands, spine, hips and knees. It causes joint pain, joint stiffness and cartilage destruction. Rheumatoid arthritis is an inflammatory, multijoint disease commonly affecting the wrists, hands, knees, feet and cervical spine. Features of these conditions relating to exercise include general morning stiffness, acute and chronic inflammation, chronic pain and loss of joint integrity. There is little difference among the various systemic forms of arthritis (osteoarthritis, rheumatoid arthritis, systemic lupus erythematosus, ankylosing spondylitis, psoriatic arthritis, gout and pseudogout) in terms of their effects on the exercise response (Minor & Kay 1997). An acute flare-up of systemic illness can blunt the exercise response due to the following reasons: (i) persons with arthritis tend to be physically less active and less fit in terms of their cardiovascular and musculoskeletal fitness; (ii) symptoms can increase the metabolic cost of physical activity by as much as 50%; (iii) the range of joint motion can be greatly restricted; and (iv) there may be an inability to perform rapid, repetitive movements.

EFFECTS OF EXERCISE TRAINING

The most immediate benefit of exercise training is a decrease in the cumulative effects of inactivity (i.e. loss of flexibility, muscle atrophy, muscle weakness, depression and general fatigue). These problems, common to all arthritic conditions, respond favourably to a *low to moderate, gradually progressive* exercise programme. However, the potential of exercise training to influence the disease process has yet to be determined.

MEDICATIONS

The major goal in the treatment of inflammatory rheumatic diseases is to control the destructive inflammatory process. Medications prescribed range from aspirin and other non-steroidal anti-inflammatory drugs (NSAIDs) to oral corticosteroids, oral and injectable gold preparations and newer immunosuppressive agents. Such agents control the inflammatory process and alleviate pain, allowing the patient to become more active. However, vigorous weight-bearing activities should be avoided for at least 1 week following local corticosteroid injections to specific joints.

RECOMMENDATIONS FOR ENDURANCE TRAINING

With arthritic diseases, there is a need to protect the affected joints by selecting low-impact activities (for example, jogging and running should be avoided when the hip and knees are involved; suitable types of activity include pool exercises, and cycle or rowing ergometry). Key components include flexibility and joint range-of-motion exercises. Programmes should be designed with an individualized progression of intensity and duration: (i) exercise should be of low intensity and short duration during the initial phase; (ii) stretch and warm-up should be continued daily even when the disease flares up; and (iii) weightlifting should be gradually incorporated. Initially, some postexercise soft tissue discomfort is to be expected.

Osteoporosis

PATHOPHYSIOLOGY

All humans, regardless of race, gender or geographical location, incur a small loss of bone mass every year, starting at about 35 years of age. Nearly all elderly men and women in industrialized countries have some degree of *osteopenia* (low bone mass). However, once osteopenia becomes severe enough to result in fractures from minimal trauma, it is clinically defined as *osteoporosis*. Women experience a 3–5-year acceleration in the rate of bone loss after the menopause, due to the superimposition of the effects of oestrogen withdrawal on the normal age-related loss. Men less frequently experience clinically significant bone loss before the age of 70. Other commonly cited risk factors for osteoporosis are: a low body mass, a lack of physical activity, chronic smoking, an excessive alcohol consumption and a low dietary calcium intake.

EFFECTS OF EXERCISE TRAINING

Osteoporosis will not alter the beneficial cardiovascular and skeletal muscle adaptations induced by exercise training. An exception to this would be any mechanical limitations imposed on the respiratory system by severe kyphosis. It is doubtful that exercise training by itself will reverse osteoporosis, but it can slow or perhaps halt the age-related decline in bone mass and delay the time at which osteopenia progresses to osteoporosis (Bloomfield 1997). Exercise alone cannot provide an effective alternative to hormone replacement therapy in preventing bone loss in the early menopausal years. However, postmenopausal women who engage in exercise training while on hormone replacement therapy (see below) are more likely to experience gains in bone mass.

MEDICATIONS

The most common prescribed medical regimen for osteoporosis is hormone replacement therapy (oestrogens with or without progestogen components in relatively low doses) in an effort to replace the endogenous hormones lost at menopause or after surgical removal of the ovaries. Oestrogen replacement therapy in postmenopausal women (when taken without progesterone) will increase plasma concentrations of HDL cholesterol and

therefore lower the risk of coronary artery disease (CAD). Other medications used to treat osteoporosis include calcitonin and biophosphates (alendronate). Biophosphates commonly produce side-effects of nausea and diarrhoea. Sodium fluoride, vitamin D and parathyroid hormone are further medications that are taken to inhibit bone resorption, but they have not yet received FDA approval.

RECOMMENDATIONS FOR ENDURANCE TRAINING

A well-balanced programme that includes both aerobic and strength-training activities should be emphasized. Strength training involving both the upper and the lower limbs helps conserve bone mass and also improves dynamic balance (thereby lowering the risk of falls). Strength training yields the best results with progression to relatively high intensities (>75% of one repetition maximum) and fewer repetitions. If multiple vertebral fractures, severe osteopenia or back pain limit an individual's ability to participate in weight-bearing exercise, the exercise mode should be shifted to swimming, walking in water, water aerobics or chair exercises. Special consideration should be given to the anxiety level many elderly persons have about falling. It is important to clear the exercise environment of hazards such as loose floor mats and exercise equipment strewn over the floor. It is also recommended that wall railings be used for standing exercises.

Lower extremity amputations

PATHOPHYSIOLOGY

This section is limited to lower extremity amputees because, unlike upper extremity amputees, the walking and running capacities of lower extremity amputees are greatly restricted, contributing to a sedentary lifestyle. The majority of amputations of the lower limbs in industrialized countries are due to peripheral vascular disease secondary to atherosclerosis or diabetes mellitus. A second important cause is vehicular or job-related trauma. Lower extremity amputations can be classified as: (i) Syme, usually involving the calcaneus bone of the foot; (ii) unilateral above-knee (transfibular) or below-knee (transfemoral) amputations; (iii) bilateral above- and below-knee amputations; and (iv) bilateral above-knee amputations. Persons with lower extremity amputations, especially those with above-knee amputations, are at increased risk of CAD, type II diabetes and hypertension due to their sedentary lifestyle. The high energy cost of walking, hair follicle infections, skin breakdown and scar tissue abscesses all contribute to reduced ambulatory activity.

EFFECTS OF EXERCISE TRAINING

Few investigators have studied the effects of exercise on lower extremity amputees. However, exercise training involving lower extremity cycling and/or the use of an ergometer involving both upper and lower extremities (e.g. Schwinn Air-Dyne) not only improves cardiovascular fitness, but also augments walking efficiency and the symmetry of prosthetic gait (James 1973; Pitetti *et al.* 1987).

MEDICATIONS/MANAGEMENT

Amputation of a lower limb does not involve specific medication other than drugs needed for pain management. For those with vascular amputations secondary to atherosclerosis or diabetes, see the sections on 'Myocardial infarction', 'Peripheral arterial disease', 'Diabetes mellitus' and 'Obesity'.

RECOMMENDATIONS FOR ENDURANCE TRAINING

The last two decades have witnessed the development of new prosthetics and new exercise machines that allow lower extremity amputees to engage in an active lifestyle, which includes endurance exercise. Improvements in prosthetic design (e.g. the Flex-Foot, Flex-Foot, Inc.) have not only made walking easier, but allow jogging and even sprinting activities. Aerobic exercise machines such as the Schwinn Air-Dyne, Stair-Master, rowing ergometers and other upper body and lower body ergometers allow lower extremity amputees many options for

endurance training. Swimming is also an excellent mode of exercise for lower extremity amputees.

Neuromuscular diseases

Stroke and head injury

PATHOPHYSIOLOGY

Stroke and head injury demonstrate a similar pathophysiology, with the following exceptions.

Stroke

A stroke arises from a cerebral vascular accident (CVA), commonly due to thrombosis, embolism or haemorrhage secondary to aneurysm. Cell death follows. The resulting neurological impairment depends on both the size and location of the involved area in the brain. Following a CVA, persons may exhibit the following: (i) impairment of motor and sensory function in the upper or lower extremities, or in both upper and lower extremities; (ii) visual field deficits; (iii) expressive and receptive aphasia (impaired ability to communicate through speech); and (iv) apraxia (impaired learning and performance of voluntary movements).

Head injury

The majority of head injuries occur as a result of vehicular accidents or gunshot wounds. Although similar to stroke with respect to the structural brain damage that may occur, head injuries are seen predominantly in young people without underlying medical problems. Although motor and sensory impairments similar to those seen in stroke are prominent, cognitive disturbances may be pre-eminent, with acute and chronic agitation, confusion, inattention, memory disturbances and learning deficits.

EFFECTS OF EXERCISE TRAINING

The impact of exercise training differs in people suffering from stroke compared to those with a head injury.

Stroke

Because of the lifestyle (i.e. little physical activity, poor diet, smoking, etc.) leading to the CVA, most patients are very deconditioned. This leaves tremendous room for improvement in physical condition. Aerobic training studies involving stroke victims who have recovered enough motor function to perform leg cycle exercise demonstrate an increase in aerobic power of over 50%. Endurance training also results in 100–150% increases in self-selected walking speeds, greater mobility and a lesser dependency on assistive walking devices (Palmer-McLean & Wilberger 1997).

Head injury

Head injury patients tend to be younger and therefore more physically fit. However, lengthy hospital bedrest may reduce the preaccident aerobic power significantly. In addition, deficits in motor capabilities can increase the energy cost of locomotion. Exercise training can improve both aerobic power and muscle strength significantly, allowing more independence in the ADL, a greater mechanical efficiency and a reduced energy cost of locomotion.

MEDICATIONS

The medical issues in and therefore the medical management of stroke and head injury differ.

Stroke

Individuals receiving vasodilator drugs (for instance, if vasospasm of the cerebral arteries is suspected) will require longer cool-down periods to prevent postexercise hypotension. Those with haemorrhagic stroke require a strict control of blood pressure. Antihypertensive medication for such individuals may lower the peak heart rate and cardiac output, and a reduced plasma fluid volume (due to administration of diuretics) may alter electrolyte balance, causing dysrhythmias.

Head injury

Intensive medical management is usually not required after acute treatment of the injury. However, anticonvulsants can be indicated for seizure-prone patients. Depression and apathy are common behavioural problems which can interfere with long-term adherence to an endurance training programme. Medications for behavioural management (particularly antidepressants) may be indicated to assist in obtaining adherence to an exercise regimen.

RECOMMENDATIONS FOR ENDURANCE TRAINING

Hypertension is one of the primary risk factors for stroke. Therefore, endurance exercise is important to reduce blood pressure as well as to increase the level of physical fitness following a stroke. Both human and animal studies have demonstrated that exercising at 40–70% of peak aerobic power can reduce blood pressure. The Schwinn Air-Dyne or other upper/lower body ergometers, cycle ergometry, treadmill walking and arm ergometry are recommended modes of exercise for stroke victims. The same modes of exercise are recommended for head injury patients.

Spinal cord injury

PATHOPHYSIOLOGY

Spinal cord injury (SCI) damages neuronal elements within the spinal cord, resulting in a loss of sensory and/or motor functions. The neurological level and completeness of injury determine the degree of impairment. Injury to the cervical segments (C1–C8) or the highest thoracic segment (T1) results in *quadriplegia* or *tetraplegia*, with functional impairment of the arms, trunk, legs and pelvic organs (bladder, bowels and sexual organs). Injury to the thoracic (T2–T12), lumbar (L1–L5), and sacral (S1–S5) segments or the cauda equina causes *paraplegia*, resulting in impairments to the trunk, legs and/or pelvic organs. These lesions cause two major physiological problems: (i) a reduced ability to perform large muscle group aerobic exercise; and (ii) a loss of sympathetic control of the cardiovascular system that reduces the ability to support high intensities of exercise. Secondary complications, especially in persons with quadriplegia, include orthostatic and exercise-induced hypotension, and an autonomic dysreflexia which can cause extreme hypertension (BP > 200/100 mmHg), headache, bradycardia, flushing, unusual sweating and nasal congestion.

EFFECTS OF EXERCISE TRAINING

Arm exercise training using arm ergometry, wheelchair ergometry, wheelchair treadmill exercise, free wheeling, swimming and wheelchair sports (e.g. wheelchair basketball, quadriplegic rugby) can all increase arm musculature strength and endurance, improving peak aerobic power by 10–20%, and enhancing the sense of well-being (Figoni 1997).

MEDICATIONS/MANAGEMENT

Management of persons with SCI is complex because of the following complications.

Skin. The risk of pressure sores and abrasions, especially in the areas of the ischial tuberosities, sacrum and coccyx, can be reduced by the use of seat cushions, and avoidance of sitting for long periods without pressure relief.

Bone. Persons with SCI have an increased risk of fractures secondary to osteoporosis. Therefore, care must be taken in making transfers from wheelchairs or exercise equipment.

Stabilization. Seat-belts or strappings are recommended for those with significant loss of trunk control/balance.

Hand-grip. The hands of those with weak or absent grip strength (e.g. quadriplegia) should be secured to ergometer handles with elastic bandages or gloves fitted with Velcro straps.

Bladder. Emptying of the bladder or leg bag before exercise is recommended to avoid bladder distension or overfilling of the bag during activity. Bladder distension may induce autonomic hyperreflexia in persons with lesions above T6.

Bowels. A regular bowel maintenance programme will avoid autonomic dysreflexic symptoms.

Hypotension. If the resting blood pressure is <80/50 mmHg, use of elastic support hose and/or an abdominal binder is recommended. Exercise should be avoided within 3 h of eating a large meal, and the blood pressure should be monitored when starting a training programme.

Pain. Overuse injuries to shoulder, wrist and hand joints are common in persons with SCI. Arm exercises that aggravate the pain in these joints should be discontinued.

Those prescribing exercise should beware of medications that induce either hypotension (e.g. Ditropan (oxybutinin chloride), Dibenyline (phenoxybenzamine hydrochloride)) or diuresis (e.g. alcohol, diuretics).

RECOMMENDATIONS FOR ENDURANCE TRAINING

Appropriate endurance training modes include arm cranking, wheelchair ergometry, wheelchair propulsion on a treadmill or rollers, and free wheeling on a track; swimming; vigorous sports such as wheelchair basketball, quadriplegic rugby, tennis and wheelchair racing (e.g. 10-km race); arm-powered cycling; and vigorous ADL such as ambulation with crutches and braces. Overuse syndromes can be prevented by varying the modes of exercise, incorporating weight training to strengthen the muscles of the upper back and posterior shoulder, and stretching exercises for the muscles of the anterior shoulder and chest. It is recommended that people with quadriplegia use a supervised and environmentally controlled, thermally neutral gym or clinic because of their limited thermoregulatory abilities.

Muscular dystrophy

PATHOPHYSIOLOGY

Muscular dystrophy (MD) comprises a family of hereditary diseases characterized by the dystrophic loss of structural protein from the muscle cells (skeletal and, in some cases, cardiac). All types of MD are characterized by a progressive deterioration of muscle strength, power and endurance. This section highlights Duchenne MD (DMD), which has the greatest prevalence. Becker MD (BMD) is also mentioned, as well as facioscapulohumeral dystrophy (FSHD). Duchenne MD progresses rapidly and is fatal. Seldom does a patient with DMD reach the third decade of life. In addition to muscle dysfunction, the patient slowly develops joint contractures due to paralysis and inactivity, especially during the wheelchair stage. In the early stages of DMD, individuals can walk, but subsequently they become wheelchair dependent and eventually bedridden. Becker MD is also progressive and fatal, but advances at a slower pace. Individuals with DMD and BMD commonly die from cardiac or pulmonary complications. FSHD affects mainly the face and upper limb muscles; it is the most benign of these three types of MD, and does not involve cardiac muscle.

EFFECTS OF EXERCISE TRAINING

Although the literature is scant, it has been reported that resistance training can slow down, and for a while slightly reverse, the deterioration in muscle function (Bar-Or 1997). Presently, there are no data on the effects of exercise training on aerobic power.

MEDICATIONS/MANAGEMENT

There is no known cure for MD. Corticosteroids, which can retard muscle weakness and prolong ambulation, have questionable efficacy in slowing muscle deterioration. Therapy (e.g. range-of-motion exercises) is aimed at maintaining the ADL (e.g. prevention of contractures). Surgery is often used for release of the Achilles tendon and stabilization of the spine. However, the bedrest that accompanies surgery (which can last for weeks) results in a precipitous decline in muscle performance. This drop in muscle function underlines the importance of physical activity following surgery. To prevent the individual from becoming overweight (due to a low level of physical activity), nutritional counselling is recommended in conjunction with physical activity.

RECOMMENDATIONS FOR ENDURANCE TRAINING

The maintenance of muscle endurance and strength or a reduction in the rate of deterioration is most important for persons with MD. Therefore, light to moderate resistance exercise should be the mainstay of the exercise programme (dystrophic muscles *do not* respond well to overload). Because of the young age of many patients, game-like 'fun' situations should be included.

Safety. In its advanced stages, DMD is often accompanied by congestive heart failure and other cardiac abnormalities. Although it is highly unlikely that a person with such advanced disease will be able to perform any exercise, maximal effort is contraindicated and exercise of minimal intensity is recommended.

Ergometry. Leg ergometers, arm ergometers or combined leg and arm ergometers are the best modes of exercise to use. However, because of muscle weakness, ergometers with breaking forces yielding power outputs as low as 5 W are needed. Additionally, the ergometer must be designed to allow for very small increments of power output (e.g. 2–3 W). Some individuals can arm crank by using only their triceps, with little contribution from the elbow flexors. The pedal shaft of the arm ergometer must be adjustable for these individuals, who can turn the crank only if the radius of the pedal shaft is small (e.g. 0.1 m instead of the standard 0.175 m).

Psychological aspects. The following quotation can be applied to many of the conditions addressed in this chapter.

Enhanced physical activity is virtually the only therapeutic modality through which a person with a debilitating disease such as MD can *actively* participate and 'take charge' (rather than be treated by others). Individuals with MD often like to take up such a challenge, even when they know that exercise and sport will not reverse the inevitable outcome of the disease. Such an effect on the person's self-esteem outweighs, in this author's opinion, any potential deleterious effect of exercise. (Bar-Or 1997)

Multiple sclerosis

PATHOPHYSIOLOGY

Multiple sclerosis (MS) is a demyelinating disease of the white matter of the central nervous system (CNS). The loss of myelin adversely affects the rapid, smooth conduction of the action potential along the neuronal pathways, interfering with smooth, rapid coordinated movements. The problems associated with MS range from minimal effects to severe disability. Symptoms that may affect exercise responses include: spasticity, incoordination, impaired balance, muscle weakness with partial paralysis, sensory numbness and dysfunction of the autonomic nervous system (e.g. reduced cardioacceleration, hypotension and loss of heat sensitivity).

EFFECTS OF EXERCISE TRAINING

Exercise training has no effect on the progression of MS. However, it can improve muscle strength, muscle endurance and aerobic power in the short term (Mulcare 1997). The individual with MS who is involved in an exercise programme should be sensitive to the following issues: muscle fatigue reducing exercise tolerance, impaired balance affecting the choice of exercise mode (e.g. a stationary cycle ergometer with foot strappings rather than a treadmill) and heat intolerance.

MEDICATIONS

Amantadine hydrochloride can temporarily reduce muscle fatigue. However, baclofen, amitriptyline hydrochloride, prednisone and hyoscyamine sulphate can all cause muscle weakness.

RECOMMENDATIONS FOR ENDURANCE TRAINING

Cycling, walking and swimming are the recommended modes of aerobic exercise, together with the use of weight machines to maintain or increase muscle strength. The progression of MS may take years, or it can progress significantly within months. Therefore, the manner in which an exercise programme progresses or regresses will vary among individuals. Daily training expectations must be flexible, to accommodate changes in medications, sleep disorders and increases in environmental temperature. In the case of progressive, non-remitting types of MS, the goal of the exercise programme is simply to slow any further physical deterioration and optimize remaining function. Some individuals with MS have either an attenuated or an absent sweating response, so the temperature of the exercise room should be kept thermally neutral (around 22°C).

Anterior poliomyelitis and post-polio syndrome

PATHOPHYSIOLOGY

Anterior poliomyelitis is an acute, self-limiting viral disease that attacks the anterior horn cells in the spinal cord. It causes flaccid paresis/paralysis and atrophy in the affected muscle groups. Approximately 40 years after contracting the disease, a quarter of the affected population develop symptoms similar to those of initial onset (e.g. fatigue, weakness, muscle and joint pain, sleep disorders and intolerance to cold). The return of these symptoms has been called collectively *post-polio syndrome* (PPS). Factors that exacerbate weakness, fatigue and pain include excessive body fat which overloads weak leg muscles and repetitive tasks which overload the smaller, remaining muscle mass.

EFFECTS OF EXERCISE TRAINING

Moderate-intensity training enhances aerobic power.

SPECIFIC POPULATION GROUPS AND ENDURANCE TRAINING

Resistance training also increases the strength of the quadriceps and hamstring muscles (Birk 1997). However, prolonged *high-intensity* training may cause joint oedema and muscle discomfort.

MEDICATIONS/MANAGEMENT

The fitting of braces/splints should allow for range of movement during exercise. The limbs may require fastening to the pedals of an ergometer. Antidepressants (e.g. amitriptiline (Elavil), nortryptiline (Pamelor), doxepin (Sinequan), fluoxetine (Prozac), sertraline (Zoloft)) are prescribed to reduce fatigue and improve sleep. These medications may increase heart rate, decrease blood pressure and, in persons with a cardiac history, cause electrocardiographic abnormalities (e.g. T-wave changes and dysrhythmias). Another side-effect of such medications is constipation, which exercise can help to correct.

RECOMMENDATIONS FOR
ENDURANCE TRAINING

Individuals with anterior poliomyelitis *without* PPS can perform a wider range of exercise intensities and duration without muscle and joint complications than those individuals *with* PPS. Intensity should be kept at 'moderate to somewhat hard' RPE, beginning at a duration of 20 min or less (2–4-min intervals), and progressing gradually to 30–40 min per session. The frequency should allow alternating rest days. Four limb ergometry, therapeutic aquatics and other non-weight-bearing modes of exercise are recommended. Sedentary individuals with PPS should consult with their physician before beginning an exercise programme.

Amyotrophic lateral sclerosis

PATHOPHYSIOLOGY

Amyotrophic lateral sclerosis (ALS) is a progressive degeneration of the lower and upper motor neurones. The average age at diagnosis is 55 years. Symptoms include progressive skeletal muscle atrophy and weakness due to involvement of the lower motor neurones, and spasticity and hyperreflexia due to degeneration of the upper motor neurones. The mean survival time after diagnosis is 2.5–3.0 years, with 20% of patients living more than 5 years and 10% longer than 10 years. Although the rate of muscle atrophy and weakness remains fairly constant over time, the rate of decline shows much inter-individual variation; some individuals lose strength very quickly, while the condition of others changes very slowly. Spasticity and hyperreflexia can interfere with coordinated movements and the range of motion, increasing the energy cost of locomotion. Pulmonary function is diminished secondary to weakness of the diaphragm and intercostal muscles. As in anterior poliomyelitis, the early phases of ALS show denervated muscle fibres which can be reinnervated by neighbouring motor units. However, such slowly formed or immature neuromuscular junctions can experience transient transmission failure, resulting in early-onset muscle fatigue. This process is transient and repairs itself after a short rest period. Thus, individuals with ALS are encouraged to stay active, but to rest frequently and avoid extreme overexertion.

EFFECTS OF EXERCISE TRAINING

As in many of the neuromuscular diseases (anterior poliomyelitis, MD, MS), exercise does not reverse or slow down the progression of ALS. However, it strengthens the healthy muscle fibres, allowing a higher level of function to be sustained for a longer time. Assisted range of motion activities help to minimize the pain associated with joint stiffness, and make it easier for health-care providers to dress, position or transfer ALS patients who can no longer care for themselves (Nau 1997).

MEDICATION/MANAGEMENT

Medications prescribed to correct for muscle spasticity, excessive saliva production, emotional problems and the discomfort of joint stiffness should not have a negative impact on the person's ability to exercise. Adaptive equipment and assistive devices can prolong the person's ability to stay active. For those with bulbar involvement (i.e. difficulty in chewing and swallowing food), nutritional supplements and/or placement of a feeding tube may be necessary.

RECOMMENDATIONS FOR ENDURANCE TRAINING

The main purpose of an exercise programme for persons with ALS is to maximize the functional capacity of healthy muscle fibres and to prevent limitations in the range of movement due to spasticity or contractures. Suggested modes of endurance exercise include treadmill walking with or without the use of handrails and recumbent cycle ergometry, in addition to active range-of-motion exercises with or without free weights, weight machines, stretching and, in time, passive range-of-motion exercises. Exercise is no longer appropriate when it results in fatigue that prevents completion of the ADL.

Cerebral palsy

PATHOPHYSIOLOGY

Unlike the previously discussed neuromuscular diseases, cerebral palsy (CP) is caused by *non-progressive* lesions of the brain that have occurred before, during or within the first few years after birth. The physical limitations for persons with CP depend on the extent and location of the lesion(s) within the brain. Manifestations of CP include spastic paralysis, ataxia, athetosis and dyskinesia. The Cerebral Palsy–International Sport and Recreation Association (CP-ISRA) has developed a classification system that is based on the individual's functional capacity and physical abilities. This system is helpful in developing a realistic exercise programme.

CP1: unable to propel a manual wheelchair due to severe spastic and athetoid quadriplegia.

CP2: can propel a wheelchair slowly and inefficiently with moderate to severe spastic quadriplegia or hemiplegia.

CP3: able to propel a wheelchair independently and may be able to ambulate, albeit poorly, with assistive devices or assistance because of moderate spastic quadriplegia or hemiplegia.

CP4: can ambulate with aid over short distances, has moderate to severe involvement of lower extremities, but minimal to near-normal function of the upper extremities.

CP5: has moderate spastic diplegia and is able to ambulate well with assistive devices and in some cases has the ability to jog.

CP6: can ambulate without assistive devices, and lower extremity function can improve from walking, jogging or cycling; good upper-extremity range of motion and strength.

CP7: minimal to mildly affected lower extremity and mild to moderately affected upper extremity.

CP8: upper and lower extremities are minimally affected.

EFFECTS OF EXERCISE TRAINING

Persons with CP benefit from regular exercise. All categories improve muscular strength and flexibility, and aerobic power improves in categories CP4–CP8. More importantly, exercise training can augment the capacity to perform the ADL and lessen the severity of symptoms such as spasticity and athetosis (Ferrara & Laskin 1997).

MEDICATIONS

Because seizures and tendencies to seizure are present in 60% or more of persons with CP, antiseizure medications are commonly prescribed (e.g. phenobarbitol, phenytoin and carbamazepine). These medications can have a depressant effect on the central nervous system, slowing the physiological responses to exercise and causing mental confusion or irritability, dizziness, nausea and weight loss. Antispasmodic and muscle relaxant medications are often prescribed; they enable the person with CP to perform physical activities with greater ease because they decrease muscle tone, but serious side-effects include drowsiness and lethargy.

RECOMMENDATIONS FOR ENDURANCE TRAINING

Arm and leg cycle ergometry exercise improves aerobic power for persons with CP. Strapping of the hands and feet to the pedals should be considered while performing such exercise. If the individual is ambulatory, treadmill walking can be performed, but safety requirements include the use of handrails on the treadmill and the presence of supervisory personnel. Such personnel must be mindful that many individuals with CP have concomitant cognitive, visual, hearing, speech and swallowing difficulties.

Parkinson's disease

PATHOPHYSIOLOGY

Parkinson's disease (PD) is associated with a reduction in the dopamine content of components of the basal ganglia of the brain. The basal ganglia are important in smooth programming of movements. The loss of dopamine results in a tremor both at rest and during physical activity, bradykinesia (i.e. a decreased ability to move the fingers, hands, arms or legs rapidly), a rigidity of the neck, shoulders, trunk and extremities that makes movement difficult, a slow and shuffling gait with decreased arm swing and difficulty in initiating a step, and postural abnormalities (increased kyphosis, flexed knees and elbows, and adducted shoulders). There are also problems in communication, due to a reduced volume and reduced clarity of speech, along with loss of facial expressions.

EFFECTS OF EXERCISE TRAINING

Aerobic training can improve, have no effect on, or reduce function in individuals with PD. This reflects the progressive nature of the disease and the impact of medications on the condition (Protos *et al.* 1997).

MEDICATIONS/MANAGEMENT

Drug management is aimed at: (i) correcting the neurochemical dopamine deficiency by the use of dopaminergics (levodopa) and monoamine oxidase type B (MAO-B) inhibitors (selegiline); and (ii) increasing the amount of circulating acetylcholines through the administration of anticholinergic drugs (benztropine, trihexyphenidyl). Common side-effects of such medication include gastroin-

testinal problems, confusion, delusional states, hallucinations, insomnia and changes in mental capacity. After long-term use (>5 years), responses to dopaminergics and MAO-B inhibitors decrease, resulting in fluctuations of motor disability. An understanding of drug absorption and metabolism is critical to the effective use of these drugs. Exercise responses depend on *consistently* exercising at the same time following medication, because: (i) plasma levels of medication can influence exercise performance, especially heart rate response; and (ii) some persons may have severe dyskinesias when drug levels peak.

RECOMMENDATIONS FOR ENDURANCE TRAINING

As with most neuromuscular disorders, approaches to exercise involve flexibility, aerobic training and muscle strengthening. The Schenkman and Butler model (1989) is recommended to distinguish functional losses resulting from the disease process from those due to physical inactivity. Because the disease interferes with motor planning and memory, repeated demonstrations with written and visual cues are necessary when learning new skills.

Cognitive and sensory disorders

Mental retardation

PATHOPHYSIOLOGY

The American Association of Mental Retardation (Luckasson *et al.* 1992) defines mental retardation as 'significantly subaverage general intellectual functioning existing concurrently with related limitations in two or more of the following adaptive skill areas: communications, self-care, home living, social skills, community use, self-direction, health and safety, functional academics, leisure and work' (Sherrill 1993). The process of classifying persons with mental retardation (MR) by IQ score is currently being replaced by a system that uses three criteria: (i) age of onset; (ii) intellectual dysfunction; and (iii) limitations in two or more adapted skill areas. However, most of the reported research on the physical fitness of persons with MR refers to levels of mental retardation according to the old classification: (i) *mild* (IQ scores ranging from 52 to 70 points, with the ability to live independently, work, marry and rear children); (ii) *moderate* (IQ scores ranging from 36 to 51 points; problems with speech and social interaction and sometimes gait problems; most individuals with Down's syndrome fall into this category); (iii) *severe and profound* (IQ scores of 20 to 33 points (severe) or 19 and lower (profound); difficulties with ADL; physical and motor disabilities; many within this category are institutionalized).

EFFECTS OF EXERCISE TRAINING

Cycle ergometry and run/walk training programmes have been successful in increasing the aerobic power of persons with MR but without Down's syndrome (Fernhall 1997). Neither run/walk exercise nor rowing increased aerobic power for persons with Down's syndrome. Circuit weight training improves muscular strength. Since motivation and task understanding are common problems, constant supervision is recommended. This population is often overweight or obese, but exercise alone is ineffective in reducing weight, indicating a need for associated dietary interventions.

MEDICATIONS/MANAGEMENT

Anticonvulsive and antidepressant medications are sometimes used, which may have an impact on the ability of persons with MR to concentrate on tasks. Exercise participation is important for this population because: (i) very low levels of physical fitness have consistently been reported; (ii) high rates of cardiovascular mortality develop at an earlier age than in the general population; and (iii) cardiovascular fitness and muscle strength are related to job performance, which in turn relates to capacity for independent living. This last factor has important economic and sociological implications.

RECOMMENDATIONS FOR ENDURANCE TRAINING

Exercise programmes that improve the overall physical fitness of the general population can be applied to persons with MR, with the following modifications: (i) it is recommended that exercise programmes always be supervised; and (ii) motivational techniques such as token rewards are particularly helpful to maintain adherence to an exercise programme.

Deafness and hardness of hearing

PATHOPHYSIOLOGY

People who are hard of hearing (i.e. those who find *difficulty* in understanding speech using the ears alone, with or without a hearing aid) or deaf (*unable* to understand speech using the ears alone, with or without a hearing aid) can participate in all types of physical activities with some minor adaptations. There are three major types of hearing loss: (i) *conduction* (the sound does not pass through the external and middle ear to reach the inner ear); (ii) *sensorineural* (an involvement of the inner ear, including the cochlea—the site of sensory receptors that convert sound waves to neural impulses, and, in some cases, the vestibular apparatus—the site of receptors determining vertical and horizontal orientation); and (iii) *mixed type* (a combination of conduction and sensorineural defects, common in the elderly).

EFFECTS OF EXERCISE TRAINING

Regular exercise produces the same positive physiological and functional benefits that are seen in persons without disabilities. Ancillary benefits include: opportunities to improve social skills; improvement in balance; and an enhancement of self-image, confidence and spatial orientation (Bloomquist 1997a).

MEDICATIONS/MANAGEMENT

The condition of hardness of hearing or deafness, in itself, requires no medications. Hearing aids are used primarily by persons with *conductive loss*. Hearing aids (there are approximately 200 types of assistive listening devices) amplify sounds, but do not make the speech clearer. Additionally, some of these devices can convert sound to light or vibration systems. Communication is the major problem when managing an exercise programme for persons who are deaf or hard of hearing. Although many deaf individuals use a variety of manual sign language systems (e.g. American Sign Language, Conceptually Accurate Signed English, Sign Essential English), an interpreter is necessary to facilitate communication. Additionally, the most astute lip readers can read only about 30% of what is said to them. If communication becomes a problem, paper and pencil communication with visual cues and concrete examples is recommended.

RECOMMENDATIONS FOR ENDURANCE TRAINING

Loss of hearing and deafness afford no physical barrier or limitation to endurance training.

Visual impairment

PATHOPHYSIOLOGY

There are two major categories of visual impairment: (i) *legal blindness* (a vision of <20/200—i.e. the ability to see at 20m what a healthy eye sees at 200m— with a limitation of acuity or of visual field (for instance, tunnel vision, where the visual field is less than 10% of normal)); and (ii) *total blindness* (the inability to recognize a strong light shone directly into the eye). In children, visual impairment is usually caused by birth defects (e.g. congenital cataracts). In elderly persons, diabetes mellitus,

macular degeneration, glaucoma and cataracts are the leading causes of visual impairment.

EFFECTS OF EXERCISE TRAINING

The positive effects of regular exercise for those with no disabilities extend to those with visual impairments. The additional benefits that exercise affords are the same as for those who are deaf or hard of hearing (Bloomquist 1997b).

MEDICATIONS/MANAGEMENT

The condition of visual impairment, in itself, requires no medications. An exception to this would be eye drops for a person with glaucoma. In some individuals, the use of corrective lenses may allow independent exercise.

RECOMMENDATIONS FOR ENDURANCE TRAINING

There are few limitations of endurance training for persons with visual impairments. Most stationary modes of exercise (i.e. Stair-Master, cycle and rowing ergometers, treadmill) as well as swimming and weight training hold no barriers for the visually impaired. Jogging or fast walking needs the assistance of a partner. The person with visual impairment is recommended to run/walk with a short tether to a partner or to hold onto the partner's upper arm. The partner should constantly give tactile and verbal cues as to changes in terrain.

References

Albright, A.L. (1997) Diabetes. In: *ACSM's Exercise Management for Persons with Chronic Diseases and Disabilities*, pp. 94–100. Human Kinetics, Champaign, IL.

American College of Sports Medicine (1995) *ACSM's Guidelines for Exercise Testing and Prescription*, 5th edn. Williams & Wilkins, Baltimore, MD.

American College of Sports Medicine (1997) *ACSM's Exercise Management for Persons with Chronic Diseases and Disabilities*. Human Kinetics, Champaign, IL.

Bar-Or, O. (1997) Muscular dystrophy. In:

ACSM's Exercise Management for Persons with Chronic Diseases and Disabilities, 180–184. Human Kinetics, Champaign, IL.

Birk, T.J. (1997) Polio and post–polio syndrome. In: *ACSM's Exercise Management for Persons with Chronic Diseases and Disabilities*, pp. 194–199. Human Kinetics, Champaign, IL.

Blair, S.N. (1993) Research lecture: physical activity, physical fitness, and health. *Research Quarterly for Exercise and Sport* 64, 365–376.

Bloomfield, S.A. (1997) Osteoporosis. In:

ACSM's Exercise Management for Persons with Chronic Diseases and Disabilities, pp. 161–166. Human Kinetics, Champaign, IL.

Bloomquist, L.E. (1997a) Deaf and hard of hearing. In: *ACSM's Exercise Management for Persons with Diseases and Disabilities*, pp. 233–236. Human Kinetics, Champaign, IL.

Bloomquist, L.E. (1997b) Visual impairment. In: *ACSM's Exercise Management for Persons with Diseases and Disabilities*, pp. 237–239. Human Kinetics, Champaign, IL.

Cerny, F.J., Pullano, T.P. & Cropp, G.J. (1982) Cardiorespiratory adaptations to exercise in cystic fibrosis. *American Review of Respiratory Diseases* **126**, 217–220.

Cooper, C.B. (1997) Pulmonary disease. In: *ACSM's Exercise Management for Persons with Chronic Diseases and Disabilities*, pp. 74–80. Human Kinetics, Champaign, IL.

Fernhall, B. (1997) Mental retardation. In: *ACSM's Exercise Management for Persons with Chronic Diseases and Disabilities*, pp. 221–226. Human Kinetics, Champaign, IL.

Ferrara, M. & Laskin, J. (1997) Cerebral palsy. In: *ACSM's Exercise Management for Persons with Chronic Diseases and Disabilities*, pp. 206–211. Human Kinetics, Champaign, IL.

Figoni, S.F. (1997) Spinal cord injury. In: *ACSM's Exercise Management for Persons with Chronic Diseases and Disabilities*, pp. 175–179. Human Kinetics, Champaign, IL.

Franklin, B.A. (1997) Myocardial infarction. In: *ACSM's Exercise Management for Persons with Chronic Diseases and Disabilities*, pp. 19–25. Human Kinetics, Champaign, IL.

Gardner, A.W. (1997) Peripheral arterial disease. In: *ACSM's Exercise Management for Persons with Chronic Diseases and Disabilities*, pp. 64–68. Human Kinetics, Champaign, IL.

Graham, T.P., Jr., Bricker, J.T., James, F.W. & Strong, W.B. (1994) Task force 1: Congenital heart disease. In: 26th Bethseda Conference: Recommendations for determing eligibility for competition in athletes with cardiovascular abnormalities. *Journal of the American College of Cardiology* **24**, 867–873.

Hahn, R.A., Teutsch, S.M., Paffenbarger, R.S. & Marks, J.S. (1990) Excess deaths from nine chronic diseases in the United States, 1986. *Journal of the American Medical Association* **24**, 2654–2659.

James, U. (1973) Effect of physical training in healthy unilateral above-knee amputees. *Scandanavian Journal of Rehabilitation Medicine* **5**, 88–101.

Luckasson, R., Caulter, D., Polloway, E., Deiss, S., Schalock, R., Snell, M., Spitalnick, D. & Stark, J. (1992) *Mental Retardation, Definition, Classification, and Systems of Support*, 9th edn. American Association of Mental Retardation, Washington, DC.

McNeil, J.M. (1993) *Americans with Disabilities: 1991–1992*. U.S. Bureau of the Census (Current Population Reports, P70–33). U.S. Government Printing Office, Washington, DC.

Minor, M.A. & Kay, D.R. (1997) Arthritis. In: *ACSM's Exercise Management for Persons with Chronic Disease and Disabilities*, pp. 149–154. Human Kinetics, Champaign, IL.

Mulcare, J.A. (1997) Multiple sclerosis. In: *ACSM's Exercise Management for Persons with Chronic Disease and Disabilities*, pp. 189–193. Human Kinetics, Champaign, IL.

Nau, K.L. (1997) Amyotrophic lateral sclerosis. In: *ACSM's Exercise Management for Persons with Chronic Disease and Disabilities*, pp. 200–205. Human Kinetics, Champaign, IL.

Nixon, P.A. (1997) Cystic fibrosis. In: *ACSM's Exercise Management for Persons with Chronic Diseases and Disabilities*, pp. 81–86. Human Kinetics, Champaign, IL.

Paffenbarger, R.S., Hyde, P.H., Wing, A.L., Lee, I.-M., Jung, D.L. & Kampert, J.B. (1993) The association of changes in physical-activity level and other lifestyle characteristics with mortality among men. *New England Journal of Medicine* **328**, 538–545.

Painter, P.L. (1997) Renal failure. In: *ACSM's Exercise Management for Persons with Chronic Diseases and Disabilities*, pp. 89–91. Human Kinetics, Champaign, IL.

Palmer-McLean, K. & Wilberger, J.E. (1997) Stroke and head injury. In: *ACSM's Exercise Management for Persons with Chronic Disease and Disabilities*, pp. 169–174. Human Kinetics, Champaign, IL.

Pitetti, K.H., Snell, P.G., Stray-Gundersen, S. & Gottschalk, F.A. (1987) Aerobic training exercise for individuals who had amputation of lower limb. *Journal of Bone and Joint Surgery* **69**, 914–921.

Protos, E.J., Stanley, R.K. & Jankovic, J. (1997) Parkinson's disease. In: *ACSM's Exercise Management for Persons with Chronic Diseases and Disabilities*, pp. 212–217. Human Kinetics, Champaign, IL.

Pyeritz, R.E. (1997) Aneurysms and Marfan syndrome. In: *ACSM's Exercise Management for Persons with Chronic Diseases and Disabilities*, pp. 69–71. Human Kinetics, Champaign, IL.

Schenkman, M. & Butler, R.B. (1989) A model for multisystem evaluation and treatment of individuals with Parkinson's disease. *Physical Therapy* **69**, 932–943.

Sherrill, C. (1993) *Adapted Physical Activity, Recreation, and Sport*, 4th edn, pp. 517–518. Brown & Benchmark, Madison, WI.

Wallace, J.P. (1997) Obesity. In: *ACSM's Exercise Management for Persons with Chronic Diseases and Disabilities*, pp. 106–111. Human Kinetics, Champaign, IL.

Wasserman, K., Hansen, J.E., Sue, K.Y., Whipp, B.J. & Casaburi, R. (1994) *Principles of Exercise Testing and Interpretation*, 2nd edn. Lea & Febiger, Philadelphia.

PART 6

ENVIRONMENTAL ASPECTS OF ENDURANCE TRAINING

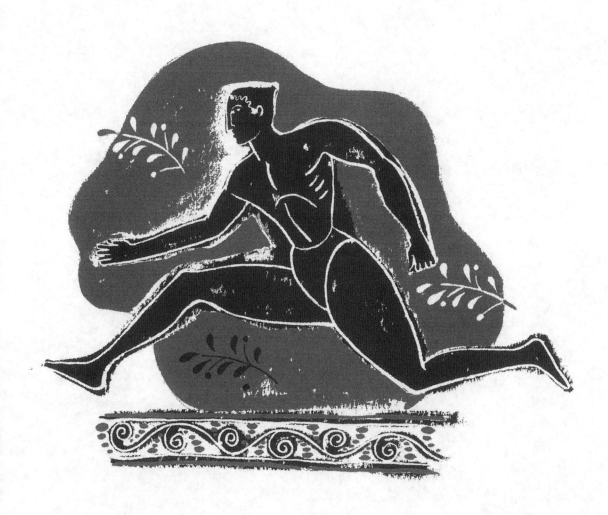

Chapter 40

Hyperthermia, Hypothermia and Problems of Hydration

TIMOTHY D. NOAKES

Introduction

It is widely believed that fluid imbalance, dehydration in particular, is the single most important factor promoting heat illnesses, including collapse, in endurance sport. We begin this chapter with a review of the origins of this particular dogma, before presenting a more complete analysis of these phenomena. This information is crucial for a more logical approach to the management of the commonly described 'heat illnesses' in sport.

The role of dehydration in the heat illnesses

Historically, athletes and their coaches have promoted the value of fluid *restriction* during both athletic training and competition (Noakes 1991, 1993). For example, the Oxford University rowing crew of 1860 were restricted to a maximum of 2 pints (about 0.9 l) of fluid each day during training. But 'outraged human nature rebelled against it; and although they did not admit it in public, there were very few men who did not rush to their waterbottles for relief, more or less often, according to the development of their conscientiousness and their obstinacy'.

A popular book on marathon running published in 1909 advised that prospective marathon runners avoid eating or drinking during the race: 'Don't get in the habit of drinking and eating in a marathon race; some prominent runners do, but it is not beneficial'.

Some famous athletes of that era, notably multiple Boston Marathon winner, Clarence de Mar, drank fluids more freely during competition, but the general practice was to restrict fluid ingestion to an absolute minimum during competition. Arthur Newton, who in the 1920s and 1930s held world records for running distances of 80–221 km and who competed in the Professional Trans-America races of 1928 and 1929, wrote: 'Even in the warmest English weather, a 26-mile run ought to be manageable with no more than a single drink, or at most two'.

Similarly, English marathoner, Jim Peters, who lowered the world record in the standard 42-km marathon by more than 9 min between 1952 and 1954 believed: 'There is no need to take any solid food at all [during a marathon race] and every effort should be made to do without liquid, as the moment food or drink is taken, the body has to start dealing with its digestion and in so doing some discomfort will almost invariably be felt'.

This conventional wisdom was enshrined in the rules of the International Amateur Athletic Federation (IAAF) governing the conduct of long-distance races at that time. The rules in force in 1953 stated that 'refreshments shall (only) be provided by the organizers of a race after 15 km or 10 miles, and thereafter every 5 km or 3 miles. No refreshment may be carried to be taken by a competitor other than that provided by the organizers'. Water was the only drink available to runners at the official refreshment stations, despite evidence that carbohydrate ingested during exercise could aid performance.

This historical review is relevant because it

establishes that, at least until 1969, competitors in endurance events, especially marathon running, were actively discouraged from drinking during exercise. The first text which actively promoted fluid ingestion during exercise was published as recently as 1979. Despite universally inadequate fluid replacement during exercise, there is no evidence that the endurance athletes of the first 70 years of the 20th century were at noticeably greater *health* risk than modern runners during exercise.

It was into this intellectual vacuum that one of the most influential studies in the modern exercise sciences exploded. The study (Wyndham & Strydom 1969) was completed as an adjunct to a larger investigation of the effects of a sucrose-supplemented diet on performance in 30-km foot races. The authors found no ergogenic effect of the high sucrose diet. However, they had also measured the rates of fluid ingestion and the levels of dehydration that developed, and it was those findings that would become so influential. The athletes drank less than they sweated; hence, all lost weight. There was a linear relationship between levels of dehydration of >3% and the athletes' postexercise rectal temperatures. Hence, the authors concluded that the level of dehydration that develops during exercise is the principal determinant of the rectal temperature during exercise, and avoidance of weight loss (dehydration) must be the most important factor preventing heat injury during exercise. But to reach this conclusion, the authors had to ignore their own published findings that the metabolic rate is also a major determinant of the rectal temperature during exercise (Wyndham *et al.* 1970).

The influence of the study came not so much from its findings but from its provocative title: *'The danger of an inadequate water intake during marathon running'*. The research neither studied nor did it identify any *dangers* of an inadequate fluid intake during marathon running. Rather, the most dehydrated runners won the races. Thus a disinterested runner might well have concluded that dehydration enhanced performance. Given this unexpected finding and the low rate of reported cases of heatstroke and other health disorders in marathon runners despite inadequate fluid intakes, a more appropriate title for that historic study might have

been: *'Remarkable resistance of marathon runners to any detrimental effects of dehydration'*.

The immediately beneficial effect of the study was to cause a review of IAAF rules governing international distance races. In 1977, rule changes allowed fluid ingestion every 2.5 km after the first 5 km of long-distance races. In 1990, the rule was again modified to allow the ingestion of water and carbohydrate every 3 km after the first 2.5 km of long-distance races. A less desirable effect of the study was to induce a dogmatic zeal amongst sports medicine practitioners to avoid the dangers of dehydration in endurance athletes. Those who were influenced by the article's title without digesting its contents seem to have adopted the following (incorrect) logic: 'Progressive dehydration during exercise causes heatstroke; hence, the most important method to prevent heatstroke during exercise is to ensure athletes ingest as much fluid as possible. Since heatstroke is also the most important cause of collapse during exercise, all persons who collapse after exercise have a heat disorder and must necessarily be dehydrated. Therefore, intravenous fluid therapy is the logical treatment for all athletes who collapse during or after exercise.'

With this background we proceed to discuss the three conditions that are classically described as exercise-related heat illnesses: heat cramps, heat exhaustion (syncope) and heatstroke. The evidence that each is indeed a real heat disorder is discussed, as is the possible role of dehydration in their causation. Hypothermia in sport is then described. Finally, a modern approach to the management of 'heat illness' is proposed.

Heat cramps

Heat cramps were probably first described among coal miners in 1923, eventually becoming known as 'miner's', 'fireman's', 'stoker's', 'cane cutter's' or, simply, 'heat' cramps. The popular modern belief is that heat cramps are caused by the severe dehydration and large sodium chloride losses that develop during exercise in hot conditions. But the original descriptions postulated that the cramps resulted from an excessive fluid intake. Fluid balance studies of patients with heat cramps failed to show that all were overhydrated. Most either lost weight during exercise or gained weight during recovery, indicating that they were dehydrated when cramps developed. However, urine outputs were high, so that severe dehydration was not a likely aetiological factor. Reductions in serum osmolality, or serum sodium or chloride concentrations were also present in some patients.

Thus, early researchers believed that heat cramps were caused by the ingestion of large volumes of water without adequate replacement of sodium chloride. However, any relationship of muscle cramps to fluid overload or development of a sodium deficit cannot be established from published data. It was generally believed that heat cramps could be prevented by adding sodium chloride to water ingested during exercise, and that they could be treated with sodium chloride infusion, but there were no controlled clinical trials to evaluate these beliefs. Two modern studies have extended our knowledge. Maughan (1986) showed that serum electrolyte concentrations and changes in plasma volume did not differ between runners who did or did not develop cramps during a 42-km marathon race. He concluded that 'exercise-induced muscle cramp may not be associated with gross disturbances of fluid and electrolyte balance'. Another study (Nicol *et al.* 1999) compared fluid balance and serum electrolyte changes during a 56-km ultramarathon foot race between runners with a history of frequent exercise-related cramps and competitors without such a history, who were competing in the same event. Again, there were no differences in either fluid balance or serum electrolyte changes between the cramp-prone group and the non-cramping controls.

In summary, there is no evidence that heat cramps are caused by dehydration or by excessive losses of sodium chloride or other electrolyte invoked by exercise. After a lifetime studying sodium balance in persons exercising in desert heat, Epstein and Sohar (1985) wrote that 'salt deficiency heat exhaustion' (and, by extension, salt deficiency heat cramps) 'is an example of christening by conjecture'. 'Such a syndrome' they concluded, 'has never been proven to exist'. Cramps can occur at rest, or during or after exercise undertaken under any environmental con-

ditions; they are specific neither to exercise, nor to exercise in the heat. The more modern hypothesis proposes that cramps are probably the result of alterations in spinal neural reflex activity activated by fatigue in susceptible individuals (Bentley 1996; Schwellnus *et al.* 1997). Persistent use of the term 'heat cramps' cannot be justified, and it continues to cloud understanding of the probable neural nature of this condition.

Heat exhaustion (heat syncope)

In current understanding, heat exhaustion or heat syncope describes a condition in which an athlete collapses during or after exercising in the heat. It is thought to be due to dehydration-induced heat retention which is insufficiently severe to cause heatstroke. Hence, heat exhaustion is described as a mild form of heatstroke caused by dehydration and which, unless correctly treated, will progress to more severe heatstroke. The errors in logic leading to these incorrect conclusions have already been traced, in part, to the study of Wyndham and Strydom (1969). Evidence that heat exhaustion is *not* a true heat disorder caused by abnormalities in heat balance and a progressive rise in core body temperature during exercise includes the following.

Firstly, rectal temperatures are not abnormally elevated in persons with 'heat exhaustion' (Holtzhausen *et al.* 1994; Roberts 1996) or in the experimental condition termed 'heat strain' (Sawka *et al.* 1992, 1996). Secondly, there is no evidence that persons with heat exhaustion will develop heatstroke if they are left untreated, or that they are more dehydrated than participants in the same events who do not develop the condition. The largest modern study of subjects who required medical attention after long-distance events showed that only a tiny proportion of participants had markedly elevated rectal temperature and few required hospitalization (Roberts 1996). These findings refute the popular belief that the majority of subjects who collapse after prolonged exercise suffer from a heat disorder that progresses inexorably to heatstroke. A third critical finding is that 85% of athletes who collapse in association with exercise, and who would therefore fulfil the diagnostic criteria for 'heat exhaustion', do so *after* they have *stopped* exercising (Irving *et al.* 1991; Holtzhausen *et al.* 1994). For reasons to be argued later in this chapter, this finding alone is incompatible with the belief that dehydration and hyperthermia are critical determinants of this condition.

A more likely explanation is that the sudden cessation of exercise induces postural hypotension by causing blood to pool in the dilated capacitance veins in the lower limb when the 'second heart' action of the lower limb musculature stops. In addition, there may be abnormal perfusion of the splanchnic circulation, with loss of a large fluid volume into the highly compliant splanchnic veins. The problem is a precipitous fall in *central* (rather than circulating) blood volume and hence, a decline in atrial filling pressure (Noakes 1988; Holtzhausen *et al.* 1994; Holtzhausen & Noakes 1995, 1997).

Historical studies of collapse in persons exposed to exercise in hot environments, cases of so-called 'heat exhaustion', emphasized that all had postural hypotension, but that rectal temperatures were not abnormally elevated. Cardiovascular instability and associated symptoms disappeared as soon as the subjects lay prone, without need for intravenous fluid therapy (Holtzhausen & Noakes 1997). Thus, these authors did not consider that dehydration contributed to the condition. For example, Adolph (1947) noted that patients with 'heat exhaustion' were 'still producing sweat and keeping cool', but showed evidence of postural hypotension. Adolph and Fulton (1924) concluded: 'The peripheral blood vessels are greatly dilated during exposure to high temperatures, and this dilatation continues indefinitely. The lack of a high resistance in the peripheral blood vessels prevents blood from returning to the heart. The heart rate increases steadily and rapidly, and is even able to increase the systolic blood pressure. In spite of this compensating activity on the part of the heart, the blood flow back to the heart finally becomes inadequate. At this point circulatory collapse or shock is complete, with faintness'. Adolph (1947) also noted that patients with this condition usually needed 'merely to lie down to feel better. The shock-like circulatory failure appears to be the crucial element in this condition'. Talbott *et al.*

(1937) also concluded that 'heat prostration is associated with vasomotor collapse. It is known that peripheral dilatation of blood vessels and tachycardia accompany exposure to high temperature. During muscle activity in high environmental temperatures, the peripheral dilatation with vasomotor collapse may approach pathological proportions'. Similarly Eichna *et al.* (1945, 1947) showed that 58% of subjects developed syncope on their first exposure to 'exhausting' exercise in the heat. The authors labelled the condition 'heat exhaustion', even though the rectal temperatures were not greatly elevated (<38°C), and indeed were similar to those measured in our subjects with exercise-associated collapse (EAC) (Holtzhausen *et al.* 1994). Others had also noted that the rectal temperature was either 'submaximal or slightly elevated' in heat exhaustion. In common with other early workers, Eichna *et al.* (1947) proposed that postural hypotension explained the syncope in subjects with 'heat exhaustion'. They concluded that the postural drop in blood pressure resulted from pooling of blood in the lower extremities on cessation of exercise, due to a work-induced venodilatation in the lower limb muscles and inactivation of the muscle pump that had aided venous return during exercise. The conclusion from these early studies must be that the terms 'heat exhaustion', 'heat prostration' or 'heat syncope' were used to describe a condition of collapse due to postural hypotension that developed in persons exercising in the heat. The terminology should not be misinterpreted to infer that the collapse is caused by an elevated body temperature due to a failure of heat regulation and that it is therefore a mild form of heatstroke. However, the possibility that postural hypotension could explain EAC has been overlooked by subsequent investigators.

These same features, particularly hypotension and tachycardia which are rapidly reversed on lying supine, are seen in athletes with EAC (Holtzhausen *et al.* 1994; Holtzhausen & Noakes 1995, 1997). Hence, we have proposed that most athletes who collapse *after* exercise have postural hypotension; this should be managed by lying supine with the legs and pelvis elevated above heart level. Such treatment has proven effective and, in our hands, has removed the need for intravenous fluid therapy in the vast majority of athletes who collapse *after* completing marathon and ultramarathon races.

Both logic and published evidence argue that heat exhaustion will not lead to heatstroke. Stopping exercise reduces the rate of heat production in subjects with 'heat exhaustion', causing them to begin cooling immediately on collapse. This contrasts to the situation in true heatstroke, in which physiological and biochemical abnormalities in skeletal muscle cause the rate of heat production to remain elevated even after the athlete stops exercising. Thus, the body temperature in heatstroke will remain in excess of 41°C unless an athlete is actively cooled to below 38°C.

Confusion about the aetiological role of dehydration in the clinically defined condition of 'heat exhaustion' in the athletic population stems from a misinterpretation of Wyndham and Strydom's study, as well as laboratory studies of the experimental condition known as 'heat strain' (Sawka *et al.* 1992, 1996). Heat strain is defined as the exhaustion that develops when persons exercise in environmental conditions specifically chosen so that thermal balance cannot be achieved, and all subjects collapse from 'heat strain' provided the exercise duration is sufficiently long. Under these extreme conditions, in which athletic competition is neither safe nor allowed, a severe pre-exercise dehydration (hypohydration) (8%) is associated with premature termination of exercise because of heat strain. Yet, and this is the point of logic that has been overlooked, *all* subjects developed heat strain even when they were fully hydrated, proving that dehydration is not an essential factor in the aetiology of heat strain. Severe hypohydration influenced only the time to onset of 'heat strain'. In that and other studies of severe environmental conditions never experienced in modern athletic competition, affected subjects terminated exercise at the same or lower rectal temperatures than when in the fully hydrated state. Hypohydration did not reduce the exercise time by increasing heat retention, as would be predicted from the expected effect of dehydration in reducing skin blood flow and the capacity for heat loss. Thus, the mechanism causing the fatigue of 'heat strain' is unknown. Perhaps 'heat strain' is

as much a misnomer as are heat cramps and heat exhaustion.

In summary, whereas dehydration affects exercise performance in the heat to varying degrees (Walsh *et al.* 1994), there is presently no evidence that the dehydration seen in endurance athletes (1–4% of body mass) (Noakes *et al.* 1988; Noakes 1993, 1995) exercising under moderate environmental conditions poses any major *health* risks or predisposes to heatstroke. Given the historical evidence, it would seem unlikely.

Classical studies of exercise dehydration performed during the Second World War (Adolph & Fulton 1924; Adolph 1947) found that military personnel forced to exercise without fluid replacement continued to exercise in hot, desert conditions until dehydration reached >7–10%. 'Dehydration exhaustion', characterized by circulatory instability with tachycardia and postural hypotension, and psychological alterations, including heightened aggression and a loss of discipline, terminated exercise. Despite levels of dehydration almost never reached by endurance athletes in modern competitions, none of the subjects lost consciousness. Loss of consciousness is *not* a characteristic of exercise-induced dehydration.

In addition, subjects were neither markedly hyperthermic nor did they show significant alterations in renal function. All recovered quickly when they lay down and ingested fluid. Recovery occurred even before any physiological effects could have resulted from fluid ingestion. On the basis of those studies, Brown (1947) concluded that dehydration posed significant health risks only at levels of dehydration of 15–20%, two to three times greater than those seen in endurance athletes (Noakes 1993). Perhaps 'dehydration exhaustion' or 'heat strain' prevents athletes from exercising to levels of dehydration that cause medical complications.

Based on the historic evidence, together with our own studies of EAC (Noakes 1988, 1995; Noakes *et al.* 1988, 1991a; Sandell *et al.* 1988; Holtzhausen *et al.* 1994; Holtzhausen & Noakes 1995, 1997) and extensive clinical experience in the management of collapsed ultramarathon runners, we have suggested that the principal pathophysiology of post-exercise collapse (EAC; heat exhaustion or heat syncopy) is a postural hypotension that develops as a result of three specific changes.

The first is an increased cutaneous blood flow in an attempt to regulate body temperature. This redistributes the central blood volume to the periphery, decreasing left atrial filling pressure and stroke volume; cardiac output is maintained by an increased heart rate. The higher the environmental temperature, the greater the cutaneous blood flow and thus the greater the peripheral location of blood volume, particularly on stopping exercise. This explains why the number of athletes who collapse during or after endurance events is linearly related to the ambient temperature (Richards & Richards 1984). Secondly, the action of the calf muscle pump helps to maintain the arterial pressure during exercise in the heat by reducing the volume of blood stored in the capacitance veins of the lower limbs. When the action of the calf muscle ceases, blood accumulates in the dilated capacitance veins, threatening arterial blood pressure.

Thirdly, training induces adaptations in the autonomic nervous system, including an increased baseline parasympathetic activity, associated with a resting bradycardia, plus an attenuated sympathetic activity, associated with a blunted vasoconstrictor response to any hypotensive stress.

If this theory is correct, the logical approach to the treatment of EAC is to elevate and cool the athlete's legs and pelvis in order to reduce the skin blood flow and the volume of blood in the cutaneous and, perhaps more importantly, the splanchnic veins. Subjects considered to be 'dehydrated' may ingest fluid. Using this form of treatment in our medical tent, we have dramatically reduced the need for intravenous fluids in collapsed ultramarathon runners, simultaneously improving medical care for those in greatest need (see Management protocols for collapsed athletes who are fully conscious).

Heatstroke

A diagnosis of heatstroke must be considered during exercise whenever a previously healthy athlete shows marked changes in mental functioning—for example, collapse with unconsciousness, a reduced level of consciousness (stupor, coma) or mental stimulation (irritability, convulsions)—in association with a rectal temperature in excess of 41°C. The factors that predispose to heatstroke are those that disturb the equilibrium between heat production and heat loss during exercise. The rate of heat loss is controlled by air temperature and humidity, the rate of wind movement across the athlete's body and the rate of sweating; the rate of heat production is determined by the athlete's mass and work rate (Noakes et al. 1991b; Wyndham et al. 1970). Thus, the rate of heat production and the risk of heatstroke are greatest in those who run the fastest and have the highest work rate, i.e. in relatively short-distance rather than marathon events. The most important causal factors are environmental conditions, the speed of running, body mass and individual susceptibility. If relatively short-distance races (6–15 km) are held under extreme environmental conditions, heat injury will occur in a significant number of competitors regardless of whether or not they become dehydrated.

The unfortunate effect of Wyndham and Strydom's study was that it established exclusive priority for one of the many factors affecting heat balance during exercise. Dehydration is certainly not the only factor and may not even be a very important factor.

Despite a decade of searching, the author has not unearthed any evidence that those who develop heatstroke during athletic competition are more dehydrated than those who complete the same races with more normal body temperatures. The absence of such information is understandable, given the very low frequency of heatstroke in modern athletic competition, especially since the introduction of suggested environmental limiting conditions beyond which competitions should not be held. It seems very unlikely that severe dehydration alone can explain why only one or two individuals develop heatstroke in races involving tens of thousands of competitors, the majority of whom become dehydrated to varying degrees without developing heatstroke. It is far more likely that, for unknown reasons, certain individuals are prone to heatstroke during exercise. Two possible explanations for the low rates of heatstroke during exercise could be that athletes develop heatstroke because of acquired conditions that occur very rarely, or that affected athletes are genetically predisposed, perhaps because of an abnormality of skeletal muscle metabolism. Malignant hyperthermia, which is usually activated by certain general anaesthetic agents, may also be triggered by other stimuli, perhaps including exercise, in susceptible individuals. The biochemical abnormality causing malignant hyperthermia is thought to reside in the ryanodine receptor in the skeletal muscle sarcoplasmic reticulum. The reticulum releases its stored calcium when exposed to a variety of triggering agents, thus activating uncontrolled skeletal muscle glycogenolysis. This in turn causes a profound acidosis, hyperthermia and ultimately an extensive and potentially fatal rhabdomyolysis. The process can be reversed only by a specific drug, dantrolene sodium, or by rapid whole-body cooling.

This contrasts to the absence of a biochemically mediated hypermetabolic state in 'heat exhaustion', in which postexercise rectal temperatures are not abnormally elevated and revert to normal without active cooling or use of any specific medications.

Summary of the heat illnesses and the role of dehydration

This search has failed to uncover any firm scientific evidence that dehydration and electrolyte imbalances are either exclusive or even important causes of heat illnesses currently described in the medical literature. This does not negate the findings that exercise-induced dehydration (i) measurably reduces skin blood flow and changes other physiological variables during exercise in the heat; and (ii) impairs exercise performance or the duration of exercise that can be sustained before the onset of 'heat strain'. Rather, this conclusion is presented simply as evidence that the aetiology of the heat illnesses is more complex than is currently believed, and that no one factor is likely to be determinative. There is no reason to believe that the prevention of 'dehydration' by encouraging athletes to drink more during exercise and the instantaneous treatment of all collapsed athletes with intravenous fluids will either prevent or cure all cases of 'heat injury' in sport.

What then is the established role of dehydration in exercise and associated 'heat disorders'? Firstly, dehydration causes important and mostly detrimental physiological changes. For example, the heart rate and rectal temperature are higher and the stroke volume and skin blood flow are lower in proportion to the level of dehydration that develops during exercise (Coyle & Montain 1993). Such changes are reduced by adequate fluid ingestion. Furthermore, performance during prolonged exercise in the heat may be impaired even at quite low levels of dehydration. However, in this author's opinion, the effect of dehydration on performance in different competitive sports has still to be quantified accurately. Too often, the relationship is dogmatically described as a documented 20–30% reduction in performance for dehydration levels of 2–5% (Saltin & Costill 1988). This seems highly improbable, given historical evidence that athletes achieved remarkable performances in endurance events in the years before regular fluid ingestion was allowed or encouraged (Noakes 1991).

It is appropriate that competitive athletes be encouraged to drink fluid during exercise, especially in the heat, in order to optimize performance and to reduce the detrimental physiological changes that develop with dehydration. However, it may not always be possible to replace all fluid lost during exercise, and some degree of dehydration may be inevitable when runners sustain sweat rates in excess of $1 l \cdot h^{-1}$. Some cyclists, on the other hand, can drink up to $2 l \cdot h^{-1}$ even during competition. But whether optimum fluid ingestion will prevent important medical complications of prolonged exercise, including heatstroke, acute renal failure and postexercise collapse, is not established (Noakes 1995). There is growing evidence that both heatstroke and acute renal failure occur in persons who are genetically predisposed to malignant hyperthermia and rhabdomyolysis in response to a variety of stresses, including prolonged exercise. This would perhaps explain (i) why true heatstroke occurs so infrequently even when large numbers of subjects compete in endurance events under unfavourable environmental conditions and, conversely, (ii) why heatstroke frequently occurs during exercise in mild environmental conditions.

Secondly, there is no good evidence proving, nor indeed any logic suggesting, that dehydration is either an important or a necessary component of the common form of EAC that occurs on cessation of exercise. Hence, intravenous fluid is not necessarily the most appropriate form of therapy for this condition. Rather, as discussed in the next section, the crucial initial step in the management of persons who collapse during or after prolonged exercise is to establish a reasonable working clinical diagnosis. This will include a clinical assessment of the patient's level of dehydration.

Thirdly, athletes can drink too much during exercise, causing hyponatraemia. This condition occurs more frequently than classical heatstroke in endurance athletes and it is potentially more dangerous; the diagnosis is made only if there is a high degree of clinical suspicion, and the treatment is more complex. As an iatrogenic condition, prevention should be relatively simple (Noakes 1992).

In summary, the assumption that dehydration is the underlying cause of heatstroke and all cases of collapse in endurance athletes is not supported by firm scientific evidence. Quite mild levels of dehydration impair exercise performance, but levels of dehydration much greater than have ever been measured in endurance athletes are necessary to produce acute renal failure and death. Hence, athletes can safely be encouraged to maintain low levels of dehydration by drinking 'enough but not too much' during exercise. But they should also be warned that very high rates of fluid ingestion ($>1.5 l \cdot h^{-1}$) sustained for many hours can lead to fluid retention and hyponatraemia, with impaired performance and a potentially fatal outcome (Irving et al. 1991). Finally, clinicians must be discouraged from assuming that all complications found in endurance athletes are heat related, are due to a severe dehydration, and should be corrected by immediate intravenous therapy. Like all patients, the collapsed athlete deserves a rational diagnosis (Noakes 1988; Holtzhausen & Noakes 1997) before therapy is initiated. If the diagnosis is not immediately apparent, there is no evidence of harm if therapy is withheld for a few minutes.

Fluid overload in prolonged exercise – the hyponatraemia of exercise

Whereas the focus of sports medicine for the past 30 years has been on the supposed dangers of dehydration, more recently it has become apparent that some athletes place their lives at much greater risk by ingesting too much fluid during prolonged exercise. This causes hyponatraemia (Noakes 1992). The possibility was first raised in a series of case reports (Noakes et al. 1985; Frizzell et al. 1986). More recently, hyponatraemia of varying severity has been reported in up to 20% of Hawaiian Ironman Triathlon competitors, including $>50\%$ of those seeking medical attention, in 18% of finishers in the New Zealand Ironman Triathlon and in 0.3–10% of ultradistance running competitors. The frequency of the condition seems to have increased substantially in the past decade (Noakes et al. 1990; Speedy et al. 1999) (Fig. 40.1). The pathogenesis remained uncertain until quite recently. Current evidence indicates that athletes with this condition ingest fluid at unusually high rates during prolonged exercise and retain fluid inappropriately. Most of the evidence comes from small retrospective studies. Three different reports (Irving et al. 1991; Speedy et al. 1999a,b) have now established that athletes with severely symptomatic hyponatraemia and postrace serum sodium concentrations below $126–128 \, mmol \cdot l^{-1}$ either gain weight during exercise or excrete a fluid excess of up to 6 l during recovery. This indicates that athletes develop the condition because they ingest an excess of fluid. Other studies have shown an inverse relationship between the postrace serum sodium concentrations and weight changes during prolonged exercise (Speedy et al. 1999). Marked overhydration causes symptomatic hyponatraemia, whereas severe dehydration causes hypernatraemia, not the reverse, as originally proposed (Hiller 1989).

In summary, a high rate of fluid ingestion during prolonged exercise leads to fluid retention in certain predisposed individuals. Fluid is retained initially in the extracellular space, but osmotic forces cause rapid diffusion into the intracellular space. Clinical symptoms develop as fluid accumulates in the brain, causing cerebral oedema. A clouding of con-

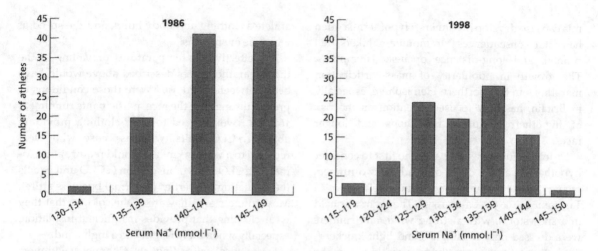

Fig. 40.1 Distribution of serum sodium concentrations in finishers in the 1986 South African Ironman Triathlon and in subjects treated in the medical facility at the finish of the 1998 Hawaiian Ironman Triathlon. Note that whereas less than 2% of all subjects in the 1986 triathlon finished with serum sodium concentrations below 135 mmol·l⁻¹ (Noakes *et al.* 1990), 54% of treated athletes in the 1998 Hawaiian race had lower values. Comparison of the two graphs shows that the overall distribution of postrace serum sodium concentrations has shifted from a median value of 140–145 mmol·l⁻¹ in the 1986 race to a median value of 130–134 mmol·l⁻¹ in athletes treated after the 1998 race. From Noakes *et al.* (1990).

sciousness is followed by progressive coma and death from respiratory or cardiac arrest if the fluid retention is not reversed.

Three possible mechanisms explain why the fluid is retained inappropriately. Firstly, high concentrations of circulating hormones may prevent an appropriate renal response to an increased blood volume and a falling serum sodium concentration. Neither vasopressin nor aldosterone concentrations are abnormally high in athletes with this condition (Irving *et al.* 1991; Speedy *et al.* 1999); hence, the nature of any hormonal imbalance has still to be identified. Secondly, the renal capacity may be inadequate to excrete fluid at high rates. This seems unlikely, as most patients with hyponatraemia excrete urine at high rates during recovery, which begins some hours after exercise. Alternatively, a transient renal failure may develop, perhaps as a result of reduced renal blood flow during exercise. This also seems unlikely, given that most cases of hyponatraemia occur in the less competitive athletes who complete their events at lower exercise intensities than their élite peers. More probably, the rate of urine production is sensitive to exercise intensity, and may be substantially reduced at quite

modest exercise intensities in some individuals. Thirdly, the rate of intestinal fluid absorption may be less than is generally believed. At high rates of fluid ingestion, unabsorbed fluid would cause reverse sodium movement from the extracellular space into the gut, creating a physiological third space. If 2 or more litres of fluid were sequestered, unabsorbed, in the intestinal lumen, hyponatraemia would develop (Noakes 1992). But the finding that fluid retention occurs in the extracellular space in some cases of hyponatraemia (Speedy *et al.* 1999a–c) argues against this possibility.

Currently, the only tested treatment is to ensure that the patient receives *no fluid* during recovery. The condition resolves spontaneously as soon as the patient begins to pass a very dilute urine, usually at rates of 400 ml·h⁻¹ or greater. Normal cerebral function usually returns before the serum sodium concentration normalizes; the latter may take 24–48 h.

Hypothermia during running

So much attention has been paid to the dangers of heatstroke during marathon running, that physicians have been slow to appreciate that hypothermia can also develop in runners. Hypothermia often has fatal consequences for mountain hikers, fell runners and long-distance open-sea swimmers. The growth in popularity of mass-participation marathons in the Northern Hemisphere, especially in Britain, has now focused attention on the risk of hypothermia during marathons and longer races.

Dr John Sutton was probably the first to consider hypothermia as the cause of death in two runners racing to the summit of Mount Wellington in Tasmania in 1903 (Noakes 1991). The event was held in a snowstorm, with a strong wind, and runners were dressed only in 'singlets and light knickers'. Soon competitors were 'lying over logs, on the ground, and under trees, too exhausted to continue'. Almost certainly, the deceased runners froze to death before they could be rescued.

The first documented case of hypothermia in a marathon was that of Ledingham *et al.* (1982), who reported a rectal temperature of 34.3°C in a runner who collapsed in the Glasgow Marathon, which on that occasion was run under dry but cold conditions (dry bulb temperature 12°C) with a wind speed of 16–40 km·h^{-1}. Maughan (1985) measured the rectal temperature of 59 runners completing the 1982 Aberdeen Marathon under more favourable weather conditions (no rain, dry bulb temperature 12°C, humidity 75%, wind speed about 26 km·h^{-1}). Four runners finished the race with rectal temperatures below 37°C. Even in the Southern Hemisphere, conditions can on occasion be sufficiently unfavourable to cause hypothermia. A study of runners admitted to the medical tent at the end of the 1985 56-km Two Oceans Marathon, run under unusually cold conditions for that region (rain, wet bulb globe temperature 19.8°C, and a wind speed of 30 km·h^{-1}), showed that eight (28%) of the collapsed runners had rectal temperatures below 37°C (Sandell *et al.* 1988). Despite maintaining a running speed in excess of 17 km·h^{-1}, one very thin élite runner collapsed on the course and was brought to the medical tent, where his rectal temperature was found to be 35.0°C.

Four factors predispose to hypothermia during distance running: the environmental conditions, the athlete's clothing and body build, and the speed at which he or she runs.

The effective air temperatures prevailing in the three marathon races described above would have been between 1 and 3°C. Were those conditions to prevail throughout the race, participants running at 16 km·h^{-1} would need to wear clothing providing about 1.1 CLO units, whereas those who were reduced to a walk (5 km·h^{-1}) would require approximately 2 CLO units of insulation (1 CLO unit equals the insulating properties of normal business attire). Most runners are unaware of the cold, so that they wear clothing that provides insufficient insulation, especially when there is rain and a high wind.

Experience with English Channel swimmers has shown that body build, especially body muscle (but also body fat) content, is a critical determinant of the rate of cooling during a long-distance swim. Probably the same applies to runners: those who have little body fat or muscle are most likely to become hypothermic. Frank Shorter, 1972 Olympic marathon gold medallist, is one such thin runner who found that he ran poorly in the cold and, conversely, rather well in the heat. Possibly this indicated that Shorter had difficulty maintaining a normally elevated body temperature when running in the cold. The thin ectomorphic African runners who currently dominate world athletics also complain of difficulty when running in cold conditions.

The role of running speed in protecting against hypothermia has already been discussed. A change from running to walking has a marked effect on the clothing needed to maintain body temperature, even at relatively mild effective temperatures. At an effective air temperature of 0°C, clothing must have four times as much insulation to maintain body temperature when resting than when running at 16 km·h^{-1}. Hypothermia is most likely in marathon runners who are lean, lightly muscled and lightly clothed, who become fatigued and who are forced to walk for prolonged periods in effective air temperatures of less than 5°C. Prevention is simply to ensure that extra clothing is available should one be forced to walk in cold conditions. Rain suits should be worn whenever an athlete begins to walk in the rain.

Guidelines for the optimum management of collapsed athletes

Conditions commonly associated with collapse during or after exercise

Table 40.1 lists the most common medical conditions encountered in competitors who collapse during or after endurance events. Contrary to the general expectation, cardiac arrest is rarely seen; it is more common in those events that attract older participants.

Certain conditions are specific to particular sports and particular environmental conditions. For example, hypothermia is likely in swim triathlons; the number of cases depends on the water temperature, the duration of the swim and whether or not wetsuits are used. Drowning and near-drowning should also be anticipated in swim events. Cycling events invariably produce high-impact bony injuries to the skull and upper limbs after accidental falls from a bicycle at high speed. Here we focus more specifically on the conditions likely to be encountered in marathon and ultramarathon foot races and in ultratriathlons of the Ironman distance (226 km).

The most frequently encountered condition in these competitions is postexercise collapse, also termed exercise-associated collapse (EAC). The characteristics of this condition have been listed as an inability to walk unassisted with or without exhaustion, nausea, cramps and normal, high or low body temperatures. In the vast majority of subjects with EAC, the rectal temperature is < 39°C. The definition specifically excludes orthopaedic conditions, which are well described and for which treatment protocols are widely standardized. For the reasons described above, we have proposed that EAC is due to the sudden onset of a progressive postural hypotension that begins immediately the athlete ceases exercise.

Symptomatic hyponatraemia, profound hypoglycaemia and exercise-induced hyperthermia (heatstroke) are three serious emergencies likely to be encountered in long-distance foot races, especially in hot environmental conditions. In cold weather conditions, hypothermia should be anticipated.

Initial management of collapsed athletes

A major deficiency in the management of collapsed athletes in the past has been the initiation of treatment before a rational differential diagnosis was determined. But the emergency treatment of life-threatening conditions, including heatstroke and hyponatraemia, can safely be delayed for 1 or 2 min while the rectal temperature is measured and a reasonable working diagnosis is established. If the rectal temperature is >41°C, cooling should commence immediately after the rectal temperature has been measured. Another obvious exception to this rule is cardiac arrest, which occurs uncommonly, but with an unambiguous diagnosis.

One reason why treatment is often initiated expeditiously is that the rate of admission to the medical facility can be extremely high. For example, close to 50% of the 14 000 competitors in the 90-km Comrades Marathon complete the race during its final hour. If 4% of those subjects collapse (Table 40.2), the average rate of admission during that period will exceed four patients per minute. Admissions are likely to be even faster in the last 10 min of the race, when the rate of finishing accelerates further.

Another reason why treatment is often initiated without a diagnosis is because of the dogma that dehydration is the sole important cause of athletic collapse. Physicians who hold this belief assume that all collapsed athletes are severely dehydrated

Table 40.1 Conditions associated with collapse during or after prolonged exercise.

Exercise-associated collapse (heat syncope/exhaustion)
Muscle cramps
Heatstroke
Hypoglycaemia
Hypothermia
Hyponatraemia
Cardiac arrest
Other medical conditions
Orthopaedic conditions including stress and frank fractures

Table 40.2 Percentage of starters treated for 'collapse' after races of different lengths.

Type of athletic event	Casualties (% of race starters)
Running (21 km)	1–5
Running (42 km)	2–20
Ultratriathlon	15–30
Cycling	5
Surf–ski paddle marathon (244 km)	0.9
Cross-country skiing	5

Table 40.3 Guidelines for determining the severity of the collapsed athlete's condition.

Non-severe	Severe
Immediate assessment	
Conscious	Unconscious or altered mental state
Alert	Confused, disorientated, aggressive
Rectal temperature < 40°C	Rectal temperature > 40°C
Systolic blood pressure > 100 mmHg	Systolic blood pressure < 100 mmHg
Heart rate < 100 beats·min^{-1}	Heart rate > 100 beats·min^{-1}
Specialized assessment	
Blood glucose 4–10 mmol·l^{-1}	Blood glucose < 4 or > 10 mmol·l^{-1}
Serum sodium 135–148 mmol·l^{-1}	Serum sodium < 135 or > 148 mmol·l^{-1}
Body weight loss 0–5%	Body weight loss > 10%
	Body weight gain > 2%

and therefore require immediate intravenous fluid. But it is possible to manage high rates of admission to the medical facility only if selected patients who require urgent, sophisticated management receive such treatment. If all collapsed athletes are treated identically, without a triage based on the nature and severity of the condition, it is very difficult to provide sufficient medical staff to cope with the high rates of admission expected when less well-trained individuals run in the heat. Thus, we need a rapid system of triage. The athlete can then be referred to the correct area of the medical facility for immediate and appropriate treatment. Criteria for determining the severity of collapse are described in Table 40.3. The initial assessment is based on the athlete's level of consciousness, and knowledge of where in the race the athlete collapsed. Patients who are seriously ill show alterations in their level of consciousness and almost always collapse before completion of the race, as discussed subsequently.

Additional helpful information is provided by measurement of rectal temperature, blood pressure and heart rate. In longer races (> 25 km) when hypoglycaemia is more likely, a glycometer should be provided. In mass events of much longer duration (> 4 h), including ultramarathons and ultratriathlons, equipment for measuring the serum sodium concentration must be available so that potentially lethal exercise-related hyponatraemia can be diagnosed expeditiously. Intravenous fluid therapy should only be considered after a serum sodium concentration > 135 mmol·l^{-1} has been demonstrated.

Diagnostic steps for the optimum management of collapsed athletes who are unconscious

If the collapsed athlete is unconscious, the initial differential diagnosis lies between a medical condition not necessarily related to exercise, for example, cardiac arrest, grand mal epilepsy, subarachnoid haemorrhage or diabetic coma, and an exercise-related disorder, especially heatstroke, hyponatraemia or severe hypoglycaemia. The latter is an uncommon cause of exercise-related coma in non-diabetic subjects. The emphasis in this chapter is not on the diagnosis of medical conditions unrelated to exercise, as the differentiation of these conditions does not usually present a problem to experienced clinicians. The critical issue in the vast majority of cases of collapse is rather the rapid differentiation of the serious from the benign, with the expeditious initiation of correct treatment for the serious conditions.

If the patient is unconscious, the crucial initial measurement is rectal temperature, followed by heart rate and blood pressure. If the rectal temperature is >41°C, the diagnosis is heatstroke, and the patient must be cooled immediately. Patients with heatstroke are also hypotensive and have a tachycardia. If the rectal temperature is <40°C in an unconscious patient, the blood pressure and pulse rate are not grossly abnormal, and there is no other obvious medical condition, the probability is that the athlete has a hyponatraemia of exercise or, rarely, another electrolyte abnormality such as hypochloraemia causing cerebral oedema. As argued earlier, there is no evidence that 'dehydration', in the range observed in endurance athletes, causes unconsciousness.

The diagnosis of hyponatraemia can be confirmed only by measuring serum sodium and chloride concentrations. If the diagnosis is suspected, there is little risk in delaying the diagnosis, provided that any intravenous fluids the patient receives have a high sodium content (3–5% saline) and are given at a very slow rate (<50ml·h^{-1}) until the diagnosis is established. In most cases, symptomatic hyponatraemia resolves spontaneously as soon as the patient begins to pass copious volumes of very dilute urine. Final correction of the serum sodium concentration may take substantially longer, usually up to 24–48h.

The measurement of heart rate and blood pressure in the supine position provides an indication of the stability of the athlete's cardiovascular status and, perhaps, an indirect indication of severe dehydration. During exercise, blood pressure and heart rate increase in proportion to the intensity of the effort. On ceasing exercise, heart rate and blood pressure initially decrease rapidly, but the heart rate may remain mildly elevated for some time, especially after prolonged exercise. The decrease in blood pressure is exaggerated when measured in the standing position, due to the development of postural hypotension, which we argue explains the majority of collapses after an athlete has completed an event.

It would be helpful if the exact level of hydration could be determined easily in all subjects, but this is not usually possible. At present, the only reliable indicators are an adequate history and clinical examination (Table 40.4), with special emphasis on the recognized clinical signs of dehydration, including loss of skin turgor, drying of the mouth and an inability to spit caused by inhibition of parotid secretions (seen at dehydration levels ≥5%). These signs are seldom present in the collapsed endurance athletes we have treated. Furthermore, changes in

Table 40.4 Helpful information required from each athlete admitted with collapse.

Pertinent history	Adequate examination
Amount of fluid ingested during the race	Level of consciousness/mental state
Amount of urine passed during the race	State of hydration (dehydration or overhydration)
Presence of vomiting and/or diarrhoea before and during the race	Rectal temperature
Amount of carbohydrate ingested before and during the race	Heart rate, supine and erect
Drugs taken during the race	Blood pressure, supine and erect
Recent intercurrent illness	Blood glucose concentration
Race preparation: heat acclimatization, training schedule, distance training	Serum sodium concentration

plasma volume and serum biochemical measures are poor indicators of dehydration in runners.

In contrast, fluid overload can be diagnosed with certainty if the athlete complains of feeling 'bloated' and 'swollen'. Another helpful sign is that rings, race identification bracelets and watchstraps feel or are demonstrably tighter. Race bracelets are helpful indicators, as these are usually loose fitting before a race.

Visible oedema over the back of the hand and in front of the tibia is also diagnostic, as is the presence of pulmonary oedema presenting either as a blood-stained sputum or auscultatory râles at the lung bases. Pulmonary oedema may also be caused by cardiac failure, which becomes an important, albeit highly unlikely, differential diagnosis. In the absence of any absolute measure of the level of hydration, persistent tachycardia and hypotension in subjects lying supine with the feet and pelvis elevated may indicate a reduced circulating blood volume, and hence a possible need for fluid replacement therapy (see the following). Any signs of overhydration are an absolute indication *not* to give intravenous fluids except by those experienced in the management of exercise hyponatraemia.

After triage, patients are sent to appropriate areas in the medical facility. These include a large area of up to 200 solid stretchers, one end of each being elevated to treat postural hypotension. EAC patients require little additional therapy. A much smaller area is set aside for the 10–20 seriously ill athletes who require highly sophisticated management.

Management protocols for unconscious athletes

HEATSTROKE

When running, metabolic rate is a function of running speed and body mass; thus the highest rectal temperatures are usually seen in the fastest runners who are competing in races of 8–21 km. In such runners, the rectal temperature may increase to ≥40.5°C without symptoms or evidence of heat-related illness (Maughan 1985; Noakes *et al.* 1991b). Higher rectal temperatures are usually associated with symptoms that include dizziness, weakness, nausea, headache, confusion, disorientation and irrational behaviour including aggressive combat-

iveness, or drowsiness progressing to coma. The combination of an elevated rectal temperature with symptoms of an altered mental state confirms the diagnosis of heatstroke and is sufficient to warrant immediate initiation of cooling. The more rapidly the rectal temperature is reduced to 38°C, the better the prognosis. The patient should be placed in a bath of ice-water for 5–10 min. The body temperature should decrease to 38°C within this time.

The theory that placing the hyperthermic athlete in ice-cold water would delay cooling by inducing cutaneous vasoconstriction should never have gained credence, given the rapid development of hypothermia in persons exposed to freezing water. A bath of ice-cold water is the most effective form of body cooling in exercise-induced hyperthermia. Rates of cooling close to $1°C \cdot min^{-1}$ can be achieved (Armstrong *et al.* 1996), with a risk of hypothermia unless care is taken. Since the rectal temperature lags behind the core temperature, active cooling must be terminated before the rectal temperature reaches normal body temperature. Shivering indicates that the core temperature has decreased to 37°C or below.

The physiological changes in heatstroke include a large reduction in peripheral vascular resistance. However, patients with heatstroke can continue to exercise vigorously almost to the moment of collapse, implying that loss of vasomotor control occurs late in the evolution of heatstroke. One possibility is that vasomotor collapse results from a sudden vasodilatation in the splanchnic area, producing a hyperkinetic circulation characterized by a very low peripheral resistance, a reduced central blood volume, a low stroke volume, tachycardia, and systolic and diastolic hypotension. A rapid reduction in body temperature reverses peripheral vasodilatation and restores the central circulation, with a reduction in heart rate and increases in central blood volume, stroke volume, and diastolic and systolic blood pressures. But if hypotension persists, myocardial damage (perhaps exacerbated by absorption of endotoxins from the ischaemic gastrointestinal tract) induces cardiac failure, with ischaemic necrosis of all major body organs. As this develops, the high output cardiac failure converts to one of low cardiac output.

As already argued, there is no evidence that

dehydration is the single critical factor causing heatstroke. Intravenous fluids are given purely to correct the expected dehydration, and to assist in stabilizing the hyperkinetic circulation. Thus ≥ 1–$1.5\,l$ of a 0.5 or 0.9% saline solution can be given initially, in part to ensure rapid venous access, should this be required. The mortality rate (10–80%) in classical (non-exercise-related) heatstroke is related directly to the duration and severity of hyperthermia, to the presence of confounding medical conditions and to the rapidity with which subsequent cooling occurs. Mortality should be zero in healthy athletes who receive prompt and appropriate cooling. Indeed, it is unusual for such athletes not to be fully recovered and ambulatory within 30–60 min of collapse, provided they are correctly and expeditiously treated.

Once the athlete's rectal temperature has been reduced to $<38°C$, it must be decided whether or not to admit the patient to hospital for further observation. A factor influencing this decision is the known tendency for rectal temperature to increase after cooling. This increase may not be noticed if the patient returns home without appropriate supervision. Any tendency for the rectal temperature to increase after the cessation of exercise and active cooling indicates the presence of ongoing heat-generating biochemical processes in muscle, unrelated to exercise and perhaps related to the biochemical abnormalities that initiate conditions like malignant hyperthermia.

In our experience, hospital admission is always required if the patient fails to regain consciousness within 30 min of appropriate therapy that returns the rectal temperature to $<38°C$. Patients who regain consciousness rapidly, whose cardiovascular system is stable, and whose rectal temperature does not increase in the first hour after active cooling ceases do not usually require hospital admission. A decision whether to admit a patient with heatstroke can therefore usually be made within 30–60 min of reaching the medical tent.

Most highly trained athletes with heatstroke recover quickly if appropriately cooled. They can usually be discharged from the medical tent, fully recovered, within 60 min of collapse. An absolute indication for hospital admission would be a failure to achieve cardiovascular stability during that time.

A persisting tachycardia and hypotension in the lying position suggest developing cardiogenic shock.

Heatstroke remains an uncommon complication during exercise, raising the possibility that factors unique to each individual may be operative (genetic predisposition, unaccustomed drug use or subclinical viral infection).

HYPOTHERMIA

The management of hypothermia requires that the patient be exposed to an external source of heating. In the medical facility this can be provided by removing the athlete's wet clothing, covering with blankets and packing with hot water bottles. Other potential sources of external heating include warm baths or electric blankets. However, the degree of hypothermia is usually quite mild in endurance athletes and simple methods of rewarming are likely to be successful.

HYPONATRAEMIA

Athletes who become unconscious during or after ultradistance running or triathlon races and whose rectal temperatures are not elevated should be considered to have symptomatic hyponatraemia until measurement of the serum sodium concentration refutes the diagnosis. Dehydration *does not* cause unconsciousness until renal failure with uraemia or hepatic failure has supervened. To achieve such a weight loss, a 50-kg athlete would require 10 h of high-intensity exercise at a sweat rate of $1\,l\cdot h^{-1}$ without any fluid replacement. It is not clear how this could occur with the modern emphasis on fluid ingestion during exercise.

All athletes with symptomatic hyponatraemia and serum sodium concentrations below $129\,mmol\cdot l^{-1}$ are overhydrated by 2–6 l (Irving *et al.* 1991; Speedy *et al.* 1999a,b). The presence of very dilute urine in a patient with an altered level of consciousness *must* alert the physician to this possible diagnosis. Under no circumstances should large volumes of fluid be given to athletes, and never to unconscious or semiconscious subjects with hyponatraemia. All unconscious hyponatraemic patients in our series recovered spontaneously, without treatment other than fluid restriction and the occasional use of diuretics. The provision of fluids to patients who are unconscious as a result of cerebral oedema delays recovery and may produce a fatal result, as appears to have happened in isolated cases during the past 5 years.

The responsibility of the medical care facility is to ensure that patients with hyponatraemia are not left in the care of anyone who is unaware that symptomatic hyponatraemia is caused by fluid overload. The race medical director must ensure that hospital physicians who are caring for athletes with hyponatraemia are aware of the correct management of this condition. The physician may have been led to believe that dehydration is the major, perhaps sole, cause of collapse. Furthermore, the hyponatraemic patient is unconscious and is not passing urine. Both factors suggest to the unwary that the patient is severely shocked, with a very low cardiac output insufficient to maintain either cerebral or renal function. In fact, unconsciousness is due to cerebral oedema, and the initially low rate of urine production is probably due to circulating antidiuretic hormones, as yet unidentified. The possibility that these patients are initially in renal failure with reduced renal perfusion and a low glomerular filtration rate has not been excluded, but it seems unlikely. Persistent hypotension and tachycardia compatible with shock have not been observed in any of the hyponatraemic athletes we, or others, have treated. Vigorously treating such patients with intravenous fluids for a perceived 'dehydration' can have fatal consequences.

The current management for this condition should include some or all of the following.

• Bladder catheterization to establish that the urine (i) is dilute, indicating a state of fluid overload, and (ii) is being passed at an ever-increasing rate during recovery. Spontaneous recovery will occur if adequate amounts of urine ($> 500\,ml \cdot h^{-1}$) are passed.

• No fluids by mouth. Salt tablets and sodium-containing foods can be given.

• High sodium (3%) solutions can be given intravenously provided they are infused slowly ($\sim 50\,ml \cdot h^{-1}$).

There is some evidence that the combined use of a diuretic with intravenous sodium replacement may expedite recovery relative to conservative, expectant management. However, there are as yet no clinical trials comparing different management protocols. Most patients have recovered spontaneously without any specific treatment except fluid restriction (Irving *et al.* 1991; Speedy *et al.* 1999a,b).

HYPOGLYCAEMIA

Exercise-induced hypoglycaemia occurs when liver glycogen depletion causes liver glucose production to lag behind the rate of glucose uptake by muscle from the blood. Hypoglycaemia occurs most commonly in events lasting $\geq 4\,h$, especially in athletes who fail to eat and drink sufficient carbohydrate before or during these events. During shorter events, the higher exercise intensity increases the probability that factors other than hypoglycaemia will initiate fatigue before liver glycogen stores are depleted.

Persons who voluntarily restrict their intake of carbohydrates (usually young women with overt or covert eating disorders) are especially at risk. The development of hypoglycaemia in unusual circumstances should raise the possibility of an eating disorder, with long-term carbohydrate restriction. A characteristic of young female athletes with eating disorders appears to be to run long-distance races without carbohydrate replacement, so that they can develop a large energy deficit.

In most cases of severe hypoglycaemia, the level of consciousness dictates that the glucose replacement be given as a 50% solution intravenously. Recovery is always rapid (within minutes) if hypoglycaemia is the sole cause of collapse. Patients who are conscious can ingest concentrated glucose solutions orally.

Management protocols for collapsed athletes who are fully conscious

EXERCISE-ASSOCIATED COLLAPSE

The term exercise-associated collapse (EAC) should be used to describe the common type of collapse that occurs in athletes who successfully complete endurance events without distress, but who suddenly develop symptoms and signs of postural hypotension when they stop exercising. This condition is analogous to the classical 'heat exhaustion' or 'heat syncope'. Although the mechanism for EAC remains to be established, EAC is benign and is not a true heat disorder, as rectal temperatures are not abnormally elevated. Furthermore, EAC does not progress inexorably to heatstroke, and there is no evidence that dehydration contributes to its aetiology.

In contrast to the benign nature of EAC, athletes who collapse *during* exercise have identifiable medical conditions, some of which are serious. These athletes require state-of-the-art interventions and highly sophisticated management.

The diagnosis of EAC can be made on the basis of a typical history, findings of a postural hypotension reversed by lying supine with the pelvis and legs elevated, and the exclusion of the readily identifiable medical syndromes already described. We postulate that EAC is nothing more serious than an exaggeration of the normal reduction in standing blood pressure that occurs after prolonged exercise. Few if any athletes with EAC are sufficiently dehydrated to show the clinical signs of dry mucous membranes, loss of skin turgor, sunken eyeballs and an inability to spit. The presence of such signs might be used to justify administration of intravenous fluids. Rather, we propose that intravenous fluid therapy should be saved for those athletes who continue to have increased heart rates (>100 beats·min^{-1}) and hypotension (systolic blood pressure <110mmHg) when lying supine with the legs and pelvis elevated above heart level. Nursing patients with EAC in the head-down position is almost always dramatically effective, producing a more stable cardiovascular system within 30–90s and, usually, instant reversal of symptoms. The symptoms of dizziness, nausea and vomiting frequently associated with this condition may result simply from a sudden reduction in blood pressure, including a dramatic fall from the elevated pressures maintained during exercise.

Subjects with EAC can be encouraged to ingest fluids orally during recovery. Sports drinks containing both glucose (5–10%) and electrolytes (Na

10–20mM) can be advocated. Fluid retention is greatest from solutions with a high sodium content (>80mM), but such solutions are generally unpalatable and are also unnecessary; when patients are correctly treated with elevation of the pelvis and legs, recovery occurs within 10–20min, and before full rehydration could have occurred. Most athletes with EAC will be able to stand and walk unaided with 10–30min of appropriate treatment, and they can be encouraged to leave the medical facility within that time. Intravenous therapy is not particularly effective, probably because the extra fluid volume delivered intravenously simply increases the volume of blood in the dilated capacitance veins in the legs and splanchnic circulations, without increasing the central blood volume or central venous pressure markedly.

MUSCLE CRAMPS

Muscle cramps are commonly seen and of varying severity. The pathophysiology is not yet determined, and as a result there is no uniform approach to treatment. Maintaining the affected muscles in the lengthened position is the only effective therapy. Icing and massage of the involved muscle groups are also used. The Boston Marathon medical team treats muscle cramps with normal saline, given intravenously. Intravenous magnesium therapy has been used in the Hawaiian Ironman Triathlon, but clinical trials of either treatment have yet to be published.

Organizing the medical facility at major endurance events

Prerace organization

Planning of the medical facility to serve competitors in endurance events depends on the predicted number of casualties, the nature of those casualties and their likely severity. Medical teams that have worked at particular events for many years are able to predict the expected number of casualties. It is vital to keep medical records for all athletes treated at any particular event and to analyse these data for historical trends.

Table 40.5 Comparison of the percentage of starters requiring medical care at the finish of foot races of different distances when run in cool or warm conditions.

Sydney-City-to-Surf, Australia 12 km		Boston, USA 42 km		Two Oceans, South Africa 56 km		Comrades, South Africa 90 km	
1984 Cool	1980 Warm	1987 Cool	1985 Warm	1990 Cool	1989 Warm	1985 Cool	1987 Warm
0.17%	0.3%	0.5%	1.3%	0.7%	3.7%	1.6%	3.6%

The total number of expected casualties is usually expressed as a percentage of the total number of race starters or entrants. This figure is determined by the nature of the race, including its length and difficulty, the nature of the participating athletes, in particular their levels of fitness and previous experience, and the environmental temperature and humidity (Table 40.5, Richards & Richards 1984). Running and triathlon events have higher casualty rates (up to 20%) than cycling events (Table 40.2), whereas shorter-distance events usually have lower casualty rates than longer events. The latter finding may be explained by the greater likelihood that prolonged events (if begun at an inappropriate time) will extend into the heat of the day.

Prerace planning to reduce the risk of collapse

Richards and Richards (1984) have shown that the number of athletes seeking medical attention in endurance running events can be dramatically reduced by continuing education programmes for the participants. The percentage of runners treated for collapse after the 12-km City-to-Surf race held annually in Sydney, Australia was linearly related to the ambient temperature on race day. However, compared with the 7-year period before 1977, the number of casualties in the next 7 years was reduced by up to 100%, with introduction of a specific education programme for race participants.

Specific prerace strategies to enhance the safety of the competitor include the following.
1 Scheduling the race at a time of year and day when the environmental conditions will not adversely affect performance or health. The medical director of the race should be given authority to cancel the race should adverse weather conditions prevail. The American College of Sports Medicine has published a position statement on acceptable ambient temperature and humidity values for safe participation in sporting activities. Adequate provision of carbohydrate-containing fluids *en route* is essential.
2 Planning the race course so that the start and finish are in an area large enough to accommodate all spectators and race finishers, medical facilities and quick get-away routes for emergency vehicles. The placing of first-aid stations along the route should be at points allowing for rapid access by emergency vehicles and should ideally be 3–5 km apart.
3 Preparticipation screening and qualification standards to ensure that unfit and inexperienced athletes do not place themselves at undue medical risk during the event as a result of their overeagerness. Most ultradistance events in South Africa require that participants have a letter signed by the secretary of their running club stating that they have achieved a satisfactory time for a given endurance event in the 6 months prior to the ultra-distance event. Cut-off times have also been introduced at the halfway mark, and athletes who fail to meet those cut-off times are removed from the race. This form of screening has greatly reduced the number of collapsed and injured athletes seeking medical attention at the race finish.
4 Prerace seminars given to participants by medical personnel can reduce the number of casualties. Advice to the athletes may include:
   • correct training (in particular, completing enough long runs in the 2 months preceding an ultramarathon);

• consumption of a high carbohydrate diet before the race;

• eating a prerace breakfast and drinking approximately 500–800 ml of fluid every hour (preferably a 5% to 10% carbohydrate solution) during the race; and

• a warning of the dangers of competing during or shortly after a pyrexial illness or while taking medication.

5 Registration forms may include questions regarding past and present medical history. This would identify, for example, athletes with diabetes, asthma and coronary artery disease. Such athletes could be sent specific information advising them on appropriate safety precautions such as having a prerace meal, carrying a steroid inhaler and wearing a medical bracelet.

6 An 'impaired competitor' policy should be implemented. Strategically positioned first-aid helpers should be given the authority to stop athletes who appear ill and unable to finish the course. Vehicles should be provided to transport 'impaired competitors' to the race finish.

7 The local hospital casualty department or other local emergency service should be advised of the forthcoming race and the likely number and nature of casualties.

8 Meetings should be held between the participating medical and allied professionals to ensure that each knows what is his or her role. A communication system on race day is vital. A two-way radio system or cellular network system can provide communication between first-aid stations on the course and the central medical facility. This system should communicate with the race organizers' computer database. Athletes that drop out of the race must be recorded as non-finishers on the database so that their whereabouts can be determined more easily.

9 An emergency transport service should be available to bring problem cases to the central medical facility, or to the nearest hospital emergency room. The use of helicopters in ultradistance events has proven invaluable in the prompt treatment and evacuation of athletes suffering from cardiac arrest and other life-threatening conditions.

Positioning and manning of first-aid stations

These are positioned *en route* at strategic positions, providing a stretch and massage facility for the treatment of cramping muscles; first aid (plasters) for chafing skin and blistered feet; and the identification of the at-risk runner who is confused or delirious. Such stations also serve as centres from which emergency cases can be transported to the central medical facility or to the nearest hospital emergency centre. Stations should be positioned in areas that have quick access to exit routes and can readily reach the central medical facility or the local hospital. The personnel manning these stations should be in direct communication with the ambulance service, so that medical emergencies can be transported swiftly to the nearest medical facility. A mobile caravan may provide the most effective solution as a first-aid station and communications centre.

Planning and equipping the medical facility at the race finish

The layout of the central medical station will depend on the facilities available to the race organizers. Figure 40.2 shows the floor plan of the medical facility at the end of the 56-km Two Oceans ultramarathon foot race held annually in Cape Town, South Africa.

The general requirements are the following.

1 Toilet facility—generally a number of portable toilets stationed behind the tent or within the facility (Fig. 40.2).

2 Chairs and tables for the computer operator at the admission area, for the laboratory technologist and diagnostic equipment, and for other medical equipment and drugs.

3 Stretchers are used in transporting collapsed athletes from the race finish to the medical facility and for athletes to lie on within the green and red zones. Such stretchers should be rigid so that the 'foot' can be elevated, and collapsed athletes can be nursed, at least initially in the head-down position.

4 A-frame stands for elevating the foot of stretchers. The A-frame can be removed once the athlete's cardiovascular status has normalized.

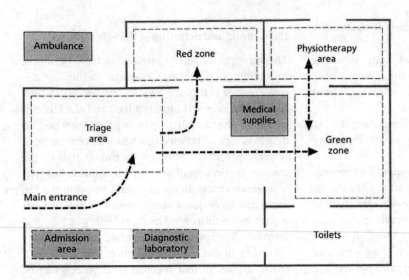

Fig. 40.2 Diagram of the floor plan for a proposed medical facility, located at the finish line, to treat athletes collapsing during or after endurance events.

Table 40.6 Basic medical and surgical equipment for the medical facility at endurance sporting events.

Diagnostic tools	*Surgical tools*
Stethoscopes	Scissors
Sphygmomanometers	Latex gloves
Rectal thermometers	Syringes (3 ml, 5 ml, 10 ml)
Torch/ophthalmoscopes	Needles (18, 21, 25 gauge)
Glucometers	Steri-strips
Reflex hammers	Adhesive bandages
Blood electrolyte analyser	Gauze pads
	Alcohol skin wipes
Resuscitation tools	Orthopaedic felt
Oral airways (sizes 6–8)	Suture sets (disposable)
Resuscitation masks (disposable)	Space blanket
Defibrillator	Fluid administration sets
	IV fluids
	Cannulas

5 Blankets—for each stretcher. These allow discreet measurement of rectal temperatures and the management of hypothermia.

6 Plastic baths sufficiently large to accommodate the torso of 40–90-kg athletes. These are filled with iced water and are used to treat heatstroke.

7 Refrigerator facility—for large races, a mobile refrigerator truck is most useful.

8 Computer terminal linked to the race finish.

9 Blood electrolyte and glucose analysers. Ideally serum sodium and potassium concentrations should be measured in all patients. This is mandatory in all subjects who are diagnosed as 'dehydrated' and in need of intravenous fluids. A serum sodium concentration of less than $130\,mmol\cdot l^{-1}$ indicates that the athlete is more likely over- rather than dehydrated (Fig. 40.1).

10 Bins for rubbish and 'sharps'.

11 Medications. Table 40.6 lists the medical equipment and Table 40.7 the medications required to cope with the expected emergency conditions. A pharmacist should be present to control the distribution and use of medications.

The quantity of each item will be determined by the number of race entrants and the predicted number of race casualties.

Table 40.7 Basic medications required in the medical facility at endurance sporting events.

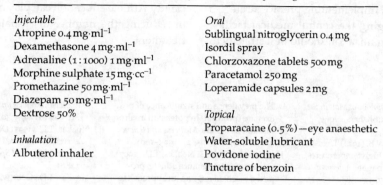

Injectable
Atropine 0.4 mg·ml^{-1}
Dexamethasone 4 mg·ml^{-1}
Adrenaline (1 : 1000) 1 mg·ml^{-1}
Morphine sulphate 15 mg·cc^{-1}
Promethazine 50 mg·ml^{-1}
Diazepam 50 mg·ml^{-1}
Dextrose 50%

Inhalation
Albuterol inhaler

Oral
Sublingual nitroglycerin 0.4 mg
Isordil spray
Chlorzoxazone tablets 500 mg
Paracetamol 250 mg
Loperamide capsules 2 mg

Topical
Proparacaine (0.5%)—eye anaesthetic
Water-soluble lubricant
Povidone iodine
Tincture of benzoin

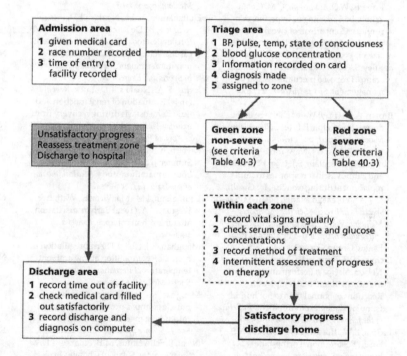

Fig. 40.3 Flow chart for the management of athletes collapsing during or after endurance events.

A study from the Melbourne City Marathon found that 62% of runners requiring medical attention needed physiotherapy for musculoskeletal complaints (Kretsch *et al.* 1984). Physiotherapy is a vital service for treating acute and chronic injuries at endurance events. Athletes make use of the physiotherapists' services both *en route* and at the race finish. At large races, we provide a separate area for the physiotherapy service, so that the central medical facility is not flooded with non-emergency cases.

Flow diagram showing how patients are managed with the different conditions

Figure 40.3 shows the management algorithm that we follow.

Conclusions

The effectiveness of medical care at ultradistance athletic events is solely dependent on an understanding of the factors that contribute to casualties in the event. An attempt should be made to avoid casualties through implementing prerace strategies and tightly managing the central medical facility. Along with this organization should be a strategy to deal with expected emergencies promptly and efficiently. Athlete education can play an important role in reducing the number of casualties that require treatment.

References

Adolph, E.F. (1947) *Physiology of Man in the Desert*. Interscience Publishers, New York.

Adolph, E.F. & Fulton, W.B. (1924) The effects of exposure to high temperatures upon the circulation in man. *American Journal of Physiology* 67, 573–588.

Armstrong, L.E., Crago, A.E., Adams, R., Roberts, W.O. & Maresh, C.M. (1996) Whole-body cooling of hyperthermic runners: Comparison of two field therapies. *American Journal of Emergency Medicine* 14, 355–358.

Bentley, S. (1996) Exercise-induced muscle cramp. Proposed mechanisms and management. *Sports Medicine* 21, 409–410.

Brown, A.H. (1947) Water shortage in the desert. In: Adolph, E.F. (ed.) *Physiology of Man in the Desert*, pp. 136–159. Interscience Publishers, New York.

Coyle, E.F. & Montain, S.J. (1993) Thermal and cardiovascular responses to fluid replacement during exercise. In: Gisolfi, C.V., Lamb, D.R. & Nadel, E.R. (eds) *Perspectives in Exercise Science and Sports Medicine, Vol. 6. Exercise, Heat, and Thermoregulation*, pp. 179–213. Cooper Publishing Group, Carmel.

Eichna, L.W., Bean, W.E., Ashe, W.F. & Nelson, N. (1945) Performance in relation to environmental temperature. Reactions of normal men to hot humid (simulated jungle) environment. *Bulletin of the Johns Hopkins Hospital* 76, 25–58.

Eichna, L.W., Horvath, S.M. & Bean, W.B. (1947) Postexertional orthostatic hypotension. *American Journal of Medical Science* 213, 641–654.

Epstein, Y. & Sohar, E. (1985) Fluid balance in hot climates: sweating, water intake, and prevention of dehydration. *Public Health Reviews* 13, 115–137.

Frizzell, R.T., Lang, G.H., Lowance, D.C. & Lathan, S.R. (1986) Hyponatraemia and ultramarathon running. *Journal of the American Medical Association* 255, 772–774.

Hiller, W.D.B. (1989) Dehydration and hyponatremia during triathlons. *Medicine and Science in Sports and Exercise* 21, S219–S221.

Holtzhausen, L.-M. & Noakes, T.D. (1995) The prevalence and significance of post-exercise (postural) hypotension in ultra-marathon runners. *Medicine and Science in Sports and Exercise* 27, 1595–1601.

Holtzhausen, L.-M. & Noakes, T.D. (1997) Collapsed ultradistance athlete: proposed mechanisms and an approach to management. *Clinical Journal of Sports Medicine* 7, 292–301.

Holtzhausen, L.-M., Noakes, T.D., Kroning, B., De Klerk, M., Roberts, M. & Emsley, R. (1994) Clinical and biochemical characteristics of collapsed ultra-marathon runners. *Medicine and Science in Sports and Exercise* 26, 1095–1101.

Irving, R.A., Noakes, T.D., Buck, R. et al. (1991) Evaluation of renal function and fluid homeostasis during recovery from exercise induced hyponatremia. *Journal of Applied Physiology* 70, 342–348.

Kretsch, A., Grogan, R., Duras, P., Allen, F., Sumner, J. & Gillam, I. (1984) 1980 Melbourne marathon study. *Medical Journal of Australia* 141, 809–814.

Ledingham, I.M., MacVicar, S., Watt, I. & Weston, G.A. (1982) Early resuscitation after marathon collapse. *Lancet* 2, 1096–1097.

Maughan, R.J. (1985) Thermoregulation in marathon competition at low ambient temperature. *International Journal of Sports Medicine* 6, 15–19.

Maughan, R.J. (1986) Exercise-induced muscle cramp: a prospective biochemical study in marathon runners. *Journal of Sports Science* 4, 31–34.

Nicol, J., Schwellnus, M.P., Noakes, T.D. & Swanevelder, S. (1999) Changes in electromyographic (EMG) activity and in serum electrolyte concentrations with clinical recovery from acute Exercise Associated Muscle Cramp (EAMC) in distance runners. *Medicine and Science in Sports and Exercise*, in press.

Noakes, T.D. (1988) Why marathon runners collapse. *South African Journal of Medicine* 73, 569–571.

Noakes, T.D. (1991) *Lore of Running*, 3rd edn. Human Kinetics, Champaign, IL.

Noakes, T.D. (1992) The hyponatremia of exercise. *International Journal of Sport Nutrition* 2, 205–228.

Noakes, T.D. (1993) Fluid balance during exercise. *Exercise and Sport Sciences Reviews* 21, 297–330.

Noakes, T.D. (1995) Dehydration during exercise: What are the real dangers? *Clinical Journal of Sports Medicine* 5, 123–128.

Noakes, T.D., Goodwin, N., Rayner, B.L., Brancken, T. & Taylor, R.K.N. (1985) Water intoxication: a possible complication during endurance exercise. *Medicine and Science in Sports and Exercise* 17, 370–375.

Noakes, T.D., Adams, B.A., Greeff, C., Lotz, T. & Nathan, M. (1988) The danger of an inadequate water intake during prolonged exercise. A novel concept. *European Journal of Applied Physiology* 47, 210–219.

Noakes, T.D., Norman, R.J., Buck, R.H., Godlonton, J., Stevenson, K. & Pittaway, D. (1990) The incidence of hyponatraemia during prolonged ultraendurance exercise. *Medicine and Science in Sports and Exercise* 22, 165–170.

Noakes, T.D., Berlinski, N., Solomon, E. & Weight, L.M. (1991a) Collapsed runners: blood biochemical changes after IV fluid therapy. *Physician and Sportsmedicine* 19 (7), 70–81.

Noakes, T.D., Myburgh, K.H., du Plessis, J., Lang, L., van der Riet, C. & Schall, R. (1991b) Metabolic rate, not percent dehydration predicts rectal temperature in marathon runners. *Medicine and Science in Sports and Exercise* 23, 443–449.

Richards, R. & Richards, D. (1984) Exertion-induced heat exhaustion and other medical aspects of the City-to-Surf fun runs, 1978–1984. *Medical Journal of Australia* 141, 799–805.

Roberts, W.O. (1996) A 12-year summary of Twin Cities Marathon injury. *Medicine and Science in Sports and Exercise* 28 (Suppl.), S123.

Saltin, B. & Costill, D.L. (1988) Fluid and electrolyte balance during prolonged exercise. In: Horton, E.S. & Terjung, R.L. (eds) *Exercise, Nutrition and Metabolism*, pp. 150–158. Macmillan, New York.

Sandell, R.C., Pascoe, M.D. & Noakes, T.D. (1988) Factors associated with collapse during and after ultramarathon footraces: a preliminary study. *Physician and Sportsmedicine* **16** (9), 86–94.

Sawka, M.N., Young, A.J., Latzka, W.A., Neufer, D.P., Quigley, M.D. & Pandolf, K.B. (1992) Human tolerance to heat strain during exercise: influence of hydration. *Journal of Applied Physiology* **73**, 368–375.

Sawka, M.N., Montain, S.J. & Latzka, W.A. (1996) Body fluid balance during exercise–heat exposure. In: Buskirk, E.R. & Phul, S.M. (eds) *Body Fluid Balance in Exercise and Sport*, pp. 139–157. CRC Press, New York.

Schwellnus, M.P., Derman, E.W. & Noakes, T.D. (1997) Aetiology of skeletal muscle 'cramps' during exercise: a novel hypothesis. *Journal of Sports Science* **15**, 277–285.

Speedy, D.B., Noakes, T.D., Rogers, I.R. *et al.* (1999) Hyponatremia in ultradistance triathletes. *Medicine and Science in Sports and Exercise* **31**, 809–815.

Talbott, J.H., Dill, D.B., Edwards, H.T., Stumme, E.H. & Consolazio, W.V. (1937) The ill effects of heat upon workmen. *Journal of Industrial Hygiene and Toxicology* **19**, 258–274.

Vrijens, D.M.J. & Rehrer, N.J. (1999) Sodium free fluid ingestion decreases plasma sodium during exercise in the heat. *Journal of Applied Physiology* **86**, 1847–1851.

Walsh, R.M., Noakes, T.D., Hawley, J.A. & Dennis, S.C. (1994) Low levels of dehydration impair exercise performance. *International Journal of Sports Medicine* **15**, 392–398.

Wyndham, C.H. & Strydom, N.B. (1969) The danger of an inadequate water intake during marathon running. *South African Medical Journal* **43**, 893–896.

Wyndham, C.H., Strydom, N.B., van Rensburg, A.J., Benade, A.J.S. & Heyns, A.J. (1970) Relation between $\dot{V}_{O_{2max}}$ and body temperature in hot humid conditions. *Journal of Applied Physiology* **29**, 45–50.

Chapter 41

Problems of High Altitude

ROY J. SHEPHARD

Introduction

From the time of the Mexico City Olympic Games (Jokl & Jokl 1968; Shephard 1974), sports physicians have frequently expressed concern about the potential risks of endurance competitions at altitudes of 2000–3000 m and higher. At its Melbourne, Australia, meeting in 1974, the Féderation Internationale de Médecine Sportive passed a resolution urging extreme caution when hosting athletic meets at altitudes above 2290 m, and they also suggested the avoidance of major competition above 3050 m. Despite such warnings, mountaineers sometimes climb for days and even weeks at much higher altitudes. They (together with older people who engage in recreational activities at mountain resorts) are probably in greater danger than the international athlete who competes in Mexico City.

Performance and safety at high altitudes are modified relative to sea-level conditions because of decreases in gravitational acceleration, wind resistance and temperature; a potential local accumulation of air pollutants in mountain valleys; high levels of solar and cosmic radiation; and above all a low partial pressure of oxygen. The impact of the low oxygen pressure on performance and health is likely to be greatest in endurance events, because the safe and successful completion of such activities depends largely on an adequate delivery of oxygen to the active tissues (see Chapter 3).

The practising sports physician should be prepared to advise officials, competitors and their coaches on a wide range of issues, including not only safety and acute changes of performance

(Goddard 1967; Margaria 1967; Jokl & Jokl 1968), but also appropriate acclimatization schedules (Goddard 1967), preventive and therapeutic use of drugs such as acetazolamide, dexamethasone and diuretics, and possible residual benefits from altitude training, real or simulated (Richardson 1974). Other forms of treatment may also be required, both for pre-existing medical conditions that are aggravated by altitude exposure, and for pathologies specific to high altitudes (such as mountain sickness, and pulmonary, cerebral and retinal oedema: Jokl & Jokl 1968; Shephard 1974; Fletcher et al. 1985; Hackett & Hornbein 1988).

The physical environment at high altitudes

Gravity

The acceleration due to gravity diminishes by about $0.3 \, cm \cdot s^{-2}$ for every 1000 m of altitude. At an altitude of 2000–3000 m, there is thus a measurable benefit to competitors (<0.1%), most obvious when cycling or running uphill. In practical terms, a much larger effect results from a latitudinal change; for instance, if the site of a competition were to be moved from the equator to near the North Pole, gravitational forces would change by >0.5%.

Wind resistance

Wind resistance accounts for a substantial component of the work performed by some classes of endurance athlete such as the distance cyclist and the speed skater (see Chapter 58). Such resistance is incurred largely as turbulent airflow over the body surface. It is thus proportional to $1/2 (A\delta v^2)$, where A is the area of the competitor and any associated equipment as projected in the direction of motion, δ is the average density of the atmosphere at a given altitude and v is the velocity of air movement relative to the competitor. The density of the atmosphere decreases in an exponential fashion as altitude increases, by a factor of 20% at 1850 m, 26% at 2500 m and 31% at 3000 m.

At sea-level, wind resistance accounts for about 11% of the energy that a runner expends in competing over a distance of 5000 m. The decrease of atmospheric density at 3000 m thus has the potential to boost a distance runner's performance by some 3.4%. The work performed against air turbulence (resistive force × distance) is proportional to the third power of relative velocity; in a racing cyclist; such work accounts for some 90% of the total energy expended, so that he or she gains a mechanical advantage of about 28% when competing at an altitude of 3000 m.

Temperature

The ambient air temperature drops by about 2°C for each 300 m increase in altitude. Wind velocities also tend to be greater at high and exposed sites, and a diminution of ground haze increases the individual's exposure to solar radiation (see below).

In general, the loss of body heat (see Chapter 17) proceeds more readily at high altitude than at sea-level. Thus, ascent to a higher altitude reduces the likelihood of heat stress in tropical latitudes, but increases the chances of hypothermia at greater latitudes. There may be significant interactions between hypoxia and cold stress, contributing to the overall picture of high-altitude deterioration (Sutton *et al.* 1987).

Air pollution

Petrol-driven vehicles operate much less efficiently as they climb to higher altitudes, and they show a corresponding increase in their emission of exhaust gases. Roads that traverse narrow mountain valleys

or pass through long tunnels may also encourage the local accumulation of pollutants.

The physiological problems encountered when exercising in a polluted environment (see Chapter 42) are exacerbated by the hypoxia of high altitude. An adverse interaction between carbon monoxide exposure and high altitudes seems particularly likely from the viewpoint of both the endurance competitor and the older exerciser with a tendency to myocardial ischaemia (Shephard 1983; Horvath *et al.* 1988).

Radiation

Direct ultraviolet radiation (at a wavelength of 295 nm) increases by as much as 35% for an ascent of 1000 m. Because the atmosphere is less hazy, there is also a decrease in the scattering of solar radiation at high altitude. At 4000 m, the ultraviolet radiation at 400 nm is increased by 147%, and that at 300 nm is increased by 250% (Heath & Williams 1989).

Cosmic radiation increases rapidly at altitudes above 1000 m (Heath & Williams 1989). At 3000 m, there is a three-fold increase over the anticipated sea-level exposure of about 24 mrad·year^{-1} (0.24 mGy·year^{-1}).

Oxygen partial pressure

The fraction of oxygen in ambient air (0.2093) does not change materially with altitude, but the partial pressure of oxygen decreases exponentially, in parallel with the decrease in atmospheric density. Nevertheless, a review of the performance of mountain climbers suggests that the pressure tables developed by the International Civil Aviation Organization (ICAO) underestimate human potential at very high altitudes. This is because simplifying assumptions have been made about ambient temperatures and humidity.

When a mountaineer reaches the summit of Mount Everest, the total atmospheric pressure, as derived from an older formula of Zuntz (250–253 mmHg), is substantially higher than the ICAO figure (235 mmHg). Moreover, this difference has important implications for human survival. Nevertheless, the widely used ICAO figures do not deviate appreciably from the true pressures at the altitudes of interest to most endurance competitors (up to 5500 m).

At an altitude of 3000 m, unit volume of air at ambient pressure contains some 31% fewer molecules of oxygen than at sea-level. Experience in Mexico City (stadium altitude about 2240 m, 24% reduction in oxygen partial pressure) has shown that, in most classes of endurance event, the adverse effects of hypoxia substantially outweigh the benefits that a competitor gains from a cooler ambient temperature, a reduced gravitational acceleration and a lower wind resistance. Thus, although world records may be set in throwing and sprint events, times for events such as 5000- and 10000-m runs are some 8% poorer at 3000 m than at sea-level (Perronet et al. 1991).

Acute effects of moderate altitudes

Moderate hypoxia produces few symptoms in a resting subject. However, sudden exposure to a very high altitude (as in the decompression of an aircraft cabin) can cause a loss of useful consciousness without any warning. When a person is undertaking vigorous exercise, the main subjective consequence of acute exposure to high altitude is severe breathlessness. Perhaps for this reason, central ratings of perceived exertion increase relative to local muscular ratings (Young et al. 1982). Both mental and physical tasks seem to require increased effort. Moreover, at least on the first day of exposure, the ability to learn a novel cognitive task is apparently impaired at altitudes as low as 1524 m (Denison et al. 1966; Crowley et al. 1992).

An altitude such as that of Mexico City has only small effects on the body's response to light exercise. The main reason for this finding is that the normal, sigmoid shape of the oxygen dissociation curve of the blood in itself offers an important defence mechanism against hypoxia (Ernsting & Shephard 1951). Indeed, until an average person reaches an altitude of 1500–2000 m, the resting arterial oxygen saturation (and thus the quantity of oxygen transported to the tissues per litre of cardiac output) remains very close to sea-level norms, despite a substantial reduction in the alveolar oxygen pressure.

On the other hand, during maximal aerobic exercise, the arterial oxygen saturation is less well protected in an endurance competitor with a large maximal cardiac output (Tucker et al. 1984; Dempsey 1986). High-performance athletes often develop some arterial unsaturation even at sea-level, and this tendency worsens as soon as the altitude is increased (Martin & O'Kroy 1993).

At rest and during submaximal exercise, a small increase of alveolar ventilation is often enough to bring the alveolar oxygen pressure to a level that will restore arterial oxygen saturation, and thus will normalize the oxygen transported per unit volume of cardiac output. However, such an adaptation may not be possible for the endurance competitor who is already developing a very large respiratory minute volume at sea-level. Moreover, any further increase in ventilation at altitude rapidly leads to hypocapnia, with resulting decreases in cerebral perfusion and an instability of both respiratory and cardiac rhythms (Lipsitz et al. 1995). If respiratory compensation is not possible, a moderate tachycardia restores oxygen transport during submaximal exercise, at the expense of some diminution in the individual's cardiac reserve (Shephard 1974). Again, the athlete who is already operating at near peak heart rates has little potential to make an adjustment of this sort, and the maximal oxygen intake is initially decreased by about 8% at an altitude such as Mexico City. Perhaps because of the diminished tissue buffering of lactate, there is also a decrease in endurance time at any given fraction of the individual's maximal oxygen intake (Horstman et al. 1980).

Exposure to high altitude usually induces a substantial endocrine response (Milledge 1994). Aldosterone secretion is suppressed, plasma levels of atrial natriuretic hormone are augmented by the effects of hypoxia on the heart and pulmonary circulation (Bärtsch et al. 1988; Milledge et al. 1989; Appenzeller & Wood 1992), and cortisol secretion is augmented, at least for the first few days in the new environment (Perhonen et al. (1995). There is also an immediate increase of blood glucose, but over a week or so this trend is countered by an increase of insulin sensitivity (Milledge 1994).

As the individual's acid–base balance adjusts to the new altitude, a greater hyperventilation can be sustained during submaximal exercise, and the tachycardia diminishes. The hormonal changes and associated losses of plasma and tissue bicarbonate also disturb the fluid balance. Perhaps as a consequence of this last change, there is a decrease of cardiac stroke volume over the first few weeks at altitude, particularly in unfit subjects (Scognamiglia *et al.* 1991). The maximal cardiac output and thus the maximal oxygen intake are depressed yet more, since there is also a decrease in maximal heart rate, and an increase of blood viscosity augments circulatory impedance. At very high altitudes, there may finally be a direct depressant effect of oxygen lack on myocardial contractility (observed by Ferretti *et al.* 1990, but not Reeves *et al.* 1987).

The pulmonary arterial pressure is increased at altitude, probably because hypoxia triggers the release of some vasoconstrictor mediator substance. Pressure increments at 2370 m amount to 18% at rest and 30% during submaximal exercise (Sime *et al.* 1974; Lockhart & Saiag 1981). This response helps to increase perfusion in the upper parts of the lungs, allowing a better matching of ventilation and perfusion, with attendant improvements in alveolar gas exchange. At first, the vascular spasm is readily reversed by administration of oxygen, but prolonged residence at altitude leads to structural changes in the pulmonary vessels and an irreversible pulmonary hypertension (Heath & Williams 1989).

The electrocardiogram of the high altitude visitor or resident reflects the increased pulmonary arterial pressures and right ventricular loading. The P wave is increased, the QT time is decreased, the electrical axis is shifted to the right and posteriorly, and in those who are most affected, there may be a right bundle branch block or T-wave inversion (Karliner *et al.* 1985).

Altitude acclimatization

If an athlete remains at altitude, the body makes a wide range of physiological and biochemical adjustments that progressively restore both the body's exercise responses and competitive performance towards sea-level values. Eventually, there is a relatively complete adjustment to altitudes of less than

4300 m (Milledge 1994). Heath and Williams (1989) found that competitors who took 8.5% longer to complete a distance run on arrival in Mexico City were running at only 5.7% less than their normal speed by the 29th day at this altitude. Likewise, after full acclimatization, the heart rate at any given power output was no greater than the values observed at sea-level.

In addition to the reduction in blood and tissue bicarbonate content discussed above, acclimatization leads to a slow but progressive increase in total body haemoglobin content. Any early decrement of blood volume is made good over the course of a few weeks. The activity of tissue enzymes is also increased (Bigard *et al.* 1991), and there are changes in muscle fibre type, fast oxidative glycolytic fibres increasing at the expense of fast glycolytic fibres (Itoh *et al.* 1990). The various processes of change each have their own characteristic time course, and any acclimatization schedule must attempt to optimize the overall response on the day of competition.

The bicarbonate content of the cerebral fluid is reduced within a few hours of moving to high altitude, and parallel adjustments of blood and tissue buffers develop over the following week. As a result, the endurance competitor can hyperventilate slightly without developing an intermittent pattern of ventilation or other signs of carbon dioxide lack. The immediate consequence of altered buffering is that the oxygen content of the arterial blood rises, and perhaps a fifth of the lost capacity to transport oxygen is restored. However, hyperventilation is a mixed blessing to an endurance competitor, because it causes cerebral vasoconstriction, and it increases the quantity of oxygen consumed by the respiratory muscles to the point where this factor may limit performance. There have been suggestions that the well-trained endurance competitor and the high-altitude native avoid this problem because their carotid bodies have a blunted sensitivity to oxygen lack. A lesser hyperventilation may be acceptable to such individuals, because the aerobic enzymes in the muscles have a higher level of activity and can function at lower partial pressures of oxygen (Zhuang *et al.* 1993; Milledge 1994).

In theory, the altitude-related decrease of tissue buffering should reduce the athlete's tolerance of lactate accumulation, so that prolonged exercise above the anaerobic threshold would become more fatiguing than at sea-level (Chapter 22). Certainly, the measurements of anaerobic capacity that are used by some laboratories become more difficult to interpret at altitude (McLellan *et al.* 1988, 1993), due in part to the influence of buffering on the transport of lactate from the muscle to the bloodstream (see Chapter 3).

The early increase in haemoglobin tends to restore the arterial oxygen content of the unit volume of blood in the face of the reduced partial pressure of oxygen in the alveoli. Early increases in red cell count and haemoglobin concentration are due almost entirely to haemoconcentration, but an increase in haemopoiesis leads to a true increase in total red cell mass over several months of exercise at high altitudes (Milledge & Coates 1985; Boutellier *et al.* 1990; Berglund 1992; Strømme & Ingjer 1994). Stimulation of erythropoiesis decreases the average age of the red cells. Their 2,3-diphosphoglycerate (DPG) levels are also increased, but this change develops rather too rapidly to be attributed to the formation of new erythrocytes (Mairbäurl 1993, 1994). The resulting rightward shift of the oxygen dissociation curve decreases the oxygen affinity of haemoglobin, and this change is presumed to help delivery of oxygen to the tissues (Mairbäurl *et al.* 1986; Mairbäurl 1994). At extreme altitudes, a very large increase in red cell count may increase the blood viscosity to such an extent as to limit maximal cardiac output, with a resulting decrease in maximal oxygen transport (Buick *et al.* 1982). A high blood viscosity also increases the risk of intravascular clotting. Winslow and Monge (1987) have thus castigated erythropoiesis as a useless adaptation to high altitudes. Nevertheless, there is growing evidence that a moderate increase in haemoglobin level can boost oxygen transport appreciably (Chapter 30).

The team physician should check both the haemoglobin concentration and the serum iron levels of competitors while they are at sea-level, because plasma volume expansion, fads of diet, poor iron absorption, iron losses in sweat, depressed red cell formation, haemorrhage and intravascular haemolysis can all predispose the endurance athlete to the unnecessary handicap of an initial anaemia or latent iron deficit while he or she is residing at high altitude. If haematology data are only obtained after a competitor has moved to high altitude, it must be remembered that, in order to be accepted as 'normal', values should be higher than those expected at sea-level (Tufts *et al.* 1985).

Other reported adaptations to high altitudes include an increase in the myoglobin content of the muscles (Reynafarje 1962), and (at moderate but not at higher altitudes) an augmentation in activity of aerobic enzyme systems in the Krebs cycle (Ward *et al.* 1989; Bigard *et al.* 1991). These tissue responses develop over 1–2 weeks.

At moderate altitudes, any initial loss of appetite is corrected once acute mountain sickness has passed, but at the altitudes encountered by many mountaineers, a negative nitrogen balance may persist (Guilland & Klepping 1985). This leads to a loss of protein from the myofibrils (Hoppeler *et al.* 1990; Hoppeler & Desplanches 1992) and a substantial overall decrease in body mass (Kayser 1994). One underlying problem is a poor absorption of food from the small bowel. There is also some evidence of a reduction in protein synthesis (Rennie *et al.* 1983). Although there is no change in the capillary network within the skeletal muscles, muscle atrophy shortens the average diffusion path, making capillary oxygen more readily available to the muscle mitochondria (Ward *et al.* 1989).

Many mountaineers have a preference for high carbohydrate diets, which increase their need for antioxidant dietary supplements (Karlsson 1997). The provision of branched-chain amino acid supplements may help to prevent protein loss in such individuals (Schena *et al.* 1992). On the basis of such markers as expired pentanes, Gerstler (1991) and van der Beek (1991) have argued that athletes also have an increased vitamin E requirement while they are at altitude.

Acclimatization must strike a reasonable balance between the development of adaptations that permit a larger respiratory minute volume and the circulatory disadvantage of a cumulative decrease in blood volume. At altitudes up to 2250 m, the respiratory gains from a sustained period of acclimatization seem to outweigh any circulatory losses, at least for the person who is training hard. Thus, where practicable, most authorities recommend a 3–4-week period of acclimatization to the altitude of competition. During this time, the athlete must be guarded against unfamiliar microorganisms, the psychological stress of living in an unfamiliar environment, and the practical risks that a well-established training plan will be interrupted by acute mountain sickness or general fatigue (Levine & Stray-Gundersen 1992).

At 3000 m, the adverse effects from a cumulative loss of plasma fluid can no longer be ignored, and it may be wise for an athlete to compete within 72 h of reaching the new altitude. Opportunity is thereby allowed for recuperation from the journey, adjustments of cerebrospinal bicarbonate levels are relatively complete, and the competitor has usually recovered from any immediate mountain sickness. However, competition is completed before there has been time for a serious fluid loss and an associated decrease in maximal cardiac output. The main disadvantage of permitting only a short pre-event stay at altitude is that the athlete has little chance to learn the peculiarities of the course and an appropriate competitive pace. In such circumstances, an early precontest visit to the site of competition can be very helpful.

Runners who are native to altitudes of 1500–2000 m have enjoyed considerable success in middle- and long-distance events, both at sea-level and at altitude, although it is still debated how far this advantage reflects long-term physiological adaptations to altitude (such as a large vital capacity and pulmonary diffusing capacity, de Meer *et al.* 1995), and how far it is due to the need for greater habitual physical activity in the less-developed societies that inhabit many such locations (Saltin *et al.* 1995). The high-altitude native experiences less early mountain sickness, and a smaller decrease in oxygen transport on returning from sea-level to high altitude (Maresh *et al.* 1983). In the 1968 Mexico City Olympic Games, the first five places in the 10 000-m event were taken by those who were either native to high altitude, or had lived at high altitude for long periods (Heath & Williams 1989). Such individuals also seem to have some advantage when endurance competitions are conducted at sea-level. Specific advantageous characteristics include a high haemo-globin concentration and (at least in some populations) a limited response of the carotid body chemoreceptors to oxygen lack (Hackett *et al.* 1980; Milledge 1986). The latter feature reduces the likelihood of hyperventilation and excessive carbon dioxide wash-out during vigorous effort. Cerebral vasoconstriction and intermittent breathing are thus avoided, and diversion of the available oxygen supply to the chest muscles is reduced.

High-altitude training camps

When compared with sea-level residents, high-altitude natives often have large vital capacities, an increased pulmonary diffusing capacity and a greater capillary density in their skeletal muscles. Further, it has been speculated that these characteristics, whether inherited or acquired over many years of residence at altitude, facilitate life in the adverse environment. Equally, these characteristics appear to confer some immediate advantage when competing at sea-level. Since sea-level residents ultimately adapt well to moderate altitudes, there has been considerable discussion of the desirability of training endurance competitors at real or simulated high altitudes, not only to enhance their performance at altitude, but also to give them an advantage in sea-level competitions.

The main negative argument is that most athletes are unwilling to spend sufficient time at altitude to induce the adaptations that are seen in permanent residents of the region. For example, the apparent polycythaemia of the first few days at altitude reflects a decrease in plasma volume (a change which is quickly reversed on return to sea-level), rather than the coveted but much more slowly developing increase of total body haemoglobin. Where prolonged high-altitude training has been adopted, the objective of the coach has usually been to time the return to sea-level so that any true, altitude-induced polycythaemia is conserved, but body buffers have had opportunity to regain their sea-level values.

An athlete's training schedule may be reduced or disrupted because of the immediate circumstances of the altitude exposure. However, it remains unclear whether the response to a given volume of training is altered if the conditioning is conducted at altitude or with an equivalent reduction in the partial pressure of inspired oxygen. Davies and Sargent (1974) found no difference of response between a leg that was trained under normobaric conditions, and the opposite limb that was trained under hypobaric conditions, but a repetition of the experiment by Melissa et al. (1997) found a greater response in the hypoxic than in the normoxic leg.

Following return to sea-level, plasma volume expansion quickly cancels out any altitude-induced haemoconcentration. Moreover, red cell production is severely depressed for the next few days, and if altitude exposure has been extreme, the suppression of haemopoiesis can be sufficient to cause a temporary anaemia (Heath & Williams 1989). There remains a theoretical possibility of gaining some advantage of oxygen transport from a persistent polycythaemia in the 4–20 days following prolonged exposure to a moderate altitude. But even this potential dividend must be set against such practical disadvantages as the likely curtailment of training, the learning of an incorrect pace while at high altitude and a reduced buffering of anaerobic metabolites (Schmidt et al. 1990).

There have been few well-controlled studies of high-altitude training programmes, but the current consensus seems to be that if athletes are in peak condition before a mountain sojourn, the net result of time spent at a high-altitude camp is no change or even a small deterioration in sea-level maximal oxygen intake, with a corresponding increase in times to complete endurance events (Roskamm et al. 1969; Shephard 1974; Adams et al. 1975; Jackson & Sharkey 1988; Terrados et al. 1988; Kuno et al. 1994; Favier et al. 1995). The one possible physiological advantage is an increase in activity of the oxidative enzymes (Kuno et al. 1994; Sundberg 1994; Melissa et al. 1997), which might allow a given level of physical activity to be sustained with less hyperventilation. There is growing evidence that athletes may gain some benefit from the alternative tactic of living at high altitude, but training at sea-level (Levine & Stray-Gundersen 1995, 1997). Most teams are now disillusioned about altitude training, except in cases where the competition must be undertaken at high

altitude and funding permits a long period of residence at an agreeable mountain resort.

A few authors have experimented with the cheaper alternative of hypoxic training at sea-level, for instance putting cyclists on ergometers in a decompression chamber (Kuno et al. 1994; Vallier et al. 1996), supplying hypoxic gas mixtures during laboratory exercise (Benoit et al. 1992), building a house where low oxygen pressures are maintained or having competitors rebreathe through long tubes during practice periods (D'Urzo et al. 1986). Notice that the last of these techniques helps to conserve tissue bicarbonate reserves and may even induce hypercarbia. Any physiological benefits from such artificial forms of altitude acclimatization have again been slight, and the impact of such tactics upon performance has generally been offset by a disruption of normal training.

High-altitude pathologies

Acute mountain sickness

Susceptibility to acute mountain sickness shows much interindividual variability (Forster 1984). During moderate recreational activity, the threshold altitude for development of the condition is in the range 2000–3000 m (Montgomery et al. 1989). In a study of people using Alpine huts, Maggiorini et al. (1990) found an overall prevalence of 9% at 2850 m, 13% at 3050 m, 34% at 3650 m and 53% at 4559 m. A high alveolar P_{CO_2} after arrival at altitude seems an early harbinger of the disorder. Perhaps because those who are fit exercise earlier and harder after ascent, such individuals seem at least as vulnerable as those who are unfit. International endurance athletes are at particular risk because of their heavy training schedules. They are thus likely to develop symptoms at a somewhat lower altitude than the average person.

Acute mountain sickness can be quite difficult to diagnose, as most of the symptoms are non-specific. Complaints are reported a few hours to 2 days following ascent to high altitude. Problems include a headache that becomes progressively more severe, insomnia, irritability and a variety of gastrointestinal disturbances. There is an increase of extracellular fluid, with a risk of progression to cerebral oedema (Ravenhill 1913), pulmonary oedema (Hackett & Hornbein 1988), generalized oedema (Malconian & Rock 1988) and (particularly in severe cases) retinal haemorrhages (Frayser *et al.* 1970; Sutton 1990, 1992). The volume and composition of the intestinal secretions is also modified, with attendant gastrointestinal disturbances (Michel *et al.* 1994). Most of these changes are secondary to hyperventilation, disturbances of acid–base balance and associated fluid shifts. At the altitudes relevant to most types of competition, the disorder usually lasts no more than 2–3 days, and most patients respond well to conservative treatment.

The best basis of prevention is to allow some acclimatization before taking heavy exercise. There have been suggestions that a high carbohydrate/low salt diet is also helpful (Porcelli & Gugelchuk 1995). Training schedules should be lightened for a couple of days, and indeed little physical activity should be taken on the first day after arriving at the new altitude. Symptomatic therapy can be given for headache and sleeplessness, although an excess of sedatives may worsen the condition by depressing respiration during sleep. Carbonic anhydrase-inhibiting diuretics such as acetazolamide (250 mg four times daily) are quite popular with mountaineers who must face severe altitudes for long periods (Ward *et al.* 1989). In such situations, there have been claims that the administration of acetazolamide conserves muscle mass and enhances physical performance (Bradwell & Coote 1987; Lassen *et al.* 1987; Coote 1995). However, at the moderate altitudes typical of international athletic competitions, carbonic anhydrase inhibitors may reduce performance (Stager *et al.* 1990) and such medications are best avoided. Although the primary symptoms are undoubtedly relieved, side-effects include diuresis and paraesthesiae. The resultant fluid loss aggravates the deterioration of endurance performance associated with acid–base disturbances and a shrinking plasma volume, and the course of natural acclimatization is slowed (Hackett *et al.* 1985; Stager *et al.* 1990). Dexamethasone may be considered for severe cases (Ferrazzini *et al.* 1987).

A persistence of mountain sickness is most unlikely at the altitudes of major competitions (2000–3000 m). If complaints continue, they usually reflect a compounding of the original episode by an intercurrent gastrointestinal infection, irrational fears of altitude, discouragement from poor track times or a progressive loss of physical condition due to the interruption of training schedules.

Chronic mountain sickness

Chronic mountain sickness seems quite distinct from the acute disorder. Chronic problems are seen in residents of high altitude. Characteristics include an extreme polycythaemia, physical and mental slowness, headaches, dizziness, difficulty in concentration, fatigue and somnolence. The problem usually resolves on going to sea-level, but recurs on return to altitude.

Cerebral oedema

Cerebral oedema is a medical emergency that usually presents as an exacerbation of acute mountain sickness. A severe headache may be accompanied by weakness, ataxia, hallucinations and incoherence, progressing to a loss of consciousness and even a stroke (Clarke 1988). Hackett and Rennie (1979) found a 1.8% prevalence of cerebral oedema among trekkers at 4243 m. Lassen (1992) suggested that an increase of cerebral blood flow was a possible aetiological factor, but Jensen *et al.* (1990) found little difference in cerebral blood flow between those who did and those who did not develop symptoms of mountain sickness. Severinghaus (1995) suggested that cellular hypoxia might attract and activate macrophages that expressed vascular endothelial growth factor; such cells could facilitate a capillary leakage of oedema fluid by dissolving the capillary basement membranes and degrading the extracellular matrix.

The most effective method of treating cerebral oedema is to evacuate the patient to a lower altitude. While awaiting evacuation, it is helpful to administer oxygen and/or to enclose the patient in a lightweight portable hyperbaric chamber (the Gamow bag, Murdoch 1992). Other components of medical treatment include administration of betamethasone (4 mg intravenously, immediately and every 4 h), acetazolamide (250 mg immediately and every 8 h), provision of an airway and general care as for an unconscious patient.

Recovery is often rapid once evacuation to a lower altitude has been completed, but sometimes there is evidence of persistent neurological damage (Houston & Dickenson 1975).

Pulmonary oedema

An intense pulmonary oedema is a medical emergency. The condition develops in 0.5–2.0% of people within 9–36 h of reaching high altitudes. The problem seems to be caused by a non-uniform pulmonary vasoconstriction. High pressures or shear forces act on those pulmonary capillaries that remain perfused, causing a disruption of the capillary endothelial layer and allowing the development of a high-permeability type of oedema (West & Mathieu-Costello 1995; West et al. 1995; Hultgren 1997). Affected individuals show a substantial leakage of high molecular weight proteins, erythrocytes, macrophages and various enzymes into the alveolar spaces (Schoene et al. 1986).

Among recreational athletes, the threshold altitude for the development of pulmonary oedema is about 2500 m, but because unusually vigorous exercise is a precipitant of the condition, endurance competitors are susceptible to pulmonary oedema at substantially lower altitudes. Circumstances predisposing to pulmonary oedema include recent respiratory infection, pulmonary venous constriction (secondary to oxygen lack), systemic peripheral vasoconstriction (secondary to hyperventilation), an increase of total blood volume and pulmonary hypertension (exacerbated by previous residence at altitude).

The syndrome is most commonly encountered in competitors with past experience of altitude. Typically, they initiate vigorous training without allowing adequate time for the body to readapt to the low partial pressure of oxygen. A poor ventilatory response to hypoxia also seems to be a risk factor (Hohenhaus et al. 1995).

The typical patient presents with acute dyspnoea, a phlegm that is blood-stained, watery and sometimes frothy, noisy breathing, chest discomfort, a cough (initially dry, but becoming wet), nausea, vomiting and a cold, clammy skin. There are the usual physical signs of alveolar exudate (including poor air entry, dullness to percussion, râles and cyanosis), tachycardia, an increased pulmonary second sound and usually a low-grade fever. The electrocardiogram shows signs of right ventricular strain, and chest radiographs reveal intense pulmonary vascular congestion, with coarse parahilar mottling (Fig. 41.1).

If neglected, pulmonary oedema can rapidly prove fatal. Prompt diagnosis is thus vital. However, there is usually a good response with bedrest, provision of oxygen at high flow rates (6–8 l·min^{-1}), use of a Gamow bag, early evacuation to a lower altitude, administration of frusemide (40 mg intravenously, immediately and every 6 h), acetazolamide (250 mg immediately and repeated every 8 h) and antibiotics (to counter secondary infection). Morphia was once administered, but is not now recommended because it leads to a further depression of ventilation (Heath & Williams 1989). The calcium channel blocker nifedipine (10 mg sublingual, plus 20 mg slow release oral preparation) may help to resolve pulmonary vasoconstriction (Oelz et al. 1989; 1992), but does not seem to affect the overall syndrome of acute mountain sickness (Hohenhaus et al. 1994).

Other forms of oedema

Occasionally, hypoxic oedema may affect the retina and other body tissues. Individuals with a prior diabetic retinopathy seem particularly vulnerable to retinal haemorrhage and oedema (Sutton 1990, 1992; Daniele & Daniele 1995).

General medical conditions

At moderate altitudes, problems of oxygen transport can often be accommodated by the simple expedient of moving a little more slowly than at sea-level. However, the athlete who attempts to sustain a normal pace of movement inevitably increases the risk of developing general medical conditions, including myocardial infarction and cardiac arrest. Even slight reductions in the arterial

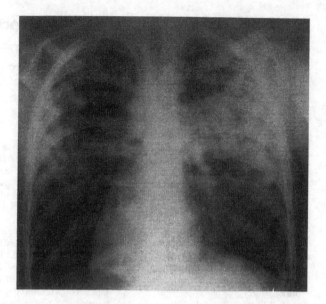

Fig. 41.1 Pulmonary oedema is one of the most serious adverse responses to high altitude and the accompanying hypoxic conditions. Radiograph courtesy of Altitude Research Division, US Air Force Research Institute of Environmental Medicine.

oxygen saturation increase the likelihood that exercise will induce cardiac dysrhythmias and such manifestations of cerebral hypoxia as central scotoma, impairment of colour vision and disturbances of coordination. The hazards remain small for a young, healthy, medically screened athlete who is competing at a moderate altitude, but must be kept in mind, particularly in events that involve Masters competitors.

Severe hypoxia can also cause the death of cerebral neurones. There have been disturbing reports of residual memory loss (Townes *et al*. 1984; Bahrke & Shukitt-Hale 1993) and other manifestations of permanent brain damage, both in habitual explorers of very high altitudes and in subjects exposed to an equivalent chamber hypoxia ('Operation Everest', Hornbein *et al*. 1989).

Black athletes should be checked for sickle cell disease, since several deaths from splenic rupture have occurred at altitudes around 2500 m. Although the condition is most common in black people, athletes of other ethnic groups are not totally exempt from a risk of splenic rupture, and the condition should be suspected in anyone who suddenly develops upper left quadrant abdominal pain (Lane & Githens 1985). Sickle cell disease seems to have an adverse effect on prolonged endurance performance (Thiriet *et al*. 1994).

Exposure to a combination of cold dry air and increased ozone concentrations makes the vulnerable contestant more liable to exercise-induced bronchospasm while at altitude. Cold exposure may also play a synergistic role in the development of pulmonary hypertension and oedema (Giesbrecht 1995).

Ultraviolet radiation is greater at altitude than at sea-level (see above), and because the air is cooler, the duration of exposure to sunlight is likely to be longer than at sea-level. Ultraviolet radiation can cause not only sunburn and cancerous skin lesions, but also blindness, particularly when such radiation is reflected from snow. Barrier creams and dark glasses with side protectors (Brandt & Malla 1982) should be used as necessary.

Conclusions

Both the practical experience of high-altitude endurance competitions and the theoretical considerations presented above support the FIMS position that medical problems attributable to altitude exposure are unlikely below 2300 m. Between 2300 and 3000 m, there is an increasing chance that the more vulnerable members of a team could develop mountain sickness, pulmonary oedema and other medical problems such as cardiac dysrhythmias and cerebral hypoxia. On present knowledge, the likelihood of occasional incidents above 3000 m is sufficient to justify both the categoric prohibition of major competitions, and the urging of caution upon recreational skiers and mountain climbers.

Acknowledgement

The studies of Dr Shephard are supported in part by research grants from the Defence and Civil Institute of Environmental Medicine, Toronto, ON.

References

Adams, W.C., Bernauer, E.M., Dill, D.B. & Bomar, J.B. (1975) Effects of equivalent sea-level and altitude training on $\dot{V}O_{2max}$ and running performance. *Journal of Applied Physiology* 39, 262–266.

Appenzeller, O. & Wood, S.C. (1992) Peptides and exercise at high and low altitudes. *International Journal of Sports Medicine* 13 (Suppl. 1), S135–S140.

Bahrke, M.S. & Shukitt-Hale, B. (1993) Effects of altitude on mood, behaviour and cognitive functioning. *Sports Medicine* 16, 97–125.

Bärtsch, P., Shaw, S., Franciolli, M., Gnadinger, M.P. & Weidmann, P. (1988) Atrial natriuretic peptide in acute mountain sickness. *Journal of Applied Physiology* 65, 1929–1937.

van der Beek, E.J. (1991) Vitamin supplementation and physical exercise performance. *Journal of Sports Sciences* 9, 77–90.

Benoit, H., Germain, M., Barthélémy, J.C. et al. (1992) Pre-acclimatization to high altitude using exercise with normobaric hypoxic gas mixtures. *International Journal of Sports Medicine* 13 (Suppl. 1), S213–S216.

Berglund, B. (1992) High altitude training. Aspects of haematological adaptation. *Sports Medicine* 4, 289–303.

Bigard, A.X., Brunet, A., Guezennec, C.Y. & Monod, H. (1991) Skeletal muscle changes after endurance training at high altitude. *Journal of Applied Physiology* 71, 2114–2121.

Boutellier, U., Dériaz, O., di Prampero, P.E. & Cerretelli, P. (1990) Aerobic performance at altitude: effects of acclimatization and haematocrit with reference to training. *International Journal of Sports Medicine* 11, S21–S26.

Bradwell, A.R. & Coote, J.H. (1987) Expedition to the Himalayas. *Postgraduate Medical Journal* 63, 165–167.

Brandt, F. & Malla, O.K. (1982) Eye problems at high altitudes. In: Brendel, W. & Zink, R.A. (eds) *High Altitude Physiology and Medicine*, pp. 212–214. Springer-Verlag, New York.

Buick, F.J., Gledhill, N., Froese, A.B. & Spriet, L.L. (1982) Red cell mass and

aerobic performance at sea level. In: Sutton, J.R., Jones, N.L. & Houston, C.S. (eds) *Hypoxia: Man at Altitude*, pp. 43–50. Thième-Stratton, New York.

Clarke, C. (1988) High altitude cerebral oedema. *International Journal of Sports Medicine* 19, 170–174.

Coote, J.H. (1995) Medicine and mechanisms in altitude sickness: recommendations. *Sports Medicine* 20, 148–159.

Crowley, J.S., Wesensten, N., Kamimori, G., Devine, J., Iwanyk, E. & Balkin, T. (1992) Effect of high terrestrial altitude and supplemental oxygen on human performance and mood. *Aviation, Space and Environmental Medicine* 63, 696–701.

D'Urzo, A.D., Liu, F.L.W. & Rebuck, A.S. (1986) Influence of supplemental oxygen on the physiological response to the P_{O_2} aerobic exerciser. *Medicine and Science in Sports and Exercise* 18, 211–215.

Daniele, S. & Daniele, C. (1995) Aggravation of laser-treated diabetic cystoid macular edema after prolonged flight: a case report. *Aviation, Space and Environmental Medicine* 66, 440–442.

Davies, C.T.M. & Sargent, A.J. (1974) Effects of hypoxic training on normoxic maximal aerobic power output. *European Journal of Applied Physiology* 33, 227–236.

Dempsey, J. (1986) Is the lung built for exercise? *Medicine and Science in Sports and Exercise* 18, 143–155.

Denison, D.M., Ledwith, F. & Poulton, E.C. (1966) Complex reaction times at simulated cabin altitudes of 5000 feet and 8000 feet. *Aerospace Medicine* 57, 1010–1013.

Ernsting, J. & Shephard, R.J. (1951) Respiratory adaptations in congenital heart disease. *Journal of Physiology (London)* 112, 332–343.

Favier, R., Spielvogel, H., Desplanches, D. et al. (1995) Training in hypoxia vs. training in normoxia in high-altitude natives. *Journal of Applied Physiology* 78, 2286–2293.

Ferrazzini, G., Maggiorini, M., Kriemler, S., Bärtsch, P. & Oelz, O. (1987) Successful treatment of acute mountain sickness

with dexamethasone. *British Medical Journal* 294, 1380–1382.

Ferretti, G., Boutellier, U., Pendergast, D.R. et al. (1990) IV. Oxygen transport system before and after exposure to chronic hypoxia. *International Journal of Sports Medicine* 11, S15–S21.

Fletcher, R.F., Wright, A.D., Jones, G.T. & Bradwell, A.R. (1985) The clinical assessment of acute mountain sickness. *Quarterly Journal of Medicine* 54, 91–100.

Forster, P. (1984) Reproducibility of individual response to exposure to high altitude. *British Medical Journal* 289, 1269.

Frayser, R., Houston, C.S., Bryan, A.C., Rennie, I.D. & Gray, G. (1970) Retinal haemorrhage at high altitude. *New England Journal of Medicine* 282, 1183–1184.

Gerstler, H. (1991) Function of Vitamin E in physical exercise: a review. *Zeitschrift für Ernahrungswissenschaft* 30, 89–97.

Giesbrecht, G.G. (1995) The respiratory system in a cold environment. *Aviation, Space and Environmental Medicine* 66, 890–902.

Goddard, R.F. (ed.) (1967) *The Effects of Altitude on Physical Performance*. Athletic Institute, Chicago.

Guilland, J.C. & Klepping, J. (1985) Nutritional alterations at high altitude in man. *European Journal of Applied Physiology* 54, 517–523.

Hackett, P.H. & Hornbein, T. (1988) Disorders of high altitude. In: Murray, J.F. & Nadel, J.A. (eds) *Textbook of Respiratory Medicine*, pp. 1646–1663. W.B. Saunders, Philadelphia.

Hackett, P.H. & Rennie, D. (1979) The incidence, importance and prophylaxis of acute mountain sickness. *Lancet* ii, 1449–1454.

Hackett, P.H., Reeves, J.T., Reeves, C.D., Grover, R.F. & Rennie, D. (1980) Control of breathing in Sherpas at low and high altitude. *Journal of Applied Physiology* 49, 374–379.

Hackett, P.H., Schoene, R.B., Winslow, R.M., Peters, R.M. & West, J.B. (1985) Acetazolamide and exercise in sojourners to 6300 meters—a preliminary study. *Medicine and Science in Sports and Exercise* **17**, 593–597.

Heath, D. & Williams, D.R. (1989) *High Altitude Medicine and Pathology*. Butterworths, London.

Hohenhaus, E., Niroomand, F., Goerre, S., Vock, P., Oelz, O. & Bärtsch, P. (1994) Nifedipine does not prevent acute mountain sickness. *American Journal of Respiratory and Critical Care Medicine* **150**, 857–860.

Hohenhaus, E., Paul, A., McCullough, R.E., Kücherer, H. & Bärtsch, P. (1995) Ventilatory and pulmonary vascular responses to hypoxia and susceptibility to high altitude pulmonary oedema. *European Respiratory Journal* **8**, 1825–1833.

Hoppeler, H. & Desplanches, D. (1992) Muscle structural modifications in hypoxia. *International Journal of Sports Medicine* **13** (Suppl. 1), S166–S168.

Hoppeler, H., Kleinert, E., Schlegel, C. *et al.* (1990) II. Morphological adaptations of human skeletal muscle to chronic hypoxia. *International Journal of Sports Medicine* **11**, S3.

Hornbein, T.F., Townes, T.B., Schoene, R.B., Sutton, J.R. & Houston, C.S. (1989) The cost to the central nervous system of climbing to extremely high altitudes. *New England Journal of Medicine* **321**, 1714–1719.

Horstman, D., Weiskopf, R. & Jackson, R.E. (1980) Work capacity during a 3-week sojourn at 4300 m: effects of relative polycythaemia. *Journal of Applied Physiology* **49**, 311–318.

Horvath, S.M., Bedi, J.F., Wagner, J.A. & Agnew, J. (1988) Maximum aerobic capacity at several ambient concentrations of CO at several altitudes. *Journal of Applied Physiology* **65**, 2696–2708.

Houston, C.S. & Dickenson, J. (1975) Cerebral form of high-altitude illness. *Lancet* ii, 758–761.

Hultgren, H.N. (1997) High altitude pulmonary oedema: hemodynamic aspects. *International Journal of Sports Medicine* **18**, 20–25.

Itoh, K., Moritani, T., Ishida, K., Hirofuji, C., Taguchi, S. & Itoh, M. (1990) Hypoxia-induced fibre type transformation in rat hind limb muscles. Histochemical and electromechanical changes. *European Journal of Applied Physiology* **60**, 331–336.

Jackson, C.G.R. & Sharkey, B.J. (1988) Altitude, training, and human performance. *Sports Medicine* **6**, 279–284.

Jensen, J.B., Wright, A.D., Lassen, N.A. *et al.* (1990) Cerebral blood flow in acute mountain sickness. *Journal of Applied Physiology* **69**, 430–433.

Jokl, E. & Jokl, P. (1968) *Exercise and Altitude*. University Park Press, Baltimore.

Karliner, J.S., Sarnquist, S.H., Graber, D.J., Peters, R.M. & West, J.B. (1985) The electrocardiogram at extreme altitude: experience on Mt. Everest. *American Heart Journal* **109**, 505–513.

Karlsson, J. (1997) *Antioxidants and Exercise*. Human Kinetics, Champaign, IL.

Kayser, B. (1994) Nutrition and energetics of exercise at altitude. Theory and possible practical implications. *Sports Medicine* **17**, 309–323.

Kuno, S., Inaki, M., Tanaka, K., Itai, Y. & Asano, K. (1994) Muscle energetics in short-term training during hypoxia in elite combination skiers. *European Journal of Applied Physiology* **69**, 301–304.

Lane, P.A. & Githens, J.H. (1985) Splenic syndrome at mountain altitudes in sickle cell trait: its occurrence in non-black persons. *Journal of the American Medical Association* **253**, 2251–2254.

Lassen, N.A. (1992) Increase of cerebral blood flow at high altitude: its possible relation to AMS. *International Journal of Sports Medicine* **13** (Suppl. 1), S47–S48.

Lassen, N.A., Friberg, L., Kastrup, J., Rizzi, D. & Jensen, J.J. (1987) Effects of acetazolamide on cerebral blood flow and brain tissue oxygenation. *Postgraduate Medical Journal* **63**, 185–187.

Levine, B.D. & Stray-Gundersen, J. (1992) A practical approach to altitude training: where to live and train for optimal performance enhancement. *International Journal of Sports Medicine* **13** (Suppl. 1), S209–S212.

Levine, B.D. & Stray-Gundersen, J. (1995) Exercise at high altitudes. In: Torg, J. & Shephard, R.J. (eds) *Current Therapy in Sports Medicine*, 3rd edn, pp. 588–593. Mosby, Philadelphia.

Levine, B.D. & Stray-Gundersen, J. (1997) 'Living high-training low': Effect of moderate altitude acclimatization with low altitude training on performance. *Journal of Applied Physiology* **83**, 102–112.

Lipsitz, L.A., Hashimoto, F., Lubowsky, L.P. *et al.* (1995) Heart rate and respiratory rhythm dynamics on ascent to high altitude. *British Heart Journal* **74**, 390–396.

Lockhart, A. & Saiag, B. (1981) Altitude and the human pulmonary circulation. *Clinical Science* **60**, 599–605.

McLellan, T., Cheung, S.S. & Meunier, M.R. (1993) The effect of normocapnic hypoxia and the duration of exposure to hypoxia on supramaximal exercise performance. *European Journal of Applied Physiology* **66**, 409–414.

McLellan, T., Jacobs, I. & Lewis, W. (1988) Acute altitude exposure and altered acid–base states. I. Effects on the exercise and blood lactate responses. *European Journal of Applied Physiology* **57**, 435–444.

Maggiorini, M., Bühler, H., Walter, M. & Oelz, O. (1990) Prevalence of acute mountain sickness in the Swiss Alps. *British Medical Journal* **301**, 853–855.

Mairbäurl, H. (1994) Red blood cell function in hypoxia at altitude and exercise. *International Journal of Sports Medicine* **15**, 51–63.

Mairbäurl, H., Schobersberger, W., Humperler, E., Haisbeler, W., Fischer, W. & Raas, E. (1986) Beneficial effects of exercising at moderate altitude on red cell oxygen transport and on exercise performance. *Pflügers Archives* **406**, 594–599.

Malconian, M.K. & Rock, P.B. (1988) Medical problems related to altitude. In: Pandolf, K.B., Sawka, M.N. & Gonzalez, R.F. (eds) *Human Performance Physiology and Environmental Medicine at Terrestrial Extremes*, pp. 545–563. Benchmark Press, Indianapolis.

Maresh, C.M., Noble, B.J., Robertson, K.L. & Sime, W.E. (1983) Maximal exercise during hypobaric hypoxia (447 Torr) in moderate altitude natives. *Medicine and Science in Sports and Exercise* **15**, 360–365.

Margaria, R. (ed.) (1967) *Exercise at Altitude*. Excerpta Medica Foundation, Amsterdam.

Martin, D. & O'Kroy, J. (1993) Effects of acute hypoxia on the $\dot{V}o_{2max}$ of trained and untrained subjects. *Journal of Sports Sciences* **11**, 37–42.

de Meer, K., Heymans, H.S. & Ziljstra, W.G. (1995) Physical adaptation of children to life at high altitude. *European Journal of Pediatrics* **154**, 263–272.

Melissa, L., MacDougall, J.D., Tarnopolsky, M.A., Cipriano, N. & Green, H.J. (1997) Skeletal muscle adaptations to training under normobaric hypoxic versus normoxic conditions. *Medicine and Science in Sports and Exercise* **29**, 238–243.

Michel, H., Larrey, D. & Blanc, P. (1994) Troubles hépato-digestifs en pratique sportive. *Presse Médicale* **23**, 479–484.

Milledge, J.S. (1986) The ventilatory response to hypoxia: how much is good for a mountaineer? *Postgraduate Medical Journal* **63**, 169–172.

Milledge, J.S. (1994) High altitude. In: Harries, M., Williams, C., Stanish, W.D. & Micheli, L.J. (eds) *Oxford Textbook of*

Sports Medicine, pp. 217–230. Oxford University Press, New York.

Milledge, J.S. & Coates, P.M. (1985) Serum erythropoietin in humans at high altitude and its relation to plasma renin. *Journal of Applied Physiology* **59**, 360–364.

Milledge, J.S., Beeley, J.M., McArthur, S. & Morice, A.H. (1989) Atrial natriuretic peptide, altitude and acute mountain sickness. *Clinical Science* **77**, 509–514.

Montgomery, A.B., Mills, J. & Luce, J.M. (1989) Incidence of acute mountain sickness at intermediate altitude. *Journal of the American Medical Association* **261**, 732–734.

Murdoch, D. (1992) The portable hyperbaric chamber for the treatment of high altitude illness. *New Zealand Medical Journal* **105**, 361–362.

Oelz, O., Maggiori, M., Ritter, M. *et al.* (1989) Nifedipine for high altitude pulmonary oedema. *Lancet* **ii**, 1241–1244.

Oelz, O., Maggiorini, M., Ritter, M. *et al.* (1992) Prevention and treatment of high altitude pulmonary oedema by a calcium channel blocker. *International Journal of Sports Medicine* **13** (Suppl. 1), S65–S68.

Perhonen, M., Takala, T., Huttunen, P. & Leppäluoto, J. (1995) Stress hormones after prolonged physical training in normo- and hypobaric conditions in rats. *International Journal of Sports Medicine* **16**, 73–77.

Perronet, F., Thibault, G. & Cousineau, D.-L. (1991) A theoretical analysis of the effect of altitude on running performance. *Journal of Applied Physiology* **70**, 399–404.

Porcelli, M.J. & Gugelchuk, G.M. (1995) A trek to the top: a review of acute mountain sickness. *Journal of the American Osteopathic Association* **95**, 718–720.

Ravenhill, T.H. (1913) Some experiences of acute mountain sickness in the Andes. *Journal of Tropical Medicine and Hygiene* **20**, 313–320.

Reeves, J.T., Groves, B.M., Sutton, J.M. *et al.* (1987) Operation Everest II: preservation of cardiac function at extreme altitude. *Journal of Applied Physiology* **63**, 531–539.

Rennie, M.J. *et al.* (1983) Effects of acute hypoxia on forearm leucine metabolism. In: Sutton, J., Houston, C.S. & Jones, N.L. (eds) *Hypoxia, Exercise and Altitude*, pp. 317–323. Liss, New York.

Reynfarje, B. (1962) Myoglobin content and enzymatic activity of muscle and altitude adaptation. *Journal of Applied Physiology* **17**, 301–305.

Richardson, R.G. (ed.) (1974) Altitude

training. *British Journal of Sports Medicine* **8**, 1–63.

Roskamm, H., Landry, F., Samek, L., Schlager, M., Weidermann, H. & Reindell, H. (1969) Effects of a standardized ergometer training program at three different altitudes. *Journal of Applied Physiology* **27**, 840–847.

Saltin, B., Larsen, H., Terrados, N. *et al.* (1995) Aerobic exercise capacity at sea level and at altitude in Kenyan boys, junior and senior runners compared with Scandinavian runners. *Scandinavian Journal of Medicine and Science in Sports* **5**, 209–221.

Schena, F., Guerrini, F., Tregnaglii, P. & Kayser, B. (1992) Branched chain amino acid supplementation during trekking at high altitude. The effects on loss of body mass, body composition and muscle power. *European Journal of Applied Physiology* **65**, 394–398.

Schmidt, W., Dahners, H.W., Correa, R., Ramirez, R., Rojas, J. & Böning, D. (1990) Blood gas transport properties in endurance-trained athletes living at different altitudes. *International Journal of Sports Medicine* **11**, 15–21.

Schoene, R.B., Hackett, P.H., Henderson, W.R. *et al.* (1986) High altitude pulmonary edema. Characteristics of lavage fluid. *Journal of the American Medical Association* **256**, 63–69.

Scognamiglia, R., Ponchia, A., Fasoli, G. & Miraglia, G. (1991) Changes in structure and function of human left ventricle after acclimatization to high altitude. *European Journal of Applied Physiology* **62**, 73–76.

Severinghaus, J.W. (1995) Hypothetical role of angiogenesis, osmotic swelling, and ischemia in high altitude cerebral edema. *Journal of Applied Physiology* **79**, 375–379.

Shephard, R.J. (1974) Altitude training camps. *British Journal of Sports Medicine* **8**, 38–45.

Shephard, R.J. (1983) *Carbon Monoxide: The Silent Killer*. C.C. Thomas, Springfield, IL.

Sime, F., Penaloza, D., Ruiz, L., Gonzalez, N., Covarrubias, E. & Postigo, R. (1974) Hypoxaemia, pulmonary hypertension and low cardiac output in newcomers to low altitude. *Journal of Applied Physiology* **36**, 561–565.

Stager, J.M., Tucker, A., Cordain, L., Engebretsen, B.J., Brechue, W.F. & Matulich, C.C. (1990) Normoxic and acute hypoxic exercise tolerance in man following acetazolamide. *Medicine and Science in Sports and Exercise* **22**, 178–184.

Strømme, S.B. & Ingjer, F. (1994) Hoydetrening (high altitude training). *Norvegische Medizin* **109**, 19–22.

Sundberg, C.J. (1994) Exercise and training during graded leg ischaemia in healthy man with special reference to effects on skeletal muscle. *Acta Physiologica Scandinavica* **615** (Suppl.), 1–50.

Sutton, J.R. (1990) Exercise at high altitudes. In: Torg, J.R., Welsh, P. & Shephard, R.J. (eds) *Current Therapy in Sports Medicine 2*, pp. 155–158. B.C. Decker, Toronto.

Sutton, J.R. (1992) Mountain sickness. *Neurology Clinics* **10**, 1015–1030.

Sutton, J.R., Houston, C.S. & Coates, G. (1987) *Hypoxia and Cold*. Praeger Publications, New York, NY.

Terrados, N., Melichna, J., Sylvén, J., Jansson, E. & Kaijser, L. (1988) Effects of training at simulated altitude on performance and muscle metabolic capacity in competitive road cyclists. *European Journal of Applied Physiology* **57**, 203–209.

Thiriet, P., Le Hesran, J.Y., Wouassi, D., Bitanga, E., Gozal, D. & Louis, F.J. (1994) Sickle cell trait performance in a prolonged race at high altitude. *Medicine and Science in Sports and Exercise* **26**, 914–918.

Townes, B.D., Hornbein, T.F., Schoene, R.B., Sarnquist, F.H. & Grant, I. (1984) Human cerebral function at extreme altitude. In: West, J.B. & Lahri, S. (eds) *High Altitude and Man*, pp. 31–36. American Physiological Society, Bethesda, MD.

Tucker, A., Stager, J.M. & Cordain, L. (1984) Arterial O_2 saturation and maximum O_2 consumption in moderate-altitude runners exposed to sea level and 3050 m. *Journal of the American Medical Association* **252**, 2867–2871.

Tufts, D.A., Haas, J.D., Beard, J.L. & Spielvogel, H. (1985) Distribution of hemoglobin and functional consequences of anemia in adult males at high altitude. *American Journal of Clinical Nutrition* **42**, 1–11.

Vallier, J.M., Chateau, P. & Guezennec, C.Y. (1996) Effects of physical training in a hypobaric chamber on the physical performance of competitive triathletes. *European Journal of Applied Physiology* **73**, 471–478.

Ward, M.P., Milledge, J.S. & West, J.B. (1989) *High Altitude Medicine and Physiology*, pp. 213–216. Chapman & Hall, London.

West, J.B. & Mathieu-Costello, O. (1995) Vulnerability of pulmonary capillaries in heart disease. *Circulation* **92**, 622–631.

West, J.B., Colice, G.L., Lee, Y.J. *et al.* (1995) Pathogenesis of high-altitude pulmonary oedema: direct evidence of stress failure of pulmonary capillaries. *European Respiratory Journal* 8, 523–529.

Winslow, R.M. & Monge, C. (1987) *Hypoxia, Polycythaemia and Acute Mountain Sickness*. Johns Hopkins University Press, Baltimore.

Young, A.J., Cymerman, A. & Pandolf, K.B. (1982) Differentiated ratings of perceived exertion are influenced by high altitude exposure. *Medicine and Science in Sports and Exercise* 14, 223–228.

Zhuang, J., Droma, T., Sun, S. *et al.* (1993) Hypoxic ventilatory responsiveness in Tibetan compared with Han residents of 3658 m. *Journal of Applied Physiology* 74, 303–311.

Chapter 42

Air Pollutants and Endurance Performance

LAWRENCE J. FOLINSBEE AND EDWARD S. SCHELEGLE

Introduction

A group of well-trained competitive distance runners prepares to step up to the starting line of a 10-km race. It is early afternoon on a warm day. As is all too common, a haze has formed over the suburban community in which the race is to be held. The runners have finished their warm-up and are prepared to start. Some of the runners notice a slight tightness in their chest that becomes greater as they try to take a deep breath in anticipation of the starter's signal. As the race begins, the runners focus on the race ahead and for a short time they ignore their mild respiratory discomfort. However, as the pack passes the 2-km mark and the racers begin to settle into their pace, the previously affected runners again notice their respiratory discomfort as it increases. Further, some of the previously unaffected runners begin to feel mild symptoms of respiratory discomfort. As the more severely affected runners pass the 5-km mark, their respiratory discomfort has intensified and their symptoms now include throat irritation and cough. These runners begin to fall off their planned race pace, as they reconsider their strategy. Some may consider dropping out of the race. These runners are pale and are unable to take a deep breath without experiencing chest discomfort and cough. Later in the race, additional runners develop moderate symptoms. Nevertheless, most of the runners with mild to moderate symptoms finish the race. At the finish line, many of the runners who experienced no symptoms wonder what their fellow runners are complaining about.

This hypothetical scenario illustrates what could happen if endurance events were held in an environment where air quality is poor. Based on both epidemiological and clinical laboratory studies, it serves to illustrate two points. There exists a wide and largely unexplained disparity in individual responsiveness to certain air pollutants. Moreover, it would appear, at first glance, that the ability of the affected runners to perform optimally in this scenario is limited by their subjective symptoms of respiratory discomfort. Whereas this may be true in part, we will examine functional limitations that also may contribute to the decrements in endurance performance of these athletes. These functional limitations depend on the composition of the ambient air pollutants that are inhaled and whether the affected athlete has a history of respiratory disease, especially asthma. We will examine the effects of three specific pollutants: ozone, sulphur dioxide and carbon monoxide.

Ozone

Ozone is the predominant oxidant found in the photochemical air pollution that is common in many urban and suburban areas. There are interactions between prolonged aerobic exercise and the effects of ozone that may be important for endurance performance. By increasing minute ventilation, aerobic exercise serves to increase the inhaled dose of ozone, thereby influencing the rate of onset as well as the magnitude of ozone-induced pulmonary symptoms and functional decrements. Secondly, if ozone-induced pulmonary symptoms and functional

628

decrements are severe enough, decrements in endurance performance and maximal oxygen intake may become apparent.

Pulmonary decrements

The primary findings in healthy human subjects exposed to ambient ozone concentrations comprise symptoms of cough and pain on deep inspiration, a decreased inspiratory capacity (IC), a mild bronchoconstriction and a rapid shallow breathing pattern during exercise. In addition, ozone increases airway hyperresponsiveness, as demonstrated by an increased physiological response to non-specific stimuli such as methacholine. The decrease in inspiratory capacity results in a decrease in forced vital capacity (FVC) and total lung capacity (TLC). In combination with the observed mild bronchoconstriction, it also contributes to a decrease in the forced expiratory volume in 1 s (FEV_1). Other consistently observed phenomena include the presence of a large intersubject variability, good intrasubject reproducibility and rather low correlations between the changes in subjective symptoms, changes in various forced expiratory endpoints and changes in airway resistance.

The majority of controlled human exposures (Adams et al. 1981; McDonnell et al. 1983; Hazucha 1987; Folinsbee 1992) have examined the effects of various ozone concentrations in healthy subjects performing continuous or intermittent exercise for variable periods of time. A large body of data regarding the interaction of ozone concentration, minute ventilation and duration of exposure is available (Fig. 42.1). The majority of controlled human exposure studies have utilized mild to moderate levels of exercise, similar to those that might be seen during a warm-up or moderate training session. However, several investigators (Adams & Schelegle 1983; Avol et al. 1984; Folinsbee et al. 1984; Gong et al. 1986) have examined the effects of ozone concentrations less than or equal to 0.21 ppm on decrements in pulmonary function during 1 h of continuous high-intensity exercise in healthy subjects. The responses observed (Table 42.1) demonstrate that ozone concentrations between 0.12 and 0.18 ppm will elicit significant symptoms and pul-

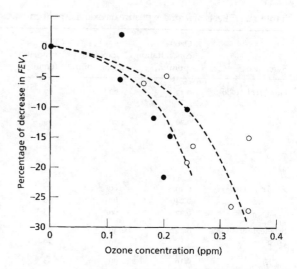

Fig. 42.1 Percentage decrease in lung function (forced expiratory volume in 1 s (FEV_1)) after 1 h of continuous exercise exposure to 0.12–0.35 ppm ozone. Response curves have been estimated for two exercise intensities, based on respiratory minute volumes of 60–70 l·min^{-1} (o) and 80–100 l·min^{-1} (●) (Folinsbee 1992).

monary function decrements in healthy humans when combined with an hour of moderate to severe intermittent or continuous exercise. Over longer exercise periods (>60 min), small effects on lung function and respiratory symptoms can be detected in trained cyclists at lower ozone concentrations (<0.09 ppm) (Brunekreef et al. 1994; Grievink et al. 1998).

Although ozone clearly causes changes in lung function and exercise breathing pattern, it does not exacerbate exercise-induced bronchoconstriction in patients with asthma (Weymer et al. 1994).

Endurance performance

Earlier epidemiological studies examining the race performance of high-school cross-country runners (Wayne et al. 1967) suggested that exercise performance was depressed by inhalation of ambient oxidant air pollutants. Wayne et al. (1967) suggested that the detrimental effects may have been related to increased airway resistance or to the associated discomfort in breathing; this could have limited the runners' motivation to perform at high levels.

Table 42.1 Effects of ozone exposure on exercise performance.

Reference	Ozone concentration (ppm)	Exposure time (min)	Exercise ventilation (l·min^{-1})	Effects on peak $\dot{V}_{O_2}$, endurance time, breathing pattern, lung function, etc.*	Subjects
Gong et al. (1986)	0.12	60	89	Reduced (−6%) FEV_1, no change in breathing pattern, peak $\dot{V}_{O_2}$ or endurance time	17 élite cyclists
	0.20	60	89	Reduced (−22%) FEV_1, decreased V_T, increased f_B, reduced (−30%) endurance time, reduced (−16%) peak $\dot{V}_{O_2}$; cough and chest tightness; 5 out of 16 failed to complete 60 min at 0.20 ppm ozone	
Avol et al. (1984)	0.16	60	57	FEV_1 reduced 6.1, 19.2 and 26.3%, respectively. Ambient air containing 0.15 ppm ozone caused 5.3% decrease in FEV_1	50 competitive cyclists
	0.24	60	60		
	0.32	60	58		
Schelegle & Adams (1986)	0.12	30	55	1 out of 10 failed to complete second 30 min	10 highly trained cyclists
		30	120		
	0.18	30	55	5 out of 10 failed to complete last 30 min; reduced (−26%) endurance time at 120 l·min^{-1}, reduced (−6%) FEV_1	
		30	120		
	0.24	30	55	7 out of 10 failed to complete last 30 min; reduced (−34%) endurance time at 120 l·min^{-1}, reduced (−11%) FEV_1	
		30	120		
Adams & Schelegle (1983)	0.20	30	52	4 out of 10 felt they could not compete maximally under these conditions; cough and shortness of breath in 7 out of 10; reduced (−6%) FEV_1	10 trained distance runners
		30	100		
	0.35	30	52	4 out of 10 failed to complete at 100 l·min^{-1}; 9 out of 10 felt they could not compete maximally under these conditions; cough and shortness of breath in 9 out of 10; reduced (−21%) FEV_1	
		30	100		
Folinsbee et al. (1984)	0.21	60	90	No reduction in endurance time; reduced (−15%) FEV_1; chest discomfort and cough; 3 out of 5 competitive cyclists felt ozone would affect their performance adversely	7 trained cyclists
Foxcroft & Adams (1986)	0.35	60	60	Reduced (−6%) peak $\dot{V}_{O_2}$, reduced (−17%) endurance time in peak $\dot{V}_{O_2}$ test, reduced (−23%) FEV_1, reduced V_T; 5 out of 8 could not perform maximally after ozone exposure	8 trained men

*FEV_1, forced expiratory volume in 1 s; V_T, tidal volume; f_B, respiratory frequency.

Numerous controlled human studies have evaluated the effects of acute ozone inhalation on exercise performance. Observations can be separated into two categories, those that have examined the effects of acute ozone inhalation on maximal oxygen intake and those that have examined the effects of acute ozone inhalation on the ability to complete strenuous continuous exercise protocols.

Adams and Schelegle (1983) exposed 10 well-trained distance runners to filtered air containing 0.20 and 0.35 ppm ozone while they exercised on a cycle ergometer at work rates simulating either a 1-h steady-state 'training' bout or a 30-min warm-up followed immediately by a 30-min 'competitive bout'. The exercise levels in the steady-state training bout were of sufficient magnitude (68% of their $\dot{V}_{O_{2max}}$) to increase mean minute ventilation to 80 l·min^{-1}. The minute ventilation averaged over the entire competitive simulation was also $80 \, l \cdot min^{-1}$, and the mean minute ventilation during the 30-min competitive bout was $105 \, l \cdot min^{-1}$. Subjective symptoms increased as a function of ozone concentration for both training and competitive protocols. In the competitive protocol, four runners who had been exposed to 0.20 ppm ozone and nine who had been exposed to 0.35 ppm ozone indicated that they could not have performed maximally. Three subjects were unable to complete both the training and competitive protocols at 0.35 ppm ozone, and a fourth failed to complete only the competitive ride.

Folinsbee et al. (1984) exposed six well-trained males and one well-trained female to 0.21 ppm ozone while they exercised continuously on a cycle ergometer for 1 h at 75% of their $\dot{V}O_{2max}$ ($\dot{V}_E = 81$ $l \cdot min^{-1}$). Following ozone exposure, the subjects reported symptoms of laryngeal and/or tracheal irritation, chest soreness and tightness upon taking a deep breath, and FVC and FEV_1 were significantly reduced. Anecdotal reports obtained from these élite competitive cyclists suggested that their performance would have been limited if they had experienced similar symptoms during an actual race.

Avol et al. (1984) exposed 50 well-conditioned cyclists to 0.0, 0.08, 0.16, 0.24 and 0.32 ppm ozone for 1 h in ambient heat (32°C) while exercising continuously ($\dot{V}_E = 57 \, l \cdot min^{-1}$). The prevalence of symptoms and reductions in FEV_1 increased in a concentration-dependent manner, being initially detected at 0.16 ppm ozone. Three and 16 cyclists, respectively, could not complete the 1-h exposure to 0.16 and 0.24 ppm ozone without a reduction in power output. Similarly, in their study of the effects of ozone exposure on $\dot{V}O_{2max}$, Gong et al. (1986) reported that five of 17 highly trained endurance cyclists were not able to complete 1 h of very heavy exercise ($\dot{V}_E = 90 \, l \cdot min^{-1}$) during exposure to 0.20 ppm ozone, although they were able to complete exercise during filtered air exposure under similar conditions ($T = 31°C$).

Schelegle and Adams (1986) extended their observations using a group of 10 highly trained endurance athletes exposed to 0.12, 0.18 and 0.24 ppm ozone while performing a similar 1-h com-

petitive protocol at a more intense work rate (about 86% of their $\dot{V}O_{2max}$; mean $\dot{V}_E = 120 \, l \cdot min^{-1}$). All subjects completed the filtered air exposure, whereas one, five and seven subjects, respectively, did not complete the 0.12, 0.18 and 0.24 ppm ozone exposures. Following 0.18 and 0.24 ppm ozone exposure, subjective symptoms increased, and FVC and FEV_1 were reduced.

Maximal oxygen intake

Of the initial studies (Folinsbee et al. 1977; Horvath et al. 1979; Savin & Adams 1979) examining the effects of acute ozone exposures on maximal oxygen intake ($\dot{V}O_{2max}$), only one showed a reduction in $\dot{V}O_{2max}$. Folinsbee et al. (1977) observed that $\dot{V}O_{2max}$ was decreased by 10.5% following 2 h of light intermittent exercise in 0.75 ppm ozone. Reductions in $\dot{V}O_{2max}$ were accompanied by a 9.5% decrease in peak work rate ($P < 0.01$), a 16% decrease in peak ventilation ($P < 0.01$) and a 6% decrease in peak heart rate ($P < 0.05$). The decrease in peak $\dot{V}_E$ was associated with a 21% decrease in tidal volume and an increase in breathing frequency. In addition, the ozone exposure resulted in subjective symptoms of cough and chest discomfort and an 18% decrease in FVC. In contrast, neither Horvath et al. (1979) nor Savin and Adams (1979) observed an effect on peak work rate or $\dot{V}O_{2max}$. The ozone exposure dose in the latter two studies produced few respiratory symptoms and little or no change in lung function.

The subsequent findings of Foxcroft and Adams (1986) and Gong et al. (1986) supported the observations of Folinsbee et al. (1977). Foxcroft and Adams (1986) observed reductions in performance time (16.7%), $\dot{V}O_{2max}$ (6.0%), peak ventilation (15.0%) and peak heart rate (5.6%) in eight aerobically trained males during a rapidly incremented $\dot{V}O_{2max}$ test following a 50-min exposure to 0.35 ppm ozone (exercise $\dot{V}_E = 60 \, l \cdot min^{-1}$). Similarly, Gong et al. (1986) found significant ($P < 0.05$) reductions in performance time (29.7%), $\dot{V}O_{2max}$ (16.4%), peak ventilation (18.5%) and peak power output (7.8%) in 17 élite endurance cyclists following 1 h exposure to 0.35 ppm ozone with very heavy exercise ($\dot{V}_E = 90 \, l \cdot min^{-1}$). In the above studies, the reductions in maximal exercise endpoints were accompanied by marked symptoms of respiratory discomfort and significant decrements in pulmonary function. Hence, it appears that maximal oxygen intake may be reduced if the test is preceded by a sufficient dose of ozone to result in respiratory symptoms and decrements in pulmonary function.

Mechanisms and interventions

Ozone exposure causes symptoms of cough, pain on deep inspiration, shortness of breath, throat irritation and wheezing in asthmatic patients. The responses observed during and following acute exposure to ozone at concentrations between 0.10 and 0.50 ppm in normal healthy human subjects include: decreases in total lung capacity (TLC), IC, FVC, FEV_1, forced expiratory flow rate between 25 and 75% of FVC ($FEF_{25-75\%}$) and tidal volume (V_T), and increases in specific airway resistance (SRaw), breathing frequency (f_B) and airway responsiveness. Ozone exposure results in airway inflammation characterized by hyperaemia and influx of neutrophils and plasma proteins. Such inflammatory responses are more pronounced in patients with asthma (Scannell et al. 1996). From this complex of responses, changes can be categorized into several general responses, including symptoms, inflammation, alterations in lung volumes, decreases in airway calibre and enhanced bronchomotor responsiveness. The mechanisms that produce these responses remain incompletely understood. The absence of consistent associations between the various responses from one individual to another suggests that the functional responses are the result of multiple interactions within the respiratory tract.

Bates et al. (1972) observed that maximum transpulmonary pressure was reduced but static compliance was unchanged, suggesting that maximal inspiratory effort was inhibited after ozone exposure. These authors speculated that inhibition may have resulted from stimulation of 'irritant receptors' located in the major bronchi.

The acute inhalation of ozone by healthy human subjects results in a concentration-dependent increase in airway resistance (Folinsbee et al. 1978; McDonnell et al. 1983; Kulle et al. 1985; Seal et al.

1993), but these changes are poorly correlated with changes in forced expiratory endpoints (McDonnell et al. 1983). Ozone-induced increases in airway resistance have a rapid onset (Beckett et al. 1985) compared with the more gradual development of decrements in forced expiratory endpoints (Kulle et al. 1985). Ozone-induced increases in airway resistance tend to be greater in subjects with atopy (McDonnell et al. 1987; Kreit et al. 1989), although this is often not the case for ozone-induced decrements in forced expiratory endpoints.

Increases in airway resistance induced by ozone can be blocked by atropine sulphate pretreatment in human subjects (Beckett et al. 1985), suggesting that the release of acetylcholine from parasympathetic postganglionic fibres innervating airway smooth muscle may play a role in this response. However, acute ozone inhalation also results in hyperresponsiveness to inhaled methacholine and acetylcholine (Holtzman et al. 1979), suggesting that the increase in sensitivity of airway smooth muscle to endogenous acetylcholine is independent of a reflex mechanism involving the cholinergic postganglionic nerves. Inhaled β-agonists can abolish ozone-induced bronchoconstriction (Beckett et al. 1985; Gong et al. 1988), suggesting that endogenously released catecholamines could modulate ozone-induced bronchoconstriction. Furthermore, patients with asthma show improvement in FEV_1 after inhalation of a β-agonist bronchodilator, indicating that bronchoconstriction plays a role in the FEV_1 response. Nevertheless, β-agonists are ineffective in modifying the decrease in FVC and other spirometric variables in non-asthmatic individuals.

Ozone-induced alterations in the pattern of breathing during exercise have been observed in dogs (Lee et al. 1979) and humans (Folinsbee et al. 1978; Adams et al. 1981; McDonnell et al. 1983; Kulle et al. 1985). In exercising humans, ozone exposure typically results in a decrease in V_T and an increase in f_B in the absence of any change in minute ventilation. The pattern of breathing appears to be most susceptible to ozone effects in the ventilation range associated with moderate to heavy submaximal exercise (i.e. approximately 45–70 l·min^{-1}) (see Folinsbee et al. 1997, p. 644). In this $\dot{V}_E$ range, V_T is approaching its typical maximal level (i.e. about 50% FVC) and any factor that reduces V_T (such as an ozone-induced decrease in IC) will lead to compensatory increases in frequency in order to maintain ventilation. There is evidence that this tachypnoeic response to ozone exposure has a behavioural as well as a reflex component. After repeated exposure to ozone, subjects tend to initiate a rapid shallow breathing pattern even before they experience restriction of inhaled volume, because they have learned that this particular breathing pattern minimizes their respiratory discomfort.

In laboratory animals, tachypnoeic responses induced by ozone can be blocked by vagal nerve cooling (Lee *et al.* 1979; Schelegle *et al.* 1993), and the activity of various vagal afferents can be examined (Coleridge *et al.* 1993). These studies indicate that non-myelinated bronchial C-fibres and rapidly adapting stretch receptors are involved in the reflex leading to rapid shallow breathing. If similar airway afferent endings are stimulated or sensitized in humans exposed to ozone, this could explain the ozone-induced rapid shallow breathing that is observed during exercise.

Bronchial C-fibres and rapidly adapting stretch receptors are known to be stimulated by prostaglandin E_2 and other lung autacoids (Coleridge *et al.* 1978). Schelegle *et al.* (1987), Eschenbacher *et al.* (1989) and Ying *et al.* (1990) have shown that pretreatment with the cyclooxygenase inhibitor indomethacin inhibits or abolishes ozone-induced pulmonary function decrements in humans. Hazucha *et al.* (1989) likewise inhibited lung function changes by pretreatment with another cyclooxygenase inhibitor, ibuprofen; they noted a concomitant reduction in levels of prostaglandin E_2 and interleukin-6. However, airway resistance changes and airway inflammatory responses were not blocked by ibuprofen, despite it being a commonly used non-steroidal anti-inflammatory agent. The hypothesis that prostaglandin E_2 or some other cyclooxygenase products may play a role in ozone-induced pulmonary function decrements is supported by the findings of McDonnell *et al.* (1990). They showed a positive correlation between pulmonary function changes and the level of prostaglandin E_2 in bronchoalveolar lavage fluid collected after ozone exposure. These studies suggest that the use of a cyclooxygenase inhibitor before strenuous exertion may minimize respiratory discomfort and pulmonary function decrements in an oxidant-polluted environment.

The mechanisms leading to the observed decrements in maximal oxygen intake and the inability to complete strenuous exercise protocols remain obscure. As stated by Åstrand and Rodahl (1977) 'the capacity for prolonged rhythmic muscular exercise is limited by an interrelated composite of cardiorespiratory, metabolic, environmental and psychological factors.' Most of the investigators cited above concluded that the reductions in exercise performance resulted from symptoms limiting the ability of their subjects to perform. However, this conclusion was reached by exclusion and not by the demonstration of a causal relationship. Symptoms of respiratory discomfort resulting from the stimulation of neural receptors in the airways may contribute to an increased 'central' rating of perceived exertion (Mihevic *et al.* 1981). Small increases in (external) resistance similar to those observed during ozone exposure generally do not alter peak $\dot{V}O_2$ and, in contrast to ozone, the effect on the respiratory pattern is then generally to increase tidal volume and decrease frequency (D'Urzo *et al.* 1987). However, inspiratory elastic loads cause a decrease in tidal volume and an increase in breathing frequency and, if large enough, they lead to a decrease in peak ventilation and peak $\dot{V}O_2$ (D'Urzo *et al.* 1985; El-Manshawi *et al.* 1986). A reflex inhibition of the ability to inspire deeply would be consistent with the reduced peak tidal volumes and peak ventilation following ozone exposure in subjects performing maximal exercise, and it would also be consistent with a physiologically induced ventilatory limitation to maximal oxygen intake.

In addition to the mitigation of some ozone effects by cyclooxygenase inhibitors, antioxidant supplements (α-tocopherol, β-carotene and ascorbic acid) can reduce the effects of ozone (Chatham *et al.* 1987; Grievink *et al.* 1998). The likely mechanism of this interaction is a reduction in formation of lipoperoxides, ozonides or oxidation products of ozone interaction.

Sulphur dioxide

Sulphur dioxide (SO_2) in the ambient air comes largely from the combustion of fossil fuels (e.g. by industries that use coal or oil as an energy source) and from certain industrial processes such as metal refining, cement manufacturing and pulp and paper production. The SO_2 from these stationary sources is the primary pollutant involved in the formation of acidic aerosols and, subsequently, acid rain (the other important constituent is nitrogen dioxide). In most developed countries, current levels of SO_2 and acid aerosols rarely, if ever, reach ambient levels that have a significant effect on lung function or exercise performance in healthy individuals. However, in some developing countries, especially in Asia, SO_2 levels can be relatively high. Although healthy endurance athletes are not likely to experience problems associated with SO_2 inhalation, patients with asthma are almost 10-fold more sensitive to SO_2 than non-asthmatics. Even brief exposures to SO_2 during exercise can lead to narrowing of the airways, or bronchoconstriction, in asthmatic individuals.

Sulphur dioxide is a highly soluble gas. As such, it tends to be removed from the inspired airstream by the moist surfaces of the upper airways, especially the nose. During resting breathing, SO_2 may be absorbed almost completely before reaching the trachea. The upper airway removal of SO_2 is decreased by breathing through the mouth, or by increased inspiratory flow rates. The breathing of dry air or cold air (with a low water content) may cause a temporary decrease in moisture on the airway surface, although cold air can lead to increased nasal secretions (Philip *et al.* 1993). The resistance of the nasal airways is typically reduced markedly during exercise (Forsyth *et al.* 1983) and the proportion of air breathed through the mouth (oral breathing) generally increases as exercise intensity increases. The poorer SO_2 scrubbing capacity of the mouth and the increased inspired flow rate lead to a greater penetration of SO_2 to the intrathoracic airways. The presence of nasal obstruction or congestion (common in allergic rhinitis) may also lead to proportionately greater oral breathing.

In the US, the prevalence of asthma in the general population is about 4–5%, but it is higher in children and adolescents, males, Puerto Rican Hispanics, and African–Americans. The prevalence rates reported in other countries may be higher; Australia, the venue for the 2000 Olympics, has a prevalence rate of greater than 10% (Bates 1995). Asthma is exacerbated by exercise in most asthmatic individuals (exercise-induced bronchospasm), and the prevalence of asthma among the athletic population (in the US) may be as high as 10–12% (Voy 1986).

Sulphur dioxide can cause exacerbation of asthmatic symptoms and lung function changes in exercising asthmatics who are exposed to concentrations of 0.25 ppm or greater for periods of only a few minutes (2–10 min). FEV_1 may drop by as much as 50–60% in the most responsive individuals. Such exposures will induce wheezing, chest tightness and dyspnoea, which in many cases are sufficient to require the use of a bronchodilator. Both cold and/or dry air and mouth breathing can exacerbate these symptoms, as explained above (US EPA 1994).

Sulphur dioxide-induced symptoms and lung function changes can be reversed rapidly by common β_2-adrenergic agonist medications (e.g. salbutamol, terbutaline) and may be prevented prophylactically by cromolyn sodium or β-agonists. Not all asthma medications are effective in this regard (e.g. ipratropium bromide). Theophylline or inhaled steroids do not significantly reduce the effects of SO_2 in asthmatics (Folinsbee 1995). Following inhalation exposure to SO_2, asthmatic individuals show a refractory period that lasts about 3–4 h, during which time the airway response to SO_2 is considerably blunted. The symptoms and lung function responses of asthmatics who are exposed to SO_2 are often self-limiting and, in many cases, undergo spontaneous reversal within an hour or so.

In an environment where significant SO_2 exposure may occur, preventive treatment with cromolyn sodium or β_2-sympathomimetics, which may be routinely used in any case, is likely to limit any potential effect of SO_2 on endurance performance. A typical precompetition warm-up may also have a prophylactic effect. The probability of exposure to

SO$_2$ levels sufficient to induce symptomatic bronchoconstriction is quite low in developed countries with effective regulation of SO$_2$ emissions. The likelihood of a significant exposure (i.e. asthmatics exercising in a high concentration of SO$_2$) is only about 2–5% annually in the general asthmatic population, although it may be higher in asthmatic endurance athletes because of their greater frequency and duration of exercise. Although there is a clear interaction between exercise and SO$_2$ exposure in causing bronchoconstriction, actual effects of SO$_2$ on exercise performance have not been tested.

Carbon monoxide

Carbon monoxide (CO) is well known as a gaseous poison that is responsible for many deaths annually, both accidental and intentional. Carbon monoxide is a by-product of incomplete combustion, especially from fires and exhaust from internal combustion engines. Because CO emissions of modern motor vehicles have been reduced significantly, the CO exposure in ambient air from this source has been much reduced except in enclosed or semienclosed spaces (e.g. parking garages, traffic tunnels, motorized vehicle events in indoor arenas). Exposure to CO indoors, from open cooking fires (e.g. barbecue grills), unvented gas or kerosene heaters or the use of gas-powered appliances or vehicles in enclosed spaces, is more likely to be of sufficient magnitude to cause biological responses. Occupational exposure to high CO levels may occur in firefighters.

Inhaled CO binds reversibly with haemoglobin, with an affinity approximately 250 times that of oxygen (Roughton & Darling 1944), to form carboxyhaemoglobin (COHb). Carbon monoxide is produced naturally in the body as a by-product of the metabolism of haemoproteins and this is primarily responsible for the background level of COHb (about 0.5–0.7%) found in healthy unexposed non-smokers. The high affinity of CO for haemoglobin prevents the accumulation of CO in tissues, but it is also responsible for the long half-time required to clear CO from the blood. When breathing a normal ambient pressure of oxygen, approximately half of the CO will be excreted every 2–4 h, the actual rate being dependent upon the inspired (ambient) concentration of CO.

Carboxyhaemoglobin levels in smokers range from 3 to 7%, depending on the numbers of cigarettes smoked in the last few hours as well as any additional ambient exposure. Because their average COHb levels are relatively high, smokers will typically excrete CO even when ambient CO levels are slightly elevated. On the other hand, non-smokers will accumulate CO at lower ambient concentrations. Carbon monoxide levels that might be encountered in vehicles in stopped traffic (40–50 ppm) could, over several hours, raise the non-smokers' COHb levels to as much as 5%, but would not increase the already elevated COHb of smokers.

Carbon monoxide reduces the oxygen-carrying capacity of the blood by binding with oxygen sites on the haemoglobin molecule. In addition, increased COHb causes a leftward shift of the oxygen–haemoglobin dissociation curve, which results in reduced unloading of oxygen at the tissue level. The decrease in oxygen-carrying capacity causes a decrease in maximal oxygen intake. The decrease in $\dot{V}o_{2max}$ is linearly related to the COHb concentration (see Fig. 42.2). However, levels below about 4% COHb have not caused a statistically significant decrement in maximal oxygen intake of healthy subjects. At COHb levels of up to about 15–20%, moderate (30–60% $\dot{V}o_{2max}$) submaximal exercise in healthy untrained individuals is unaffected because increased cardiac output can compensate for the decreased oxygen-carrying capacity of the blood. At heavy (65–85% $\dot{V}o_{2max}$) submaximal exercise intensities, or at lower intensities in highly trained individuals, the cardiovascular system may be unable to compensate for the loss of oxygen-carrying capacity. Ability to sustain maximal exercise also may be impaired by elevated COHb levels as low as 3–5%.

Despite the reduced oxygen-carrying capacity of the blood, the increased COHb does not alter ventilation levels at exercise intensities below the lactic acid threshold (LAT). However, increased COHb also lowers the LAT. At work intensities above the LAT, ventilation and lactate levels are increased, and end-tidal CO$_2$ is decreased (Koike et al. 1991).

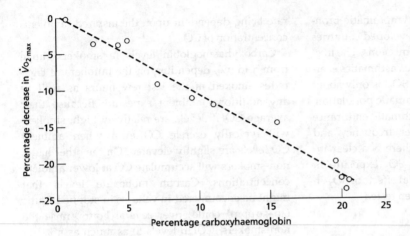

Fig. 42.2 Effect of increase in carboxyhaemoglobin (COHb) level on maximum oxygen intake in healthy subjects. The data point at $\dot{V}_{O_{2max}} = 0$ represents the non-exposed, nonsmoker healthy population mean for COHb (modified from Folinsbee 1992 by the addition of data from Koike *et al.* 1991).

Reduced inspired P_{O_2} (altitude) and increased COHb reduce maximum oxygen intake by different mechanisms. Hypoxia leads to a reduction in haemoglobin saturation, whereas carbon monoxide reduces the number of oxygen-carrying sites available. In residents at moderate altitude (1.5–2.5 km), the effect of minor increases of COHb (<6%) on peak $\dot{V}_{O_2}$ is similar to that in sea-level residents. At higher altitudes and higher COHb concentrations, the combination of the two stressors may cause effects in hypoxia-sensitive tissues.

Summary

Air pollutant exposure can affect exercise performance. Ozone causes symptomatic airway injury and inflammation. Pain on deep inspiration reduces vital capacity, which leads in turn to alterations in the breathing pattern. These and other respiratory symptoms also lead to reduced performance. These effects can be minimized by antioxidant supplementation and prophylactic use of non-steroidal anti-inflammatory medication.

Carbon monoxide reduces the oxygen-carrying capacity of the blood, thus reducing maximum oxygen intake and anaerobic threshold. The best preventive measure is to avoid exposure for at least 3–4 h prior to endurance competition.

Sulphur dioxide leads to bronchoconstriction in asthmatic individuals and could cause a ventilatory limitation in performance. The effects of SO_2 can be mitigated by the prophylactic use of either cromolyn sodium or a β_2-sympathomimetic medication (e.g. salbutamol). β_2-Sympathomimetics can also be used to reverse SO_2-induced bronchoconstriction.

References

Adams, W.C. & Schelegle, E.S. (1983) Ozone and high ventilation effects on pulmonary function and endurance performance. *Journal of Applied Physiology* **55**, 805–812.

Adams, W.C., Savin, W.M. & Christo, A.E. (1981) Detection of ozone toxicity during continuous exercise via the effective dose concept. *Journal of Applied Physiology* **51**, 415–422.

Åstrand, P.-O. & Rodahl, K. (1977) *Textbook of Work Physiology: Physiological Bases of Exercise*, 2nd edn, p. 465. McGraw-Hill Book Company, New York.

Avol, E.L., Linn, W.S., Venet, T.G., Shamoo, D.A. & Hackney, J.D. (1984) Comparative respiratory effects of ozone and ambient oxidant pollution exposure during heavy exercise. *Journal of the Air Pollution Control Association* **34**, 804–809.

Bates, D.V. (1995) Observations on asthma. *Environmental Health Perspectives* **103** (Suppl. 6), 243–247.

Bates, D.V., Bell, G.M., Burnham, C.D. *et al.* (1972) Short-term effects of ozone on the lung. *Journal of Applied Physiology* **32**, 176–181.

Beckett, W.S., McDonnell, W.F., Horstman, D.H. & House, D.E. (1985) Role of the parasympathetic nervous system in acute lung response to ozone. *Journal of Applied Physiology* **59**, 1879–1885.

Brunekreef, B., Hoek, G., Breugelmans, O. & Leentvaar, M. (1994) Respiratory effects of low-level photochemical air pollution in amateur cyclists. *American Journal of Respiratory and Critical Care Medicine* **150**, 962–966.

Chatham, M.D., Eppler, J.H. Jr, Sauder, L.R., Green, D. & Kulle, T.J. (1987) Evaluation of the effects of vitamin C on ozone-induced bronchoconstriction in normal subjects. *Annals of the New York Academy of Sciences* **498**, 269–279.

Coleridge, H.M., Coleridge, J.C.G., Baker, D.G., Ginzel, K.H. & Morrison, M.A. (1978) Comparison of the effects of histamine and prostaglandin on afferent C-fiber endings and irritant receptors in the intrapulmonary airways. *Advances in Experimental Medicine and Biology* **99**, 291–305.

Coleridge, J.C.G., Coleridge, H.M., Schelegle, E.S. & Green, J.F. (1993) Acute inhalation of ozone stimulates bronchial C-fibers and rapidly adapting receptors in dogs. *Journal of Applied Physiology* **74**, 2345–2352.

D'Urzo, A.D., Chapman, K.R. & Rebuck, A.S. (1985) Effect of elastic loading on ventilatory pattern during progressive exercise. *Journal of Applied Physiology* **59**, 34–38.

D'Urzo, A.D., Chapman, K.R. & Rebuck, A.S. (1987) Effect of inspiratory resistive loading on control of ventilation during progressive exercise. *Journal of Applied Physiology* **62**, 134–140.

El-Manshawi, A., Killian, K.J., Summers, E. & Jones, N.L. (1986) Breathlessness during exercise with and without resistive loading. *Journal of Applied Physiology* **61**, 896–905.

Eschenbacher, W.L., Ying, R.L., Kreit, J.W. & Gross, K.B. (1989) Ozone-induced lung function changes in normal and asthmatic subjects and the effect of indomethacin. In: Schneider, T., Lee, S.D., Wolters, G.J.R. & Grant, L.D. (eds) *Atmospheric Ozone Research and its Policy Implications: Proceedings of the 3rd US–Dutch International Symposium, May 1988, Nijmegen, the Netherlands*, pp. 493–499. Elsevier Science Publishers, Amsterdam.

Folinsbee, L.J. (1992) Human health effects of air pollution. *Environmental Health Perspectives* **100**, 45–56.

Folinsbee, L.J. (1995) Sulfur oxides: controlled human exposure studies. In: Lee, S.D. & Schneider, T. (eds) *Comparative Risk Analysis and Priority Setting for Air Pollution Issues: Proceedings of the 4th US–Dutch International Symposium, June 1993, Keystone, CO*, pp. 326–334. Air & Waste Management Association, Pittsburgh.

Folinsbee, L.J., Silverman, F. & Shephard, R.J. (1977) Decrease of maximum work performance following ozone exposure. *Journal of Applied Physiology* **42**, 531–536.

Folinsbee, L.J., Drinkwater, B.L., Bedi, J.F. & Horvath, S.M. (1978) The influence of exercise on the pulmonary function changes due to exposure to low concen-

trations of ozone. In: Folinsbee, L.J., Wagner, J.A., Borgia, J.F., Drinkwater, B.L., Gliner, J.A. & Bedi, J.F. (eds) *Environmental Stress: Individual Human Adaptations*, pp. 125–145. Academic Press, New York.

Folinsbee, L.J., Bedi, J.F. & Horvath, S.M. (1984) Pulmonary function changes after 1 h continuous heavy exercise in 0.21 ppm ozone. *Journal of Applied Physiology* **57**, 984–988.

Folinsbee, L.J., Kim, C.S., Kehrl, H.R., Prah, J.D. & Devlin, R.B. (1997) Methods in human inhalation toxicology. In: Massaro, E.J. (ed.) *Handbook of Human Toxicology*, pp. 607–670. CRC Press, Boca Raton.

Forsyth, R.D., Cole, P. & Shephard, R.J. (1983) Exercise and nasal patency. *Journal of Applied Physiology* **55**, 860–865.

Foxcroft, W.J. & Adams, W.C. (1986) Effects of ozone exposure on four consecutive days on work performance and $\dot{V}o_{2max}$. *Journal of Applied Physiology* **61**, 960–966.

Gong, H. Jr, Bradley, P.W., Simmons, M.S. & Tashkin, D.P. (1986) Impaired exercise performance and pulmonary function in élite cyclists during low-level ozone exposure in a hot environment. *American Review of Respiratory Disease* **134**, 726–733.

Gong, H. Jr, Bedi, J.F. & Horvath, S.M. (1988) Inhaled albuterol does not protect against ozone toxicity in nonasthmatic athletes. *Archives of Environmental Health* **43**, 46–53.

Grievink, L., Jansen, S.M.A., van't Veer, P. & Brunekreef, B. (1998) Acute effects of ozone on pulmonary function of cyclists receiving antioxidant supplements. *Occupational and Environmental Medicine* **55**, 13–17.

Hazucha, M.J. (1987) Relationship between ozone exposure and pulmonary function changes. *Journal of Applied Physiology* **62**, 1671–1680.

Hazucha, M.J., Bates, D.V. & Bromberg, P.A. (1989) Mechanism of action of ozone on the human lung. *Journal of Applied Physiology* **67**, 1535–1541.

Holtzman, M.J., Cunningham, J.H., Sheller, J.R., Irsigler, G.B., Nadel, J.A. & Boushey, H.A. (1979) Effect of ozone on bronchial reactivity in atopic and nonatopic subjects. *American Review of Respiratory Diseases* **120**, 1059–1067.

Horvath, S.M., Gliner, J.A. & Matsen-Twisdale, J.A. (1979) Pulmonary function and maximum exercise responses following acute ozone exposure. *Aviation, Space, and Environmental Medicine* **50**, 901–905.

Koike, A., Wasserman, K., Armon, Y. & Weiler-Ravell, D. (1991) The work rate-dependent effect of carbon monoxide on ventilatory control during exercise. *Respiration Physiology* **85**, 169–183.

Kreit, J.W., Gross, K.B., Moore, T.B., Lorenzen, T.J., D'Arcy, J. & Eschenbacher, W.L. (1989) Ozone-induced changes in pulmonary function and bronchial responsiveness in asthmatics. *Journal of Applied Physiology* **66**, 217–222.

Kulle, T.J., Sauder, L.R., Hebel, J.R. & Chatham, M.D. (1985) Ozone response relationships in healthy nonsmokers. *American Review of Respiratory Disease* **132**, 36–41.

Lee, L.-Y., Dumont, C., Djokic, T.D., Menzel, T.E. & Nadel, J.A. (1979) Mechanism of rapid, shallow breathing after ozone exposure in conscious dogs. *Journal of Applied Physiology* **46**, 1108–1114.

McDonnell, W.F., Horstman, D.H., Hazucha, M.J. *et al.* (1983) Pulmonary effects of ozone exposure during exercise: dose–response characteristics. *Journal of Applied Physiology* **54**, 1345–1352.

McDonnell, W.F., Horstman, D.H., Abdul-Salaam, S., Raggio, L.J. & Green, J.A. (1987) The respiratory responses of subjects with allergic rhinitis to ozone exposure and their relationship to nonspecific airway reactivity. *Toxicology and Industrial Health* **3**, 507–517.

McDonnell, W., Koren, H., Devlin, R., Abdul-Salaam, S., Ives, P. & O'Neil, J. (1990) Biochemical and cellular correlates of changes in pulmonary functions and symptoms in humans exposed to ozone. *American Review of Respiratory Diseases* **141**, A72.

Mihevic, P.M., Gliner, J.A. & Horvath, S.M. (1981) Perception of effort and respiratory sensitivity during exposure to ozone. *Ergonomics* **24**, 365–374.

Philip, G., Jankowski, R., Baroody, F.M., Naclerio, R.M. & Togias, A.G. (1993) Reflex activation of nasal secretion by unilateral inhalation of cold dry air. *American Review of Respiratory Diseases* **148**, 1616–1622.

Roughton, F.J.W. & Darling, R.C. (1944) The effect of carbon monoxide on the oxyhemoglobin dissociation curve. *American Journal of Physiology* **141**, 17–31.

Savin, W.M. & Adams, W.C. (1979) Effects of ozone inhalation on work performance and $\dot{V}o_{2max}$. *Journal of Applied Physiology* **46**, 309–314.

Scannell, C.H., Chen, L.L., Aris, R. *et al.* (1996) Greater ozone-induced inflammatory responses in subjects with asthma.

American Journal of Respiratory and Critical Care Medicine **154**, 24–29.

Schelegle, E.S. & Adams, W.C. (1986) Reduced exercise time in competitive simulations consequent to low level ozone exposure. *Medicine and Science in Sports and Exercise* **18**, 408–414.

Schelegle, E.S., Adams, W.C. & Siefkin, A.D. (1987) Indomethacin pretreatment reduces ozone-induced pulmonary function decrements in human subjects. *American Review of Respiratory Diseases* **136**, 1350–1354.

Schelegle, E.S., Carl, M.L., Coleridge, H.M., Coleridge, J.C.G. & Green, J.F. (1993) Contribution of vagal afferents to respiratory reflexes evoked by acute inhalation of ozone in dogs. *Journal of Applied Physiology* **74**, 2338–2344.

Seal, E. Jr, McDonnell, W.F., House, D.E. *et al.* (1993) The pulmonary response of white and black adults to six concentrations of ozone. *American Review of Respiratory Diseases* **147**, 804–810.

US EPA (1994) *Supplement to the second addendum (1986) to air quality criteria for particulate matter and sulfur oxides (1982): assessment of new findings on sulfur dioxide acute exposure health effects in asthmatic individuals.* Report no. EPA-600/FP-93/002, US Environmental Protection Agency, Research Triangle Park, NC. Available at www.epa.gov/ncepihom/nepishom.

Voy, R.O. (1986) The US Olympic Committee experience with exercise-induced bronchospasm, 1984. *Medicine and Science in Sports and Exercise* **18**, 328–330.

Wayne, W.S., Wehrle, P.F. & Carroll, R.E. (1967) Oxidant air pollution and athletic performance. *Journal of the American Medical Association* **199**, 151–154.

Weymer, A.R., Gong, H. Jr, Lyness, A. & Linn, W.S. (1994) Pre-exposure to ozone does not enhance or produce exercise-induced asthma. *American Journal of Respiratory and Critical Care Medicine* **149**, 1413–1419.

Ying, R.L., Gross, K.B., Terzo, T.S. & Eschenbacher, W.L. (1990) Indomethacin does not inhibit the ozone-induced increase in bronchial responsiveness in human subjects. *American Review of Respiratory Disease* **142**, 817–821.

Chapter 43

Endurance Performers and Time-Zone Shifts

THOMAS REILLY, GREG ATKINSON AND JIM WATERHOUSE

Introduction

Sport competitions, particularly those requiring endurance, are distributed throughout the world. This widespread availability of competition has been facilitated by television and commercial sponsorship, as well as the ease of human transportation by air. Tournaments for team sports have assumed a more global representation than in previous decades, and games players regularly travel overseas in seeking international competition.

Travel is nowadays an accepted feature of the habitual activity of endurance athletes and games players. It may entail travelling internally within the same country, for example interstate competitions in North America or Australia, or across multiple national boundaries within the continents of Europe or Asia. Such journeys can be disruptive, causing tiredness and boredom, particularly in experienced travellers for whom air travel is no longer exhilarating. Travel fatigue may be further compounded if the journey is overnight and prevents normal sleep. Furthermore, long-haul flights may be associated with a gradual dehydration due to ambient conditions on board the aircraft, particularly the low water vapour content in cabin air.

Residual effects of the flight itself can be ameliorated once the destination is reached. This applies to air travel from North America to South America or from Western European countries to South Africa, for example, where the journey does not entail crossing multiple transmeridian boundaries. Stiffness from being too long in a cramped posture may be offset by periodically walking along the cabin aisle, performing light stretching exercises or isometric contractions. Such activity may also reduce the risk of deep vein thrombosis associated with being seated in a cramped posture for many hours. Drinking copiously, preferably avoiding coffee and alcohol because of their diuretic effects, helps to avoid the dehydration that can cause discomfort after disembarkation. A postflight shower or light exercise session can then have positive recuperative effects. Flying eastwards or westwards across different time zones presents a unique set of problems for the travelling endurance athlete, in that such time shifts disturb the body's circadian rhythms. The desynchronization of human circadian timekeepers causes the phenomenon known as jet lag.

The human body clock

The human circadian rhythm is controlled by the suprachiasmatic cells of the hypothalamus. The major determinant of the timing of circadian rhythms is the spin of the Earth about its vertical axis. The associated alternation of environmental darkness and light is matched by the sleep–activity cycle in humans. Information about the alternation of light and dark is transmitted directly to the suprachiasmatic nuclei from the eyes. There is another less direct route, via melatonin. The pineal gland deep within the brain is sensitive to changes in light intensity during the day, and it possesses important time-keeping functions. The hormone melatonin is synthesized from serotonin in the pineal gland, and there is a secondary source of melatonin within the retina. Human melatonin

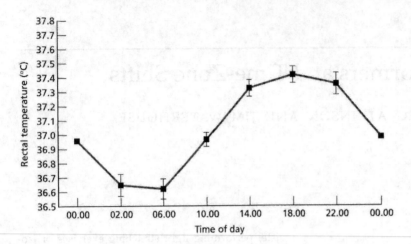

Fig. 43.1 The normal circadian rhythm in rectal temperature.

levels are not measurable during the day, but increase rapidly around dusk and stay at an elevated level through the night. The rise in melatonin accompanies a fall in body temperature of around 0.8°C from its highest point at about 18.00 h to a nadir in the early morning (Fig. 43.1). The changing levels of melatonin and the time information they contain are monitored by the suprachiasmatic nuclei.

Many components of team game performance demonstrate a circadian rhythm that approximates the circadian curve in body temperature. These measures include muscle strength and power, joint flexibility, and circulatory and metabolic responses to submaximal exercise (Reilly 1990). Ventilation also exhibits a circadian rhythm during low to moderate exercise and, at least at the start of sustained exercise, the ventilatory equivalent for oxygen ($\dot{V}_E/\dot{V}_{O_2}$) is low when core temperature is at its trough (Fig. 43.2).

The pace at which individuals choose to commence sustained exercise depends on the time of day; speed is lowest in the early morning (Fig. 43.3) and highest in the evening (Atkinson *et al.* 1993a). A preference for evening exercise was evident in the work rate of soccer players during indoor four-a-side games that were sustained for 4 days (Reilly & Walsh 1981). The pace of play reached a peak at 18.00 h and a trough 12 h later, closely conforming to the curve in body temperature. Feelings of fatigue

were correlated negatively with levels of physical activity.

Individual factors influence circadian rhythm characteristics. Introverts tend to be better performers in the morning, whereas extroverts reach a peak later in the day and stay alert for longer in the evening. Whilst such differences may be relevant when the direction of a time-zone shift is considered, the difference in the acrophase (timing of the peak) of body temperature between these personality types is only about 1 h. Individual differences in chronotypes have been described in terms of morningness–eveningness, that is, 'morning types' and 'evening types'. The preference for timing of diurnal activity is thought to be more important than personality in determining responses to circadian phase shifts, 'morning types' having the advantage on travelling eastwards and being disadvantaged by a westward flight.

The control of circadian rhythms in physiological and performance variables is affected by age (Reilly *et al.* 1997c). Older subjects show a reduced amplitude and a tendency towards morningness in their circadian cycles. Veteran cyclists plan greater amounts of their training for morning sessions than do young adults, and in endurance time trials they are relatively closer to their peak evening times than are their younger counterparts. The flatter circadian rhythm does not benefit older individuals, who tend to suffer more extreme symptoms and may take

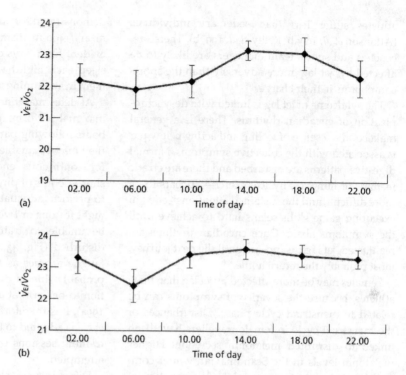

Fig. 43.2 The circadian rhythm in $\dot{V}_E/\dot{V}_{O_2}$ in response to (a) light and (b) moderate exercise on a cycle ergometer.

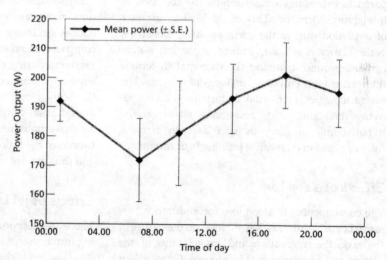

Fig. 43.3 The self-chosen exercise intensity demonstrates a circadian function.

longer than younger people to recover following long-haul flights across multiple time zones.

Jet lag

The symptoms of jet lag include periodic fatigue during the day and yet inability to sleep at night, difficulty in concentrating, mental confusion and disorientation, increased irritability and loss of vigour. Symptoms are generally more severe and last longer following a flight eastwards compared to a flight westwards, and they are more intense the more time zones that have been traversed. Younger people suffer less than older individuals and athletes suffer less than sedentary individuals (Atkinson *et al.* 1993b; Reilly *et al.* 1997b). Therefore, coaches and sports team managers are likely to be affected by 'jet lag' more adversely than the sports competitors in their charge.

The syndrome of jet lag is linked with desynchronization of circadian rhythms. There is a general malaise, and a sense of feeling and acting below par is associated with the collective symptoms. Normal digestive patterns are disturbed and there are erratic feelings of hunger. Physical exercise appears to be more difficult, and the sustained attention needed in executing game skills seems hard to achieve until the symptoms abate. Once circadian rhythms are readjusted, jet lag disappears until the next journey, most probably the return home.

Females may be more affected by jet lag than male athletes, because the severity of symptoms can be related to menstrual cycle phase. Disturbances of the menstrual cycle in female travellers have been linked to disrupted melatonin secretion. Higher melatonin levels in the Scandinavian winter compared to values in summer inhibit the secretion of luteinizing hormone. This could lead to absence of ovulation during the corresponding menstrual cycle (Harma *et al.* 1994). Indeed, secondary amenorrhoea is more common than normal in female flight attendants employed on long-haul flights. The extent to which menstrual disturbances accompanying time-zone shifts accentuate stress on the hypothalamic–pituitary–ovarian axis in females fully engaged in endurance training is uncertain.

Effects of sleep loss

The consequences of sleep loss for endurance performance are complex; they depend on the nature of the task, the motivation and expectations of the subject and environmental influences. Gross motor performances may be unaffected by partial sleep deprivation for 2–3 days, whereas performances that depend on mental decision-making can be affected adversely by one night when sleep is restricted to 3 h (Reilly & Deykin 1983). The magnitude of the time of day effect on muscle performance is greater than that due to restricting sleep to 3 h only (Reilly & Hales 1988). This has also been demonstrated for swimming performance over 100-m and 400-m distances; the time of day effect is evident for 3 days of partial sleep deprivation (3 h sleep each night) without any significant impairment in swimming times (Sinnerton & Reilly 1992).

Athletes may find themselves capable of normal maximal performance in single short-term exercise bouts following partial sleep loss, but nevertheless they may be unable to maintain the effort required for continuous endurance exercise or repetitive shorter bouts of physical activity. They may be able to perform adequately if sleep is restricted to 3 h a night for one or two nights, but thereafter they will be unable to train maximally if sleep remains disturbed (Fig. 43.4). In typical training sessions, fatigue accrues as the training session progresses, probably due to difficulty in maintaining motivation to perform at a high intensity (Reilly & Piercy 1994). It is therefore important that the sleep–wake cycle is adapted to the new environment before full training sessions or competitive engagements are attempted.

Difficulties in sleeping after crossing multiple time zones are eventually self-correcting. Disturbances are likely to last longer following eastward compared to westward flight. Napping at times of tiredness during the new local day is to be avoided, since a prolonged nap may retard adjustment of the body clock to the new time zone (Minors & Waterhouse 1981a). Furthermore, sedative drugs can have potential hangover effects on muscle performance the following morning (Zinzen *et al.* 1994) and thus are not recommended.

Effects of jet lag on performance

There are methodological difficulties in demonstrating impairments in sport performance due to jet lag. To show such changes in performance, it is necessary to identify circadian characteristics of the performance rhythm as it is being re-established. This is practically impossible for endurance sport, due to likely residual effects of repetitive testing. Thus inferences about the influence of jet lag on endurance performance or games play must rely on retrospective analyses of competitive matches or research on selected components of performance.

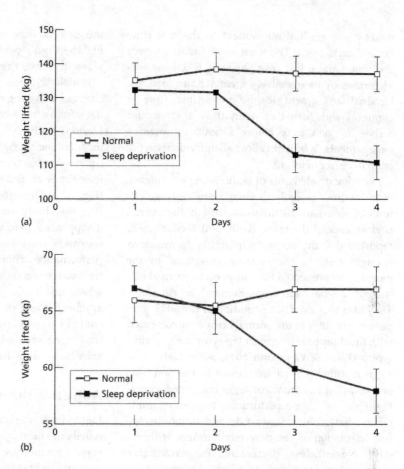

Fig. 43.4 Maximum leg-press (b) and maximum deadlift (a) over 4 days of sleep deprivation and during 4 days of normal sleep ($n = 8$).

Deleterious effects of jet lag have been demonstrated in American footballers after travelling coast-to-coast. Teams travelling from western to central or eastern zones were detrimentally affected except when matches were played at night. West-coast teams playing at home in the evening were found to have an advantage (Jehue *et al.* 1993). When going eastwards, overall mean performance was depressed more and the peak performance declined more than was the case when teams travelled westwards. This is compatible with the fact that the 'body clock' adjusts more easily to a lengthening rather than a shortening of the day, its innate period being marginally in excess of 24 h when observed under free running conditions. Modifying training times for a few days before departure to reflect the time of competition in the other time zone was of some benefit to American footballers (Jehue

et al. 1993). Similar trends are likely to apply to Australian athletes travelling from coast to coast or to Europeans moving across continental time zones for competitive engagements.

Whilst team performance is determined by a host of factors, retrospective analysis of competitive results permits investigation of how robust the effects of jet lag may be. The effects of jet lag on American footballers after the coast-to-coast trips reported by Jehue *et al.* (1993) have been corroborated by others. Teams from the west coast of the US competing against opponents from the east coast in Monday night football games (start time 21.00 h) had an advantage by virtue of the greater proximity of the start time to their circadian rhythm acrophase at 18.00 h (Smith *et al.* 1997). Observations made on the former USSR volleyball team during consecutive competitions in Japan were interpreted as evidence of gradual adjustment to the new time zone (Sasaki 1980). The team lost its matches over the first 3 days, but over the next 6 days it was victorious by progressively greater point margins. Gradual adjustment to the new time zone is common with teams on tour; thus, they should arrive in good time before serious competitive engagements, in order to allow all individuals in the team to be free of jet lag.

Focusing on elements of endurance performance in individuals is likely to yield more sensitive criteria of circadian disturbances than is the overall performance of the team. Reilly and Mellor (1988) reported that the normal superiority in muscular strength tests in the evening compared to the morning was reversed for 5 days on the arrival of a Rugby League team from England in Australia. They also showed that restoration of the body temperature rhythm to the normal acrophase coincided with the disappearance of jet lag symptoms. Klein's group (Klein & Wegmann 1974, 1980; Klein et al. 1977) reported a 3–4% decrement in reaction time and complex psychomotor tasks compared to pre-flight values. Those performing the more simple tasks adjusted at a faster rate and demonstrated full adaptation to the new environment within 3 days. Nevertheless, decrements in performance were evident for 5 days postflight. Decrements in arm strength, elbow flexor strength and sprint times (6–13% lower than preflight baselines) were reported for 81 military personnel following a flight eastwards across six time zones (Wright et al. 1983). Following air travel, there were significant reductions in the endurance performance of elbow flexor

muscles and time for a 2.8-km run. Five days following the flight, perceived exertion during exercise was still greater than normal.

British Olympic male gymnasts demonstrated changes in a range of performance measures for 5 days following a trip from London to Tallahassee, Florida (Reilly et al. 1997a). The dependent variables included leg strength, back strength, choice reaction time and subjective jet lag symptoms, all monitored four times each day on alternate days for a week (Fig. 43.5). The sleep–wake cycle was re-established first, then body temperature; jet lag symptoms also disappeared before rhythms in the performance measures were completely stabilized. Whilst the performance criteria were essentially short term, they are nevertheless relevant to games contexts where anaerobic effects are superimposed on an acyclic pattern of aerobic demands. It was concluded that an allowance of 1 day to adapt for each time zone crossed was insufficient to permit all subjects to adjust fully to the new local time.

Adjusting the body clock

Left to itself, the body clock would run with a periodicity of about 25 h compared to the 24 h needed to stay in harmony with the night–day cycle of darkness and light (Minors & Waterhouse 1981b). Under normal circumstances, the body clock is adjusted in the same way as a watch that keeps time poorly — by external signals. Several signals adjust circadian rhythms, and making use of them helps the body adjust to time-zone transitions.

The main signal is exposure to light, particularly

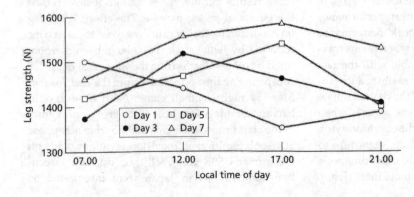

Fig. 43.5 Re-establishment of normal circadian rhythm of leg strength in a group of 17 subjects following a westward flight across five time zones.

direct sunlight out of doors. This acts both directly and via the rhythm of melatonin (see above). Additional factors that may promote adjustment include: (i) the pattern of sleep and activity (including exercise); (ii) the timing and type of meals; and (iii) exposure to social influences.

The necessity to adjust the body clock is demonstrated in Fig. 43.6. The biological clock is clearly at odds with environmental cues. Any attempt to

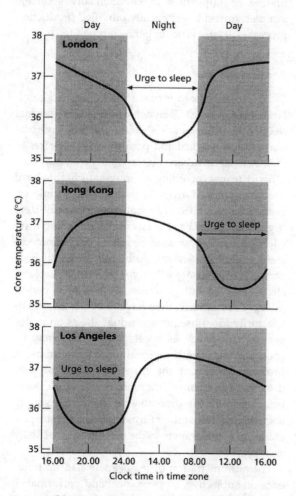

Fig. 43.6 Diagrammatic representation of the circadian rhythm of the core (rectal) temperature in an individual who sleeps generally 24.00–08.00 h and is mainly sedentary during the day. The curves demonstrate how the core temperature is out of harmony with the urge to sleep after travelling eastwards (to Hong Kong) and westwards (to Los Angeles).

promote adjustment must consider whether a phase delay or a phase advance is required.

Promoting adjustment of the body clock

The process of adjustment

Complete adjustment of the body clock takes several days. The aim is to speed up this process as much and as safely as possible, since peak performance will only be restored when the athlete is fully adjusted to the new time zone. This applies to training as well as to competition. Until the circadian rhythm is normalized, it is more difficult for an individual to produce maximal effort. While adjustment is taking place, the characteristics of the rhythm are changed. It displays a lower amplitude, a lower peak value and a lower average value overall (Reilly et al. 1997b).

A practice frequently adopted by athletes prior to flying overseas in a westward direction is to go to bed some hours later than normal each night and to get up a similar amount of time later each morning. It may not always be possible to do this, but its main benefit is to encourage thinking ahead about times in the country of destination. In contrast, those going eastwards bring forward getting to bed and getting up by some hours. It is not useful to try to adjust fully to the time-zone transition before the journey, since this would interrupt training schedules and lifestyle too much and it may not have a large effect on the body clock (Reilly & Maskell 1989). This advice applies to both a phase delay (getting to sleep later) and a phase advance (getting to bed earlier). Nocturnal shift-workers, for example, are unlikely to reverse their circadian rhythms fully when working nights, since the natural alternations of daytime light and night-time darkness remain unchanged.

Where there is a choice of flight times and airports, the player or team manager should select a schedule that facilitates adjustments of circadian rhythm. A flight that gets the European traveller to the US destination in the evening, for example, would be helpful. For trips that entail crossing eight time zones or more, it can be beneficial to plan an overnight stopover midway; this avoids the severe symptoms that are experienced if the journey is completed without a break. The ideal travel schedule is seldom possible, but at least available alternatives should be considered.

Possibilities for speeding adjustment

Athletes and coaches must acknowledge the disturbance of the body's circadian rhythms that follows rapid travel across time zones if they are to take steps to accelerate adjustment to the new time zone. Several strategies have been proposed (Waterhouse *et al.* 1997), differing in their practicality and in their potential side-effects. They embrace nutritional, pharmacological, environmental and behavioural measures.

Timing and composition of meals

It has been suggested that high protein breakfasts promote alertness and that high carbohydrate evening meals (vegetables, potatoes, rice, bread, pasta, desserts, and so on) promote sleep (Graeber *et al.* 1981). The theory is that such meals affect plasma amino acids and, thence, the uptake of amino acids into the brain, their incorporation into neurotransmitters and the release of neurotransmitters. High protein meals (meat, cheese, eggs, etc.) raise plasma tyrosine concentrations, but whether this elevation promotes the release of catecholamines by the activating systems of the brain, and so increases alertness, is less clear. Similarly, high carbohydrate meals elevate the concentration of plasma tryptophan, but whether this rise stimulates the raphé nucleus and sleep is uncertain (Leathwood 1989).

Studies of electroencephalographic (EEG) waves during sleep have shown some changes in athletes on a carbohydrate-rich diet (Francart *et al.* 1995), but effects on sleep latency or on the quality of sleep have not been demonstrated. The two-phase dietary method (alternating feeding and fasting) was marketed in the US under the title 'President Reagan's antijet lag-diet', but its benefits have not been confirmed experimentally.

Only small improvements in sleep and mental performance were observed when the efficacy of dietary manipulation was examined in military per-

sonnel (Graeber 1989), but studies have been few and poorly designed. A variant of this proposal comprises two types of pill, one to be taken in the morning and the other in the evening. Each pill contains a mixture of substances; the morning pill includes tyrosine, and the evening one tryptophan. The accompanying marketing literature does not enable a judgement to be made on the scientific value of these preparations. Besides, L-tryptophan achieved adverse publicity in 1990 owing to the finding of impurities in commercially available samples, linked to genetically modified production processes. Its use is no longer recommended.

Sedatives

Disturbance of sleep is one of the unwanted corollaries of jet lag. Resynchronizing the normal sleep–wakefulness cycle seems to precede a restoration of physiological and performance measures to their normal circadian rhythm (Reilly *et al.* 1997a).

Sport teams travelling on long-haul flights have used various sedatives to induce sleep while on board the aircraft (Reilly 1990). Minor tranquillizers (e.g. temazepam) have been employed to help travellers get to sleep, so as to be refreshed for immediate activities on arrival. Although drugs such as benzodiazepines are effective in getting people to sleep, they do not guarantee a prolonged period asleep. Furthermore, they have not been tested satisfactorily for subsequent residual effects on motor performance, such as sports skills. They may be counterproductive if given at an incorrect time. A prolonged sleep at the time an individual feels drowsy (presumably when he or she would have been asleep in the time zone of departure) simply anchors rhythms at their former phases and so operates against adjustment to the new time zone (Reilly *et al.* 1997b).

The administration of temazepam had no influence on subjective, physiological and performance measures following a westward flight across five time zones (Reilly *et al.* 1997a). The circadian rhythms of athletes differed from those of sedentary subjects, although neither group benefited from the medication. Whether short-acting hypnotics such as zolpidem, which has a shorter half-life than most benzodiazepines, would be effective in such cases and in adjustment to more extreme phase shifts remains to be clarified.

Melatonin

In normal circumstances, melatonin from the pineal gland is secreted into the bloodstream between about 21.00 and 07.00 h. It can be regarded as a 'dark pulse' or 'internal time cue' for the body clock (Atkinson et al. 1997). Some studies have shown that if melatonin capsules are taken in the evening of the new time zone they reduce the symptoms of 'jet lag' (Arendt et al. 1987). Whilst this is an important finding, there are some caveats:

1 Jet lag was assessed subjectively in these studies. It is not known if there would also be improvements in mental and physical performance, and in motivation to train hard—or even if these variables would show further decrements.

2 It is not clear if melatonin produces its effect by promoting adjustment of the body clock or by some other means (increasing a sense of well-being or the ability to sleep, for example). Whilst recent work suggests that melatonin can adjust the body clock, a beneficial effect requires careful timing of ingestion according to whether the need is to advance or delay the clock.

3 Melatonin lowers body temperature and this may account for its hypnotic action.

4 Melatonin is only just becoming commercially available (largely in the US) and the results from many clinical trials are still awaited. The commercially available capsules contain supraphysiological dosages, which may account for its transient unpleasant subjective effects.

More information is required before melatonin can be recommended. It is freely available in the US, but is not licensed for therapeutic use in Australia or Europe. Systematic monitoring of athletes voluntarily taking it during long-haul flights and days afterwards is needed to establish its effects. Nevertheless some endurance athletes currently use melatonin in attempts to shift their body clock and overcome jet lag more quickly. The following points need to be taken into consideration (Reilly et al. 1998):

1 It is impossible to predict the effect on the body's rhythms unless the timing of the body clock is known. The athlete must have spent some days in a local time zone and slept normally. Once travelling, it becomes very difficult to predict the phase of the body clock. If melatonin is given at the wrong 'body time', it may delay rather than accelerate adjustment to local time zones. When given prior to the trough of the circadian rhythm in body temperature, it advances the body clock, irrespective of local time. In contrast, when given following the trough of body temperature, it delays the timing of the body clock.

2 Sleepiness, headache, nausea and mild confusion are side-effects from ingesting melatonin capsules. An allergic reaction occurs in 1 in 240 individuals.

3 There is no proper control of ingredients when melatonin capsules are purchased in the US, and not all preparations are pure. There is particular danger in buying a product containing cow pineal gland. The tablets in most of the commercially available jars contain 3 mg melatonin. The warnings on the bottle must be taken seriously.

4 Plasma levels may vary by 25-fold in different individuals after a 5-mg dose, so effects are unpredictable.

Maintaining alertness

One approach towards combating jet lag is to use pharmacological means to promote and maintain alertness. Drugs used for this purpose include amphetamines, caffeine, modafinil (an α_1-adrenoceptor antagonist) and pemoline (a drug with dopamine-like properties). Although these drugs improve performance in several tasks, they affect the ability to initiate and sustain sleep adversely (Akerstedt & Ficca 1997). These effects could be counterproductive following time-zone transitions. Besides, their effects on physical performance relevant to endurance sport have not been adequately addressed, and their use could contravene doping regulations.

Bright light exposure and exercise

Bright light (that is, of an intensity found during natural daylight, but not normally indoors) can adjust the body clock. The timing of exposure is crucially important (Minors et al. 1991) and is the opposite of that for melatonin ingestion; thus, bright light in the morning (05.00–11.00 h according to body time) advances the clock and bright light in the evening (21.00–03.00 h on body time) delays it. It is important to avoid light exposure at times which produce a shift of the body clock in the opposite direction to that desired. Table 43.1 indicates times when light should be sought or avoided after different time-zone transitions; the appropriate timing varies as the body clock adjusts (see below).

Even though 'bright light' (>8000 lux) is of an intensity normally not achieved in domestic or interior lighting (normally <350 lux), commercial light boxes and visors that produce a light source sufficient in intensity are now available commercially (Waterhouse et al. 1998). Light visors, in particular, may prove useful. A modern ring of make-up lights produces 3000 lux, which is certainly enough, but the contemporary view is that bright indoor lighting (>1000 lux) is also valuable.

Since outdoor lighting is the obvious choice, it would be natural to consider training outdoors—for example, an easy training session—when light is required, and to relax indoors when it should be avoided. This raises the question whether physical exercise and inactivity can, in some way, add to the effects of light and dark, respectively. Current evidence is not conclusive.

For the first few days in the new time zone, maximal exercise should be avoided during training sessions. Skills requiring fine coordination are likely to be impaired, which could lead to accidents or injuries if players were to conduct training sessions or matches too strenuously. Where a series of tournament engagements is scheduled, it helps to have at least one friendly match during the initial period, that is, before the end of the first week in the overseas country. Subject to these caveats, exercise is recommended for sport participants. It helps adjust the body clock and also aids athletes in their mental preparations for competition.

In practice, therefore, to combine exposure to bright light and exercise, and to combine dim light and relaxation, would seem practicable. There is little research evidence to suggest that exercise by itself alters the speed of adjustment of the body clock in humans.

It might seem that to adjust as fully as possible to the *lifestyle and habits* of the new time zone would be the best remedy. This is not always the case on the first day or so after the flight. In the case of a westward flight through eight time zones, to delay the clock requires bright light at 21.00–03.00 h body time and its avoidance at 05.00–11.00 h. By new local time, this becomes equal to 13.00–19.00 h for bright light and 21.00–03.00 h for dim light (see Table 43.1). Natural daylight and darkness at night would provide this combination. Consider, by contrast, a flight to the east through eight time zones. Now light is required at 05.00–11.00 h body time (13.00–19.00 h local time) and should be avoided 21.00–03.00 h body time (05.00–11.00 h local time). That is, morning light for the first day or so *would be*

Table 43.1 The use of bright light to adjust the body clock after time-zone transitions.

	Bad local times for exposure to bright light	Good local times for exposure to bright light
Time zones to the west		
4 h	01.00–07.00*	17.00–23.00†
8 h	21.00–03.00*	13.00–19.00†
12 h	17.00–23.00*	09.00–15.00†
Time zones to the east		
4 h	01.00–07.00†	09.00–15.00*
8 h	05.00–11.00†	13.00–19.00*
10–12 h	Treat this as 12–14 h to the west‡	

* Will advance the body clock; † will delay the body clock; ‡ note that this is because the body clock adjusts to delays more easily than advances.

unhelpful and tend to make the clock adjust in the wrong direction (although light in the afternoon and in the evening is fine). The timing of exposure to bright light is critical on the first days after the flight (Table 43.1). After a couple of days, when partial adjustment has occurred, it is then advisable to change the timing of the light exposure towards that of the local inhabitants, so that the visitors' habits become synchronized with those of the local inhabitants.

Conclusions

Circadian rhythms must be taken into account when endurance or team game participants travel across multiple time zones to compete in sport. Deleterious effects of jet lag are exacerbated if there are additional environmental stressors, such as heat or altitude. Performance can be adversely affected even when flights are within one country, coast-to-coast in the US or Australia, for example. Whilst jet lag symptoms persist, even if only periodically during the day, it is recommended that training be kept to a low intensity to reduce possibilities of errors and injuries. Teams may be more vulnerable to defeat at the hands of home-based opponents in the early rounds of tournaments, unless the need to readjust first to the new time zone is taken into account when the 'tour' itinerary is being planned.

References

Akerstedt, T. & Ficca, G. (1997) Alertness-enhancing drugs as a countermeasure to fatigue in irregular work hours. *Chronobiology International* 14, 145–158.

Arendt, J., Aldhous, M., English, J. *et al.* (1987) Some effects of jet-lag and their alteration by melatonin. *Ergonomics* 3, 1379–1394.

Atkinson, G., Coldwells, A., Reilly, T. & Waterhouse, J. (1993a) Circadian rhythmicity in self-chosen work-rate. In: Gutenbrunner, C., Hildebrandt, G. & Moog, R. (eds) *Chronobiology and Chronomedicine: Basic Research and Applications*, pp. 478–484. Peter Lang, Frankfurt.

Atkinson, G., Coldwells, A., Reilly, T. & Waterhouse, J. (1993b) A comparison of circadian rhythms in work performance between physically active and inactive subjects. *Ergonomics* 36, 273–281.

Atkinson, G., Reilly, T., Waterhouse, J. & Winterburn, S. (1997) Pharmacology and the travelling athlete. In: Reilly, T. & Orme, M. (eds) *The Clinical Pharmacology of Sport and Exercise*, pp. 293–301. Elsevier, Amsterdam.

Francart, A.L., Davenne, D., François, T., Renaud, A. & Garnier, A. (1995) Influence du régime dissocié 'Scandinavian' sur la structure du sommeil des sportifs. *Comptes Rendues de la Société de Biologie* 183, 467–473.

Graeber, R.C. (1989) Jet lag and sleep disruption. In: Krugger, M.H., Roth, T. & Dement, C. (eds) *Principles and Practice in Sleep Medicine*, pp. 324–331. W.B. Saunders, Philadelphia.

Graeber, R., Sing, H. & Cuthbert, B. (1981) The impact of transmeridian flight on deploying soldiers. In: Johnson, L., Tepas, D. & Colquhoun, P. (eds) *Biological Rhythms, Sleep and Shiftwork*, pp. 513–537. MIT Press, Lancaster.

Harma, M., Laitinen, J., Partinen, M. & Savanto, S. (1994) The effect of four-day round trip flights over 10 time zones on the circadian variation of salivary melatonin and cortisol in air-time flight attendants. *Ergonomics* 37, 1479–1489.

Jehue, R., Street, D. & Huizenga, R. (1993) Effect of time zone and game time changes on peak performance: National Football League. *Medicine and Science in Sports and Exercise* 25, 127–131.

Klein, K.E. & Wegmann, H.M. (1974) The resynchronization of human circadian rhythms after transmediterranean flights as a result of flight direction and mode of activity. In: Scheving, L.E. Halberg, F. & Pauly, J.F. (eds) *Chronobiology*, pp. 564–570. Igaku Shoin, Tokyo.

Klein, K.E. & Wegmann, H.M. (1980) *Significance of Circadian Rhythms in Aerospace Operations*. Nato Agard (no. 247), Neuilly-sur-Seine.

Klein, K.E., Hermann, R., Kuklinski, P. & Wegmann, H.M. (1977) Circadian performance rhythms: experimental studies in air conditions. In: Mackie, R.R. (ed.) *Vigilance: Theory, Operational Performance and Physiological Correlates*, pp. 111–132. Plenum Press, New York.

Leathwood, P. (1989) Circadian rhythms of plasma amino acids, brain neurotransmitters and behaviour. In: Arendt, J., Minors, D. & Waterhouse, J. (eds) *Biological Rhythms in Clinical Practice*, pp. 131–159. John Wright, Bristol.

Minors, D.S. & Waterhouse, J.M. (1981a) Anchor sleep as a synchroniser of abnormal routines. *International Journal of Chronobiology* 7, 165–168.

Minors, D.S. & Waterhouse, J.M. (1981b) *Circadian Rhythms and the Human*. John Wright, Bristol.

Minors, D., Waterhouse, J. & Wirz-Justice, A. (1991) A human phase–response curve to light. *Neuroscience Letters* 133, 36–40.

Reilly, T. (1990) Human circadian rhythms and exercise. *Critical Reviews in Biomedical Engineering* 18, 165–180.

Reilly, T. & Deykin, T. (1983) Effects of partial sleep loss on subjective states, psychomotor and physical peformance tests. *Journal of Human Movement Studies* 9, 157–170.

Reilly, T. & Hales, A.J. (1988) Effects of partial sleep deprivation on performance measures in females. In: Megaw, E.D. (ed.) *Contemporary Ergonomics 1988*, pp. 509–514. Taylor & Francis, London.

Reilly, T. & Maskell, P. (1989) Effects of altering the sleep–wake cycle on human circadian rhythms and motor performance. *Proceedings of the First IOC Congress on Sports Sciences*, pp. 106–107. US Olympic Committee, Colorado Springs, CO.

Reilly, T. & Mellor, S. (1988) Jet-lag in student Rugby League players following a near-maximal time-zone shift. In: Reilly, T., Lees, A., Davids, K. & Murphy, W. (eds) *Science and Football*, pp. 249–256. E. & F. N. Spon, London.

Reilly, T. & Piercy, M. (1994) The effect of partial sleep deprivation on weight lifting performance. *Ergonomics* 37, 106–115.

Reilly, T. & Walsh, T.J. (1981) Physiological, psychological and performance measures during an endurance record for 5-a-side soccer play. *British Journal of Sports Medicine* 15, 122–128.

Reilly, T., Atkinson, G. & Budgett, R. (1997a) Effects of temazepam on physiological and performance variables following a westerly flight across five time zones. *Journal of Sports Sciences* 15, 62.

Reilly, T., Atkinson, G. & Waterhouse, J. (1997b) *Biological Rhythms and Exercise.* Oxford University Press, Oxford.

Reilly, T., Waterhouse, J. & Atkinson, G. (1997c) Aging, rhythms of physical performance and adjustments to changes in the sleep–activity cycle. *Occupational and Environmental Medicine* 54, 812–816.

Reilly, T., Maughan, R. & Budgett, R. (1998) Melatonin: a position statement of the British Olympic Association. *British Journal of Sports Medicine* 32, 99–100.

Sasaki, T. (1980) Effect of jet-lag on sports performances. In: Scheving, L.E. & Halberg, F. (eds) *Chronobiology: Principles and Applications to Shifts in Schedules,* pp. 417–431. Sijthoff & Noordhoff, Rockville, MD.

Sinnerton, S. & Reilly, T. (1992) Effects of sleep loss and time of day in swimmers. In: MacLaren, D., Reilly, T. & Lees, A. (eds) *Biomechanics and Medicine in Swimming: Swimming Science V,* pp. 399–404. E. & F. N. Spon, London.

Smith, R.S., Guilleminault, C. & Efron, B. (1997) Circadian rhythms and enhanced athletic performance in the National Football League. *Sleep* 20, 362–365.

Waterhouse, J., Reilly, T. & Atkinson, G. (1997) Jet-lag. *Lancet* 350, 1611–1616.

Waterhouse, J., Minors, D., Folkard, S. *et al.* (1998) Light of domestic intensity produces phase shifts of the circadian oscillator in humans. *Neuroscience Letters* 245, 97–100.

Wright, J.E., Vogel, J.A., Sampson, J.T., Knapik, J.J., Patton, J.F. & Daniels, W.L. (1983) Effects of travel across time zones (jet lag) on exercise capacity and performance. *Aviation, Space and Environmental Medicine* 54, 132–137.

Zinzen, E., Clarys, J.P., Cabri, J., Vanderstappen, D. & Van den Berg, T.J. (1994) The influence of triazolam and flunitrazepam on isokinetic and isometric muscle performance. *Ergonomics* 37, 69–78.

PART 7

CLINICAL ASPECTS OF ENDURANCE TRAINING

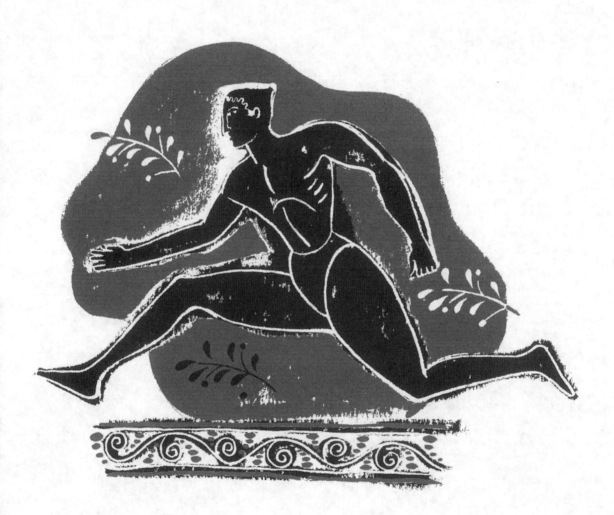

Chapter 44

Medical Surveillance of Endurance Sport

ROY J. SHEPHARD

Introduction

From the standpoint of medical surveillance, endurance activities fall into three broad categories: international endurance competitions such as a 10 000-m run or the Tour de France cycle race, mass participation events (marathon races, 'fun runs', triathlons and ski-hikes such as the Vasa Loppet) and epic expeditions such as an ascent of Mount Everest or a transpolar ski trek. Differing principles govern the provision of medical coverage for each of these categories of activity.

International competition

Most international competitions include some endurance events, and the general arrangements made for medical screening, preparation and care of the participants (Dirix *et al.* 1988) need only slight modifications to accommodate the special needs of the endurance competitor.

Preliminary screening

Preliminary medical screening should focus particularly upon the function of the cardiorespiratory system, looking for evidence of exercise-induced bronchospasm and conditions that might be harbingers of sudden cardiac death (Shephard 1989, 1995). A watch must also be kept for other previously unrecognized medical disorders, for example early diabetes and (in winter sports contestants) unusual sensitivity to cold. Finally, note should be taken of musculoskeletal problems that might be exacer-

bated by prolonged training (for example, differences of leg length or a poor limb alignment).

Respiratory allergies and exercise-induced bronchospasm are likely to impair endurance performance if they remain untreated (Shephard 1977). Moreover, poor counselling may cause the athlete unwittingly to take medication that will lead to disqualification from competition. Permitted treatments of exercise-induced bronchospasm include cromoglycate, theophylline, beclomethasone dipropionate (inhalation therapy only) and (again by inhalation only) such β_2-agonists as salbutamol, terbutaline, metaproterenol, orciprenaline and rimiterol. However, inhaled fenoterol is prohibited, because this drug is readily metabolized to 4-hydroxyamphetamine (Cowan 1994). Adrenaline, ephedrine and isoprenaline are also prohibited (Fitch & Morton 1988), and the systemic administration of all β-agonists is banned, in part because such drugs have been used to increase the body mass of athletes (Delbeke *et al.* 1995; Spann & Winter 1995).

In the young competitor, disorders that predispose to sudden death (Shephard 1989, 1995; Goodman 1995; Maron 1996; Van Camp *et al.* 1995; see Chapter 48) include conditions increasing myocardial oxygen demand (pulmonary stenosis, aortic stenosis or regurgitation, Marfan's syndrome, mitral valve prolapse and regurgitation, hypertension, phaeochromocytoma and hypertrophic cardiomyopathy), impairments of coronary blood flow (anomalous origin of coronary artery, or coronary atheroma), anaemia (related to poor nutrition or sickle cell disease), abnormalities of cardiac rhythm (conduction block, premature ventricular

653

contractions, Wolff–Parkinson–White syndrome) and episodes of syncope (hypoglycaemia, hypocapnia, epilepsy, reversal of intracardiac shunt, hypertrophic cardiomyopathy or Stokes–Adams attacks). In Masters competition, many of the same considerations arise; dominant causes of myocardial ischaemia are now coronary atherosclerosis, cardiomyopathy, hypertension and aortic stenosis or regurgitation. Additional potential disturbances of rhythm include atrial fibrillation and flutter. Syncope may arise from a poor venous tone (varicosities or the use of hypotensive drugs), malfunction of a prosthetic valve or pacemaker, the sick sinus syndrome and supraventricular or ventricular tachycardia. Excessive dyspnoea during exercise may reflect poor myocardial function.

A standard history and clinical examination of the heart will be complemented as necessary by resting and stress electrocardiography, echocardiography, an evaluation of the blood pressure response during a symptom-limited treadmill test and Holter monitoring for significant dysrhythmias (Venerando et al. 1988). However, mass laboratory screening for cardiovascular abnormalities is not recommended in the absence of specific signs and symptoms (Maron 1996; Shephard 1996). Even the supposed most common cause of sudden death in young athletes (hypertrophic cardiomyopathy) is rarely detected prior to death. A family history of sudden death at an early age is probably the only useful indicator of this particular risk. Echocardiographic measurements of ventricular dimensions can be particularly misleading in an endurance competitor (Shephard 1996), and since false-positive test results are frequent, the widespread use of echocardiography causes much unnecessary expense, anxiety and exclusion from competition.

Many endurance and ultra-endurance events, including some team sports, carry normal participants close to hypoglycaemia (Noakes et al. 1985; Ekblom 1986; Shephard 1990). Problems of blood glucose regulation are naturally more severe if there is a tendency to diabetes. If insulin is already being administered to an athlete, there is a danger that the metabolic demands of endurance exercise may provoke a hypoglycaemic crisis by reducing the need for insulin, but at the same time increasing the

rate of absorption of injected hormone from an intramuscular depot (Leon 1992).

Frostbite is always a potential danger in prolonged winter sports events, and a person who has an unusual vascular sensitivity to cold must be advised to take extra precautions on days when the wind chill is high.

Finally, endurance events place an extended strain on some segments of the musculoskeletal system, and the active body parts should receive a thorough clinical examination. Older competitors are more likely to have musculoskeletal problems than their younger counterparts.

Preparation

During preparation of an athlete for major competition, the physician can contribute advice on sound nutrition (Burke & Read 1989) and the avoidance of overtraining (Kuipers & Keizer 1988; Verde et al. 1992; see Chapter 34). Some physicians monitor immunoglobulin levels or carry out intradermal tests of the immune response, and if immune function appears to be flagging they may administer immunoglobulins or other immunomodulating drugs (Liesen et al. 1989; Liesen & Uhlenbruck 1992).

The physician should also develop a good rapport with the athlete, offering minor psychotherapy and appropriate counsel against doping as required.

NUTRITION

The physician should be prepared to offer sound advice, both on the overall food needs of an endurance athlete and on more specific aspects of nutritional preparation for competition, including such topics as glycogen loading and the needs for glutamine, mineral and vitamin supplements during and after an event (Grandjean & Ruud 1994; Maughan 1994; Williams 1994; Butterfield 1995; Noakes et al. 1995; Chapter 29).

Some endurance athletes (particularly contestants in distance-running competitions: Deuster et al. 1986; Fogelholm 1989) seem to have an inadequate total intake of food relative to their energy expenditure. Thus, it is important to monitor body mass during periods of intensive training, to ensure that an energy deficit does not develop (Wheeler *et al.* 1986). Other possible explanations of an apparent energy deficit include a decrease in the energy cost of running with training and errors in estimating the amount of food consumed (Grandjean & Ruud 1994).

An energy expenditure as high as 83 MJ was estimated during one 24-h cycling event (White *et al.* 1984), and on mountainous stretches of the Tour de France, figures of 32.4 MJ·day^{-1} have been recorded (Saris *et al.* 1989). Others have noted average expenditures of 31 MJ·day^{-1} over 7 days of walking (Thomas & Reilly 1975), 29 MJ over 7 h of cross-country skiing (Hedman 1957) and approaching 22 MJ·day^{-1} in triathletes (Green *et al.* 1989). In some events, such as cross-Canada runs, expenditures of 30–40 MJ·day^{-1} may continue for several months (Mertens *et al.* 1996). It is useful for those contemplating very prolonged activities to increase their body fat stores by perhaps 10 kg (this will provide a reserve approaching 300 MJ of food energy). If physical activity is continued over the entire day throughout several weeks, it becomes necessary to find (largely by trial and error) preparations that allow the individual concerned to ingest a substantial amount of energy while exercising (Shephard *et al.* 1977). There were rumours at a recent Tour de France that coaches to one team of cyclists had endeavoured to deal with this issue by administering free fatty acids intravenously. The practice came to light when the fat became rancid and the athletes showed a correspondingly adverse reaction!

Glycogen loading augments an intramuscular reserve of fuel that can be metabolized under both aerobic and anaerobic conditions (Costill 1988; Hasson & Barnes 1989). Perhaps because heavy mechanical loading of the quadriceps occludes the local blood supply, causing work to become anaerobic, glycogen loading is particularly effective in overcoming fatigue among distance cyclists (Williams 1994). Benefit is smaller for distance runners than for cyclists, and in some studies runners have shown only insignificant gains in endurance times after glycogen loading (Brewer *et al.* 1988; Madsen *et al.* 1990).

By sustaining blood glucose concentration, glyco-

gen loading also helps to maintain cerebral performance. This gives a significant advantage in team sports, and in events requiring quick tactical decisions, such as orienteering (Kujala *et al.* 1989) and dinghy sailing (Niinimaa *et al.* 1977).

The traditional approach to glycogen loading (Saltin & Hermansen 1967) involved an initial bout of exhausting exercise, followed by 3 days on a low carbohydrate diet and then 3 days on a high carbohydrate diet. Such tactics led to irritability, hypoglycaemia and an interruption of training during the first 3 days of the regimen. However, an equally effective 'supercompensation' of glycogen reserves is possible if the 3 days of low carbohydrate diet are omitted (Sherman *et al.* 1981).

The rate of replenishment of glycogen stores can be critical to performance (for example, if a soccer team must play a succession of matches over the course of several days). Full restocking of the muscle fibres takes about 48 h. It is helped by a high carbohydrate diet, and often the athlete's diet is less than optimal from this viewpoint (Shephard & Leatt 1987). Nevertheless, prolonged or repeated use of a high carbohydrate diet can eventually lead to a deficit of essential fatty acids (linoleic and linolenic acids, essential components of cell membranes) and fat-soluble vitamins (A, D, E and K). This in turn increases the athlete's susceptibility to muscle damage from free radicals (Karlsson 1997).

Periodic claims are made for the performance-enhancing value of branched-chain amino acids. These substances compete with tryptophan, restricting transport of the latter substance into the brain. This then reduces brain serotonin levels, and could delay the onset of central fatigue (Blomstrand *et al.* 1991). However, it has yet to be demonstrated conclusively that branched-chain amino acids have a beneficial effect on endurance performance. Indeed, Wagenmakers *et al.* (1991) have argued that, by depleting the citric acid cycle intermediate 2-oxoglutarate, branched-chain amino acids can have a negative influence on performance.

Because endurance events depend on oxygen transport, it is important to maximize an athlete's haemoglobin concentration. Endurance competitors are in theory vulnerable to anaemia because of iron loss in sweat, intravascular haemolysis, occasional bleeding in the bladder and intestines, and a poor absorption of iron from the intestines (Haymes & Lamanca 1989; Miller 1990). Iron therapy may be helpful in selected individuals, particularly if blood tests show that the iron saturation of ferritin is low, but it is important not to be misled by plasma volume expansion and a resulting pseudoanaemia (Green et al. 1984; Newhouse & Clement 1988). In general, an athlete who is consuming a well-balanced diet does not require mineral supplements (Clarkson 1991). Some teams have attempted to increase blood haemoglobin levels by training or living at high altitudes (Chapter 30).

Although body mineral stores are substantial, if preparation of the athlete is followed by a prolonged series of competitions in a hot and humid environment, a cumulative depletion of key minerals can develop. Simple evidence of such losses can be obtained (Wyndham & Strydom 1972) by a monitoring of body mass; as salt is lost by sweating, fluid reserves become depleted, and the body weight falls.

By increasing the rate of lactate clearance from muscle (Chapter 22), bicarbonate administration enhances performance over events lasting up to 7.5 min. The effective dose is about $0.3\,g{\cdot}kg^{-1}$, taken 2–3 h before an event. However, in many competitors the advantage gained from increased lactate buffering is offset by gastrointestinal discomfort, vomiting and diarrhoea.

The need for B-group vitamins is proportional to total energy consumption. Demand is thus high in an endurance athlete (Shephard 1984). Nevertheless, if a good mixed diet is provided, the intake of vitamins usually rises to match energy expenditure (van der Beek 1991). It has been argued that vitamin C can protect against injuries and/or speed the healing of tendons. Both vitamin C and vitamin E supplements have also been advocated to counter the accumulation of free radicals during strenuous exercise. Although a deficient intake of these vitamins can undoubtedly cause health problems, including an increased susceptibility to viral infections, there is only limited evidence of benefit from vitamin supplements in well-nourished individuals (Peters et al. 1996).

OVERTRAINING

On the principle that if a little training is good, more training must be better, many athletes reach a state of overtraining (Kuipers & Keizer 1988; O'Brien 1988; Verde et al. 1992), with adverse consequences for both performance and health (Chapter 34).

The affected individual feels fatigued and lacks motivation for further training or competition. There are complaints of a loss of appetite, weight loss and disturbed sleep. The waking pulse rate is elevated, and blood samples may show an elevation of serum enzyme levels (creatine phosphokinase, lactate dehydrogenase and serum glutamic oxaloacetic transaminase; Noakes 1987). In male competitors, a predominance of catabolism is shown by a decrease in the ratio of testosterone to cortisone, associated with a high level of sex hormone-binding globulins (Adlercreutz et al. 1986).

The athlete often becomes accident prone, and overuse injuries of muscle and bone are common in affected individuals. Immune responses are impaired, both at rest and immediately following a bout of exercise (Verde et al. 1992) (Chapter 50). Concentrations of immunoglobulins in saliva and plasma fall, lymphocyte proliferation is reduced (perhaps because of a decreased concentration of an important lymphocyte nutrient, plasma glutamine), natural killer cell counts decrease, and the cytolytic activity of individual natural killer cells may also be reduced by the accumulation of prostaglandins. Moreover, the ratio of T-helper to T-suppressor cells decreases (Shephard 1997). As a consequence of these various changes, the affected individual becomes more vulnerable to viral infections (Nieman et al. 1990; Brenner et al. 1994; Shephard & Shek 1995). Recently, it has been suggested that the deaths of a number of top Swedish orienteers were attributable to a viral myocarditis, precipitated by overtraining and a resulting immune suppression (Wesslen et al. 1996); such incidents ceased when competitors were checked more closely for viral infections.

Before reaching a diagnosis of overtraining, it is important to rule out any more serious cause of symptoms, such as a haemolytic streptococcal infection or glandular fever. The condition is best prevented by developing an appropriate 'tapering' of training prior to competition, in discussion with the coach and the athlete. Psychotherapy is also important both in prevention and in treatment, given growing evidence that 'stress' has an adverse effect upon immune function (LaPerrière *et al.* 1994). Once the syndrome of overtraining is fully developed, the athlete requires a substantial period of complete rest. Sometimes, full recovery requires the cessation of training for several weeks or even months.

DOPING

The sports physician has an important role to play in protecting the competitor against the abuse of performance-enhancing drugs, through a combination of appeals to fair play and warnings against the dangers of self-prescribed medication (Chapter 31). The medical adviser must ensure that all team members are thoroughly familiar with the list of banned drugs, so that prohibited substances are not taken inadvertently during prescribed or self-treatment of minor ailments. Competitors and their coaches should be asked to present for checking any 'over-the-counter' medications that they may have purchased.

At one time, amphetamines were popular drugs of abuse among endurance competitors. These compounds were valued partly for their cerebral stimulating effects, and partly because they diverted blood flow from skin to muscle (Puffer 1986). Reputedly, the illegal administration of such drugs caused a number of heatstroke fatalities among international competitors during the 1960s. Side-effects of the amphetamines include irregularities of heart rhythm, a dangerous rise of core temperature and a masking of fatigue that predisposes to collapse, heat exhaustion and stroke (Bell & Doege 1987). However, drugs of this class are readily detected by the doping control technology of modern competitions, and they are now rarely used by endurance athletes.

Caffeine remains a popular stimulant, particularly for long-distance cyclists, although the associated diuresis can be an embarrassment. Caffeine stimulates the brain, reduces cerebral and possibly muscular fatigue, and mobilizes fat. High blood concentrations were discovered in some athletes at the Montreal Olympic Games. In 1984, the International Olympic Committee (IOC) prohibited urinary caffeine levels in excess of $15 \, mg \cdot l^{-1}$, and in 1986 this threshold was reduced to $12 \, mg \cdot l^{-1}$ (Bell & Doege 1987). The latter ceiling corresponds to a dose of some 400 mg. Permitted levels are substantially higher than would be reached by the drinking of customary daily amounts of coffee (a total intake of perhaps 200 mg).

A third abuse admitted by some long-distance competitors is blood doping (Chapter 30). Recently, there have been suspicions that synthetic preparations of erythropoietin have been administered in order to stimulate haemoglobin production. There are many risks associated with standard blood transfusions (Dirix *et al.* 1988), including allergic reactions, acute haemolysis leading to kidney damage, delayed transfusion reactions with fever and jaundice, transmission of diseases such as viral hepatitis and human immunodeficiency virus (HIV), a possible overloading of the circulation and metabolic shock. Some of these dangers are avoided by an autologous transfusion of the competitor's stored blood, but the athlete then faces a substantial interval when training is disrupted by the loss of blood (Eichner 1987). Unfortunately, there is as yet no good test for blood doping, although procedures are being developed, based upon blood concentrations of haemoglobin, bilirubin, iron and erythropoietin (Berglund 1988).

The abuse of anabolic steroids was once thought to be a problem only among competitors in power sports, but recently a growing number of cases have been identified among endurance competitors. Presumably, the intent is to stimulate erythropoiesis, although there is no good evidence that any significant increase of aerobic power results from this type of treatment. In other instances, there has been an abuse of various peptide hormones (chorionic gonadotrophic hormone, human growth hormone and adrenocorticotrophic hormone), presumably with similar objectives in mind (Kicman & Cowan 1992).

Local or intra-articular injection of certain anaesthetics (procaine, xylocaine and carbocaine, but not cocaine) is permitted when medically justified, but diagnosis, dose and route of administration must be reported immediately to the IOC. Corticosteroids may also be administered locally or intra-articularly, but again must be detailed to the IOC, since some athletes have abused corticosteroids in an attempt to overcome lethargy and tiredness.

Preliminary site visit

It is desirable that the team physician make an early visit to the competitive locale in order to inspect the athletic facilities, to establish liaison with local medical committees (including any necessary accreditation of the medical team), to determine the adequacy of available medical facilities, equipment and living quarters, to discuss the provision of medical insurance coverage for team members, to determine any specific environmental and sanitary hazards, and to relate the World Health Organization's recommended schedule of prophylactic immunizations and vaccinations to the current experience of local public health agencies.

In IOC-sponsored events, the basic minimum standards for both athletic and medical facilities have been specified (Hanneman 1988), but it is useful to ascertain local regulations governing the import and export of any additional equipment that the sports physician may desire.

Potential environmental hazards include extremes of heat and cold (see Chapter 40), together with pollution of ambient air (see Chapter 42), water and ground. It may be necessary to exert pressure on local organizers to ensure that events do not proceed in the midday heat in order to provide television crews with good natural lighting and large crowds. Appropriate agreement should also be reached on environmental conditions that require the cancellation or delaying of a competition. On the basis of site observations, competitors can be given a suitable acclimatization schedule, and told where and when to exercise in order to minimize exposure to local environmental hazards.

In a developing country, water can be a potent route for the transmission of bacteria (leptospirosis, salmonella, shigella and cholera), viruses (particularly poliomyelitis and enteroviral infections) and parasitic infections such as amoebiasis and schistosomiasis (Diop Mar 1988). Drinking stations along the course of an event must use water of adequate quality (if necessary, bottled, boiled or chemically treated), and the athlete should be warned against eating seafood or other produce which has been washed in dirty water. Ice and ice-cream of unknown quality must also be avoided. In events such as the triathlon and cross-country runs, further risks arise from swimming on polluted beaches or wading through polluted streams. If a competition takes place on contaminated ground, there is a potential for injuries to become infected with the microorganisms that cause gas gangrene and tetanus. Finally, in some countries residents are exposed to serious insect-borne diseases such as malaria and encephalitis. Malaria, indeed, remains the most important hazard for those travelling to developing countries. In West Africa, for example, the incidence of malaria in visitors who fail to take prophylactic medication is 24 000 cases per month, with an alarming 480 fatalities per month (Steffen 1991).

Measures to prevent such infections include: (i) a careful check on the nature and timing of required vaccinations and immunizations; (ii) ensuring that contestants take a full course of chloroquine or another potent antimalarial drug during and following visits to those parts of the world where malaria is prevalent; and (iii) prescribing such other forms of chemoprophylaxis as may be recommended by local public health agencies (Diop Mar 1988).

Immediate preparation

The athlete should be examined briefly immediately before departure for an event. Such examination may reveal conditions such as an injury that requires close monitoring or even precludes competition. The examination offers a further opportunity for confidence-building discussion between the doctor and the athlete. Medical records should be updated, and if the competition will take the athlete away from the main treatment facility, a summary of the medical history, including details of medication, vaccinations and immunizations, allergies and the like should be prepared, either to travel with the athlete, or to be available over the internet. Any medications that the athlete is currently receiving should be checked relative to the current antidoping regulations of the particular competition and, where necessary, legitimate drug needs should be discussed with the monitoring committee.

Protection of both athletes and the accompanying medical team against hepatitis B or C and HIV infection is a growing concern. In fact, there are at most isolated incidents where trauma sustained in contact sports may have caused the spread of either type of infection. Medical staff should be instructed to wear gloves and protective glasses when giving treatments that involve bleeding wounds or contact with body secretions. All waste material should be burnt, and all potentially contaminated equipment and surfaces treated with bleach. Any open injuries should be covered if a contestant returns to play. However, all members of an athletic team must understand that the most likely sources of cross-infection are unprotected sex and such practices as the sharing of drinking bottles, razors, toothbrushes and the needles used for 'doping' or other forms of drug abuse.

Arrangements to speed immediate adjustment to the new environment should be reviewed with both athletes and coaches. Advice may be needed on the time needed to compensate for shifts in circadian rhythms (Chapter 43), increases in altitude (Chapter 41) and changes of climate (Chapter 40).

Counsel can also be offered on the optimal choice of fluids and food in the periods immediately before and during competition (Costill 1988) (Chapter 29). It seems best to take a carbohydrate-containing meal 3–4 h before an event. If large amounts of glucose are given in the hour immediately before competition, some have argued that this may provoke a massive secretion of insulin, with a fall of blood glucose and a deterioration of performance during competition (Costill 1988; Hasson & Barnes 1989). However, there may be some advantage in taking a small amount of glucose or fructose 5 min before a race begins. Likewise, a limited pre-event loading with fluid (to 500 ml) may be helpful, although if larger amounts of fluid are ingested and the day is cold the athlete may face an embarrassing diuresis. During competition, thirst provides a poor guide to fluid needs. If the day is warm and the rules of competition allow, an attempt should be made to drink 150 ml of fluid every 15 min, either as pure water, or as a dilute glucose–electrolyte solution.

Medical supervision during competition

The medical requirements of the athlete are usually quite limited, during both attendance at an event and actual participation. The largest number of treatments are for minor respiratory and gastrointestinal infections, sunburn, minor skin complaints, minor psychological problems and minor musculoskeletal problems. Nevertheless, the supervising physician must remain constantly vigilant, and must be prepared to deal with more serious problems, including hyperthermia (in summer endurance events and team sports), hypothermia (in swimming, sailing, mountaineering and winter events) and cardiac catastrophes in competitors and officials alike.

Most respiratory infections resolve spontaneously, but analgesics, antihistamines and decongestants may provide symptomatic relief. A throat swab should be taken to determine if there is any secondary bacterial infection and, if so, to identify its sensitivity to antibiotics. Eichner (1993) has suggested that if there is no fever, and symptoms are limited to the head and neck, there is no need to halt training. However, fever, myalgia, tachycardia and premature ventricular contractions are all warnings to rest (Shephard & Shek 1995).

Traveller's diarrhoea affects a third or more of visitors to developing countries (Pasvol 1994). The most likely cause is infection with an unfamiliar strain of *Escherichia coli*. The resultant diarrhoea may lead to a marked fluid loss, with a resulting deterioration in endurance performance. Care in the selection of clean, hygienic food can often prevent such infections, but it is difficult to maintain dietary restrictions throughout a prolonged visit to a foreign country. An affected individual should take soup and salted glucose or sugar solution, potassium-containing fruit juices and soft drinks *ad libitum* in order to restore fluid and electrolyte losses. The use of codeine and morphine has been banned by the IOC, but diphenoxylate (5 mg four times daily) or loperamide (4 mg, and a further 2 mg after the passage of each unformed stool, to a maximum of 16 mg·day^{-1}) can be taken for the relief of painful spasms. An oral preparation containing trimethoprim (160–200 mg) and sulphamethoxazole (800 mg) administered twice daily will usually effect a rapid cure. Ciprofloxacin (500 mg b.d.) has sometimes been used for prophylaxis. However, this is not recommended. It alters the bacterial flora of the gut, which can in itself cause diarrhoea. Moreover, there is a risk of developing resistant strains of bacteria by the repeated use of such drugs.

A combination of a sustained increase of body temperature and glandular enlargement may herald either a form of glandular fever (infectious mononucleosis, toxoplasmosis or cytomegalovirus infection), or occasionally the primary seroconversion illness of an HIV infection (the latter is frequently accompanied by a rash). The glandular fevers are important because of the associated risks of splenic rupture and myocarditis. They may also predispose to the postviral fatigue syndrome (Pasvol 1994). Diagnosis is based on a combination of clinical findings, the presence of >15% atypical lymphocytes in peripheral blood and positive antibody tests. Total bedrest seems to delay recovery (Dalrymple 1964; Haines 1987). The rate of return to training is gauged from the exercise tolerance of the patient, but contact sports should be avoided, particularly if there is splenic enlargement (Pasvol 1994).

Chronic fatigue is sometimes related to overtraining, and sometimes follows a viral illness. One study found a psychiatric disorder in as many as 70% of those affected. A further 5% had some medical precipitant, but in the remainder of patients the condition remained unexplained (Manu *et al.* 1988). There is no effective pharmaceutical treatment. Reassurance, support and graded exercise within the patient's tolerance seem the best tactics to speed recovery.

Medical supervision of mass participation events

The potential medical problems associated with mass participation events such as a marathon, a 'fun run', a triathlon or a large-scale cross-country ski competition (Table 44.1) are in many respects greater than those associated with major international competition. The number of participants to be supervised is very much larger. Competitors also cover a much wider spectrum of ages from quite young children to senior citizens. They vary widely in their initial level of training and experience. Moreover, a number are affected by chronic medical conditions, some of which as yet unrecognized. Treatment must usually be offered from makeshift facilities, using limited equipment, and because the event is less prestigious than a major international competition, few medical and paramedical personnel may offer their time for emergency care.

Nevertheless, many of the general principles of preparation, both preventive and therapeutic, are similar to those already discussed for the top-level athlete (Tunstall-Pedoe 1984; Dobbin 1986; Robertson 1988).

Initial preparations

A medical committee should be established at an early stage in preparations for the event. This should include not only interested local physicians, but also representatives of other paramedical disciplines whose help will be sought in dealing with casualties—physiotherapists, podiatrists, nurses, the St John's Ambulance Brigade and the Red Cross or Red Crescent. A reasonable level of staffing for a marathon run includes 20 first-aiders, three nurses, one physiotherapist, one podiatrist and one doctor for every 1000 registrants (Tunstall-Pedoe 1984).

Table 44.1 Distribution of casualties seeking medical aid during Seattle's Emerald City Marathon from 1983 to 1987. Data from Robertson (1988), with permission.

Injury*	%
Muscle cramps or strains	22
Blisters	20
Other orthopaedic injuries	23
Exhaustion or dehydration	17
Thermal injuries	14
Other medical problems	4

*Total injuries 2.0–5.5% of finishers.

Although the number of admissions to local hospitals is unlikely to be large, contact should be made with appropriate emergency departments to ensure that they know of the event and are familiar with the treatment of possible emergencies, particularly hyperthermia and hypothermia. Training should also be offered to those of the paramedical team who have not had previous experience in dealing with a mass participation event. All members of the team should advise disorientated individuals to withdraw from competition.

Liaison should be established with both the race organizers and local ambulance and police units to ensure adequate control of crowds and traffic. Sufficient vehicles must be available to evacuate the anticipated number of casualties from treatment stations, to collect stragglers who fail to complete the event because of thermal problems or general exhaustion, and to return all of these individuals to the finish line.

Waiver clauses in the initial application form should clarify that competitors in an athletic event: (i) compete at their own risk; and (ii) accept the responsibility of seeking medical advice if they are uncertain about their fitness to participate. The early circulation of a medical advice sheet can substantially reduce the incidence of casualties during an event. In particular, registrants should be given information about minimal training requirements, techniques of heat acclimatization (Murphy 1979) and protection against cold, methods of avoiding musculoskeletal problems, general factors increasing cardiovascular risks (Tunstall-Pedoe 1983), and potentially serious dangers such as hyperthermia, hypothermia and hypoglycaemia. Participants should be warned that thirst is not a good guide to fluid needs, that those who do not drink regularly are likely to drop out of competition (Holmich et al. 1988), and that alcohol on the night before an event can lead to both dehydration and impaired thermal regulation (Maughan 1984, 1994). Registrants should also be told categorically not to participate if they are unwell, and not to persist in competition if they are feeling faint or exhausted. Because heat stress often impairs judgement, it is wise to assign partners who will run at a similar pace and will monitor each other's condition over the event. Casualties may be too confused to indicate even

their names after a collapse has occurred. As with international competition, all participants should therefore carry information sheets giving their name, the name and address of their personal physician and a brief medical history. The process of public education can be reinforced if the chairperson of the medical committee offers practical advice in prior presentations to the local newspaper, radio and television stations.

Early decisions need to be taken on any lower or upper age limits for participation, and on the desirability of admitting to events those with known disabilities. Although quite young children often complete an event such as a marathon run without harm, the involvement of preadolescents in prolonged competition is to be discouraged. The prolonged training that is required can have adverse effects on immature bones, time is taken from normal psychosocial development, and an exhausted child may face excessive pressures to complete the actual event from ambitious parents or coaches (Chapter 35).

Detailed planning

The route for the event should be surveyed in detail. Any obstacles and bottlenecks must be either eliminated or at least clearly marked. Provision must also be made for an adequate number of drink, first-aid and toilet stations.

Fluid ingestion is encouraged by keeping the stomach well filled. In events that cover a distance of 16 km and more, drinks should therefore be provided every 3–4 km. The design of a drinking station needs careful thought, so that runners do not slip on discarded paper cups and fruit peelings, or collide with others who have stopped. Cups should be large enough that participants can drink about 150 ml of fluid from a container that is no more than half-filled. This minimizes the spillage of fluid. Participants should be told how drinks will be passed to them, and where to discard their cups after use. Some companies now manufacture quite exotic beverages for the athlete, but the prime need is to replenish body water reserves. It is better to have a sufficient supply of clean water than a limited volume of a commercial drink that is more palatable, but is quickly depleted by the first wave of competitors. It was once thought that the rate of fluid absorption was increased by chilling the beverage that was provided but this view has now been discredited (Sun *et al.* 1988; McArthur & Feldman 1989; Lambert & Maughan 1992). An excessive intake of water over an ultramarathon run or similar event is undesirable, since it can sometimes cause hyponatraemia (Noakes *et al.* 1985; Frizell *et al.* 1986). If glucose–electrolyte solutions are provided, these must be freshly prepared, as they provide an excellent culture medium for bacteria. Some commercially available preparations also contain rather a high concentration of glucose (>5%); this slows gastric emptying and thus limits the absorption of water. The sponging or hosing of participants is not recommended as a general measure. Although it gives participants a psychological boost, it may also increase heat stress by causing a vasoconstriction of the cutaneous blood vessels (Bassett *et al.* 1987).

First-aid stations should be sited immediately beyond the drinking stations. Tents or trailers may be used for accommodation. They should be protected from wet ground, and should have at least a minimum of telephone communication with a nearby ambulance. In cool conditions, there should be sufficient heating of the first-aid station to prevent the development of hypothermia in exhausted runners, and in warm weather, fans or air-conditioners will be required to avoid heat stress in both staff and patients.

Some participants who have overhydrated excessively before a race may develop a diuresis, and others may be affected by the 'runner's trots'. Well-marked toilets should therefore be provided at strategic points along the runners' route.

Immediately beyond the finishing line, there should be a large recovery area, where all participants can change into warm, dry clothing, eat and sit until they have recovered sufficiently to make the homeward journey. The medical treatment section within the recovery area should be large enough to accommodate at least 5% of the anticipated number of participants (Tunstall-Pedoe 1984; Robertson 1988). Simple facilities for each sex should include reserves of dry clothing, camp beds, pillows and blankets, adequate fresh water and ice, dressings, waste buckets and vomit bowls. Medical equipment

should include stretchers, splints, dressings, oxygen cylinders, blood pressure cuffs, stethoscopes, rectal thermometers, transfusion sets with drip stands, the standard array of emergency drugs and, if possible, a portable defibrillator.

If wheelchair athletes are to be included as participants in a distance-running event (Marshall 1984), suitably adapted toilet facilities must be organized at appropriate intervals along the route. Wheelchairs can reach speeds of $60 \text{km} \cdot \text{h}^{-1}$. It is thus important to ensure that the course has no steep hills or sharp bends, and that there is adequate space to allow those in wheelchairs to overtake tired runners. Notice also that, because they reach very high speeds and have impaired thermoregulation, wheelchair participants are particularly vulnerable to hypothermia.

Immediate preparations

A substantial number of registrants often decide themselves to withdraw from competition some 2 weeks before an endurance event because of pregnancy, injury or infection (Clough *et al.* 1987). A much clearer idea of the size of the field can thus be obtained if participation is confirmed in the final week before an event.

The anticipated weather conditions along the route should be discussed with the local meteorological station on the morning of the event. Participants should be advised if particular care is needed to avoid heat stress, frostbite or hypothermia (Richards *et al.* 1979; Hanson 1985). If conditions exceed a wet bulb temperature of 28°C, if the wind chill is more severe than −35°C or if there is black ice, races should be cancelled (American College of Sports Medicine 1984; Tunstall-Pedoe 1984). If conditions are warm, a slowing of pace should be recommended to participants (England *et al.* 1982), and a clothing check should be instituted if starting temperatures are below 15°C (Robertson 1988).

At the start of the race, participants should be reminded of the information given in the advice sheet, and warned against competing if they feel unwell. Registration in the following year should be offered to all who decide to withdraw from competition for health reasons.

Plan of treatment

The entrances to first-aid and medical stations should be guarded, to allow the logging of casualties as they are admitted, and to exclude press, television crews and relatives. Authorized personnel should be given suitable identification badges.

The proportion of participants seeking medical help ranges widely between 0.1 and 12.5% in different events (Williams *et al.* 1981; Tunstall-Pedoe 1984; Robertson 1988), depending largely upon weather conditions. A preliminary triage should divide casualties between those who are to be treated by podiatrists (mainly blisters and subungual haematomas), those appropriate to physiotherapists (for instance, cases of severe cramps) and the rare cases needing immediate and intensive medical care (intravenous fluids or resuscitation).

Most of the complaints encountered over the course of an endurance event are minor in nature (Table 44.1). They include blisters, chafing and even nipple bleeding from nylon running shorts and vests, muscle cramps and general exhaustion. Depending on environmental conditions, a proportion of competitors (mainly the less fit individuals) may develop various heat pathologies (Wyndham & Strydom 1972) or hypothermia (Pugh 1972; see Chapter 40). Rectal temperatures should thus be recorded immediately on all those who have collapsed. Oral temperatures should be avoided, since gross errors can arise in an athlete due to cooling of the tongue by inspired air, and lack of control over the recent drinking of hot or cold fluids. In no circumstances should a participant who is dazed, disorientated or having problems of thermoregulation be allowed to return to competition. Nevertheless, at the end of the event, many participants who seem confused and ill respond well to a monitored warm-down that includes slow walking and the administration of oral fluids (Robertson 1988).

Major cardiac events are surprisingly rare in mass participation events. For instance, there is about one death per million person-hours in cross-country skiing (Williams *et al.* 1981; Tunstall-Pedoe 1983, 1984; Sadaniantz & Thompson 1990; Vuori 1995). Nevertheless, it is important that aggressive participants be discouraged from denying prodromal

symptoms (Northcote & Ballantyne 1984), and that those providing medical care are thoroughly familiar with techniques of cardiac resuscitation. It is also important that hospitals receiving casualties do not confuse a race-induced release of serum creatine kinase from the active skeletal muscles with the cardiac enzyme release that accompanies myocardial infarction (Young 1984; Noakes 1987).

Many of the minor problems of mass competition can be avoided by simple preventive measures. Clothing should be comfortable, preferably of natural fibre that 'breathes' and does not chafe, and capable of adjustment to allow a variation in thermal protection over a long day. A hat should be added in bright sunlight, and most women will be more comfortable wearing a brassière. In cold weather, heat loss is substantially reduced by wearing a hat and gloves (Maughan 1984). Shoes should have been 'broken in', but still able to provide adequate ankle support. Socks should be well-fitting woollen or cotton rather than nylon. The application of zinc oxide powder, plaster and petroleum jelly at friction points will minimize skin problems (Hölmich *et al.* 1988).

Thermal emergencies are less likely if events are cancelled in extreme conditions and care is taken with the hydration of participants when the weather is warm. Cardiac catastrophes are also unlikely if participants are encouraged not to persist in an event beyond the point of exhaustion.

Most events are repeated on an annual basis. It is thus important to call a final meeting of the medical committee after the event, to review successes in both prevention and treatment, and to learn any necessary lessons for future years. If the experience has been adverse because of apparent negligence, national associations may wish to consider exercising some sanctions against the organizers of the event (Robertson 1988).

Medical emergencies in wilderness expeditions

Where possible, those contemplating a mountain expedition, a long wilderness canoe trip or an arctic ski-trek should recruit a physician to their numbers. However, the extreme nature of the environment and the very limited facilities only allow the provision of minimal emergency care during the trip.

The specific example of climbing is considered in Chapter 62. Prudence would suggest a thorough medical examination and extensive training before an expedition, but in practice some mountaineering and transarctic teams have included older individuals who were relatively unfit and had known medical problems (Pugh 1972; Shephard 1991; Shephard & Rode 1992).

A physician who is joining a wilderness expedition must be thoroughly familiar with the likely problems of a particular habitat, but probably her or his most important function will be to decide when a casualty should be evacuated. Arrangements should be made for the airlifting of emergency supplies and for evacuation before the trip is begun, and radio communication with base should be maintained throughout.

Acknowledgements

Dr Shephard's studies are supported in part by research grants from the Defence and Civil Institute of Environmental Medicine, Toronto, ON.

References

Adlercreutz, H., Harkonen, M., Kuop-pasalmi, K. *et al.* (1986) Effects of training on plasma anabolic and catabolic steroid hormones and their response during physical exercise. *International Journal of Sports Medicine* 7, 27–28.

American College of Sports Medicine (1984) Prevention of thermal injuries during distance running. *Sports Medicine Bulletin* 19 (3), 8.

Bassett, D., Nagle, F., Mookerjee, S. *et al.* (1987) Thermoregulatory response to skin wetting during prolonged treadmill running. *Medicine and Science in Sports and Exercise* 19, 28–32.

van der Beek, E.J. (1991) Vitamin supplementation and physical exercise performance. *Journal of Sports Sciences* 9 (Suppl.), 77–90.

Bell, A.J. & Doege, C.T. (1987) Athletes use and abuse of drugs. *Physician and Sportsmedicine* 15 (3), 99–108.

Berglund, B. (1988) Development of techniques for the detection of blood doping in sport. *Sports Medicine* 5, 127–135.

Blomstrand, E., Hassmen, P., Ekblom, B. & Newsholme, E.A. (1991) Administration of branch-chained amino acids during sustained exercise —effects on performance and on plasma concentration of some amino acids. *European Journal of Applied Physiology* 63, 83–88.

Brenner, I.K.M., Shek, P.N. & Shephard, R.J. (1994) Infection in athletes. *Sports Medicine* 17, 86–107.

Brewer, J., Williams, C. & Patton, A. (1988) The influence of high carbohydrate diets on endurance running performance. *European Journal of Applied Physiology* 57, 698–706.

Burke, L.M. & Read, R.S.D. (1989) Sports nutrition: approaching the nineties. *Sports Medicine* 8, 80–100.

Butterfield, G. (1995) Dietary requirements of the athlete. In: Torg, J. & Shephard, R.J. (eds) *Current Therapy in Sports Medicine*, pp. 512–517. Mosby, Philadelphia.

van Camp, S.P., Bloor, C.M., Mueller, F.O., Cantu, R.C. & Olson, H.G. (1995) Nontraumatic sports death in high school and college athletes. *Medicine and Science in Sports and Exercise* 27, 641–647.

Clarkson, P.M. (1991) Minerals: exercise performance and supplementation in athletes. *Journal of Sports Sciences* 9 (Suppl.), 91–116.

Clough, P.J., Dutch, S., Maughan, R.J. & Shepherd, J. (1987) Pre-race drop-out in marathon runners: reasons for withdrawal and future plans. *British Journal of Sports Medicine* 21, 148–149.

Costill, D.L. (1988) Nutrition and dietetics. In: Dirix, A., Knuttgen, H.G. & Tittel, K. (eds) *The Olympic Book of Sports Medicine*, pp. 603–634. Blackwell Scientific Publications, Oxford.

Cowan, D. (1994) Drug abuse. In: Harries, M., Williams, C., Stanish, D. & Micheli, L.J. (eds) *Oxford Textbook of Sports Medicine*, pp. 314–329. Oxford Medical Publications, New York.

Dalrymple, W. (1964) Infectious mononucleosis—II. Relationship of bedrest and activity to prognosis. *Postgraduate Medical Journal* 35, 345–349.

Delbeke, F.T., Desmet, N. & Debackere, M. (1995) The abuse of doping agents in competing body builders in Flanders (1988–93). *International Journal of Sports Medicine* 16, 66–70.

Deuster, P.A., Kyle, S.B., Moser. P.B.,

Vigersky, R.A., Singh, A. & Schoomaker, E.B. (1986) Nutritional survey of highly trained women runners. *American Journal of Clinical Nutrition* 44, 956–962.

Diop Mar, I. (1988) Infectious diseases in tropical climates. In: Dirix, A., Knuttgen, H.G. & Tittel, K. (eds) *The Olympic Book of Sports Medicine*, pp. 583–588. Blackwell Scientific Publications, Oxford.

Dirix, A., Knuttgen, H.G. & Tittel, K. (1988) *The Olympic Book of Sports Medicine*. Blackwell Scientific Publications, Oxford.

Dobbin, S. (1986) Providing medical services for fun runs and marathons in North America. In: Sutton, J. & Brock, R.C. (eds) *Sports Medicine for the Mature Athlete*, pp. 193–203. Benchmark Press, Indianapolis.

Eichner, E.R. (1987) Blood doping: results and consequences from the laboratory and the field. *Physician and Sportsmedicine* 15 (1), 120–129.

Eichner, R. (1993) Infection, immunity and exercise. What to tell patients. *Physician and Sportsmedicine* 21 (1), 125–135.

Ekblom, B. (1986) Applied physiology of soccer. *Sports Medicine* 3, 50–60.

England, A., Fraser, D., Hightower, A. *et al.* (1982) Preventing heat injury in runners: suggestions from the 1979 Peachtree road race experience. *Annals of Internal Medicine* 97, 196–201.

Fitch, K.D. & Morton, A.R. (1988) Respiratory disease. In: Dirix, A., Knuttgen, H.G. & Tittel, K. (eds) *The Olympic Book of Sports Medicine*, pp. 531–541. Blackwell Scientific Publications, Oxford.

Fogelholm, M. (1989) Estimated energy expenditure, diet and iron status of male Finnish endurance athletes: a cross-sectional study. *Medicine and Science in Sports and Exercise* **11**, 59–63.

Frizell, R., Lang, G., Lowance, D. & Lathan, S. (1986) Hyponatremia and ultramarathon running. *Journal of the American Medical Association* **255**, 772–774.

Goodman, J. (1995) Exercise and sudden cardiac death: etiology in apparently healthy individuals. *Sport Sciences Review* **4** (2), 14–30.

Grandjean, A.C. & Ruud, J.S. (1994) Energy intake of athletes. In: Harries, M., Williams, C., Stanish, W.D. & Micheli, L.J. (eds) *Oxford Textbook of Sports Medicine*, pp. 53–65. Oxford Medical Publications, New York.

Green, D.R., Gibbons, C., O'Toole, M. & Hiller, W.B.O. (1989) An evaluation of dietary intakes of triathletes: are recommended dietary allowances being met? *Journal of the American Dietetic Association* **89**, 1653–1654.

Green, H.J., Thomson, J.A., Ball, M.E. *et al.* (1984) Alterations in blood volume following short-term supramaximal exercise. *Journal of Applied Physiology* **56**, 145–149.

Haines, J. (1987) When to resume sports after infectious mononucleosis. How soon is safe? *Postgraduate Medicine* **81**, 331–333.

Hanneman, D. (1988) Standardization of medical care during international sports events. In: Dirix, A., Knuttgen, H.G. & Tittel, K. (eds) *The Olympic Book of Sports Medicine*, pp. 646–652. Blackwell Scientific Publications, Oxford.

Hanson, P. (1985) Marathon medicine. *Emergency Medicine* **17** (15), 62–92.

Hasson, S.M. & Barnes, W.S. (1989) Effect of carbohydrate ingestion on exercise of varying intensity and duration. Practical implications. *Sports Medicine* **8**, 327–334.

Haymes, E. & Lamanca, J.J. (1989) Iron losses in runners during exercise: implications and recommendations. *Sports Medicine* **7**, 277–285.

Hedman, R. (1957) The available glycogen in man and the connection between the rate of oxygen intake and carbohydrate usage. *Acta Physiologica Scandinavica* **40**, 305–321.

van Helder, W. (1995) Exercise and diabetes. In: Torg, J. & Shephard, R. J. (eds) *Current Therapy in Sports Medicine*, pp. 684–685. Mosby, Philadelphia.

Hölmich, P., Darre, E., Jahnsen, F. & Hartvig-Jensen, T. (1988) The elite marathon runner: problems during and after competition. *British Journal of Sports Medicine* **22**, 19–21.

Karlsson, J. (1997) *Antioxidants and Exercise.* Human Kinetics, Champaign, IL.

Kicman, A.T. & Cowan, D.A. (1992) Peptide hormones and sport: misuse and detection. *British Medical Bulletin* **48**, 496–517.

Kuipers, H. & Keizer, H.A. (1988) Overtraining in elite athletes. Review and directions for the future. *Sports Medicine* **6**, 79–92.

Kujala, U.M., Heinonen, O.J., Kvist, M.L. *et al.* (1989) Orienteering performance and ingestion of glucose and glucose polymers. *British Journal of Sports Medicine* **23**, 105–108.

Lambert, C.P. & Maughan, R.J. (1992) Effect of temperature of ingested beverages on the rate of accumulation in the blood of an added tracer for water uptake. *Scandinavian Journal of Medicine and Science in Sports* **2**, 76–78.

LaPerrière, A., Ironson, G., Antoni, M.T. *et al.* (1994) Exercise and psychoneuroimmunology. *Medicine and Science in Sports and Exercise* **26**, 182–190.

Leon, A.S. (1992) The role of exercise in the prevention and treatment of diabetes mellitus and blood lipid disorders. In: Shephard, R.J. & Miller, H. (eds) *Exercise and the Heart in Health and Disease*, pp. 299–368. Marcel Dekker, New York.

Liesen, H. & Uhlenbruck, G. (1992) Sports immunology. *Sport Sciences Review* **1**, (1) 94–116.

Liesen, H., Riedel, H., Widenmayer, W., Order, U., Mücke, S. & Geist, S. (1989) Substitution and preventive treatment in top athletes. In: Böning, D., Braumann, K.M., Busse, M.W., Maassen, N. & Schmidt, W. (eds) *Sport — Rettung Oder Risiko für die Gesundheit?*, pp. 531–538. Deutscher Ärzteverlag, Köln.

McArthur, K.E. & Feldman, M. (1989) Gastric secretion, gastrin release, and gastric temperature in humans as affected by liquid meal temperature. *American Journal of Clinical Nutrition* **49**, 51–54.

Madsen, K., Pedersen, P.K., Rose, P. & Richter, E.A. (1990) Carbohydrate supercompensation and muscle glycogen utilization during exhaustive running in highly trained athletes. *European Journal of Applied Physiology* **61**, 467–472.

Manu, P., Lane, T. & Matthews, D. (1988) The frequency of chronic fatigue syndrome in patients with chronic fatigue. *Annals of Internal Medicine* **109**, 554–556.

Maron, B.J. (chair) (1996) Cardiovascular preparticipation screening of competitive athletes. *Medicine and Science in Sports and Exercise* **28**, 1445–1452.

Marshall, T. (1984) Wheelchairs and marathon road racing. *British Journal of Sports Medicine* **18**, 301–304.

Maughan, R. (1984) Temperature regulation during marathon competition. *British Journal of Sports Medicine* **18**, 257–260.

Maughan, R. (1994) Fluid and electrolyte loss and replacement in exercise. In: Harries, M., Williams, C., Stanish, W.D. & Micheli, L.J. (eds) *Oxford Textbook of Sports Medicine*, pp. 82–93. Oxford Medical Publications, New York, NY.

Mertens, D.J., Rhind, S., Berkhoff, F. *et al.* (1996) Nutritional, immunologic and psychological responses to a 7250 km run. *Journal of Sports Medicine and Physical Fitness* **36**, 132–138.

Miller, B.J. (1990) Haematological effects of running: a brief review. *Sports Medicine* **9**, 1–6.

Murphy, R. (1979) Heat illness and athletics. In: Strauss, R. (ed.) *Sports Medicine and Physiology*, pp. 320–326. W.B. Saunders, Philadelphia.

Newhouse, I.J. & Clement, D. (1988) Iron status in athletes. An update. *Sports Medicine* **5**, 337–352.

Nieman, D.C., Johanssen, L.M., Lee, J.W. & Arabatzis, K. (1990) Infectious episodes in runners before and after the Los Angeles marathon. *Journal of Sports Medicine and Physical Fitness* **30**, 316–328.

Niinimaa, V., Wright, G.R., Shephard, R.J. & Clarke, J. (1977) Characteristics of the successful dinghy sailor. *Journal of Sports Medicine and Physical Fitness* **17**, 83–96.

Noakes, T.D. (1987) Effect of exercise on serum enzyme activities in humans. *Sports Medicine* **4**, 245–267.

Noakes, T.D., Nathan, M., Irving, R.A. *et al.* (1985) Physiological and biochemical measurements during a 4-day surf-ski marathon. *South African Medical Journal* **67**, 212–216.

Noakes, T.D., Hawley, J.A. & Dennis, S.C. (1995) Fluid and energy replacement during prolonged exercise. In: Torg, J. & Shephard, R.J. (eds) *Current Therapy in Sports Medicine*, pp. 517–520. Mosby, Philadelphia.

Northcote, R.J. & Ballantyne, D. (1984) Reducing the prevalence of exercise-related cardiac death. *British Journal of Sports Medicine* **18**, 288–292.

O'Brien, M. (1988) Overtraining and sports psychology. In: Dirix, A., Knuttgen, H.G. & Tittel, K. (eds) *The Olympic Book of Sports Medicine*, pp. 635–645. Blackwell Scientific Publications, Oxford.

Pasvol, G. (1994) Infections in sports medicine. In: Harries, M., Williams, C.,

Stanish, W.D. & Micheli, L.J. (eds) *Oxford Textbook of Sports Medicine*, pp. 305–314. Oxford Medical Publications, New York.

Peters, E.M., Goetzsche, J.M., Joseph, L.E. & Noakes, T.D. (1996) Vitamin C as effective as combinations of anti-oxidant nutrients in reducing the incidence of upper respiratory tract infections in ultra-distance runners. *South African Journal of Sports Medicine* 4, 23–27.

Puffer, C.J. (1986) The use of drugs in swimming. *Clinical Sports Medicine* 5, 77–89.

Pugh, L.G.C.E. (1972) Accidental hypothermia among hillwalkers and climbers in Britain. In: Cumming, G.R., Snidal, D. & Taylor, H.W. (eds) *Environmental Effects on Work Performance*, pp. 41–55. Canadian Association of Sport Sciences, Ottawa.

Richards, R., Richards, D., Schofield, P., Ross, V. & Sutton, J. (1979) Reducing the hazards in Sydney's the Sun-to-Surf runs 1971–79. *Medical Journal of Australia* 2, 453–457.

Robertson, J.W. (1988) Medical problems in mass participation runs. Recommendations. *Sports Medicine* 6, 261–270.

Sadaniantz, A. & Thompson, P.D. (1990) The problem of sudden death in athletes as illustrated by case studies. *Sports Medicine* 9, 199–204.

Saltin, B. & Hermansen, L. (1967) Glycogen stores and prolonged severe exercise. In: Blix, G. (ed.) *Nutrition and Physical Activity*, p. 32. Almqvist & Wiksell, Uppsala.

Saris, W.H.M., van Erp-Baart, M.A., Brouns, F. *et al.* (1989) Study on food intake and energy expenditure during extreme sustained exercise: the Tour de France. *International Journal of Sports Medicine* 10, S26–S31.

Shephard, R.J. (1977) Exercise-induced bronchospasm: a review. *Medicine and Science in Sports and Exercise* 9, 1–10.

Shephard, R.J. (1984) *Biochemistry of Physical Activity*. C.C Thomas, Springfield, IL.

Shephard, R.J. (1989) Cardiovascular aspects of sports medicine. In: Teitz, C. (ed.) *Scientific Foundations of Sports Medicine*, pp. 27–57. B.C. Decker, Burlington, ON.

Shephard, R.J. (1990) Meeting carbohydrate and fluid needs in soccer. *Canadian Journal of Sports Sciences* 15, 165–171.

Shephard, R.J. (1991) Some consequences of polar stress; data from a trans polar ski trek. *Arctic Medical Research* 50, 25–29.

Shephard, R.J. (1995) Exercise and sudden death: an overview. *Sport Sciences Review* 4 (2), 1–13.

Shephard, R.J. (1996) The athlete's heart: Is big beautiful? *British Journal of Sports Medicine* 30, 5–10.

Shephard, R.J. (1997) *Physical Activity, Training and the Immune Response*. Cooper Publications, Carmel, IN.

Shephard, R.J. & Leatt, P. (1987) Carbohydrate and fluid needs of the soccer player. *Sports Medicine* 4, 164–176.

Shephard, R.J. & Rode, A. (1992) *Observations on the Soviet/Canadian Transpolar Ski Trek*. Karger, Basel.

Shephard, R.J. & Shek, P.N. (1995) Infectious disease in athletes: New interest for an old problem. *Journal of Sports Medicine and Physical Fitness* 34, 11–22.

Shephard, R.J., Conway, S., Thomson, M., Anderson, G.H. & Kavanagh, T. (1977) Nutritional demands of sub-maximum work: marathon and trans-Canada events. In: Pavluk, J. (ed.) *International Symposium on Athletic Nutrition*, pp. 42–58. Polska Federacja Sportu, Warsaw.

Sherman, W.M., Costill, D.L., Fink, W.J. & Miller, J.M. (1981) Effect of exercise–diet manipulation on muscle glycogen and its subsequent utilization during performance. *International Journal of Sports Medicine* 2, 114–118.

Spann, C. & Winter, M.E. (1995) Effect of clenbuterol on athletic performance. *Annals of Pharmacotherapy* 29, 75–77.

Steffen, R. (1991) Travel medicine—prevention-based epidemiological data. *Transactions of the Royal Society of Tropical Medicine and Hygiene* 85, 156–162.

Sun, W.M., Houghton, L.A., Read, N.W. *et al.* (1988) Effect of meal temperature on gastric emptying of liquids in man. *Gut* 29, 302–305.

Thomas, V. & Reilly, T. (1975) Circulatory, psychological and performance variables during 100 hours of paced continuous exercise under conditions of controlled energy intake and work output. *Journal of Human Movement Studies* 1, 149.

Tunstall-Pedoe, D.S. (1983) Cardiological problems in sport. *British Journal of Hospital Medicine* 29, 213–220.

Tunstall-Pedoe, D.S. (1984) Popular marathons, half-marathons and long-distance runs: recommendations for medical support. *British Medical Journal* 288, 1355–1359.

Venerando, A., Zeppilli, P. & Caselli, G. (1988) Cardiovascular disease. In: Dirix, A., Knuttgen, H.G. & Tittel, K. (eds) *The Olympic Book of Sports Medicine*, pp. 505–530. Blackwell Scientific Publications, Oxford.

Verde, T., Thomas, S. & Shephard, R.J. (1992) Potential markers of overtraining in the endurance athlete. *British Journal of Sports Medicine* 26, 167–175.

Vuori, I. (1995) Sudden death and exercise: effects of age and type of activity. *Sport Sciences Review* 4 (2), 46–84.

Wagenmakers, A.J.M., Beckerw, E.J., Brouns, F. *et al.* (1991) Carbohydrate supplementation, glycogen depletion and amino acid metabolism during exercise. *American Journal of Physiology* 260, E883–E890.

Wesslen, L., Pahlson, C., Linquist, O. *et al.* (1996) An increase in sudden unexpected deaths among young Swedish orienteers during 1979–1992. *European Heart Journal* 17, 902–910.

Wheeler, G.D., Wall, S.R., Belcastro, A.N., Conger, P. & Cumming, D. (1986) Are anorexic tendencies prevalent in the habitual runner? *British Journal of Sports Medicine* 20, 77–81.

White, J.A., Ward, C. & Nelson, H. (1984) Ergogenic demands of a 24 hour cycling event. *British Journal of Sports Medicine* 18, 165–171.

Williams, C. (1994) Diet and sports performance. In: Harries, M., Williams, C., Stanish, W.D. & Micheli, L.J. (eds) *Oxford Textbook of Sports Medicine*, pp. 65–82. Oxford Medical Publications, New York, NY.

Williams, R.S., Schocken, D.D., Morey, M. & Koisch, F.P. (1981) Medical aspects of competitive distance running. *Postgraduate Medicine* 70, 41–44.

Wyndham, C.H. & Strydom, N.B. (1972) Körperliche Arbeit bei höher Temperatur. In: Hollmann, W. (ed.) *Zentrale Themen der Sportmedizin*, pp. 131–149. Springer-Verlag, Berlin.

Young, A. (1984) Plasma creatine kinase after the marathon—a diagnostic dilemma. *British Journal of Sports Medicine* 18, 269–272.

Chapter 45

Considerations for Preparticipation Cardiovascular Screening in Young Competitive Athletes

BARRY J. MARON

Sudden deaths of competitive athletes are personal tragedies with great impact on the lay and medical communities (Maron 1993). They are usually due to a variety of previously unsuspected cardiovascular diseases (James *et al.* 1967; Thompson *et al.* 1979, 1982; Maron *et al.* 1980, 1986a, 1996a; Waller & Roberts 1980; Tsung *et al.* 1982; Virmani *et al.* 1982; Furlanello *et al.* 1984; Topaz & Edwards 1985; Thiene *et al.* 1988; Corrado *et al.* 1990; Burke *et al.* 1991; Drory *et al.* 1991; McCaffrey *et al.* 1991; van Camp *et al.* 1995; Liberthson 1996). Particularly in young people, such events often assume a high public profile, due to the widely held perception that trained athletes constitute the healthiest element of our society. The occasional deaths of well-known élite athletes exaggerate this visibility (Maron 1993; Maron & Garson 1994). Athletic field catastrophes have also substantially increased interest in the role and efficacy of preparticipation screening (Maron *et al.* 1996a).

This chapter considers: (i) the benefits and limitations of preparticipation screening for early detection of cardiovascular abnormalities in competitive athletes; (ii) cost-efficiency and feasibility issues, as well as the medical–legal implications of screening; and (iii) US consensus recommendations and guidelines for the most prudent, practical and effective screening procedures and strategies, based on a recent American Heart Association consensus panel (Maron *et al.* 1996a). Given the large number of competitive athletes in most developed countries and recent public health initiatives on physical activity and exercise, these issues have become particularly relevant.

Definitions and background

This chapter focuses on the competitive athlete, previously described as one who participates in an organized team or individual sport requiring systematic training and regular competition against others, while placing a high premium on athletic excellence and achievement (Maron & Mitchell 1994a; Maron & Mitchell 1994b). The purpose of screening, as described here, is to provide medical clearance for participation in competitive sport through routine and systematic evaluations intended to identify clinically relevant and pre-existing cardiovascular abnormalities and thereby reduce the risks associated with organized sport. It should, however, be emphasized that raising the possibility of a cardiovascular abnormality on a standard screening examination is only the first tier of recognition, after which referral to a specialist for further diagnostic investigation will probably be required. When a definitive cardiovascular diagnosis is made, the US consensus panel guidelines of Bethesda Conference #26 (Maron & Mitchell 1994a) should be utilized to formulate recommendations for continued participation or disqualification from competitive sport.

The American Heart Association guidelines (Maron *et al.* 1996a) (Table 45.1) focus primarily on the potential for population-based screening of high-school and collegiate student athletes rather than individual clinical assessments of athletes. They are designed to apply to competitors of all ages and both genders. The recommendations may also be extrapolated to athletes in youth, middle-school,

Table 45.1 American Heart Association consensus panel recommendations for preparticipation screening.

Family history: premature sudden death or heart disease in surviving relatives

Personal history: heart murmur, systemic hypertension, fatiguability, syncope, exertional dyspnoea or chest pain, as well as parental verification of the history

Physical examination: heart murmur*, femoral pulses, stigmata of Marfan syndrome and blood pressure measurement

---

*Precordial auscultation is recommended in both supine/sitting and standing positions to identify heart murmurs consistent with left ventricular outflow tract obstruction.

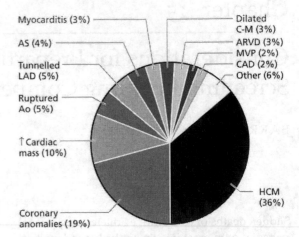

Fig. 45.1 Causes of sudden cardiac death in young competitive athletes (median age 17 years), based on systematic tracking of 158 athletes in the US, primarily 1985–95. ↑, increased; Ao, aorta; ARVD, arrythmogenic right ventricular dysplasia; AS, aortic stenosis; CAD, coronary artery disease; C-M, cardiomyopathy; HCM, hypertrophic cardiomyopathy; LAD, left anterior descending; MVP, mitral valve prolapse. Adapted with permission of the American Heart Association from Maron *et al.* (1996a).

masters or professional sports, and in some instances to participants in intense recreational sporting activities. It is also recognized that the overall preparticipation screening process extends well beyond the considerations described here (which are limited to the cardiovascular system), involving many other organ systems and medical issues.

The American Heart Association screening recommendations are predicated on the probability that intense athletic training is likely to increase the risk for sudden cardiac death (or disease progression) in trained athletes with clinically important underlying structural heart disease, although presently it is not possible to quantify that risk. Certainly, the vast majority of young athletes who die suddenly do so during athletic training or competition (Maron *et al.* 1980, 1996b; van Camp *et al.* 1995). These observations support the proposition that physical exertion is an important trigger for sudden death, given the presence of certain underlying cardiovascular diseases. Finally, the early detection of clinically significant cardiovascular disease through preparticipation screening may, in many instances, permit timely therapeutic interventions that prolong life.

Causes of sudden death in athletes

A variety of cardiovascular abnormalities are the most common causes of sudden death in competitive athletes (James *et al.* 1967; Thompson *et al.* 1979,

1982; Maron *et al.* 1980, 1986a, 1996a; Waller & Roberts 1980; Tsung *et al.* 1982; Virmani *et al.* 1982; Furlanello *et al.* 1984; Topaz & Edwards 1985; Thiene *et al.* 1988; Corrado *et al.* 1990; Burke *et al.* 1991; Drory *et al.* 1991; McCaffrey *et al.* 1991; van Camp *et al.* 1995; Liberthson 1996). The responsible lesions differ considerably with regard to age. In younger athletes (less than about 35 years of age) the vast majority of incidents are due to a variety of cardiac malformations largely congenital in origin (Figs 45.1–45.3) (James *et al.* 1967; Maron *et al.* 1980, 1986a, 1996a; Tsung *et al.* 1982; Furlanello *et al.* 1984; Topaz & Edwards 1985; Thiene *et al.* 1988; Corrado *et al.* 1990; Burke *et al.* 1991; Drory *et al.* 1991; McCaffrey *et al.* 1991; van Camp *et al.* 1995; Liberthson 1996). Virtually any disease capable of causing sudden death in young people may potentially do so in young competitive athletes. These cardiovascular diseases may be relatively common among young athletes who die suddenly, but they are uncommon in the general population. The lesions that are responsible for sudden death do not all occur with the same frequency, most being responsible for ≤5%

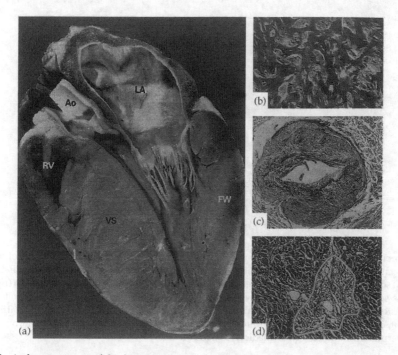

Fig. 45.2 Morphological components of the disease process in hypertrophic cardiomyopathy (HCM), the most common cause of sudden death in young competitive athletes. (a) A gross heart specimen sectioned in a cross-sectional plane similar to that of the echocardiographic (parasternal) long axis. Left ventricular wall thickening shows an asymmetrical pattern, confined primarily to the ventricular septum (VS), which bulges prominently into the left ventricular outflow tract. The left ventricular cavity appears reduced in size. FW, left ventricular free wall. (b–d) Histological features characteristic of left ventricular myocardium in HCM: (b) markedly disordered architecture, with hypertrophied cardiac muscle cells arranged at perpendicular and oblique angles; (c) an intramural coronary artery with thickened wall, due primarily to medial hypertrophy, and apparently narrowed lumen; (d) replacement fibrosis in an area of ventricular myocardium adjacent to an abnormal intramural coronary artery. Ao, aorta; LA, left atrium; RV, right ventricle. From Maron (1997), reproduced with permission of *The Lancet*.

of all such deaths (Fig. 45.1). Such deaths occur most commonly in intense team sports, such as basketball and football, which also have high levels of participation, particularly in North America.

The single most common cardiovascular abnormality causing sudden death in young athletes is hypertrophic cardiomyopathy (HCM), usually in its non-obstructive form (Maron *et al.* 1980, 1986a, 1987b, 1996a; Tsung *et al.* 1982; Drory *et al.* 1991; Wigle *et al.* 1985; Burke *et al.* 1991; Louie & Edwards 1994; van Camp *et al.* 1995; Klues *et al.* 1995; Liberthson 1996; Maron 1997; Spirito *et al.* 1997). HMC accounts for about 35% of these deaths (Maron *et al.* 1996a) (Figs 45.1 & 45.2). HCM is a primary and familial cardiac disease with heterogeneous expres-

sion, complex pathophysiology and diverse clinical course. Several disease-causing mutations in genes encoding proteins of the cardiac sarcomere have been identified (Geisterfer-Lowrance *et al.* 1990; Thierfelder *et al.* 1994; Marian & Roberts 1995; Schwartz *et al.* 1995; Watkins *et al.* 1995), including abnormalities affecting the β-myosin heavy chain, cardiac troponin T and troponin I, α-tropomyosin and myosin-binding protein C and α-actin. Within the general population, HCM is a relatively uncommon malformation occurring in about 0.2% of people (Maron *et al.* 1995a).

The next most frequent causes of sudden death are a variety of congenital coronary anomalies, particularly anomalous origin of the left main coronary

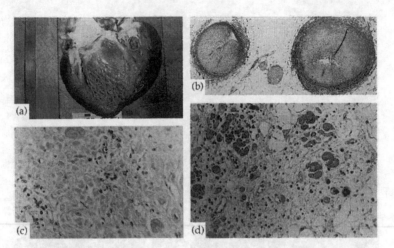

Fig. 45.3 Cardiac morphological findings at autopsy in four competitive athletes who died suddenly of causes other than HCM. (a) Gross specimen from an athlete with greatly enlarged ventricular cavities, consistent with dilated cardiomyopathy. (b) Histological section of the left anterior descending coronary artery (left) and a diagonal branch (right), showing severe (>95%) cross-sectional luminal narrowing by atherosclerotic plaque. (c) Foci of inflammatory cells consistent with myocarditis. (d) Histological section of right ventricular wall showing islands of myocytes within a matrix of fatty and fibrous replacement, characteristic of arrhythmogenic right ventricular dysplasia. Adapted from Maron *et al.* (1996a); reproduced with permission of the American Medical Association.

artery from the right (anterior) sinus of Valsalva (Cheitlin *et al.* 1974; Roberts 1987; Gaither *et al.* 1991; Maron *et al.* 1991; Jureidini *et al.* 1994). Less common causes include myocarditis (Fig. 45.3), dilated cardiomyopathy (Fig. 45.3), Marfan syndrome with aortic rupture, arrhythmogenic right ventricular dysplasia (Fig. 45.3), sarcoidosis, mitral valve prolapse, aortic valve stenosis, atherosclerotic coronary artery disease (Fig. 45.3), long QT syndrome and possibly intramural (tunnelled) coronary arteries (James *et al.* 1967; Maron *et al.* 1980, 1986a, 1996a; Tsung *et al.* 1982; Topaz & Edwards 1985; Thiene *et al.* 1988; Corrado *et al.* 1990; Burke *et al.* 1991; Drory *et al.* 1991; McCaffrey *et al.* 1991; Moss *et al.* 1991; Vincent *et al.* 1992; McKenna *et al.* 1994; van Camp *et al.* 1995; Liberthson 1996; Roden *et al.* 1996). Occasionally, athletes dying suddenly demonstrate no evidence of structural cardiovascular disease, even after careful gross and microscopic examination of the heart. In such instances (about 2% of one series) (Maron *et al.* 1996b), it may be difficult either to exclude non-cardiac factors (e.g. drug abuse) or to know whether careful serial sectioning of the specialized conducting system and associated

vasculature (not a part of the standard medical examiners' protocol) would have revealed occult but clinically relevant abnormalities (James *et al.* 1967; Thiene *et al.* 1983; Bharti & Lev 1986). One can only speculate on the potential aetiology in many such deaths, but it is possible that some episodes are due to a primary dysrhythmia in the absence of cardiac morphological abnormalities (Benson *et al.* 1983), previously unidentified Wolff–Parkinson–White syndrome, rare diseases in which structural abnormalities of the heart are characteristically lacking at necropsy (such as long QT or Brugade syndromes or possibly exercise-induced coronary spasm) or undetected segmental right ventricular dysplasia.

Middle-aged and older athletes (over the age of 35 years) are largely involved in competitive long-distance running. The vast majority of deaths in such athletes are due to atherosclerotic coronary artery disease (Thompson *et al.* 1979, 1982; Waller & Roberts 1980; Virmani *et al.* 1982); only rarely are congenital cardiovascular diseases such as HCM or coronary artery anomalies responsible for cardiac incidents in this age group.

Since this chapter focuses on the cardiovascular evaluation of athletes, other related medical problems that may occasionally cause sudden death in the young competitor, such as cerebral aneurysm, sickle cell trait (Kark *et al.* 1987), non-penetrating blunt chest impact (Maron *et al.* 1995b) or bronchial asthma, have been excluded from consideration. Also, issues related to drug screening are not part of this discussion, although ingestion of agents such as cocaine may have important adverse cardiovascular consequences (Isner *et al.* 1986; Virmani *et al.* 1988; Kloner *et al.* 1992). Screening for systemic hypertension has been addressed, although this disease is not regarded as an important cause of sudden unexpected death in young athletes (Kaplan *et al.* 1994).

Prevalence and scope of the problem

Relevant to the design of any screening strategy is the fact that sudden cardiac death in young athletes is a devastating but rather infrequent event; only a small proportion of participants in organized sports are at risk (Maron *et al.* 1998b). Indeed, each of the lesions with potential to cause sudden death in young athletes occurs infrequently in the general population, ranging from the relatively common (i.e. HCM) to apparently very rare conditions (e.g. coronary artery anomalies, arrhythmogenic right ventricular dysplasia, long QT syndrome or Marfan syndrome). It is a reasonable estimate that all congenital malformations relevant to athletic screening together may have a prevalence of <0.5% in the general athletic population.

The large reservoir of competitive athletes also constitutes a major obstacle to screening tactics (van Camp *et al.* 1995; Maron *et al.* 1996a, 1998a). In the US, for example, there are approximately 5–6 million competitive athletes at the high-school level (grades 9–12), in addition to lesser numbers of university (500000) and professional (5000) athletes. This total does not include an unspecified number of youth, middle-school and masters level competitors for which reliable estimates are not presently available. In any given year, there are probably as many as 8–10 million trained athletes in the US.

The prevalence of athletic field deaths due to cardiovascular disease is not known with certainty, but it appears to be approximately 1 per 200000 athletes of high-school age per year, and disproportionately more frequent in males than in females (Maron *et al.* 1998b). Given this relatively low prevalence, the heightened public awareness and intense interest in sudden deaths among athletes, often fuelled by the news media, are disproportionate to their actual numerical impact as a public health problem.

Ethical considerations in screening

Within a benevolent society, physicians have a responsibility to initiate prudent efforts to identify life-threatening diseases in athletes, in order to minimize the cardiovascular risks associated with sport and protect the health of participants (Maron *et al.* 1987a, 1996a; Maron & Mitchell 1994a,b; Pelliccia & Maron 1995). There is also an implicit ethical obligation on educational institutions (e.g. high schools and universities) to implement cost-effective strategies to assure that student-athletes are not exposed to unacceptable and avoidable medical risks (Maron *et al.* 1996b). The present author does not accept the libertarian view that high-school and university athletes should be permitted to assume any specifically disclosed cardiovascular risk associated with sport, as part of the overall uncertainty and risk of living. Despite sufficient resources, the motivation to implement cardiovascular screening in professional sports does not presently exist, due to the economic pressures in such sports environments, where athletic participation represents a vocation and remuneration for services is often substantial.

The extent to which preparticipation screening can be supported at any level is mitigated by cost-efficiency considerations, practical limitations and an awareness that 'zero risk' cannot be achieved in competitive sports (Maron *et al.* 1994; Mitten & Maron 1994). Indeed, there is often an implied acceptance of risk by athletes; as a society, we permit or condone many sporting activities known to have intrinsic risks that cannot be controlled absolutely — for example, motor racing and mountain climbing, as well as more traditional sports such as football in which the possibility of serious traumatic injury exists.

Legal considerations

Although educational institutions and professional teams are required to use reasonable care in conducting their athletic programmes, there is currently no clear legal precedent regarding their duty to conduct preparticipation screening of athletes to detect medically significant cardiovascular abnormalities in the US (Mitten 1993; Maron *et al.* 1996a). As yet, no lawsuits have apparently been brought forward alleging negligence through failure to perform cardiovascular screening or diagnose cardiac disease in young competitive athletes. In the absence of binding requirements established by state law or athletic governing bodies, most institutions and teams presently rely on the team physician (or other medical personnel) to determine appropriate medical screening procedures.

A physician who has medically cleared an athlete to participate in competitive sport is not necessarily legally liable for an injury or death caused by an undetected cardiovascular condition. Malpractice liability for failure to discover a latent, asymptomatic cardiovascular condition requires proof that a physician was negligent, deviating from customary or accepted medical practice in his (or her) specialty in performing preparticipation screening of athletes, and furthermore that utilization of established diagnostic criteria and techniques would have disclosed the medical condition.

The law permits the medical profession to establish the appropriate nature and scope of preparticipation screening based on use of its collective medical judgement. This necessarily involves the development of reliable diagnostic procedures in the light of cost–benefit and feasibility factors. The American Heart Association recommendations for cardiovascular preparticipation screening of athletes described here (Maron *et al.* 1996a) represent a viewpoint on the proper standard of medical care; however, these guidelines will establish the legal standard of care only if they are generally accepted or customarily followed by physicians, or are relied upon by courts in determining the nature and scope of the legal responsibility borne by sponsors of competitive athletes (Mitten 1993; Mitten & Maron 1994; Maron *et al.* 1998a,b).

Preparticipation examinations in US high schools and universities occur largely at the discretion of the examining physician and as customary practice. A considerably different situation has existed in Italy since 1971 in the form of government legislation ('Medical Protection of Athletic Activities Act'); this requires preventive medical evaluations for all competitive athletes (Pelliccia & Maron 1995). Unique to Italy, all citizens (ages 12–40) who are engaged in organized sport must undergo annual medical clearance by an approved physician, stipulating that the athlete is free of cardiovascular abnormalities that could unacceptably increase the risk of sudden cardiac death during training or competition. Since 1982, more detailed guidelines have been formulated for these preparticipation examinations; they include as a minimum, history and physical examination, a 12-lead electrocardiograph (ECG) and exercise and pulmonary function tests. Echocardiography has been specifically required (since 1994) only in selected professional sports (soccer, boxing and cycling). Under Italian law, the examining physician is primarily responsible for the accuracy of this clinical assessment, and stands as the final arbiter of eligibility for sport, issuing official certification of medical clearance. In the event that an incorrect or incomplete medical diagnosis leads directly to impaired health or death of an athlete, the physician responsible for sanctioning the athletic competition can be held accountable in the criminal (as well as civil) court.

Current customary practice in the US

It is important to acknowledge the limitations of the preparticipation screening process currently in place for student athletes in the US and most other countries. Only in this way can an informed public be created which might otherwise harbour important misconceptions regarding the principles and efficacy of athletic screening. Currently, universally accepted standards for the screening of high school and university athletes are lacking, and there are no approved certification procedures for the professionals who perform such screening examinations (Glover & Maron 1998). Some form of medical clearance by a physician or other trained health-care worker, usually consisting of a history and physical examination, is customary for high-school athletes. However, there is no agreement among US states as to the precise format of such preparticipation medical evaluations (Fig. 45.4). Eight US states (16%) have no approved history and physical examination questionnaires to guide examiners, and one of these states has no formal screening requirement. In the remaining 43 US states, several items relevant to cardiac-related problems have frequently been omitted from questionnaires. For example, exertional dyspnoea or chest pain, prior restriction from sport participation and family history of heart disease or Marfan syndrome were included in 0–56% of the state forms. Specific cardiovascular items regarding the physical examination were included in forms from only 5–37% of states, including documentation of a heart murmur, irregular heart rhythm, peripheral pulses or stigmata of Marfan syndrome. Seventeen (40%) out of 43 states had history and physical questionnaires that met at least nine of the 13 recommendations of the 1996 American Heart Association (Table 45.1), whereas 12 states (28%) covered four or fewer of these recommended items (Fig. 45.4). Therefore 40% of all US states do not formally require this process, do not have approved standard history and physical examination questionnaires to serve as guidelines for examiners (some require only a signature to provide medical clearance), or use approved forms that are

judged inadequate (Glover & Maron 1998) when evaluated against the specific screening recommendations proposed by the American Heart Association consensus panel (Maron *et al.* 1996a) (Table 45.1). These findings emphasize that at present it is not possible to assume that medical clearance for high-school sport precludes the possibility of underlying, potentially lethal cardiovascular disease. Existing guidelines regarding the examiners for preparticipation screening are also worthy of consideration. In a substantial proportion of US states, non-physician health-care workers are sanctioned to administer preparticipation screening, including practitioners with limited cardiovascular training (such as chiropractors in nine states) and nurse practitioners or physician assistants (in 20 states each) (Fig. 45.5).

We recently assessed the status of preparticipation cardiovascular screening in some 1000 US colleges and universities and found similar limitations in the screening process (Pfister *et al.* 1998). For example, about 25% of the colleges surveyed had inadequate history and physical questionnaires to guide the examiners (Fig. 45.6). Important omissions from the history forms in 40% or more of the athletic programmes included a history of premature sudden death in the family, exertional chest pain/shortness of breath, excessive fatigue and a family history of Marfan syndrome.

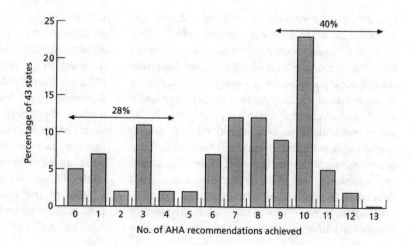

Fig. 45.4 Combined assessment of history and physical examination cardiovascular questionnaires used in 43 states, judged with respect to inclusion of the 13 specific 1996 American Heart Association (AHA) recommendations for preparticipation screening of high-school athletes; 28% of 43 states met four or fewer recommendations and 40% met nine or more recommendations. Eight other US jurisdictions had no formal questionnaires. From Glover and Maron (1998); reproduced with permission of the American Medical Association.

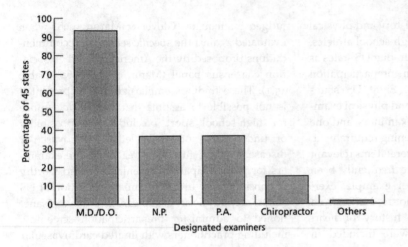

Fig. 45.5 Approved examiners for preparticipation screening of athletes in US high schools. Individual states may have approved more than one category of examiner. D.O., Doctor of osteopathy; N.P., nurse practitioner; P.A., physician assistant.

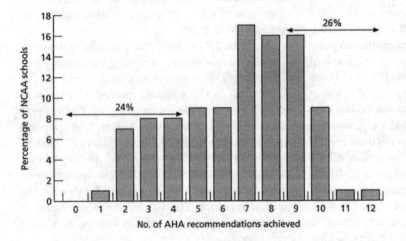

Fig. 45.6 Combined assessment of history and physical examination cardiovascular questionnaires used in 879 US colleges and universities, judged with respect to inclusion of 12 specific and relevant 1996 American Heart Association (AHA) recommendations for preparticipation screening; 24% of the institutions met four or fewer recommendations and 26% met nine or more recommendations.

Expectations of screening strategies

Preparticipation screening by history and physical examination alone (without non-invasive testing) does not possess sufficient power to guarantee detection of many critical cardiovascular abnormalities in large populations of young trained athletes in high school or university. Haemodynamically significant congenital aortic valve stenosis is the lesion most likely to be detected reliably during routine screening, due to its characteristically loud heart murmur. Detection of HCM by the standard screening history or physical examination is unreliable, because most patients have the non-obstructive form of this disease, characteristically expressed with no or only a soft heart murmur

(Wigle *et al.* 1985; Maron *et al.* 1987b, 1996a,b; Louie & Edwards 1994; Maron 1997). Furthermore, the majority of athletes with HCM do not experience syncope or have a family history of premature sudden death. This disease is also not easily detected by a preparticipation personal history (Wigle *et al.* 1985; Maron *et al.* 1987a, 1996b; Louie & Edwards 1994; Maron 1997). When symptoms such as chest pain or impaired consciousness are involved, the standard personal history has a low specificity for the detection of many cardiovascular abnormalities that lead to sudden cardiac death in young athletes.

Most of the lesions being considered here as potentially responsible for sudden death in young athletes are challenging to detect, even when echocardiography, ECG or other non-invasive tests are incorporated into the standard screening process—e.g. a variety of congenital coronary anomalies (particularly anomalous origin of the left main coronary artery from the right sinus of Valsalva). Despite these major limitations, a standard history and physical examination screening are theoretically of value by virtue of their ability to identify (or raise the suspicion of) cardiovascular abnormalities in some at-risk athletes. For example, genetic diseases such as HCM and Marfan syndrome and some cases of arrhythmogenic right ventricular dysplasia and premature atherosclerotic coronary artery disease can be suspected from the family history or by virtue of transient symptoms; physical examination may identify the stigmata of Marfan syndrome, lesions associated with left ventricular outflow obstruction (aortic valvular stenosis and some patients with HCM) by a loud heart murmur, and systemic hypertension by a routine measurement of blood pressure.

There are no prospective data to permit a direct assessment of the efficacy of large-scale athletic screening. A recent retrospective analysis of 134 young athletes who died suddenly from a variety of cardiovascular diseases showed that only 3% of those individuals who had been exposed to standard preparticipation screening were suspected of having cardiac disease, and less than 1% ultimately received an accurate diagnosis (Maron *et al.* 1996a) (Fig. 45.7).

Based on these observations, the preparticipation screening process as currently structured and carried out in US high schools appears to lack sufficient power to recognize clinically important cardiovascular abnormalities consistently. In contrast, preparticipation cardiovascular screening of competitive athletes in Italy (which routinely includes a 12-lead ECG, as well as a standard history and physical examination) identified a not inconsequential number of HCM cases (*n* = 22) over a 7-year period among 33735 consecutive athletes, a prevalence of 0.07% (Corrado *et al.* 1998) (Fig. 45.8). Each of the 22 HCM athletes was disqualified from competitive sports upon diagnosis, and each survived over an 8.2 ± 5 year follow-up.

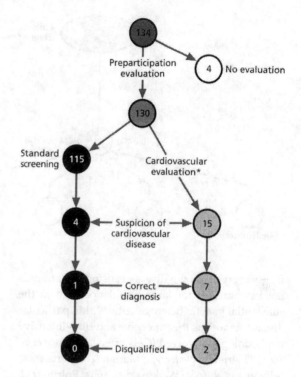

Fig. 45.7 Flow diagram showing impact of preparticipation medical history and physical examinations on the detection of structural cardiovascular disease (and causes of sudden death). *, Cardiovascular evaluation with testing (independent of standard school or institutional preparticipation screening), performed in 15 athletes because of symptoms, family history, cardiac murmur or physical findings suggestive of heart disease. From Maron *et al.* (1996b); reproduced with permission of the American Medical Association.

Potential efficacy and limitations of non-invasive screening tests

The addition of non-invasive diagnostic tests to the screening process has the potential to enhance detection of certain cardiovascular defects in young athletes. The two-dimensional echocardiogram is the principal diagnostic tool for clinical recognition of HCM, demonstrating an otherwise unexplained asymmetrical left ventricular wall thickening, the *sine qua non* of this disease (Maron & Epstein 1979; Wigle *et al.* 1985; Maron *et al.* 1987; Louie & Edwards 1994; Klues *et al.* 1995; Maron 1997). Comprehensive and routine screening for HCM by genetic testing

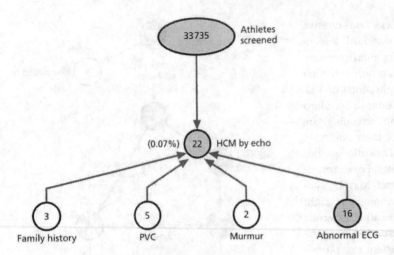

Fig. 45.8 Evidence from national Italian preparticipation screening programme (Padua, Italy; Centre for Sports Medicine 1979–96) showing that hypertrophic cardiomyopathy (HCM) was a detectable (and disqualifying) condition, identified most commonly by abnormalities on the routine 12-lead ECG which led to diagnostic echocardiography. PVC, premature ventricular contraction. Adapted from Corrado *et al.* (1998).

for a variety of known disease-causing mutations is not yet practical for large populations, given the substantial genetic heterogeneity of this particular disease, as well as the expensive and time-intensive methodologies involved (Geisterfer-Lowrance *et al.* 1990; Thierfelder *et al.* 1994; Marian & Roberts 1995; Schwartz *et al.* 1995; Watkins *et al.* 1995; Spirito *et al.* 1997).

Echocardiography could also be expected to detect other relevant abnormalities associated with sudden death in young athletes, such as valvular heart disease (e.g. mitral valve prolapse and aortic valvular stenosis), aortic root dilatation and left ventricular dysfunction (associated with myocarditis or dilated cardiomyopathy). However, such diagnostic testing cannot guarantee recognition of all important lesions, and some relevant cardiovascular diseases may be beyond detection with any screening methodology. Identification of many congenital coronary artery anomalies requires sophisticated laboratory examination, including coronary arteriography, although in selected young athletes echocardiography may raise a strong suspicion of important anomalies such as origin of the left main coronary artery from the right sinus of Valsalva (Gaither *et al.* 1991; Maron *et al.* 1991; Jureidini *et al.* 1994). Arrhythmogenic right ventricular dysplasia cannot usually be diagnosed reliably by echocardiography and ECG; the best available non-invasive test for this disease is probably magnetic resonance imaging, which unfortunately is expensive and not

universally available (Ricci *et al.* 1992; McKenna *et al.* 1994).

Cost-efficiency issues are important when assessing the feasibility of applying expensive non-invasive testing to the screening of large athletic populations (Risser *et al.* 1985; Lewis *et al.* 1989; Feinstein *et al.* 1993; Murry *et al.* 1995; Weidenbener *et al.* 1995). In the vast majority of instances, adequate financing and personnel are lacking for such endeavours. In those situations in which the full expense of testing would be the responsibility of administrative bodies such as a school, university or team, the costs are probably prohibitive (in the US, an average of about $600). Even if the prevalence of HCM in a young athletic population were assumed to be 1 : 500 (Maron *et al.* 1995a), at $600 per study it would theoretically cost $300 000 to detect one previously undiagnosed case.

Screening protocols incorporating non-invasive testing at greatly reduced cost have been described (Risser *et al.* 1985; Murry *et al.* 1995; Weidenbener *et al.* 1995). However, these efforts have involved unique circumstances in which echocardiographic equipment was donated and professional expenses were waived for all but technician-related costs. Also, some investigators have suggested an inexpensive shortened-format echocardiogram for population screening (limited to parasternal views; about 2 min in duration) (Murry *et al.* 1995; Weidenbener *et al.* 1995). Although such initiatives should not be discouraged, public service projects based largely on volunteers cannot usually be sustained on a consistent basis.

An important limitation of preparticipation screening with two-dimensional echocardiography is the potential for false-positive or false-negative test results. False-positive results arise from the assignment of borderline values for left ventricular wall thicknesses (or particularly enlarged cavity size). It is necessary to make a differential diagnosis between the normal but extreme physiological adaptations of the athlete's heart (Chapter 48; Huston et al. 1985; Maron 1986; Pelliccia et al. 1991, 1996b) and pathological conditions such as HCM or other cardiomyopathies (Maron et al. 1995b). Such clinical dilemmas (which cannot always be resolved conclusively in individual athletes) generate emotional, financial and medical burdens for the athlete, family, team and institution by virtue of the uncertainty that is created and the requirement for additional testing. False-negative screening results may occur in athletes with HCM if testing by echocardiography occurs when phenotypic expression is incomplete (Maron et al. 1986b). Left ventricular hypertrophy is often absent or mild in athletes with HCM who are younger than 13–15 years. In such individuals, the echocardiographic findings may not be diagnostic at preparticipation screening.

The 12-lead ECG has been proposed as a more practical and cost-efficient alternative to routine echocardiography for population-based screening (Maron et al. 1987a; LaCorte et al. 1989; Zehender et al. 1990; Corrado et al. 1998). The ECG is abnormal in about 95% of patients with HCM (Maron et al. 1983), and it may also be abnormal in other potentially lethal structural lesions. It usually identifies the important (but uncommon) long QT syndrome (Moss et al. 1991; Vincent et al. 1992; Roden et al. 1996). However, a proportion of genetically affected relatives in families with long QT syndrome may not have phenotypic expression on the ECG (Vincent et al. 1992).

The ECG suffers as a primary screening test, in comparison to the echocardiogram, because it lacks an imaging capability for recognition of structural cardiovascular malformations. The ECG also has a relatively low specificity as a screening test in ath-

letic populations, because of the high frequency with which ECG alterations develop as a normal physiological adaptation to training (Zehender et al. 1990; Pelliccia et al. 1996a). Such false-positive ECG test results substantially complicate the use of the 12-lead ECG as a primary screening tool in athletic populations. About 20–25% of athletes examined in the context of preparticipation screening have ECG patterns that ultimately stimulate echocardiographic study (Maron et al. 1987a). Élite athletes not infrequently demonstrate abnormal ECG patterns consistent with pathological conditions (Pelliccia et al. 1996a), even in the absence of structural heart disease and without increased cardiac dimensions due to training. Nevertheless, experience gained with the systematic preparticipation screening programme in Italy suggests that the routine ECG can detect athletes with previously unsuspected and underlying cardiovascular disease, particularly HCM (Corrado et al. 1998).

To date, there have been relatively few published reports of cardiovascular screening efforts in large athletic populations (Maron et al. 1987a; Lewis et al. 1989; Feinstein et al. 1993; Murry et al. 1995; Weidenbener et al. 1995; Fuller et al. 1997). Most of these studies have implemented non-invasive testing (i.e. conventional or limited echocardiographic examination or 12-lead ECG) in young high-school or university athletes. The populations ranged in size from 250 to 2000 athletes, and were usually studied over a 1-year period. In general, very few potentially lethal cardiovascular abnormalities were detected.

Perspectives on race and gender

Hypertrophic cardiomyopathy is an important cause of sudden death in young African–American athletes and there is preliminary evidence that such catastrophes may be more common in black athletes than in their white counterparts (Maron et al. 1996b, 1997). The substantial occurrence of HCM-related sudden death in young black male athletes (Fig. 45.9) contrasts sharply with the very infrequent reports of black patients with HCM in hospital- and clinic-based populations from tertiary referral centres (Wigle et al. 1985; Maron et al. 1987b; Louie &

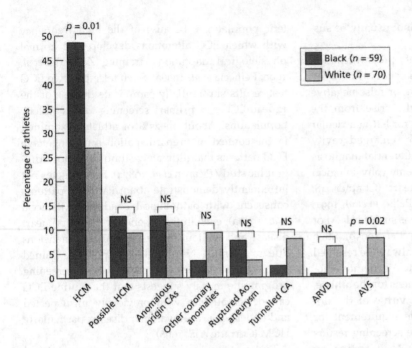

Fig. 45.9 Impact of race on cardiovascular causes of sudden death in competitive athletes. Ao, aorta; ARVD, arrythmogenic right ventricular dysplasia; AVS, aortic valve stenosis; CA, coronary arteries; HCM, hypertrophic cardiomyopathy.

Edwards 1994; Klues *et al.* 1995; Maron 1997; Spirito *et al.* 1997). In African–Americans, HCM is most frequently encountered when the disease results in sudden and unexpected death during competitive athletics. These data emphasize the disproportionate access to subspecialty health care between the black and white communities in the US, making it less likely for young black male athletes to receive a relatively sophisticated cardiovascular diagnosis such as HCM. Consequently, African–American athletes with HCM are less likely to be identified or disqualified from competition, in accordance with the recommendations of Bethesda Conference #26 (Maron & Mitchell 1994a).

Sudden death on the athletic field is uncommon in young women (Maron *et al.* 1980, 1986a, 1996a; van Camp *et al.* 1995), who comprise only about 10% of all such deaths; the low prevalence in women may be explained by lower participation rates or

less severe training demands and cardiac adaptation (Pelliccia *et al.* 1996b); further, HCM is less commonly recognized clinically in women (Wigle *et al.* 1985; Maron *et al.* 1987b; Louie & Edwards 1994; Klues *et al.* 1995; Maron 1997). This suggests the possibility that gender itself confers some protection against sudden death. Nevertheless, available data do not provide a compelling justification to construct specific screening algorithms based on gender, race or demographic subgrouping.

Acknowledgements

Portions of the present text are adapted from the American Heart Association Medical/Scientific Statement, 'Cardiovascular Preparticipation Screening of Competitive Athletes' (Maron *et al.* 1996a) with the permission of the American Heart Association.

References

Benson, D.W., Benditt, D.G., Anderson, R.W. *et al.* (1983) Cardiac arrest in young, ostensibly healthy patients: clinical, hemodynamic and electrophysiologic findings. *American Journal of Cardiology* **52**, 65–69.

Bharti, S. & Lev, M. (1986) Congenital abnormalities of the conduction system in sudden death in young adults. *Journal of the American College of Cardiology* **8**, 1096–1104.

Burke, A.P., Farb, V., Virmani, R., Goodin, J.

& Smialek, J.E. (1991) Sports-related and non-sports-related sudden cardiac death in young adults. *American Heart Journal* **121**, 568–575.

van Camp, S.P., Bloor, C.M., Mueller, F.O., Cantu, R.C. & Olson, H.G. (1995) Non-traumatic sports death in high school and college athletes. *Medicine and Science in Sports and Exercise* **27**, 641–647.

Cheitlin, M.D., De Castro, C.M. & McAllister, H.A. (1974) Sudden death as a complication of anomalous left coronary origin from the anterior sinus of Valsalva. A not-so-minor congenital anomaly. *Circulation* **50**, 780–787.

Corrado, D., Thiene, G., Nava, A., Rossi, L. & Pennelli, N. (1990) Sudden death in young competitive athletes: clinico-pathologic correlations in 22 cases. *American Journal of Medicine* **89**, 588–596.

Corrado, D., Basso, C., Schiavon, M. & Thiene, G. (1998) Screening for hypertrophic cardiomyopathy in young athletes. *New England Journal of Medicine* **339**, 364–369.

Drory, Y., Turetz, Y., Hiss, Y. *et al.* (1991) Sudden unexpected death in persons <40 years of age. *American Journal of Cardiology* **68**, 1388–1392.

Feinstein, R.A., Colvin, E. & Oh, M.K. (1993) Echocardiographic screening as part of a preparticipation examination. *Clinical Journal of Sports Medicine* **3**, 149–152.

Fuller, C.M., McNulty, C.M., Spring, D.A. *et al.* (1997) Prospective screening of 5615 high school athletes for risk of sudden cardiac death. *Medicine and Science in Sports and Exercise* **29**, 1131–1138.

Furlanello, F., Bettini, R., Cozzi, F. *et al.* (1984) Ventricular arrhythmias and sudden death in athletes. *Annals of the New York Academy of Science* **427**, 253–279.

Gaither, N.S., Rogan, K.M., Stajduhar, K. *et al.* (1991) Anomalous origin and course of coronary arteries in adults: identification and improved imaging utilizing transesophageal echocardiography. *American Heart Journal* **122**, 69–75.

Geisterfer-Lowrance, A.A.T., Kass, S., Tanigawa, G. *et al.* (1990) A molecular basis for familial hypertrophic cardiomyopathy: a β-cardiac myosin heavy chain gene missense mutation. *Cell* **62**, 999–1006.

Glover, D.W. & Maron, B.J. (1998) Profile of preparticipation cardiovascular screening for high school athletes. *Journal of the American Medical Association* **279**, 1817–1819.

Huston, T.P., Puffer, J.C. & Rodney, Mc. W.

(1985) The athlete heart syndrome. *New England Journal of Medicine* **4**, 24–32.

Isner, J.M., Estes, N.A.M. III, Thompson, P.D. *et al.* (1986) Acute cardiac events temporally related to cocaine abuse. *New England Journal of Medicine* **315**, 1438–1443.

James, T.N., Froggatt, P. & Marshall, T.K. (1967) Sudden death in young athletes. *Annals of Internal Medicine* **67**, 1013–1021.

Jureidini, S.B., Eaton, C., Williams, J., Nouri, S. & Appleton, R.S. (1994) Transthoracic two-dimensional and color flow echocardiographic diagnosis of aberrant left coronary artery. *American Heart Journal* **127**, 438–440.

Kaplan, N.M., Deveraux, R.B. & Miller, H.S. Jr (1994) Systemic hypertension. Task Force 4. In: Maron, B.J. & Mitchell, J.H. (eds) 26th Bethesda Conference, Recommendations for Determining Eligibility for Competition in Athletes with Cardiovascular Abnormalities. *Journal of the American College of Cardiology* **24**, 885–888.

Kark, J.A., Posey, D.M., Schumacher, H.R. & Ruehle, C.J. (1987) Sickle-cell as a risk factor for sudden death in physical training. *New England Journal of Medicine* **317**, 781–787.

Kloner, R.A., Hale, S., Alkekr, K. & Rezkalla, S. (1992) The effects of acute and chronic cocaine use on the heart. *Circulation* **85**, 407–419.

Klues, H.G., Schiffers, A. & Maron, B.J. (1995) Phenotypic spectrum and patterns of left ventricular hypertrophy in hypertrophic cardiomyopathy: morphologic observations and significance as assessed by two-dimensional echocardiography in 600 patients. *Journal of the American College of Cardiology* **26**, 1699–1708.

LaCorte, M.A., Boxer, R.A., Gottesfeld, I.B., Singh, S., Strong, M. & Mandell, L. (1989) EKG screening program for school athletes. *Clinical Cardiology* **12**, 41–44.

Lewis, J.F., Maron, B.J., Diggs, J.A., Spencer, J.E., Mehrotra, P.P. & Curry, C.L. (1989) Preparticipation echocardiographic screening for cardiovascular disease in a large, predominantly black population of collegiate athletes. *American Journal of Cardiology* **64**, 1029–1033.

Liberthson, R.R. (1996) Sudden death from cardiac causes in children and young adults. *New England Journal of Medicine* **334**, 1039–1044.

Louie, E.K. & Edwards, L.C. (1994) Hypertrophic cardiomyopathy. *Progress in Cardiovascular Diseases* **36**, 275–308.

McCaffrey, F.M., Braden, D.S. & Strong,

W.B. (1991) Sudden cardiac death in young athletes: a review. *American Journal of Diseases of Childhood* **145**, 177–183.

McKenna, W.J., Thiene, G., Nava, A. *et al.* (1994) Diagnosis of arrhythmogenic right ventricular dysplasia/cardiomyopathy. *British Heart Journal* **71**, 215–218.

Marian, A.J. & Roberts, R. (1995) Recent advances in the molecular genetics of hypertrophic cardiomyopathy. *Circulation* **91**, 532–540.

Maron, B.J. (1986) Structural features of the athlete heart as defined by echocardiography. *Journal of the American College of Cardiology* **7**, 190–203.

Maron, B.J. (1993) Sudden death in young athletes: lessons from the Hank Gathers affair. *New England Journal of Medicine* **329**, 55–57.

Maron, B.J. (1997) Hypertrophic cardiomyopathy. *Lancet* **350**, 127–133.

Maron, B.J. & Epstein, S.E. (1979) Hypertrophic cardiomyopathy: a discussion of nomenclature. *American Journal of Cardiology* **43**, 1242–1244.

Maron, B.J. & Garson, A. (1994) Arrhythmias and sudden cardiac death in élite athletes. *Cardiology Reviews* (Zipes, D. ed.) **2** (1), 26–32.

Maron, B.J. & Mitchell, J.H. (1994a) 26th Bethesda Conference. Recommendations for determining eligibility for competition in athletes with cardiovascular abnormalities. *Journal of the American College of Cardiology* **24**, 845–899.

Maron, B.J. & Mitchell, J.H. (1994b) Revised eligibility recommendations for competitive athletes with cardiovascular abnormalities. (Introduction to Bethesda Conference #26.) *Journal of the American College of Cardiology* **24**, 848–850.

Maron, B.J., Roberts, W.C., McAllister, H.A., Rosing, D.R. & Epstein, S.E. (1980) Sudden death in young athletes. *Circulation* **62**, 218–229.

Maron, B.J., Wolfson, J.K., Ciró, E. & Spirito, P. (1983) Relation of electrocardiographic abnormalities and patterns of left ventricular hypertrophy identified by two-dimensional echocardiography in patients with hypertrophic cardiomyopathy. *American Journal of Cardiology* **51**, 189–194.

Maron, B.J., Epstein, S.E. & Roberts, W.C. (1986a) Causes of sudden death in competitive athletes. *Journal of the American College of Cardiology* **7**, 204–214.

Maron, B.J., Spirito, P., Wesley, Y.E. & Arce, J. (1986b) Development and progression of left ventricular hypertrophy in children with hypertrophic cardiomyopathy. *New England Journal of Medicine* **315**, 610–614.

Maron, B.J., Bodison, S.A., Wesley, Y.E., Tucker, E. & Green, K.J. (1987a) Results of screening a large group of intercollegiate competitive athletes for cardiovascular disease. *Journal of the American College of Cardiology* **10**, 1214–1221.

Maron, B.J., Bonow, R.O., Cannon, R.O., Leon, M.B. & Epstein, S.E. (1987b) Hypertrophic cardiomyopathy: interrelation of clinical manifestations, pathophysiology, and therapy. *New England Journal of Medicine* **316**, 780–789 and 844–852.

Maron, B.J., Leon, B.J., Swain, J.A., Cannon, R.O. III & Pelliccia, A. (1991) Prospective identification by two-dimensional echocardiography of anomalous origin of the left main coronary artery from the right sinus of Valsalva. *American Journal of Cardiology* **68**, 140–142.

Maron, B.J., Brown, R.W., McGrew, C.A., Mitten, M.J. Jr, Caplan, A.L. & Hutter, A.M. Jr (1994) Ethical, legal and practical considerations affecting medical decision-making in competitive athletes. In: Maron, B.J. & Mitchell, J.H. (eds) 26th Bethesda Conference. Recommendations for Determining Eligibility for Competition in Athletes with Cardiovascular Abnormalities. *Journal of the American College of Cardiology* **24**, 854–860.

Maron, B.J., Gardin, J.M., Flack, J.M., Gidding, S.S. & Bild, D. (1995a) Assessment of the prevalence of hypertrophic cardiomyopathy in a general population of young adults: echocardiographic analysis of 4111 subjects in the CARDIA Study. *Circulation* **92**, 785–789.

Maron, B.J., Poliac, L., Kaplan, J.A. & Mueller, F.O. (1995b) Blunt impact to the chest leading to sudden death from cardiac arrest during sports activities. *New England Journal of Medicine* **333**, 337–342.

Maron, B.J., Pelliccia, A. & Spirito, P. (1995c) Cardiac disease in young trained athletes: insights into methods for distinguishing athlete's heart from structural heart disease with particular emphasis on hypertrophic cardiomyopathy. *Circulation* **91**, 1596–1601.

Maron, B.J., Thompson, P.D., Puffer, J.C. *et al.* (1996a) Cardiovascular preparticipation screening of competitive athletes. *Circulation* **94**, 850–856.

Maron, B.J., Shirani, J., Poliac, L.C., Mathenge, R., Roberts, W.C. & Mueller, F.O. (1996b) Sudden death in young competitive athletes: clinical, demographic and pathological profiles.

Journal of the American Medical Association **276**, 199–204.

Maron, B.J., Poliac, L.C. & Mathenge, R. (1997) Hypertrophic cardiomyopathy as an important cause of sudden cardiac death on the athletic field in African–American athletes (abstract). *Journal of the American College of Cardiology* **29** (Suppl. A), 462A.

Maron, B.J., Mitten, M.J., Quandt, E.F. & Zipes, D.P. (1998a) Competitive athletes with cardiovascular disease — the case of Nicholas Knapp. *New England Journal of Medicine* **339**, 1632–1635.

Maron, B.J., Gohman, T.E. & Aeppli, D. (1998b) Prevalence of sudden cardiac death during competitive sports activities in high school athletes. *Journal of the American College of Cardiology* **32**, 1881–1884.

Mitten, M.J. (1993) Team physicians and competitive athletes: allocating legal responsibility for athletic injuries. *University of Pittsburgh Literary Review* **55**, 129–169.

Mitten, M.J. & Maron, B.J. (1994) Legal considerations that affect medical eligibility for competitive athletes with cardiovascular abnormalities and acceptance of Bethesda Conference recommendations. *Journal of the American College of Cardiology* **24**, 861–863.

Moss, A.J., Schwartz, P.J., Crampton, R.S. *et al.* (1991) The long QT syndrome: prospective longitudinal study of 328 families. *Circulation* **84**, 1136–1144.

Murry, P.M., Cantwell, J.D., Heith, D.L. & Shoop, J. (1995) The role of limited echocardiography in screening athletes. *American Journal of Cardiology* **76**, 849–850.

Pelliccia, A. & Maron, B.J. (1995) Preparticipation cardiovascular evaluation of the competitive athlete: perspectives from the 30 year Italian experience. *American Journal of Cardiology* **75**, 827–831.

Pelliccia, A., Maron, B.J., Spataro, A., Proschan, M.A. & Spirito, P. (1991) The upper limit of physiologic cardiac hypertrophy in highly trained élite athletes. *New England Journal of Medicine* **324**, 295–301.

Pelliccia, A., Cullasso, F., Di Paolo, F.M. *et al.* (1996a) Clinical significance of abnormal electrocardiographic patterns in élite athletes: the impact of gender and cardiac morphologic adaptations to training (abstract). *Circulation* **94**, I-326.

Pelliccia, A., Maron, B.J., Culasso, F., Spataro, A. & Caselli, G. (1996b) Athlete's heart in women: echocardiographic characterization of highly

trained élite female athletes. *Journal of the American Medical Association* **276**, 211–215.

Pfister, G.C., Puffer, J.C. & Maron, B.J. (1998) Is preparticipation screening adequate for the detection of cardiovascular disease in competitive student-athletes in United States colleges and universities? *Circulation* **98** (Suppl. I), I-187.

Ricci, C., Longo, R., Pagnan, L. *et al.* (1992) Magnetic resonance imaging in right ventricular dysplasia. *American Journal of Cardiology* **70**, 1589–1595.

Risser, W.L., Hoffman, H.M., Gordon, B.G. Jr & Green, L.W. (1985) A cost–benefit analysis of preparticipation sports examination of adolescent athletes. *Journal of School Health* **55**, 270–273.

Roberts, W.C. (1987) Congenital coronary arterial anomalies unassociated with major anomalies of the heart or great vessels. In: Roberts, W.C. ed. *Adult Congenital Heart Disease*, pp. 583–615. FA Davis Co., Philadelphia.

Roden, D.M., Lazzara, R., Rosen, M., Schwartz, P.J., Towbin, J. & Vincent, G.M. (1996) Multiple mechanisms in the long-QT syndrome: current knowledge, gaps, and future directions. *Circulation* **94**, 1996–2012.

Schwartz, K., Carrier, L., Guicheney, P. & Komajda, M. (1995) Molecular basis of familial cardiomyopathies. *Circulation* **91**, 532–540.

Spirito, P., Seidman, C.E., McKenna, W.J. & Maron, B.J. (1997) The management of hypertrophic cardiomyopathy. *New England Journal of Medicine* **336**, 775–785.

Thiene, G., Pennelli, N. & Rossi, L. (1983) Cardiac conduction system abnormalities as a possible cause of sudden death in young athletes. *Human Pathology* **14**, 706–709.

Thiene, G., Nava, A., Corrado, D., Rossi, L. & Penelli, N. (1988) Right ventricular cardiomyopathy and sudden death in young people. *New England Journal of Medicine* **318**, 129–133.

Thierfelder, L., Watkins, H., MacRae, C. *et al.* (1994) α-Tropomyosin and cardiac troponin T mutations cause familial hypertrophic cardiomyopathy: a disease of the sarcomere. *Cell* **77**, 701–712.

Thompson, P.D., Stern, M.P., Williams, P., Duncan, K., Haskell, W.L. & Wood, P.D. (1979) Death during jogging or running. A study of 18 cases. *Journal of the American Medical Association* **242**, 1265–1267.

Thompson, P.D., Funk, E.J., Carleton, R.A. & Sturner, W.Q. (1982) Incidence of death during jogging in Rhode Island from 1975 through 1980. *Journal of the*

American Medical Association **247**, 2535–2538.

Topaz, O. & Edwards, J.E. (1985) Pathologic features of sudden death in children, adolescents and young adults. *Chest* **87**, 476–482.

Tsung, S.H., Huang, T.Y. & Chang, H.H. (1982) Sudden death in young athletes. *Archives of Pathology and Laboratory Medicine* **106**, 168–170.

Vincent, G.M., Timothy, K.W., Leppert, M. & Keating, M. (1992) The spectrum of symptoms and QT intervals in carriers of the gene for the long-QT syndrome. *New England Journal of Medicine* **327**, 846–852.

Virmani, R., Robinowitz, M. & McAllister,

H.A. Jr (1982) Nontraumatic death in joggers: a series of 30 patients at autopsy. *American Journal of Medicine* **72**, 874–882.

Virmani, R., Robinowitz, M., Smialek, J.E. & Smyth, D.F. (1988) Cardiovascular effects of cocaine: an autopsy study of 40 patients. *American Heart Journal* **115**, 1068–1076.

Waller, B.F. & Roberts, W.C. (1980) Sudden death while running in conditioned runners aged 40 years or over. *American Journal of Cardiology* **45**, 1292–1300.

Watkins, H., Conner, D., Thierfelder, L. *et al.* (1995) Mutations in the cardiac myosin binding protein-C gene on chromosome 11 cause familial hypertrophic

cardiomyopathy. *Nature Genetics* **11**, 434–437.

Weidenbener, E.J., Krauss, M.D., Waller, B.F. & Taliercio, C.P. (1995) Incorporation of screening echocardiography in the preparticipation exam. *Clinical Journal of Sports Medicine* **5**, 86–89.

Wigle, E.D., Sasson, Z., Henderson, M.A. *et al.* (1985) Hypertrophic cardiomyopathy: the importance of the site and extent of hypertrophy — a review. *Progress in Cardiovascular Diseases* **28**, 1–83.

Zehender, M., Meinertz, T., Keul, J. & Just, H. (1990) ECG variants and cardiac arrhythmias in athletes: clinical relevance and prognostic importance. *American Heart Journal* **119**, 1378–1391.

Chapter 46

Lung Fluid Movements in Endurance Sport

NIELS H. SECHER

Introduction

A surprising insight into fluid movement during endurance training was generated from the evaluation of pulmonary diffusing capacity ($\dot{D}Lco$) following exercise (Rasmussen *et al.* 1992; Hanel *et al.* 1997). $\dot{D}Lco$ is reduced for many hours after exercise, and this limitation of $\dot{D}Lco$ is explained not so much by an effect of exercise on the lungs, as by the redistribution of blood from the lungs to the previously exercising muscles. The resulting decrease in central blood volume leaves less haemoglobin available to bind with oxygen (or, as it is usually determined, with carbon monoxide, CO), and $\dot{D}Lco$ decreases.

Although the postexercise reduction in $\dot{D}Lco$ is of little consequence for oxygen transport during a second bout of exercise (Hanel *et al.* 1994; McKenzie *et al.* 1999), a smaller than normal pulmonary blood volume is of interest because the central blood volume is a regulated variable. In the first few hours after exercise, thirst and minimal urine production compensate for the decreased central blood volume and this in turn enhances the total blood volume of the athlete (Secher *et al.* 1997).

Blood volume

Most physiological variables respond to regular bouts of physical activity. For plasma volume, the response is an increase which is especially fast and prominent (Fellmann 1992). After only 2 h of endurance training each day for 3 days, plasma volume increases by about 20% (Green *et al.* 1989,

1990). If training is discontinued, there is a corresponding reduction in plasma volume within a few days (Coyle *et al.* 1986). The increase in red cell volume is much slower; an increase can only be detected after about 3 weeks of training (Schmidt *et al.* 1988). The earliest sign of erythropoiesis is an increased number of newly formed red cells (reticulocytes) in the blood. An increase in the number of reticulocytes can be detected in peripheral blood after only 2 days of training (Schmidt *et al.* 1988).

An enlarged blood volume as a response to training is a teleologically predictable outcome of training. Endurance training enhances oxygen transport to skeletal muscle and maximal oxygen intake is related to the red cell mass rather than to the concentration of haemoglobin in the blood. In recent years, the importance of red cell mass has been emphasized by the increased maximal oxygen intake and work capacity of athletes after the reinfusion of previously collected and stored blood ('blood doping', see Chapter 30). The importance of the red cell volume for exercise capacity is pertinent to the current discussion on administration of erythropoietin (EPO), not only to patients with kidney disease, but also to athletes.

Changes in plasma volume bear no direct relationship to aerobic power, but the training-induced increase in plasma volume increases cardiac output during exercise (Green *et al.* 1990) and reduces the catecholamine response (Green *et al.* 1989). Thus, in untrained as opposed to trained humans, cardiac output during exercise is preload limited (Hopper *et al.* 1988).

Central blood volume

The central blood volume controls the total body blood volume and it is the central blood volume which is tightly regulated by neural and hormonal mechanisms. The central circulation is innervated by numerous nerve fibres, both unmyelinated and myelinated, that provide the central nervous system with information about distension of the central vessels and the heart (Mark & Manica 1983). As an example, sympathetic activity increases in response to a reduced central blood volume, despite unchanged or even an elevated blood pressure, as occurs during the first minutes of head-up tilt (Pedersen *et al*. 1995).

The activity of afferent nerves from the central circulation can be assessed only indirectly in humans. However, the release of atrial natriuretic peptide (ANP) can be readily determined in plasma. Reflecting ANP release from the right atrium in particular, the pulmonary artery concentration is about twice as high as the arterial concentration, which in turn is higher than the venous concentration; nevertheless, the three concentrations vary in parallel (Perko *et al*. 1994). It is often considered that ANP is released into the blood in response to an enhanced atrial pressure as well as an increase in volume. However, when the right atrial pressure is increased by maintaining a positive end-expiratory pressure, the atrium is compressed by the external pressure and the plasma level of ANP decreases. In other words, the release of ANP occurs in proportion to filling of the central blood volume, rather than in response to an increase in right atrial pressure.

The importance of the central blood volume in total blood volume regulation is illustrated by the influence of gravity on the circulation. During a period of bedrest, the relative increase in central blood volume compared to the fraction of the total blood volume found in the lower limbs results in a rapid decrease of plasma volume. The decrease is greater in trained compared to untrained individuals (0.9 versus 0.5 l over 24 h; Convertino 1998). Similarly, a spaceflight is associated with a marked reduction in plasma volume; in this situation, the blood volume becomes distributed equally throughout the body, making even facial oedema

prevalent. These observations support the view that the reduced central blood volume associated with the upright posture produces the signal which maintains the 'normal' or prevailing plasma volume.

Central blood volume during exercise

The central blood volume increases during exercise. A direct relationship can be established between cardiac output and the central blood volume, ranging from the extremes of hypovolaemic shock to intense dynamic exercise. This indicates the importance of Starling's 'law' of the heart. During exercise, the 'venous pump' provides a force redistributing blood towards the thoracic vessels, as elegantly demonstrated by Beecher *et al*. (1936). The elevated central blood volume results in an increase in plasma ANP (Freund *et al*. 1988; Ray *et al*. 1990b) and an increase in left ventricular end-diastolic volume (Ray *et al*. 1990a). Ray *et al*. (1993) demonstrated that sympathetic nerve activity decreases in response to exercise in the upright position. In contrast, during supine exercise, the central blood volume reservoirs are already filled before activity begins, and there is minimal change in plasma ANP concentration with activity. In both body positions, sympathetic nerve activity increases as 'waste products' accumulate in the working muscles.

Given that the total blood volume is reduced after bedrest and spaceflight (both situations ensuring maintenance of a large central blood volume), it is not easy to explain how the elevation of central blood volume during exercise leads to an increase in total blood volume. However, as mentioned earlier, recordings of $\dot{D}L_{CO}$ postexercise offer an explanation of the enlarged blood volume of endurance athletes (Rasmussen *et al*. 1992; Hanel *et al*. 1997).

Pulmonary diffusing capacity

In contrast to most links in the oxygen transport chain from the atmosphere to skeletal muscle (Chapter 3), the lungs appear to be remarkably stable components. The pulmonary ventilation increases with training, the heart and blood volume adapt to changes in physical activity, the number of muscle capillaries and the size of the mitochondria increase, as do the enzyme activities in the Krebs cycle. Only the lungs remain unaffected by habitual physical activity, whether evaluated by standard tests such as forced expiratory volume in one second (FEV_1) and vital capacity (VC), or whether assessed from determinations of resting $\dot{D}Lco$. Accordingly, the anatomical lung size is an important determinant of oxygen exchange (Secher 1983; Hopkins *et al.* 1998).

The stability of lung physiology with endurance training does not indicate that lung function is uninfluenced by exercise. Pulmonary function is evaluated by $\dot{D}Lco$ which expresses the rate of diffusion of CO across the alveolar–capillary membrane (Krogh 1914). The diffusing capacity is determined using CO rather than oxygen, because the 'back pressure' or partial pressure of CO in the capillary blood can be assumed to be close to zero (the affinity of CO to haemoglobin is about 200 times that for oxygen and little CO is present in the blood of normal non-smoking humans). Yet, as elucidated by Roughton and Forster (1957), the pulmonary diffusing capacity is determined not only by the characteristics of the alveolar–capillary membrane, but also by the number of red cells, and thus the amount of haemoglobin, present in the pulmonary capillaries and available to equilibrate with CO (and normally oxygen). Thus Roughton and Forster (1957) distinguished between the membrane component ($\dot{D}_m$) and the capillary blood volume component (V_c) of the oxygen diffusion barrier.

Although the pulmonary area available for diffusion and also the characteristics of the alveolar–capillary membrane remain fairly constant over time, the central blood volume is highly variable in humans, due to transitions from a supine to a standing posture. When standing, the dependent veins are immediately filled and the central blood volume is correspondingly reduced. Prolonged standing causes a further reduction of central blood volume by filtration of fluid in dependent regions of the body and an equal mobilization of water from regions of the upper body. Changes in distribution of blood volume are described in relation to 'an indifference point', that is the region of the body where no fluid displacement occurs on standing.

This indifference point (or plane) is located between the umbilicus and the iliac crest (Perko *et al.* 1993). As more blood is presented to the lungs when the subject is supine than when standing, the $\dot{D}Lco$ is larger in the supine position.

During exercise, a redistribution of blood occurs, blood from the exercising legs being moved centrally by the venous pump. The resultant increase in pulmonary capillary blood volume explains, in part, the increase in $\dot{D}Lco$. However, during the first hour following exercise, $\dot{D}Lco$ returns to its resting level; it decreases further, to about 10% below the resting level, from 2 to at least 6 h after exercise (Rasmussen *et al.* 1986; Caillaud *et al.* 1993; McKenzie *et al.* 1999) (Fig. 46.1). The postexercise decrease in $\dot{D}Lco$ does not depend on the intensity of exercise (Hanel *et al.* 1993), and it is of similar magnitude in both trained and untrained subjects (Sheel *et al.* 1998). Although a decrease of $\dot{D}_m$ is the predominant cause of the limitation of $\dot{D}Lco$ immediately after exercise (Miles

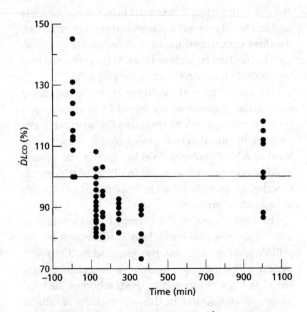

Fig. 46.1 Pulmonary diffusing capacity ($\dot{D}Lco$) after 'all-out' rowing on an ergometer. Immediately after rowing $\dot{D}Lco$ increases markedly, due to an augmentation of central blood volume. When cardiac output has returned to the prerowing value, $\dot{D}Lco$ decreases for up to at least 6 h. The horizontal line indicates the prerowing value. Individual data from Rasmussen *et al.* (1986, 1992) and Hanel *et al.* (1994, 1997).

et al. 1983; Manier *et al.* 1991, 1993), the subsequent prolonged reduction in $\dot{D}L$CO is attributable to an effect on V_c (Hanel *et al.* 1994; Sheel *et al.* 1998). V_c is elevated immediately after exercise, but after 1 h it has returned to the resting level, and it then continues to decrease for at least 6 h (Fig. 46.2).

Central blood volume after exercise

The distribution of blood in the body can be followed surprisingly easily by determination of electrical impedance. The reduced central blood volume induced by a head-up tilt (Matzen *et al.* 1991) or lower body negative pressure (Perko *et al.* 1996) is reflected in an elevated thoracic impedance. Impedance values closely match directly determined central blood volumes (Pawelczyk *et al.* 1994) and changes in plasma ANP levels (Perko *et al.* 1994). After exercise, the changes in thoracic impedance support the view that the central blood volume is

reduced. The thoracic impedance is increased by about 4 ohms at the time when the $\dot{D}L$CO is reduced (Rasmussen *et al.* 1992; Hanel *et al.* 1997). Conversely, electrical impedance is reduced by about 4 ohms over the legs, suggesting that the blood content of the previously exercising muscles is augmented. More direct evidence supporting a redistribution of the blood volume after exercise comes from the use of technetium-labelled erythrocytes (Hanel *et al.* 1997). Postexercise, when $\dot{D}L$CO is reduced, there appears to be about 7% less blood in the thorax and about 3% more blood in the leg muscles.

The changes in blood volume distribution after exercise are large enough to be detected by the volume-regulating hormones of the body, notably by ANP. Hanel *et al.* (1997) detected a 22% reduction in plasma ANP when $\dot{D}L$CO was reduced postexercise (Fig. 46.3). Measuring an ANP fragment (pro-ANP (1–30)) with a shorter plasma half-life, the reduction is about seven times more pronounced (H.B. Nielsen, personal communication). Other

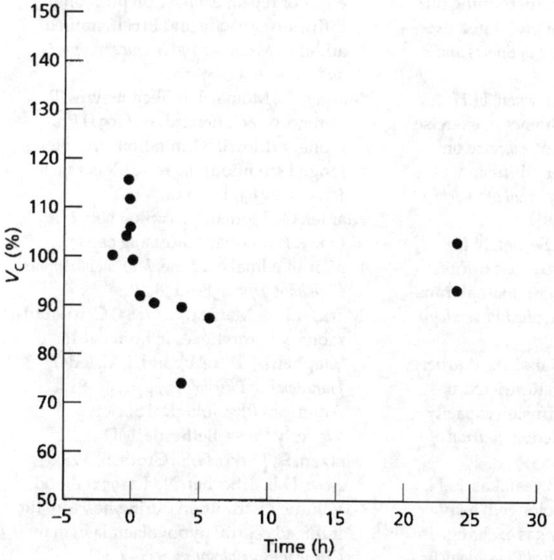

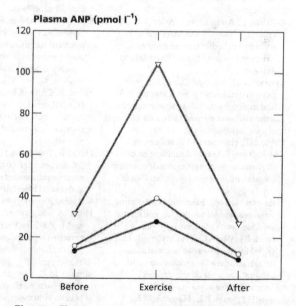

Fig. 46.2 The central blood volume after exercise. Values are expressed relative to rest and are derived from the capillary blood volume (V_c) as determined by pulmonary diffusion for carbon monoxide. Data are average values from studies by Miles *et al.* (1983), Manier *et al.* (1991, 1993), Hanel *et al.* (1994) and Sheel *et al.* (1998). The central blood volume is elevated for the first hour of recovery from exercise, but then decreases for at least 6 h.

Fig. 46.3 Plasma atrial natriuretic peptide (ANP) before, during and after exercise. Values represent the median and range for eight subjects (Hanel *et al.* 1997). Although ANP is elevated during exercise, it decreases to below the resting values 2 h after exercise.

hormonal variables offer some explanation as to why the elevated ANP of exercise is not associated with diuresis. During exercise, plasma vasopressin increases to high values (55-fold; $50\,pmol\cdot l^{-1}$; Hanel *et al.* 1997) which would have a significant antidiuretic effect.

Conclusion

Although adaptations to repeated bouts of physical exercise are numerous and teleologically predictable, it has been difficult to establish cause and effect relationships. The model here presented of blood volume regulation during training offers such a relationship. This model is unique in that it is based on recovery phenomena rather than on the perturbations taking place during exercise. When the blood volume is elevated for relatively brief periods of exercise during a 24-h period, urine production and sodium excretion are inhibited by elevated plasma concentrations of antidiuretic hormone and aldosterone, respectively. Conversely, in the hours following recovery from exercise, the central blood volume is reduced, as a larger fraction of the total blood volume is encompassed within the vascular bed of previously exercising muscles. There is much evidence to suggest that the central blood volume is the regulated fraction of the total blood volume. Over a day, endurance training results, on average, in a reduced central blood volume that acts as a stimulus to up-regulate blood volume. Changes in the distribution of the blood volume after exercise do not depend on exercise intensity, making exercise as important for blood volume regulation in a normal person as it is in athletes.

References

Beecher, H.K., Field, M.E. & Krogh, A. (1936) The effect of walking on the venous pressure at the ankle. *Skandinavisches Archives für Physiologie* **73**, 133–141.

Caillaud, C., Anselme, F., Mercier, J. & Préfaut, C. (1993) Pulmonary gas exchange in highly trained athletes. *European Journal of Applied Physiology* **67**, 431–437.

Convertino, V.A. (1998) Changes in peak oxygen uptake and plasma volume in fit and unfit subjects following exposure to a simulation of microgravity. *Acta Physiologica Scandinavica* **164**, 251–257.

Coyle, E.F., Hemmert, M.K. & Coggan, A.R. (1986) Effects of detraining on cardiovascular responses to exercise: role of blood volume. *Journal of Applied Physiology* **60**, 95–99.

Fellmann, N. (1992) Hormonal and plasma volume alterations following endurance exercise. *Sports Medicine* **13**, 37–49.

Freund, B.J., Wade, C.E. & Claybaugh, J.R. (1988) Effect of exercise on atrial natriuretic factor: release mechanisms and implications for fluid homeostasis. *Sports Medicine* **6**, 364–376.

Green, H.J., Jones, L.L., Houston, M.E., Ball-Burnett, M.E. & Farrance, B.W. (1989) Muscle energetics during prolonged cycling after exercise hypervolemia. *Journal of Applied Physiology* **66**, 622–631.

Green, H.J., Jones, L.L. & Painter, D.C. (1990) Effects of short-term training on cardiac function during prolonged exercise. *Medicine and Science in Sports and Exercise* **22**, 488–493.

Hanel, B., Gustafsson, F., Larsen, H.H. & Secher, N.H. (1993) Influence of exercise intensity and duration of exercise on post-exercise pulmonary diffusion capacity. *International Journal of Sports Medicine* **14**, S11–S14.

Hanel, B., Clifford, P.S. & Secher, N.H. (1994) Restricted post exercise diffusion capacity does not impair maximal transport for O_2. *Journal of Applied Physiology* **77**, 2408–2412.

Hanel, B., Teunissen, I., Rabøl, A., Warberg, J. & Secher, N.H. (1997) Restricted post-exercise pulmonary diffusion capacity and central blood depletion. *Journal of Applied Physiology* **83**, 11–17.

Hopkins, S.R., Gavin, T.P., Siafakas, N.N. *et al.* (1998) Effect of prolonged, heavy exercise on pulmonary gas exchange in athletes. *Journal of Applied Physiology* **85**, 1523–1532.

Hopper, M.K., Coggan, A.R. & Coyle, E.F. (1988) Exercise stroke volume relative to plasma volume expansion. *Journal of Applied Physiology* **64**, 404–408.

Krogh, M. (1914) Diffusion of gases through the lungs of man. *Journal of Physiology (London)* **49**, 271–300.

McKenzie, D.C., Lama, I.L., Potts, J.E.,

Sheel, A.W. & Coutts, K.D. (1999) The effect of repeat exercise on pulmonary diffusion capacity and EIH in trained athletes. *Medicine and Science in Sports and Exercise* **31**, 99–104.

Manier, G., Moinard, J., Techoueyres, P., Varene, N. & Guenard, H. (1991) Pulmonary diffusion limitation after prolonged strenuous exercise. *Respiration Physiology* **83**, 143–154.

Manier, G., Moinard, J. & Stoicheff, H. (1993) Pulmonary diffusing capacity after maximal exercise. *Journal of Applied Physiology* **75**, 2580–2585.

Mark, A.L. & Manica, G. (1983) Cardiopulmonary baroreflexes in humans. In: Shepherd, J.T. & Abboud, F.M. (eds) *Handbook of Physiology*, pp. 795–813. American Physiological Society, Waverly Press, Bethesda, MD.

Matzen, S., Perko, G.E., Groth, S., Friedman, D.B. & Secher, N.H. (1991) Blood volume distribution during head-up tilt induced central hypovolaemia in man. *Clinical Physiology* **11**, 411–422.

Miles, D.S., Doerr, C.E., Schonfeld, S.A., Sinks, D.E. & Gotshall, R.W. (1983) Changes in pulmonary diffusing capacity and closing volume after running a marathon. *Respiration Physiology* **52**, 349–359.

Pawelczyk, J.A., Matzen, S., Friedman, D.B. & Secher, N.H. (1994) Cardiovascular and hormonal responses to central hypovolaemia in humans. In: Secher, N.H., Pawelczyk, J.A. & Ludbrook, J. (eds) *Blood Loss and Shock*, pp. 25–36. Edward Arnold, London.

Pedersen, M., Madsen, P., Klokker, M., Olesen, H.L. & Secher, N.H. (1995) Sympathetic influence on cardiovascular responses to sustained head-up tilt in humans. *Acta Physiologica Scandinavica* **155**, 435–444.

Perko, G., Payne, G. & Secher, N.H. (1993) An indifference point for electrical impedance in humans. *Acta Physiologica Scandinavica* **148**, 143–151.

Perko, G., Payne, G., Linkis, P. *et al.* (1994) Thoracic impedance and pulmonary atrial natriuretic peptide during head-up tilt induced hypovolaemic shock in humans. *Acta Physiologica Scandinavica* **150**, 449–459.

Perko, G., Schmidt, J.F., Warberg, J. & Secher, N.H. (1996) Regional electrical impedance during pharmacological intervention and lower body negative pressure. *European Journal of Applied Physiology* **73**, 459–464.

Rasmussen, B., Hanel, B., Jensen, K., Serup, B. & Secher, N.H. (1986) Decrease in pulmonary diffusion capacity after maximal exercise. *Journal of Sports Science* **4**, 185–188.

Rasmussen, J., Hanel, B., Saunamaki, K. & Secher, N.H. (1992) Recovery of pulmonary diffusing capacity after maximal exercise. *Journal of Sports Science* **10**, 525–531.

Ray, C.A., Cureton, K.J. & Ouzts, H.G. (1990a) Postural specificity of cardiovascular adaptations to exercise training. *Journal of Applied Physiology* **69**, 2202–2208.

Ray, C.A., Delp, M.D. & Hartle, D.K. (1990b) Interactive effects of body posture on exercise-induced atrial natriuretic peptide release. *American Journal of Physiology* **258**, E775–E779.

Ray, C.A., Rea, R.F., Clary, M.P. & Mark, A.L. (1993) Muscle sympathetic nerve response to dynamic one-legged exercise: effect of posture. *American Journal of Physiology* **264**, H1–H7.

Roughton, F.J.W. & Forster, R.E. (1957) Relative importance of diffusion and chemical reaction rates in determining rate of exchange of gases in the human lung, with special reference to true diffusing capacity of pulmonary membrane and volume of blood in the lung capillaries. *Journal of Applied Physiology* **11**, 290–302.

Schmidt, W., Massen, N., Troest, F. & Boning, D. (1988) Training induced effects on blood volume, erythrocyte turnover and haemoglobin oxygen binding properties. *European Journal of Applied Physiology* **57**, 490–498.

Secher, N.H. (1983) The physiology of rowing. *Journal of Sports Science* **1**, 23–43.

Secher, N.H., Nielsen, H.B. & Madsen, P. (1997) Fluid volume homeostasis: acute effects of exercise and adaptation to training. *Berichte der ÖGKC (Österreichische Gesellschaft für Klinische Chemie)* 27–29.

Sheel, A.W., Coutts, K.D., Potts, J.E. & McKenzie, D.C. (1998) The time course of pulmonary diffusing capacity for carbon monoxide following short duration high intensity exercise. *Respiration Physiology* **111**, 271–281.

Chapter 47

Cardiovascular Benefits of Endurance Exercise

AARON R. FOLSOM AND MARK A. PEREIRA

Introduction

Diseases of the cardiovascular system, in particular high blood pressure, coronary heart disease and stroke, are among the leading causes of morbidity and mortality in most industrialized countries. Although there is no rigorous experimental proof that endurance exercise prevents cardiovascular disease, evidence from observational (non-experimental) epidemiological studies indicates convincingly that this is the case. This chapter summarizes the cardiovascular benefits of endurance exercise, the possible mechanisms of its effects and the frequency, intensity, duration and type of exercise needed to produce such effects.

Methodological issues in research on exercise and health

The demonstration of a causal relation between lack of exercise and cardiovascular diseases has been hampered by several methodological issues. The strongest aetiological proof would be offered by experimental studies in which healthy subjects would be randomized to either endurance exercise or no exercise conditions and both groups would then be followed to observe the respective incidence of cardiovascular disease. Such experiments have not proven feasible, because of their long duration, the large sample sizes required and the high proportion of drop-outs or non-compliers from experimental groups. There have been several successful trials of endurance exercise in patients who have had established hypertension or who have sustained a

myocardial infarction, but these tertiary prevention trials offer only indirect information on disease aetiology. Medical scientists therefore have had to rely on evidence from observational studies, measuring cardiovascular disease incidence in relation to self-determined exercise patterns. Unfortunately, healthy or fitter individuals may tend to select themselves to high exercise levels and sicker individuals may select lower exercise levels, potentially overestimating the association between exercise and prevention of disease. Another problem is the relatively homogeneous distribution of exercise in most industrialized populations. The small difference between 'high' and 'low' exercise categories hampers the detection of possible relationships between exercise and cardiovascular disease (LaPorte *et al.* 1984).

The accurate measurement of habitual endurance activity is another major methodological challenge to epidemiological investigations. For reasons of safety, practicality and cost, objective measures of exercise or fitness have not been used extensively. Questionnaire estimates of habitual exercise have, at best, only moderate reliability and validity. This has led to misclassification of exercise levels in many studies. Misclassification is also likely if a determination of occupational exercise is based on job title alone, or if leisure exercise is estimated from a single questionnaire. Other errors arise in the diagnosis of cardiovascular disease.

Yet another methodological challenge to epidemiological studies is the control of confounding factors relating to both exercise and cardiovascular disease. Confounders are extraneous factors that can distort real associations. For example, in studies of coronary heart disease incidence, it is usually important to take into account other coronary risk factors, such as age, smoking habits and intake of saturated fat, to determine the 'independent' effect of exercise on disease. Fortunately, in recent years epidemiologists have paid more attention to these methodological issues, conducting studies with better designs and analyses.

Exercise and high blood pressure

High blood pressure is a highly prevalent cardiovascular disease. Depending on criteria of hypertension and measurement techniques, it is estimated to affect up to 40% of adults in industrialized countries (Stamler *et al.* 1993; Frohlich 1994; Burt *et al.* 1995). It is also a major risk factor for macrovascular (coronary heart disease and stroke) and microvascular (renal and retinal disease) diseases. Clinical studies suggest that exercise may lower blood pressure directly, through various physiological mechanisms, and indirectly through reduction of body fat. Therefore, regular aerobic exercise, in conjunction with die-tary modification, is recommended for the primary and secondary prevention of high blood pressure (National High Blood Pressure Education Program Working Group 1993).

As demonstrated in human and animal experiments, the most likely mechanisms through which endurance exercise helps to control blood pressure are attenuation of adrenergic sympathetic activity and reduction of total peripheral vascular resistance (Tipton 1991; Arakawa 1993; Reid *et al.* 1994). For example, in a randomized, parallel group, crossover study, Reid *et al.* (1994) reported significant reductions in total peripheral resistance and mean arterial pressure despite no change in body mass after a 12-week aerobic exercise programme at 70% of maximal aerobic power for 30 min, 3 days per week. The change in blood pressure was –7/–6 (systolic blood pressure/diastolic blood pressure) mmHg.

Several meta-analyses of randomized trials have consistently reported that aerobic exercise programmes reduce blood pressure in adults with either normal or high blood pressure (Fagard 1993; Kelley & McClellan 1994; Kelley 1995; Halbert *et al.*

1997). The range in the estimated difference of blood pressure between exercise and control groups was 3–10 mmHg, depending on the extent of hypertension in the study population, characteristics of the exercise programme and the methodological rigour of the experiments. The meta-analysis by Kelley and McClellan (1994) reported net exercise effects of –7/–6 mmHg from studies of hypertensive adults. The meta-analysis by Kelley (1995) yielded a pooled effect approximately 50% smaller (–3/–3 mmHg) for normotensive subjects than for hypertensive subjects. The meta-analysis performed by Fagard (1993) also demonstrated effects of –3/–3, –6/–7 and –10/–8 mmHg for studies of normotensive, borderline hypertensive and hypertensive subjects, respectively. These blood pressure effects appear to be independent of age and body mass change.

The effect of physical activity on blood pressure may have an intensity threshold. Independent of weight loss, randomized clinical studies have consistently demonstrated that low- to moderate-intensity activities are as effective, and perhaps more effective in reducing blood pressure than are high-intensity physical activities (Hagberg *et al.* 1989; Matsusaki *et al.* 1992; Marceau *et al.* 1993; Braith *et al.* 1994). For example, Marceau *et al.* (1993) found similar 24-h blood pressure reductions in response to moderate (50% maximal aerobic power) and vigorous (70% maximal aerobic power) training intensities in adults with mild to moderate hypertension, whereas only the low-intensity training regimen lowered daytime blood pressures. These findings are consistent with some animal models (Tipton 1991). Two independent literature reviews have concluded that more studies of low-intensity training reported significant blood pressure-lowering effects than did studies of higher-intensity training (Hagberg 1990; Tipton 1991).

Prospective epidemiological investigations (Table 47.1) are in agreement with the clinical studies, demonstrating that regular physical activity or physical fitness is associated with a reduced risk of developing high blood pressure in white men (Paffenbarger *et al.* 1983, 1991; Blair *et al.* 1984; Haapanen *et al.* 1997; Pereira *et al.* 1999). Only one study included black people, and this reported no association for black women and men (Pereira *et al.* 1999).

Table 47.1 Epidemiological studies of leisure-time exercise and incidence of high blood pressure. The definition of exercise or fitness varies across studies. The dark diamonds indicate point estimates of the relative risks, the horizontal lines the 95% confidence intervals. The studies included from top to bottom were Paffenbarger *et al.* (1983), Blair *et al.* (1984), Folsom *et al.* (1990), Paffenbarger *et al.* (1991), Haapanen *et al.* (1997) and Pereira *et al.* (1999).

Study design, population	No. of cases	Degree of adjustment	Relative risk and 95% confidence intervals
Prospective studies of hypertension incidence			
Harvard male alumni	681		
Light vs. no sports		+	
Vigorous vs. no vigorous sport		+	
Texas health center men and women			
Highest fit vs. lowest fit	240	++	
Iowa women	978		
Moderate vs. low leisure activity		+	
High vs. low leisure activity		+	
U. Penn male alumni	739		
Light vs. no sports		+	
Vigorous and light vs. no sports		+	*p* for trend < 0.01
Vigorous vs. no sports		+	
Northeastern Finland			
Vigorous activity 1+ vs. <1 times/week			
Men	142	+	
Women	117	+	
Four US communities			
High vs. low leisure activity			
White men	485	+++	
White women	482	+++	
Black men	130	+++	
Black women	205	+++	

Relative risk axis: 0.1   0.25   0.5   1.0   2.0   4.0   10.0

+ Age only; ++ Age and some risk factors; +++ Age and major risk factors.

One potential reason for the lack of association in black people and women may be the use of physical activity questionnaires that were designed primarily for white men. Another reason may be that the range of moderate activity necessary for blood pressure effects is not as broad in women and black people as in white men. The null findings in women could also be due to an increased variability in blood pressure from menstrual cycle effects, menopausal status or hormone use.

The salient epidemiological features of the associations between endurance exercise and prevention of high blood pressure, addressing criteria for causality, are as follows.

1 *Strength*: for white men (Table 47.1) there is an approximately 30% lower incidence of high blood pressure for physically active versus inactive individuals.

2 *Consistency*: all six studies in Table 47.1 have reported an inverse association between physical activity or fitness and high blood pressure. However, two studies reported results for men and women separately and both found that physical activity was associated with a lower incidence of high blood pressure in men but not in women (Haapanen *et al.* 1997; Pereira *et al.* 1999).

3 *Dose–response*: four studies in Table 47.1 have evaluated more than two exercise groups (Paffenbarger *et al.* 1983, 1991; Folsom *et al.* 1990; Pereira *et al.* 1999) and all have reported dose–response associations between low levels of physical activity and the incidence of high blood pressure. The trends in the studies by Paffenbarger *et al.* (1983, 1991) and Folsom *et al.* (1990) (Table 47.1) demonstrate lower relative risks for vigorous exercise than moderate- or low-intensity exercise. Although these findings appear to contradict the evidence from clinical studies of an exercise intensity threshold for blood pressure effects, closer examination of the epidemiological studies is necessary to address this issue. Haapanen *et al.* (1997) found that vigorous physical activity was no longer an important predictor of hypertension risk after controlling for the total physical activity level in men. Paffenbarger *et al.* (1991) found that the reduction in risk of hypertension was greatest in college alumni reporting participation in vigorous sports 1–2 h per week, whereas those participating in vigorous sports for longer durations had relative risks closer to 1.0. Additionally, stronger associations of hypertension incidence have been demonstrated with non-sport leisure activity, such as bicycling and walking, than with sports and exercise typically performed at higher intensity levels by white men (Pereira *et al.* 1999).

4 *Temporality*: studies included in Table 47.1 are prospective; physical activity was measured before the onset of high blood pressure.

5 *Independence*: although most epidemiological studies have assessed high blood pressure by self-report and controlled for few potential confounders, we (Pereira *et al.* 1999) measured blood pressure clinically and adjusted our data for age, education, parental history of high blood pressure, blood pressure level at baseline, smoking, alcohol intake, dietary intake, body mass index and waist–hip ratio, and found a monotonic inverse association between physical activity and incident hypertension that was similar to the results of the other studies for white men.

6 *Generalizability*: to date, few epidemiological studies have reported associations between physical activity and high blood pressure in women or non-whites. Therefore, the conclusions pertain to populations of white middle-aged men, but generalizations to women and non-white ethnicities remain unsubstantiated.

Moderate-intensity endurance exercise appears to be efficacious in the control of blood pressure, either through a reduction in body fat or direct physiological effects on the sympathetic and cardiovascular systems. This supports public health recommendations of regular aerobic exercise, such as walking, cycling and swimming. When not contraindicated, physicians should prescribe regular physical activity to all patients and tailor the prescription depending on hypertensive status. There is a need for more clinical and epidemiological research using physical activity intervention and assessment methods designed for women, black people and other ethnic groups.

Exercise and coronary heart disease

Coronary heart disease is caused by atherosclerotic narrowing of the coronary arteries. Its ischaemic manifestations—angina, myocardial infarction and sudden death—result from a compromised coronary circulation. This is most commonly due to rupture of an atherosclerotic plaque and attendant coronary arterial thrombosis and occlusion (Fuster *et al.* 1992a,b). Major risk factors for coronary heart disease include hypercholesterolaemia, high blood pressure, cigarette smoking and diabetes mellitus.

The role of exercise in preventing coronary heart disease has been investigated extensively and reviewed frequently. Powell *et al.* (1987) summarized 54 published investigations of exercise and coronary heart disease incidence. These and a few additional studies have been summarized further in a second meta-analysis (Berlin & Colditz 1990). Additional studies through the mid-1990s were reviewed in the United States Surgeon General's Report on Physical Activity and Health (US Department of Health and Human Services 1996b). At least 27 additional original reports on exercise and coronary heart disease were not included in the original review, although some of them were updates of earlier studies (Pekkanen *et al.* 1987; Fraser *et al.* 1992; Paffenbarger *et al.* 1993; Prineas *et al.* 1993; Simonsick *et al.* 1993; Stender *et al.* 1993; Lakka *et al.* 1994; Sherman *et al.* 1994a; Eaton *et al.* 1995; Lee *et al.* 1995; Lemaitre *et al.* 1995; O'Connor *et al.* 1995; Haapanen *et al.* 1996; Kaplan *et al.* 1996; Lissner *et al.* 1996; Mensink *et al.* 1996; Folsom *et al.* 1997; Fraser & Shavlik 1997; Hedblad *et al.* 1997; Kushi *et al.* 1997; Leon *et al.* 1997; Rosengren & Wilhelmsen 1997; Tunstall-Pedoe *et al.* 1997; Bijnen *et al.* 1998; Hakim *et al.* 1998; Kujala *et al.* 1998; Wannamethee *et al.* 1998). Taking all of the published data together leads fairly convincingly to the conclusion that lack of endurance exercise is a contributory cause of coronary heart disease.

Table 47.2 summarizes the outcome of the meta-analysis of Berlin and Colditz (1990), based on Powell *et al.* (1987). The salient epidemiological features of the association between endurance exercise and prevention of coronary heart disease are as follows.

1 *Strength*: the risk of coronary heart disease in subjects who undertake high levels of exercise is a half to two-thirds that of subjects with low exercise levels (Table 47.2). The relative risk of physical inactivity therefore is somewhat less than the relative risks of coronary disease ascribed to hypercholes-

terolaemia, high blood pressure or cigarette smoking. Nevertheless, it is substantial.

2 *Consistency*: the association between exercise and a reduction in the risk of coronary disease is generally consistent. About two-thirds of all studies show that exercise is associated with a significant reduction in risk (Powell *et al.* 1987; Berlin & Colditz 1990). Occupational and leisure-time exercise studies seem equally consistent in demonstrating an effect. This effect extends to both fatal and non-fatal coronary events (Table 47.2). Studies with the best methodologies generally show the strongest relationships.

3 *Dose–response*: two-thirds of the studies that measured exercise at two or more levels demonstrated a dose–response relation (Powell *et al.* 1987); that is, the greater the level of exercise, the lower the risk of coronary heart disease. The summary estimates demonstrating dose–response are shown in the bottom two rows of Table 47.2.

4 *Temporality*: the majority of studies have been prospective, thereby demonstrating that activity level appropriately predates the onset of coronary heart disease. Recent studies have documented that subjects who report an *increase* in exercise levels have a further reduction in the risk of coronary heart disease over those reporting no change in exercise

Table 47.2 Pooled relative risk (RR)* (95% confidence interval (CI)) for leisure-time exercise and coronary heart disease (CHD) events.

Exercise levels compared	CHD		CHD death		Myocardial infarction		Myocardial infarction or sudden death	
	RR	95% CI	RR	95% CI	RR	95% CI	RR	95% CI
Two groups								
High versus low	0.63	0.55–0.77	0.53	0.29–1.0	0.77	0.59–1.0	0.43	0.28–0.67
Three groups								
High versus moderate			0.77	0.57–1.0	0.71	0.59–0.91		
High versus sedentary			0.63	0.45–0.83	0.34	0.22–0.53		

*Adapted from Berlin and Colditz (1990) by taking reciprocals of relative risks for lack of exercise. Based on studies reviewed by Powell *et al.* (1987).

level (Paffenbarger *et al.* 1993; Wannamethee *et al.* 1998).

5 *Independence*: most studies that measured other coronary risk factors simultaneously have reported that exercise was independently associated with reduced coronary heart disease occurrence.

6 *Generalizability*: most studies have focused on middle-aged, white men. Evidence is less available but suggestive that exercise also protects older men (Morris *et al.* 1980; Donahue *et al.* 1988; Simonsick *et al.* 1993; Sherman *et al.* 1994a; LaCroix *et al.* 1996; Fraser & Shavlik 1997; Bijnen *et al.* 1998), non-white men (Cassel *et al.* 1971; Garcia-Palmieri *et al.* 1982; Donahue *et al.* 1988; Folsom *et al.* 1997) and women (Table 47.3).

The association between exercise and coronary

disease is even stronger for studies that have measured coronary heart disease incidence or mortality rates in relation to endurance *fitness* (exercise capacity as measured during treadmill or cycle ergometer exercise). Indeed, all prospective studies of fitness report lower coronary heart disease incidence rates in fit versus unfit subjects (Table 47.4). The relative risk of coronary heart disease in fit adults is one-third to one-half of that for unfit adults. Furthermore, people who improve their level of fitness reduce their coronary heart disease risk over those who make no change in fitness (Blair *et al.* 1995). Unfortunately, only one of the fitness studies involved women, and none involved a large sample of non-whites. Furthermore, levels of fitness are to a substantial degree determined by heredity (Chapter 15), implying that the observed associations do not reflect simply a beneficial effect of exercise.

Table 47.3 Epidemiological studies of leisure-time exercise and cardiovascular disease occurrence in women. Only one cardiovascular endpoint per study is depicted. The definition of exercise varies across studies. The dark diamonds indicate point estimates of the relative risks, the horizontal lines the 95% confidence intervals. The studies included from top to bottom were Salonen *et al.* (1982), Lapidus and Bengtsson (1986), Sherman *et al.* (1994b), Tunstall-Pedoe *et al.* (1997), Lissner *et al.* (1996), Kushi *et al.* (1997), Mensink *et al.* (1996), Fraser *et al.* (1992), Magnus *et al.* (1979), Scragg *et al.* (1987), Lemaitre *et al.* (1995) and O'Connor *et al.* (1995).

Study design, population	No. of cases	Degree of adjustment	Relative risk and 95% confidence intervals (highest vs. lowest exercise groups)
Prospective studies of CHD incidence			
North Karelia, Finland	63	+++	
Gothenberg, Sweden	23	+	
Framingham, MA		+++	
Scotland	177	+	
4 US communities	85	+++	
Prospective studies of CVD mortality			
Gothenberg, Sweden	22	+++	
Iowa	258	++	
Germany	16	+++	
US adventists	139	++	
Case–control studies			
Netherlands		++	
Auckland, New Zealand	121	+	
Seattle, WA	268	+++	
Boston, MA	74	+++	

+ Age only; ++ Age and some risk factors; +++ Age and major risk factors. CHD, coronary heart disease; CVD, cardiovascular disease.

Table 47.4 Epidemiological studies of endurance fitness and cardiovascular disease occurrence. Only one cardiovascular endpoint per study is depicted. The definition of exercise varies across studies. The dark diamonds indicate point estimates of the relative risks, the horizontal lines the 95% confidence intervals. The studies included from top to bottom were Peters *et al.* (1983), Sobolski *et al.* (1987), Erikssen (1986), Bruce *et al.* (1983), Wilhelmsen *et al.* (1981), Lakka *et al.* (1994), Slattery and Jacobs (1988), Ekelund *et al.* (1988), Hein *et al.* (1992), Sandvik *et al.* (1993) and Blair *et al.* (1996).

Study design, population	No. of cases	Degree of adjustment	Relative risk and 95% confidence intervals (highest vs. lowest exercise groups)
Prospective studies of CHD incidence			
Los Angeles, CA men	29	+++	
Belgian men	19	+++	$p = 0.02$
Norwegian men		o	Inverse association
Seattle, WA men		o	
	202		
Seattle, WA women		o	
Gothenberg, Sweden men	55	+++	Inverse association
Kuopio, Finland men	42	+++	
Prospective studies of CVD or CHD mortality			
US male railroad workers	258	+++	
North American men		+++	
Copenhagen, Denmark men	266	++	
Oslo, Norway men	143	+++	
Texas health center men	111	+++	
Texas health center women	11	+++	

(Relative risk scale: 0.1 0.25 0.5 1.0 2.0 4.0 10.0)

o None; + Age only; ++ Age and some risk factors; +++ Age and major risk factors. CHD, coronary heart disease; CVD, cardiovascular disease.

In addition to reducing the incidence of coronary heart disease, endurance exercise appears to reduce the risk of death following myocardial infarction. Several randomized, controlled trials of exercise in postmyocardial infarction patients have been conducted. Unfortunately, these tertiary prevention trials have all been relatively small; they have been conducted only in men, and they have sometimes involved other interventions besides exercise. Only one trial showed a significant benefit by itself, but pooled data from postinfarction trials indicate that survival is improved among patients who exercise (Shephard 1986; O'Connor *et al.* 1989). O'Connor *et al.* (1989) performed a meta-analysis of 22 randomized exercise trials involving a total of 4554 postinfarction patients followed for an average of 3 years after randomization. The relative risks in the pooled exercise group versus the pooled comparison group were significantly reduced for *total mor-*

tality (relative risk = 0.80), *cardiovascular mortality* (0.78) and *fatal reinfarction* (0.75). *Sudden death* was significantly reduced in exercisers at 1 year (relative risk = 0.63), but not at 2 and 3 years. There was no observable effect of exercise on the rate of *non-fatal reinfarctions*. Thus, existing data suggest that endurance exercise in patients who survive a myocardial infarction results in a 20% reduction in the overall mortality rate, due to a decreased risk of cardiovascular mortality, fatal reinfarctions and early sudden death. Recommendations have been published for prescribing exercise in the clinical setting to prevent and rehabilitate cardiovascular diseases (Harris *et al.* 1989; American College of Sports Medicine 1994; American Heart Association 1994; American Association of Cardiovascular and Pulmonary Rehabilitation 1995; NIH Consensus Development Panel on Physical Activity and Cardiovascular Health 1996).

Table 47.5 Biological mechanisms by which exercise may contribute to the primary or secondary prevention of coronary heart disease*. From Haskell *et al.* (1992).

Maintains or increases myocardial oxygen supply
Delays progression of coronary atherosclerosis (possible)
   Improves lipoprotein profile (increases HDL-C/LDL-C ratio) (probable)
   Improves carbohydrate metabolism (increases insulin sensitivity) (probable)
   Decreases platelet aggregation and increases fibrinolysis (probable)
   Decreases adiposity (usually)
Increases coronary collateral vascularization (unlikely)
Increases epicardial artery diameter (possible)
Increases coronary blood flow (myocardial perfusion) or distribution (possible)

Decreases myocardial work rate and oxygen demand
Decreases heart rate at rest and in submaximal exercise (usually)
Decreases systolic and mean systemic arterial pressure during submaximal exercise (usually) and at rest (possible)
Decreases cardiac output during submaximal exercise (probable)
Decreases circulating plasma catecholamine levels (decrease of sympathetic tone) at rest (probable) and at submaximal exercise (usually)

Increases myocardial function
Increases stroke volume at rest and in submaximal and maximal exercise (likely)
Increases ejection fraction at rest and during exercise (likely)
Increases intrinsic myocardial contractility (possible)
Increases myocardial function resulting from decreased 'afterload' (probable)
Increases myocardial hypertrophy (probable); but this may not reduce CHD risk

Increases electrical stability of myocardium
Decreases regional ischaemia or ischaemia at submaximal exercise (possible)
Decreases catecholamines in myocardium at rest (possible) and at submaximal exercise (probable)
Increases ventricular fibrillation threshold due to reduction of cyclic AMP (possible)

---

*Expression of likelihood that effect will occur for an individual participating in endurance-type training programme for 16 weeks or longer at 65–80% of functional capacity for 25 min or longer (1.25 MJ per session) for three or more sessions per week ranges from unlikely, possible, likely, probable to usually.
AMP, adenosine monophosphate; CHD, coronary heart disease; HDL-C, high density lipoprotein cholesterol; LDL-C, low density lipoprotein cholesterol.

Haskell *et al.* (1992) summarized biological mechanisms by which endurance exercise may reduce coronary heart disease incidence or mortality rates (Table 47.5). The four broad categories of benefit are: (i) improved myocardial oxygen supply; (ii) decreased myocardial work and oxygen demand; (iii) increased myocardial function; and (iv) increased electrical stability of the myocardium.

Atherosclerosis is most likely to be reduced by the beneficial effects of exercise on coronary risk factors. Exercise clearly can improve blood pressure, reduce body mass, modify blood lipids and increase insulin sensitivity. These effects are discussed elsewhere in this chapter. In addition, exercise may lead indi-rectly to reductions in psychological stress (US Department of Health and Human Services 1996b) and smoking (Folsom *et al.* 1985). Exercise might also reduce atherogenesis directly. For example, a randomized, controlled exercise trial of angina patients followed by coronary angiography suggested that 30 min per day of exercise at 75% of maximal aerobic power was sufficient to reduce atherosclerosis progression (Hambrecht *et al.* 1993). Although difficult to demonstrate in humans, exercise has prevented the initial development of coronary atheroma in a controlled trial where non-human primates were fed an atherogenic diet (Kramsch *et al.* 1981). Exercise may reduce the risk of coronary thrombosis when atherosclerosis is present, by increasing fibrinolysis (Williams *et al.* 1980; Schuit *et al.* 1997) and possibly by reducing platelet aggregability (Rauramaa *et al.* 1986). Effects of exercise on fibrinogen, however, are inconsistent (El-Sayed 1996).

In animals, exercise can increase the calibre of the coronary arteries, enhance the collateral circulation and increase coronary blood flow (Laughlin 1994). However, such adaptations of the coronary vasculature are undocumented in humans. Exercise can reduce heart rate and blood pressure, both major determinants of myocardial oxygen demand (Maskin 1986). The lengthening of the diastolic phase may also enhance myocardial perfusion. These adaptations may lead to reduced circulating levels of noradrenaline (Cooksey *et al.* 1978) and increased resistance to ventricular fibrillation (Billman *et al.* 1984). Correspondingly, humans who exercise regularly appear to have a reduced risk of cardiac arrest compared with those who are sedentary, even though the overall risk of cardiac arrest is somewhat higher during exercise than during rest (Siscovick *et al.* 1982, 1984; Mittleman *et al.* 1993).

Exercise and stroke

Cerebrovascular stroke is a major cause of mortality and disability, especially among the elderly. There are several aetiologies of stroke, the two most prevalent being thromboembolic stroke, which most often results from atherosclerosis of the cerebral or precerebral arteries, and intracerebral haemorrhage. High blood pressure is the most important risk factor for stroke, and most other risk factors for atherosclerosis increase the risk of stroke.

The role of endurance exercise in reducing the risk of stroke is not as well established as for coronary heart disease, in part because stroke is a rarer event and studies are smaller. We have identified 30 published epidemiological studies of exercise and stroke. Of these, 12 included a comparison of active occupations with less active occupations: four reported a statistically significant negative association between strenuous work and risk of stroke (Pomrehn *et al.* 1982; Salonen *et al.* 1982; Lapidus & Bengtsson 1986; Gillum *et al.* 1996); three found

some evidence of a positive or U-shaped association (Komachi *et al.* 1971; Tanaka *et al.* 1982; Nakayama *et al.* 1997); and the remainder found no association (Paffenbarger *et al.* 1970; Okada *et al.* 1976; Menotti & Seccareccia 1985; Menotti *et al.* 1990; Håheim *et al.* 1993). Stroke studies that included primarily estimates of leisure-time exercise—presumably mostly endurance activity—are shown in Table. 47.6. They fulfil the criteria for causality in the following way:

1 *Strength*: the median relative risk (RR) was 0.69 for the group with the highest level of exercise, defined by each study, versus the least active group. Many individual relative risk estimates, however, were not statistically significant as reflected by confidence intervals overlapping 1.0 (Table 47.6). Case–control studies (median RR ≈ 0.5, RR range = 0.24–0.88) tended to indicate more benefit than prospective studies (median RR ≈ 0.70), suggesting some degree of bias in the case–control data. In general, however, the association for stroke is nearly as strong as that observed for coronary heart disease.

2 *Consistency*: with only four exceptions, estimated relative risks in Table 47.6 were less than 1.0, demonstrating good consistency for an association between endurance exercise and a reduced risk of stroke.

3 *Dose–response*: of the 14 studies that could quantify exercise at two or more levels, nine (Herman *et al.* 1983; Paffenbarger *et al.* 1984; Paganini-Hill *et al.* 1988; Wannamethee & Shaper 1992; Håheim *et al.* 1993; Abbott *et al.* 1994b; You *et al.* 1995; Gillum *et al.* 1996; Bijnen *et al.* 1998) observed a dose–response pattern of lower stroke occurrence at successively greater exercise levels.

4 *Temporality*: most studies were prospective, thus verifying that exercise level was assessed before the onset of stroke.

5 *Independence*: most investigators adjusted for other atherosclerotic risk factors, to examine the independent association between exercise and stroke.

Table 47.6 Epidemiological studies of leisure-time exercise and stroke occurrence. Only one stroke endpoint per study is depicted. The definition of exercise varies across studies. The dark diamonds indicate point estimates of the relative risks, the horizontal lines the 95% confidence intervals. The studies included from top to bottom were Salonen *et al.* (1982), Lapidus and Bengtsson (1986), Harmsen *et al.* (1990), Wannamethee and Shaper (1992), Håheim *et al.* (1993), Simonsick *et al.* (1993), Abbott *et al.* (1994a), Lindenstrøm *et al.* (1993), Kiely *et al.* (1994), Gillum *et al.* (1996), Paffenbarger *et al.* (1984), Paganini-Hill *et al.* (1988), Folsom *et al.* (1990), Lindsted *et al.* (1991), Bijnen *et al.* (1998), Herman *et al.* (1983), Ellekjaer *et al.* (1992), Shinton and Sagar (1993), You *et al.* (1995), You *et al.* (1997) and Sacco *et al.* (1998).

Study design, population	No. of cases	Degree of adjustment	Relative risk and 95% confidence intervals (highest vs. lowest exercise groups)
Prospective studies of stroke incidence			
Finnish men	71	+++	
Finnish women	56	+++	
Swedish women	13	+	
Swedish men	230	+	
British men	128	+++	
Oslo men	81	+++	
Boston, MA elderly	—	++	
New Haven, CT elderly	—	++	
Iowa elderly	—	++	
Hawaii Japanese men	48	+++	
Copenhagen women	265	++	
Framingham men	107	+++	
Framingham women	127	+++	
US blacks, 45–74	104	+++	
US white men, 45–64	69	+++	
US white men, 65–74	201	+++	
US white women, 45–64	53	+++	
US white women, 65–74	196	+++	
Prospective studies of stroke mortality			
Male college alumni	103	+++	$p = 0.001$
Californian elderly	63	?	Inverse $p = 0.001$
Iowa women	218	+++	
Male 7th-day adventists	410	++	
Elderly Dutch men	47	+++	
Case–control studies			
Dutch men & women	132	+++	
Norwegian men & women	134	+	
English men & women	65	++	
Australian men & women	203	+++	
Australian young adults	201	+++	
Manhattan, NY men & women	369	+++	

Scale: 0.1 0.25 0.5 1.0 2.0 4.0 10.0

+ Age only; ++ Age and some risk factors but not high BP; +++ Age and major risk factors including high BP.

Despite a growing number of studies of exercise and stroke, gaps remain. Few investigators have studied women or non-whites; current data reassuringly do not show a different pattern of findings for these subgroups. Few studies have had sufficient numbers of cases to compare subtypes of stroke (Harmsen *et al.* 1990; Abbott *et al.* 1994b; Gillum *et al.* 1996). Likewise, there apparently have been no investigations of the relationship between stroke occurrence and levels of physical fitness.

In summary, existing evidence suggests that endurance exercise probably reduces the risk of cerebrovascular stroke, but the findings are not conclusive. The probable mechanisms include a reduction of blood pressure, reduced atherosclerosis and/or reduced thrombosis of the cerebral and precerebral arteries. However, additional research is needed to clarify the causality and generalizability of these findings, as well as the duration, frequency and intensity of exercise that are required to prevent stroke.

Exercise and metabolic cardiovascular risk factors

Obesity

Obesity is an important risk factor for atherosclerotic diseases and high blood pressure (Rexrode et al. 1996). Excess energy intake relative to energy utilization is the cause of obesity. Controlled trials show unequivocally that exercise programmes reduce excess weight in obese patients (Ballor & Keesey 1991; Garrow & Summerbell 1995; Miller et al. 1997). Furthermore, reduction of body fat is more easily achieved and maintained when exercise is part of a weight-loss programme (Miller et al. 1997). Clinicians should certainly recommend exercise to overweight patients in whom there is no medical contraindication.

Blood lipids and lipoproteins

The incidence of coronary heart disease and thrombotic stroke is associated directly with plasma concentrations of total cholesterol, low density lipoprotein (LDL) cholesterol and triglycerides, and inversely with high density lipoprotein (HDL) cholesterol concentrations (Castelli et al. 1977; Austin et al. 1998). Recent clinical trials have demonstrated clearly that lowering of elevated plasma LDL cholesterol reduces the incidence of coronary heart disease (Gould et al. 1998) and stroke (Crouse et al. 1997). Raising HDL cholesterol concentrations may

also reduce coronary disease incidence (Manninen et al. 1988).

The numerous studies of the effects of acute and long-term exercise on lipid metabolism in normolipaemic and hyperlipaemic subjects have been thoroughly reviewed (Durstine & Haskell 1994; Stefanick & Wood 1994; Superko 1995). Proper interpretation of these results is difficult, due to the presence of many confounding factors that affect blood lipid values, including energy intake, dietary composition and changes of body mass. In general, prospective studies and clinical trials have shown little independent effect of endurance exercise on total or LDL cholesterol, or on the atherogenic moiety lipoprotein(a). Prospective studies in subjects with hypertriglyceridaemia or normolipaemia generally have shown a significant reduction in serum triglycerides after exercise training. The decrease in triglycerides has usually been tied to exercise-induced weight loss.

Regular exercise often increases HDL cholesterol concentrations in a dose-dependent manner, although findings are less consistent for women than for men. In addition, the ratio of HDL subfractions, HDL_2/HDL_3, may increase beneficially with exercise without necessarily altering the total HDL cholesterol concentration (Rauramaa et al. 1984).

One of the best-designed experimental studies to date is that of Wood et al. (1983). In a randomized, controlled 1-year trial of running in 81 men, they found a correlation between exercise level and increased HDL cholesterol, but there was a threshold effect: a significant increase in HDL cholesterol was detected only in those men whose running distance during the last 7 months of the trial exceeded an average of 12.9 km (8 miles) per week. Furthermore, an exercise-induced loss of body mass was an essential element of the HDL cholesterol response. Wood et al. (1988) subsequently showed that HDL cholesterol and triglyceride changes with a decrease of body mass were comparable whether they were achieved through exercise or diet.

In summary, evidence suggests that exercise training probably has beneficial effects on the levels of triglycerides and HDL cholesterol, to a large degree indirectly through an exercise-mediated decrease of body fat. The most likely direct mechanisms for these effects are exercise-induced alterations in lipolytic enzymes, such as lipoprotein lipase and hepatic lipase (Lithell *et al.* 1979; Herbert *et al.* 1984; Kantor *et al.* 1984). Clinicians may wish to recommend exercise as part of a complete regimen for control of dyslipidaemias.

Glucose intolerance and insulin sensitivity

Diabetes mellitus is an important coronary heart disease risk factor, and recent evidence suggests hyperinsulinaemia may be also (Ruige *et al.* 1998). Prospective studies suggest that, independent of body mass, exercise is associated with a reduced incidence of type 2 diabetes (Manson *et al.* 1991, 1992; Helmrich *et al.* 1994; Burchfiel *et al.* 1995). Exercise and physical conditioning appear to influence insulin and glucose regulation in normal subjects (Holloszy *et al.* 1986; King *et al.* 1987) and in patients with type 2 diabetes (Björntorp 1982; Kemmer & Berger 1983; Rauramaa 1984; Krotkiewski *et al.* 1985; Richter & Galbo 1986). Exercise has been shown to increase insulin receptor density, enhance insulin sensitivity and improve glucose utilization (LeBlanc *et al.* 1979; Soman *et al.* 1979; Pedersen *et al.* 1980; Schneider *et al.* 1984; Ronnemaa *et al.* 1986). A reduction of adiposity accompanying exercise is an important factor contributing to efficient glucose metabolism, although exercise may also have an independent effect. Recent evidence suggests that non-vigorous as well as vigorous activity may increase insulin sensitivity (Mayer-Davis *et al.* 1998).

In summary, exercise has important beneficial effects on glucose tolerance and insulin utilization and in the prevention of diabetes. These health effects may play an important role in the cardiovascular effects of exercise. Clinicians should strongly consider recommending appropriate exercise to obese patients and colleagues at risk of type 2 diabetes as well as to those who have diabetes. Exercise, however, must be undertaken cautiously in diabetics at risk of hypoglycaemia, such as those who are insulin dependent.

Exercise recommendations for cardiovascular health

The minimal and optimal levels of physical activity for health benefits are not known, and this topic is a current research priority. The recommendation '. . . adults should accumulate 30min or more of moderate-intensity activity on most, preferably all, days of the week' set forth by the Centers for Disease Control and Prevention and the American College of Sports Medicine (Pate *et al.* 1995) was an arbitrary guideline based on observational epidemiological data and a few small clinical studies which fall short of providing unequivocal scientific evidence to support an absolute level of physical activity required to achieve health benefits. Although this recommendation may be an appropriate message to initiate behaviour change in the large percentage of sedentary adults, the efficacy of this pattern of physical activity for health benefit is not known. This uncertainty was highlighted by: (i) letters published in response to the recommendation (Williams 1995; Winett 1995); (ii) conservative language used in the Surgeon General's Report (which is an evidence-based document) regarding the new recommendation; and (iii) an article that discussed the controversies surrounding the recommendation and the disparity of opinions held by the authors of the recommendation (Barinaga 1997).

Given the complexity of physical activity, with many components that may affect the health endpoint of interest (Caspersen 1989), and the dependence of the measured associations on the distribution of physical activity and the risk factor in the population of interest, it is not surprising that there is no consensus on the minimal or optimal type, duration, frequency and intensity of exercise necessary to achieve *health benefits*. We emphasize health benefits, to distinguish from the amount of physical activity necessary for improvements in physiological fitness. The epidemiological data are not precise enough to tease out the independent effects of different types and quantities of activity, and they are limited by the difficulty in recalling physical activities of low to moderate intensity. Therefore, there is a need for more appropriately designed clinical trials to determine the optimal components and doses of exercise for favourable effects on cardiovascular disease risk. It has been suggested that the physical activity epidemiology literature indicates that most of the reduction in risk of chronic diseases and all-cause mortality may be observed at the low end of the physical activity spectrum, between the least active and low to moderately active individuals, with more, but proportionately less, health benefit conferred by moving from a moderate level of activity to a higher level (Pate *et al.* 1995). However, not all studies support this non-linear dose–response relationship between physical activity and health (Kannel & Sorlie 1979; Paffenbarger *et al.* 1984; Lee *et al.* 1995).

Probably the most useful data pertaining to the nature of the dose–response curve between physical activity and cardiovascular risks are the comprehensive reviews of physical activity and coronary heart disease by Powell *et al.* (1987) and Berlin and Colditz (1990). The medians of pooled relative risks for various heart disease endpoints (Table 47.2) indicate that the relationship with physical activity displays a dose–response effect, with no indication that the curve is not linear. However, this conclusion is a tenuous one, due to the limited number of activity categories, the inconsistent methodologies across studies, and some heterogeneity of relative risks among studies. Also, at the time of these reviews there were few studies including older individuals or women, and therefore the results pertain primarily to middle-aged men. Nevertheless, recent epidemiological studies have consistently demonstrated that moderate-intensity activity (primarily walking) reduces the risk of cardiovascular disease and mortality in older men and women (LaCroix *et al.* 1996; Kushi *et al.* 1997; Hakim *et al.* 1998).

The beneficial effects of physical activity probably depend on the type, frequency, duration and intensity of the activity, as well as on the specific risk factor or clinical endpoint of interest. There is much overlap among the components comprising the spectrum of physical activity in the prevention of cardiovascular disease. For example, total energy expenditure is a critical component for body weight maintenance and therefore important in the prevention of such conditions as hypertension, low HDL cholesterol, high LDL cholesterol and hyperinsulinaemia, all of which have potentially atherogenic effects. Earlier in this chapter we discussed examples of potentially threshold-dependent physiological effects of exercise. To increase HDL cholesterol, a negative energy balance and loss of body fat or stimulation of lipoprotein lipase may be required through a critical total volume (frequency × duration × intensity) of exercise (Schwartz 1987; Williams *et al.* 1990). For blood pressure, the dose–response curve may have a threshold toward the lower end, as moderate-intensity exercise appears sufficient to maximize the benefit for this risk factor. Although dose–response curves for specific risk factors may vary according to the underlying physiological mechanisms, the overall impact of physical activity on cardiovascular health probably follows a monotonic linear pattern. Therefore, the exercise type (endurance activities with large muscle groups such as walking and jogging), frequency (daily) and duration (at least 20 min) are all probably important for preventing cardiovascular disease through various mechanistic pathways related to energy balance, dyslipidaemia, high blood pressure and other less traditional risk factors.

Exercise recommendations by health organizations

The available data on exercise and health have been translated into policy recommendations for both individuals and populations. The evolution of US guidelines on exercise for individuals, which has been thoroughly reviewed (US Department of Health and Human Services 1996a), serves as an excellent example of exercise policy development. Until the mid-1990s, most guidelines recommended at least 30 min of vigorous endurance exercise at >60% cardiorespiratory capacity, on 3 or more days per week. However, several groups have recently advised that exercise intensity need only be moderate or greater, based on the dose–response data discussed earlier and on the difficulty for most people in complying with vigorous exercise recommendations (Pate *et al.* 1995; NIH Consensus Development Panel on Physical Activity and Cardiovascular Health 1996).

A large proportion of the population in most industrialized countries does not exercise regularly. In the US, approximately 25% of the adult population is totally sedentary (US Department of Health and Human Services 1996c). Only about 15–20% of US adults participate in regular, sustained endurance activity. As a result, the US Department of Health and Human Services set population-wide exercise objectives for the year 2000 (US Department of Health and Human Services 1995). Two of the primary Year 2000 goals for exercise are that at least 30% of US citizens aged 6 years and older will participate regularly, preferably daily, in light to moderate physical activities for at least 30 min, and at least 20% of adults and 75% of children will engage in vigorous activities, 3 or more days per week, for 20 min or more per occasion. Population strategies for exercise promotion are reviewed elsewhere (US Department of Health and Human Services 1996d).

If lack of exercise is a true cause of cardiovascular disease, then the estimated effect of increasing exercise on a population-wide basis can be predicted. If it is assumed that a lack of moderate to vigorous exercise carries a relative risk for cardiovascular disease of 1.5, then an increase in the population-wide prevalence of exercise from 20% to 40% might reduce cardiovascular disease rates by 7%. An increase in exercise prevalence from 20% to 60% might reduce cardiovascular disease rates by a sizeable 14%.

Implications for the endurance competitor

Endurance athletes have markedly better cardiovascular fitness and risk factor levels than non-athletes (Seals *et al.* 1984; Darga *et al.* 1989; Pratley *et al.* 1995). In fact, some masters athletes may have similar or even more favourable cardiovascular disease risk factor profiles than much younger non-athletes (Seals *et al.* 1984). There is a direct linear relationship between weekly running distance, up to approximately 80 km per week, and HDL cholesterol concentration in both men (Williams 1997) and women (Williams 1996). Furthermore, exercise intensity as determined by self-reported 10-km racing speed, was found to relate more strongly than running dis-

tance with systolic blood pressure in men and women and waist circumference in men (Williams 1998a). Large prospective studies have demonstrated that physical activity akin to conditioning sports or cardiovascular endurance activity reduces cardiovascular disease risk (Paffenbarger *et al.* 1978, 1984; Lakka *et al.* 1994; Kujala *et al.* 1998). These apparent cardiovascular benefits have also been demonstrated in adults in their seventh decade of life and older (Siscovick *et al.* 1997; Williams 1998b).

Although the studies described above suggest that the increased risk of cardiovascular disease associated with the ageing process can be attenuated by participation in competitive endurance sport, these are all observational studies of individuals who elected to take up sport. As such, there may be a selection bias related to a genetic predisposition for fitness and health and a confounding bias related to other lifestyle habits and characteristics of athletes versus non-athletes. Thus, the common caveat of all these studies is that they were not randomized experiments. It is not feasible to randomize someone to be an endurance athlete or a non-athlete. However, extrapolation from observational studies strongly suggests that endurance sport confers considerable protection from cardiovascular disease. Additionally, many trials of endurance exercise, although below the level of competitive athletics, have demonstrated improvements in cardiovascular disease risk profile (e.g. Wood *et al.* 1988). Nevertheless, the cardiovascular benefits of endurance sport must be weighed against the increased risk of injury from extreme levels of competitive sport. It is likely that a point of diminishing health returns is reached at a certain threshold level of sport or exercise participation.

Conclusion

Endurance exercise is clearly important in the primary, secondary and tertiary prevention of coronary heart disease. It also appears to contribute to the prevention and control of high blood pressure and cerebrovascular stroke. Evidence on the frequency, intensity, duration and type of exercise required for cardiovascular benefits is incomplete.

Exercise for cardiovascular health can certainly be recommended to most individuals, but additional research is needed to refine specific recommenda- tions for subgroups of the population. How to moti- vate individuals to adopt endurance exercise as a lifelong habit remains a challenge.

References

Abbott, R.D., Behrens, G.R., Sharp, D.S. *et al.* (1994a) Body mass index and throm- boembolic stroke in nonsmoking men in older middle age: the Honolulu Heart Program. *Stroke* **25**, 2370–2376.

Abbott, R.D., Rodriguez, B.L., Burchfiel, C.M. & Curb, J.D. (1994b) Physical activ- ity in older middle-aged men and reduced risk of stroke: the Honolulu Heart Program. *American Journal of Epi- demiology* **139**, 881–893.

American Association of Cardiovascular and Pulmonary Rehabilitation (1995) *Guidelines for Cardiac Rehabilitation Pro- grams*, 2nd edn. Human Kinetics, Champaign, IL.

American College of Sports Medicine (1994) Position stand: exercise for patients with coronary artery disease. *Medicine and Science in Sports and Exercise* **26**, i–v.

American Heart Association (1994) Cardiac rehabilitation programs: a state- ment for healthcare professionals from the American Heart Association. *Circula- tion* **90**, 1602–1610.

Arakawa, K. (1993) Antihypertensive mechanism of exercise. *Journal of Hyper- tension* **11**, 223–229.

Austin, M.A., Hokanson, J.E. & Edwards, K.L. (1998) Hypertriglyceridemia as a cardiovascular risk factor. *American Journal of Cardiology* **81**, 7B–12B.

Ballor, D.L. & Keesey, R.E. (1991) A meta- analysis of the factors affecting exercise- induced changes in body mass, fat mass and fat-free mass in males and females. *International Journal of Obesity* **15**, 717–726.

Barinaga, M. (1997) How much pain for cardiac gain? *Science* **276**, 1324–1327.

Berlin, J.A. & Colditz, G.A. (1990) A meta- analysis of physical activity in the pre- vention of coronary heart disease. *American Journal of Epidemiology* **132**, 612–628.

Bijnen, F.C.H., Caspersen, C.J., Feskens, E.J.M., Saris, W.H.M., Mosterd, W.L. & Kromhout, D. (1998) Physical activity and 10-year mortality from cardiovascu- lar diseases and all causes: the Zutphen Elderly Study. *Archives of Internal Medi- cine* **158**, 1499–1505.

Billman, G.E., Schwartz, P.J. & Stone, H.L.

(1984) The effects of daily exercise on susceptibility to sudden cardiac death. *Circulation* **69**, 1182–1189.

Björntorp, P.M. (1982) Effects of physical training on diabetes mellitus, Type II. In: Bostrom, H. & Ljungstedt, N. (eds) *Recent Trends in Diabetes Research*, pp. 115–125. Almqvist & Wiksell Interna- tional, Stockholm, Sweden.

Blair, S.N., Goodyear, N.N., Gibbons, L.W. & Cooper, K.H. (1984) Physical fitness and incidence of hypertension in healthy normotensive men and women. *Journal of the American Medical Association* **252**, 487–490.

Blair, S.N., Kohl, H.W. III, Barlow, C.E., Paffenbarger, R.S. Jr, Gibbons, L.W. & Macera, C.A. (1995) Changes in physical fitness and all-cause mortality: a prospective study of healthy and unhealthy men. *Journal of the American Medical Association* **273**, 1093–1098.

Blair, S.N., Kampert, J.B., Kohl, H.W. III *et al.* (1996) Influences of cardiorespira- tory fitness and other precursors on car- diovascular disease and all-cause mortality in men and women. *Journal of the American Medical Association* **276**, 205–210.

Braith, R.W., Pollock, M.L., Lowenthal, D.T., Graves, J.E. & Limacher, M.C. (1994) Moderate- and high-intensity exercise lowers blood pressure in nor- motensive subjects 60–79 years of age. *American Journal of Cardiology* **73**, 1124–1128.

Bruce, R.A., Hossack, K.F., DeRouen, T.A. & Hofer, V. (1983) Enhanced risk assess- ment for primary coronary heart disease events by maximal exercise testing: 10 years' experience of Seattle Heart Watch. *Journal of the American College of Cardiol- ogy* **2**, 565–573.

Burchfiel, C.M., Sharp, D.S., Curb, J.D. *et al.* (1995) Physical activity and incidence of diabetes: the Honolulu Heart Program. *American Journal of Epidemiology* **141**, 360–368.

Burt, V.L., Culter, J.A., Higgins, M. *et al.* (1995) Trends in prevalence, awareness, treatment, and control of hypertension in the adult US population—data from the health examination surveys, 1960 to 1991. *Hypertension* **26**, 60–69.

Caspersen, C.J. (1989) Physical activity epidemiology: concepts, methods, and applications to exercise science. In: Holloszy, J.O. (ed.) *Exercise and Sport Sci- ences Reviews*, Vol. 17, pp. 423–473. Williams & Wilkins, Baltimore, MD.

Cassel, J., Heyden, S., Bartel, A.G. *et al.* (1971) Occupation and physical activity and coronary heart disease. *Archives of Internal Medicine* **128**, 920–928.

Castelli, W.P., Doyle, J.T., Gordon, T. *et al.* (1977) HDL cholesterol and other lipids in coronary heart disease. The Coopera- tive Lipoprotein Phenotyping Study. *Circulation* **55**, 767–772.

Cooksey, J.D., Reilly, P., Brown, S., Bromze, H. & Cryer, P.E. (1978) Exercise training and plasma catecholamines in patients with ischemic heart disease. *American Journal of Cardiology* **42**, 372–376.

Crouse, J.R. III, Byington, R.P., Hoen, H.M. & Furberg, C.D. (1997) Reductase inhibitor monotherapy and stroke pre- vention. *Archives of Internal Medicine* **157**, 1305–1310.

Darga, L.L., Lucas, C.P., Spafford, T.R., Schork, M.A., Illis, W.R. & Holden, N. (1989) Endurance training in middle- aged physicians. *Physician and Sportsmedicine* **17** (7), 85–101.

Donahue, R.P., Abbott, R.D., Reed, D.M. & Yano, K. (1988) Physical activity and coronary heart disease in middle-aged and elderly men: the Honolulu Heart Program. *American Journal of Public Health* **78**, 683–685.

Durstine, J.L. & Haskell, W.L. (1994) Effects of exercise training on plasma lipids and lipoproteins. *Exercise and Sport Sciences Reviews* **22**, 477–521.

Eaton, C.B., Medalie, J.H., Flocke, S.A., Zyzanski, S.J., Yaari, S. & Goldbourt, U. (1995) Self-reported physical activity predicts long-term coronary heart disease and all-cause mortalities. Twenty-one-year follow-up of the Israeli Ischemic Heart Disease Study. *Archives of Family Medicine* **4**, 323–329.

Ekelund, L.G., Haskell, W.L., Johnson, J.L., Whaley, F.S., Criqui, M.H. & Sheps, D.S. (1988) Physical fitness as a predictor of cardiovascular mortality in asympto- matic North American men. The Lipid Research Clinic's Mortality Follow-up

Study. *New England Journal of Medicine* **319**, 1379–1384.

Ellekjaer, E.F., Wyller, T.B., Sverre, J.M. & Holmen, J. (1992) Lifestyle factors and risk of cerebral infarction. *Stroke* **23**, 829–834.

El-Sayed, M.S. (1996) Fibrinogen levels and exercise: is there a relationship? *Sports Medicine* **21**, 402–408.

Erikssen, J. (1986) Physical fitness and coronary heart disease morbidity and mortality. A prospective study in apparently healthy, middle aged men. *Acta Medica Scandinavica* **711** (Suppl.), 189–192.

Fagard, R.H. (1993) Physical fitness and blood pressure. *Journal of Hypertension* **11** (Suppl. 5), S47–S52.

Folsom, A.R., Caspersen, C.J., Taylor, H.L. et al. (1985) Leisure time physical activity and its relationship to coronary risk factors in a population-based sample. *American Journal of Epidemiology* **121**, 570–579.

Folsom, A.R., Prineas, R.J., Kaye, S.A. & Munger, R.G. (1990) Incidence of hypertension and stroke in relation to body fat distribution and other risk factors in older women. *Stroke* **21**, 701–706.

Folsom, A.R., Arnett, D.K., Hutchinson, R.G., Liao, F., Clegg, L.X. & Cooper, L.S. (1997) Physical activity and incidence of coronary heart disease in middle-aged women and men. *Medicine and Science in Sports and Exercise* **29**, 901–909.

Fraser, G.E. & Shavlik, D.J. (1997) Risk factors for all-cause and coronary heart disease mortality in the oldest-old. The Adventist Health Study. *Archives of Internal Medicine* **157**, 2249–2258.

Fraser, G.E., Strahan, T.M., Sabaté, J., Beeson, W.L. & Kissinger, D. (1992) Effects of traditional coronary risk factors on rates of incident coronary events in a low-risk population. The Adventist Health Study. *Circulation* **86**, 406–413.

Frohlich, E.D. (1994) Hypertension. In: Pearson, T.A., Criqui, M.H., Luepker, R.V., Oberman, A. & Winston, M. (eds) *Primer in Preventive Cardiology*, pp. 131–142. American Heart Association, Dallas, TX.

Fuster, V., Badimon, L., Badimon, J.J. & Chesebro, J.H. (1992a) The pathogenesis of coronary artery disease and the acute coronary syndromes (1). *New England Journal of Medicine* **326**, 242–250.

Fuster, V., Badimon, L., Badimon, J.J. & Chesebro, J.H. (1992b) The pathogenesis of coronary artery disease and the acute

coronary syndromes (2). *New England Journal of Medicine* **326**, 310–318.

Garcia-Palmieri, M.R., Costas, R. Jr, Cruz-Vidal, M., Sorlie, P.D. & Havlik, R.J. (1982) Increased physical activity. A protective factor against heart attacks in Puerto Rico. *American Journal of Cardiology* **50**, 749–755.

Garrow, J.S. & Summerbell, C.D. (1995) Meta-analysis: effect of exercise, with or without dieting, on the body composition of overweight subjects. *European Journal of Clinical Nutrition* **49**, 1–10.

Gillum, R.F., Mussolino, M.E. & Ingram, D.D. (1996) Physical activity and stroke incidence in women and men: the NHANES I Epidemiologic Follow-up Study. *American Journal of Epidemiology* **143**, 860–869.

Gould, A.L., Rossouw, J.E., Santanello, N.C., Heyse, J.F. & Furberg, C.D. (1998) Cholesterol reduction yields clinical benefit: impact of statin trials. *Circulation* **97**, 946–952.

Haapanen, N., Miilunpalo, S., Vuori, I., Oja, P. & Pasanen, M. (1996) Characteristics of leisure time physical activity associated with decreased risk of premature all-cause and cardiovascular disease mortality in middle-aged men. *American Journal of Epidemiology* **143**, 870–880.

Haapanen, N., Milunpalo, S., Vuori, I., Oja, P. & Pasanen, M. (1997) Association of leisure time physical activity with the risk of coronary heart disease, hypertension and diabetes in middle-aged men and women. *International Journal of Epidemiology* **26**, 739–747.

Hagberg, J.M. (1990) Exercise, fitness, and hypertension. In: Bouchard, C., Shephard, R.J., Stephens, J.R. & McPherson, B.D. (eds) *Exercise, Fitness, and Health: a Consensus of Current Knowledge*, pp. 455–466. Human Kinetics, Champaign, IL.

Hagberg, J.M., Montain, S.J., Martin, W.H. III & Ehsani, A.A. (1989) Effect of exercise training in 60- to 69-year-old persons with essential hypertension. *American Journal of Cardiology* **64**, 348–353.

Håheim, L.L., Holme, I., Hjermann, I. & Leren, P. (1993) Risk factors of stroke incidence and mortality: a 12-year follow-up of the Oslo Study. *Stroke* **24**, 1484–1489.

Hakim, A.A., Petrovitch, H., Burchfiel, C.M. et al. (1998) Effects of walking on mortality among nonsmoking retired men. *New England Journal of Medicine* **338**, 94–99.

Halbert, J.A., Silagy, C.A., Finucane, P.,

Withers, R.T., Hamdorf, P.A. & Andrews, G.R. (1997) The effectiveness of exercise training in lowering blood pressure: a meta-analysis of randomised controlled trials of 4 weeks or longer. *Journal of Human Hypertension* **11**, 641–649.

Hambrecht, R., Niebauer, J., Marburger, C. et al. (1993) Various intensities of leisure time physical activity in patients with coronary artery disease: effects on cardiorespiratory fitness and progression of coronary atherosclerotic lesions. *Journal of the American College of Cardiology* **22**, 468–477.

Harmsen, P., Rosengren, A., Tsipogianni, A. & Wilhelmsen, L. (1990) Risk factors for stroke in middle-aged men in Göteborg, Sweden. *Stroke* **21**, 223–229.

Harris, S.S., Caspersen, C.J., DeFriese, G.H. & Estes, E.H. Jr (1989) Physical activity counseling for healthy adults as a primary preventive intervention in the clinical setting. Report for the U.S. Preventive Services Task Force. *Journal of the American Medical Association* **261**, 3588–3598.

Haskell, W.L., Leon, A.S., Caspersen, C.J. et al. (1992) Cardiovascular benefits and assessment of physical activity and physical fitness in adults. *Medicine and Science in Sports and Exercise* **24** (Suppl. 6), S201–S220.

Hedblad, B., Ogren, M., Isacsson, S.O. & Janzon, L. (1997) Reduced cardiovascular mortality risk in male smokers who are physically active. Results from a 25-year follow-up of the prospective population study of men born in 1914. *Archives of Internal Medicine* **157**, 893–899.

Hein, H.O., Suadicani, P. & Gyntelberg, F. (1992) Physical fitness or physical activity as a predictor of ischaemic heart disease? A 17-year follow-up in the Copenhagen Male Study. *Journal of Internal Medicine* **232**, 471–479.

Helmrich, S.P., Ragland, D.R. & Paffenbarger, R.S. Jr (1994) Prevention of non-insulin-dependent diabetes mellitus with physical activity. *Medicine and Science in Sports and Exercise* **26**, 824–830.

Herbert, P.N., Bernier, D.N., Cullinane, E.M., Edelstein, L., Kantor, M.A. & Thompson, P.D. (1984) High density lipoprotein metabolism in runners and sedentary men. *Journal of the American Medical Association* **252**, 1034–1037.

Herman, B., Schmitz, P.I.M., Leyten, A.C.M. et al. (1983) Multivariate logistic analysis of risk factors for stroke in Tilburg, the Netherlands. *American Journal of Epidemiology* **118**, 514–525.

Holloszy, J.O., Schultz, J., Kusnierkiewicz,

J., Hagberg, J.M. & Ehsani, A.A. (1986) Effects of exercise on glucose tolerance and insulin resistance. *Acta Medica Scandinavica* **711** (Suppl.), 55–65.

Kannel, W.B. & Sorlie, P. (1979) Some health benefits of physical activity: the Framingham Study. *Archives of Internal Medicine* **139**, 857–861.

Kantor, M.A., Cullinane, E.M., Herbert, P.N. & Thompson, P.D. (1984) Acute increase in lipoprotein lipase following prolonged exercise. *Metabolism* **33**, 454–457.

Kaplan, G.A., Strawbridge, W.J., Cohen, R.D. & Hungerford, L.R. (1996) Natural history of leisure-time physical activity and its correlates: associations with mortality from all causes and cardiovascular disease over 28 years. *American Journal of Epidemiology* **144**, 793–797.

Kelley, G.A. (1995) Effects of aerobic exercise in normotensive adults: a brief meta-analytic review of controlled trials. *Southern Medical Journal* **88**, 42–46.

Kelley, G. & McClellan, P. (1994) Antihypertensive effects of aerobic exercise: a brief meta-analytic review of randomized controlled trials. *American Journal of Hypertension* **7**, 115–119.

Kemmer, F.W. & Berger, M. (1983) Exercise and diabetes mellitus: physical activity as part of daily life and its role in the treatment of diabetic patients. *International Journal of Sports Medicine* **4**, 77–88.

Kiely, D.K., Wolf, P.A., Cupples, L.A., Beiser, A.S. & Kannel, W.B. (1994) Physical activity and stroke risk: the Framingham Study. *American Journal of Epidemiology* **140**, 608–620.

King, D.S., Dalsky, G.P., Staten, M.A., Clutter, W.E., Van Houten, D.R. & Holloszy, J.O. (1987) Insulin action and secretion in endurance-trained and untrained humans. *Journal of Applied Physiology* **63**, 2247–2252.

Komachi, Y., Iida, M., Shimamoto, T., Chikayama, Y. & Takahashi, H. (1971) Geographic and occupational comparisons of risk factors in cardiovascular diseases in Japan. *Japanese Circulation Journal* **35**, 189–207.

Kramsch, D.M., Aspen, A.J., Abramowitz, B.M., Kreimendahl, T. & Hood, W.B. Jr (1981) Reduction of coronary atherosclerosis by moderate conditioning exercise in monkeys on an atherogenic diet. *New England Journal of Medicine* **305**, 1483–1489.

Krotkiewski, M., Lonnroth, P., Mandroukas, K. *et al.* (1985) The effects of physical training on insulin secretion and effectiveness and on glucose metabolism in obesity and type 2 (non-insulin-

dependent) diabetes mellitus. *Diabetologia* **28**, 881–890.

Kujala, U.M., Kaprio, J., Sarna, S. & Koskenvuo, M. (1998) Relationship of leisure-time physical activity and mortality: the Finnish twin cohort. *Journal of the American Medical Association* **279**, 440–444.

Kushi, L.H., Fee, R.M., Folsom, A.R., Mink, P.J., Anderson, K.E. & Sellers, T.A. (1997) Physical activity and mortality in postmenopausal women. *Journal of the American Medical Association* **277**, 1287–1292.

LaCroix, A.Z., Leveille, S.G., Hecht, J.A., Grothaus, L.C. & Wagner, E.H. (1996) Does walking decrease the risk of cardiovascular disease hospitalizations and death in older adults? *Journal of the American Geriatric Association* **44**, 113–120.

Lakka, T.A., Venäläinen, J.M., Rauramaa, R., Salonen, R., Tuomilehto, J. & Salonen, J.T. (1994) Relation of leisure-time physical activity and cardiorespiratory fitness to the risk of acute myocardial infarction in men. *New England Journal of Medicine* **330**, 1549–1554.

Lapidus, L. & Bengtsson, C. (1986) Socioeconomic factors and physical activity in relation to cardiovascular disease and death: a 12-year follow-up of participants in a population study of women in Gothenburg, Sweden. *British Heart Journal* **55**, 295–301.

LaPorte, R.E., Adams, L.L., Savage, D.D., Brenes, G., Dearwater, S. & Cook, T. (1984) The spectrum of physical activity, cardiovascular disease, and health: an epidemiologic perspective. *American Journal of Epidemiology* **120**, 507–517.

Laughlin, M.H. (1994) Effects of exercise training on coronary circulation: introduction. *Medicine and Science in Sports and Exercise* **26**, 1226–1229.

LeBlanc, J., Nadeau, A., Boulay, M. & Rousseau-Migneron, S. (1979) Effects of physical training and adiposity on glucose metabolism and ^{125}I-insulin binding. *Journal of Applied Physiology* **46**, 235–239.

Lee, I.-M., Hsieh, C.-C. & Paffenbarger, R.S. Jr (1995) Exercise intensity and longevity in men. The Harvard Alumni Health Study. *Journal of the American Medical Association* **273**, 1179–1184.

Lemaitre, R.N., Heckbert, S.R., Psaty, B.M. & Siscovick, D.S. (1995) Leisure-time physical activity and the risk of nonfatal myocardial infarction in postmenopausal women. *Archives of Internal Medicine* **155**, 2302–2308.

Leon, A.S., Myers, M.J. & Connett, J. (1997) Leisure time physical activity and the 16-year risks of mortality from coronary

heart disease and all-causes in the Multiple Risk Factor Intervention Trial (MRFIT). *International Journal of Sports Medicine* **18** (Suppl. 3), S208–S215.

Lindenstrøm, E., Boysen, G. & Nyboe, J. (1993) Lifestyle factors and risk of cerebrovascular disease in women. The Copenhagen City Heart Study. *Stroke* **24**, 1468–1472.

Lindsted, K.D., Tonstad, S. & Kuzma, J.W. (1991) Self-report of physical activity and patterns of mortality in Seventh-Day Adventist men. *Journal of Clinical Epidemiology* **44**, 355–364.

Lissner, L., Bengtsson, C., Björkelund, C. & Wedel, H. (1996) Physical activity levels and changes in relation to longevity. *American Journal of Epidemiology* **143**, 54–62.

Lithell, H., Orlander, J., Schele, R., Sjodin, B. & Karlsson, J. (1979) Changes in lipoprotein–lipase activity and lipid stores in human skeletal muscle with prolonged heavy exercise. *Acta Physiologica Scandinavica* **107**, 257–261.

Magnus, K., Matroos, A. & Strackee, J. (1979) Walking, cycling, or gardening, with or without seasonal interruption, in relation to acute coronary events. *American Journal of Epidemiology* **110**, 724–733.

Manninen, V., Elo, M.O., Frick, M.H. *et al.* (1988) Lipid alterations and decline in the incidence of coronary heart disease in the Helsinki Heart Study. *Journal of the American Medical Association* **260**, 641–651.

Manson, J.E., Rimm, E.B., Stampfer, M.J. *et al.* (1991) Physical activity and incidence of non-insulin-dependent mellitus in women. *Lancet* **338**, 774–778.

Manson, J.E., Nathan, D.M., Krolewski, A.S., Stampfer, M.J., Willett, W.C. & Hennekens, C.H. (1992) A prospective study of exercise and incidence of diabetes among US male physicians. *Journal of the American Medical Association* **268**, 63–67.

Marceau, M., Kouame, N., Lacourciere, Y. & Cleroux, J. (1993) Effects of different training intensities on 24-hour blood pressure in hypertensive subjects. *Circulation* **88**, 2803–2811.

Maskin, C.S. (1986) Aerobic exercise training and cardiopulmonary disease. In: Weber, K.T. & Janicki, J.S. (eds) *Cardiopulmonary Exercise Training*, pp. 317–332. W.B. Saunders, Philadelphia, PA.

Matsusaki, M., Ikeda, M., Tashiro, E. *et al.* (1992) Influence of workload on the antihypertensive effect of exercise. *Clinical and Experimental Pharmacology and Physiology* **19**, 471–479.

Mayer-Davis, E.J., D'Agostino, R., Karter, A.J. *et al.* (1998) Intensity and amount of physical activity in relation to insulin sensitivity. The Insulin Resistance Atherosclerosis Study. *Journal of the American Medical Association* **279**, 669–674.

Menotti, A. & Seccareccia, F. (1985) Physical activity at work and job responsibility as risk factors for fatal coronary heart disease and other causes of death. *Journal of Epidemiology and Community Health* **39**, 325–329.

Menotti, A., Keys, A., Blackburn, H. *et al.* (1990) Twenty-year stroke mortality and prediction in twelve cohorts of the Seven Countries Study. *International Journal of Epidemiology* **19**, 309–315.

Mensink, G.B.M., Deketh, M., Mul, M.D.M., Schuit, A.J. & Hoffmeister, H. (1996) Physical activity and its association with cardiovascular risk factors and mortality. *Epidemiology* **7**, 391–397.

Miller, W.C., Koceja, D.M. & Hamilton, E.J. (1997) A meta-analysis of the past 25 years of weight loss research using diet, exercise or diet plus exercise intervention. *International Journal of Obesity and Related Metabolic Disorders* **21**, 941–947.

Mittleman, M.A., Maclure, M., Tofler, G.H., Sherwood, J.B., Goldberg, R.J. & Muller, J.E. (1993) Triggering of acute myocardial infarction by heavy physical exertion. Protection against triggering by regular exertion. Determinants of Myocardial Infarction Onset Study Investigators. *New England Journal of Medicine* **329**, 1677–1683.

Morris, J.N., Everitt, M.G., Pollard, R., Chave, S.P. & Semmence, A.M. (1980) Vigorous exercise in leisure-time: protection against coronary heart disease. *Lancet* **ii**, 1207–1210.

Nakayama, T., Date, C., Yokoyama, T., Yoshiike, H., Yamaguchi, M. & Tanaka, H. (1997) A 15.5-year follow-up study of stroke in a Japanese Provincial City: the Shibata Study. *Stroke* **28**, 45–52.

National High Blood Pressure Education Program Working Group (1993) National High Blood Pressure Working Group report on primary prevention of hypertension. *Archives of Internal Medicine* **153**, 186–208.

NIH Consensus Development Panel on Physical Activity and Cardiovascular Health (1996) Physical activity and cardiovascular health. *Journal of the American Medical Association* **276**, 241–246.

O'Connor, G.T., Buring, J.E., Yusuf, S. *et al.* (1989) An overview of randomized trials of rehabilitation with exercise after myocardial infarction. *Circulation* **80**, 234–244.

O'Connor, G.T., Hennekens, C.H., Willett, W.C. *et al.* (1995) Physical exercise and reduced risk of nonfatal myocardial infarction. *American Journal of Epidemiology* **142**, 1147–1156.

Okada, H., Horibe, H., Ohno, Y., Hayakawa, N. & Aoki, N. (1976) A prospective study of cerebrovascular disease in Japanese rural communities, Akabane and Asahi. Part 1: Evaluation of risk factors in the occurrence of cerebral hemorrhage and thrombosis. *Stroke* **7**, 599–607.

Paffenbarger, R.S. Jr, Laughlin, M.E., Gima, A.S. & Black, R.A. (1970) Work activity of longshoremen as related to death from coronary heart disease and stroke. *New England Journal of Medicine* **282**, 1109–1114.

Paffenbarger, R.S. Jr, Wing, A.L. & Hyde, R.T. (1978) Physical activity as an index of heart attack risk in college alumni. *American Journal of Epidemiology* **108**, 161–175.

Paffenbarger, R.S. Jr, Wing, A.L., Hyde, R.T. & Jung, D.L. (1983) Physical activity and incidence of hypertension in College Alumni. *American Journal of Epidemiology* **117**, 245–257.

Paffenbarger, R.S. Jr, Hyde, R.T., Wing, A.L. & Steinmetz, C.H. (1984) A natural history of athleticism and cardiovascular health. *Journal of the American Medical Association* **252**, 491–495.

Paffenbarger, R.S. Jr, Jung, D.L., Leung, R.W. & Hyde, R.T. (1991) Physical activity and hypertension: an epidemiological view. *Annals of Medicine* **23**, 319–327.

Paffenbarger, R.S. Jr, Hyde, R.T., Wing, A.L., Lee, I.-M., Jung, D.L. & Kampert, J.B. (1993) The association of changes in physical activity level and other lifestyle characteristics with mortality among men. *New England Journal of Medicine* **328**, 538–545.

Paganini-Hill, A., Ross, R.K. & Henderson, B.E. (1988) Postmenopausal oestrogen treatment and stroke: a prospective study. *British Medical Journal* **297**, 519–522.

Pate, R.R., Pratt, M., Blair, S.N. *et al.* (1995) Physical activity and public health. A recommendation from the Centers for Disease Control and Prevention and the American College of Sports Medicine. *Journal of the American Medical Association* **273**, 402–407.

Pedersen, O., Beck-Nielsen, H. & Heding, L. (1980) Increased insulin receptors after exercise in patients with insulin-dependent diabetes mellitus. *New England Journal of Medicine* **302**, 886–892.

Pekkanen, J., Marti, B., Nissinen, A., Tuomilehto, J., Punsar, S. & Karvonen, M.J. (1987) Reduction of premature mortality by high physical activity: a 20-year follow-up of middle-aged Finnish men. *Lancet* **1**, 1473–1477.

Pereira, M.A., Folsom, A.R., McGovern, P.G. *et al.* (1999) Physical activity and incident hypertension in black and white adults: The Atherosclerosis Risk in Communities (ARIC) Study. *Preventive Medicine* **28**, 304–312.

Peters, R.K., Cady, L.D. Jr, Bischoff, D.P., Bernstein, L. & Pike, M.C. (1983) Physical fitness and subsequent myocardial infarction in healthy workers. *Journal of the American Medical Association* **249**, 3052–3056.

Pomrehn, P.R., Wallace, R.B. & Burmeister, L.F. (1982) Ischemic heart disease mortality in Iowa farmers: the influence of life-style. *Journal of the American Medical Association* **248**, 1073–1076.

Powell, K.E., Thompson, P.D., Caspersen, C.J. & Kendrick, J.S. (1987) Physical activity and the incidence of coronary heart disease. *Annual Reviews of Public Health* **8**, 253–287.

Pratley, R.E., Hagberg, J.M., Rogus, E.M. & Goldberg, A.P. (1995) Enhanced insulin sensitivity and lower waist-to-hip ratio in master athletes. *American Journal of Physiology* **268**, E484–E490.

Prineas, R.J., Folsom, A.R. & Kaye, S.A. (1993) Central adiposity and increased risk of coronary artery disease mortality in older women. *Annals of Epidemiology* **3**, 35–41.

Rauramaa, R. (1984) Relationship of physical activity, glucose tolerance, and weight management. *Preventive Medicine* **13**, 37–46.

Rauramaa, R., Salonen, J.T., Kukkonen-Harjula, K. *et al.* (1984) Effects of mild physical exercise on serum lipoproteins and metabolites of arachidonic acid: a controlled randomised trial in middle-aged men. *British Medical Journal* **288**, 603–606.

Rauramaa, R., Salonen, J.T., Seppanen, K. *et al.* (1986) Inhibition of platelet aggregability by moderate-intensity physical exercise: a randomized clinical trial in overweight men. *Circulation* **74**, 939–944.

Reid, C.M., Dart, A.M., Dewar, E.M. & Jennings, G.L. (1994) Interactions between the effects of exercise and weight loss on risk factors, cardiovascular haemodynamics and left ventricular structure in overweight subjects. *Journal of Hypertension* **12**, 291–301.

Rexrode, K.M., Manson, J.E. & Hennekens, C.H. (1996) Obesity and cardiovascular disease. *Current Opinions in Cardiology* 11, 490–495.

Richter, E.A. & Galbo, H. (1986) Diabetes, insulin and exercise. *Sports Medicine* 3, 275–288.

Ronnemaa, T., Mattila, K., Lehtonen, A. & Kallio, V. (1986) A controlled randomized study on the effect of long-term physical exercise on the metabolic control in type 2 diabetic patients. *Acta Medica Scandinavica* 220, 219–224.

Rosengren, A. & Wilhelmsen, L. (1997) Physical activity protects against coronary death and deaths from all causes in middle-aged men. Evidence from a 20-year follow-up of the primary prevention study in Goteborg. *Annals of Epidemiology* 7, 69–75.

Ruige, J.B., Assendelft, W.J., Dekker, J.M., Kostense, P.J., Heine, R.J. & Bouter, L.M. (1998) Insulin and risk of cardiovascular disease: a meta-analysis. *Circulation* 97, 996–1001.

Sacco, R.L., Gan, R., Boden-Albala, B. *et al.* (1998) Leisure-time physical activity and ischemic stroke risk. The Northern Manhattan Stroke Study. *Stroke* 29, 380–387.

Salonen, J.T., Puska, P. & Tuomilehto, J. (1982) Physical activity and risk of myocardial infarction, cerebral stroke and death: a longitudinal study in Eastern Finland. *American Journal of Epidemiology* 115, 526–537.

Sandvik, L., Erikssen, J., Thaulow, E., Erikssen, G., Mundal, R. & Rodahl, K. (1993) Physical fitness as a predictor of mortality among healthy, middle-aged Norwegian men. *New England Journal of Medicine* 328, 533–537.

Schneider, S.H., Amorosa, L.F., Khachadurian, A.K. & Ruderman, N.B. (1984) Studies on the mechanism of improved glucose control during regular exercise in type 2 (non-insulin-dependent) diabetes. *Diabetologia* 26, 355–360.

Schuit, A.J., Schouten, E.G., Kluft, C., de Maat, M., Menheere, P.P.C.A. & Kok, F.J. (1997) Effect of strenuous exercise on fibrinogen and fibrinolysis in healthy elderly men and women. *Thrombosis and Haemostasis* 78, 845–851.

Schwartz, R.S. (1987) The independent effects of dietary weight loss and aerobic training on high density lipoprotein and apolipoprotein A-I concentrations in obese men. *Metabolism* 36, 165–171.

Scragg, R., Stewart, A., Jackson, R. & Beaglehole, R. (1987) Alcohol and exercise in myocardial infarction and sudden coronary death in men and women. *American Journal of Epidemiology* 126, 77–85.

Seals, D.R., Allen, W.K., Hurley, B.F., Dalsky, G.P., Ehsani, A.A. & Hagberg,

J.M. (1984) Elevated high-density lipoprotein cholesterol levels in older endurance athletes. *American Journal of Cardiology* 54, 390–393.

Shephard, R.J. (1986) Exercise in coronary heart disease. *Sports Medicine* 3, 26–49.

Sherman, S.E., D'Agostino, R.B., Cobb, J.L. & Kannel, W.B. (1994a) Does exercise reduce mortality rates in the elderly? Experience from the Framingham Heart Study. *American Heart Journal* 128, 965–972.

Sherman, S.E., D'Agostino, R.B., Cobb, J.L. & Kannel, W.B. (1994b) Physical activity and mortality in women in the Framingham Heart Study. *American Heart Journal* 128, 879–884.

Shinton, R. & Sagar, G. (1993) Lifelong exercise and stroke. *British Medical Journal* 307, 231–234.

Simonsick, E.M., Lafferty, M.E., Phillips, C.L. *et al.* (1993) Risk due to inactivity in physically capable older adults. *American Journal of Public Health* 83, 1443–1450.

Siscovick, D.S., Weiss, N.S., Hallstrom, A.P., Inui, T.S. & Peterson, D.R. (1982) Physical activity and primary cardiac arrest. *Journal of the American Medical Association* 248, 3113–3117.

Siscovick, D.S., Weiss, N.S., Fletcher, R.H., Schoenbach, V.J. & Wagner, E.H. (1984) Habitual vigorous exercise and primary cardiac arrest: effect of other risk factors on the relationship. *Journal of Chronic Diseases* 37, 625–631.

Siscovick, D.S., Fried, L., Mittelmark, M., Rutan, G., Bild, D. & O'Leary, D.H. (1997) Exercise intensity and subclinical cardiovascular disease in the elderly. The Cardiovascular Health Study. *American Journal of Epidemiology* 145, 977–986.

Slattery, M.L. & Jacobs, D.R. Jr (1988) Physical fitness and cardiovascular disease mortality. The US Railroad Study. *American Journal of Epidemiology* 127, 571–580.

Sobolski, J., Kornitzer, M., DeBacker, G. *et al.* (1987) Protection against ischemic heart disease in the Belgian Physical Fitness Study: physical fitness rather than physical activity? *American Journal of Epidemiology* 125, 601–610.

Soman, V.R., Koivisto, V.A., Deibert, D., Felig, P. & DeFronzo, R.A. (1979) Increased insulin sensitivity and insulin binding to monocytes after physical training. *New England Journal of Medicine* 301, 1200–1204.

Stamler, J., Stamler, R. & Neaton, J.D. (1993) Blood pressure, systolic and diastolic, and cardiovascular risks. US population data. *Archives of Internal Medicine* 153, 598–615.

Stefanick, M.L. & Wood, P.D. (1994) Physical activity, lipid and lipoprotein metabolism, and lipid transport. In: Bouchard, C., Shephard, R.J. & Stephens, T. (eds) *Physical Activity, Fitness, and Health: International Proceedings and Consensus Statement*, pp. 417–431. Human Kinetics, Champaign, IL.

Stender, M., Hense, H.W., Doring, A. & Keil, U. (1993) Physical activity at work and cardiovascular disease risk: results from the MONICA Augsburg study. *International Journal of Epidemiology* 22, 644–650.

Superko, H.R. (1995) Exercise and lipoprotein metabolism. *Journal of Cardiovascular Risk* 2, 310–315.

Tanaka, H., Ueda, Y., Hayashi, M. *et al.* (1982) Risk factors for cerebral hemorrhage and cerebral infarction in a Japanese rural community. *Stroke* 13, 62–73.

Tipton, C.M. (1991) Exercise, training and hypertension: an update. In: Holloszy, J.O. (ed.) *Exercise and Sport Sciences Reviews*, Vol. 19, pp. 447–504. Williams & Wilkins, Baltimore, MD.

Tunstall-Pedoe, H., Woodward, M., Tavendale, R., A'Brook, R. & McClusky, M.K. (1997) Comparison of the prediction by 27 different factors of coronary heart disease and death in men and women of the Scottish heart health study: cohort study. *British Medical Journal* 315, 722–729.

US Department of Health and Human Services (1995) *Healthy People 2000: Mid-course Review and 1995 Revisions*. US Department of Health and Human Services, Public Health Service, Washington, D.C.

US Department of Health and Human Services (1996a) Chapter 2: Historical background, terminology, evolution of recommendations, and measurement. In: *Physical Activity and Health: A Report of the Surgeon General*, pp. 9–57. US Department of Health and Human Services, Centers for Disease Control and Prevention, National Center for Chronic Disease Prevention and Health Promotion, Atlanta, GA.

US Department of Health and Human Services (1996b) Chapter 4: The effects of physical activity on health and disease. In: *Physical Activity and Health: A Report of the Surgeon General*, pp. 81–172. US Department of Health and Human Services, Centers for Disease Control and Prevention, National Center for Chronic Disease Prevention and Health Promotion, Atlanta, GA.

US Department of Health and Human Services (1996c) Chapter 5: Patterns and trends in physical activity. In: *Physical Activity and Health: A Report of the Surgeon General*, pp. 173–207. US Department of Health and Human Services, Centers for Disease Control and Prevention, National Center for Chronic Disease Prevention and Health Promotion, Atlanta, GA.

US Department of Health and Human Services (1996d) Chapter 6: Understanding and promoting physical activity. In: *Physical Activity and Health: A Report of the Surgeon General*, pp. 209–259. US Department of Health and Human Services, Centers for Disease Control and Prevention, National Center for Chronic Disease Prevention and Health Promotion, Atlanta, GA.

Wannamethee, G. & Shaper, A.G. (1992) Physical activity and stroke in British middle-aged men. *British Medical Journal* 304, 597–601.

Wannamethee, G., Shaper, A.G. & Walker, M. (1998) Changes in physical activity, mortality, and incidence of coronary heart disease in older men. *Lancet* 351, 1603–1608.

Wilhelmsen, L., Bjure, J., Ekstrom-Jodal, B. *et al.* (1981) Nine years' follow-up of a maximal exercise test in a random population sample of middle-aged men. *Cardiology* 68 (Suppl. 2), 1–8.

Williams, P.T. (1995) Letter to the editor. *Journal of the American Medical Association* 274, 533–534.

Williams, P.T. (1996) High-density lipoprotein cholesterol and other risk factors for coronary heart disease in female runners. *New England Journal of Medicine* 334, 1298–1303.

Williams, P.T. (1997) Relationship of distance run per week to coronary heart disease risk factors in 8283 male runners. The National Runners' Health Study. *Archives of Internal Medicine* 157, 191–198.

Williams, P.T. (1998a) Relationships of heart disease risk factors to exercise quantity and intensity. *Archives of Internal Medicine* 158, 237–245.

Williams, P.T. (1998b) Coronary heart disease risk factors of vigorously active sexagenarians and septuagenarians. *Journal of the American Geriatric Society* 46, 134–142.

Williams, P.T., Krauss, R.M., Vranizan, K.M. & Wood, P.D. (1990) Changes in lipoprotein subfractions during diet-induced and exercise-induced weight loss in moderately overweight men. *Circulation* 81, 1293–1304.

Williams, R.S., Logue, E.E., Lewis, J.G. *et al.* (1980) Physical conditioning augments the fibrinolytic response to venous occlusion in healthy adults. *New England Journal of Medicine* 302, 987–991.

Winett, R.A. (1995) Letter to the editor. *Journal of the American Medical Association* 274, 534–535.

Wood, P.D., Haskell, W.L., Blair, S.N. *et al.* (1983) Increased exercise level and plasma lipoprotein concentrations: a one-year, randomized, controlled study in sedentary, middle-aged men. *Metabolism* 32, 31–39.

Wood, P.D., Stefanick, M.L., Dreon, D.M. *et al.* (1988) Changes in plasma lipids and lipoproteins in overweight men during weight loss through dieting as compared with exercise. *New England Journal of Medicine* 319, 1173–1179.

You, R., McNeil, J.J., O'Malley, H.M., Davis, S.M. & Donnan, G.A. (1995) Risk factors for lacunar infarction syndromes. *Neurology* 45, 1483–1487.

You, R.X., McNeil, J.J., O'Malley, H.M., Davis, S.M., Thrift, A.G. & Donnan, G.A. (1997) Risk factors for stroke due to cerebral infarction in young adults. *Stroke* 28, 1913–1918.

Chapter 48

Cardiovascular Risks of Endurance Sport

ROY J. SHEPHARD

The heart of the endurance athlete has interested physiologists because of its large size and very slow resting rate of contraction. The first characteristic is a reflection of myocardial hypertrophy, and the second an expression of the altered autonomic balance induced by endurance training. Clinicians noted these same features (particularly in rowers, cyclists and distance runners) from the earliest days of sports medicine (Osler 1892). Many physicians regarded such hypertrophy as a healthy response to prolonged exercise. Others worried about the bradycardia and associated electrocardiographic features, or drew a parallel to the large hearts observed in various cardiac pathologies. In particular, concern was expressed that the cardiac enlargement was responsible for the occasional incidents of sudden cardiac death during endurance competition. It was suggested that the large heart 'indicates undue strain or . . . the danger of eventual degeneration' (Keys & Friedell 1938), and in some instances training was restrained or even forbidden because of myocardial hypertrophy.

This chapter looks critically at the concepts of myocardial hypertrophy and cardiomyopathy, noting that the distinction between a normal and a pathological enlargement of the heart is difficult to make using such criteria as clinical examination, electrocardiography and echocardiography. The causes of sudden death during endurance exercise are examined briefly, and the rarity of such events is emphasized. Finally, the danger of an overdiagnosis of pathological cardiomyopathies is stressed.

Development of the concept of 'athlete's heart'

Awareness of cardiac hypertrophy among endurance competitors increased as examination of postero-anterior (PA) radiographs of the chest began to supplement such simple clinical indices of cardiac size as thoracic percussion and detection of a prominent, displaced apical impulse or a right ventricular lift. Sports physicians quickly found that the cardiothoracic ratios of many athletes exceeded the supposed normal limit of 0.50 (Keys & Friedell 1938). Use of both PA and lateral radiographs allowed observers to make crude estimates of the external volume of the heart (Reindell *et al.* 1966). Values averaged about 700 ml (10–11 ml·kg^{-1} body mass) in sedentary young men, but were as large as 1000–1100 ml (14–15 ml·kg^{-1}) in well-trained endurance athletes. As the quality of electrocardiograms (ECGs) improved, these, also, were interpreted in a quantitative sense (Bramwell & Ellis 1931). Left ventricular hypertrophy was diagnosed if the sum of the S wave in lead V_1 and the R wave in lead V_5 exceeded 35 mm (3.5 mV). Likewise, right ventricular hypertrophy was diagnosed if the sum of the R wave in lead V_1 and the S wave in lead V_5 exceeded 10.5 mm (1.05 mV) (Sokolow & Lyon 1949a,b). Other investigators developed more complicated methods for evaluation of the ECG (Romhilt & Estes 1968; Scott 1973). However, correlations of the electrocardiographic findings with radiography, echocardiography or ultimate post-mortem evaluation remained poor. This is perhaps not surprising, since hypertrophy of the chest muscles (typical of rowers and other prime candidates for ventricular hypertrophy) often attenuated ECG voltages (Park & Crawford 1985), and radiographs measured only the external dimensions of the heart, not distinguishing myocardial hypertrophy from a large ventricular cavity. One might anticipate a distinction between the firm, rounded radiographic contours of a heart with physiological hypertrophy, the sagging, distended form of a failing myocardium (Shephard 1969), and the irregular contours of a heart with what is generally an asymmetrical pathological hypertrophic cardiomyopathy (Klues et al. 1995). But in practice the two ventricles and the atria make varying contributions to the cardiac silhouette, depending on the axis of the heart, and it is not easy to distinguish the left ventricle from the other chambers of the heart. Perhaps the most important method of differentiating physiological from pathological enlargement of the heart is functional. If the cardiac enlargement is due to rheumatic valvular disease or a hypertrophic cardiomyopathy, the cardiac ejection fraction is poor and the patient shows a limited effort tolerance. In contrast, if the cardiac hypertrophy reflects a physiological response to endurance training, there is a large ejection fraction and an outstanding peak power output.

Use and misuse of echocardiographic and magnetic resonance imaging

Interest in cardiac enlargement as a possible cause of sudden, exercise-related death increased as wide-angle, two-dimensional echocardiography (Morganroth et al. 1975; Maron et al. 1981) and magnetic resonance imaging (Milliken et al. 1988; Fleck et al. 1989) became widely available. Rost and Hollmann (1992) suggested that overenthusiastic use of the echocardiogram led to much overdiagnosis of abnormalities, and they termed hypertrophic myocardiopathy an 'ultrasound-specific' disease. However, warnings against the dangers of 'athlete's heart' have continued until quite recently (Sandric 1980; Brandenburg 1990; Nienhaber et al. 1990).

The main advantage of the new techniques was that the cardiologist could measure the thicknesses of the ventricular walls and interventricular septum, as well as the internal dimensions of the ventricular chambers. Important differences were noted between the hearts of endurance and resistance athletes. In the former, thick ventricular walls seemed an adaptation to volume loading of the heart, but in the latter, thickening of the free walls and interventricular septum was not accompanied by any increase in left ventricular end-diastolic diameter (Morganroth et al. 1975; Snoeckx et al. 1982; George et al. 1991; Urhausen & Kindermann 1992).

The new technology also held the potential to distinguish endurance hypertrophy from both the distended heart of cardiac failure and the irregularly hypertrophied cardiomyopathic heart. Unfortunately, this potential has not always been realized, because the limits of resolution for echocardiography, typically 2 mm for an individual dimension (Perreault & Turcotte 1994), are of a similar order to many of the differences that distinguish the cardiac dimensions of young endurance athletes from those associated with pathological enlargements of the heart. As recently as 1991, Pelliccia et al. suggested that the distinction between physiological and pathological hypertrophy 'depends largely on the judgement whether the magnitude of the left ventricular wall thickness exceeds that expected as a result of athletic training alone'. Nevertheless, the choice of dividing line remains contentious. The originally specified ceiling for physiological hypertrophy was a posterior wall diastolic thickness of 11 mm. It was quickly discovered that up to 60% of endurance athletes exceeded this limit. Pelliccia et al. (1991) opted for a value of 13 mm; 7% of rowers, canoeists and cyclists in their series had a wall thickness greater than 13 mm. All of the individuals thus identified also had enlarged left ventricular end-diastolic dimensions, in the range 55–63 mm, a useful point of contrast with pathological hypertrophy (where the cavity is usually either normal or smaller than normal). Other investigators have further revised the normal limits for wall thickness upward to 16 mm (Shapiro 1984; Spirito et al. 1994; Williams & Bernhardt 1995), 18 mm (Van Camp et al. 1995) or even 19 mm (Reguero et al. 1995). Plainly, the new standards leave little margin to distinguish physiological hypertrophy from the 17–18-mm wall thickness typical of pathological pressure (aortic stenosis, hypertension) or volume (aortic or mitral regurgitation) overload (George *et al.* 1991). The new ceiling still offers a small margin to distinguish some cases of hypertrophic cardiomyopathy; this abnormality is commonly associated with a ventricular thickness of 20 mm or more, although some patients in this diagnostic category have readings in the range 13–15 mm (Maron *et al.* 1995).

The large heart of the endurance athlete arises mainly from rigorous training, but competitive selection is also a factor. Individuals are selected for endurance sport because they have inherited hearts that are large when untrained and hypertrophy readily in response to endurance training (see Chapter 15). The overall size of the competitor is a further consideration. In endurance sports such as rowing, large competitors have a substantial advantage, and such individuals necessarily have large hearts; indeed, according to most dimensional theorists, heart volume is proportional to the third power of stature (Asmussen & Christensen 1967). Thus, if volumes are expressed per unit of lean body mass, the 'large' hearts of resistance athletes often become 'normal' (Longhurst *et al.* 1980; Snoeckx *et al.* 1982; Van Camp *et al.* 1995) and in endurance competitors only the thickness of the interventricular septum is greater than in control subjects (Hagan *et al.* 1985).

Perhaps the most effective method of distinguishing between physiological and pathological hypertrophy is to collect data over several weeks or months of reduced training. A pathological enlargement of the heart remains unchanged in response to such a tactic, but the heart of the endurance competitor quickly regresses towards 'normal' sedentary values once training ceases (Ehsani *et al.* 1978).

Ratio of thickness of interventricular septum to dimensions of ventricular cavity

Some cardiologists have expressed concern about a possible pathological cardiac enlargement if the ratio of interventricular septum to left posterior ventricular wall thickness exceeds 1.3 : 1 (Huston *et al.* 1985). Such ratios can rise as high as 2.0 in athletes, much higher than in patients with pathological pressure or volume overload (Roeske *et al.* 1976;

Menapace *et al.* 1982; Shapiro 1984), but do not, in themselves, appear to be either dangerous or pathological (Huston *et al.* 1985); 60% of basketball players (Roeske *et al.* 1976) and 83% of child swimmers (Allen *et al.* 1976) have septal thicknesses that exceed accepted norms for the sedentary population. One case report described an athlete with a ratio of 1.5; 4 years after cessation of training, both the ECG and the echocardiogram had returned to 'normal' limits (Oakley & Oakley 1982).

Other cardiologists have argued that the ratio of septal thickness to left ventricular end-systolic or end-diastolic diameter is the most useful diagnostic feature of the echocardiogram. The upper limit of normality for the septal thickness/end-systolic diameter ratio has been set somewhat arbitrarily at 0.48 (3 s.d. above normal values) (Huston *et al.* 1985); this choice is debatable, given that some cardiorespiratory characteristics of international endurance competitors are four or more s.d. above the population average. A discrepancy between cardiac dimensions and ergometric performance (Urhausen & Kindermann 1992) and abnormalities of cardiac rhythm are other helpful indicators that enlargement is pathological.

Hypertrophy and myocardial ischaemia

Although ventricular hypertrophy is important to success in endurance competition, there have been fears that it might predispose to myocardial ischaemia and thus sudden cardiac death during exercise. There might be a propensity to sudden death if hypertrophy altered the pathway for conduction of electrical signals within the heart, or predisposed to myocardial ischaemia by increasing the diffusion distance from the coronary vessels to myocardial mitochondria; subvalvular hypertrophy might also restrict ventricular ejection (thus increasing cardiac work rate), and other abnormalities of ventricular structure might limit diastolic filling. Such problems arise mainly, if not exclusively, in a small group of individuals with congenital myocardial dystrophy. This abnormality can cause a disturbance of electrical conduction (Pye & Cobbe 1992; Maron *et al.* 1994), mitral regurgitation (Shapiro 1984), limited ventricular compliance, poor diastolic filling (Dickhuth *et al.* 1983) and/or hypotension (McKenna & Camm 1989; Maron 1993).

However, a physiological increase in heart size does not necessarily predispose to myocardial ischaemia in the healthy athlete. With physiological hypertrophy, there is a parallel development of the myocardial capillaries, as in hypertrophied skeletal muscle; thus, the myocardial blood supply of the endurance competitor remains at least as good as that found in the hypotrophic heart of a sedentary person. Moreover, the determinants of myocardial oxygen pressures include: (i) the relationship of myocardial work rate to myocardial oxygen supply; (ii) the tension developed in the ventricular wall; and (iii) the relative duration of the systolic phase of the cardiac cycle.

Myocardial work rate

The myocardial work rate is approximated by the double product (heart rate × systolic blood pressure). Plasma volume expansion, myocardial hypertrophy and enhanced ventricular contractility allow the endurance athlete to sustain a larger stroke volume than a less well-trained person during vigorous exercise. A given external task can thus be performed at a lower heart rate and a lower cardiac work rate than in a sedentary individual.

This does not necessarily protect the athlete during competition; during all-out effort, the cardiac work rate of the endurance performer is likely to be substantially greater than that of a sedentary person. Nevertheless, the athlete's myocardial oxygen consumption is reduced at a given external work rate, so that during ordinary daily life the risk of myocardial ischaemia is much less than in a sedentary person of similar age.

Ventricular wall tension

According to the law of LaPlace (as modified for a thick-walled structure), the total tension exerted by the ventricular wall is approximately proportional to the product of intraventricular pressure and the average ventricular radius (Shephard 1982).

The large average radius of the athlete's ventricle may cause some increase of tension for a given arterial pressure. However, because the ventricular wall is much thicker in an endurance competitor than in a sedentary person, the force exerted per unit of cross-section at any given intraventricular pressure is lower in the endurance competitor than in the untrained person (Shephard 1982).

Relative duration of systolic phase

A high tension is developed in the ventricular wall during systole, irrespective of a person's training status, and this tends to occlude the coronary vasculature (particularly the perforating branches that supply the critical subendocardial region). Myocardial perfusion thus occurs largely during the diastolic phase of the cardiac cycle. This gives an important advantage to the endurance athlete; rapid ventricular emptying and a slow heart rate lead to an increase in the diastolic phase of the cardiac cycle.

Exercise and sudden death

Exercise-related death is a rare event in young endurance athletes, but nevertheless it usually attracts great publicity because the individual is well known, and may be performing in front of a large crowd. A pathological cardiac hypertrophy is often invoked to explain such deaths, and sometimes it is inferred that the condition should have been detected at preparticipation examination (Dickhuth *et al.* 1994; Smith 1994; Winget *et al.* 1994; American Heart Association 1996). However, there is growing evidence that such screening is not cost effective (Fleck *et al.* 1989; Chapter 45). Moreover, in the great majority of instances where cardiomyopathy is detected at post-mortem examination, exhaustive laboratory screening has failed to detect the abnormality.

Exercise-related deaths in endurance athletes have many causes (Chillag *et al.* 1980; Rosenzweig *et al.* 1991; Winget *et al.* 1994; Goodman 1995; Torg 1995; American Heart Association 1996). A number of recent catastrophes in long-distance cyclists have been attributed to a high red cell count, induced by doping with erythropoietin; conceivably, prolonged training at actual or simulated high altitude could have a similar effect. Other incidents are due to mechanical injury or heat stress. Sometimes, there is rupture of a congenital aneurysm in the circle of Willis. Occasionally, there is an acute myocarditis due to recent influenza or some other viral infection (Drory *et al.* 1991; McCaffrey *et al.* 1991; Francis 1995); a series of incidents in Scandinavian orienteers was thought to arise from a combination of infection with overtraining (Ilbäck *et al.* 1989; Kiel *et al.* 1989), and there were no further deaths when greater care was taken to reduce training during viral infections. Sometimes, there is evidence of a fatal myocardial ischaemia; in older athletes, the commonest cause is coronary atheroma, but in young competitors the usual cause is a previously undetected congenital anomaly such as an abnormal origin of the coronary vessels (Cheitlin *et al.* 1974; Roberts *et al.* 1982; Menke *et al.* 1985; Rosenzweig *et al.* 1991). In some instances, no obvious pathology can be found. Blame then tends to be attributed to myocardial hypertrophy. It is alleged that this is pathological in type or extent and that it has caused myocardial ischaemia, or has led to a fatal dysrhythmia. However, it is increasingly recognized that there is little relationship between ventricular hypertrophy and sudden death in the absence of an inherited dystrophy with disarray of the myocardial fibres (McKenna & Camm 1989). In endurance competitors, the problem thus becomes one of distinguishing a congenital, dystrophic hypertrophy from a physiological hypertrophy.

Hypertrophic cardiomyopathy has often been diagnosed on the post-mortem finding of an interventricular septal thickness that is 'excessive' relative to arbitrary normal standards. However, the verdict is then heavily loaded in favour of 'proving' that septal hypertrophy is responsible for an exercise-induced death, since training thickens both the ventricular wall and the interventricular septum, and post-mortem examinations are being performed on individuals who have died during endurance competition. In order to establish that septal thickening had pathological significance, it would be necessary either to make a prospective comparison of outcomes between endurance athletes with supposedly normal septa and those with thickened septa, or alternatively to carry out a blind post-mortem comparison between competitors who died on the sports field and colleagues who had reached a similar level of training but were killed in traffic accidents. Neither type of trial is likely to take place for logistic reasons, since sudden death on the sports field is a very rare event. No one group of investigators could accumulate sufficient incidents to conduct either type of study. Moreover, although details of training programmes would probably be available for a top competitor who died during competition, it would be much more difficult to obtain reliable information on the regimens followed by those who had been involved in traffic accidents, or indeed to match personal lifestyle and other cardiac risk factors between competitors.

Hypertrophic cardiomyopathy and sudden death

It is frequently stated that hypertrophic cardiomyopathy is the 'commonest cause of death' in young athletes (Maron *et al.* 1980; Spirito *et al.* 1989; Brandenburg 1990; Nienhaber *et al.* 1990; Van Camp *et al.* 1995; American Heart Association 1996). However, this viewpoint must be examined in the perspective of the minuscule total number of exercise-related deaths: around 100 incidents per year in young US athletes (Winget *et al.* 1994), and one death per 11 million hours of physical activity in Finnish men aged 20–39 years (Vuori 1995). A retrospective study of 215 413 marathon runners disclosed only four exercise-related deaths; three of the four fatalities were in runners aged 32–58 years, and all of these had evidence of coronary atherosclerotic disease. The one young runner in this series was aged 19 years, and in his case post-mortem examination disclosed an anomalous coronary artery (Maron *et al.* 1996).

Likewise, a computerized search of the US literature (Chillag *et al.* 1980) covering a 50-year period revealed only *four* incidents where an exercise-related death was thought to have been due to hypertrophic cardiomyopathy.

The view that hypertrophic cardiomyopathy is a 'common' cause of exercise-related death can probably be traced to a paper by Maron *et al.* (1980). This report covered a 4-year period; it summarized case histories on 29 US athletes who had died between the ages of 13 and 30 years. Nineteen of the 29 individuals were said to have hypertrophic cardiomyopathy, although the septal/free wall ratio met even the minimum diagnostic criterion of 1.3 : 1.0 in only eight of the 19 cases. It is unlikely that all of these eight individuals had hypertrophic cardiomyopathy; indeed, in the absence of a documented family history and histopathology, a substantial fraction of them could have had a physiological rather than a pathological hypertrophy. Thus, the whole hypothesis that hypertrophic cardiomyopathy is a common cause of exercise-related death seems to have been founded on a maximum of two *possible* cases per year across the US. Spirito *et al.* (1989) have further pointed out that almost all reports concerning hypertrophic cardiomyopathy derive from two reference laboratories. The view of widespread prevalence arises, at least in part, from a repeated description of the supposed 19 cases of Maron *et al.* (1980) in a minimum of 25 independent publications. One recent estimate of prevalence (1 in 500 athletes, American Heart Association 1996) seems likely to prove a gross overestimate.

Maron *et al.* (1996) accumulated reports on 158 sudden exercise-related deaths in US athletes under 35 years of age; the study covered a 10-year period. The cardiovascular system was responsible for 134 of the 158 incidents, and perhaps because of the US context, the non-endurance sports of basketball and American football accounted for 92 of the 134 episodes (68%). The diagnostic criteria were relatively weak: a hypertrophied and non-dilated ventricle, with only one other supporting clinical or morphological feature. Nevertheless, only a third of the group were said to be 'probable' or 'definite' cases of hypertrophic cardiomyopathy. Even accepting that all of the 'probable' or 'definite' diagnoses were correct, hypertrophic cardiomyopathy would have caused only four or five exercise-related deaths per year in the US.

Other reports have further confused the issue by using even less satisfactory diagnostic criteria; for example, Van Camp *et al.* (1995) classified as 'probable hypertrophic cardiomyopathy' all deaths where the cardiac mass exceeded 400 g in the absence of other systemic, valvular or cardiac disorders. But despite the broad inclusiveness of the diagnostic net, the total incidence among US athletes was apparently only about five cases per year.

The foregoing comments in no way deny the existence of a rare inherited malformation of the ventricular wall, based on molecular abnormalities in the genes encoding protein molecules of the sarcomeres (Marian *et al.* 1994; Klues *et al.* 1995; Roberts 1997). A few of the athletes who die while exercising *may* be affected by such a condition. However, the diagnosis of ventricular cardiomyopathy requires a clear family history, reinforced by such evidence as cardiac symptoms on exertion, abnormal patterns of left ventricular filling (Maron *et al.* 1993) and failure of the cardiac enlargement to regress out of season (Maron *et al.* 1994), preferably accompanied by carefully blinded histopathology and demonstration of the characteristic gene structure. Moreover, there is no particular reason why this particular disorder should affect endurance athletes; indeed, because of myocardial dysfunction, an exceptional performance seems unlikely, precluding participation in major competition.

Benefits of cardiac hypertrophy

Any remote dangers of exercise for the person with ventricular hypertrophy must be weighed carefully against the known benefits of a moderate increase in heart size. The cardiac hypertrophy seen in many endurance competitors is associated with a large stroke volume, and thus a large maximal cardiac output and peak oxygen transport. In consequence, the athlete can undertake any given physical task at a smaller fraction of maximal oxygen intake than would a sedentary person. Many aspects of exercise-related strain, from the increase of systemic blood pressure to a sense of personal fatigue, are thus less for the person who has trained to the point of developing a large heart and a large maximal oxygen intake.

If cardiac hypertrophy is advantageous for the young adult, it becomes even more important for an older individual. Maximal oxygen intake decreases progressively over the span of adult life. In a sedentary person, the rate of loss averages about $500\,\mu l\cdot kg^{-1}\cdot min^{-1}$ per year (Shephard 1997). By the age of 75–80 years, he or she often lacks sufficient aerobic power to climb even a slight slope without becoming excessively breathless. Soon, even the minor chores of daily life become very fatiguing, and the last 10 years of life are spent in growing institutional dependency.

It is difficult to determine the true, inherent rate of ageing of cardiorespiratory function in an endurance athlete, because competitors tend to reduce their volume of training and increase their body fat mass as they become older. Nevertheless, cross-sectional comparisons between young athletes and older individuals who have maintained their training programmes suggest a somewhat slower rate of functional loss than in sedentary subjects (Kavanagh *et al.* 1989; Shephard 1997). Given a much higher initial aerobic power, and possibly a slightly slower rate of ageing, elderly endurance competitors have a large advantage of maximal oxygen intake, equivalent to a 10–20-year reduction in biological age (Shephard 1997). This provides the functional capacity to live independently to 90 or even 100 years of age, in contrast with the institutional support needed by sedentary individuals around 80 years of age. Although regular exercise reduces the overall risk of premature death, it has only a minor impact upon survival prospects in old age (Pekkanen *et al.* 1987; Paffenbarger *et al.* 1994). Thus, endurance competitors are likely to die of acute intercurrent disease before their physical condition has deteriorated to the point where institutional support is required.

Overall health impact of ventricular hypertrophy

Although death on the sports field attracts much attention, the critical issue from the viewpoint of health policy is the impact of prolonged endurance training on the individual's overall survival prospects and quality of life.

In terms of survival, epidemiological data show that although endurance athletes on average have a larger heart than sedentary individuals, their life expectancy compares favourably with that of the general population. Sarna *et al.* (1993) made a retrospective examination of 2613 athletes who had rep-

resented Finland in either the Olympic games or the world or European championships between 1920 and 1965. The endurance athletes survived to an average age of 75.6 years, compared with 69.9 years in a sample of 1712 sedentary adults, and 71.5 years for those who had been Finnish champions in power sports. There was thus no evidence that endurance competition had shortened the lifespan—indeed, survival appeared to be enhanced. Nevertheless, not all of their 6-year advantage can be attributed to endurance training, since personal lifestyle, particularly cigarette consumption, is likely to have differed between the endurance athletes and the general population. On the other hand, the true impact of endurance training may have been larger than suggested by the mortality statistics, since it is uncertain whether all of the athletes continued training in the long interval between competition and their average age at death.

Because independence is prolonged by endurance training, the athlete's quality of life, also, is likely to be enhanced relative to that of a sedentary person. Physicians have worried excessively about the one in 10-million chance that endurance sport might cause sudden death, while neglecting the major public health problem presented by the millions of sedentary senior citizens who require full-time geriatric care. Health policy must be assessed not simply in terms of survival, but also in terms of quality-adjusted life expectancy (Shephard 1996); and in such terms, a large, hypertrophied heart offers a statistically important advantage to the sport participant.

Need for detailed prescreening of competitors

International competition places heavy physical demands on the heart, accompanied by a massive release of stress hormones, and this may reveal a minor cardiac abnormality that would not have been apparent in a sedentary young adult. Nevertheless, it is plain from the foregoing discussion that the risk of any type of cardiac death during competition is *extremely* small, and current evidence suggests that endurance training reduces rather than increases the overall risk of sudden death. Many sports physicians still feel that an exercise-related death is a reflection on the quality of care that they have given, and they continue to cherish hopes that some miraculous laboratory test will enable them to detect vulnerable individuals and offer meaningful warnings against major competition. However, a consideration of Bayes theorem shows that any mass screening process is doomed to failure, given the very small number of individuals with pathological hearts.

The recent position statement of the American Heart Association (1996) seems ambivalent about the need for mass echocardiographic examination of athletes. Although pointing to the major problems of high screening costs and false-positive diagnoses, it still states that: 'This viewpoint, however, is not intended to actively discourage all efforts at population screening'. Nevertheless, the best practical advice for the young athlete seems to be to avoid any preparticipation cardiac screening beyond a standard clinical examination, whether the ventricle appears normal or increased in its dimensions. The routine performance of echocardiography and other sophisticated laboratory examinations is likely to do little more than precipitate a chain of costly invasive procedures, with attendant cardiac phobias, unnecessary medical costs, premature cessation of sport involvement and loss of life insurance coverage (Franklin & Kahn 1995). Maron *et al.* (1996) noted that most of the young athletes who died while exercising had been screened, but cardiovascular disease had been diagnosed in only 5% of those examined, and the diagnosis had been correct in less than 1% of the sample! Specifically, only one of 48 suspected cases of hypertrophic cardiomyopathy had been diagnosed prior to death! Likewise, there is no evidence as yet that the much vaunted mandatory screening of Italian athletes (Chapter 45) has influenced the risk of exercise-induced deaths favourably.

Conclusions

Although ventricular hypertrophy is sometimes suggested as the commonest cause of sudden, exercise-related death in the young adult, the total number of exercise-induced deaths is very small, and their relationship to either ventricular hypertrophy in general or cardiomyopathy in particular is far from established. There is a rare inherited form of myocardial dystrophy that predisposes to sudden death, but this is not peculiar to athletes. Indeed, because those affected have a low physical work capacity, they are unlikely to have become involved in endurance sport. Mass preparticipatory laboratory screening of endurance athletes currently leads to an unacceptable toll of false-positive diagnoses, and detailed examination of an athlete's heart is warranted only if there is a strong family history of early cardiac death. In general, the 'athlete's heart' should be viewed as a beneficial adaptation to endurance training that increases overall survival and quality-adjusted life expectancy, enhancing physical work capacity and reducing the likelihood of dependency in old age.

References

Allen, H.D., Goldberg, S.J., Sahn, D., Schy, N. & Wojcik, R. (1976) A quantitative echocardiographic study of champion childhood swimmers. *Circulation* 55, 142–155.

American Heart Association (1996) Cardiovascular preparticipation screening of competitive athletes. *Medicine and Science in Sports and Exercise* 28, 1445–1452.

Asmussen, E. & Christensen, E.H. (1967) *Kompendium: Legem sölvelsernes Specielle Teori.* Kobenhavns Universitets Fond til Tilverbringelse af Läremidler, Copenhagen.

Bramwell, C. & Ellis, R. (1931) Some observations on the circulatory mechanism in marathon runners. *Quarterly Journal of Medicine* 24, 329–346.

Brandenburg, R.O. (1990) Syncope and sudden death in hypertrophic cardiomyopathy. *Journal of the American College of Cardiology* 15, 962–964.

Cheitlin, M., DeCastro, C. & McAllister, H. (1974) Sudden death as a complication of anomalous left coronary origin from the anterior sinus of Valsalva. *Circulation* 50, 780–787.

Chillag, S., Bates, M., Voltin, R. & Jones, D. (1980) Sudden death: Myocardial infarction in a runner with normal coronary arteries. *Physician and Sportsmedicine* 18 (3), 89–94.

Dickhuth, H.H., Jakob, E., Staiger, L. & Keul, J. (1983) Two dimensional echocardiographic measurements of left ventricular volume and stroke volume of endurance athletes and untrained subjects. *International Journal of Sports Medicine* 4, 21–26.

Dickhuth, H.H., Röcker, K., Hipp, A., Heitkamp, H.C. & Keul, J. (1994) Echocardiographic findings in endurance athletes with hypertrophic non-obstructive cardiomyopathy (HNCM) compared to non-athletes with HNCM and to physiological hypertrophy (Athlete's Heart). *International Journal of Sports Medicine* **15**, 273–277.

Drory, Y., Kramer, M.R. & Lev, B. (1991) Exertional sudden death in soldiers. *Medicine and Science in Sports and Exercise* **23**, 147–151.

Ehsani, A.A., Hagberg, J.M. & Hickson, R.C. (1978) Rapid changes in left ventricular dimensions and mass in response to physical conditioning and deconditioning. *American Journal of Cardiology* **42**, 52–56.

Fleck, S.J., Henke, C. & Wilson, W. (1989) Cardiac MRI of élite junior Olympic weightlifters. *International Journal of Sports Medicine* **10**, 329–333.

Francis, G.S. (1995) Viral myocarditis. Detection and management. *Physician and Sportsmedicine* **23** (7), 63–83.

Franklin, B. & Kahn, J.K. (1995) Detecting the individual prone to exercise-related sudden cardiac death. *Sport Sciences Review* **4** (2), 85–105.

George, K.P., Wolfe, L.A. & Burggraf, G.W. (1991) The 'Athletic Heart Syndrome'. *Sports Medicine* **11**, 300–331.

Goodman, J.M. (1995) Exercise and sudden cardiac death. Etiology in apparently healthy individuals. *Sport Sciences Review* **4** (2), 14–30.

Hagan, R.D., Laird, W.P. & Gettman, L.R. (1985) The problems of per-surface area and per-weight standardization indices in the determination of cardiac hypertrophy in endurance-trained athletes. *Journal of Cardiopulmonary Rehabilitation* **5**, 554–560.

Huston, T.P., Puffer, J.C. & Rodney, W.M. (1985) The athlete heart syndrome. *New England Journal of Medicine* **313**, 24–32.

Ilbäck, N.G., Fohlman, J. & Friman, G. (1989) Exercise in Coxsackie B3 myocarditis: effect on heart lymphocyte subpopulations and the inflammatory reaction. *American Heart Journal* **117**, 1298–1302.

Kavanagh, T., Mertens, D.J., Matosevic, V., Shephard, R.J. & Evans, B. (1989) Health and aging of Masters athletes. *Clinical Sports Medicine* **1**, 72–88.

Keys, A. & Friedell, H.L. (1938) Size and stroke of the heart in young men in relation to physical activity. *Science* **88**, 456–458.

Kiel, R.J., Smith, F.E., Chason, J., Khatib, R. & Reyes, M.D. (1989) Coxsackie virus B3 myocarditis in C3H/HeJ mice: Description of an inbred model and the effect of

exercise on the virulence. *European Journal of Epidemiology* **5**, 348–350.

Klues, H.G., Schiffers, A. & Maron, B.J. (1995) Phenotypic spectrum and patterns of left ventricular hypertrophic cardiomyopathy: morphologic observations and significance as assessed by two dimensional echocardiography in 600 patients. *Journal of the American College of Cardiology* **26**, 1699–1708.

Longhurst, J.C., Kelly, A.R., Gonyea, W.J. & Mitchell, J.H. (1980) Echocardiographic left ventricular masses in distance runners and weight-lifters. *Journal of Applied Physiology* **48**, 154–162.

McCaffrey, F.M., Braden, D.S. & Strong, W.B. (1991) Sudden cardiac death in young athletes: a review. *American Journal of Diseases of Children* **145**, 177–183.

McKenna, W.J. & Camm, A.J. (1989) Sudden death in hypertrophic cardiomyopathy. Assessment of patients at high risk. *Circulation* **80**, 1489–1492.

Marian, A.J., Kelly, D., Mares, A. *et al.* (1994) A missense mutation in the beta-myosin heavy chain gene is a predictor of premature sudden death in patients with hypertrophic cardiomyopathy. *Journal of Sports Medicine and Physical Fitness* **34**, 1–10.

Maron, B.J. (1993) Hypertrophic cardiomyopathy in athletes: catching a killer. *Physician and Sportsmedicine* **21** (9), 83–91.

Maron, B.J., Roberts, W.C., McAllister, H.A., Rosing, D.R. & Epstein, S.E. (1980) Sudden death in young athletes. *Circulation* **62**, 218–229.

Maron, B.J., Gottdiener, J., Bonow, R.O. & Epstein, S.E. (1981) Hypertrophic cardiomyopathy: cardiomyopathy with unusual localizations of left ventricular hypertrophy undetectable by M-mode echocardiography. *Circulation* **63**, 409–418.

Maron, B.J., Pellicia, A., Spataro, A. & Granata, M. (1993) Reduction in left ventricular wall thickness after deconditioning in highly trained Olympic athletes. *British Heart Journal* **69**, 125–128.

Maron, B.J., Isner, J.M. & McKenna, W.J. (1994) Hypertrophic cardiomyopathy, myocarditis and other myopericardial diseases. *Medicine and Science in Sports and Exercise* **26**, S261–S267.

Maron, B.J., Pellicia, A. & Spirito, P. (1995) Cardiac disease in young trained athletes: insights into methods for distinguishing athlete's heart from structural heart disease, with particular emphasis on hypertrophic cardiomyopathy. *Circulation* **91**, 1596–1601.

Maron, B.J., Shirani, J., Poliac, L.C., Mathenge, R., Roberts, W.C. & Mueller, F.C. (1996) Sudden death in young competitive athletes. *Journal of the American Medical Association* **276**, 199–204.

Menapace, F.J., Hammer, W.J., Ritzer, T.F. *et al.* (1982) Left ventricular size in competitive weight-lifters: an echocardiographic study. *Medicine and Science in Sports and Exercise* **14**, 72–75.

Menke, D., Waller, B. & Pless, J. (1985) Hypoplastic coronary arteries and high take-off position of the right coronary ostium: a fatal combination of congenital artery anomalies in an amateur athlete. *Chest* **88**, 299–301.

Milliken, M.C., Stray-Gundersen, J., Pesjock, R.M., Katz, J. & Mitchell, J.H. (1988) Left ventricular mass as determined by magnetic resonance imaging in male endurance athletes. *American Journal of Cardiology* **62**, 301–305.

Morganroth, J., Maron, B.J., Henry, W.L. & Epstein, S.E. (1975) Comparative left ventricular dimensions in athletes. *Annals of Internal Medicine* **82**, 521–524.

Nienhaber, C.A., Hiller, S., Spielmann, R.P., Geiger, M. & Kuck, H. (1990) Syncope in hypertrophic cardiomyopathy: multivariate analysis of prognostic determinants. *Journal of the American College of Cardiology* **15**, 948–955.

Oakley, D.G. & Oakley, C.M. (1982) Significance of abnormal electrocardiograms in highly trained athletes. *American Journal of Cardiology* **50**, 985–989.

Osler, W. (1892) *The Principles and Practice of Medicine*, p. 635. Appleton, New York.

Paffenbarger, R.S., Hyde, R.T., Wing, A.L., Lee, I.-M. & Kampert, J.B. (1994) Some interrelations of physical activity, physiological fitness, health and longevity. In: Bouchard, C., Shephard, R.J. & Stephens, T. (eds) *Physical Activity, Fitness and Health*, pp. 119–133. Human Kinetics, Champaign, IL.

Park, R.C. & Crawford, M.H. (1985) Heart of the athlete. *Current Problems in Cardiology* **10**, 1–73.

Pekkanen, J., Marti, B., Nissinen, A., Tuomilehto, J., Punsar, S. & Karvonen, M.J. (1987) Reduction of premature mortality by high physical activity: a 20-year follow-up of middle-aged Finnish men. *Lancet* **i**, 1473–1477.

Pelliccia, A., Maron, B.J., Spataro, A., Proschan, M.A. & Spirito, P. (1991) The upper limit of physiologic cardiac hypertrophy in highly trained élite athletes. *New England Journal of Medicine* **324**, 295–301.

Perreault, H. & Turcotte, R.A. (1994)

Exercise-induced cardiac hypertrophy. Fact or fallacy? *Sports Medicine* **17**, 288–308.

Pye, M.P. & Cobbe. S.M. (1992) Mechanisms of ventricular arrhythmias in cardiac failure. *Cardiovascular Research* **26**, 740–750.

Reguero, J.J.R., Cubero, G.I., de la Iglesia, J.L. *et al.* (1995) Prevalence and upper limit of cardiac hypertrophy in professional cyclists. *European Journal of Applied Physiology* **70**, 375–378.

Reindell, H., König, K. & Roskamm, H. (1966) *Functionsdiagnostik Des Gesunden und Kranken Herzens*. Thieme, Stuttgart.

Roberts, R. (1997) Molecular genetics and its application to cardiac muscle disease. *Sports Medicine* **23**, 1–10.

Roberts, W., Siegel, R. & Zipes, D. (1982) Origin of the right coronary artery from the left sinus of Valsalva and its functional consequences: analysis of ten necropsy patients. *American Journal of Cardiology* **49**, 863–868.

Roeske, W.R., O'Rourke, R.A., Klein, H., Leopold, G. & Karliner, J.S. (1976) Noninvasive evaluation of ventricular hypertrophy in professional athletes. *Circulation* **53**, 286–292.

Romhilt, D.W. & Estes, E.H. (1968) Point score system for the ECG diagnosis of left ventricular hypertrophy. *American Heart Journal* **75**, 752–758.

Rosenzweig, A., Watkins, H., Hwang, D.-S. *et al.* (1991) Preclinical diagnosis of familial hypertrophic cardiomyopathy by genetic analysis of blood lymphocytes. *New England Journal of Medicine* **325**, 1753–1760.

Rost, R. & Hollmann, W. (1992) Cardiac problems in endurance sports. In: Shephard, R.J. & Åstrand, P.-O. (eds) *Endurance in Sport*, pp. 438–451. Blackwell Science, Oxford.

Sandric, S. (1980) Echocardiography in sports medicine: clinical diagnostic possibilities and limitations. In: Lubich, T. & Venerando, A. (eds) *Sports Cardiology*, pp. 707–716. Aulo Gaggi, Bologna.

Sarna, S., Sahi, T., Koskwenvuo, M. & Kaprio, J. (1993) Increased life expectancy of world class male athletes. *Medicine and Science in Sports and Exercise* **25**, 237–244.

Scott, R.C. (1973) Ventricular hypertrophy. *Cardiovascular Clinics* **5**, 219–254.

Shapiro, L.M. (1984) Physiological left ventricular hypertrophy. *British Heart Journal* **52**, 130–135.

Shephard, R.J. (1969) *Endurance Fitness*, 1st edn. University of Toronto Press, Toronto.

Shephard, R.J. (1982) *Physiology and Biochemistry of Exercise*. Praeger Publishing, New York.

Shephard, R.J. (1996) Habitual physical activity and quality of life. *Quest* **48**, 354–365.

Shephard, R.J. (1997) *Aging, Physical Activity and Health*. Human Kinetics, Champaign, IL.

Smith, D.M. (1994) Pre-participation physical evaluations. Development of uniform guidelines. *Sports Medicine* **18**, 293–300.

Snoeckx, L.H.E.H., Abeling, H.F.M., Lambregts, J.A.C., Schmitz, J.J.F., Verstappen, F.T.J. & Reneman, R.S. (1982) Echocardiographic dimensions in athletes in relation to their training programs. *Medicine and Science in Sports and Exercise* **14**, 428–434.

Sokolow, M. & Lyon, T.P. (1949a) The ventricular complex in left ventricular hypertrophy as obtained by unipolar precordial and limb leads. *American Heart Journal* **37**, 161–186.

Sokolow, M. & Lyon, T.P. (1949b) The ventricular complex in right ventricular hypertrophy as obtained by unipolar precordial and limb leads. *American Heart Journal* **38**, 273–294.

Spirito, P., Chiarella, F., Carratino, L., Berisso, M.Z., Bellotti, P. & Vecchio, C. (1989) Clinical course and prognosis of hypertrophic cardiomyopathy in an outpatient population. *New England Journal of Medicine* **320**, 749–755.

Spirito, P., Pelliccia, A., Proschan, M.A. *et al.* (1994) Morphology of the 'athlete's heart' assessed by echocardiography in 9476 élite athletes representing 27 sports. *American Journal of Cardiology* **74**, 802–806.

Torg, J. (1995) Sudden cardiac death in the athlete. In: Torg, J. & Shephard, R.J. (eds) *Current Therapy in Sports Medicine 3*, pp. 8–10. Mosby/Yearbook, Philadelphia.

Urhausen, A. & Kindermann, W. (1992) Echocardiographic findings in strength and endurance-trained athletes. *Sports Medicine* **13**, 270–284.

Van Camp, S.P., Bloor, C.M., Mueller, F.O., Cantu, R. & Olson, H.G. (1995) Nontraumatic sports death in high school and college athletes. *Medicine and Science in Sports and Exercise* **27**, 641–647.

Vuori, I. (1995) Sudden death and exercise: effects of age and type of activity. *Sport Sciences Review* **4** (2), 46–84.

Williams, C.C. & Bernhardt, D.T. (1995) Syncope in athletes. *Sports Medicine* **19**, 223–234.

Winget, J.P., Capeless, M.A. & Ades, P.A. (1994) Sudden death in athletes. *Sports Medicine* **18**, 375–383.

Chapter 49

Reproductive Changes and the Endurance Athlete

ANNE B. LOUCKS

Introduction

The high prevalence of menstrual disorders in women athletes has been well known for more than 20 years, and the skeletal damage in amenorrhoeic athletes has been known for 15 years (Otis *et al.* 1997). Although investigators have speculated about the basis of these disorders from the beginning, no cause has yet been proven, and no mediating physiological mechanism has yet been demonstrated. This review begins by citing the clinical consequences of menstrual disorders in athletes. It then provides a basic introduction to regulation of the reproductive system. This is followed by a brief summary of extensive descriptive information characterizing amenorrhoeic athletes, regularly menstruating athletes and regularly menstruating sedentary women. For comparison, the corresponding information characterizing male athletes is also summarized. The chapter then discusses the most prominent hypotheses about the cause of menstrual disorders in athletes, and proceeds to describe several controlled experiments that have investigated some of these hypotheses by attempting to disrupt the reproductive cycle in regularly menstruating women. Finally, the results of these experiments are interpreted and some generalizations are made.

Clinical consequences of menstrual disorders in athletes

Infertility is the first consequence of amenorrhoea, since amenorrhoeic women are not developing egg cells that can be fertilized. Infertility may also be a hazard in regularly menstruating, physically active women who neither display nor experience any signs of menstrual disorders. Hormone measurements reveal a suppression of progesterone secretion and a shortening of the luteal phase in an extraordinarily large proportion of these women. In one sample of regularly menstruating female runners, 48% of the women displayed evidence of luteal phase deficiency in the first menstrual cycle studied and 79% did so within 3 months (De Souza *et al.* 1998).

Paradoxically, unintended pregnancies may be another consequence of menstrual disorders. Many physically active women experience irregular menstrual cycles. If such irregularly menstruating women practise unprotected sex, they are especially unlikely to guess correctly every time the days on which they are fertile.

Perhaps the most hazardous clinical consequence of menstrual disorders is osteoporosis. As in postmenopausal women, low oestrogen levels in amenorrhoeic and irregularly menstruating athletes lead directly to a progressive demineralization of the skeleton (Otis *et al.* 1997; Tomten *et al.* 1998), perhaps via a nitric oxide-dependent mechanism (Stacey *et al.* 1998). The resulting low bone mineral densities raise the risk of fractures both during an athlete's competitive years and later in her life. Osteoporotic spinal fractures result in permanent disabilities and chronic pain. Among young women, bone mineral density declines in proportion to the number of menses that have been missed (Drinkwater *et al.* 1990). Moreover, repeat measurements on athletes first examined 8 years previously indicate that the bone loss in amenorrhoeic athletes is irreversible, even if the athletes recover regular menses or begin oestrogen therapy (Keen & Drinkwater 1997). Thus, early detection and intervention appear to be critical in minimizing permanent skeletal damage due to menstrual disorders. Steroid replacement therapy in the form of low-dose oral contraceptives or conjugated oestrogens and progesterones is specifically recommended to prevent further bone loss (Committee on Sports Medicine of the American Academy of Pediatrics 1989; Shangold *et al.* 1990).

A third clinical consequence of amenorrhoea may be an impairment of skeletal muscle oxidative metabolism and athletic performance. In amenorrhoeic athletes, phosphocreatinine recovers more slowly after exercise (Harber *et al.* 1998). In regularly menstruating women, physical training speeds the phosphocreatinine recovery rate, which depends on the presence of normal thyroid hormone levels. Since thyroid hormones are suppressed in amenorrhoeic athletes (Loucks *et al.* 1992), such individuals may be at a physiological disadvantage in their ability to perform repeated exercise bouts compared to their regularly menstruating competitors.

Regulation of the menstrual cycle

The regulation of the menstrual cycle by the hypothalamic–pituitary–ovarian (HPO) axis includes both negative and positive feedback mechanisms, as well as inputs from the central nervous system and other systems at various levels within the axis. The glands of the HPO axis secrete their hormones rhythmically. Indeed, the secretion of gonadotrophin-releasing hormone (GnRH) pulses into the pituitary portal blood by neurones within the hypothalamus must occur at an optimal frequency if the axis as a whole is to function normally. Although the pituitary portal blood is not accessible for measurement of GnRH in humans, the GnRH pulses are reflected by a pulsatile secretion of luteinizing hormone (LH) from the pituitary gland into the blood, and this LH can be measured in peripheral blood samples. If blood is sampled every 10 min for 24 h, it is possible to study the frequency and amplitude of the LH pulses.

Given a proper pulsatile and monthly rhythmic stimulation by LH and pituitary follicle-stimulating hormone (FSH), clusters of ovarian cells ('ovarian follicles') grow and secrete oestrogen, the serum concentration of which rises. Gradually one of the follicles becomes dominant. Eventually, the rising concentration of oestrogen exerts a positive feedback on LH secretion. In response, the pituitary gland secretes a surge of LH into the blood, causing the dominant follicle to rupture, and thereby releasing an egg cell for potential fertilization. The remaining cells of the dominant follicle then undergo rapid chemical and morphological change to form the corpus luteum, which begins secreting both progesterone and oestrogen into the blood. The interval in which a dominant follicle develops, from menses until ovulation, is known as the follicular phase of the menstrual cycle. If fertilization does occur, the interval from ovulation until the next menses, when the corpus luteum is active, is known as the luteal phase of the cycle.

Oestrogen and progesterone have profound influences on the uterine endometrium. Oestrogen stimulates endometrial proliferation, whereas progesterone causes it to become highly vascularized. These are necessary, hospitable conditions for the successful implantation of a fertilized egg. If no fertilization occurs after several days, the ability of the corpus luteum to secrete progesterone becomes exhausted, the structural integrity of the endometrium collapses, and menstruation ensues. Under normal circumstances, the secretory capacity of the corpus luteum is sustained long enough for the rapidly dividing cells derived from a fertilized egg to become implanted in the endometrium 6 or 7 days after fertilization. Under some conditions, however, the secretory capacity of the corpus luteum is exhausted too soon, and the endometrium sloughs off before implantation can occur. The likelihood of this rises when the luteal phase is shorter than 10 days. Thus, infertility can result from failure of the ovary to release an egg for fertilization or from failure of a fertilized egg to become properly implanted in the endometrium.

The length and regularity of the menstrual cycle vary considerably both across populations and during a woman's reproductive years (Treolar *et al.*

1967). During adolescence, the median length of the menstrual cycle amongst North American females is 33 days, and the median standard deviation of the variation in length from month to month is 7 days. By the age of 20, the median length and median standard deviation have decreased to 29 days and 4 days, respectively. Both of these numbers continue to decline slowly through to the age of 40 years. Both numbers increase greatly again during the years preceding menopause, when menstruation ceases permanently.

The average age of menarche has fallen dramatically over the past 150 years in all western societies—from an average of 17 years to less than 13 years (Styne & Grumbach 1991). What activates the reproductive system at puberty is unknown, and what deactivates the reproductive system in infancy and again at menopause is also unknown (Loucks 1996). Since we know so little about the normal development and senescence of the reproductive system, it is not surprising that we know little about its abnormal disruption.

Characterization of eumenorrhoeic and amenorrhoeic athletes

The study of menstrual disorders amongst athletes begins by excluding subjects whose disorders can be explained by extraneous factors such as pregnancy, eating disorders, hyperprolactinaemia, hyperandrogenism, depression and organic diseases that are known to disrupt menstrual function. Many cases remain to be explained after this has been done. Among amenorrhoeic athletes, hormonal abnormalities cannot be attributed simply to athletic training, because amenorrhoeic athletes differ from regularly menstruating sedentary women in two respects: they are athletes and they are amenorrhoeic. To distinguish the independent influences of these two factors it is necessary to compare both types of women to a third type: regularly menstruating athletes. Differences between regularly menstruating sedentary women and athletes can then be attributed to athletic training, and differences between regularly menstruating and amenorrhoeic athletes can be attributed to amenorrhoea.

To ensure that fair comparisons are made, amen-orrhoeic and regularly menstruating women must be carefully selected to exclude women with irregular cycles. Hormone concentrations vary from day to day around the menstrual cycle, and it is impossible to know which days to compare when the length of the cycle is unpredictable. In our own studies (Loucks *et al.* 1989, 1992), we selected only those amenorrhoeic athletes who had not menstruated in the previous 6 months. For regularly menstruating athletes and sedentary women, we selected only those who had recorded menstrual cycles occurring at intervals of 26–32 days for 6 months prior to the study, and in whom we had confirmed ovulation in the immediately preceding cycle by showing a midcycle surge of LH.

To ensure that we detected any effect of athletic training if one existed, we chose competitive runners, swimmers and triathletes who had earned at least 200 aerobic points per week throughout the previous 6 months of training (Cooper 1977); on average, they had earned approximately 350 points per week. Sedentary women had earned less than 30 points per week, which is the minimum recommended for improving cardiovascular fitness.

Observations on the ovarian axis

Amenorrhoeic competitive athletes (AA) display a complete absence of follicular development, ovulation and luteal function (Fig. 49.1) (Loucks *et al.* 1989; Pirke *et al.* 1990). By contrast, eumenorrhoeic competitive athletes (CA) display regular menstrual cycles of 26–32 days' duration that are indistinguishable from those of eumenorrhoeic sedentary women. Nevertheless, closer examination of the eumenorrhoeic athletes reveals extended follicular phases and shorter luteal phases, with progesterone concentrations that are blunted by 50% (Fig. 49.1) (Loucks *et al.* 1989) relative to eumenorrhoeic sedentary women (Fig. 49.1, CS) (Loucks *et al.* 1989). Similar observations have been made in eumenorrhoeic women running recreationally as little as 20 km per week (Ellison & Lager 1986; Brookes *et al.* 1990; Pirke *et al.* 1990).

The proximal cause of these disruptions of ovarian function in athletes is a disturbance of the GnRH pulse generator in the hypothalamus of the

Fig. 49.1 Urinary oestrone-glucuronide (E_1G, an oestradiol metabolite) and pregnanediol-glucuronide (PdG, a progesterone metabolite) over an entire menstrual cycle in eumenorrhoeic sedentary women (CS) and eumenorrhoeic athletes (CA), and over an entire month in amenorrhoeic athletes (AA). The mass of each metabolite (ng E_1G and µg PdG) excreted in overnight urine samples is normalized to the mass (mg) of creatinine (CR) excreted in the same samples. The black and shaded bars at the bottom of the figure indicate the days of menses in the CS and CA women, respectively, at the beginning and end of the cycle of observation. From Loucks *et al.* (1989), with permission.

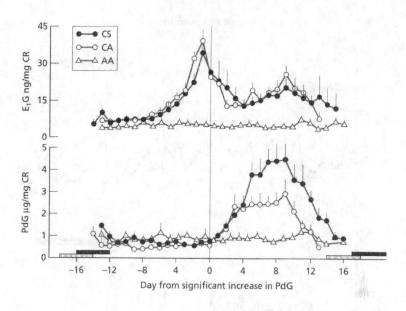

brain. This, in turn, disrupts the pulsatile rhythm of serum LH concentrations upon which ovarian function critically depends (Veldhuis *et al.* 1985; Yahiro *et al.* 1987; Loucks *et al.* 1989; Laughlin & Yen 1996). Mechanisms linking behaviour and environmental conditions to the GnRH pulse generator are the focus of much current research.

In a eumenorrhoeic sedentary young woman, the 24-h LH profile in the early follicular phase is characterized by regular, high-frequency pulses of low amplitude (Fig. 49.2, Loucks *et al.* 1989). During sleep, the frequency slows and the amplitude increases (Loucks *et al.* 1989). Eumenorrhoeic athletes display a slower, but still regular rhythm of larger pulses (Fig. 49.2, Loucks *et al.* 1989). Amenorrhoeic athletes display even fewer pulses, at irregular intervals (Fig. 49.2, Loucks *et al.* 1989).

Associations

We were unable to distinguish between the dietary and exercise habits and histories of the amenorrhoeic and eumenorrhoeic athletes. Both groups of athletes reported that their body weights were similar and stable, despite dietary energy intakes that were similar to those of sedentary women (Loucks *et al.* 1989). That is, their dietary energy intake was much less than would be expected for

an athlete's level of physical activity, a feature commonly observed amongst athletic women (Drinkwater *et al.* 1984; Marcus *et al.* 1985; Nelson *et al.* 1986; Kaiserauer *et al.* 1989; Myerson *et al.* 1991). The apparent inconsistency between a stable body mass and an unexpectedly low reported dietary energy intake is controversial.

Others have noted that a stable body mass is *not* necessarily proof of energy sufficiency, because behaviour modification and endocrine-mediated alterations in resting metabolic rate can counteract the potential influences of dietary energy excess or deficiency on body mass (Leibel *et al.* 1995). Furthermore, both energy intake and energy expenditure are very difficult to measure reliably. Some investigators have attributed the apparent discrepancy between energy intake and expenditure in athletic women to an underreporting of their dietary intake (Wilmore *et al.* 1992; Edwards *et al.* 1993). Underreporting of dietary intake is common in all populations (Mertz *et al.* 1991), but it does not account for the metabolic substrate and hormone indications of energy deficiency that are observed in athletes.

Amenorrhoeic athletes display low blood glucose levels during the feeding phase of the day (Laughlin & Yen 1996), low insulin and high insulin-like growth factor-binding protein I (IGFBP-I) over the entire 24 h (Laughlin & Yen 1996), loss of the leptin

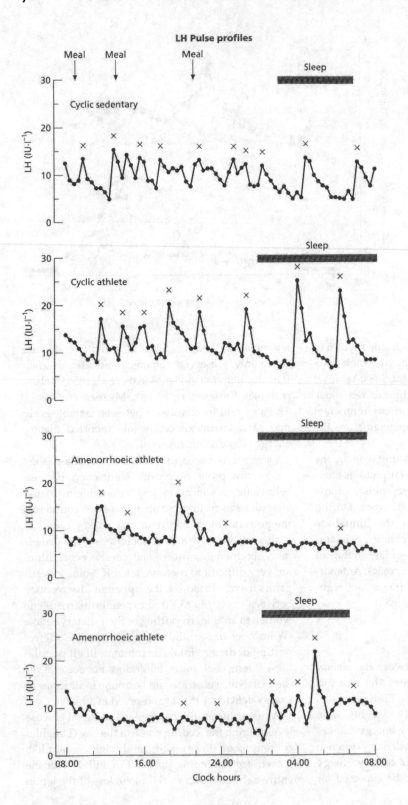

Fig. 49.2 The 24-h pulsatile luteinizing hormone (LH) rhythms of a eumenorrhoeic sedentary woman (CS), a eumenorrhoeic athlete (CA) and two amenorrhoeic athletes (AA) (from Loucks *et al.* 1989, with permission). Blood samples were drawn at 20-min intervals.

diurnal rhythm (Laughlin & Yen 1997), and low tri-iodothyronine (T_3) levels in the morning (Myerson et al. 1991; Loucks et al. 1992). All of these abnormalities are signs of energy deficiency. T_3 regulates basal metabolic rate, and low T_3 levels occur in numerous conditions, from fasting to cancer, in which dietary energy intake is insufficient to meet metabolic demand. In addition, eumenorrhoeic and amenorrhoeic athletes both display low insulin and high IGFBP-I levels during the feeding phase of the day, as well as low leptin (Laughlin & Yen 1997) and elevated growth hormone levels over 24 h (Laughlin & Yen 1996). IGFBP-I is a hepatic protein which is thought to modulate the growth-promoting actions of insulin-like growth factor I (IGF-I), which has been proposed as a signal interfacing fuel availability to reproductive control at the hypothalamus or the ovary (Jenkins et al. 1993).

Amenorrhoeic athletes also display mildly elevated resting serum levels of the classic stress hormone cortisol (Ding et al. 1988; Loucks et al. 1989; De Souza et al. 1991, 1994a; Laughlin & Yen 1996), and this observation is the basis for attributing their amenorrhoea to stress. Mild increases of serum cortisol are also associated with amenorrhoea in patients with functional hypothalamic amenorrhoea (Suh et al. 1988) and anorexia nervosa (Gold et al. 1986). Proponents of the stress hypothesis choose not to emphasize, though, that cortisol is a glucoregulatory hormone which is activated by low blood glucose levels. Thus, elevated cortisol levels may simply be a sign of chronic energy deficiency.

Observations in male athletes

Reproductive disorders are less obvious in men than in women, since men do not have the opportunity to notice symptoms such as menstrual abnormalities. Even when clinical measurements are made, reproductive disorders seem less common and less extreme in male than they are in female athletes. To be sure, many of these measurements have been misguided. For example, many have reported that mean levels of LH are not reduced in endurance-trained men compared to sedentary controls, but very little can be concluded from such observations, because it is the pulsatility of LH, not

its mean level, that is disrupted in female athletes and it is the pulsatility which regulates gonadal function in both men and women. No 24-h studies of LH pulsatility in male athletes have been published to date. Shorter, less reliable studies have reported inconsistent results (MacConnie et al. 1986; Seidman et al. 1990; Wheeler et al. 1991). Reduced total and/or free testosterone levels have been reported by many cross-sectional and prospective studies of endurance-trained male athletes (Frey et al. 1983; Wheeler et al. 1984, 1991; Ayers et al. 1985; Strauss et al. 1985; Urhausen et al. 1987; Hackney et al. 1988; Hakkinen et al. 1989; McColl et al. 1989; De Souza et al. 1994b; Roemmich & Sinning 1997), but not all (Remes et al. 1979; Peltonen et al. 1981; Lucia et al. 1996). Only one pair of investigators (Roemmich & Sinning 1997) has reported levels as below the normal range. Nor have any investigators reported observations of semen quality outside the normal range (Ayers et al. 1985; Bagatell & Bremner 1990; Griffith et al. 1990; Arce et al. 1993; De Souza et al. 1994b; Lucia et al. 1996). Where statistically significant reductions in reproductive system measurements have been noted, these have been found in the most intensively training athletes (MacConnie et al. 1986; McColl et al. 1989; De Souza et al. 1994b). Consequently, the consensus is that clinical expression of reproductive dysfunction with exercise is uncommon in men, and the long-term physiological suppression of the hypothalamic–pituitary–testicular axis in men probably does not have major significance (Cumming & Wheeler 1994; Lucia et al. 1996).

Hypotheses

Since cross-sectional data can contradict but cannot demonstrate causality, comparisons between amenorrhoeic and eumenorrhoeic athletes and sedentary women lead to two ambiguities concerning the mechanism of menstrual disorders in athletes. Firstly, do the mildly elevated cortisol levels seen in amenorrhoeic women indicate that their amenorrhoea is caused by stress or by energy deficiency? Secondly, would the luteal suppression of eumenorrhoeic athletes progress to amenorrhoea if their athletic training regimen were more severe, or are some women simply more robust than others, so that the disruption of reproductive function has a different endpoint in them? Controlled experiments are needed to resolve such ambiguities. In this field of study, as in others, competing explanations have emerged.

Body composition

The body composition hypothesis holds that the ovarian axis is disrupted when the amount of energy stored in the body as fat declines below some critical level (Frisch & McArthur 1974). For several years, this was the most widely publicized explanation outside the research community, and the least widely believed within the research community. Despite early associations of menarche and amenorrhoea with body composition (Frisch & McArthur 1974), later observations on athletes have not consistently verified this association (e.g. Crist & Hill 1990), nor have they found the appropriate temporal relationship between changes in body composition and menstrual function (for reviews, see Scott & Johnson 1982; Loucks & Horvath 1985; Sinning & Little 1987; Bronson & Manning 1991). Eumenorrhoeic and amenorrhoeic athletes span a common range of body compositions (Loucks et al. 1984) which is leaner than most eumenorrhoeic sedentary women. Furthermore, if the growth and sexual development of young animals are blocked by dietary restriction, normal LH pulsatility resumes only a few hours after normal feeding is permitted, and long before any change in body mass or composition occurs (Bronson 1986).

Energy availability

Although Warren (1980) suggested that the reproductive function of dancers is disrupted by an 'energy drain', an empirically testable hypothesis was first clearly stated in terms of brain energy availability by Winterer et al. (1984). This hypothesis holds that failure to provide sufficient metabolic fuels to meet the energy requirements of the brain causes an alteration in brain function that disrupts the GnRH pulse generator.

At the organismal level, the energy availability hypothesis recognizes that mammals partition energy amongst five major metabolic activities: cellular maintenance, thermoregulation, locomotion, growth and reproduction (Wade & Schneider 1992); thus, the expenditure of energy in one function, such as locomotion, makes it unavailable for others, such as reproduction.

Considerable data from biological field trials support the hypothesis that mammalian reproductive function depends on energy availability, particularly in females (for reviews, see Bronson & Manning 1989; Wade & Schneider 1992; Bronson & Heideman 1994; Wade et al. 1996). Anoestrus has been induced in Syrian hamsters by food restriction, the administration of pharmacological blockers of carbohydrate and fat metabolism, insulin administration (which shunts metabolic fuels into storage) and cold exposure (which consumes metabolic fuels in thermogenesis) (Wade & Schneider 1992). Disruptive effects on the reproductive system were independent of body size and composition. Amenorrhoea has been induced in monkeys by training them to run voluntarily on a motorized treadmill for prolonged periods. The menstrual cycles of these animals were restored by dietary supplementation, without any moderation of their exercise regimen (Cameron et al. 1990).

Among women distance runners, energy balance is a better predictor of oestradiol levels ($r = 0.88$) than are body mass index ($r = 0.42$) or percentage body fat ($r = 0.48$) (Zanker & Swaine 1998).

Exercise stress

The stress hypothesis holds that exercise activates the adrenal axis, which disrupts the GnRH pulse generator by various intermediary mechanisms. To be meaningfully independent of the energy availability hypothesis, however, the stress hypothesis further implies that the adrenal axis is activated by some aspect of exercise other than its energy cost.

Certainly, there are central and peripheral mechanisms by which the adrenal axis can disrupt the ovarian axis (Rivier & Rivest 1991), and prolonged aerobic exercise without glucose supplementation does activate the adrenal axis. Furthermore, Selye (1939) induced anoestrus and ovarian atrophy in rats by abruptly forcing them to run strenuously for prolonged periods. Others, too, have induced anoestrus in rats by forced swimming (Asahina *et al.* 1959; Axelson 1987), by forced running (Chatterton *et al.* 1990) and by requiring animals to run further and further for smaller and smaller food rewards (Manning & Bronson 1989, 1991). Elevated cortisol levels in such studies were interpreted as signs of stress, and the induced reproductive disorders were widely interpreted as evidence that 'exercise stress' had a counter-regulatory influence on the female reproductive system.

However, it is not known whether the adrenal axis mechanisms that disrupt the ovarian axis in such animal experiments operate in voluntarily exercising women. Nor is it known whether these mechanisms are independent of energy availability. Furthermore, glucose supplementation during exercise prevents the cortisol response in both rats (Slentz *et al.* 1990) and men (Tabata *et al.* 1991). Until recently, all animal and human investigations of the influence of the 'activity stress paradigm' on reproductive function confounded the stress of exercise with the stress of forcing animals to exercise and/or with energy deficiency. Consequently, there is as yet no unconfounded experimental evidence that the stress of exercise disrupts reproductive function. The mild increase of serum cortisol seen in amenorrhoeic athletes may simply be part of a multifaceted endocrine response to energy deficiency.

Results of prospective experiments

Long-term experiments

Several investigators have attempted to induce menstrual disorders through exercise training, but most (Boyden *et al.* 1983; Bullen *et al.* 1984; Bonen 1992; Rogol *et al.* 1992) have applied only a moderate volume of exercise, or have increased the volume of exercise gradually over several months, and diet has been uncontrolled or unquantified. In the most recent of such studies (Rogol *et al.* 1992), subjects appear to have been physically trained and luteally suppressed before the investigation began (Loucks *et al.* 1993; Rogol *et al.* 1993).

Only one experiment has successfully induced menstrual disorders in regularly menstruating women. That experiment (Bullen *et al.* 1985) imposed a high volume of aerobic exercise abruptly, in imitation of Selye (1939); it caused a large proportion of menstrual disorders in the first month, and an even larger proportion in the second. Disorders were more prevalent in a subgroup fed a controlled weight-loss diet than in another subgroup fed for weight maintenance. Even the weight maintenance subgroup may have been underfed, though, since body mass is an unreliable indicator of energy balance (Leibel *et al.* 1995).

Short-term experiments

We (Loucks *et al.* 1994, 1995, 1998) and others (Williams *et al.* 1995) have performed short-term studies seeking to modify LH pulsatility experimentally. Williams *et al.* (1995) found that the combination of increased exercise and dietary restriction disrupted LH pulsatility.

Our own experiments (Loucks *et al.* 1994, 1995, 1998) examined the independent effects of exercise stress and energy availability on LH pulsatility. We defined and controlled energy availability as dietary energy intake minus exercise energy expenditure, and exercise stress as everything associated with exercise except its energy cost. We found that low energy availability disrupted LH pulsatility, whereas exercise stress did not. LH pulsatility was suppressed regardless of whether energy availability was reduced by extreme dietary energy restriction alone, by extreme exercise energy expenditure alone, or by a combination of moderate dietary energy restriction and moderate exercise energy expenditure (Fig. 49.3). LH pulsatility was unaffected when the diet was supplemented to meet the energy cost of exercise. Low energy availability also suppressed plasma glucose, insulin, IGF-I, leptin and T_3, while raising growth hormone and cortisol levels, all of these effects being reminiscent of the abnormalities in metabolic substrates and hormones seen in amenorrhoeic athletes.

Interpretations and generalizations

Our short-term experiments have demonstrated

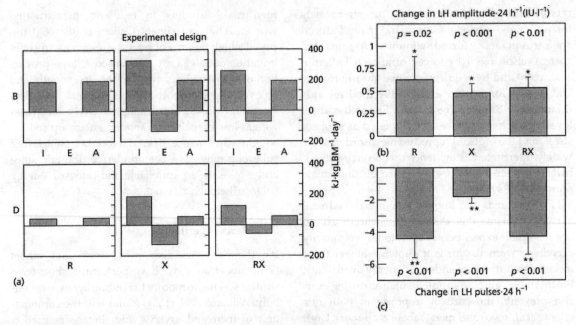

Fig. 49.3 (a) Experimental design. Energy availability (A) was defined as dietary energy intake (I) minus exercise energy expenditure (E). Balanced (B = 45 kcal·kgLBM^{-1}·day^{-1} = 188 kJ·kgLBM^{-1}·day^{-1}) and deficient (D = 10 kcal·kgLBM^{-1}·day^{-1} = 42 kJ·kgLBM^{-1}·day^{-1}) energy availability treatments were administered through severe dietary energy restriction alone (R), through severe exercise energy expenditure alone (X: E = 30 kcal·kgLBM^{-1}·day^{-1} = 126 kJ·kgLBM^{-1}·day^{-1} = 1300 kcal·day^{-1} = 5.44 MJ·day^{-1} at 70% $\dot{V}O_{2max}$), and through the combination (RX) of moderate dietary restriction (I = 25 kcal·kgLBM^{-1}·day^{-1} = 105 kJ·kgLBM^{-1}·day^{-1}) and moderate exercise energy expenditure (E = 15 kcal·kgLBM^{-1}·day^{-1} = 63 kJ·kgLBM^{-1}·day^{-1} = 650 kcal·day^{-1} = 2.72 MJ·day^{-1} at 70% $\dot{V}O_{2max}$) for 4 days in the early follicular phase. (b) Effects of low energy availability on luteinizing hormone (LH) pulse amplitude. LH pulse amplitude was increased by all three treatments. (c) Effects of low energy availability on LH pulse frequency. LH pulse frequency was reduced by all three treatments. From Loucks *et al.* (1994, 1995, 1998), with permission.

that exercise has no suppressive effect on LH pulsatility in women beyond the effect of its energy cost on energy availability. This suggests that low energy availability, not stress, disrupts LH pulsatility in women athletes. If this suggestion is verified by longer-term experiments, then athletic women will know that they can prevent or reverse menstrual disorders by dietary supplementation without moderating their exercise regimen.

In this regard, it is noteworthy that amongst our experimental subjects, dietarily restricted women reported that they felt hungry, but exercising women, who were equally energy deficient on only a normal sedentary diet, reported that they did not feel hungry. Meanwhile, exercising women whose diets were supplemented to maintain energy balance indicated that they felt overfed and that

they had to force themselves to eat when they were not hungry. This suggests that appetite may be an inadequate indicator of energy balance during athletic training, just as thirst is an inadequate indicator of water balance during competition.

In the general population, there is probably a continuum of dietary and exercise combinations that disrupt LH pulsatility, from dietary restriction alone in some women to exercise energy expenditure alone in others. In addition to dietary restriction and exercise, other conditions that have been thought to disrupt reproductive function by stress may actually do so by impairing energy availability. These include surgery, burns and infection, which all reduce energy availability physiologically, and melancholic depression which impairs energy availability psychologically and behaviourally through reduced appetite, decreased emphasis on feeding and sustained anorexia (Rivier & Rivest 1991; Chrousos & Gold 1992). In animal studies of the effect of immobilization stress on LH pulsatility, immobilization is accompanied by a 60% suppression of *ad libitum* dietary energy intake (Shibasaki *et al.* 1988). Therefore, future controlled experiments analogous to ours may show that other stressors also have no suppressive effect on LH pulsatility beyond their impact on energy availability.

Acknowledgements

This research was supported in part by the US Army Medical Research Acquisition Activity (USAMRAA) grant #DAMD 17-95-1-5053, and in part by Grant Mo1 RR00034 from the General Clinical Research Branch, Division of Research Resources, NIH. The content of the information presented in this chapter does not necessarily reflect the position or the policy of the government, and no official endorsement should be inferred.

References

Arce, J.C., De Souza, M.J., Pescatello, L.S. & Luciano, A.A. (1993) Subclinical alterations in hormones and semen profile in athletes. *Fertility and Sterility* **59**, 398–404.

Asahina, K., Kitahara, F., Yamanaka, M. & Akiba, T. (1959) Influences of excessive exercise on the structure and function of rat organs. *Japanese Journal of Physiology* **9**, 322–326.

Axelson, J.F. (1987) Forced swimming alters vaginal estrous cycles, body composition, and steroid levels without disrupting lordosis behavior or fertility in rats. *Physiology of Behavior* **41**, 471–479.

Ayers, J.W., Komesu, Y., Romani, T. & Ansbacher, R. (1985) Anthropomorphic, hormonal, and psychologic correlates of semen quality in endurance-trained male athletes. *Fertility and Sterility* **43**, 917–921.

Bagatell, C.J. & Bremner, W.J. (1990) Sperm counts and reproductive hormones in male marathoners and lean controls. *Fertility and Sterility* **53**, 688–692.

Bonen, A. (1992) Recreational exercise does not impair menstrual cycles: a prospective study. *International Journal of Sports Medicine* **13**, 110–120.

Boyden, T.W., Pamenter, R.W., Stanforth, P., Rotkis, T. & Wilmore, J.H. (1983) Sex steroids and endurance running in women. *Fertility and Sterility* **39**, 629–632.

Bronson, F.H. (1986) Food-restricted, prepubertal, female rats: rapid recovery of luteinizing hormone pulsing with excess food, and full recovery of pubertal development with gonadotropin-releasing hormone. *Endocrinology* **118**, 2483–2487.

Bronson, F.H. & Heideman, P.D. (1994) Seasonal regulation of reproduction in mammals. In: Knobil, E. & Neill, J.D. (eds) *The Physiology of Reproduction*,

Vol 2, pp. 541–583. Raven Press, New York.

Bronson, F.H. & Manning, J. (1989) Food consumption, prolonged exercise, and LH secretion in the peripubertal female rat. In: Pirke, K.M., Wuttke, W. & Schweiger, U. (eds) *The Menstrual Cycle and its Disorders*, pp. 42–49. Springer-Verlag, Berlin.

Bronson, F.H. & Manning, J.M. (1991) The energetic regulation of ovulation: a realistic role for body fat. *Biology of Reproduction* **44**, 945–950.

Brookes, A., Pirke, K.M., Schweiger, U. *et al.* (1990) Cyclic ovarian function in recreational athletes. *Journal of Applied Physiology* **68**, 2083–2086.

Bullen, B.A., Skrinar, G.S., Beitins, I.Z. *et al.* (1984) Endurance training effects on plasma hormonal responsiveness and sex hormone excretion. *Journal of Applied Physiology* **56**, 1453–1463.

Bullen, B.A., Skrinar, G.S., Beitins, I.Z., von Mering, G., Turnbull, B.A. & McArthur, J.W. (1985) Induction of menstrual disorders by strenuous exercise in untrained women. *New England Journal of Medicine* **312**, 1349–1353.

Cameron, J.L., Nosbisch, C., Helmreich, D.L. & Parfitt, D.B. (1990) Reversal of exercise-induced amenorrhea in female cynomolgus monkeys (*Macaca fascicularis*) by increasing food intake. *72nd Annual Meeting of the Endocrine Society*, abstract 1042, Endocrine Society, Bethesda, MD, USA.

Chatterton, R.T. Jr, Hartman, A.L., Lynn, D.E. & Hickson, R.C. (1990) Exercise-induced ovarian dysfunction in the rat. *Proceedings of the Society for Experimental Biology and Medicine* **193**, 220–224.

Chrousos, G.P. & Gold, P.W. (1992) The concepts of stress and stress system dis-

orders. *Journal of the American Medical Association* **267**, 1244–1252.

Committee on Sports Medicine of the American Academy of Pediatrics (1989) Amenorrhea in adolescent athletes. *Pediatrics* **84**, 394–395.

Cooper, K.H. (1977) *The Aerobics Way*. Bantam Books, New York.

Crist, D.M. & Hill, J.M. (1990) Diet and insulin like growth factor I in relation to body composition in women with exercise-induced hypothalamic amenorrhea. *Journal of the American College of Nutrition* **9**, 200–204.

Cumming, D.C. & Wheeler, G.D. (1994) Exercise, training, and the male reproductive system. In: Bouchard, C., Shephard, R.J. & Stephens, T. (eds) *Physical Activity, Fitness, and Health, International Proceedings and Consensus Statement*, pp. 980–992. Human Kinetics, Champaign, IL.

De Souza, M.J., Maguire, M.S., Maresh, C.M., Kraemer, W.J., Rubin, K.R. & Loucks, A.B. (1991) Adrenal activation and the prolactin response to exercise in eumenorrheic and amenorrheic runners. *Journal of Applied Physiology* **70**, 2378–2387.

De Souza, M.J., Luciano, A.A., Arce, J.C., Demers, L.M. & Loucks, A.B. (1994a) Clinical tests explain blunted cortisol responsiveness but not mild hypercortisolism in amenorrheic runners. *Journal of Applied Physiology* **76**, 1302–1309.

De Souza, M.J., Arce, J.C., Pescatello, L.S., Scherzer, H.S. & Luciano, A.A. (1994b) Gonadal hormones and semen quality in male runners. A volume threshold effect of endurance training. *International Journal of Sports Medicine* **15**, 383–391.

De Souza, M.J., Miller, B.E., Loucks, A.B. *et al.* (1998) High frequency of luteal phase deficiency and anovulation in recreational women runners: Blunted elevation in FSH observed during luteal–follicular transition. *Journal of Clinical Endocrinology and Metabolism* **83**, 4220–4232.

Ding, J.-H., Scheckter, C.B., Drinkwater, B.L., Soules, M.R. & Bremner, W.J. (1988) High serum cortisol levels in exercise-associated amenorrhea. *Annals of Internal Medicine* **108**, 530–534.

Drinkwater, B.L., Nilson, K., Chesnut, C.H., Bremner, W.J., Shainholtz, S. & Southworth, M.B. (1984) Bone mineral content of amenorrheic and eumenorrheic athletes. *New England Journal of Medicine* **311**, 277–281.

Drinkwater, B.L., Bruemner, B. & Chesnut, C.H. III (1990) Menstrual history as a determinant of current bone density in young athletes. *Journal of the American Medical Association* **263**, 545–548.

Edwards, J.E., Lindeman, A.K., Mikesky, A.E. & Stager, J.M. (1993) Energy balance in highly trained female endurance runners. *Medicine and Science in Sports and Exercise* **25**, 1398–1404.

Ellison, P.T. & Lager, C. (1986) Moderate recreational running is associated with lowered salivary progesterone profiles in women. *American Journal of Obstetrics and Gynecology* **154**, 1000–1003.

Frey, M.A.B., Doerr, B.M., Srivastava, L.S. & Glueck, C.J. (1983) Exercise training, sex hormones and lipoprotein relationships in men. *Journal of Applied Physiology* **54**, 757–762.

Frisch, R.E. & McArthur, J.W. (1974) Menstrual cycles: fatness as a determinant of minimum weight for height necessary for their maintenance or onset. *Science* **185**, 949–951.

Gold, P.W., Gwirtsman, H., Avgerinos, P.C. et al. (1986) Abnormal hypothalamic–pituitary–adrenal function in anorexia nervosa: pathophysiologic mechanisms in underweight and weight-corrected patients. *New England Journal of Medicine* **314**, 1335–1342.

Griffith, R.O., Dressendorfer, R.H., Fullbright, C.D. & Wade, C.E. (1990) Testicular function during exhaustive training. *Physician and Sportsmedicine* **18**, 54–64.

Hackney, A.C., Sinning, W.E. & Bruot, B.C. (1988) Reproductive hormone profiles of endurance-trained and untrained males. *Medicine and Science in Sports and Exercise* **20**, 60–65.

Hakkinen, K., Keskinen, K.L., Alen, M., Komi, P.V. & Kauhanen, H. (1989) Serum hormone concentrations during prolonged training in élite endurance-trained and strength-trained athletes.

European Journal of Applied Physiology **59**, 233–238.

Harber, V.J., Petersen, S.R. & Chilibeck, P.D. (1998) Thyroid hormone concentrations and muscle metabolism in amenorrheic and eumenorrheic athletes. *Canadian Journal of Applied Physiology* **23**, 293–306.

Jenkins, P.J., Ibanez-Santos, X., Holly, J. et al. (1993) IGFBP-1: a metabolic signal associated with exercise-induced amenorrhea. *Neuroendocrinology* **57**, 600–604.

Kaiserauer, S., Snyder, A.C., Sleeper, M. & Zierath, J. (1989) Nutritional, physiological, and menstrual status of distance runners. *Medicine and Science in Sports and Exercise* **21**, 120–125.

Keen, A.D. & Drinkwater, B.L. (1997) Irreversible bone loss in former amenorrheic athletes. *Osteoporosis International* **7**, 311–315.

Laughlin, G.A. & Yen, S.S.C. (1996) Nutritional and endocrine–metabolic aberrations in amenorrheic athletes. *Journal of Clinical Endocrinology and Metabolism* **81**, 4301–4309.

Laughlin, G.A. & Yen, S.S.C. (1997) Hypoleptinemia in women athletes: absence of diurnal rhythm with amenorrhea. *Journal of Clinical Endocrinology and Metabolism* **82**, 318–321.

Leibel, R.L., Rosenbaum, M. & Hirsch, J. (1995) Changes in energy expenditure resulting from altered body weight. *New England Journal of Medicine* **332**, 621–628.

Loucks, A.B. (1996) The reproductive system. In: Bar-Or, O., Lamb, D.R. & Clarkson, P.M. (eds) *Exercise and the Female—a Life Span Approach*, pp. 41–71. Cooper Publishing Company, Carmel, IN.

Loucks, A.B. & Horvath, S.M. (1985) Athletic amenorrhea: a review. *Medicine and Science in Sports and Exercise* **17**, 56–72.

Loucks, A.B., Horvath, S.M. & Freedson, P.S. (1984) Menstrual status and validation of body fat prediction in athletes. *Human Biology* **56**, 383–392.

Loucks, A.B., Mortola, J.F., Girton, L. & Yen, S.S.C. (1989) Alterations in the hypothalamic–pituitary–ovarian and hypothalamic–pituitary–adrenal axes in athletic women. *Journal of Clinical Endocrinology and Metabolism* **68**, 402–411.

Loucks, A.B., Laughlin, G.A., Mortola, J.F., Girton, L., Nelson, J.C. & Yen, S.S.C. (1992) Hypothalamic–pituitary–thyroidal function in eumenorrheic and amenorrheic athletes. *Journal of Clinical Endocrinology and Metabolism* **75**, 514–518.

Loucks, A.B., Cameron, J.L. & De Souza, M.J. (1993) Subject assignment may have biased experimental results. *Journal of Applied Physiology* **74**, 2045–2046.

Loucks, A.B. & Heath, E.M. (1994) Dietary restriction reduces luteinizing hormone (LH) pulse frequency during waking hours and increases LH pulse amplitude during sleep in young menstruating women. *Journal of Clinical Endocrinology and Metabolism* **78**, 910–915.

Loucks, A.B., Brown, R., King, K., Thuma, J.R. & Verdun, M. (1995) A combined regimen of moderate dietary restriction and exercise training alters luteinizing hormone pulsatility in regularly menstruating young women. *77th Annual Meeting of the Endocrine Society*, abstract #P3–360, Endocrine Society, Bethesda, MD, USA.

Loucks, A.B., Verdun, M. & Heath, E.M. (1998) Low energy availability, not the stress of exercise, alters LH pulsatility in exercising women. *Journal of Applied Physiology* **84**, 37–46.

Lucia, A., Chicharro, J.L., Perez, M., Serratosa, L., Bandres, F. & Legido, J. (1996) Reproductive function in male endurance athletes: sperm analysis and hormone profile. *Journal of Applied Physiology* **81**, 2627–2636.

McColl, E.M., Wheeler, G.D., Gomes, P., Bhambhani, Y. & Cumming, D.C. (1989) The effects of acute exercise on pulsatile LH release in high-mileage male runners. *Clinical Endocrinology* **31**, 617–621.

MacConnie, S.E., Barkan, A., Lampman, R.M., Lampman, R.M., Schork, M.A. & Beitins, I.Z. (1986) Decreased hypothalamic gonadotropin-releasing hormone secretion in male marathon runners. *New England Journal of Medicine* **315**, 411–417.

Manning, J.M. & Bronson, F.H. (1989) Effects of prolonged exercise on puberty and luteinizing hormone secretion in female rats. *American Journal of Physiology* **257**, R1359–R1364.

Manning, J.M. & Bronson, F.H. (1991) Suppression of puberty in rats by exercise: effects on hormone levels and reversal with GnRH infusion. *American Journal of Physiology* **260**, R717–R723.

Marcus, R., Cann, C., Madvig, P. et al. (1985) Menstrual function and bone mass in élite women distance runners. *Annals of Internal Medicine* **102**, 158–163.

Mertz, W., Tsui, J.C., Judd, J.T. et al. (1991) What are people really eating? The relation between energy intake derived from estimated diet records and intake determined to maintain body weight. *Ameri-*

can *Journal of Clinical Nutrition* **54**, 291–295.

Myerson, M., Gutin, B., Warren, M.P. *et al.* (1991) Resting metabolic rate and energy balance in amenorrheic and eumenorrheic runners. *Medicine and Science in Sports and Exercise* **23**, 15–22.

Nelson, M.E., Fisher, E.C., Catsos, P.D., Meredith, C.N., Turksoy, R.N. & Evans, W.J. (1986) Diet and bone mineral status in amenorrheic runners. *American Journal of Clinical Nutrition* **43**, 910–916.

Otis, C.L., Drinkwater, B.L., Johnson, M., Loucks, A. & Wilmore. J. (1997) ACSM position stand on the female athlete triad. *Medicine and Science in Sports and Exercise* **29**, i–ix.

Peltonen, P., Marniemi, J., Hietanen, E., Vuori, I. & Ehnholm, C. (1981) Changes in serum lipids, lipoproteins and heparin releasable lipolytic enzymes during moderate physical training in man: a longitudinal study. *Metabolism* **30**, 518–526.

Pirke, K.M., Schweiger, U., Broocks, A., Tuschl. R.J. & Laessle, R.G. (1990) Luteinizing hormone and follicle stimulating hormone secretion patterns in female athletes with and without menstrual disturbances. *Clinical Endocrinology* **33**, 345–353.

Remes, K., Kuoppasalmi, K. & Adlercreutz, H. (1979) Effects of longterm physical training on plasma testosterone, androstenedione, luteinizing hormone, and sex hormone binding globulin capacity. *Scandinavian Journal of Clinical and Laboratory Investigation* **39**, 743–749.

Rivier, C. & Rivest, S. (1991) Effect of stress on the activity of the hypothalamic–pituitary–gonadal axis: peripheral and central mechanisms. *Biology of Reproduction* **45**, 523–532.

Roemmich, J.N. & Sinning, W.E. (1997) Weight loss and wrestling training: effects on growth-related hormones. *Journal of Applied Physiology* **82**, 1760–1764.

Rogol, A.D., Weltman, A., Weltman, J.Y. *et al.* (1992) Durability of the reproductive axis in eumenorrheic women during 1 year of endurance training. *Journal of Applied Physiology* **72**, 1571–1580.

Rogol, A.D., Evans, W.S., Weltman, J.Y., Veldhuis, J.D. & Weltman, A.L. (1993) Reply to 'Subject assignment may have biased experimental results.'. *Journal of Applied Physiology* **74**, 2046–2047.

Scott, E.C. & Johnson, F.E. (1982) Critical fat, menarche, and the maintenance of menstrual cycles: a critical review. *Journal of Adolescent Health Care* **2**, 249–260.

Seidman, D.S., Dolev, E., Deuster, P.A., Burstein, R., Arnon, R. & Epstein, Y. (1990) Androgenic responses to long-term physical training in male subjects. *International Journal of Sports Medicine* **11**, 421–424.

Selye, H. (1939) The effect of adaptation to various damaging agents on the female sex organs in the rat. *Endocrinology* **25**, 615–624.

Shangold, M., Rebar, R.W., Colston-Wentz, A. & Schiff, I. (1990) Evaluation and management of menstrual dysfunction in athletes. *Journal of the American Medical Association* **263**, 1665–1669.

Shibasaki, T., Yamauchi, N., Kato, Y. *et al.* (1988) Involvement of corticotropin-releasing factor in restraint stress-induced anorexia and reversion of the anorexia by somatostatin in the rat. *Life Sciences* **43**, 1103–1110.

Sinning, W.E. & Little, K.D. (1987) Body composition and menstrual function in athletes. *Sports Medicine* **4**, 34–45.

Slentz, C.A., Davis, J.M., Settles, D.L., Pate, R.R. & Settles, S.J. (1990) Glucose feedings and exercise in rats: glycogen use, hormone responses, and performance. *Journal of Applied Physiology* **69**, 989–994.

Stacey, E., Korkia, P., Hukkanen, M.V., Polak, J.M. & Rutherford, O.M. (1998) Decreased nitric oxide levels and bone turnover in amenorrheic athletes with spinal osteopenia. *Journal of Clinical Endocrinology and Metabolism* **83**, 3056–3061.

Strauss, R.H., Lanese, R.R. & Malarkey, W.B. (1985) Weight loss in amateur wrestlers and its effect on testosterone levels. *Journal of the American Medical Association* **254**, 3337–3338.

Styne, D.M. & Grumbach, M.M. (1991) Disorders of puberty in the male and female. In: Yen, S.S.C. & Jaffe, R.B. (eds) *Reproductive Endocrinology*, pp. 511–544. W.B. Saunders Co., Philadelphia.

Suh, B.Y., Liu, J.H., Berga, S.L., Quigley, M.E., Laughlin, G.A. & Yen, S.S.C. (1988) Hypercortisolism in patients with functional hypothalamic amenorrhea. *Journal of Clinical Endocrinology and Metabolism* **66**, 733–739.

Tabata, I., Ogita, F., Miyachi, M. & Shibayama, H. (1991) Effect of low blood glucose on plasma CRF, ACTH, and cortisol during prolonged physical exercise. *Journal of Applied Physiology* **71**, 1807–1812.

Tomten, S.E., Falch, J.A., Birkeland, K.I., Hemmersbach, P. & Hostmark, A.T. (1998) Bone mineral density and menstrual irregularities. A comparative

study on cortical and trabecular bone structures in runners with alleged normal eating behavior. *International Journal of Sports Medicine* **19**, 92–97.

Treolar, A.E., Boynton, R.E., Behn, B.G. & Brown, B.W. (1967) Variation of the human menstrual cycle through reproductive life. *International Journal of Fertility* **12**, 77–126.

Urhausen, A., Kullmer, T. & Kinderman, W. (1987) A 7-week follow-up study of the behavior of testosterone and cortisol during the competition period in rowers. *European Journal of Applied Physiology* **56**, 528–533.

Veldhuis, J.D., Evans, W.S., Demers, L.M., Thorner, M.O., Wakat, D. & Rogol, A.D. (1985) Altered neuroendocrine regulation of gonadotropin secretion in women distance runners. *Journal of Clinical Endocrinology and Metabolism* **61**, 557–563.

Wade, G.N. & Schneider, J.E. (1992) Metabolic fuels and reproduction in female mammals. *Neuroscience and Biobehavioral Reviews* **16**, 235–272.

Wade, G.N., Schneider, J.E. & Li, H.-Y. (1996) Control of fertility by metabolic cues. *American Journal of Physiology* **270** (*Endocrinology and Metabolism* **33**), E1–E19.

Warren, M.P. (1980) The effects of exercise on pubertal progression and reproductive function in girls. *Journal of Clinical Endocrinology and Metabolism* **51**, 1150–1157.

Wheeler, G.D., Wall, S.R., Belcastro, A.N. & Cumming, D.C. (1984) Reduced serum testosterone and prolactin levels in male distance runners. *Journal of the American Medical Association* **252**, 514–516.

Wheeler, G.D., Singh, M., Pirce, W.D., Epling, W.F. & Cumming, D.C. (1991) Endurance training decreases serum testosterone levels in men without change in luteinizing hormone pulsatile release. *Journal of Clinical Endocrinology and Metabolism* **72**, 422–425.

Williams, N.I., Young, J.C., McArthur, J.W., Bullen, B., Skrinar, G.S. & Turnbull, B. (1995) Strenuous exercise with caloric restriction: effect on luteinizing hormone secretion. *Medicine and Science in Sports and Exercise* **27**, 1390–1398.

Wilmore, J.H., Wambsgans, K.C., Brenner, M. *et al.* (1992) Is there energy conservation in amenorrheic compared with eumenorrheic distance runners? *Journal of Applied Physiology* **72**, 15–22.

Winterer, J., Cutler, G.B. Jr & Loriaux, D.L. (1984) Caloric balance, brain to body ratio, and the timing of menarche. *Medical Hypotheses* **15**, 87–91.

Yahiro, J., Glass, A.R., Fears, W.B., Ferguson, E.W. & Vigersky, R.A. (1987) Exaggerated gonadotropin response to luteinizing hormone-releasing hormone in amenorrheic runners. *American Journal of Obstetrics and Gynecology* **156**, 586–591.

Zanker, C.L. & Swaine, I.L. (1998) The relationship between oestradiol concentration and energy balance in young women distance runners. *International Journal of Sports Medicine* **19**, 104–108.

Chapter 50

Endurance Exercise and the Immune Response

DAVID C. NIEMAN

Introduction

Publications on the topic of exercise immunology date from late in the 19th century, but it was not until the mid-1980s that a significant number of investigators world-wide devoted their resources to this area of research endeavour. From 1900 to 1999, just over 1000 papers on exercise immunology were published, with 80% of these appearing in the 1990s (Hjertman & Nieman 1999). In this chapter, emphasis will be placed on reviewing literature published since 1990 on four current topics that have practical application to endurance athletes: (i) the contrast in immune function between athletes and non-athletes; (ii) acute immune changes that occur following prolonged and intensive exercise; (iii) the role of nutritional supplements in attenuating exercise-induced changes in immunity; and (iv) practical recommendations for athletes.

Key points that will be emphasized in this chapter include the following.
• The immune systems of athletes and non-athletes when measured in the resting state are more similar than disparate. Even when significant differences in resting immune function have been observed in athletes, investigators have had little success in linking these to a higher incidence of infection and illness.
• Many components of the immune system exhibit adverse change after prolonged, heavy exertion. During this 'open window' of impaired immunity (which may last between 3 and 72 h, depending on the immune measure), viruses and bacteria may gain a foothold, increasing the risk of subclinical and clinical infection.

• The influence of nutritional supplements, primarily zinc, vitamin C, glutamine and carbohydrate, on the acute immune response to prolonged exercise has been measured in endurance athletes. Vitamin C and glutamine have received much attention, but the data thus far are inconclusive. The most impressive results have been reported with carbohydrate supplementation.
• Carbohydrate beverage ingestion has been associated with higher plasma glucose levels, an attenuated cortisol and growth hormone response, fewer perturbations in blood immune cell counts, a lesser granulocyte and monocyte phagocytosis and oxidative burst activity, and a diminished pro- and anti-inflammatory cytokine response. Overall, these data indicate that the physiological stress to the immune system is reduced when endurance athletes use carbohydrate beverages before, during and after prolonged and intense exertion.

Immune function in endurance athletes and non-athletes

Among élite athletes and their coaches, a common perception is that prolonged and intense exertion lowers resistance and predisposes to upper respiratory tract infection (URTI) (Nieman 1994, 1997a). In a 1996 survey conducted by the Gatorade Sports Science Institute, 89% of 2700 high school and college coaches and athletic trainers checked 'yes' to the question 'Do you believe overtraining can compromise the immune system and make athletes sick?' (Gatorade Sports Science Institute, Barrington, IL, personal communication). Several studies using epidemiological designs have verified that URTI risk is elevated during periods of heavy training and in the 1–2-week period following participation in competitive endurance races (Nieman *et al.* 1990a; Peters *et al.* 1993, 1996; Peters-Futre 1997; Foster 1998). Foster (1998) showed that a high percentage of illnesses occurred when élite athletes exceeded individually identifiable training thresholds, mostly related to the strain of training. Animal studies have generally supported the finding that one or two periods of exhaustive exercise following inoculation lead to a more frequent appearance of infection and a higher fatality rate (although results vary depending on the pathogen) (Chao *et al.* 1992; Cannon 1993).

In contrast, a common belief among fitness enthusiasts is that regular exercise confers resistance against infection. In a survey of 170 non-élite marathon runners (personal best time, an average of 3 h 25 min) who had been training for and participating in marathons for an average of 12 years, 90% reported that they definitely or mostly agreed with the statement that they 'rarely get sick' (unpublished observations). A survey of 750 Masters athletes (ranging in age from 40 to 81 years) showed that 76% perceived themselves as less vulnerable to viral illnesses than their sedentary peers (Shephard *et al.* 1995). Three randomized exercise training studies have demonstrated that near-daily exercise is associated with a significant reduction in URTI (Nieman *et al.* 1990b, 1993, 1998b).

Do the immune systems of endurance athletes and non-athletes function differently? Although the URTI epidemiological data suggest that disparities should exist, attempts thus far to compare resting immune function in athletes and non-athletes have failed to provide compelling evidence that athletic endeavour is linked to clinically important changes in immunity (Pedersen *et al.* 1996b; Mackinnon 1997; Nieman 1998a).

Adaptive immunity

In the resting state, the adaptive immune system (i.e. the function of T and B cells which produce specific reactions and immunological memory to each infectious agent when they are activated) appears to be largely unaffected by intensive and prolonged exercise training, although results may vary according to training status, the assay method and age (Tvede *et al.* 1991; Baj *et al.* 1994; Nieman *et al.* 1995b, 1995c, 1999b).

Baj *et al.* (1994) compared mitogen-induced lymphocyte proliferative responses (the typical *in vitro* laboratory test for T- and B-cell function) in 16 untrained males and 15 élite male cyclists during periods of both low- and high-volume training. No significant difference between groups was measured while the cyclists engaged in low-volume training. However, during a period of high-volume training, two of four mitogen assays were elevated 35–50% in the endurance athletes. One other comparison reported no difference in mitogen induced lymphocyte proliferative responses between controls and élite cyclists during periods of either low- or high-volume training (Tvede *et al.* 1991). A comparison of non-athletes and élite female rowers 3 months prior to the world championships found a slight elevation in mitogen-induced lymphocyte proliferation when using a whole blood culture, but not with separated mononuclear cells (Nieman *et al.* 1999b). Highly conditioned females have been reported to have a significantly greater proliferative response compared to their sedentary elderly peers, a finding confirmed in comparisons of trained and untrained elderly males (Nieman *et al.* 1993; Shinkai *et al.* 1995) (see Fig. 50.1). Together, these data suggest that T- and B-cell functions are not consistently altered by athletic endeavour except in older adults.

Innate immunity

The innate immune system (i.e. immune cells which act as a first line of defence against infectious agents) appears to respond differentially to the chronic stress of intensive exercise, with natural killer cell activity (NKCA) tending to be enhanced while neutrophil function is suppressed (especially during periods of high-volume training).

Natural killer (NK) cells are large granular lymphocytes that can mediate cytolytic reactions against a variety of neoplastic and virally infected cells. NK cells also exhibit key non-cytolytic func-

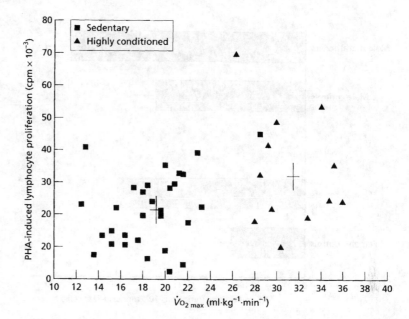

Fig. 50.1 Phytohemagglutin (PHA)-induced lymphocyte proliferation was 56% higher ($P < 0.05$) in 12 highly conditioned compared to 30 sedentary elderly women. Crosses represent mean ± s.d. for each group. Data are from Nieman *et al.* (1993).

tions, and can inhibit microbial colonization and the growth of certain viruses, bacteria, fungi and parasites. NKCA is measured with a 4-h ^{51}Cr release assay, in which certain types of cancer or virally infected cells are mixed with blood lymphocytes and monocytes. NK cells, which represent about 10–15% of blood lymphocytes, respond quickly and, within 4 h, can lyse a significant proportion of the ^{51}Cr-labelled target cells. The released ^{51}Cr is collected into filters, and then measured with a gamma counter.

Most but not all cross-sectional studies have shown an enhanced NKCA in endurance athletes when compared to non-athletes (Pedersen *et al.* 1989; Tvede *et al.* 1991; Nieman *et al.* 1993, 1995b, 1995c, 1999b; Shinkai *et al.* 1995). Trained rodents also demonstrate a greater NKCA (Jonsdottir *et al.* 1997; Hoffman-Goetz 1998). Figure 50.2 summarizes the data from two studies comparing 22 male marathoners and 18 non-athletes, and 20 female élite rowers and 19 non-athletes (Nieman *et al.* 1995c, 1999b).

The data of Tvede *et al.* (1991) support a higher NKCA in élite cyclists during the summer (their intensive training period) compared to the winter (their low training period). Several prospective

studies utilizing moderate endurance training regimens of 8–15 weeks' duration have reported no significant elevation in NKCA relative to sedentary controls (both young and older adults) (Nieman *et al.* 1990b, 1993, 1998b). Together, these data imply that endurance exercise may have to be intensive and prolonged (i.e. at athletic levels) before NKCA is chronically elevated.

Neutrophils are an important component of the innate immune system, aiding in the phagocytosis of many bacterial and viral pathogens, and the release of immunomodulatory cytokines (Smith & Pyne 1997). Neutrophils are considered to be the body's most effective phagocytes, and are critical in the early control of invading infectious agents. Neutrophil function can be expressed either as a measure of the ability to engulf pathogens (phagocytosis), or the facility to kill the pathogens once engulfed (the oxidative burst).

No researcher has reported an elevation in neutrophil function (either phagocytic ability or oxidative burst) among athletes when compared to non-athletes (Smith *et al.* 1990; Baj *et al.* 1994; Hack *et al.* 1994; Pyne *et al.* 1995; Nieman *et al.* 1999b). Neutrophil function has been reported to be suppressed in athletes, but only during periods of

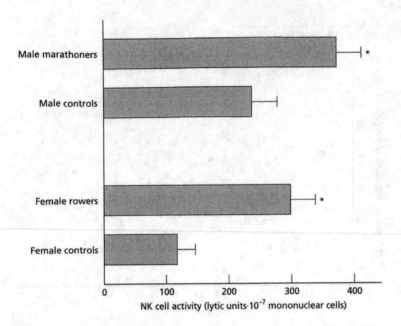

Fig. 50.2 Natural killer (NK) cell activity was significantly higher in 22 male marathoners compared to 18 controls, and in 20 élite female rowers compared to 19 controls. Data from Nieman *et al.* (1995c, 1999b). *, $P < 0.05$.

high-intensity training (Smith & Pyne 1997; Pyne & Gleeson 1998). This is especially apparent in the studies by Hack *et al.* (1994) and Baj *et al.* (1994), where neutrophil function in athletes was similar to controls during periods of low-volume training, but was significantly suppressed during the summer months of intensive training. Nieman *et al.* (1999b) reported no difference in neutrophil/monocyte phagocytosis or oxidative burst activity between non-athletes and élite female rowers 3 months prior to the world championships.

Clinical implications

Even when significant changes in the concentration and functional activity of immune parameters have been observed in athletes, investigators have had little success in linking these to a higher incidence of infection and illness (Lee *et al.* 1992; Pedersen & Bruunsgaard 1995; Shephard & Shek 1996; Mackinnon *et al.* 1997; Gabriel *et al.* 1998; Nieman 1998a; Nieman *et al.* 1999b). In one report, élite swimmers undertaking intensive training had significantly lower neutrophil oxidative activity at rest than age- and sex-matched sedentary individuals, and function was further suppressed during the period of strenuous training prior to national-level competition (Pyne *et al.* 1995). None the less, URTI rates did not differ between the swimmers and sedentary controls. Nieman *et al.* (1999b) reported that URTI rates were similar in female élite rowers and non-athletes during a 2-month winter/spring period despite higher NKCA and T-cell function (whole blood assay) in the rowers.

Two studies indicate that salivary immunoglobulin A (IgA) concentration warrants further research as a marker of potential infection risk in athletes. Mackinnon *et al.* (1993) demonstrated that élite squash and hockey athletes with low salivary IgA concentrations experienced higher rates of URTI. This was later confirmed in a study of élite swimmers (Gleeson *et al.* 1996). Salivary IgA levels measured in swimmers before individual training sessions showed significant correlations with infection rates, and the number of infections observed in the swimmers was predicted by the preseason and the mean pretraining salivary IgA levels.

In general, but with one exception (NKCA), the immune systems (resting state) of athletes and non-athletes appear to be more similar than disparate. Of the various immune function tests that show some change with athletic endeavour, only salivary IgA has emerged as a potential marker of infection risk (Shephard & Shek 1998a). Future research should concentrate on this immune measure using large groups of athletes and non-athletes to demonstrate its clinical usefulness.

The acute immune response: the 'open window' theory

In the light of the mixed results regarding the effect of chronic, intensive training on resting immune function and host protection, several authors have theorized that each bout of prolonged exercise leads to transient but clinically significant changes in immune function (Hoffman-Goetz & Pedersen 1994; Pedersen et al. 1996a; Nieman 1997b, 1998b). During this 'open window' of altered immunity (which may last between 3 and 72 h, depending on the immune measure), viruses and bacteria may gain a foothold, increasing the risk of subclinical and clinical infection.

Although this is an attractive hypothesis, no serious attempt has been made by investigators to demonstrate that athletes showing the most extreme immunosuppression following heavy exertion are those that contract an infection during the following 1–2 weeks (Shephard & Shek 1998a). This link must be established before the 'open window' theory can be wholly accepted.

Many components of the immune system exhibit change after prolonged, heavy exertion (Nieman & Nehlsen-Cannarella 1991; Nieman 1997b, 1998a; Pedersen et al. 1998b).

High neutrophil and low lymphocyte blood counts, induced by high plasma cortisol

Exercise is associated with an extensive perturbation of white blood cell counts, with prolonged, high-intensity endurance exercise leading to the greatest degree of cell trafficking (an increase in blood granulocyte and monocyte counts, and a decrease in blood lymphocytes) (Haq et al. 1993; Shephard & Shek 1996; Nieman et al. 1999a). Several mechanisms appear to be involved, including exercise-induced changes in stress hormone and cytokine concentrations, body temperature changes, increases in blood flow, lymphocyte apoptosis and dehydration (Haq et al. 1993; Cross et al. 1996; Pedersen et al. 1996a; Gannon et al. 1997; Nieman 1997b; Brenner et al. 1998; Mars et al. 1998). Following prolonged running at high intensity, the concentration of serum cortisol is significantly elevated above control levels for several hours, and this has been related to many of the immunosuppressive and cell trafficking changes experienced during recovery (Pedersen et al. 1996a; Nieman 1997b). The mode of exercise appears to have little effect on the pattern of change in blood leucocyte subsets when intensity and duration are similar. In one study of 10 triathletes, for example, 2.5 h of high-intensity running or cycling (~75% $\dot{V}O_{2max}$) both caused a sustained increase in the neutrophil/lymphocyte ratio (Nieman et al. 1998c; see Fig. 50.3).

Increase in blood granulocyte and monocyte phagocytosis, but a decrease in nasal neutrophil phagocytosis

Following prolonged, high-intensity running, substances released from injured muscle cells initiate an inflammatory response (Belcastro et al. 1996; Ostrowski et al. 1998; Raj et al. 1998). Monocytes and neutrophils invade the inflamed area and phagocytose debris. The increase in blood granulocyte and monocyte phagocytosis may therefore represent a part of the inflammatory response to acute muscle injury. Phagocyte specimens collected from the peripheral blood, however, may react differently from those taken from the respiratory tract. Using nasal lavage samples, Müns (1993) showed that compared to controls, the capacity of phagocytes to ingest Escherichia coli was significantly suppressed in athletes for more than 3 days after running a 20-km road race (see Fig. 50.4).

Decrease in nasal and salivary IgA concentration

The secretory immune system of the mucosal tissues of the upper respiratory tract is considered the first barrier to colonization by pathogens, with IgA the major effector of host defence. Secretory IgA

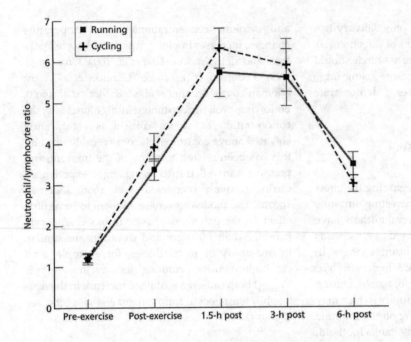

Fig. 50.3 The neutrophil/lymphocyte ratio rose to a similar degree in 10 triathletes following 2.5 h of cycling or running at ~75% $\dot{V}O_{2max}$. Data from Nieman *et al.* (1998c).

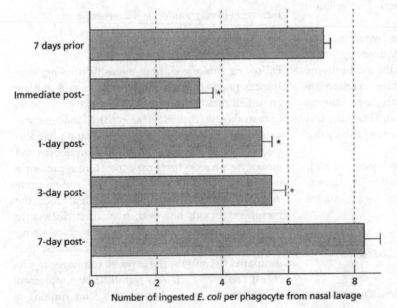

Fig. 50.4 Number of ingested *Escherichia coli* per phagocyte taken from nasal lavage samples from runners before and after a 20-km race. Data from Müns (1993). *, $P < 0.05$.

inhibits attachment and replication of pathogens, preventing their entry into the body. Data from Müns *et al.* (1989) have shown that IgA concentration in nasal secretions is decreased by nearly 70% for at least 18 h after racing 31 km. Following strenu- ous prolonged exercise, salivary secretion rates fall, decreasing the level of IgA-mediated immune protection at the mucosal surface (Mackinnon *et al.* 1987; Ljungberg *et al.* 1997). Steerenberg *et al.* (1997) reported that salivary flow rate and total salivary

IgA output were reduced in 42 triathletes following an Olympic-distance triathlon.

Decrease in nasal mucociliary clearance

In one study of 12 runners and 10 controls, nasal mucociliary transit time was significantly prolonged after a marathon race (17.1 versus 8.9 min, athletes versus controls), and returned to prerace levels after several days (Müns *et al.* 1995). The decrement in nasal mucociliary clearance rate appeared to be caused in part by abnormally functioning ciliated cells. These data, combined with the impairment in nasal neutrophil function and nasal/salivary IgA secretion rates, suggest that host protection in the upper airway passages is suppressed for a prolonged time after endurance running races.

Decrease in granulocyte and macrophage oxidative burst activity (killing activity)

Following sustained, heavy exertion, granulocytes have a reduced oxidative burst capacity (Nieman 1997a; Ortega *et al.* 1996; Smith & Pyne 1997). The decrease in granulocyte oxidative burst may represent a reduced killing capacity by blood neutrophils

(on a per-cell basis) due to stress and overloading (Smith & Pyne 1997). Davis *et al.* (1997) have shown that, in mice, alveolar macrophage antiviral resistance is suppressed following prolonged strenuous exercise to fatigue, an effect due in part to adrenal catecholamines (Kohut *et al.* 1998).

Decrease in natural killer cell cytotoxic activity

Following intensive and prolonged endurance exercise, NKCA is decreased 40–60% for at least 6 h (Shinkai *et al.* 1993; Nieman *et al.* 1995a, 1997c, 1999a) (see Fig. 50.5). This decrease is greater and longer lasting than has been reported for exercise of less than 1 h duration (Nieman 1997b, 1998a; Woods *et al.* 1999). The decrease in NKCA appears to be related to the cortisol-induced redistribution of blood NK lymphocytes from the blood compartment to other tissues (Nieman 1997b). In fact, the decrease in NKCA closely parallels the drop in blood NK cell concentration, implying that each NK cell retains normal function. It has not yet been determined where the blood NK cells go to, and whether the decreased NKCA in the blood compartment represents what is occurring in other lymphoid tissues, or is linked with URTI risk.

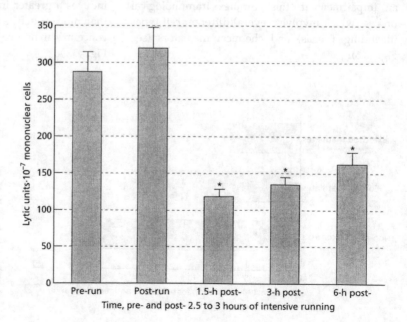

Fig. 50.5 Natural killer cell activity response to 2.5 h of intensive running in 62 marathoners. Data from Nieman (1997b); Nieman *et al.* (1995a). *, $P < 0.05$.

Decrease in mitogen-induced lymphocyte proliferation

Compared to resting non-athletic controls, whole blood Concanavalin A-induced lymphocyte proliferation falls 30–40% (unadjusted for changes in T-cell number) for more than 3h following 2.5h of intensive running (Nieman *et al.* 1995d). Others have reported an even greater decrease after endurance race events (Eskola *et al.* 1978; Shinkai *et al.* 1993). The decrease in T-cell function is more prolonged than has been described after exercise of less than 1h duration (Nieman 1997b). Except for the immediate postrun time point, the decrease in T-cell function parallels the drop in blood T-cell concentration (Nieman *et al.* 1995d; Nieman 1997b).

Decrease in the delayed-type hypersensitivity skin response

Bruunsgaard *et al.* (1997b) examined the effect of competing in a half-Ironman triathlon (mean time, 6.5h) on *in vivo* cell-mediated immunity through use of a skin test with seven antigens. The delayed-type hypersensitivity (DTH) reaction was suppressed 60% 2 days after the competition in the triathletes when compared to controls, indicating an impairment in this complex immunological process which involves several different cell types (including T cells) and chemical mediators (see Fig. 50.6).

Increase in plasma concentrations of pro- and anti-inflammatory cytokines

Cytokines are low molecular weight proteins and peptides which help control and mediate interactions among cells involved in immune responses. Exercise bouts which induce muscle cell injury cause a sequential release of the pro-inflammatory cytokines tumour necrosis factor-α (TNF-α), interleukin (IL)-1β and IL-6, followed very closely by anti-inflammatory cytokines such as IL-4, IL-10 and IL-1ra (Northoff *et al.* 1994; Drenth *et al.* 1995; Bury *et al.* 1996; Bruunsgaard *et al.* 1997a; Gannon *et al.* 1997; Nehlsen-Cannarella *et al.* 1997; Rohde *et al.* 1997; Weinstock *et al.* 1997; Nieman *et al.* 1998a; Ostrowski *et al.* 1998; Smits *et al.* 1998). TNF-α and IL-1β stimulate the production of IL-6, which induces the acute phase response and the production of IL-1ra. Recent work using muscle biopsies and urine samples has shown more clearly the intimate link between all of these cytokines (Ostrowski *et al.* 1998). The inflammatory cytokines help regulate a rapid migration of neutrophils and then later, monocytes, into areas of injured muscle cells and other metabolically active tissues to initiate repair (Belcastro *et al.* 1996). Endurance exercise associated with muscle soreness (e.g. marathon running) induces a greater inflammatory cytokine response than modes such as cycling or rowing that are more concentric in nature (Nieman *et al.* 1998a, 1999a) (see Fig. 50.7).

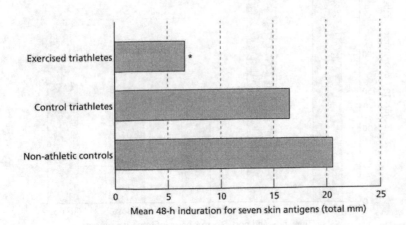

Fig. 50.6 A reduced delayed-type hypersensitivity (DTH) skin test response was measured in 22 male triathletes 48h after competing in a half-Ironman triathlon competition compared to controls (11 non-exercising triathletes and 22 moderately trained males). Data from Bruunsgaard *et al.* (1997b). *, $P < 0.05$.

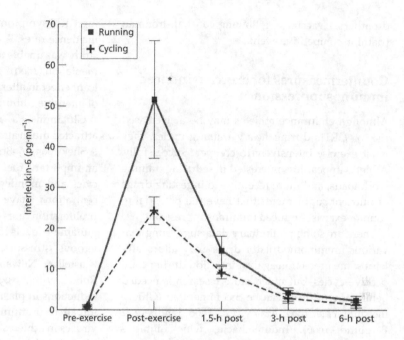

Fig. 50.7 Plasma concentrations of IL-6 were significantly higher following 2.5 h of running compared to cycling at ~75% $\dot{V}_{O_{2max}}$ in 10 triathletes. Data from Nieman *et al.* (1998a).

Decrease in ex vivo *production of cytokines (interferon-γ, IL-1 and IL-6) in response to mitogens and endotoxin*

Several investigators have reported that the mitogen-induced release of various cytokines (in particular, TNF-α, IL-1, IL-2, IL-6, IL-10 and interferon-γ) is suppressed after prolonged and strenuous exercise (Baum *et al.* 1997; Weinstock *et al.* 1997; Smits *et al.* 1998).

Blunted major histocompatibility complex (MHC) II expression in macrophages

The MHC antigens are essential for reactions of immune recognition. Class I MHC antigens play a role in self- and non-self recognition, while class II MHC antigens, found on antigen-presenting cells such as macrophages, assist in the process of cell-mediated immune responses. After phagocytosis and antigen processing, small antigenic peptides are bound to MHC II and presented to T lymphocytes, an important step in adaptive immunity. Woods *et al.* (1997) have demonstrated that exhaustive exercise (2–4 h per day for 7 days) significantly suppresses the expression of MHC II in mice

macrophages, an effect due in part to elevated cortisol levels. These data imply that heavy exertion can blunt macrophage expression of MHC II, negatively affecting the process of antigen presentation to T lymphocytes, and thus their ability to respond to an antigenic challenge (e.g. DTH).

Taken together, these data suggest that the immune system is suppressed and stressed, albeit transiently, following prolonged endurance exercise (Pedersen *et al.* 1998a). Thus it makes sense (but still remains unproven) that URTI risk may be increased when the endurance athlete goes through repeated cycles of heavy exertion, has been exposed to novel pathogens and has experienced other stressors to the immune system including lack of sleep, severe mental stress, malnutrition or weight loss.

Several studies have shown that despite altered immunity following prolonged and intensive exercise, the ability of the immune system to mount an antibody response to vaccination over the 2–4 week postexercise period is not affected. In a study by Bruunsgaard *et al.* (1997b), male triathletes when compared to sedentary controls had normal antibody production to pneumococcal, tetanus and diphtheria vaccines following a half-Ironman triathlon competitive event.

Countermeasures for exercise-induced immunosuppression

Although endurance athletes may be at increased risk of URTIs during heavy training cycles, they must exercise intensively to compete successfully. Athletes appear less interested in reducing training work loads, and more receptive to ingesting drugs or nutrient supplements that have the potential to counter exercise-induced immunosuppression.

There are some preliminary data suggesting that various immunomodulator drugs may afford athletes some protection against infection during competitive cycles, but much more research is needed before any of these can be recommended (Ghighineishvili et al. 1992; Atalay et al. 1996; Lindberg & Berglund 1996). Indomethacin, which inhibits prostaglandin production, has been administered to athletes prior to exercise, or used in vitro to determine whether the drop in NKCA can be countered. Although some success has been reported following 1h of intensive cycling (Pedersen et al. 1996a), indomethacin has had no significant effect in countering the steep drop in NKCA following 2.5h of running (Nieman et al. 1995a).

Investigators have measured the influence of nutritional supplements, primarily zinc (Singh et al. 1994), dietary fat (Venkatraman & Pendergast 1998), vitamin C (Peters et al. 1993, 1996; Nieman et al. 1997b), glutamine (Rowbottom et al. 1995; Castell et al. 1996; Mackinnon & Hooper 1996; Castell & Newsholme 1997; Rohde et al. 1998a) and carbohydrate (Gleeson et al. 1998; Henson et al. 1998, 1999; Nieman 1998b), on the immune and infection response to intense and prolonged exercise (Shephard & Shek 1995, 1998b; Pedersen et al. 1998a).

Several double-blind placebo studies of South African ultramarathon runners have demonstrated that 3 weeks of vitamin C supplementation (doses of about 600 mg·day^{-1}) are related to fewer reports of URTI symptoms (Peters et al. 1993, 1996; Peters-Futre 1997). This has not been replicated, however, by other research teams, and the method of reporting URTI symptoms resulted in unrealistically high incidence rates. A double-blind, placebo-controlled study was unable to establish that vitamin C supplementation (1000 mg·day^{-1} for 8 days) had any significant effect in altering the immune response to 2.5 h of intensive running (Nieman et al. 1997b).

Glutamine, a non-essential amino acid, has attracted much attention by investigators (Shephard & Shek 1995, 1998b; Rohde et al. 1998a). Glutamine is an important fuel along with glucose for lymphocytes and monocytes, and decreased plasma concentrations have a direct effect in lowering proliferation rates of lymphocytes. Reduced plasma glutamine levels have been observed in response to various stressors, including prolonged exercise (Castell & Newsholme 1997; Gleeson et al. 1998; Rohde et al. 1998b). Whether exercise-induced reductions in plasma glutamine levels are linked to impaired immunity and host protection against viruses in athletes is still unsettled, but the majority of studies have not favoured such a relationship (Mackinnon & Hooper 1996; Shewchuk et al. 1997; Rohde et al. 1998a).

Carbohydrate supplementation has been reported to attenuate certain immune changes following prolonged and heavy exertion (Nieman 1998b). Earlier research had established that a reduction in blood glucose levels was linked to hypothalamic–pituitary–adrenal activation, an increased release of adrenocorticotrophic hormone and cortisol, increased plasma growth hormone, decreased insulin and a variable effect on blood epinephrine levels (Murray et al. 1991). Given the link between stress hormones and immune responses to prolonged and intensive exercise, carbohydrate administration was hypothesized to maintain plasma glucose concentrations, attenuate increases in stress hormones and thereby diminish changes in immunity relative to placebo ingestion (Nieman 1998b) (see Fig. 50.8).

This hypothesis was first tested in a group of 30 experienced marathon runners (Nehlsen-Cannarella et al. 1997; Nieman et al. 1997a; Henson et al. 1998). A double-blind, placebo-controlled, randomized study investigated the effect of carbohydrate fluid ingestion on the immune response to 2.5 h of running. In a subsequent study of 10 triathletes, carbohydrate ingestion was studied for its effect on the immune response to 2.5 h of running and cycling (Henson *et al.* 1998, 1999; Nieman *et al.* 1998a). During four sessions, subjects ran on treadmills

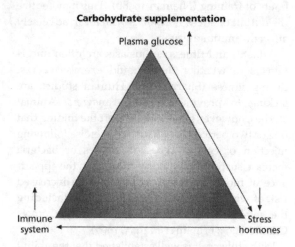

Carbohydrate supplementation

Fig. 50.8 This model suggests that carbohydrate supplementation during prolonged and intensive exercise maintains or elevates plasma glucose concentrations, attenuating the normal rise in stress hormones, and thereby countering negative immune changes.

or cycled using their own bicycles on electro-magnetically braked tripod trainers for 2.5 h at ~75% $\dot{V}o_{2max}$.

Data from these studies indicated that carbo-hydrate beverage ingestion before, during (about $1 \, l \cdot h^{-1}$) and after 2.5 h of exercise was associated with higher plasma glucose levels, an attenuated cortisol and growth hormone response, fewer perturbations in blood immune cell counts, a lesser granulocyte and monocyte phagocytosis and oxidative burst activity, and a diminished pro- and anti-inflammatory cytokine response (Nieman 1998b) (see Fig. 50.9). Overall, the hormonal and immune responses to carbohydrate compared to placebo ingestion suggested that the physiological stress was diminished. Some immune variables were affected slightly by carbohydrate ingestion (for example, granulocyte and monocyte function), whereas others were strongly influenced (e.g. plasma cytokine levels and blood cell counts).

The clinical significance of these carbohydrate-induced effects on the endocrine and immune systems awaits further research. At this point, the data indicate that athletes ingesting carbohydrate beverages before, during and after prolonged and

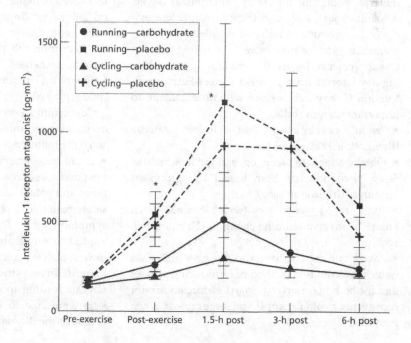

Fig. 50.9 The pattern of change in plasma IL-1 receptor antagonist over time was influenced by carbo-hydrate versus placebo ingestion ($F_{4,36} = 4.80$, $P = 0.003$). *, $P < 0.05$, change from pre-exercise, carbo-hydrate versus placebo.

intensive exercise should experience less physiological stress. Research to determine whether carbohydrate ingestion will improve host protection against viruses in endurance athletes during periods of intensified training or following competitive endurance events is warranted.

Practical recommendations

Although policy recommendations must be considered tentative, the data on the relationship between moderate exercise and lowered risk of URTI are consistent with guidelines urging the general public to engage in near-daily brisk walking (Nieman 1997a). There is reason to believe that endurance athletes who engage in normal training cycles also experience a reduced URTI risk (Shephard et al. 1995).

For athletes undergoing intensive training or engaging in long endurance race events, there is a risk of immune suppression and viral infection. Several lifestyle practices may help to serve as countermeasures (Nieman 1997a).

• Keep other life stresses to a minimum. Mental stress in and of itself has been linked to an increased risk of URTI (Cohen et al. 1991).

• Eat a well-balanced diet to keep vitamin and mineral pools in the body at optimal levels (Chandra 1991). Although there is insufficient evidence to recommend nutrient supplements, ultramarathon runners may benefit by taking vitamin C supplements before ultramarathon races (600 mg·day^{-1} for at least 1 week) (Peters-Futre 1997). Vitamin C may help reduce oxidative damage to important immune cells.

• Avoid overtraining and chronic fatigue (Rowbottom et al. 1995).

• Obtain adequate sleep on a regular schedule. Sleep disruption has been linked to suppressed immunity (Irwin et al. 1992).

• Avoid rapid weight loss (which has also been linked to adverse immune changes) (Nieman et al. 1998b).

• Avoid putting the hands to the eyes and nose (which is a common method of introducing viruses into the body) (Ansari et al. 1991). Before important race events, avoid ill people and large crowds when possible.

• For athletes competing during the winter months, influenza vaccination is recommended (Nieman 1994, 1997a).

• Use carbohydrate beverages before, during and after marathon-type race events or unusually heavy bouts of training (Nieman 1998b). This may reduce the output of stress hormones which can adversely affect the immune system.

Athletes and fitness enthusiasts are often uncertain as to whether they should exercise or rest during illness (Sharp 1989). Human studies are lacking to provide definitive answers. Animal studies, however, generally support the finding that one or two periods of exhaustive exercise following injection of certain types of viruses or bacteria increase susceptibility to infection, with the appearance of more severe symptoms, and an increased risk of widespread infection of the body including the myocardium (Friman & Ilbäck 1992, 1998; Cannon 1993; Friman et al. 1995, 1997).

With athletes, it is well established that the ability to compete is reduced during illness. Also, case histories have shown that sudden and unexplained downturns in athletic performance can sometimes be traced to a recent bout of illness (Sharp 1989). In some athletes, exercising when unwell can lead to a severely debilitated state known as the 'postviral fatigue syndrome' (Behan et al. 1993; Maffulli et al. 1993; Parker et al. 1996). The symptoms of this condition can persist for several months, and include weakness, inability to train hard, easy fatiguability, frequent infections and depression (Budgett 1998).

Concerning exercising when unwell, clinical authorities recommend (Sharp 1989; Friman et al. 1997) the following.

• If one has common cold symptoms (e.g. runny nose and sore throat without fever or general body aches and pains), intensive exercise training may be safely resumed a few days after the resolution of symptoms.

• Mild to moderate exercise (e.g. walking) when unwell with the common cold does not appear to be harmful. In two studies using nasal sprays of a rhinovirus leading to common cold symptoms, subjects were able to engage in exercise during the course of the illness without any adverse effects on either the severity of symptoms or performance capability (Weidner *et al.* 1997, 1998).

• If there are symptoms of fever, extreme tiredness, muscle aches and swollen lymph glands, 2–4 weeks should probably be allowed before resumption of intensive training (Sharp 1989; Friman *et al.* 1997).

Possible indicators of overtraining include immunosuppression with loss of motivation for training and competition, depression, poor performance and muscle soreness. However, at this time, there are no practical markers of immunosuppression (other than infection) that coaches and clinicians can use to indicate that an athlete is overtrained (Shephard & Shek 1998a).

References

Ansari, S.A., Springthorpe, V.S., Sattar, S.A., Rivard, S. & Rahman, M. (1991) Potential role of hands in the spread of respiratory viral infections: studies with human parainfluenza virus 3 and rhinovirus 14. *Journal of Clinical Microbiology* **29**, 2115–2119.

Atalay, M., Marnila, P., Lilius, E.M., Hanninen, O. & Sen, C.K. (1996) Glutathione-dependent modulation of exhausting exercise-induced changes in neutrophil function of rats. *European Journal of Applied Physiology* **74**, 342–347.

Baj, Z., Kantorski, J., Majewska, E. *et al.* (1994) Immunological status of competitive cyclists before and after the training season. *International Journal of Sports Medicine* **15**, 319–324.

Baum, M., Muller-Steinhardt, M., Liesen, H. & Kirchner, H. (1997) Moderate and exhaustive endurance exercise influences the interferon-gamma levels in whole-blood culture supernatants. *European Journal of Applied Physiology* **76**, 165–169.

Behan, P.O., Behan, W.M., Gow, J.W., Cavanagh, H. & Gillespie, S. (1993) Enteroviruses and postviral fatigue syndrome. *Ciba Foundation Symposium* **173**, 146–159.

Belcastro, A.N., Arthur, G.D., Albisser, T.A. & Raj, D.A. (1996) Heart, liver, and skeletal muscle myeloperoxidase activity during exercise. *Journal of Applied Physiology* **80**, 1331–1335.

Brenner, I., Shek, P.N., Zamecnik, J. & Shephard, R.J. (1998) Stress hormones and the immunological responses to heat and exercise. *International Journal of Sports Medicine* **19**, 130–143.

Bruunsgaard, H., Galbo, H., Halkjaer-Kristensen, J., Johansen, T.L., MacLean, D.A. & Pedersen, B.K. (1997a) Exercise-induced increase in serum interleukin-6 in humans is related to muscle damage. *Journal of Physiology (London)* **499** (3), 833–841.

Bruunsgaard, H., Hartkopp, A., Mohr, T. *et al.* (1997b) *In vivo* cell-mediated immunity and vaccination response following prolonged, intense exercise. *Medicine and Science in Sports and Exercise* **29**, 1176–1181.

Budgett, R. (1998) Fatigue and underperformance in athletes: the overtraining syndrome. *British Journal of Sports Medicine* **32**, 107–110.

Bury, T.B., Louis, R., Radermecker, M.F. & Pirnay, F. (1996) Blood mononuclear cell mobilization and cytokines secretion during prolonged exercises. *International Journal of Sports Medicine* **17**, 156–160.

Cannon, J.G. (1993) Exercise and resistance to infection. *Journal of Applied Physiology* **74**, 973–981.

Castell, L.M. & Newsholme, E.A. (1997) The effects of oral glutamine supplementation on athletes after prolonged, exhaustive exercise. *Nutrition* **13**, 738–742.

Castell, L.M., Poortmans, J.R. & Newsholme, E.A. (1996) Does glutamine have a role in reducing infections in athletes? *European Journal of Applied Physiology* **73**, 488–490.

Chandra, R.K. (1991) 1990 McCollum award lecture. Nutrition and immunity: lessons from the past and new insights into the future. *American Journal of Clinical Nutrition* **53**, 1087–1101.

Chao, C.C., Strgar, F., Tsang, M. & Peterson, P.K. (1992) Effects of swimming exercise on the pathogenesis of acute murine *Toxoplasma gondii* Me49 infection. *Clinical Immunology and Immunopathology* **62**, 220–226.

Cohen, S., Tyrrell, D.A. & Smith, A.P. (1991) Psychological stress and susceptibility to the common cold. *New England Journal of Medicine* **325**, 606–612.

Cross, M.C., Radomski, M.W., Vanhelder, W.P., Rhind, S.G. & Shephard, R.J. (1996) Endurance exercise with and without a thermal clamp: effects on leukocytes and leukocyte subsets. *Journal of Applied Physiology* **81**, 822–829.

Davis, J.M., Kohut, M.L., Colbert, L.H., Jackson, D.A., Ghaffar, A. & Mayer, E.P.

(1997) Exercise, alveolar macrophage function, and susceptibility to respiratory infection. *Journal of Applied Physiology* **83**, 1461–1466.

Drenth, J.P., Van Uum, S.H.M., Van Deuren, M., Pesman, G.J., Van Der Ven-Jongekrijg, J. & Van Der Meer, J.W.M. (1995) Endurance run increases circulating IL-6 and IL-1ra but down regulates *ex vivo* TNF-α and IL-1β production. *Journal of Applied Physiology* **79**, 1497–1503.

Eskola, J., Ruuskanen, O., Soppi, E. *et al.* (1978) Effect of sport stress on lymphocyte transformation and antibody formation. *Clinical and Experimental Immunology* **32**, 339–345.

Foster, C. (1998) Monitoring training in athletes with reference to overtraining syndrome. *Medicine and Science in Sports and Exercise* **30**, 1164–1168.

Friman, G. & Ilbäck, N.G. (1992) Exercise and infection—interactions, risks and benefits. *Scandinavian Journal of Medicine and Science in Sports* **2**, 177–189.

Friman, G. & Ilbäck, N.G. (1998) Acute infection: metabolic responses, effects on performance, interaction with exercise, and myocarditis. *International Journal of Sports Medicine* **19** (Suppl. 3), S172–S182.

Friman, G., Wesslen, L., Karjalainen, J. & Rolf, C. (1995) Infectious and lymphocytic myocarditis: epidemiology and factors relevant to sports medicine. *Scandinavian Journal of Medicine and Science in Sports* **5**, 269–278.

Friman, G., Larsson, E. & Rolf, C. (1997) Interaction between infection and exercise with special reference to myocarditis and the increased frequency of sudden deaths among young Swedish orienteers 1979–92. *Scandinavian Journal of Infectious Disease* **104** (Suppl.), 41–49.

Gabriel, H.H., Urhausen, A., Valet, G., Heidelbach, U. & Kindermann, W. (1998) Overtraining and immune system: a prospective longitudinal study in endurance athletes. *Medicine and Science in Sports and Exercise* **30**, 1151–1157.

Gannon, G.A., Rhind, S.G., Suzui, M., Shek, P.N. & Shephard, R.J. (1997) Circulating levels of peripheral blood leucocytes and cytokines following competitive cycling. *Canadian Journal of Applied Physiology* 22, 133–147.

Ghighineishvili, G.R., Nicolaeva, V.V., Belousov, A.J. *et al.* (1992) Correction by physiotherapy of immune disorders in high-grade athletes. *Clinica Terapeutica* 140, 545–550.

Gleeson, M., Pyne, D.B., McDonald, W.A. *et al.* (1996) Pneumococcal antibody responses in élite swimmers. *Clinical and Experimental Immunology* 105, 238–244.

Gleeson, M., Blannin, A.K., Walsh, N.P., Bishop, N.C. & Clark, A.M. (1998) Effect of low- and high-carbohydrate diets on the plasma glutamine and circulating leukocyte responses to exercise. *International Journal of Sport Nutrition* 8, 49–59.

Hack, V., Strobel, G., Weiss, M. & Weicker, H. (1994) PMN cell counts and phagocytic activity of highly trained athletes depend on training period. *Journal of Applied Physiology* 77, 1731–1735.

Haq, A., Al-Hussein, K., Lee, J. & Al-Sedairy, S. (1993) Changes in peripheral blood lymphocyte subsets associated with marathon running. *Medicine and Science in Sports and Exercise* 25, 186–190.

Henson, D.A., Nieman, D.C., Parker, J.C.D. *et al.* (1998) Carbohydrate supplementation and the lymphocyte proliferative response to long endurance running. *International Journal of Sports Medicine* 19, 1–7.

Henson, D.A., Nieman, D.C., Blodgett, A.D. *et al.* (1999) Influence of mode and carbohydrate on the immune response to long endurance exercise. *International Journal of Sport Nutrition*, in press.

Hjertman, J.M.E. & Nieman, D.C. (1999) *Compendium of the Exercise Immunology Literature, 1997–99*. International Society of Exercise and Immunology, Paderborn, Germany.

Hoffman-Goetz, L. (1998) Influence of physical activity and exercise on innate immunity. *Nutrition Reviews* 56, S126–S130.

Hoffman-Goetz, L. & Pedersen, B.K. (1994) Exercise and the immune system: a model of the stress response? *Immunology Today* 15, 382–387.

Irwin, M., Smith, T.L. & Gillin, J.C. (1992) Electroencephalographic sleep and natural killer activity in depressed patients and control subjects. *Psychosomatic Medicine* 54, 10–21.

Jonsdottir, I.H., Johansson, C., Asea, A. *et al.* (1997) Duration and mechanisms of the increased natural cytotoxicity seen after chronic voluntary exercise in rats. *Acta Physiologica Scandinavica* 160, 333–339.

Kohut, M.L., Davis, J.M., Jackson, D.A. *et al.* (1998) The role of stress hormones in exercise-induced suppression of alveolar macrophage antiviral function. *Journal of Neuroimmunology* 81, 193–200.

Lee, D.J., Meehan, R.T., Robinson, C., Mabry, T.R. & Smith, M.L. (1992) Immune responsiveness and risk of illness in US Air Force Academy cadets during basic cadet training. *Aviation, Space, and Environmental Medicine* 63, 517–523.

Lindberg, K. & Berglund, B. (1996) Effect of treatment with nasal IgA on the incidence of infectious disease in world-class canoeists. *International Journal of Sports Medicine* 17, 235–238.

Ljungberg, G., Ericson, T., Ekblom, B. & Birkhed, D. (1997) Saliva and marathon running. *Scandinavian Journal of Medicine and Science in Sports* 7, 214–219.

Mackinnon, L.T. (1997) Immunity in athletes. *International Journal of Sports Medicine* 18 (Suppl. 1), S62–S68.

Mackinnon, L.T. & Hooper, S.L. (1996) Plasma glutamine and URTI during intensified training in swimmers. *Medicine and Science in Sports and Exercise* 28, 285–290.

Mackinnon, L.T., Chick, T.W., Van As, A. & Tomasi, T.B. (1987) The effect of exercise on secretory and natural immunity. *Advances in Experimental Medicine and Biology* 216A, 869–876.

Mackinnon, L.T., Ginn, E.M. & Seymour, G.J. (1993) Temporal relationship between decreased salivary IgA and URTI in élite athletes. *Australian Journal of Science and Medicine in Sport* 25, 94–99.

Mackinnon, L.T., Hooper, S., Jones, S., Gordon, R. & Bachmann, A. (1997) Hormonal, immunological, and hematological responses to intensified training in élite swimmers. *Medicine and Science in Sports and Exercise* 29, 637–645.

Maffulli, N., Testa, V. & Capasso, G. (1993) Post-viral fatigue syndrome. A longitudinal assessment in varsity athletes. *Journal of Sports Medicine and Physical Fitness* 33, 392–399.

Mars, M., Govender, S., Weston, A., Naicker, V. & Chuturgoon, A. (1998) High intensity exercise: a cause of lymphocyte apoptosis? *Biochemical and Biophysical Research Communications* 249, 366–370.

Müns, G. (1993) Effect of long-distance running on polymorphonuclear neutrophil phagocytic function of the upper airways. *International Journal of Sports Medicine* 15, 96–99.

Müns, G., Liesen, H., Riedel, H. & Bergmann, K.-Ch. (1989) Einfluß von Langstreckenlauf auf den IgA-gehalt in Nasensekret und Speichel. *Deutsche Zeitschrift für Sportmedizin* 40, 63–65.

Müns, G., Singer, P., Wolf, F. & Rubinstein, I. (1995) Impaired nasal mucociliary clearance in long-distance runners. *International Journal of Sports Medicine* 16, 209–213.

Murray, R., Paul, G.L., Seifent, J.G. & Eddy, D.E. (1991) Responses to varying rates of carbohydrate ingestion during exercise. *Medicine and Science in Sports and Exercise* 23, 713–718.

Nehlsen-Cannarella, S.L., Fagoaga, O.R., Nieman, D.C. *et al.* (1997) Carbohydrate and the cytokine response to 2.5 hours of running. *Journal of Applied Physiology* 82, 1662–1667.

Nieman, D.C. (1994) Exercise, infection, and immunity. *International Journal of Sports Medicine* 15, S131–S141.

Nieman, D.C. (1997a) Exercise immunology: practical applications. *International Journal of Sports Medicine* 18 (Suppl. 1), S91–S100.

Nieman, D.C. (1997b) Immune response to heavy exertion. *Journal of Applied Physiology* 82, 1385–1394.

Nieman, D.C. (1998a) Effects of athletic training on infection rates and immunity. In Kreider, R.B., Fry, A.C. & O'Toole, M. (eds) *Overtraining in Sport*, pp. 193–217. Human Kinetics, Champaign, IL.

Nieman, D.C. (1998b) Influence of carbohydrate on the immune response to intensive, prolonged exercise. *Exercise Immunology Review* 4, 64–76.

Nieman, D.C. & Nehlsen-Cannarella, S.L. (1991) The effects of acute and chronic exercise on immunoglobulins. *Sports Medicine* 11, 183–201.

Nieman, D.C., Johanssen, L.M., Lee, J.W., Cermak, J. & Arabatzis, K. (1990a) Infectious episodes in runners before and after the Los Angeles Marathon. *Journal of Sports Medicine and Physical Fitness* 30, 316–328.

Nieman, D.C., Nehlsen-Cannarella, S.L., Markoff, P.A. *et al.* (1990b) The effects of moderate exercise training on natural killer cells and acute URTIs. *International Journal of Sports Medicine* 11, 467–473.

Nieman, D.C., Henson, D.A., Gusewitch, G. *et al.* (1993) Physical activity and immune function in elderly women. *Medicine and Science in Sports and Exercise* 25, 823–831.

Nieman, D.C., Ahle, J.C., Henson, D.A. *et*

al. (1995a) Indomethacin does not alter the natural killer cell response to 2.5 hours of running. *Journal of Applied Physiology* **79**, 748–755.

Nieman, D.C., Brendle, D., Henson, D.A. *et al.* (1995b) Immune function in athletes versus nonathletes. *International Journal of Sports Medicine* **16**, 329–333.

Nieman, D.C., Buckley, K.S., Henson, D.A. *et al.* (1995c) Immune function in marathon runners versus sedentary controls. *Medicine and Science in Sports and Exercise* **27**, 986–992.

Nieman, D.C., Simandle, S., Henson, D.A. *et al.* (1995d) Lymphocyte proliferative response to 2.5 hours of running. *International Journal of Sports Medicine* **16**, 404–408.

Nieman, D.C., Fagoaga, O.R., Butterworth, D.E. *et al.* (1997a) Carbohydrate supplementation affects blood granulocyte and monocyte trafficking but not function following 2.5 hours of running. *American Journal of Clinical Nutrition* **66**, 153–159.

Nieman, D.C., Henson, D.A., Butterworth, D.E. *et al.* (1997b) Vitamin C supplementation does not alter the immune response to 2.5 hours of running. *International Journal of Sport Nutrition* **7**, 174–184.

Nieman, D.C., Henson, D.A., Garner, E.B. *et al.* (1997c) Carbohydrate affects natural killer cell redistribution but not activity after running. *Medicine and Science in Sports and Exercise* **29**, 1318–1324.

Nieman, D.C., Nehlsen-Cannarella, S.L., Fagoaga, O.R. *et al.* (1998a) Influence of mode and carbohydrate on the cytokine response to heavy exertion. *Medicine and Science in Sports and Exercise* **30**, 671–678.

Nieman, D.C., Nehlsen-Cannarella, S.L., Henson, D.A., Butterworth, D.E., Fagoaga, O.R. & Utter, A. (1998b) Immune response to exercise training and/or energy restriction in obese women. *Medicine and Science in Sports and Exercise* **30**, 679–686.

Nieman, D.C., Nehlsen-Cannarella, S.L., Henson, D.A., Butterworth, D.E., Fagoaga, O.R. & Utter, A. (1998c) Influence of carbohydrate ingestion and mode on the granulocyte and monocyte response to heavy exertion in triathletes. *Journal of Applied Physiology* **84**, 1252–1259.

Nieman, D.C., Nehlsen-Cannarella, S.L., Fagoaga, O.R. *et al.* (1999a) Immune response to two hours of rowing in female élite rowers. *International Journal of Sports Medicine*, in press.

Nieman, D.C., Nehlsen-Cannarella, S.L.,

Fagoaga, O.R. *et al.* (1999b) Immune function in female élite rowers and nonathletes. *Medicine and Science in Sports and Exercise*, in press.

Northoff, H., Weinstock, C. & Berg, A. (1994) The cytokine response to strenuous exercise. *International Journal of Sports Medicine* **15**, S167–S171.

Ortega, E., Rodriguez, M.J., Barriga, C. & Forner, M.A. (1996) Corticosterone, prolactin and thyroid hormones as hormonal mediators of the stimulated phagocytic capacity of peritoneal macrophages after high-intensity exercise. *International Journal of Sports Medicine* **17**, 149–155.

Ostrowski, K., Rohde, T., Zacho, M., Asp, S. & Pedersen, B.K. (1998) Evidence that interleukin-6 is produced in human skeletal muscle during prolonged running. *Journal of Physiology (London)* **508** (3), 949–953.

Parker, S., Brukner, P. & Rosier, M. (1996) Chronic fatigue syndrome and the athlete. *Sports Medicine, Training and Rehabilitation* **6**, 269–278.

Pedersen, B.K. & Bruunsgaard, H. (1995) How physical exercise influences the establishment of infections. *Sports Medicine* **19**, 393–400.

Pedersen, B.K., Tvede, N., Christensen, L.D., Klarlund, K., Kragbak, S. & Halkjær-Kristensen, J. (1989) Natural killer cell activity in peripheral blood of highly trained and untrained persons. *International Journal of Sports Medicine* **10**, 129–131.

Pedersen, B.K., Bruunsgaard, H., Klokker, M. *et al.* (1996a) Exercise-induced immunomodulation: possible roles of neuroendocrine and metabolic factors. *International Journal of Sports Medicine* **18** (Suppl. 1), S2–S7.

Pedersen, B.K., Rohde, T. & Zacho, M. (1996b) Immunity in athletes. *Journal of Sports Medicine and Physical Fitness* **36**, 236–245.

Pedersen, B.K., Ostrowski, K., Rohde, T. & Bruunsgaard, H. (1998a) Nutrition, exercise and the immune system. *Proceedings of the Nutrition Society* **57**, 43–47.

Pedersen, B.K., Rohde, T. & Ostrowski, K. (1998b) Recovery of the immune system after exercise. *Acta Physiologica Scandinavica* **162**, 325–332.

Peters, E.M., Goetzsche, J.M., Grobbelaar, B. & Noakes, T.D. (1993) Vitamin C supplementation reduces the incidence of postrace symptoms of upper respiratory tract infection in ultramarathon runners. *American Journal of Clinical Nutrition* **57**, 170–174.

Peters, E.M., Goetzsche, J.M., Joseph, L.E.

& Noakes, T.D. (1996) Vitamin C as effective as combinations of anti-oxidant nutrients in reducing symptoms of upper respiratory tract infection in ultramarathon runners. *South African Journal of Sports Medicine* **11** (3), 23–27.

Peters-Futre, E.M. (1997) Vitamin C, neutrophil function, and URTI risk in distance runners: the missing link. *Exercise Immunology Review* **3**, 32–52.

Pyne, D.B. & Gleeson, M. (1998) Effects of intensive exercise training on immunity in athletes. *International Journal of Sports Medicine* **19** (Suppl. 3), S183–S191.

Pyne, D.B., Baker, M.S., Fricker, P.A., McDonald, W.A. & Nelson, W.J. (1995) Effects of an intensive 12-wk training program by élite swimmers on neutrophil oxidative activity. *Medicine and Science in Sports and Exercise* **27**, 536–542.

Raj, D.A., Booker, T.S. & Belcastro, A.N. (1998) Striated muscle calcium-stimulated cysteine protease (calpain-like) activity promotes myeloperoxidase activity with exercise. *Pflügers Archives—European Journal of Physiology* **435**, 804–809.

Rohde, T., MacLean, D.A., Richter, E.A., Kiens, B. & Pedersen, B.K. (1997) Prolonged submaximal eccentric exercise is associated with increased levels of plasma IL-6. *American Journal of Physiology* **273** (1 Pt 1), E85–E91.

Rohde, T., Krzywkowski, K. & Pedersen, B.K. (1998a) Glutamine, exercise, and the immune system—is there a link? *Exercise Immunology Review* **4**, 49–63.

Rohde, T., MacLean, D.A. & Pedersen, B.K. (1998b) Effect of glutamine supplementation on changes in the immune system induced by repeated exercise. *Medicine and Science in Sports and Exercise* **30**, 856–862.

Rowbottom, D.G., Keast, D., Goodman, C. & Morton, A.R. (1995) The haematological, biochemical and immunological profile of athletes suffering from the overtraining syndrome. *European Journal of Applied Physiology* **70**, 502–509.

Sharp, J.C.M. (1989) Viruses and the athlete. *British Journal of Sports Medicine* **23**, 47–48.

Shephard, R.J. & Shek, P.N. (1995) Heavy exercise, nutrition and immune function: is there a connection? *International Journal of Sports Medicine* **16**, 491–497.

Shephard, R.J. & Shek, P.N. (1996) Impact of physical activity and sport on the immune system. *Reviews on Environmental Health* **11**, 133–147.

Shephard, R.J. & Shek, P.N. (1998a) Acute and chronic over-exertion: do depressed immune responses provide useful markers? *International Journal of Sports Medicine* **19**, 159–171.

Shephard, R.J. & Shek, P.N. (1998b) Immunological hazards from nutritional imbalance in athletes. *Exercise Immunology Review* **4**, 22–48.

Shephard, R.J., Kavanagh, T., Mertens, D.J., Qureshi, S. & Clark, M. (1995) Personal health benefits of Masters athletics competition. *British Journal of Sports Medicine* **29**, 35–40.

Shewchuk, L.D., Baracos, V.E. & Field, C.J. (1997) Dietary L-glutamine does not improve lymphocyte metabolism or function in exercise-trained rats. *Medicine and Science in Sports and Exercise* **29**, 474–481.

Shinkai, S., Kurokawa, Y., Hino, S. *et al.* (1993) Triathlon competition induced a transient immunosuppressive change in the peripheral blood of athletes. *Journal of Sports Medicine and Physical Fitness* **33**, 70–78.

Shinkai, S., Kohno, H., Kimura, K. *et al.* (1995) Physical activity and immune senescence in men. *Medicine and Science in Sports and Exercise* **27**, 1516–1526.

Singh, A., Failla, M.L. & Deuster, P.A. (1994) Exercise-induced changes in immune function: effects of zinc supplementation. *Journal of Applied Physiology* **76**, 2298–2303.

Smith, J.A. & Pyne, D.B. (1997) Exercise, training, and neutrophil function. *Exercise Immunology Review* **3**, 96–117.

Smith, J.A., Telford, R.D., Mason, I.B. & Weidemann, M.J. (1990) Exercise, training and neutrophil microbicidal activity. *International Journal of Sports Medicine* **11**, 179–187.

Smits, H.H., Grunberg, K., Derijk, R.H., Sterk, P.J. & Hiemstra, P.S. (1998) Cytokine release and its modulation by dexamethasone in whole blood following exercise. *Clinical and Experimental Immunology* **111**, 463–468.

Steerenberg, P.A., van Asperen, I.A., van Nieuw Amerongen, A., Biewenga, A., Mol, D. & Medema, G.J. (1997) Salivary levels of immunoglobulin A in triathletes. *European Journal of Oral Science* **105**, 305–309.

Tvede, N., Steensberg, J., Baslund, B., Kristensen, J.H. & Pedersen, B.K. (1991) Cellular immunity in highly-trained élite racing cyclists and controls during periods of training with high and low intensity. *Scandinavian Journal of Sports Medicine* **1**, 163–166.

Venkatraman, J.T. & Pendergast, D. (1998) Effect of the level of dietary fat intake and endurance exercise on plasma cytokines in runners. *Medicine and Science in Sports and Exercise* **30**, 1198–1204.

Weidner, T.G., Anderson, B.N., Kaminsky, L.A., Dick, E.C. & Schurr, T. (1997) Effect of a rhinovirus-caused upper respiratory illness on pulmonary function test and exercise responses. *Medicine and Science in Sports and Exercise* **29**, 604–609.

Weidner, T.G., Cranston, T., Schurr, T. & Kaminsky, L.A. (1998) The effect of exercise training on the severity and duration of a viral upper respiratory illness. *Medicine and Science in Sports and Exercise* **30**, 1578–1583.

Weinstock, D., Konig, D., Harnischmacher, R., Keul, J., Berg, A. & Northoff, H. (1997) Effect of exhaustive exercise stress on the cytokine response. *Medicine and Science in Sports and Exercise* **29**, 345–354.

Woods, J.A., Ceddia, M.A., Kozak, C. & Wolters, B.W. (1997) Effects of exercise on the macrophage MHC II response to inflammation. *International Journal of Sports Medicine* **18**, 483–488.

Woods, J.A., Nieman, D.C., Smith, J. & Davis, J.M. (1999) The innate immune response to exercise. *Medicine and Science in Sports and Exercise*, **31**, 57–66.

Chapter 51

Other Health Benefits of Physical Activity

ROY J. SHEPHARD

Introduction

Discussion of the health benefits of sport participation often focuses on the potential of endurance activity to reduce susceptibility to fatal heart attacks, with a resulting extension of longevity in active individuals (Paffenbarger *et al.* 1986, 1994a; Pekkanen *et al.* 1987; Powell *et al.* 1987). From the viewpoint of maximizing lifespan, involvement in sport seems somewhat more effective than participation in other types of endurance activity. The optimal volume of leisure energy expenditure has been estimated at about 8 MJ per week (Paffenbarger *et al.* 1986, 1994a; Chapter 47). If a person initiates such an energy expenditure at the age of 35 years, there is an apparent likelihood that their lifespan will be extended by about 2 years. However, participants in many sports are selected in part on body build, and it is difficult to evaluate how far this may have biased life expectancy (Wilson *et al.* 1990). Sarna *et al.* (1993) found that Finnish endurance athletes lived 5.7 years longer than the general Finnish population, but those who engaged in power sports that demanded a mesomorphic body type had an advantage of only 1.6 years.

Furthermore, the magnitude of any benefit depends on the age when the activity is begun, since the mortality curves for active and sedentary groups tend to come together around 80 years of age (Pekkanen *et al.* 1987). Thus, the initiation of endurance activity at an age of 70 years extends lifespan by only a few months (Paffenbarger *et al.* 1994a), and in the oldest age categories vigorous

exercise may actually shorten a person's lifespan (Linsted *et al.* 1991).

The importance of extending life expectancy by the adoption of regular endurance activity should not be minimized. Nevertheless, such activity yields many other health benefits, some of which are at least as useful as the extension of lifespan. Potential gains may be categorized into conditions where benefit is well established (Table 51.1), those where current evidence of benefit is suggestive (Table 51.2), and those where the evidence is equivocal (Table 51.3) (Shephard 1995a).

In addition to decreasing risks of ischaemic heart disease, hypertension and obesity, a regular programme of moderate physical activity is likely to improve perceived health, to augment respiratory and musculoskeletal function, to extend the period of independence and self-care as a senior citizen, to decrease susceptibility to humoral disorders and neoplasms, to boost immune function and to enhance various aspects of psychological function (Shephard 1985, 1994a; US Surgeon General 1996). Regular exercise may also have a favourable influence on certain aspects of personal lifestyle (Shephard 1989), improving the individual's prospects for future good health. Against these benefits must be weighed some potential negative consequences, seen especially in the athlete who is preparing for very high levels of competition: an increased risk of musculoskeletal injuries, particularly in sports that involve physical contact, a suppression of immune function with an increased risk of infections, and a heavy commitment of time, which in younger competitors

Table 51.1 Conditions where the beneficial effect of regular physical activity is well established.

Coronary heart disease
Hypertension
End-stage renal disease
Type II diabetes mellitus
Osteoporosis
Certain types of neoplasm (colon, breast, reproductive tract)
Surgical trauma
Depression
Anxiety

Table 51.2 Conditions where current evidence is suggestive of a beneficial effect of regular physical activity.

Peripheral vascular disease
Obesity
Chronic phases of rheumatoid and osteoarthritis
Chronic lung disease

Table 51.3 Conditions where evidence concerning the effect of regular physical activity is equivocal.

Cerebrovascular accidents
Type I diabetes
Low back problems
Bladder problems
Immune function
Neuromuscular disorders
Substance abuse
Pregnancy

can have negative consequences for psychosocial development.

Unfortunately, we have relatively little information on the optimal intensity, frequency and duration of conditioning needed to maximize the various potential gains and avoid the negative effects of excessive training (Shephard 1994a, 1997d; US Surgeon General 1996). Often, the competitive athlete may realize greater benefits than the recreational exerciser, because he or she is undertaking a more rigorous programme. However, in some instances, the amount of training that is demanded by international competition may exceed a personal optimum, bringing adverse consequences for both immediate and long-term health (Verde *et al.* 1992).

Quality of life and perceived health

Concept of quality-adjusted lifespan

A person's health-related quality of life is a *Gestalt* that reflects physical, social, emotional and cognitive functioning, personal productivity and intimacy (Shumaker *et al.* 1990). For most people, the integrated product of lifespan and quality of life (the quality-adjusted lifespan) is of more concern than any mere extension of life (Shephard 1982b, 1996b).

Involvement in regular physical activity is particularly effective in increasing a person's quality-adjusted lifespan (Rejeski *et al.* 1996; Shephard 1996b). Personal justification of involvement in a prolonged training programme is made more commonly in terms of 'feeling better' than in anticipation of a simple prolongation of lifespan (Shephard 1994b). Factors contributing to the improved mood state of an exerciser include an enhanced self-concept, a greater sense of self-esteem, perceptions of better physical functioning and an augmented effort tolerance (McAuley 1994; McAuley & Rudolph 1995).

Concept of perceived health

Every person lives at some point on a biological continuum that extends from a state of complete physical, mental and social health to overt illness (Herzlich 1973; Fig. 51.1).

Perceptions of health on a given day, the impact of such perceptions on competitive performance and the likelihood that medical services will be sought all depend on the person's current location along the health–illness continuum. Perceived health has an important bearing on medical costs, since most physician consultations reflect a worsening of perceived health rather than the development of some specific organic disease (Shephard 1986a). Controlled studies of the general population have documented that regular involvement in a moderate endurance training programme reduces the demands for both physician and hospital services,

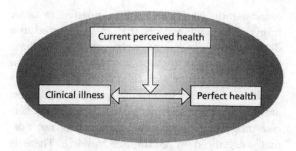

Fig. 51.1 Diagram illustrating the concept of perceived health. An individual lies at some point on a continuum extending from perfect health to clinical illness. The location on this continuum influences the likelihood of symptoms and the demand for medical services. Appropriate amounts of exercise or success in competition, by elevating mood state, may displace perceived health to the right. Conversely, if the demands of the coach exceed the capacity of the individual or the rewards of training seem disappointing, perceived health may be displaced to the left.

with parallel reductions in absenteeism from work and the purchase of non-prescribed medications (Shephard 1986a, 1996a). Moreover, these responses occur within a few months of initiating an exercise programme; thus, they seem likely to reflect an improvement in perceived health, rather than a reduction in the prevalence of organic illness.

Quality of life in endurance athletes

Perceptions of the current quality of life in athletes are shaped by the personal and social gains realized through participation in competitive events, as well as by the more general changes in perceived health and mood state that occur in the recreational exerciser.

Regular endurance exercise and/or competitive success usually displaces personal perceptions of health rightward, in a positive direction (Shephard 1994a), and most competitors regard their health as better than that of their sedentary peers (Shephard et al. 1995). Nevertheless, international athletes are under extreme pressure to produce outstanding performances. Thus, some competitors make strident demands for medical services if they sense even a minor leftward displacement of perceived or objective health, in the direction of clinical illness.

A secretion of β-endorphins contributes to the elevation of mood that is associated with prolonged endurance activity. This has been termed the 'runner's high'. It has the potential to become a dangerous addiction in susceptible individuals (Harber & Sutton 1984; Shephard 1992). The β-endorphin response depends on the intensity and duration of effort. Plasma endorphin levels are thus likely to be much greater in the international athlete than in the recreational exerciser.

Other factors having a positive effect upon arousal and thus mood state during vigorous endurance exercise include a secretion of catecholamines and an increase of neural traffic in the reticular formation of the brain.

As the season develops, both personal satisfaction (a sense of accomplishment and 'self-actualization') and the praise of significant others (such as the coach or team-mates) can further enhance perceived health in a successful competitor. In contrast, if athletic preparation has been pursued to the point of overtraining (Chapter 34), with a decrease in competitive performance, musculoskeletal injuries and a suppression of immune function, then both the perceived and the objectively determined health of the athlete may deteriorate (Verde et al. 1992).

Practical consequences of changes in perceived health

It is difficult to conduct objective studies to examine and interpret changes in an athlete's perceived health.

Some competitors enjoy dangerous pursuits, and in consequence have a high injury rate (Nicholl et al. 1991). But even if it were shown that international competitors made less than average demands for medical services, it could be argued that this advantage had arisen because particularly healthy individuals elected to participate in high-level competition, rather than because endurance training had enhanced perceived or objective health.

Regular participation in moderate endurance activity probably does have a favourable effect on perceived health. On the other hand, overtraining is associated with a higher than normal level of consultations for upper respiratory infections (Nieman *et al.* 1990; Verde *et al.* 1992; Brenner *et al.* 1994), and it may also predispose to more serious conditions, including acute myocarditis (Wesslen *et al.* 1996).

Respiratory function

Many endurance athletes—particularly swimmers and other contestants in events that use the chest muscles—have a very large vital capacity. This is attributable in part to athletic selection, but it also reflects a specific, training-induced strengthening of the thoracic muscles.

Since a person's maximal oxygen transport is usually limited by the pumping ability of the heart rather than by lung capacities (Shephard 1994a; Chapter 3), a large vital capacity might be thought to have no great significance for health. On the other hand, in some old people, the symptom that limits a bout of vigorous exercise is the development of an unacceptable level of breathlessness (Shephard 1993a). Dyspnoea tends to develop when the tidal volume exceeds 50% of a person's vital capacity, so that the individual who has a large vital capacity can tolerate a larger-than-average respiratory minute volume before complaining of dyspnoea. Moreover, if such an individual has the misfortune to contract a chronic respiratory disease, the above-average initial lung capacity may ultimately be important in limiting the extent of disability and the shortening of lifespan.

Still, in too many people, cigarette smoking and a resultant chronic bronchitis or obstructive lung disease cause a substantial decline in vital capacity and other important markers of lung function over the course of adult life. Participation in endurance exercise encourages a lifelong abstinence from cigarettes (Morgan *et al.* 1976; Shephard 1989; Shephard *et al.* 1995), and in part for this reason the age-related decrease of lung function tends to be smaller in athletes than in the general population.

Endurance exercise is a useful form of therapy in chronic respiratory diseases such as asthma, cystic fibrosis and chronic obstructive lung disease. Swimming is particularly helpful for the asthmatic, partly because it teaches breathing control, and partly because it offers physical activity in a humid environment. The moist ambient air helps to loosen mucus and reduces the probability of exercise-induced bronchospasm relative to other forms of physical activity that are performed in a drier atmosphere. Some swimmers with asthma have reached the highest levels of international competition (Morton & Fitch 1990).

Although the symptoms of chronic chest disease are alleviated by participation in a progressive exercise programme, respiratory function is not normally enhanced by endurance training. There is no evidence that rehabilitation programmes that develop cardiovascular or muscular endurance can restore damaged lung tissue. Mechanisms of any observed benefit include: (i) an increase in the mechanical efficiency of physical activity, which reduces the oxygen demands of both limb and chest muscles; (ii) a strengthening of the limb muscles, facilitating their perfusion; this reduces the production of anaerobic metabolites, and thus curbs the respiratory minute volume induced by a given intensity of effort; (iii) a strengthening of the chest muscles; this allows a more rapid inspiration and a slower expiration, reducing the risk of expiratory collapse of the airway; (iv) the postural drainage and encouragement of expectoration associated with vigorous body movements; and (v) psychological factors (including a breaking of the vicious cycle of dyspnoea, fear of exercise, muscular weakness and yet greater dyspnoea) (Shephard 1976; O'Donnell & Webb 1995).

Musculoskeletal factors

Muscle strength

For a number of years, experts in preventive medicine recommended that middle-aged adults should develop cardiovascular endurance, but that they should avoid all forms of exercise designed to strengthen the skeletal muscles.

Several arguments were advanced against muscle-building programmes: (i) the resulting increase in body mass would boost cardiac work rate and overall energy expenditures during most tasks; this in turn would impair athletic performance and predispose to myocardial ischaemia; (ii) the heavy isotonic or isometric straining of a muscle-building regimen might in itself precipitate a heart attack; and (iii) the inclusion of muscle-strengthening exercises would limit the response to an aerobic training programme (Dudley & Fleck 1987).

Some people took the interdiction of muscular conditioning very literally. All of their efforts were concentrated on endurance activities such as distance running. A common consequence of this approach was a weakening of muscles that did not contribute directly to the competitive performance.

Certainly, the athlete who has developed a large lean mass must perform more work than a lighter competitor when it is necessary to displace the body weight against gravity. But if the limb muscles have been strengthened by appropriate muscular training, then the desired body movements can be accomplished with a lesser rise of blood pressure than would be seen in a weaker individual. Since blood pressure is in turn the main determinant of cardiac work rate, the loading of the heart may actually be smaller in a well-muscled subject than in a person whose muscles have been weakened by an exclusive focus upon cardiovascular training. Muscle loss is particularly likely to occur if an athlete is worried about becoming too fat or failing to make a desired weight category (Marquart & Sobal 1994). Gymnasts and ballet dancers are especially vulnerable groups (Davis & Kennedy 1995).

The blood pressure rises progressively during either a sustained isometric contraction or a series of heavy isotonic efforts (Fig. 51.2) (MacDougall *et al.* 1985). However, muscles can be strengthened by quite brief contractions, with extended rest intervals. If such a pattern of training is adopted, and care is taken to avoid straining against a closed glottis, then muscle-building exercise offers little risk to older competitors.

Tendons, ligaments and cartilage

Muscle-training programmes increase the strength not only of muscles, but also of tendons and ligaments (Fig. 51.3). The latter can then withstand larger forces without rupturing or tearing from their points of insertion (Tipton *et al.* 1975). On the other hand, if a ligament or joint capsule has been damaged repeatedly by athletic trauma, it becomes vulnerable to reinjury.

Articular cartilage responds to training in an analogous manner to the tendons. The immediate effect of endurance activity is to decrease the water content of the cartilage and thus its thickness. With repeated bouts of exercise, the cartilage increases in thickness, becoming more resistant to compression, and less vulnerable to tears. On the other hand, both overtraining and repeated local trauma increase the individual's vulnerability to osteoarthritis.

The risk of developing osteoarthritis is highest among participants in team sports that involve

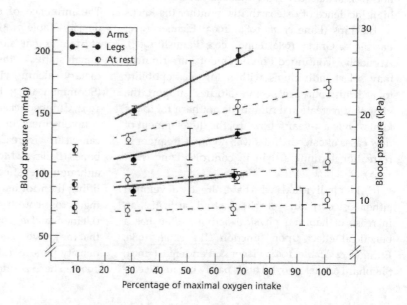

Fig. 51.2 Rise of arterial systolic, mean and diastolic pressures in response to selected intensities of endurance work performed with the arms or the legs and at rest. Data obtained from femoral artery catheterization. From Åstrand and Rodahl (1986), with permission.

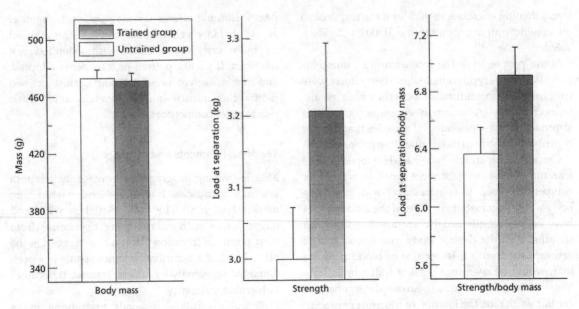

Fig. 51.3 The influence of endurance training on the junctional strength of the medial collateral ligament of rats. The diet of untrained animals was restricted so that the animals in trained and untrained groups were of equal mass. From Tipton *et al.* (1975), with permission.

much body contact (Panush 1994). Runners who are competing at the highest levels of competition may also be vulnerable to subsequent osteoarthritis (Marti *et al.* 1988; Kujala *et al.* 1995). However, retrospective studies of recreational runners do not suggest that such individuals have an unusually high incidence of osteoarthritis in either the knees or the hips (Lane *et al.* 1986, 1993; Eichner 1989; Pascale & Grana 1989; Lane 1992; Panush 1994). Arguably, continued involvement in running may select individuals with a low susceptibility to arthritis, but prospective studies support the view that recreational running is not harmful to the joints. Over a 5-year follow-up, the development of new cases of osteoarthritis was no more frequent in recreational runners than in controls (Lane *et al.* 1993).

In older individuals who have already developed either osteoarthritis or rheumatoid arthritis, an increase of habitual physical activity often has a beneficial effect upon function (Ike *et al.* 1989; Ettinger & Afable 1994; Fisher & Pendergast 1994; Shephard & Shek 1997). This is partly because it cor-

rects muscular weakness associated with over-protection of the patient, and partly because the patient's tolerance of discomfort is increased.

Bone density

The influence of endurance training upon bone density (Table 51.4) depends in part on the volume of training that is undertaken, and in part on nutritional status. Other important variables include dietary calcium, vitamin D and hormonal balance (Suominen 1993; Drinkwater 1994; Loucks *et al.* 1994; Chilibeck *et al.* 1995).

Involvement in moderate recreational activities can clearly increase the density of weight-bearing bones (Bailey & McCulloch 1990; Drinkwater 1994), although the effect is much greater for weight-lifting than for aerobic activities such as orienteering, cross-country skiing, cycling and running (Heinonen *et al.* 1993; Hamdy *et al.* 1994). Provided that the activity is sustained, an above-average bone density persists into old age (Suominen & Rahkila 1991). There is often a specific local strengthening of bone architecture where muscle contractions are resisted (for example, in the playing arm of tennis competitors). In contrast, weight-supported activities such as swimming are sometimes associated with quite low bone densities (Risser *et al.* 1990; Grimston *et al.* 1993).

If conditioning is pursued to the point of developing a negative energy balance, with a reduction in lean tissue mass (Nichols *et al.* 1995) and sex hormone levels (Prior 1990; Smith & Rutherford 1993), then there can be a decrease of bone density, particularly in the vertebrae (Drinkwater *et al.* 1986, 1990; Louis *et al.* 1991). Moreover, such changes may be sufficient to increase susceptibility to stress fractures (Myburgh *et al.* 1990). The adverse effects of heavy training seem more likely to be reversed if normal sex hormone concentrations are restored. However, the precise benefits and risks of specific hormonal supplements (Drinkwater 1994) remain the subject of debate. If oestradiol levels are low, then supplements of calcium and vitamin D alone are not sufficient to prevent adverse changes in bone mineral density (Baer *et al.* 1992). However, the decrease in density of the lumbar spine can be at least partially reversed by intensive exercise (Wolman *et al.* 1990).

Prolongation of independence

The typical senior citizen spends about 10 years with some limitation of daily activity, and a final year of life when a relative or an institution must provide almost total support (Health & Welfare, Canada 1982; Shephard 1997a). There are many reasons for the final years of dependency, sociological, psychological and medical. In some instances, the immediate cause is a clinical catastrophe—a sudden stroke, or the onset of blindness (Robine & Ritchie 1991). But often, the underlying problem is physiological: oxygen transport, muscular strength or flexibility has declined to a level where the individual lacks sufficient residual function to sustain independent living (Bassey *et al.* 1992; Guralnik *et al.* 1993). Much also depends on motivation and the nature of the living environment. Highly motivated seniors whose homes have been well adapted to their needs can continue living

alone despite severe physical handicaps (Shephard 1997a).

The influence of physiological factors may be illustrated by the age-related decline in maximal oxygen intake. Regular endurance training has a substantial impact on the magnitude of this variable. Many of the lighter tasks of daily living require an energy expenditure which is three or four times the resting metabolic rate (3–4 METS, equivalent to an oxygen consumption of 11–14 $ml \cdot kg^{-1} \cdot min^{-1}$). Independence is thus likely to be threatened by severe fatigue if a senior cannot sustain this minimum of oxygen transport (Shephard 1997a).

The average person finds difficulty in maintaining their full maximal oxygen intake for more than a few minutes. It remains possible to deploy about 70% of the maximum value for an hour of vigorous activity, but fatigue develops over an 8-h day if energy demands exceed 40% of maximal aerobic power (Shephard 1994a).

Comparison between endurance athletes and the general population does not suggest that continued participation in endurance sports slows the intrinsic rate of ageing to any great extent (Shephard 1988, 1997a). The rate of loss of aerobic power amounts to 3–4 $ml \cdot kg^{-1} \cdot min^{-1}$ for every 10 years of adult life, both in continuing athletes, compared with about 5 $ml \cdot kg^{-1} \cdot min^{-1}$ in sedentary adults (Kavanagh *et al.* 1989; Shephard 1988). On the other hand, at any given age an appropriately graded programme of endurance sports can increase a person's maximal oxygen intake by up to 10 $ml \cdot kg^{-1} \cdot min^{-1}$, equivalent to some 20 years of rejuvenation in terms of this particular variable (Sidney & Shephard 1978; Shephard 1997a; Fig. 51.4). The physiological status of the endurance athlete at any given age is further enhanced relative to an average person because of initial selection. Thus, in terms of oxygen transport, the endurance competitor should have the functional resources to live independently for many more years than a sedentary individual.

In the age range where the capacity for independent living is likely to be an important practical issue (80 years and above), endurance activity increases overall longevity by no more than a few

Table 51.4 Cross-sectional studies showing influence of sports participation on bone mass. For details of references see primary source, Schoutens et al. (1989), with permission.

Reference	No. of subjects/type of exercise	Sex/mean age (years) of subjects (range) [SD]	Bone studied (technique)*	Results
Tennis players				
Huddlestone et al. (1980)	35 senior tennis players	M (70–84)	Radius (SPA)	Playing side + 11%
Jones et al. (1977)	44 professional tennis players 23 professional tennis players	M/27 (18–50) F/24 (14–34)	Humerus, 11 cm proximal to distal end (X-ray): cortical thickness	Playing side + 34.9% (M); + 28.4% (F)
Montoye (1980)	61 senior tennis players	M/64 [4.4]	Hand-wrist and hand (X-ray) Radius, ulna, humerus (SPA)	Bone width and mineral content greater in dominant limb
Physical activity				
Aloia et al. (1978)	30 marathon runners; 16 controls	M/42 (30–60) [7.7]	Total body calcium (NAA); radius, distal (SPA)	Total body calcium + 11% in marathon runners; radius no difference
Brewer et al. (1983)	42 with history of running > 2 years; 38 physically inactive	F/39 (30–49) [5.8] premenopausal	Phalanx 5th finger, os calcis (X-ray). Radius, distal + midshaft (SPA)	Bone mineral in marathon runners greater in finger and midshaft radius; equal in distal radius; less in os calcis
Cann et al. (1984)	11 amenorrhoeic athletes; 26 premature ovarian failure; 50 controls	F/41.6 (16–49)	Lumbar spine (CT); radius, distal one-third (SPA)	Amenorrhoeic athletes (vs. controls): spinal trabecular bone −24%; radial cortical bone not significantly low

Reference	Subjects	Sex/age	Site (technique)*	Results
Drinkwater et al. (1984)	25 marathon runners: 11 amenorrhoeic (67 km·week⁻¹); 14 cyclic (40 km·week⁻¹)	F/25 [4,5]	Lumbar spine (DPA); radius, 2 sites (SPA)	Bone density L1-L4: cyclic > amenorrhoeic; radius no difference
Laval-Jeantet et al. (1984)	136; five grades of physical activity	F/90 aged 28-40; 17 aged 41 to menopause; 27 menopausal	Vertebra L3 (CT)	Activity level influences vertebral density (especially level 4)
Marcus et al. (1985)	17 marathon runners (less than 3 h), >65 km·week⁻¹; no oestrogen therapy: 11 secondary amenorrhoea; 6 regular menses	F/(20-29)	Lumbar spine (CT); radius (SPA)	Mineral density lumbar spine: menstruating athletes > amenorrhoeic runners. Mineral density radius normal in both groups
Nilsson & Westlin (1971)	9 top rank athletes; 55 athletes; 24 controls exercising; 15 controls	M/22	Femur, distal end (SPA)	Bone density top rank > athletes > controls exercising > controls. Weightlifters + throwers + runners > soccer players + swimmers
Stillman et al. (1986)	19 low activity (mean age 51.5 years); 36 moderate activity (age 53.2 years); 28 high activity (age 43.1 years); no individual > 60 years	F/(30-85)	Radius; distal one-third (SPA)	Bone mineral/bone width adjusted for age and menstrual status: high activity > moderate > low

*Technique for bone mass measurement: CT, computed tomography; DPA, double photon absorptiometry; NAA, neutron activation analysis; SPA, single photon absorptiometry.

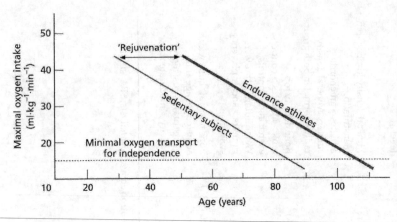

Fig. 51.4 The influence of regular endurance training on the ageing of maximal oxygen intake. The rate of loss of oxygen transport is about $3-4\,ml\cdot kg^{-1}\cdot min^{-1}$ for each 10 years of adult life in both athletes and about $5\,ml\cdot kg^{-1}\cdot min^{-1}$ in their sedentary peers, but regular training can enhance oxygen transport by $10\,ml\cdot kg^{-1}\cdot min^{-1}$, equivalent to a rejuvenation of 20 years with respect to this particular variable. Initial selection further enhances the physiological status of the competitive athlete at any given age.

months (Paffenbarger *et al.* 1986, 1994a; Pekkanen *et al.* 1987). A more important effect of sports participation or vigorous leisure activity is to increase the likelihood that a person will remain in good functional health until close to the time of death. Retrospective questioning of the institutionalized elderly has offered some confirmation of this hypothesis; Shephard and Montelpare (1988) showed that those who were currently unable to care for themselves had a low level of physical activity at the age of 50 years.

Similar arguments may be advanced with regard to the loss of function in other body systems. For example, the independence of an elderly person may be threatened by an inability to lift the body mass from a chair or a toilet seat, or the loss of flexibility in a major joint may make it impossible to dress without assistance (Shephard 1997a). Again, there is good evidence that an appropriate pattern of regular physical exercise can sustain advantages of strength and flexibility equivalent to 10–20 years of rejuvenation (Shephard 1997a).

In the frail elderly, the quality of life can be substantially increased by involvement in a regular exercise programme. However, excessive muscle strengthening may have a less than expected impact on the individual's age of dependency. Indeed, a large lean body mass can lead to a relatively low

peak oxygen transport per unit of body mass, and thus a poor cardiovascular endurance.

Any advantage of flexibility that is shown by an endurance competitor tends to be localized to the joints that are used in a given type of sport. For example, if a competitor has sustained no local injuries or dislocations, involvement in swimming may conserve very flexible shoulder joints to an advanced age.

Metabolic factors and the incidence of humoral disorders

Obesity

Obesity was classically attributed to overeating, but more recent observations have suggested that regular endurance exercise makes an important contribution to the avoidance of obesity. Cross-sectional studies have linked a low body mass index and/or low skinfold readings with reported levels of habitual physical activity or aerobic fitness (Voorips *et al.* 1992; Williamson *et al.* 1993; French *et al.* 1994; DiPietro 1995; Shephard & Bouchard 1995). Moreover, regular physical activity is inversely associated with the undesirable centripetal pattern of fat distribution (Tremblay *et al.* 1990; Seidell *et al.* 1991; Slattery *et al.* 1992). However, cross-sectional associations do not indicate causality, and based on this evidence alone, it might be argued that slimness encouraged physical activity rather than the converse. Most (Klesges *et al.* 1992; French *et al.* 1994; Ching *et al.* 1996) but not all (Williamson *et al.* 1993) longitudinal studies support a causal inference, showing an inverse association between the extent of leisure activity and subsequent weight gain.

Many ways can be suggested whereby participation in endurance exercise might contribute to the avoidance of obesity. In particular: (i) the greater self-esteem of an athlete may avoid the need to seek consolation in snacks and energy-rich 'treats'; (ii) pride may develop in maintaining a trim body form, and this tendency may be reinforced by the advice of a coach; and (iii) large amounts of energy are undoubtedly consumed, both by the performance of prolonged endurance exercise and by the subsequent postexercise stimulation of metabolism (Bielinski *et al.* 1985; Bahr *et al.* 1987; Sedlock 1994).

If a fat-rich diet is consumed (as is commonly the case for American football players), this may discourage overeating, and a smaller percentage of the ingested energy will be absorbed from the intestines. Many endurance competitors prefer to eat a diet that is rich in carbohydrate rather than fat, because they are seeking repeatedly to replenish or to boost their muscle glycogen stores. Nevertheless, a high proportion of energy needs is met by the metabolism of fat in those classes of athlete who pursue individual bouts of exercise to significant glycogen depletion and who exercise for long periods at intensities below the anaerobic threshold.

Some male long-distance runners carry as little as 5% body fat, compared with 20–25% in a sedentary young man. The adverse health consequences of a substantial (20–25 kg) accumulation of body fat have been well documented by actuarial statistics (Society of Actuaries 1959; Metropolitan Life 1983; Andres 1994). The person whose weight for height is much above average (20–30-kg excess) has an increased risk of diabetes, circulatory diseases, pneumonia, influenza, digestive diseases and renal diseases (Society of Actuaries 1959; Metropolitan Life 1983; Andres 1994).

The health impact of smaller accumulations of fat is less clear cut, particularly if body fat content is gauged from weight-for-height tables. Endurance athletes generally have a low weight for height, but some types of competitor have an increased weight for height because they accumulate unusual quantities of lean tissue. In contrast, smokers often have a below-average body mass, and (at least in the general population) a low weight for height may reflect a suboptimal lean tissue mass rather than a low body fat content.

Blood lipids

Regular endurance exercise can have favourable effects on the blood lipid profile. Nevertheless, in practice many endurance training programmes have only a limited impact on blood cholesterol levels, particularly if body mass is held constant. Among possible explanations: (i) the body can alter the amounts of cholesterol excreted via the bile and reabsorbed from the intestines; and (ii) the liver is capable of synthesizing substantial quantities of cholesterol from the normal building blocks of metabolism (acetyl coenzyme A (CoA) and acetyl CoA). However, the very prolonged bouts of running associated with marathon training increase serum concentrations of the useful, scavenging high density lipoprotein (HDL) fraction of cholesterol (particularly the HDL_2 subfraction and its associated apoprotein A-I), while decreasing the concentration of the undesirable low density lipoprotein (LDL) fraction and speeding the clearance of chylomicrons from the circulation (Williams *et al.* 1982; Kavanagh *et al.* 1983; Haskell 1984; Durstine & Haskell 1994; Stefanick & Wood 1994).

These changes seem to be related in part to an increase of lipoprotein lipase (LPL) and lecithin cholesterol acyltransferase (LCAT) activity, with a greater breakdown of triglycerides (Young & Steinhardt 1993; Stefanick & Wood 1994). A decrease of body mass may also be involved, since LDL cholesterol is particularly low in very lean long-distance runners.

Diabetes mellitus

Regular endurance exercise seems helpful in both the prevention (Helmrich *et al.* 1991; Manson *et al.*

1991, 1992) and the treatment of many patients with diabetes mellitus (Leon 1992). Nevertheless, 'diabetes mellitus' is a heterogeneous collection of metabolic disorders, and only certain types of diabetes profit directly from an increase of physical activity.

In the young adult with the autoimmune type I diabetes mellitus, there is a deficiency in circulating insulin, and it is not clearly established that an increase in physical activity can help the course of this form of the disease. It remains quite possible for those with mild diabetes to participate in vigorous endurance sport, but care must be taken to ensure that exercise does not cause a worsening of hyperglycaemia and ketosis. The uptake of insulin from an intramuscular depot may also be accelerated by exercise, and when coupled with an increased rate of carbohydrate usage, this can provoke a hypoglycaemic crisis during or immediately following sustained physical activity. Other immediate dangers of vigorous exercise include retinal detachment, infection of superficial injuries and an increased susceptibility to myocardial infarction. The main value of regular exercise for the young diabetic is in reducing the likelihood of late complications (particularly atherosclerotic heart disease).

In the older person, diabetes mellitus may reflect a decreased sensitivity of the tissues to insulin, or a decreased pancreatic output of insulin. Vigorous endurance exercise is particularly helpful in those with a reduced sensitivity to insulin (Helmrich et al. 1991), and it is most effective before the disease has progressed to the point where insulin treatment is required. Involvement in endurance sport can lower resting blood sugar and increase insulin sensitivity (Gudat et al. 1994; Hespel et al. 1995), in part because of an increased muscle blood flow and an increased transport of glucose into the muscle sarcoplasm during activity (Harris et al. 1987), and in part because of changes in body composition (particularly a reduction in intra-abdominal fat stores). An increase in habitual physical activity reduces and sometimes abolishes the need for insulin injections (Holm & Krotkiewski 1985; Leon 1992; Barnard et al. 1994). However, the glucose tolerance curve is not necessarily normalized as a result of endurance training.

Neoplasms

There has been much discussion about the possible impact of sports participation on the risk of developing a neoplasm (Shephard 1986b, 1993b, 1995b; Lee 1995; US Surgeon General 1996). Divergent conclusions have reflected the wide range of potential neoplasms and the differing categories of athlete that have been investigated.

In some specific situations, the athlete may be at an increased risk of malignancy. Swimmers, dinghy sailors and other participants in water sports have a high exposure to ultraviolet radiation, and thus an above-average risk of skin tumours. Likewise, athletes who have required repeated radiographs because of recurrent injuries may develop neoplasms attributable to local X-irradiation. On the other hand, the endurance competitor is usually at a reduced risk of several types of tumour because of lifelong abstinence from cigarettes.

The end result for the endurance competitor is that the overall risk of malignancy is a little lower than in the general population. One particular component of the reduced risk that has been consistently documented is a reduced incidence of colonic cancers. This could reflect simply differing dietary preferences in an active person with a 'healthy' lifestyle (Willett et al. 1990), but several studies that showed a favourable effect of endurance exercise controlled for diet (US Surgeon General 1996). The main explanation of benefit is probably a prostaglandin-related increase in gastrointestinal motility that is associated with endurance exercise (Cordain et al. 1986) (the 'runner's trots'). As a consequence of increased gastrointestinal motility, toxic materials remain in the large intestine for a shorter time period than would be likely in a sedentary individual.

Some authors have also reported reduced risks of breast, uterine and prostatic cancers among those who engage in endurance activity (Bernstein et al. 1994; Lee 1995; Shephard 1995b; Oliveria et al. 1996). For such lesions, the findings are less unanimous. Possible explanations of any benefit include an exercise-induced decrease in the secretion of sex hormones (particularly as a young adult), and a reduction in body fat depots where carcinogenic oestrones can be synthesized.

Immune function

The acute effect of strenuous and prolonged physical activity is a temporary suppression of immune function. Manifestations include a decrease in the circulating natural killer cell count and activity and a reduction in mucosal levels of immunoglobulin A (IgA) (Pedersen 1997; Shephard 1997b). This response is exacerbated if an athlete faces the added emotional stress of top-level international competition (Laperrière et al. 1994). There is some evidence that the depression of immune response can be sufficient to decrease resistance to infections, at least temporarily (Nieman et al. 1990; Brenner et al. 1994; Peters-Futre 1997). In theory, at least, there might also be a transient increase in susceptibility to neoplasia (Shephard & Shek 1995).

Nevertheless, repeated bouts of endurance exercise reduce the vulnerability of an individual to a given intensity of effort, so that the immune system of a well-trained athlete may be somewhat superior to that of a sedentary individual, both at rest and at a fixed intensity of submaximal exercise (Shephard 1997b). The potential gains of endurance training can be negated if the competitor is perceiving the demands of either training or competition as stressful. Overtraining is also associated with a marked depression of immune function (Verde et al. 1992).

Psychological function

The potential of sport involvement to improve mood state has already been noted. Various cross-sectional population studies have shown associations between physical activity and well-being (Stephens 1988), with a low incidence of depression and anxiety among regular exercisers (Stephens 1988; Weyerer 1992). However, it could be argued that low levels of physical activity were the consequence rather than the cause of impaired psychological health. The beneficial effect of exercise has been less clearly demonstrated in intervention studies, particularly if the subjects have initially been in good psychological health (King et al. 1993;

Landers & Petruzello 1994; Paffenbarger et al. 1994b; Brown et al. 1995).

Participation in endurance sport may induce an increase of self-esteem, because of (i) the approval of significant others (the coach, team-mates, spectators, friends or relatives) or (ii) the satisfaction of personal goals (self-actualization). The first of these influences seems more likely to operate in team and spectator sports than in individual types of physical activity. At the same time, bouts of prolonged vigorous exercise tend to increase the level of cerebral arousal through both an increase of proprioceptive stimulation and an increased output of catecholamines. Finally, prolonged exercise may increase the output of β-endorphins (the 'runner's high'), with a positive influence upon mood state (Harber & Sutton 1984; Shephard 1992).

There have been reports that regular physical activity improves the intellectual performance of young children (Shephard 1997c) and slows the deterioration of neural function in seniors (Shephard & Leith 1990). In young children, the enhanced academic performance has been linked to an increase of body awareness, including a more accurate perception of body dimensions, a better appreciation of the vertical and more accurate finger recognition, in accord with the classical French concept of a linkage between motor and intellectual development (Shephard 1982a). Nevertheless, a number of alternative explanations of the findings remain possible (Shephard 1997c). The optimal pattern of sport for inducing any such an effect has yet to be defined, but if the French hypothesis is well founded, gains of academic performance might be greater in forms of sport that require highly skilled movements than in the repetitive movements typical of many endurance activities.

In older adults, it has been speculated that exercise may help cerebral performance by periodically raising the systemic blood pressure and thus increasing the perfusion of the brain. If this hypothesis is true, the greatest response might be anticipated from sports that demand vigorous muscular straining. However, the exercise-induced rise of blood pressure is usually quite short-lived. Moreover, elderly subjects have shown gains of cerebration in response to cardiovascular endurance-type activities, although increases in cardiorespiratory fitness are not essential to psychological benefit (Landers & Petruzzello 1994). The true explanation of the findings may thus be an increase of arousal, a greater awareness of the surrounding environment, or even an increased interest in life associated with membership of a sports club, rather than an improvement of cerebral perfusion (Dustman *et al.* 1984; Shephard & Leith 1990).

Personal lifestyle

It seems likely that involvement in endurance sport could have a beneficial influence on various aspects of personal lifestyle, such as diet, the consumption of cigarettes, the abuse of alcohol and other drugs, sleep patterns and other variables (Shephard 1989). In practice, the overall impact of sport on lifestyle and thus the risk of future disease is surprisingly small. However, a greater effect has been seen when endurance sports have been distinguished from activities with a strong social context (Perrier 1979).

Some studies suggest that athletes have an above-average tendency to die violent deaths. This has been attributed to their leadership in war, their quest for vertiginous stimulation and their willingness to take risks when driving a vehicle (Polednak 1978).

In the US, there have also been suggestions that by the time that they reach middle-age, former 'major letter' winners are more likely than their non-competitive peers to be overweight, heavy smokers and heavy consumers of alcohol (Montoye *et al.* 1956). This reflects the social nature of many 'major letter' sports, and the relatively short period of active participation. In contrast, cross-country skiers continue vigorous participation to an advanced age, and Scandinavian studies suggest that relatively few members of this group become addicted to cigarettes. In part because they maintain a favourable lifestyle, but also because of an ecto-morphic body build, the cross-country skiers lived several years longer than their sedentary counterparts (Fig. 51.5, Table 51.5, Karvonen *et al.* 1974). Masters athletes (mainly swimmers and distance runners) are also unlikely to be current smokers, although the cessation of smoking in members of this group often antedates their involvement in sport (Shephard *et al.* 1995). Smoking withdrawal

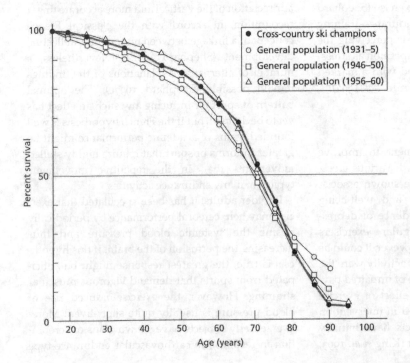

Fig. 51.5 Survival of Finnish male cross-country ski champions (median year of death 1947) compared with three cohorts of the general Finnish male population: 1931–35, 1946–50 and 1956–60. From Karvonen *et al.* (1974), with permission.

Table 51.5 Numbers of Finnish male cross-country skiers surviving at various ages compared with three cohorts of the general Finnish population. Compare with Fig. 51.5. From Karvonen *et al.* (1974), with permission.

Age (years)	Skiers	Total male population		
		1931–35	1946–50	1956–60
15–19	1000	1000	1000	1000
20–24	1000	981	988	995
25–29	982	953	967	987
30–34	963	928	946	976
35–39	945	901	925	964
40–44	917	871	901	946
45–49	872	836	870	923
50–54	847	793	826	887
55–59	800	738	765	832
60–64	738	666	685	753
65–69	672	578	583	646
70–74	527	478	465	515
75–79	397	372	341	368
80–84	224	273	238	228
85–89	113	203	144	120
90–94	38	164	100	63
95–99	38	—	—	43

and sport involvement seem to be expressions of an inherent above-average interest in health (Kavanagh *et al.* 1989).

Conclusion

Involvement in endurance sport induces changes in various body systems that intuitively seem to have a positive value for health. Such a response supplements the well-accepted gains in cardiovascular function with endurance conditioning. However, the dose–response relationship is non-linear, and in high-performance athletes a careful watch must be kept to avoid overtraining. Excessive training not only negates the anticipated gains, but can also have a strongly negative effect upon overall health.

Acknowledgement

The studies of Dr Shephard are supported in part by research grants from the Defence and Civil Institute of Environmental Medicine, Toronto, ON.

References

Andres, R. (1994) Mortality and obesity: the rationale for age-specific height–weight tables. In: Hazzard, W.R., Bierman, E.L., Blass, J.P., Ettinger, W.E. & Halter, J.B. (eds) *Principles of Geriatric Medicine and Gerontology*, pp. 847–853. McGraw-Hill, New York.

Åstrand, P.O. & Rodahl, K. (1986) *Textbook of Work Physiology*, 3rd edn. McGraw-Hill, New York.

Baer, J.T., Taper, L.J., Gwazdaukas, F.G. *et al.* (1992) Diet, hormonal and metabolic factors affecting bone mineral density in adolescent amenorrheic and eumenorrheic female runners. *Journal of Sports Medicine and Physical Fitness* **32**, 51–58.

Bahr, R., Ingnes, I., Vaage, O., Sejersted, O.M. & Newsholme, E.A. (1987) Effect of duration of exercise on excess postexercise O_2 consumption. *Journal of Applied Physiology* **62**, 485–490.

Bailey, D.A. & McCulloch, R.G. (1990) Bone tissue and physical activity. *Canadian Journal of Sport Sciences* **15**, 229–239.

Barnard, R.J., Jung, T. & Inkeles, S.B. (1994)

Diet and exercise in the treatment of NIDDM: the need for early emphasis. *Diabetes Care* **17**, 1469–1472.

Bassey, E.J., Fiatarone, M.J., O'Neill, E.F., Kelly, M., Evans, W.J. & Lipsitz, L.A. (1992) Leg extensor power and functional performance in very old men and women. *Clinical Science* **82**, 321–327.

Bernstein, L., Henderson, B.E., Hamisch, R., Sullivan-Halley, J. & Ross, R.K. (1994) Physical exercise and reduced risk of breast cancer in young women. *Journal of the National Cancer Institute* **86**, 1403–1408.

Bielinski, R., Schutz, Y. & Jéquier, E. (1985) Energy metabolism during the postexercise recovery in man. *American Journal of Clinical Nutrition* **42**, 69–82.

Brenner, I.K.M., Shek, P.N. & Shephard, R.J. (1994) Infection in athletes. *Sports Medicine* **17**, 86–107.

Brown, D.R., Wang, Y., Ward, A. *et al.* (1995) Chronic psychologic effects of exercise and exercise plus cognitive change strategies. *Medicine and Science in Sports and Exercise* **27**, 765–775.

Chilibeck, P.D., Sale, D.G. & Webber, C.E. (1995) Exercise and bone mineral density. *Sports Medicine* **19**, 103–122.

Ching, P.L.Y.H., Willett, W.C., Rimm, E.B., Coldlitz, G.A., Gortmaker, S.L. & Stampfer, M.J. (1996) Activity level and risk of overweight in male health professionals. *American Journal of Public Health* **86**, 25–30.

Cordain, L., Latin, R.W. & Behnke, J.J. (1986) The effects of an aerobic running program on bowel transit time. *Journal of Sports Medicine and Physical Fitness* **26**, 101–104.

Davis, C. & Kennedy, S.H. (1995) Eating disorders in athletes. In: Torg, J. & Shephard, R.J. (eds) *Current Therapy in Sports Medicine 3*, pp. 540–543. B. C. Decker, Toronto.

DiPietro, L. (1995) Physical activity, body weight, and adiposity: an epidemiological perspective. *Exercise and Sport Sciences Reviews* **23**, 275–303.

Drinkwater, B.L. (1994) Physical activity, fitness and osteoporosis. In: Bouchard, C., Shephard, R.J. & Stephens, T. (eds) *Physical Activity, Fitness and Health*, pp.

724–736. Human Kinetics, Champaign, IL.

Drinkwater, B., Nilson, K., Ott, S. & Chestnut, C.H. (1986) Bone mineral density after resumption of menses in amenorrheic athletes. *Journal of the American Medical Association* **256**, 380–382.

Drinkwater, B., Bruemmer, B. & Chestnut, C.H. (1990) Menstrual history as a determinant of current bone density in young athletes. *Journal of the American Medical Association* **263**, 545–548.

Dudley, G.A. & Fleck, S.J. (1987) Strength training and endurance training. *Sports Medicine* **4**, 79–85.

Durstine, J.L. & Haskell, W.L. (1994) Effects of exercise training on plasma lipids and lipoproteins. *Exercise and Sport Sciences Reviews* **22**, 477–521.

Dustman, R.E., Ruhling, R.O., Russell, E.M. *et al.* (1984) Aerobic exercise and improved neuropsychological function of older individuals. *Neurobiology of Aging* **5**, 35–42.

Eichner, E.R. (1989) Does running cause osteoarthritis? An epidemiological perspective. *Physician and Sportsmedicine* **17** (3), 147–154.

Ettinger, W.H. & Afable, R.F. (1994) Physical disability from knee osteoarthritis: the role of exercise as an intervention. *Medicine and Science in Sports and Exercise* **26**, 1435–1440.

Fisher, N.M. & Pendergast, D.R. (1994) Effects of a muscle exercise program on exercise capacity in subjects with osteoarthritis. *Archives of Physical Medicine and Rehabilitation* **75**, 792–797.

French, S.A., Jeffery, R.W., Forster, J.L., McGovern, P.G., Kelder, S.H. & Baxter, J.E. (1994) Predictors of weight change over two years among a population of working adults: the Healthy Worker Project. *International Journal of Obesity* **18**, 145–154.

Grimston, S.K., Willows, N.D. & Hanley, D.A. (1993) Mechanical loading regime and its relationship to bone mineral density in children. *Medicine and Science in Sports and Exercise* **25**, 1203–1210.

Gudat, U., Berger, M. & Lefèbvre, P. (1994) Physical activity, fitness, and non-insulin dependent (type II) diabetes mellitus. In: Bouchard, C., Shephard, R.J. & Stephens, T. (eds) *Physical Activity, Fitness and Health*, pp. 669–683. Human Kinetics, Champaign, IL.

Guralnik, J.M., LaCroix, A.Z., Abbot, R.D. *et al.* (1993) Maintaining mobility in late life. *American Journal of Epidemiology* **137**, 845–857.

Hamdy, R.C., Anderson, S., Whalen, K.E. & Harvill, L.M. (1994) Regional differences in bone density of young men involved in different exercises. *Medicine and Science in Sports and Exercise* **26**, 884–888.

Harber, V.J. & Sutton, J.O. (1984) Endorphins and exercise. *Sports Medicine* **1**, 154–171.

Harris, M.I., Hadden, W.C., Knowler, W.C. & Bennett, P.H. (1987) Prevalence of diabetes and impaired glucose tolerance and plasma glucose levels in US population aged 20–74 yr. *Diabetes* **36**, 523–534.

Haskell, W.L. (1984) The influence of exercise on the concentration of triglyceride and cholesterol in the plasma. *Exercise and Sport Sciences Reviews* **12**, 205–244.

Health & Welfare, Canada (1982) *Canada Health Survey*. Health & Welfare, Canada, Ottawa.

Heinonen, A., Oja, P., Kannus, P., Sievänen, H., Mänttäri, A. & Vuori, I. (1993) Bone mineral density of female athletes in different sports. *Bone and Mineral* **23**, 1–14.

Helmrich, S.P., Ragland, D.R., Leung, R.W. & Paffenbarger, R.S. (1991) Physical activity and reduced occurrence of non-insulin dependent diabetes mellitus. *New England Journal of Medicine* **325**, 147–152.

Herzlich, C. (1973) *Health and Illness*. Academic Press, London.

Hespel, P., Vergauwen, L., Vandenberghe, K. & Richter, E.A. (1995) Important role of insulin and blood flow in stimulating glucose uptake in contracting skeletal muscle. *Diabetes* **44**, 210–215.

Holm, G.A.L. & Krotkiewski, M.J. (1985) Exercise in the treatment of diabetes mellitus. In: Welsh, P. & Shephard, R.J. (eds) *Current Therapy in Sports Medicine*, pp. 105–108. B. C. Decker, Burlington, ON.

Ike, R.W., Lampmann, R.M. & Castor, C.W. (1989) Arthritis and aerobic exercise: a review. *Physician and Sportsmedicine* **17** (2), 128–139.

Karvonen, M.J., Klemola, H., Virkajarvi, J. & Kekkonen, A. (1974) Longevity of endurance skiers. *Medicine and Science in Sports* **6**, 49–51.

Kavanagh, T., Shephard, R.J., Lindley, L.J. & Pieper, M. (1983) Influence of exercise and lifestyle variables upon high density lipoprotein cholesterol after myocardial infarction. *Arteriosclerosis* **3**, 249–259.

Kavanagh, T., Mertens, D. & Shephard, R.J. (1989) Health and aging of Masters athletes. *Clinical Sports Medicine* **1**, 72–88.

King, A.C., Taylor, C.B. & Haskell, W.L. (1993) Effects of differing intensities and formats of 12 months of exercise training on psychological outcomes in older adults. *Health Psychology* **12**, 292–300.

Klesges, R.C., Klesges, L.M., Haddock, C.K. & Eck, L.H. (1992) A longitudinal analysis of the impact of dietary intake and physical activity on weight change in adults. *American Journal of Clinical Nutrition* **55**, 818–822.

Kujala, U.M., Kettunen, J., Paananen, H. *et al.* (1995) Knee osteoarthritis in former runners, soccer players, weight lifters, and shooters. *Arthritis and Rheumatism* **38**, 539–546.

Landers, D.M. & Petruzello, S.J. (1994) Physical activity, fitness and anxiety. In: Bouchard, C., Shephard, R.J. & Stephens, T. (eds) *Physical Activity, Fitness and Health*, pp. 868–882. Human Kinetics, Champaign, IL.

Lane, N.E. (1992) Exercise and osteoarthritis. *Bulletin of Rheumatic Diseases* **41**, 5–7.

Lane, N.E., Bloch, D.A., Jones, N.H. *et al.* (1986) Long-distance running, bone density and osteoarthritis. *Journal of the American Medical Association* **255**, 1147–1151.

Lane, N., Michel, B., Bjorkengren, A. *et al.* (1993) The risk of osteoarthritis with running and aging: a 5 year longitudinal study. *Journal of Rheumatology* **20**, 461–468.

Laperriere, A., Ironson, G., Antoni, M.T., Schneiderman, N., Klimas, N. & Fletcher, M.A. (1994) Exercise and psychoneuroimmunology. *Medicine and Science in Sports and Exercise* **26**, 182–190.

Lee, I.-M. (1995) Exercise and physical health: cancer and immune function. *Research Quarterly* **66**, 286–291.

Leon, A.S. (1992) The role of exercise in the prevention and management of diabetes mellitus and blood lipid disorders. In: Shephard, R.J. & Miller, H. (eds) *Exercise and the Heart in Health and Disease*, pp. 299–368. Marcel Dekker, New York.

Linsted, K.D., Tonstad, S. & Kuzma, J.W. (1991) Self-report of physical activity and patterns of mortality in Seventh-Day Adventist men. *Journal of Clinical Epidemiology* **44**, 355–364.

Loucks, A.B. (1994) Physical activity, fitness and female reproductive morbidity. In: Bouchard, C., Shephard, R.J. & Stephens, T. (eds) *Physical Activity, Fitness and Health*, pp. 943–954. Human Kinetics, Champaign, IL.

Louis, O., DeMeirleir, K., Kalender, W. *et al.* (1991) Low vertebral bone density values in young non-élite female runners. *International Journal of Sports Medicine* **12**, 214–217.

McAuley, E. (1994) Physical activity and psychosocial outcomes. In: Bouchard, C., Shephard, R.J. & Stephens, T. (eds) *Physical Activity, Fitness and Health*, pp.

551–568. Human Kinetics, Champaign, IL.

McAuley, E. & Rudolph, D. (1995) Physical activity, aging and psychological well-being. *Journal of Aging and Physical Activity* **3**, 67–96.

MacDougall, J.D., Tuxen, D., Sale, D.G., Moroz, J.R. & Sutton, J.R. (1985) Arterial blood pressure response to heavy resistance exercise. *Journal of Applied Physiology* **58**, 785–790.

Manson, J.E., Rimm, E.B., Stamfer, M.J. *et al.* (1991) Physical activity and incidence of non-insulin dependent diabetes mellitus in women. *Lancet* **338**, 774–778.

Manson, M.E., Nathan, D.M., Krolewski, A.S. *et al.* (1992) A prospective study of exercise and incidence of diabetes among U.S. male physicians. *Journal of the American Medical Association* **268**, 63–67.

Marquart, L.F. & Sobal, J. (1994) Weight loss beliefs, practices and support systems for high school wrestlers. *Journal of Adolescent Health* **15**, 410–415.

Marti, B., Vader, J.P., Minder, C.E. & Abelin, T. (1988) On the epidemiology of running injuries: the 1984 Bern Grand Prix study. *American Journal of Sports Medicine* **16**, 285–294.

Metropolitan Life (1983) Metropolitan height and weight tables. *Statistical Bulletin of the Metropolitan Life Insurance Co* **64** (2, January–June).

Montoye, H.J., van Huss, W.D., Olson, H., Hudec, A. & Mahoney, E. (1956) Study of longevity and morbidity of college athletes. *Journal of the American Medical Association* **162**, 1132–1134.

Morgan, P., Gildiner, M. & Wright, G. (1976) Smoking reduction in adults who take up exercise: a survey of running clubs for adults. *Canadian Association of Health, Physical Education and Recreation Journal* **42** (5), 39–43.

Morton, A. & Fitch, K. (1990). Exercise-induced bronchial obstruction. In: Torg, J., Welsh, P. & Shephard, R.J. (eds) *Current Therapy in Sports Medicine 2*, pp. 53–59. B. C. Decker, Toronto.

Myburgh, K.H., Hutchins, J., Fataar, A.B., Hough, S.F. & Noakes, T.D. (1990) Low bone density is an etiological factor for stress fractures in athletes. *Annals of Internal Medicine* **113**, 754–759.

Nicholl, J.P., Coleman, P. & Williams, B.T. (1991) Pilot study of the epidemiology of sports injuries and exercise-related morbidity. *British Journal of Sports Medicine* **25**, 61–66.

Nichols, D.L., Sanborn, C.F., Bonnick, S.L., Gench, B. & DiMarco, N. (1995) Relationship of regional body composition to bone mineral density in college females. *Medicine and Science in Sports and Exercise* **27**, 178–182.

Nieman, D.C., Johanssen, L.M., Lee, J.W. & Arabatzis, K. (1990) Infectious episodes in runners before and after the Los Angeles marathon. *Journal of Sports Medicine and Physical Fitness* **30**, 316–328.

O'Donnell, D.E. & Webb, K.A. (1995) Exercise reconditioning in patients with chronic airflow limitation. In: Torg, J. & Shephard, R.J. (eds) *Current Therapy in Sports Medicine 3*, pp. 678–682. B. C. Decker, Toronto.

Oliveria, S.A., Kohl, H.W., Trichopoulos, D. & Blair, S.N. (1996) The association between cardiorespiratory fitness and prostate cancer. *Medicine and Science in Sports and Exercise* **28**, 97–104.

Paffenbarger, R.S., Hyde, R.T., Wing, A.L. & Hsich, C.C. (1986) Physical activity, all-cause mortality and longevity of college alumni. *New England Journal of Medicine* **314**, 606–613.

Paffenbarger, R.S., Hyde, R.T., Wing, A.L., Lee, I.M. & Kampert, J.B. (1994a) Some interrelations of physical activity, physiological fitness, health and longevity. In: Bouchard, C., Shephard, R.J. & Stephens, T. (eds) *Physical Activity, Fitness and Health*, pp. 119–133. Human Kinetics, Champaign, IL.

Paffenbarger, R.S., Lee, I.-M. & Leung, R. (1994b) Physical activity and personal characteristics associated with depression and suicide in American college men. *Acta Psychiatrica Scandinavica* (Suppl. 377), 16–22.

Panush, R.S. (1994) Physical activity, fitness and osteoarthritis. In: Bouchard, C., Shephard, R.J. & Stephens, T. (eds) *Physical Activity, Fitness and Health*, pp. 712–723. Human Kinetics, Champaign, IL.

Pascale, M. & Grana, W.A. (1989) Does running cause osteo-arthritis? An orthopedic perspective. *Physician and Sports Medicine* **17** (3), 156–166.

Pedersen, B.K. (1997) *Exercise Immunology*. R. G. Landes, Georgetown, Texas.

Pekkanen, J., Marti, B., Nissinen, A., Tuomilehto, J., Punsar, S. & Karvonen, M.J. (1987) Reduction of premature mortality by high physical activity: a 20-year follow-up of middle-aged Finnish men *Lancet* **i**, 1473–1477.

Perrier (1979) *The Perrier Study: Fitness in America*. Author, New York.

Peters-Futre, E. (1997) Vitamin C, neutrophil function, and upper respiratory tract infection risk in distance runners: the missing link. *Exercise Immunology Review* **3**, 32–52.

Polednak, A.P. (1978) *The Longevity of Athletes*. C.C. Thomas, Springfield, IL.

Powell, K.E., Thompson, P.D., Caspersen, C.J. & Kendrick, J.S. (1987) Physical activity and the incidence of coronary heart disease. *Annual Reviews of Public Health* **8**, 253–287.

Prior, J.L. (1990) Reproduction: exercise-related adaptations and the health of women and men. In: Bouchard, C., Shephard, R.J., Stephens, T., Sutton, J. & McPherson, B. (eds) *Exercise, Fitness and Health*, pp. 661–676. Human Kinetics, Champaign, IL.

Rejeski, W.J., Brawley, L.R. & Schumaker, S.A. (1996) Physical activity and health-related quality of life. *Exercise and Sport Sciences Reviews* **24**, 71–108.

Risser, W.L., Lee, E.J., LeBlanc, A., Poindexter, H.B., Risser, J.M. & Schneider, V. (1990) Bone density in eumenorrheic female college athletes. *Medicine and Science in Sports and Exercise* **22**, 570–574.

Robine, J.M. & Ritchie, K. (1991) Healthy life expectancy: evaluation of a global indicator of change in population health. *British Medical Journal* **302**, 457–460.

Sarna, S., Sahi, T., Koskenvuo, M. & Kaprio, J. (1993) Increased life expectancy of world class male athletes. *Medicine and Science in Sports and Exercise* **25**, 237–244.

Schoutens, A., Laurent, E. & Poortmans, J.R. (1989) Effect of inactivity and exercise on bone. *Sports Medicine* **7**, 71–81.

Sedlock, D.A. (1994) Fitness level and post-exercise energy expenditure. *Journal of Sports Medicine and Physical Fitness* **34**, 336–342.

Seidell, J.C., Cigolini, M., Deslypere, J.-P., Charzewska, J., Ellsinger, B.-M. & Cruz, A. (1991) Body fat distribution in relation to physical activity and smoking habits in 38-year-old European men. *American Journal of Epidemiology* **133**, 257–265.

Shephard, R.J. (1976) Exercise and chronic obstructive lung disease. *Exercise and Sport Sciences Reviews* **4**, 263–296.

Shephard, R.J. (1982a) *Physical Activity and Growth*. Year Book Publishers, Chicago.

Shephard, R.J. (1982b) Are we asking the right questions? *Journal of Cardiac Rehabilitation* **2**, 21–26.

Shephard, R.J. (1985) The value of physical fitness in preventive medicine. In: Evered, D. & Whelan, J. (eds) *The Value of Preventive Medicine*, pp. 164–182. CIBA Foundation Symposium, Pitman, London.

Shephard, R.J. (1986a) *The Economic Benefits of Endurance Fitness*. Human Kinetics, Champaign, IL.

Shephard, R.J. (1986b) Exercise and malignancy. *Sports Medicine* 3, 235–241.

Shephard, R.J. (1987) *Physical Activity and Aging*. Croom Helm, London.

Shephard, R.J. (1988) The ageing of cardiovascular function. In: Spirduso, W. & Eckert, H.M. (eds) *The Academy Papers. Physical Activity and Aging*, pp. 175–185. Human Kinetics, Champaign, IL.

Shephard, R.J. (1989) Exercise and lifestyle change. *British Journal of Sports Medicine* 23, 11–22.

Shephard, R.J. (1992) Exercise addiction: a dangerous euphoria? In: Shephard, R.J., Anderson, J.A., Eichner, E.R., George, F.J., Sutton, J.R. & Torg, J.S. (eds) *1992 Year Book of Sports Medicine*, pp. xvii–xxvi. Year Book Publishers, Chicago.

Shephard, R.J. (1993a) Aging, respiratory function and exercise. *Journal of Aging and Physical Activity* 1, 59–83.

Shephard, R.J. (1993b) Exercise in the prevention and treatment of cancer: an update. *Sports Medicine* 15, 258–280.

Shephard, R.J. (1994a) *Physical Activity, Fitness and Health*. Human Kinetics, Champaign, IL.

Shephard, R.J. (1994b) Determinants of exercise in people aged 65 years and older. In: Dishman, R. (ed.) *Advances in Exercise Adherence*, pp. 343–360. Human Kinetics, Champaign, IL.

Shephard, R.J. (1995a) Physical activity, fitness and health: the current consensus. *Quest* 47, 288–303.

Shephard, R.J. (1995b) Exercise and cancer: linkages with obesity? *International Journal of Obesity* 19, S63–S68.

Shephard, R.J. (1996a) Financial aspects of employee fitness programs. In: Kerr, J., Griffiths, A. & Cox, T. (eds) *Workplace Health: Employee Fitness and Exercise*, pp. 29–54. Taylor & Francis, London.

Shephard, R.J. (1996b) Physical activity and quality-adjusted lifespan. *Quest* 48, 354–365.

Shephard, R.J. (1997a) *Physical Activity, Aging and Health*. Human Kinetics, Champaign, IL.

Shephard, R.J. (1997b) *Physical Activity, Immune Function and Health*. Cooper Publications, Carmel, IN.

Shephard, R.J. (1997c) Curricular physical activity and academic performance. *Pediatric Exercise Science* 9, 113–126.

Shephard, R.J. (1997d) What is the optimal type of physical activity to enhance health? *British Journal of Sports Medicine* 31, 277–284.

Shephard, R.J. & Bouchard, C. (1995) Relationship between perceptions of physical activity and health-related fitness. *Journal of Sports Medicine and Physical Fitness* 35, 149–158.

Shephard, R.J. & Leith, L. (1990) Physical activity and cognitive changes with aging. In: Howe, M.L., Stones, M.J. & Brainerd, C.J. (eds) *Cognitive and Behavioral Performance Factors in Atypical Aging*, pp. 153–180. Springer-Verlag, New York.

Shephard, R.J. & Montelpare, W.M. (1988) Geriatric benefits of exercise as an adult. *Journals of Gerontology* 43, M86–M90.

Shephard, R.J. & Shek, P.N. (1995) Cancer, immune function and physical activity. *Canadian Journal of Applied Physiology* 20, 1–25.

Shephard, R.J. & Shek, P.N. (1997) Autoimmune disorders, physical activity and training, with particular reference to rheumatoid arthritis. *Exercise Immunology Review* 3, 53–67.

Shephard, R.J., Kavanagh, T. & Mertens, D.J. (1995) Personal health benefits of Master's athletic competition. *British Journal of Sports Medicine* 29, 35–40.

Shumaker, S.A., Anderson, R.T. & Czajkowski, S.M. (1990) Psychological tests and scales. In: Spilker, B. (ed.) *Quality of Life Assessments in Clinical Trials*, pp. 95–113. Raven Press, New York.

Sidney, K.H. & Shephard, R.J. (1978) Frequency and intensity of exercise training for elderly subjects. *Medicine and Science in Sports* 10, 125–131.

Slattery, M.L., McDonald, A., Bild, D.E. *et al.* (1992) Associations of body fat and its distribution with dietary intake, physical activity, alcohol, and smoking in blacks and whites. *American Journal of Clinical Nutrition* 55, 943–950.

Smith, R. & Rutherford, O.M. (1993) Spine and total body bone mineral density and serum testosterone levels in male athletes. *European Journal of Applied Physiology* 67, 330–334.

Society of Actuaries (1959) *Build and Blood Pressure Study*. Society of Actuaries, Chicago.

Stefanick, M.L. & Wood, P.D. (1994) Physical activity, lipid and lipoprotein metabolism, and lipid transport. In: Bouchard, C., Shephard, R.J. & Stephens, T. (eds) *Physical Activity, Fitness and Health*, pp. 417–431. Human Kinetics, Champaign, IL.

Stephens, T. (1988) Physical activity and mental health in the United States and Canada: evidence from four population surveys. *Preventive Medicine* 17, 35–47.

Suominen, H. (1993) Bone mineral density and long-term exercise. An overview of cross-sectional athlete studies. *Sports Medicine* 16, 316–330.

Suominen, H. & Rahkila, P. (1991) Bone mineral density of the calcaneus in 70- to 81-yr-old male athletes and a population sample. *Medicine and Science in Sports and Exercise* 23, 1227–1233.

Tipton, C.M., Matthes, R.D., Maynard, J.A. & Carey, R.A. (1975) The influence of physical activity on ligaments and tendons. *Medicine and Science in Sports* 7, 165–175.

Tremblay, A., Després, J.-P., Leblanc, C. *et al.* (1990) Effect of intensity of physical activity on body fatness and fat distribution. *American Journal of Clinical Nutrition* 51, 153–157.

US Surgeon General (1996) *Physical Activity and Health*. US Department of Health and Human Services, Washington, DC.

Verde, T., Thomas, S. & Shephard, R.J. (1992) Potential markers of overtraining in the distance athlete. *British Journal of Sports Medicine* 26, 167–175.

Voorips, L.E., Meijers, J.H.H., Sol, P., Seidell, J.C. & van Staveren, W.A. (1992) History of body weight and physical activity of elderly women differing in current physical activity. *International Journal of Obesity* 16, 199–205.

Wesslen, L., Pahlson, C., Linquist, O. *et al.* (1996) An increase of unexpected cardiac deaths among young Swedish orienteers during 1979–1992. *European Heart Journal* 17, 902–910.

Weyerer, S. (1992) Physical inactivity and depression in the community: evidence from the Upper Bavarian field study. *International Journal of Sports Medicine* 13, 492–496.

Willett, W.C., Stampfer, M.J., Coldlitz, G.A., Rosner, B.A. & Speizer, F.E. (1990) Relation of meat, fat and fiber intake to the risk of colon cancer in a prospective study among women. *New England Journal of Medicine* 323, 1664–1672.

Williams, P.T., Wood, P.D., Haskell, W.L. & Vranizan, K. (1982) The effects of running mileage and duration on plasma lipoprotein levels. *Journal of the American Medical Association* 247, 2672–2679.

Williamson, D.F., Madans, J., Anda, R.F., Kleinman, J.C., Kahn, H.S. & Byers, T. (1993) Recreational physical activity and ten-year weight change in a US National Cohort. *International Journal of Obesity* 17, 279–286.

Wilson, B.R.A., Olson, H.W., Sprague, H.A., van Huss, W.D. & Montoye, H.J. (1990) Somatotype and longevity of former University athletes and non-athletes. *Research Quarterly* **61**, 1–6.

Wolman, R.L., Clark, P., McNally, E., Harries, M. & Reeve, J. (1990) Menstrual state and exercise as determinants of spinal trabecular bone density in female athletes. *British Medical Journal* **301**, 516–518.

Young, D.R. & Steinhardt, M.A. (1993) The importance of physical fitness versus physical activity for coronary artery disease risk factors: a cross-sectional analysis. *Research Quarterly* **64**, 377–384.

Chapter 52

Overuse Syndromes

ANDREW J. MALLOCH AND JACK E. TAUNTON

Introduction

Endurance athletes aim to train in a way that allows an optimal improvement in performance without any harmful effects. The modern athlete, though, often treads a fine line between maximal beneficial training and overtraining.

A negative response to training may manifest as the more generalized overtraining syndrome or as localized overuse injuries. Overuse injuries from repetitive stress to bone, muscle or tendon result in microtrauma. If the stressful activity continues, damage is cumulative and may exceed the affected tissue's ability to repair.

Over 50% of all sporting injuries are due to overuse (James *et al.* 1978), with most affecting the lower limb. The knee is the commonest site of injury in runners, and patellofemoral pain syndrome (PFPS) is the commonest diagnosis (Clement *et al.* 1981; Macintyre *et al.* 1991; Baquie & Brukner 1997). In team sports, such as soccer, overuse injuries may account for 35% of all injuries seen in a season; they tend to occur mostly during preseason training and at the end of the season (Engstrom *et al.* 1990). Common running-related overuse injuries include PFPS, iliotibial band friction syndrome, tibial stress syndrome, Achilles tendinitis, plantar fasciitis, patellar tendinitis, metatarsal stress syndrome (and stress fractures), tibial stress fracture, tibialis posterior tendinitis and peroneal tendinitis (Clement *et al.* 1981). Examples of non-running overuse injuries include supraspinatus tendinitis, biceps tendinitis and lateral epicondylitis.

As overuse injuries are common and potentially serious, prevention is the ideal. Failing this, early diagnosis and prompt appropriate treatment will nearly always improve prognosis. Treatment is aimed at getting the athlete back to full activity as soon as is appropriate. Unfortunately, recurrence of overuse injuries is common, so the treatment plan should include an assessment of the likely causes of the current injury and of any factors that may make recurrence more likely. The preparticipation sports examination should also include such an assessment and a 'prehabilitation' plan where appropriate.

Prevention of overuse injuries centres on a properly designed training programme as well as the correction of injury-specific risk factors. In this chapter we discuss the principles of training, before moving on to discuss the diagnosis, treatment and prevention of some of the common and more interesting overuse injuries seen in the sports medicine clinic.

Training principles

Training errors have been implicated in many overuse injuries (James *et al.* 1978; Matheson *et al.* 1987; Clement *et al.* 1993), but a properly designed progressive training programme should avoid such hazards.

When an athlete trains, each training stimulus causes protein breakdown, but with some degree of rest, resynthesis and adaptation of the tissue can occur: i.e. hypertrophy of muscle and tendon and an increased bone mass in exercise-specific locations. It is essential therefore for any training programme to incorporate planned rest periods, absolute or relative, as well as variation of training type, intensity and volume if adaptation rather than injury is to result. For the same reason, an individual should not increase his or her training load by more than 10% per week, so that any increase in workload is gradual.

Because each athlete will respond to training at a different rate and each sport has different demands, training programmes should be individualized and sport specific (Kibler & Chandler 1994). Ideally, training should be divided into phases to prepare the athlete for training and competition. Kibler and Chandler (1994) describe the objectives and phases of an optimal training programme as follows.

Objectives

1 General athletic fitness—which lays the foundation for the next training objective.
2 Sport-specific fitness—concentrating on sport-specific muscle flexibility, strength and balance, as well as the patterns of exercise relevant to the sport concerned.
3 Aerobic and/or anaerobic fitness—each sport places different energy demands on the athlete and these can be recreated during training so that the appropriate energy systems are trained. Speed, agility, balance and other skills are also emphasized.

Phases

Volume, intensity and type of work are varied throughout the training cycle. The purpose is to allow the athlete to peak for specific competitions or specific times in the season. Kibler and Chandler (1994) describe five phases in the ideal training cycle:
1 active rest;
2 off-season (general preparation);
3 preseason (specific preparation);
4 early in-season; and
5 late in-season (peaking).

The components and objectives of each phase are described in detail elsewhere (Kibler & Chandler 1994).

Other important areas that should be addressed as part of a complete training package include the training surface and/or environment, shoes (equipment), sport technique and nutrition, abnormalities of which have been implicated in causing overuse injuries. How these factors relate to specific injuries will be discussed below.

Stress fractures

A stress fracture can be defined as a partial or complete fracture of bone that results from repeated application of a stress lower than that required to fracture the bone in a single loading, but in excess of that bone's capacity for repair (Martin & McCulloch 1987).

Stress fractures are common and, in some cases, career-threatening. Therefore, early and accurate diagnosis is important. The injury should be suspected in any athlete presenting with exercise-related pain relieved by rest. The lower limb is the commonest site for stress fractures (Matheson et al. 1987; Clement et al. 1993; Brukner et al. 1996); running and/or jumping are the causal activities in most cases. Stress fractures are also seen in other parts of the body, notably the lower back (Micheli & Wood 1995).

Incidence

Prospective studies of stress fractures are few. One recent study found a stress fracture incidence of 21.1% (or 0.7/1000 training hours) in competitive track and field athletes (Bennell et al. 1996a), whilst another found an incidence of 19% in collegiate track athletes (Johnson et al. 1994). Zernicke et al. (1993) found an incidence (of tibial stress fractures only) of 20% in élite collegiate female runners. Other retrospective studies (Brubaker & James 1974; James et al. 1978; Clement et al. 1981) have found that up to 15% of all injuries to runners are stress fractures.

Many studies of military recruits have shown a higher number of stress fractures in females than in males, but this has not been demonstrated convincingly in athletic populations (Bennell et al. 1996a, reviewed in Brukner & Bennell 1997).

Some stress fractures are common in particular sports:
- femur—more common in runners (Clement *et al.* 1993; Brukner *et al.* 1996);
- tibia and fibula—more common in distance runners (Bennell *et al.* 1996a; Brukner *et al.* 1996);
- navicular—more common in basketball players, sprinters, jumpers and hurdlers (Bennell *et al.* 1996a; Brukner *et al.* 1996);
- pars interarticularis—more common in younger athletes (Micheli & Wood 1995; Brukner *et al.* 1996), especially gymnasts and dancers.

Age and gender patterns are also seen. Stress fractures of the tibia and fibula are more common in younger athletes, whilst fractures of the femur and tarsal bones are more common in older athletes (Matheson *et al.* 1987). Metatarsal fractures are more common in females (Bennell *et al.* 1996a; Brukner *et al.* 1996), but this may be due in part to the high rate of metatarsal fractures in ballerinas who dance *en pointe*; their male counterparts, who do not rise above *demi-pointe*, avoid metatarsal stress fractures (Harrington *et al.* 1993).

In most studies (Taunton *et al.* 1981; Matheson *et al.* 1987; Bennell *et al.* 1996a) the tibia is the commonest site of stress fracture. Other commonly affected bones include the metatarsals, tarsals, femur, fibula, pelvis and spine.

Aetiology

Stress fractures are the result of repetitive, cyclic loading of bone in excess of its functional capacity. Stress is defined as force or load/area, where the force is the sum of internal (muscle) and external (ground reaction) forces. Stress can be either compression or tension, so that in theory, there are several ways to exceed the critical point at which a stress fracture will occur.

1 *The force applied to bone is increased.* Bad technique, increased training load, biomechanical problems or muscle inflexibility may all increase the direct muscle pull across bone, causing a load sufficient to result in stress fracture (Frankel 1978). Muscle fatigue or weakness may lead to decreased shock absorption in the lower limb, resulting in an increased load applied directly to bone (Clement 1975; Frankel 1978).

Running and jumping are both high-impact activities in which increased muscle activity and ground reaction forces apply loads of up to 10 × body weight to the lower limb (Scully & Besterman 1982). These loads can be further increased by changing to a hard running surface or running in inappropriate footwear.

2 *The number of stresses to bone is increased.* The increased number of stresses to bone if running distance is increased too quickly may have a cumulative negative effect, resulting in microfractures which, unless there is a rest period, may progress to stress fracture. A slower increase in training distance allows bone remodelling to occur without damage—an adaptive response.

3 *The surface area over which load is distributed is decreased.* The normal adaptive response of bone to stress involves remodelling such that new bone is deposited in a manner that distributes load efficiently, i.e. form follows function (Wolff's law). Osteoclasts first resorb bone and then osteoblasts lay down new bone in a process that may take 90 days to complete (Johnson 1963). When cortical bone is stressed, the eventual outcome is the laying down of new bone on the compression side of the bone and resorption of bone on the tension side. In the long term this enables bone to handle increased stress, but during remodelling the bone is weakened; resorption temporarily decreases the surface area over which load is distributed, until new bone is laid down. Continued loading may result in microinjury, which may then progress to a stress fracture.

Gradually progressive and varied training programmes with planned rest periods should prevent damage from occurring, and instead allow adaptation (Clement 1987). This point is illustrated by studies which show increased radionuclide uptake in the bones of athletes, representing active, painless remodelling of bone in response to stress (Matheson *et al.* 1987).

Usually, the cause of a stress fracture is multifactorial, with a combination of some or all of the above factors playing some part. Training errors, a change to new shoes and 'alignment problems' would appear to be important in increasing the stress to bone in training athletes (Taunton *et al.* 1981; Matheson *et al.* 1987).

Female athletes suffering from the triad of disordered eating, amenorrhoea and subsequent osteoporosis are at a greatly increased risk of stress fracture (Bennell *et al.* 1996b). Other significant risk factors for stress fractures in female athletes are a lower bone density, a history of menstrual disturbance, less lean mass in the lower limb, a low fat diet and a leg length discrepancy. All of these factors could result in an increased force applied to bone and/or a reduced surface area over which that force is applied.

Anatomical considerations

Some studies suggest that problems such as pes cavus, pronation, lateral tibial torsion, tibia vara, genu varum, genu valgus, subtalar varus, subtalar valgus, leg length discrepancy and Morton's toe increase susceptibility to stress fractures (Taunton *et al.* 1981; Matheson *et al.* 1987; Harrington *et al.* 1993, reviewed in Krivickas 1997). Unfortunately most of these studies are retrospective, and causal relationships are difficult to prove. However, one prospective study did find that leg length discrepancy in females was a significant risk factor (Bennell *et al.* 1996b).

Clinical experience suggests that the above anatomical abnormalities increase stress to bone in a variety of ways, leading to a stress fracture in some individuals, who often have other risk factors (discussed above).

Diagnosis

HISTORY

Exercise-related pain relieved by rest is the usual presenting complaint. At first the pain is a dull ache after exercise, which disappears quickly in the immediate postexercise period. If activity is repeated at the same level, the pain will be slower to resolve postexercise and will also begin to appear during physical activity, at first appearing during the warm-up only. The pain then persists throughout activity and takes longer to settle, adversely affecting athletic performance. Eventually, the pain is present during everyday activities, will not settle with rest, and the athlete starts to limp.

In many cases the pain is well localized to the site of injury, but in some it may be less well so. A stress fracture of the neck of the femur may present as anterior thigh, hip or groin pain in a runner (Clement *et al.* 1993), and a navicular stress fracture as a vague medial arch pain in a sprinter, hurdler or jumper (Clement 1987).

Night pain can occur, but this feature and others such as unexpected weight loss or night sweats should alert the clinician to the possibility of more sinister pathology.

Training errors, inappropriate footwear and a change to a harder training surface may all contribute to the development of a stress fracture, so that a full training history is essential.

There may be a past history or family history of stress fractures, and in females there may be a history of menstrual disturbance, eating disorder or osteoporosis. Nutritional status should be ascertained (especially calcium intake) and past medical history detailed.

EXAMINATION

On examination there will usually be a well-localized tender area overlying the injured bone, with some overlying soft tissue swelling, and occasionally some erythema (Matheson *et al.* 1987). Rarely, callus may be palpable, especially if the presentation is late.

The range of motion at adjacent joints is usually normal, as is muscle power on testing, unless there is related disuse muscle atrophy. There may be a gait disturbance, and pain on hopping if the fracture is of a lower limb bone.

A useful test, especially in stress fractures of the tibia, is the tuning fork test; a tuning fork placed on the skin near a suspected stress fracture will exacerbate pain at the fracture site.

A biomechanical screen may uncover abnormalities which predispose to stress fracture. If a functional biomechanical problem is suspected, the gait and running technique can be assessed directly by the clinician or by video analysis, or it can be assessed indirectly by looking at the wear pattern on the athlete's running shoes.

At-risk stress fractures

Stress fractures of the tibia, fibula and metatarsal shafts can usually be diagnosed on history and physical findings alone, as these bones are easily palpable and the history is relatively straightforward. There are, however, a group of at-risk stress fractures which may present more vaguely; in these, complications are more common, so that a missed diagnosis could prove disastrous.

FEMUR

Femoral stress fractures occur in runners. They may present with vague pain, most commonly in the anterior thigh, but also in the hip or groin (Clement *et al.* 1993). A past history of stress fracture is common. On examination there may be no soft tissue or bony tenderness, and the range of motion at the hip and hip muscle power are usually normal. Hopping on the ipsilateral leg will reproduce the athlete's pain in up to 70% of cases and it may be the only abnormality on examination (Clement *et al.* 1993). Late presentation or delayed diagnosis could result in non-union, malunion, a displaced fracture or avascular necrosis of the femoral head, depending on the site of fracture.

A high index of suspicion is required, and early investigation with bone scan may minimize the risk of missing the diagnosis. Magnetic resonance imaging (MRI) may become the investigation of choice in future. A recent study showed MRI to be as sensitive as but much more specific than bone scan in the diagnosis of hip injuries in athletes (Shin *et al.* 1996).

Treatment will usually involve a period of non-weight-bearing rest, with cautious reintroduc-

tion of weight-bearing as pain and check radiographs dictate. Non-weight-bearing should continue until radiographs show healing is complete. Distraction or tension side fractures of the femur, non-healing compression side fractures and displaced fractures may require internal fixation.

ANTERIOR TIBIA

The tibia is the commonest site for stress fractures. The majority affect the proximal and distal thirds on the compression, or posteromedial, side of the bone. These fractures heal well with conservative treatment.

Some tibial fractures occur in the middle third of the tibia, on the anterior aspect, or tension side of the bone. Pain is usually well localized, with tenderness and overlying soft tissue swelling at the site of fracture. Anterior cortical fracture at this site (the 'dreaded black line') may take a long time to heal, and may progress to complete fracture even with early diagnosis and appropriate conservative treatment. Some authors therefore advocate early operative treatment to prevent complete fracture, especially in élite athletes.

We, however, have seen clinical improvement in these fractures using electromagnetic stimulation 8 h daily for 4–6 weeks.

NAVICULAR

Navicular stress fractures are rare, but should be excluded in any athlete, particularly a sprinter, hurdler or jumper, who complains of medial foot pain. The pain is usually rather vague and gradual in onset, and the athlete often presents late. On examination there may be tenderness over the dorsum of the foot, along the medial side of the longitudinal arch or over the navicular bone itself.

The navicular bone has a zone of relative avascularity in its middle third, which is vulnerable to the repeated loading of running and jumping (Clement 1987). This means that, if a stress fracture occurs, the risks of non-union and/or necrosis are greatly increased, so that a neglected or misdiagnosed fracture could have serious consequences. Unless there is a high index of suspicion with medial foot pain, the diagnosis can easily be missed.

Treatment involves a prolonged period of non-weight-bearing rest and prolonged absence from sport.

Follow-up computerized tomography (CT) scan is important in assessing the severity of the fracture. Those athletes with a complete fracture will require bone grafting and possibly internal fixation.

FIFTH METATARSAL

A fracture of the base of the fifth metatarsal 5 mm distal to the insertion of the peroneus brevis tendon, at the junction of the metaphysis and diaphysis, is termed a Jones' fracture. This fracture is seen mostly in jumpers. It presents with acute or gradual onset lateral foot pain and tenderness near, or over, the base of the fifth metatarsal.

The diagnosis should be suspected and excluded early, so that the common complication of non-union can be avoided (Clement 1987). Internal fixation of this injury is often recommended.

SESAMOIDS

The great toe sesamoids are the other site of stress fractures in the foot. As the sesamoids are weight-bearing points of the forefoot, they are prone to injury. The medial sesamoid is usually involved, and fracture may be associated with a 'turf toe' injury. Presentation is with pain at the first metatarsophalangeal joint. If acute, the injury can mimic gout or cellulitis, with swelling, pain and erythema (Clement 1987). If chronic, the swelling and redness are minimal, but there is still pain with weight-bearing activity.

Conservative treatment using an orthotic with a cut-out under the sesamoids is often useful. However, should non-union occur despite conservative treatment, excision or bone grafting may be required.

PARS INTERARTICULARIS

Away from the lower limb, fracture of the pars interarticularis (spondylolysis) usually of the L5 verte-bra, but also of L3 and L4, is a common cause of back pain in non-endurance athletes, but it is also seen in those involved in endurance sports. This fracture is particularly common in gymnastics and other sports that involve repetitive hyperextension of the lumbar spine. Fast bowlers in cricket often have a unique unilateral pars stress fracture.

The injury is a frequent cause of back pain in athletes 18 years and younger, causing 47% of low back pain in one group of young athletes, compared with only 5% of back pain in adult athletes (Micheli & Wood 1995). Unilateral or bilateral (the problem is commonly bilateral) low back pain which is worse on hip extension while standing on the contralateral leg should prompt investigation to exclude this diagnosis.

Bone scan is positive early in injury, and early diagnosis may prevent progression to a stress fracture. After a positive bone scan, a CT scan is indicated to confirm the diagnosis and characterize any fracture, allowing precise diagnosis and treatment (Congeni *et al.* 1997).

Treatment may involve rest, avoiding painful activities, bracing for a 'prefracture' stress injury or a painful fracture, and strengthening the abdominal musculature.

Differential diagnosis

The differential diagnosis of activity-related bone pain depends on the site of pain but may include such diverse pathologies as sarcoma (and other malignancies), osteomyelitis, osteoid osteoma, compartment syndrome, shin splints, synovitis, Morton's neuroma and a lumbar disc lesion. Sinister pathology is fortunately rare, but must not be forgotten.

Investigation

IMAGING

Plain radiography of the affected area is the first step in investigating a possible stress fracture. Unfortunately, plain radiography has a sensitivity of only 30–70% for all stress fractures (Matheson *et al.* 1987), but as low as 11% (Clement 1987; Matheson *et al.*

1987) in tarsal stress fractures and 24% in femoral stress fractures (Clement *et al.* 1993). Specificity, however, is much higher.

Changes typically seen on plain radiography include new periosteal bone formation, sclerosis, callus formation and a fracture line. Unfortunately it can take up to 3 months for these changes to appear, so that negative initial radiographs do not rule out a stress fracture. One of the benefits of plain radiographs is exclusion of many of the differential diagnoses discussed above. If changes indicative of stress fracture are present, radiography is very specific, so if the fracture is straightforward and does not involve an area prone to complications, investigation may stop with a positive X-ray.

However, many élite athletes are under pressure to perform, and if initial plain radiographs are negative and symptoms do not resolve quickly further investigation is indicated.

The next step is a bone scan. This is almost 100% sensitive in the diagnosis of stress fractures, although it is much less specific (Taunton *et al.* 1981). A bone scan will be positive within 6–72 h of injury, and in some cases early prefracture changes are apparent, allowing intervention and fracture prevention (Matheson *et al.* 1987).

A bone scan involves the intravenous injection of technetium-99 m methylene diphosphonate, which is taken up in rapidly remodelling bone and incorporated into calcium hydroxyapatite crystals. The pattern of uptake is scanned during three phases of uptake—the angiogram, blood pool and delayed static phases.

In stress fracture, all three phases of the bone scan are positive. The characteristic pattern is a focal, ovoid-shaped zone of increased uptake, usually involving one cortex of the bone at the site of pain. Different patterns are seen with soft tissue injuries: for example, in periostitis the increased uptake is more linear, more diffuse and present in the delayed static phase only, whilst other soft tissue injuries show increased uptake in the angiogram and blood pool phases only. Also, old and new lesions can be differentiated on bone scan.

As previously mentioned, the bone scan is less specific than a plain X-ray. Diagnoses such as sarcoma, osteoid osteoma and osteomyelitis cannot be ruled out by bone scan alone, so in many cases further characterization of the lesion is wise if not mandatory.

In many clinics, the next investigation performed after a positive bone scan will be a CT scan, although in some centres MRI is becoming the investigation of choice.

CT scan allows the clinician to look at the injury in greater detail, differentiating a stress reaction from a stress fracture and excluding more sinister pathologies such as osteomyelitis, osteoid osteoma and malignancies. Characteristic signs of stress fracture seen on CT include a linear cortical defect, focal cortical lucency, periosteal new bone, cortical bridging and focal sclerosis. Where radiography has been negative and the bone scan is positive, CT is particularly good at delineating the fracture line in stress fractures of the middle third of the tibia, the navicular and the pars interarticularis region. Accurate diagnosis is essential, as the rehabilitation of a stress injury is very different from that of a stress fracture.

MRI allows finer detail to be seen, but it is expensive and access to MRI is limited; in many centres it may not be an option. However, it is becoming apparent that MRI has much to offer in the diagnosis of stress fractures. Typical changes seen in stress fracture include periosteal and marrow oedema, as well as a fracture line. In some injuries, such as stress fracture of the base of the second metatarsal, MRI is becoming the investigation of choice (Harrington *et al.* 1993), because more detail can be seen (Shin *et al.* 1996; Slocum *et al.* 1997). It is likely that MRI will become the overall investigation of choice in the future.

Other investigations discussed in the literature, such as thermography, are of little use in practice (Matheson *et al.* 1987).

BIOCHEMICAL INVESTIGATIONS

If the history suggests metabolic bone disease or the female athlete triad, bone biochemistry, thyroid function, ovarian function and prolactin levels should be checked, and bone densitometry studies considered.

Treatment

Most stress fractures respond well to conservative treatment, with return to full activity in 6–8 weeks, although longer rest may be required for some fractures. The aim of treatment is to reintroduce sport at a rate that is within the functional capacity of bone, enabling it to meet the required physical stresses. The basic principles of treatment are as follows (Clement 1987; Reeder et al. 1996).

PHASE 1

Pain control
 Physiotherapy
 Non-steroidal anti-inflammatory drugs (NSAIDs)
 Ice massage
 Crutches if pain is very severe
 Pneumatic leg brace in tibial fractures (Swenson et al. 1997)
Physical modalities
 Electromagnetic bone stimulation and ultrasound may aid healing
Modified rest
 Avoiding the causal activity—weight-bearing allowed as pain dictates, but no running or jumping
Maintenance of fitness
Cycling, swimming, running in water
Non-weight-bearing sport-specific skills
Stretching/flexibility/range-of-motion exercises
Local muscle strengthening and retraining.

PHASE 2 FOLLOWS PHASE 1 AFTER 10–14 PAIN-FREE DAYS

Graded reintroduction of the causal activity can now start, initially on alternate days. At first only low-intensity activity is allowed, for example, brisk walking in a runner, but progression to jogging and eventually to running and sprinting is allowed as pain dictates. Once able to run painlessly for 30–45 min, the athlete may progress to functional activities such as hopping and jumping and then onto sport-specific drills.

Frequent assessment is necessary, checking for bony tenderness. Pain at any stage requires rest for 1–2 days and then resumption of rehabilitation at a lower level, before resuming the planned progression of activity. Pain is the guide and controls the rate of progression.

Modification of risk factors such as nutritional deficiency, menstrual disturbance, eating disorder, osteoporosis, biomechanical abnormalities and training errors may help prevent fracture recurrence. Calcium supplementation and hormonal replacement therapy may protect the athlete with osteoporosis from a recurrence.

Treatment of at-risk stress fractures

Treatment of at-risk stress fractures is less straightforward, because of the risk of complications. Successful treatment will often be more aggressive, involving more prolonged non-weight-bearing and earlier surgical intervention. Treatment varies from conservative to surgical, and opinion as to which is most appropriate for a given injury varies from specialist to specialist. What is certain, however, is that all at-risk stress fractures merit specialist care.

Prevention

Prevention of stress fractures involves avoiding the aetiological factors discussed above, if possible.

The importance of an individualized, sport-specific training programme cannot be overemphasized. Exercise loads should be increased only gradually, and rest periods planned. Muscle stretching and strengthening should be part of the training routine, unnecessarily hard running surfaces should be avoided, and appropriate running shoes worn. Fortunately, well-designed training programmes are now the rule rather than the exception.

Education of athletes as to the symptoms of stress fractures, the importance of early diagnosis and the dangers of late presentation may shorten the time to diagnosis.

Biomechanical abnormalities such as pronation and a pes cavus foot may predispose to stress fracture, and their negative effects may be reduced by orthotics and appropriate running shoes. Off-the-shelf orthotics may be sufficient, or made-to-measure orthotics may be required. Most running shoe manufacturers now produce motion control shoes which limit pronation; they may be all that is required for some individuals who overpronate. Leg length discrepancy can be corrected with a heel lift.

The female athlete triad of eating disorder, amenorrhoea and osteoporosis is relatively common. Coaches, athletes and health workers should be aware of this syndrome and its significance, so that affected athletes can be identified and helped to compete safely. The successful management of this difficult problem may include nutritional, hormonal and psychological therapy, as well as training modification (see Chapter 36).

Bennell *et al.* (1996a) suggest that it may be possible to identify female athletes at risk for stress fracture by using age at menarche and calf girth as predictors of risk. Use of this model in their cohort of track and field athletes would have assigned athletes correctly to fracture and non-fracture groups in 80% of cases. Further studies are required to validate this approach.

Conclusion

Stress fractures are common injuries in endurance athletes. A high index of suspicion and early appropriate investigation will improve the prognosis, and in some instances may prevent progression to fracture. Most fractures respond well to conservative treatment, allowing return to full activity in 6–8 weeks.

There is a group of at-risk fractures in which the risks of complications such as non-union, malunion, avascular necrosis and displaced fracture are greatly increased. Awareness of these fractures is necessary to allow early diagnosis and referral for specialist treatment.

Patellofemoral pain syndrome

Patellofemoral pain syndrome (PFPS) is an overuse injury of the knee extensor mechanism, and it is the commonest single overuse injury seen in runners (Clement *et al.* 1981; Macintyre *et al.* 1991; Baquie & Brukner 1997). However, its pathophysiology is not well understood. Previously PFPS was called chondromalacia patellae, but arthroscopic studies have shown that chondromalacia is not present in most cases. The pain of PFPS can be disabling, and can lead to prolonged absence from sport.

Anatomy and aetiology

Most authorities agree that anatomical factors are important in the aetiology of PFPS.

The rectus femoris and vastus lateralis, intermedius and medialis muscles combine to form the quadriceps which is the extensor mechanism of the knee. The quadriceps tendon encases the proximal patella, with retinacula and retinacular thickenings (the patellofemoral ligaments) acting together to guide the patella through the femoral groove during knee flexion and extension.

Quadriceps pull during contraction is oblique, in line with the femoral shaft, and it tends to draw the patella laterally. This lateral pull is countered by the forward prominence of the lateral femoral condyle, the medial patellar retinaculum and the lower fibres of vastus medialis. Vastus medialis is opposed by the lateral pull of the iliotibial tract and the lateral patellar retinaculum, so that if there is an insufficiency of vastus medialis, the patella will be drawn laterally over the lateral femoral condyle during quadriceps contraction. Abnormal tracking over the lateral condyle is thought to result in irritation of the patellar undersurface, and pain. The same effect will be seen with a tight lateral retinaculum or any other factor which alters the angle of pull on the patella during activity. Femoral anteversion, subtalar pronation of the foot, increased Q angle, patella alta, ligamentous laxity and increased height in men have all been implicated in PFPS (reviewed in Krivickas 1997), but there are many studies which find no association between these anatomical factors and PFPS (reviewed in Krivickas 1997).

Training errors such as a sudden increase in training distance/intensity, running on a cambered surface, repetitive hill running, a single severe training session or competition (e.g. running a marathon) and running in inappropriate shoes have all been associated with the development of PFPS (Clement *et al.* 1981).

Diagnosis

HISTORY

The athlete usually presents with gradual onset, rather vague anterior knee pain which appears to be coming from behind the patella. Pain is usually present with activity, and tends to vary in intensity. When running, pain is worse on hills, and walking up or down stairs may also be painful. Pain on standing after a period of sitting (the 'theatre-goer's sign') is often volunteered by the patient as a prominent symptom.

As the condition progresses, the knee may swell from time to time, it may feel unstable and may buckle occasionally as a result of painful reflex inhibition of the knee extensor mechanism. Subluxation, or even dislocation of the patella may occur.

A full training history should be taken to exclude training errors.

EXAMINATION

The athlete should be assessed standing initially, with the observer looking specifically for any increased Q angle, femoral anteversion, genu varum or valgum, foot type, pronation and abnormal tracking of the patella during single leg squatting or stepping. Pelvic tilt when standing should be noted, as it may signify leg length discrepancy or pelvic rotation, both of which can be checked for later in the examination. Hopping and/or squatting may reproduce the athlete's pain. The athlete's running or sports shoes may be examined for abnormal wear patterns, in which case, gait analysis is appropriate. Wasting of the ipsilateral thigh muscles may be apparent with the athlete standing.

If the patient lies supine, thigh girth can be measured and compared with the normal side. Differences of 10 mm represent significant quadriceps wasting (Doxey 1987). Alignment and leg length may also be assessed best with the athlete lying supine. Patellar height may then be assessed, looking for patella alta, or the rarer patella baja. The knee is then examined for signs of effusion; this is rare, but when present may inhibit vastus medialis obliques (VMO) function increasing the tendency of the patella to track laterally.

Patellar tracking can be assessed with the patient lying supine and flexing the knee to 90° from full extension and back again. The patella should track straight through the femoral groove, but in PFPS may track laterally. Crepitation may or may not be present, and this sign correlates poorly with symptoms.

Palpation of the lateral and medial patellar facets and of the lateral retinaculum at its attachment along the lateral patellar border may reproduce the patient's pain. The inferior pole of the patella and patellar tendon should then be palpated, and if tender signify patellar tendinitis. Tenderness of the superior patellar pole is more unusual, but it implies quadriceps tendinitis. If the patella is compressed onto the femur with downward pressure, this may also reproduce the patient's pain. Patellar orientation and glide can be assessed simply (reviewed in Fredericson 1996). Next, the clinician should check for apprehension by trying forcibly to displace the patella laterally while moving the knee from 90 degrees of flexion to full extension. If this manoeuvre gives the patient the sensation of impending dislocation, it is a positive test for apprehension and indicates abnormal patellar mobility.

Meniscal damage, ligamentous laxity and tender plicae should all be looked for and excluded. The hips, lower back and lower limb neurovascular system should also be examined to exclude referred pain as the cause, noting any decreased range of motion, muscle weakness or asymmetry in the lower limb.

Differential diagnosis

Tumour, meniscal injury, quadriceps tendinitis, patellar tendinitis, plica syndrome, osteochondritis dissecans, arthritis, Sinding–Larsen–Johansson and Osgood–Schlatter syndrome in the young and referred pain are all included in the differential diagnosis of anterior knee pain.

Investigation

Plain radiographs of the knee in PFPS are frequently normal, but are indicated if conservative treatment is not quickly effective. Standard anteroposterior (AP), lateral and patellar views allow assessment of the knee joint, patellofemoral joint and the patella, as well as excluding some more sinister pathologies such as a bone tumour. Degenerative change in the knee joint may be seen on the AP views, while degenerative changes in the patellofemoral joint and osteochondritis of the patella may be apparent on the patellar view. Patella alta or baja can be seen in the lateral view.

There is no place for CT or MRI in the investigation of uncomplicated PFPS.

Treatment

Treatment depends on the amount of pain the athlete is experiencing. It may include the following.

Pain-relieving measures. Ice, NSAIDs, taping, physical therapy and physical modalities.

Activity modification. For example, a decrease in training load, avoidance of hills or other aggravating factors.

Quadriceps strengthening. Strengthening of vastus medialis obliques using closed kinetic chain, eccentric drop squats is the cornerstone of treatment in our clinic. The programme we use is 3 × 20 squats daily, starting with slow concentric squats for 5 days, progressing to eccentric drop squats for 5 days. Weight is then added; initially, the athlete carries 2.3 kg (5 lb) in each hand while performing the drop squats. The weight carried is increased by 2.3 kg (5 lb) on each side every 5 days to a usual maximum of 9 kg (20 lb) in each hand. Some pain is likely to be experienced by the athlete initially, so ice, NSAIDs and patellar taping are useful in the early stages of rehabilitation. Increasing pain with the squats may require a day or two of rest before restarting the programme at a lower level. After this 30-day programme, patients move to a maintenance programme which entails doing 3 × 20 drop squats with 9 kg (20 lb) in each hand on alternate days for a number of months.

Knee extensions may be particularly aggravating in PFPS and should be avoided.

Proximal muscle strengthening. Weakness of the gluteus medius can lead to a tight iliotibial band on the affected side. This in turn may cause increased lateral patellar tracking and pain. Lateral leg raises, 3 × 10 daily, with the patient lying on his or her side, raising the leg to the horizontal, increasing the ankle weight by 1/2 kg every 3–5 days to a maximum of 4 kg, will improve gluteus medius strength. The exercise should also be performed on the contralateral side.

Any other proximal muscle weakness uncovered during the examination should be corrected with specific strengthening exercises.

Stretching. Hamstring, calf and iliotibial band stretches are the most important (Fredericson 1996).

Fitness training. Maintenance of cardiovascular fitness is essential for any athlete unable to train normally. Swimming and/or pool running may be all that can be tolerated initially, but cycling may be possible as rehabilitation progresses.

Orthotics. The role of orthotics in the management of PFPS is controversial. Whilst functional orthotics reduce rear foot movement, they have little effect on knee alignment during activity (Smith *et al.* 1986, reviewed in Kilmartin & Wallace 1994), although changes in patellar positioning at rest have been shown (Klingman *et al.* 1997).

Patellar stabilizing brace. Bracing may be useful in individuals with marked lateral tracking and a hypermobile patella that fails to respond to the above measures. However, one recent review concluded that knee braces and sleeves should be avoided in PFPS treatment (Arroll *et al.* 1997).

Surgical treatment. Lateral retinacular release is only indicated when there is a tight lateral retinaculum in intractable PFPS. Exceptionally, more extensive surgery may be required for severe angular or rotational patellar malalignment.

Prevention

Specific measures are unproven, but it seems likely that general measures such as the avoidance of training errors, the correction of biomechanical abnormalities and preseason strengthening may all help prevent PFPS.

Achilles tendon overuse injuries

Any athlete involved in activity which involves repeated lower limb impact loading is at risk of developing an Achilles tendon injury. Frequencies of between 4.7 and 18% (James *et al.* 1978; Krissoff & Ferris 1979; Clement *et al.* 1984; Macintyre *et al.* 1991) have been reported. In one series of 109 runners, training errors were identified as the primary aetiological factor in over 75% of cases (Clement *et al.* 1984).

Treatment of Achilles injuries can be very frustrating for patient and physician alike. The response to treatment in individual patients with seemingly identical injuries is very variable. Prolonged convalescence is not unusual, and recurrence is common.

Anatomy

The Achilles tendon is the common tendon of the gastrocnemius and soleus muscles. It inserts into the posterior superior calcaneus. The gastrocnemius lies superficially in the calf, originating proximally for the medial and lateral femoral condyles as two heads which unite distally and join the tendon of soleus. The soleus arises from the posterior surface of the head and proximal third of the fibula, from the line of the soleus muscle on the tibia and from the tendinous arch between the head of the fibula and the tibia. The plantaris is a small, delicate muscle belly, which originates near the lateral head of gastrocnemius, with a long terminal tendon. Its tendon runs between gastrocnemius and soleus, and inserts

into the medial edge of the Achilles tendon. The plantaris is absent in 5–10% of people.

These three muscles are collectively described as the triceps surae. It is the prime ankle plantar flexor.

There are two bursae which lie near the insertion of the Achilles: the subcutaneous bursa between skin and the tendon, and the retrocalcaneal bursa between the tendon and the calcaneus.

Tendon structure

Tendons are comprised of densely packed collagen and elastic fibres, and proteoglycans. The collagen fibres are grouped into primary bundles which in turn are grouped together to form fascicles. Fascicles are grouped together, forming tertiary bundles which are surrounded by loose connective tissue called the endotenon. This holds the tertiary bundles together, allowing them to move relative to each other, as well as carrying blood vessels, nerves and lymphatics. The entire tendon, comprising tertiary bundles covered by endotenon, is encased by a fine connective tissue sheath, the epitenon. In the Achilles tendon, the epitenon is surrounded by paratenon and the two are collectively referred to as the peritendon. There is a thin layer of fluid between the epitenon and peritenon which reduces friction with tendon movement. The paratenon is replaced by a synovial sheath at various friction or pressure points.

Blood supply to most of the Achilles tendon is good. It derives from small vessels arising from the posterior tibial and peroneal arteries. There is a region of relative avascularity in the Achilles tendon in the area 20–60mm proximal to its insertion (Hastad *et al.* 1959; Lagergren & Lindholm 1959).

Classification of tendon injuries

The following classification was adapted from Puddu *et al.* (1976) and Clancy (1990) by Leadbetter (1993).

PARATENONITIS

Paratenonitis refers to inflammation of the paratenon. It presents as diffuse discomfort within the tendon. In the acute form, there is a swollen, oedematous tendon, associated crepitus and overlying warmth. In chronic cases the paratenon is inflamed and thickened, often being adherent to the underlying tendon.

TENDINOSIS

Tendinosis is characterized by atrophic intratendinous degeneration, which may be caused by microtrauma, ageing or vascular compromise. Unlike paratenonitis, the process is non-inflammatory and is characterized histologically by intratendinous collagen degeneration and fibre disorientation, hypocellularity, scattered vascular ingrowth and occasional local necrosis or calcification. Clinically, there is usually a tendon nodule which may be asymptomatic or point tender, but there is no sheath swelling. Tendinosis may be asymptomatic or painful and may present with tendon rupture.

PARATENONITIS WITH TENDINOSIS

Paratenonitis may be present with tendinosis. The presentation is similar to that of paratenonitis alone, but often there is a palpable tendon nodule.

TENDINITIS

Tendinitis refers to acute overload and some degree of tendon failure. The injury may be anything from an interstitial microinjury to complete rupture of the tendon. Degenerative changes are seen in nearly all ruptured tendons, so it seems likely that tendon failure is the clinical endpoint of a degenerative process (Jarvinen et al. 1997).

Aetiology

The aetiology of tendon injuries is multifactorial, with some or all of the following factors implicated.

AGE

Achilles tendon overuse injuries are commoner in older athletes, perhaps due to decreased local blood flow (Hastad et al. 1959).

BIOMECHANICAL FACTORS

Forefoot and rear foot varus and tibia vara may all cause excessive and prolonged pronation. This produces a whipping action or bowstring effect in the Achilles tendon (Smart et al. 1980). It can cause microtears, resulting in a tendinosis and/or paratenonitis which may eventually lead to partial or complete tendon rupture.

Prolonged pronation also increases internal tibial rotation. This conflicts with the external tibial rotation which occurs as body weight passes over the foot during running. This generates torsional forces which are transmitted through the Achilles tendon, perhaps causing vascular compromise through a 'wringing out' of the tendon vasculature (Smart et al. 1980) in the region of relative avascularity (Hastad et al. 1959; Lagergren & Lindholm 1959). This situation is aggravated in individuals with poor calf flexibility, who compensate for this by increasing pronation still further (Bates et al. 1979).

In a series of 109 patients with Achilles tendon injuries functional overpronation was seen in 56% (Clement et al. 1984).

TRAINING ERRORS

Excessive or sudden increases in training intensity or volume may result in loads in excess of the Achilles tendon's functional capacity. Uphill running also increases Achilles strain. Training errors were found to be the primary aetiological factor in over 75% of cases in one series of 109 Achilles tendon injuries (Clement et al. 1984).

TRAINING SURFACES

Cambered surfaces, uneven terrain, hard surfaces and all-weather tracks have all been implicated in Achilles tendon injury.

SHOE DESIGN

Appropriate footwear is essential to avoid overuse injuries in any sport involving running and/or jumping. For Achilles tendon injuries, the shoe heel is especially important. Ideally, a good shoe should have a firm, well-fitting heel counter and a moderately flared heel.

Inadequate heel wedging may increase the strain in the Achilles tendon; the heel wedge should ideally be maintained at 12–15 mm (Smart *et al.* 1980). Athletes who suddenly change from training shoes to flatter competitive running shoes often experience Achilles problems.

The other important area in the running shoe is under the metatarsal heads. Here, shoe flexibility is essential; otherwise, the lever arm from the ankle is extended out to the forefoot, further increasing Achilles strain.

Motion control shoes are often effective in reducing moderate degrees of pronation.

INDIRECT VIOLENCE

Three types of indirect violence capable of rupturing the Achilles tendon have been identified (Lindholm & Arner 1959):
1 pushing off with the weight-bearing foot while extending the knee, e.g. starting a sprint;
2 unexpected ankle dorsiflexion, where the heel suddenly sinks down, e.g. slipping down a hole in the ground; and
3 violent dorsiflexion of a plantar flexed foot, e.g. jumping and then landing with the foot in plantar flexion.

INACTIVITY

Achilles injuries are common in sedentary individuals who take part in sport sporadically. Such individuals may have a relatively poor basal circulation in the Achilles tendon, so that the region of relative hypovascularity (Hastad *et al.* 1959; Lagergren & Lindholm 1959) is even more vulnerable to ischaemic insult and injury during activity (Jarvinen *et al.* 1997).

IATROGENIC FACTORS

Steroids may interfere with tendon healing and, by relieving symptoms, allow athletes to train with tendon injuries. Both of these effects increase the chance of further injury or tendon rupture.

Fluoroquinilone antibiotics may rarely cause tendon degeneration and rupture, although it is not yet known why this happens.

RHEUMATIC CONDITIONS

Gout, pseudogout, heterotopic ossification, Sever's disease, rheumatoid collagenolysis and ankylosing spondylitis have all been implicated in Achilles tendon disease, causing about 2% of chronic injuries (Jarvinen *et al.* 1997).

Other seronegative arthropathies such as those associated with psoriasis and inflammatory bowel disease can result in an insertional Achilles tendinitis, often with accompanying plantar fasciitis.

HEREDITARY DISEASES WITH DISTURBED COLLAGEN METABOLISM

Conditions such as Ehlers–Danlos syndrome, Marfan syndrome and homocystinuria cause approximately 1% of chronic tendon complaints (Jarvinen *et al.* 1997).

Pathogenesis

Just how the above aetiological factors cause tendon injury is not clear, although it seems that repetitive mechanical loading of the tendon results in a remodelling, or adaptive, response. If the response is insufficient, the remodelling phase results in temporary weakness (Zamora & Marini 1988). If loading continues, this may result in degenerative and inflammatory changes within the tendon, ultimately resulting in an overuse injury (Archambault *et al.* 1995). All of the above-mentioned aetiological factors either increase tendon loading or weaken tendon structure, increasing the chance of injury, rather than successful adaptation for a given exercise load.

The zone of relative hypovascularity 20–60 mm proximal to the Achilles insertion may be further compromised by torsional forces related to increased pronation. Poor perfusion may cause ischaemia–reperfusion injury (Gordon 1991) and increased core tendon temperatures (Wilson & Goodship 1994) during exercise, both of which may result in tendon damage.

Many studies have found that the region of hypovascularity is the commonest site for Achilles tendon rupture (Lindholm & Arner 1959; Gillespie & George 1969; Ralston & Schmidt 1971; Shields *et al.* 1976) so relative ischaemia may well be important in the development of tendon injury. However, two recent studies conflict with this theory, showing uniform blood flow throughout the Achilles tendon (Astrom & Westlin 1994a) and increased blood flow in Achilles tendinopathy (Astrom & Westlin 1994b).

More studies are required before the pathogenesis of overuse Achilles tendon injury is fully understood.

Diagnosis

HISTORY

From the above classification, it is clear that overuse Achilles tendon injuries can present acutely with partial or complete tendon failure, or the process may present only when sporting activity is compromised.

In the latter scenario, the onset of Achilles tendon pain may be insidious and rather poorly localized, rarely stopping the athlete from training in its initial stages. Often, the athlete will complain of pain and stiffness first thing in the morning, and pain after activity which settles quickly. At this stage there are no physical signs. If activity continues, the pain may increase and be present at the beginning of activity, but the athlete can run through the pain and can still continue with normal training/competition. The pain is still present after activity and takes longer to settle.

As things progress, the pain becomes more prominent, appearing during activity and lasting for days despite rest. Any return to activity is thwarted by the recurrence of pain. Finally, the pain is present with ordinary daily activities, may be present at rest and is commonly present at night. The athlete is unable to train or compete.

If the athlete presents acutely, the pain is usually constant and relatively severe, with the athlete unable to train normally. Just walking may be difficult if a partial or complete rupture has occurred.

A detailed training history including the types of training surface may give clues to diagnosis and aeti-

ology. A past medical history is essential to exclude those systemic illnesses listed as aetiological factors above. Previous injuries and past treatment with steroids are also important factors to ask about.

EXAMINATION

With the patient standing, pronation can be assessed, if present, and gross swelling of the Achilles tendon may be apparent. A biomechanical screen may reveal other abnormalities. The athlete's running shoes should be checked for abnormal wear and, if indicated, a gait analysis should be performed.

Gross structure and function are best assessed by comparing the injured with the contralateral tendon. Palpation for crepitus, nodules and local or generalized tenderness should be through a full range of motion. Gastrocnemius and soleus flexibility is best assessed with the patient sitting. A minimum of 10° of dorsiflexion is a prerequisite for running activities.

Paratenonitis and paratenonitis with tendinosis are characterized by inflammation and thickening of the paratenon, often accompanied by crepitus.

Tendinosis is characteristically asymptomatic, with no abnormal physical findings until partial or complete tendon rupture occurs. However, in some patients tendinosis results in the formation of palpable nodules, which can be painful and tender to touch.

Insertional tendinitis is characterized by tenderness at the Achilles insertion. It is often accompanied by retrocalcaneal bursitis and prominence of the posterosuperior aspect of the calcaneus. The pain of bursitis can be elicited by compressing the region between the Achilles tendon insertion and the os calcis between two fingers.

Partial tendon rupture is often painful, with stabbing pain during activity. Local areas of tendon thickening or nodules are often palpable on examination.

Complete rupture is often painless in the initial stages, but the patient may report an audible snap or a sensation of being 'shot' in the back of the leg at the time of injury. Initially, a gap in the tendon may be palpable, but after 24 h or so the gap becomes obscured by swelling. The patient can often plantar flex to some degree, due to the action of the secondary plantar flexors, but powerful plantar flexion is usually impossible. If the patient can walk, he or she may do so with a flat-footed gait and with no 'toe-off' from the stance phase (Hoppenfeld 1976). Thompson's squeeze test is abnormal. For this test the patient is asked to kneel on a seat, with both feet suspended over the edge, while facing away from the examiner who then squeezes the medial and lateral heads of gastrocnemius together. Usually this test results in plantar flexion, but in rupture of the Achilles tendon plantar flexion will be absent or greatly reduced in the affected limb.

Differential diagnosis

The differential diagnosis includes tumour, calcaneal pain (e.g. bone bruise, stress fracture or exostosis), Sever's disease, plantar fasciitis, retrocalcaneal and subcutaneous bursitis, nerve entrapment, rupture of soleus or the medial head of gastrocnemius, tibial stress fractures and posterior tibial stress syndrome.

Investigation

The diagnosis is primarily clinical.

Plain radiography is usually normal, occasionally showing a Haglund's deformity (a posterosuperior calcaneal prominence).

Ultrasound is the investigation of choice in our clinic. It can be used to image Achilles tendon disease accurately, allowing precise diagnosis and optimum treatment (Mafulli *et al.* 1987).

In centres with ready access to MRI, it is also a valuable diagnostic tool.

Treatment

PARATENONITIS AND PARATENONITIS WITH TENDINOSIS

Activity modification

If the pain is very severe and/or chronic, crutch immobilization and complete rest may be required initially. Modified rest should continue until the athlete has been asymptomatic for 7–10 days, with gradual return to preinjury activity levels thereafter. Too early a return to activity may cause a relapse (Clement *et al.* 1984).

Cast immobilization should be avoided.

Fitness training

It is important for the athlete to maintain cardiovascular fitness while he or she is unable to train normally. This is usually achieved by swimming, pool running or cycling if tolerated. Most can pool run comfortably and cycle comfortably on the flat until they are able to start a walk–run programme. Cycling should be performed with the heel rather than the toes in contact with the pedal in order to avoid Achilles stress (Clement *et al.* 1984).

Pain control

Ice massage is very effective at reducing pain and swelling, both in the acute phase and throughout rehabilitation (Knight 1990). Physical modalities such as ultrasound may also decrease inflammation in the acute phase of injury, but scientific evidence supporting such treatment is scant (Kvist 1994).

Oral or topical NSAIDs may reduce pain and inflammation very effectively, especially in the early phase of treatment. Prolonged use is not recommended.

Stretching

Wall leans with the knee in full flexion and then in 30–45° of flexion will stretch both gastrocnemius and soleus effectively. Stretching and a warm-up (e.g. cycling) should precede the muscle strengthening drills described below.

Night splint

For those patients with morning stiffness as a prominent symptom a tension night splint, as used for plantar fasciitis, can be beneficial.

Eccentric strengthening

Eccentric muscle strengthening of the triceps surae is the cornerstone of management (Curwin &

Stanish 1984). In our clinic a progressive heel drop programme is used. The patient performs three sets of 20 heel drops daily, initially with both feet together on the edge of a stair, dropping down slowly to below the level of the stair (full dorsiflexion) and then slowly coming back up to a fully plantarflexed position. After 5 days, the patient progresses to one foot at a time, moving slowly down and slowly up. The next progression, after a further 5 days, is to a fast drop down to the dorsiflexed position and then slowly back up into full plantar flexion with both feet together. After 5 days of this, progress is to fast drop down, slow up, one foot at a time. Weight carried in a rucksack can be added at 5-day intervals in 2.3-kg (5-lb) increments up to a usual maximum of 9 kg (20 lb). Some pain is expected with this programme, but if progressive pain occurs at any point the patient should drop back a stage or may even have to rest for a day or two. Stretching before and after exercise is important, and postexercise icing for 10 min or so may greatly reduce pain and inflammation.

Niesen-Vertommen *et al.* (1992) found that patients using such a rehabilitation programme (eccentric rather than concentric exercise) experienced less pain than patients using a concentric exercise programme.

Deep transverse friction and deep friction massage

Both are advocated, especially in chronic Achilles injury where postinflammatory adhesions have formed (Cyriax 1980).

Orthotics

Heel lifts worn in both shoes will reduce strain on the Achilles tendon in the initial stages of rehabilitation (Clement *et al.* 1984). Custom-made insoles are effective in reducing prolonged pronation if this is present (Bates *et al.* 1979); they decrease both maximal pronation and the velocity of rear foot movement (Smith *et al.* 1986).

Education

Correction of training errors, sport technique and

inadequacies of equipment (shoes) may prevent injury recurrence.

Steroid injection

Steroid injection may cause tendon rupture. It has no place in the management of tendon injury. The only indication is persistent retrocalcaneal bursitis, and even then great care must be taken not to inject the Achilles tendon.

Surgery

Surgical treatment is reserved for those patients who fail to respond to at least 6 months of conservative treatment. Surgery may involve release and excision of diseased posterior paratenon (the anterior paratenon carries the blood supply to the tendon), excision of devitalized tendon and excision of the retrocalcaneal bursa. Occasionally, when the os calcis impinges on the Achilles tendon near its insertion, the posterior superior angle of the os calcis is excised. Cast immobilization is rarely used in the postoperative period (Schepsis *et al.* 1994). Early range-of-motion and stretching exercises are emphasized. Light jogging is rarely started sooner than 2–3 months postoperatively. The athlete returns to competitive activity levels 5–6 months after the operation. Satisfactory results are obtained in 87–95% of patients who are treated operatively (Anderson *et al.* 1992; Schepsis *et al.* 1994).

Return to sport

When the patient has been pain free for 7–10 days, is non-tender, has a full range of motion in the ipsilateral ankle joint and has at least 75% of normal plantar flexor strength, return to running can start. The patient progresses through walking, to running/walking, to running as pain allows. Once he or she is running painlessly for 30–45 min, tempo intervals can be introduced in the middle of a run and progressed eventually to sprinting, jumping and other sport-specific drills such as cutting.

TENDON TEARS AND RUPTURE

Partial tears of the Achilles tendon will require surgery if conservative treatment, including cast immobilization, fails. If the tear is significant, it may be appropriate to consider early surgery rather than waiting to see if conservative treatment is effective. In patients with chronic tears requiring surgery, those with proximal tears (more than 30 mm above the calcaneus) have an operation in which devitalized tendon tissue is removed, whereas those with more distal lesions often also undergo excision of the retrocalcaneal bursa and the posterior superior angle of the calcaneus. 'Satisfactory' long-term results are achieved in only two-thirds of cases (Morberg et al. 1997).

Complete rupture of the Achilles tendon may be managed conservatively or surgically. Conservative treatment takes two forms. The first comprises 6–8 weeks of cast immobilization, followed by lengthy rehabilitation. The second involves 'supervised neglect' of long-standing ruptures discovered by chance in the elderly. According to Waterston et al. (1997) regular review is all that is required and such patients rarely need further treatment. Although safe, non-surgical treatment carries a higher risk of rerupture (reviewed in Waterston et al. 1997).

Surgery involves some risks, and is probably inappropriate for non-athletes or older patients. For athletes, surgery offers the best hope of returning to preinjury performance and carries a lower risk of rerupture (Waterston et al. 1997).

Prevention

Prevention of Achilles tendon injuries centres on the avoidance of training errors. Training programmes should ideally be sport and athlete specific, have programmed rest periods and avoid large increases in intensity or volume. Stretching should be routine, and preseason conditioning may well reduce the risk of injury.

Other aetiological factors such as inappropriate training surfaces and running shoes should be addressed. Biomechanical problems such as excess pronation may be neutralized with orthotics and motion control running shoes.

Steroid injections are contraindicated in the treatment of Achilles tendon injuries and treatment with fluoroquinilone antibiotics should probably be avoided if possible.

Patellar tendinitis

Patellar tendinitis, otherwise known as jumper's knee, is the other common lower limb overuse tendon injury. It is especially prevalent in basketball players, but also affects those in other sports including volleyball, soccer and running. Patellar tendinitis is the commonest overuse injury seen in volleyball players (Watkins & Green 1992), and causes about 5% of all running injuries (Macintyre et al. 1991).

The injury tends to recur, and prolonged absence from sport is common (Cook et al. 1997).

Anatomy

The patellar tendon is the continuation of the quadriceps tendon, the superficial fibres of which run over the patella before inserting into the tibial tubercle. The deep fibres of the patellar tendon originate at the inferior patellar pole before they, too, insert into the tibial tubercle.

Pathology

Pathologically, patellar tendinitis is usually localized to the bone–tendon junction at the inferior patellar pole. The changes seen are usually those of tendinosis, the features of which are discussed in the Achilles tendon section above.

Classification

Anterior knee pain is the commonest symptom of patellar tendinitis. The following widely used classification, proposed by Blazina et al. (1973) and later modified by Roels et al. (1978), is based on the pain experienced by the patient.

Phase 1 Pain after activity.
Phase 2 Pain during warm-up that disappears after the warm-up is complete only to reappear after activity.

Phase 3 Pain during and after minimal activity which prevents sport participation.

Phase 4 Complete tendon rupture.

Aetiology

Training errors are important in the aetiology of patellar tendinitis. In sports in which patellar tendinitis is common, jumping which results in recurrent eccentric loading of the knee extensor mechanism is a major part of the game. Athletes involved in these sports spend a considerable amount of training time working on their jumping (Briner & Kacmar 1997). The athletes who can jump quickest and highest are the very ones at increased risk of developing patellar tendinitis (Lian *et al.* 1996), prompting some to suggest that such athletes should decrease the time they spend jump training (Briner & Kacmar 1997). Harder training surfaces increase ground reaction forces, have been implicated in patellar tendinitis (Ferretti 1986) and should be avoided when possible.

Volleyball players who play more than four times a week, have been playing for 2–5 years and who are aged 20–25 are at the greatest risk of patellar tendinitis (Ferretti *et al.* 1984). Cook *et al.* (1997) found that 56% of patients with patellar tendinitis developed their first symptoms before they were 20 years old.

Since high forces during jumping (high and fast jumpers, and hard surfaces), excessive training, playing volumes, and age seem important aetiological factors, this supports the view that patellar tendinitis is an overuse injury caused by repetitive eccentric loading.

Various anatomical factors may contribute to patellar tendinitis: patella alta, leg length discrepancy and tight hamstrings (Kujala *et al.* 1986); rectus femoris inflexibility (Smith *et al.* 1991); and increased Q angle (Ferretti 1986).

Diagnosis

HISTORY

The athlete complains of anterior knee pain, worse with activity (especially when landing or stopping suddenly) and he or she can usually localize pain to the inferior patellar pole. Initially, the pain is present only before or after sport, but it often progresses to the point where everyday activities are painful and pain is constantly present.

A training history may reveal training errors such as excessive jump training or training on inappropriate surfaces.

EXAMINATION

Initially the athlete is examined standing, thus allowing the clinician to screen for abnormalities such as leg length discrepancy, patella alta and increased Q angle. Hopping and/or squatting may reproduce the athlete's pain, and wasting of the ipsilateral thigh muscles may be apparent. Running shoes should be checked for abnormal wear patterns.

With the athlete lying supine, the knee can be examined fully. There may be pain at the inferior patellar pole on forced flexion, limiting flexion. The inferior patellar pole is best palpated by gently tilting the superior pole posteriorly; the inferior pole then tilts anteriorly, allowing the clinician to palpate the undersurface where the deep fibres of the patellar tendon originate. This is usually the site of maximal tenderness, but the tendon may also be tender distally and at its insertion into the tibial tuberosity. The patella should also be checked for pain on patellar grinding, maltracking and instability, whilst the knee should be examined fully to exclude other diagnoses.

The hips are examined for range of motion, the iliotibial band, hamstrings and quadriceps are assessed for flexibility and all muscle groups acting on the hips and knees are tested for power.

Differential diagnosis

The differential diagnosis includes Sinding–Larsen–Johansson syndrome, Osgood–Schlatter syndrome, PFPS, fat pad inflammation, bursitis, arthritis of the patellofemoral or knee joints, meniscal injury, osteochondral injury of the femoral condyles and tumour.

Investigation

The diagnosis is usually made clinically, but the injury can be clearly visualized with diagnostic ultrasound.

The characteristic abnormalities seen on ultrasound are either a hypoechoic zone in the tendon or a fusiform swelling of the tendon at the site of tenderness. These abnormalities may be present in asymptomatic subjects, and they may resolve completely with time (Cook *et al.* 1997). Ultrasound is thus used to confirm the clinical diagnosis and not as a screening tool.

Plain radiography may show tendon calcification. It also excludes some of the differential diagnoses listed above.

MRI has also been used effectively in the diagnosis of patellar tendinitis (Bodne *et al.* 1988).

Treatment

As with other tendon injuries the management depends on whether the injury is acute or chronic.

For the acute injury, initial management focuses on pain relief with active rest, ice, NSAIDs and physical treatment modalities. Painful activities are avoided, but fitness can be maintained with swimming, pool running and cycling if tolerated. These fitness activities should continue throughout the entire rehabilitative programme.

If the injury is no longer acute, treatment can start with lower limb stretches, range-of-motion exercises progressing to concentric and then eccentric strengthening of the quadriceps muscle–tendon unit as pain allows. In our clinic the drop squat programme, described above, is used for eccentric strengthening. Specific attention should be paid to any flexibility or strength deficits uncovered during the initial examination.

Once pain decreases and strength and flexibility have improved, a graduated return to sport can start. A walk–run programme is used and once the athlete is able to run for 30 min or more without pain, sport-specific drills such as cutting, jumping and kicking can commence, the volume and intensity of training increasing gradually as pain dictates.

Up to a third of patients are unable to participate in their sport for 6 months or more, because of continuing symptoms (Cook *et al.* 1997). Those patients who have not responded to conservative treatment should be considered for surgery (Cook *et al.* 1997). Steroid injections should be avoided.

We have had success in utilizing a special patellar stabilization brace and more recently are utilizing lithotripsy, extracorporeal shock wave therapy with encouraging results. Similar results have been seen with this treatment of achilles tendinopathy and plantar fasciitis. Surgery usually involves excision of devitalized tendon. The median time to return to sport after surgery is 7–12 months (Cook *et al.* 1997).

Prevention

Varied training, planned rest and individualized and sport-specific training are as important in the prevention of patellar tendinitis as for other overuse injuries. Specific measures such as heel lifts for leg length discrepancy, hamstring and quadriceps stretching and limiting jump training are likely to be helpful in prevention, although all these measures are unproven.

Plantar fasciitis

Plantar fasciitis is a strain or tearing of the plantar aponeurosis. It is a common overuse injury seen in athletes participating in any sport that involves running, with reported frequencies of 4.7–8.5% (James *et al.* 1978; Gudas 1980; Taunton *et al.* 1982; Macintyre *et al.* 1991). The injury is often disabling, and often requires a long rehabilitation.

Anatomy

The plantar fascia runs forwards from the medial tuberosity of the calcaneus as three slips, of which the central slip is the thickest. These slips divide further and insert into the proximal phalanxes of each toe. The plantar aponeurosis assists in maintaining the medial longitudinal arch of the foot, helps with shock absorption during weight-bearing and aids locking of the midtarsal bones prior to push-off (Taunton *et al.* 1982).

The treatment of plantar fasciitis often involves prolonged rehabilitation.

Aetiology

Plantar fasciitis is most commonly an overuse injury, although it can be caused by direct trauma to the fascia. Any factor which increases the stretch on the fascia during the gait cycle will increase the likelihood of injury. Similarly any increase in the number or magnitude of stresses may result in injury.

PRONATION

Pronation has been implicated as a causal factor. With pronation, there is increased stretch on the plantar fascia when standing (Krivickas 1997). Excessive pronation that persists into the push-off phase of the gait cycle results in an unstable foot and an overstretched plantar fascia; this may cause forces beyond its functional capacity, resulting in injury (Taunton *et al*. 1982).

Leg length discrepancy may result in pronation on the shorter leg side (Krivickas 1997) increasing the chance of plantar fasciitis on that side (Taunton *et al*. 1982).

ACHILLES TENDON TIGHTNESS

Achilles tendon tightness may cause compensatory pronation and abnormal stretching of the plantar fascia. Kibler *et al*. (1991) found that the majority of athletes with plantar fasciitis lack more than 5° of ankle dorsiflexion with the knee extended (20° is normal), and Taunton *et al*. (1982) found poor ankle dorsiflexion in 20% of patients with plantar fasciitis.

PES CAVUS FOOT TYPE

Plantar fasciitis is also seen in athletes with a pes cavus-type foot. This is thought to predispose to plantar fasciitis by causing an increased stretch on the plantar fascia at heel strike (Taunton *et al*. 1982) and, because of decreased shock absorption, excessive transmission of weight-bearing forces to soft tissues such as the plantar fascia (James *et al*. 1978; Lutter 1981).

Potentially, both of these mechanisms render the plantar fascia more vulnerable to overuse injury.

TRAINING ERRORS

Training errors commonly associated with plantar fasciitis (James *et al*. 1978; Taunton *et al*. 1982) include excessive training intensity or duration, a recent sudden increase in training volume or intensity, an inappropriate running surface, too much hill running and no 'rest' weeks in the training routine.

FOOTWEAR

Running shoes ideally absorb shock, control pronation, are flexible at the metatarsophalangeal joints and provide good arch support to prevent unnecessary strain on the plantar fascia. A good shoe should also have an adequate heel wedge to prevent excessive pronation. Old or inappropriate footwear may contribute to the development of plantar fasciitis (Taunton *et al*. 1982).

Diagnosis

HISTORY

Heel pain and medial arch pain, worse in the morning and with activity, are the classic features of plantar fasciitis, but morning stiffness may also be a prominent feature.

At first the pain is worse on rising and tends to ease off with initial activity, increasing again later in the day with weight-bearing. Going up stairs or up on the toes may be especially painful. During sporting activity, the pain may initially disappear after warm-up, only to reappear after activity but, as the injury progresses pain is present throughout activity and may progress to the stage where sporting activity is impossible and everyday activities are painful.

Very acute onset of pain in athletes may signal rupture of the plantar fascia.

The history should include a full training history

with the emphasis on the training errors mentioned above.

EXAMINATION

The athlete's gait, foot type, alignment and calf flexibility should be assessed. Muscle power throughout the lower limb should be examined and imbalances noted. An examination of the athlete's training footwear may reveal abnormal wear.

The examiner can then move down to the problem area. There is often exquisite tenderness over the medial calcaneal tubercle, extending along the entire medial plantar fascia. Occasionally tenderness may be confined solely to the midportion of the medial slip of the plantar fascia (Taunton *et al.* 1982). Often, pain may be elicited on stressing the fascia by passively dorsiflexing the toes. Sometimes nodules may be palpable in the fascia.

Swelling may be visible, and there may be a palpable defect in the fascia if rupture has occurred. Rarely, if there has been a complete rupture of the plantar fascia, a ball of retracted fascia may be palpable.

Differential diagnosis

The differential diagnosis includes: tarsal tunnel syndrome (entrapment of the medial calcaneal branch of the posterior tibial nerve), stress fracture of the calcaneum, Sever's disease, neuroma, heel bursitis, calcaneal periostitis (heel bruise), rheumatoid arthritis, Reiter's syndrome, gout, osteoathritis of the ankle and referred pain (Taunton *et al.* 1982).

Investigation

PLAIN RADIOGRAPHY

X-rays are very often completely normal, although often a calcaneal spur (present in 15–25% of the population) is seen, and resorption (implying acute inflammation) may be observed at the calcaneal origin (Newell & Miller 1977). Calcaneal spur formation is thought due to a combination of periosteal detachment, subsequent haemorrhage and osteoblastic activity (Taunton *et al.* 1982), but calcaneal spurs are commonly seen in asymptomatic individuals (Newell & Miller 1977).

Diagnoses such as tumour and stress fracture of the calcaneus can be ruled out by plain radiography.

BONE SCINTIGRAPHY

A bone scan is rarely indicated in plantar fasciitis, but it will be positive in up to 95% of patients with a calcaneal spur and 33% of those without a spur (Tudor *et al.* 1997). The main indication for bone scan is if a stress fracture of the calcaneus is suspected.

OTHER IMAGING

Ultrasound may visualize the changes in the plantar fascia accurately and non-invasively (Cardinal *et al.* 1997), but will rarely alter management.

MRI is also a very effective diagnostic tool in the investigation of heel pain (reviewed in DiMarcangelo & Yu 1997), but its relative inaccessibility and expense make it an unrealistic option in most settings.

Treatment

Initial treatment is the same as for other overuse injuries, with the emphasis on pain relief, activity modification, NSAIDs, ice massage, low-dye taping, physical therapeutic modalities and, sometimes, heel lifts or cups. Fitness maintenance with cycling, swimming and pool running is important. When pain allows, gentle stretching, range-of-motion exercises and calf stretches can be instituted (as described for Achilles tendinitis). Tension splints which maintain a stretch on the plantar fascia at night, and can be easily manufactured in the office, improve treatment outcome (Batt *et al.* 1996).

A recent study (Gudeman *et al.* 1997) suggests that iontophoresis of 0.4% dexamethasone is effective in reducing pain in the initial stages of treatment if combined with the above measures, although it does not affect the eventual outcome. This early improvement may be especially useful in the treatment of élite athletes, allowing an earlier return to sport.

Once the acute symptoms have abated, strengthening of ankle flexors, extensors, everters and invertors can begin, using simple band exercises. The patient can be progressed from low- to high-resistance bands as pain allows. The small muscles of the foot can be strengthened with towel curls and bottle rolls. The ankle drop protocol (as described for Achilles injuries) is started early. If other adaptive weaknesses or inflexibilities in the lower limb have been uncovered, these should also be addressed.

The patient should be symptom free, have a full range of motion at the ankle, be non-tender and have at least 75% of normal dorsiflexor strength before progressing to the walk–run programme (as described above). Once running is painless, sport-specific exercises can be started. Return to sport may be as quick as 6 weeks (Clancy 1982; Chandler & Kibler 1993).

Some athletes will not respond to conservative treatment, and will require steroid injection. This may give dramatic resolution of symptoms (Taunton et al. 1982). Steroid injections are, however, associated with fat pad atrophy and rupture of the plantar fascia (Leach et al. 1987) which may take many months to heal (Acevedo & Beskin 1998). Steroid injections should be used sparingly.

Surgical release of the fascia is indicated only in those rare cases where all other treatment has failed.

Prevention

Advice on appropriate footwear, orthotics (to correct pronation or accommodate a cavus foot) and heel lifts (to correct leg length discrepancy), together with Achilles stretches, calf strengthening and correction of training errors, may all be useful in plantar fasciitis prevention.

Muscle overuse injuries

We know much less about muscle injuries than we do about tendon and bone injuries. Muscle injuries are very common and tend to recur. The hamstrings are perhaps most commonly injured in sports that involve sprinting, such as soccer, American and Australian football, rugby and basketball (Eckstrand & Gillquist 1983).

Other muscles prone to injury include the medial gastrocnemius and rectus femoris (which both cross two joints and are therefore susceptible to strain injury), and the adductor longus muscle.

Generally, muscle strain injuries occur when the muscle is passively stretched or activated during stretch (Garrett 1996), i.e. during eccentric contraction.

Incidence

Macintyre et al. (1991) found that muscle strains accounted for 6% of injuries to runners seen in one clinic over a 4-year period: adductor strains were commonest, followed by gastrocnemius, gluteus, hamstring and quadriceps strains. Bennell and Crossley (1996) studied a group of 95 track and field athletes, finding that hamstring strains were the cause of 14% of all injuries sustained over a 12-month period. In a recent study of all injuries presenting to a sports medicine centre (Baquie & Brukner 1997) 4.1% of patients had muscle strains. However, it is likely that many more people experience minor muscle strains; these cause absence from sport, but resolve without necessitating a visit to a sports injury clinic. For example, a study looking at hamstring injuries in élite Australian footballers (Orchard et al. 1997) found an incidence of 16% over the course of a season, and Watson (1996) found that hamstring injuries constituted 6.5% of all injuries in adolescent Gaelic football players. Eckstrand and Gillquist (1983) found that the hamstrings were the most commonly injured muscle group in a cohort of soccer players.

Experimental findings and aetiology of muscle injuries

A brief look at experimental findings (reviewed in Garrett 1996) may be helpful in understanding how and why muscle injuries occur.

1 Experimentally, muscle activation alone is not enough to cause an injury. There has to be an element of stretch before injury occurs, because the

force required is several times larger than that produced during maximal isometric contraction. This is why most muscle injuries occur during an eccentric muscle contraction e.g. sprinting or kicking a ball. Muscle inflexibility will increase vulnerability to such an injury.

2 When a muscle is stretched to failure, it tends to fail near the muscle–tendon junction, with some muscle tissue still attached to the tendon.

3 Within the muscle, the passive elements (connective tissue and muscle fibres) absorb strain, but activation of the muscle increases this absorptive ability by 100%. Thus if muscle activation is in any way compromised, the ability to absorb strain is reduced, increasing the vulnerability of the muscle. Two common causes of decreased muscle activation are muscle fatigue and pre-existing injury.

4 When a disruptive muscle injury occurs, there is an initial haemorrhage, followed 1–2 days later by inflammation. By day 7, fibrous tissue begins to replace the inflammatory reaction, with scar tissue being laid down (Nikolau *et al.* 1987). Initially there is a decrease in the muscle's ability to develop tension, dropping to 70% of normal immediately after injury, declining to 50% of normal within 24 h and then improving to 90% of normal by day 7 postinjury. In non-disruptive muscle injury, at 7 days postinjury, the muscle can develop only 77% of its normal tension (Obremsky *et al.* 1994). In either injury therefore there is a definite period of postinjury weakness when a return to previous activity levels risks reinjury.

Hamstring injuries

Hamstring injuries are common. They occur most often during sprinting or when kicking a ball. Both of these activities involve ballistic hip flexion and knee extension, during which the hamstrings contract eccentrically, i.e. they contract while lengthening. In some cases the resulting load will exceed the functional capacity of the muscle and result in injury.

Anatomy

The hamstrings comprise the semimembranosus,

semitendinosus and biceps femoris muscles. The semimembranosus, semitendinosus and long head of the biceps femoris originate from the ischial tuberosity, whereas the short head of the biceps femoris originates from the posterolateral femur at the lateral border of the linea aspera.

The biceps femoris inserts into the fibular head, whereas the semimembranosus and semitendinosus insert into the medial aspect of the proximal tibia.

The principal actions of the hamstrings are to assist in hip extension and knee flexion.

Diagnosis

The long head of biceps femoris is the most commonly injured hamstring muscle in runners and, as predicted experimentally, injuries tend to occur at the muscle–tendon junction (Garrett 1996). Injuries may vary from minor strains to complete avulsion of the muscle origin, but the typical injury is a partial tear (Garrett 1996).

HISTORY

The athlete with a hamstring injury will complain of sudden onset pain over the proximal hamstrings, classically occurring during sprinting or kicking. There may be an accompanying popping or tearing sensation at the site of injury. Usually, but not always, this will prevent the athlete from finishing the run or match. There may be a history of a similar injury in the past.

EXAMINATION

There is tenderness over the site of the strain or tear. This is usually near the ischial tuberosity, but may be anywhere in the hamstring muscles. Stretching and resisted contraction of the hamstrings may elicit pain, and straight leg raising may be limited on the affected side.

Haematoma formation is common. It may be intramuscular, where the muscle fascia remains intact and limits haematoma size, or intermuscular, where the fascia is torn and the haematoma may become very large, with associated extensive ecchymosis. Large tears and avulsion injuries of the hamstrings may result in quite dramatic bleeding.

In avulsion of the hamstring at its origin, or a large tear, a defect may be palpable. In the case of an avulsion, retraction of the detached muscle belly may also be palpable.

A full lower limb biomechanical screen, including a shoe check, should be carried out and the lower limb musculature should be assessed for flexibility and strength deficits and/or imbalances.

Differential diagnosis

The diagnosis of a hamstring injury is usually straightforward, but if the history is atypical, other diagnoses should be considered, including tumour, the referred pain of sciatica or a lumbar disc lesion, neurological or vascular claudication and compartment syndrome (Kujala *et al.* 1997).

Investigation

Cybex strength testing often reveals an eccentric rather than concentric weakness in those with chronic hamstring problems.

The diagnosis of hamstring injury is usually made clinically, but if there is diagnostic doubt, or if the injury fails to respond to treatment, further investigation may be appropriate.

Plain radiography may reveal a bony avulsion injury, and may exclude some other possible diagnoses.

MRI, CT and ultrasound may help to determine the degree of injury and the response to treatment in complicated cases or in the élite athlete under pressure to return to sport.

Treatment

Initial treatment should include ice (for 15–20 min every 30–60 min during the first day), compression, elevation and immobilization to limit pain, bleeding and inflammation. Crutches are advisable initially for all but minor injuries, in order to reduce the chances of a reinjury and further bleeding. However, mobilization should start early enough to prevent muscle atrophy, but late enough to prevent

further injury and allow formation of the granulation tissue matrix. A short course of NSAIDs may be useful in reducing initial pain levels.

Therapeutic ultrasound is often used in the initial stages to reduce pain and to promote healing, although there is no proof that it improves outcome.

The purpose of the above measures is to control symptoms, to limit bleeding and inflammation, and to prevent further injury. After the first 2–3 days, an assessment of muscle function should be carried out to ascertain the degree of damage. A decrease in muscle power may indicate total muscle rupture or a large haematoma. In such cases further investigation with ultrasound (or CT/MRI) is indicated, because some injuries will require surgical intervention.

If the injury is adjudged to be minor, then gentle compression, mobilization, stretching and progressive strengthening exercises should commence and proceed as pain allows. Exercises should start with isometric training, progressing to concentric exercises, then eccentric drills and (after about 2 weeks) sport-specific drills.

The athlete is able to return to sport when pain free and when there is normal strength, flexibility and range of motion of the injured muscle. Too early a return to sport risks reinjury.

Failure to respond to treatment for more than 3–4 weeks is an indication for further investigation to exclude a large haematoma or substantial tear (Garrett 1996).

A late complication of muscle haematoma formation is heterotopic calcification, also known as myositis ossificans. Calcification at the site of the haematoma may result in disabling pain and will require surgical removal of the affected tissue once the calcification process is complete (i.e. once the bone scan is 'cold'). Unfortunately, this condition may recur after surgery.

SURGICAL TREATMENT

If there is complete muscle origin rupture, persistent pain or persistent tightness, surgery may be indicated to relieve symptoms and improve functional outcome.

Surgery may also be indicated for the hamstring syndrome, characterized by fibrotic shortening in the hamstring tendons near their origin, with accompanying chronic gluteal pain. This may be an overuse injury, resulting from repetitive microtrauma to bone, periosteum or muscle–tendon near the origin. The pain is usually relieved by partial division of the biceps insertion (Puranen & Orava 1988).

Hamstring compartment syndrome has been described in long-distance runners. It improves with fasciotomy (Kujala *et al.* 1997).

Prevention

Pre-exercise stretching and warm-ups may help to decrease muscle tension, which in turn reduces the load on the muscle tendon unit at any given length, thus protecting the tissue from injury (Garrett 1996). Conversely, prior injury (Garrett 1996) and/or fatigue (Mair *et al.* 1996) increase muscle tension, increasing injury risk. In consequence, the majority of hamstring injuries occur near the beginning or end of matches and practices (Dorman 1971). Stretching should be carried out after warm-up. Each muscle group should be stretched repeatedly, as this is known to reduce muscle resistance to stretching (Garrett 1996).

Proper conditioning is also important in preventing injury. A conditioned athlete is less likely to become fatigued, and is less likely to suffer from muscle weakness or imbalance, both of which may cause injury (Orchard *et al.* 1997). These authors advocate preseason isokinetic testing of hamstring strength as a means of identifying athletes who need a preventive strengthening programme.

A recent minor hamstring injury may increase the risk of major injury if there is no rest or rehabilitative period (Eckstrand & Gillquist 1983). Athletes should therefore be discouraged from returning prematurely to sport.

Upton *et al.* (1996) found that thermal pants may have a role in preventing recurrent hamstring injuries. The use of thermal pants to prevent recurrent hamstring injuries is widespread. Interestingly, though, the investigators felt that insufficient preseason training and inadequate rehabilitation were much more important causes of hamstring injury than any failure to wear thermal pants.

Groin pain

Groin injuries are often complex. They are frequently difficult to diagnose and slow to respond to treatment, resulting in prolonged absence from sport. Sports like soccer and ice hockey are particularly vulnerable to such injuries. Renstrom and Peterson (1980) reported that 5% of all soccer injuries are groin injuries, and Smodlaka (1980) found that up to 28% of soccer players had a past history of groin injury.

Overuse adductor injuries often become chronic and such injuries are the commonest cause of groin pain in athletes. Other less common causes such as osteitis pubis and sports hernia are more difficult to diagnose, but they must be considered along with the many other conditions listed below. Multiple pathologies commonly coexist in athletes with groin pain (Ekberg *et al.* 1988).

Differential diagnosis

The following conditions should be considered in an athlete with groin pain.
Tears or strains of the adductors, rectus abdominis, iliopsoas or rectus femoris muscles
Osteitis pubis
Inguinal or femoral hernia
Sports hernia
Hip conditions including Perthe's disease, slipped capital femoral epiphysis, stress fracture of the neck of the femur, arthritis and bursitis of the hip
Ilioinguinal or obturator neuropathy
Stress fracture of the pubic ramus or symphysis
Osteomyelitis of the pubic ramus or symphysis
Iliopsoas bursitis
Prostatitis, urethritis, epididymitis
Referred pain from the spine, e.g. radiculopathy at L1 or L2 level.

Diagnosis

A thorough history should be taken to include, where appropriate, the injury mechanism, training history, pain pattern, presence or absence of paraesthesia and past medical history.

The athlete should be examined both standing and supine.

An abnormal gait, pain on hopping or leg length discrepancy may indicate hip pathology. Decreased hip rotation with tenderness over the symphysis pubis implies a diagnosis of osteitis pubis, whereas tenderness over the adductors and pain on passive abduction and active adduction suggest an adductor injury.

A visible or palpable mass in the groin, tenderness around the superficial inguinal ring and a cough impulse suggest a femoral or inguinal hernia, whilst tenderness at, or just superior and medial to, the pubic tubercle with associated pain on resisted sit-ups suggests a diagnosis of sports hernia.

Ilioinguinal neuralgia should be suspected if there is decreased or altered sensation over the medial groin, pain with hip hyperextension and tenderness over the nerve close to the anterior superior iliac spine, where it penetrates the abdominal wall and can become entrapped. The diagnosis can be confirmed with a nerve block at this site.

The other nerve that may become entrapped and cause groin pain is the obturator nerve (Bradshaw & McCrory 1997). Adductor weakness and medial thigh paraesthesia on the affected side are characteristic features and the diagnosis can be confirmed by nerve block and EMG.

Iliopsoas bursitis or muscle injury may present with deep anterior thigh or groin pain. This is difficult to localize, but may be reproduced by resisted hip flexion or stretching of the hip flexors such as occurs during a lunge. Femoral stress fractures may present in a similar way, but the hop test will be positive in up to 70% of femoral stress fractures (Clement et al. 1993).

In males, prostatitis is a commonly missed cause of groin pain, and some authorities suggest that a rectal examination should be part of the routine groin examination (Karlsson et al. 1994).

Investigation

Investigation of groin pain may include plain radiography, ultrasound, herniography, bone scan, MRI,

CT and EMG, depending on the suspected diagnosis or diagnoses.

Treatment

The management of adductor strains, osteitis pubis and sports hernia are discussed below. The management of all the other causes of groin pain is beyond the scope of this chapter, but is excellently reviewed in Karlsson et al. (1994) and Fricker (1997).

Adductor injuries

Overuse adductor strain injuries, usually of the adductor longus, are the commonest cause of groin pain in athletes, with repetitive minor injuries over a period of time resulting in chronic pain. Less commonly, the initial injury may be an acute contusion or strain, but usually by the time the clinician is consulted the injury has become chronic. The commonest mechanism of adductor injury is forced abduction of the leg, as often occurs in soccer, football and ice hockey.

Diagnosis

HISTORY

The injury usually results in well-localized pain over the adductor longus, the most commonly affected muscle–tendon unit. Activities involving rapid adduction at the hip, such as kicking a ball, may aggravate the pain. There may be a history of a similar injury in the past.

EXAMINATION

Tenderness may be elicited over the site of injury, the adductor tendon, tendon insertion or muscle belly; the distinction is important because the site of injury determines the treatment. The muscle–tendon junction and the tendon itself are the commonest sites of injury, and the pain is reproduced by actively adducting and/or by passively abducting the thigh. If the site of injury is in the muscle belly, a haematoma may be felt and bruising may be evident.

An assessment of lower limb biomechanics, muscle power and flexibility should be carried out.

Investigation

The diagnosis is usually made clinically, but adductor lesions can be visualized with ultrasound, CT or MRI if there is any diagnostic doubt, or if further information is required.

Treatment

Initially, as with other muscular injuries, pain control and control of bleeding are important. Rest, ice and NSAIDs are used initially, but after 24–48 h mobilization and range-of-motion exercises are commenced as pain allows. Some pain is expected during treatment, but increasing pain implies a negative response; in such cases, a day or so of rest may be required before recommencing treatment at a lower level.

Stretching and strengthening exercises start early and progress gradually as pain allows. General fitness should be maintained, with upper body weights and swimming (not breast stroke) initially. As treatment progresses, the athlete may be able to cycle and/or pool run, again shifting gradually from low volume and intensity to higher work rates. Groin-specific strengthening can begin, progressing through isometric to concentric and then to eccentric drills.

Any strength and flexibility deficits uncovered during the initial examination should be addressed with appropriate strengthening and stretching exercises.

Once strength and range of motion improve, exercise load, volume, intensity and speed should be increased and sport-specific drills introduced. Gradual return to sport can then commence.

A minority of injuries fail to respond to treatment and may require surgical intervention. Surgery may involve removal of devitalized tendon, repair of the tendon, or tenotomy. If the initial injury is a complete tear or a partial tear accompanied by a large haematoma (which may interfere with healing), early surgery should be contemplated.

Prevention

Preseason strength training, proper prematch warm-ups and pre- and postmatch stretching are important in preventing groin injuries. Treatment of seemingly minor groin injuries may prevent lesions becoming chronic.

Osteitis pubis

Osteitis pubis is an overuse injury of the symphysis pubis. It is seen most commonly in athletes who participate in running, soccer, Australian Rules football, rugby, ice hockey and tennis. It is more commonly seen in men and can run a course of many years (Fricker *et al.* 1991). Osteitis pubis may also be associated with pelvic surgery, urinary tract infection, rheumatological conditions and pregnancy (Coventry & Mitchell 1961; Fricker *et al.* 1991).

Diagnosis

HISTORY

Characteristically the pain of osteitis pubis is of gradual onset and is felt at the symphysis. The pain may migrate from side to side, and may radiate to the upper adductors, rectus abdominis and scrotum. It may be provoked by kicking, running and pivoting on one leg (Fricker *et al.* 1991), and typically the athlete cannot run at more than 80% of normal speed (Ekberg *et al.* 1988). Osteitis pubis may present acutely or as a chronic condition.

EXAMINATION

The patient is usually tender over the symphysis pubis, and the pain is reproduced by active adduction or passive abduction of the thigh. There may be evidence of associated sacroiliac joint dysfunction and/or decreased range of motion of one or both hips. Limitation of hip rotation (usually internal rotation) and a resultant increase in stress across the symphysis pubis is thought to be a causal factor (Williams 1978). Muscle power of all the lower limb muscle groups should be assessed, as should lower limb biomechanics.

Investigation

Plain radiography may demonstrate symphyseal instability on a flamingo view (where the patient stands on one leg and then the other). Instability is present if more than 2 mm of shift across the symphysis is apparent on the films. Also on plain radiography, there may be erosions at either symphysis margin, with widening of the cleft.

Bone scan shows increased uptake at the symphysis on the delayed views. Bone scans are very sensitive but lack specificity, so that a stress fracture of the pubic rami or osteomyelitis of the pubic symphysis cannot be ruled out by bone scan alone. A normal plain X-ray may help to exclude these possibilities, although blood culture, needle aspiration or even open biopsy of the symphysis may be required to make the diagnosis of osteomyelitis (Karpos et al. 1995).

Treatment

Treatment of sports-related osteitis pubis may be frustrating for patient and clinician alike. However, osteitis pubis is a self-limiting disorder which will settle with time, and the patient can be reassured that he or she will get better. The average time to recovery is 9–10 months (Fricker 1997).

Fitness should be maintained with swimming, pool running and cycling, taking care to avoid anything that aggravates the pain. Severe pain may prevent any activity in the initial stage, in which case pain relief is the priority. Stretching to improve flexibility of the hips and strengthening of the muscles around the pelvis and hips are important and should be started as early as pain allows.

Malalignment issues, such as pelvic rotation, and muscle weakness and/or imbalance should be addressed, as should any anatomical abnormalities, such as leg length discrepancy.

Some athletes may benefit from NSAIDs and thermal protector shorts, and some authors advocate injection of corticosteroid into the pubic symphysis as a means of speeding recovery (Holt et al. 1995). However, the use of corticosteroid injections is still controversial.

Sports hernia

Some athletes experience groin pain that originates in the lower abdominal wall. It represents an overuse disruption of the muscles of the inguinal canal, but there is no clinically detectable hernia. The problem has been termed 'sports hernia' (Hackney 1993) or 'sportsman's hernia' (Malycha & Lovell 1992). Usually the pain does not settle with conservative treatment and often it prevents the athlete from competing. Because there is little to find on examination, the diagnosis is often made at surgery, when a deficiency of the lower abdominal musculature is found. Several different muscular lesions have been described, but the presentation of all of them is similar. Differences in the precise lesion may simply be a function of the particular sport concerned. Athletes in sports that involve twisting and turning at speed, such as soccer, rugby, ice hockey, Australian Rules football and tennis, are prone to sports hernia. This injury is also being seen increasingly in professional basketball players, where it is often associated with a high adductor strain. The number of sports hernia injuries seen in the US National Basketball Association (NBA) has been increasing in recent years.

Sports hernias may be bilateral, and can be associated with osteitis pubis and adductor tenoperiostitis.

Anatomical considerations

Malycha and Lovell (1992) described a syndrome of undiagnosed chronic groin pain associated with a distension of the medial posterior inguinal wall (transversalis fascia) apparent only at operation; they called it the sportsman's hernia.

Hackney (1993) described an injury characterized by a weakened transversalis fascia which had become separated from the conjoint tendon; he called it the sports hernia. Both Malycha and Lovell (1992) and Hackney (1993) felt that these injuries represented an early or incipient direct inguinal hernia. Inguinal hernia repair produced excellent results in both of the groups of athletes described.

However, Gilmore (1992) described an injury primarily of the anterior inguinal canal wall characterized by a torn external oblique aponeurosis, subsequent dilatation of the superficial inguinal ring, a torn conjoint tendon and a dehiscence between the conjoint tendon and the inguinal ligament.

Simonet *et al.* (1995) described a group of 10 icehockey players with chronic groin pain in whom the lesion was a tear of the internal oblique muscle.

Lacroix *et al.* (1998) reported a lesion characterized by extensive tearing of the external oblique aponeurosis in the direction of its fibres and a lateral tear of the superficial inguinal ring associated with ilioinguinal nerve entrapment. The conjoint tendon remained intact, and there appeared to be no weakening of the transversalis fascia and no associated hernia sac. All the athletes in this study were ice-hockey players suffering from chronic groin pain.

Pinney *et al.* (unpublished study) described 16 icehockey players in whom the lesion was an attenuation, defect or deficiency of the transversalis fascia.

The term 'sports hernia' could reasonably be used to describe all of these lesions.

Aetiology

The aetiology of sports hernia is unknown, but it is likely that inadequate eccentric strength of the muscles that stabilize the pelvis during rotation is a major aetiological factor.

Diagnosis

HISTORY

Few athletes are able to pinpoint a specific traumatic incident which started the pain. Runners tend to report an insidious onset, whilst soccer, rugby and ice-hockey players report either an acute or a chronic onset of symptoms (Hackney 1993). The pain feels 'muscular' (a dull ache) and is worsened by activity, especially sudden movements, ipsilateral hip extension, contralateral rotation of the upper body and sit-ups (Taylor *et al.* 1991; Lacroix *et al.* 1998). The pain is usually well localized over the conjoint tendon, but may radiate to the groin, scrotum, hip or back, and will often be severe enough to prevent sporting activity.

EXAMINATION

Resisted sit-ups may reproduce the groin pain, as may coughing, sneezing and Valsalva's manoeuvre. Most patients are tender at the superficial inguinal ring or pubic tubercle, and the superficial inguinal ring may be dilated. By definition, no hernia is palpable on examination, although a mild cough impulse can be felt in some patients. Midinguinal tenderness is often present.

Lower limb muscle power, flexibility and biomechanics should be assessed so that any abnormalities may be addressed during rehabilitation.

Investigation

The sports hernia is often diagnosed at operation, although there is usually a strong clinical suspicion of the condition prior to going to the operating theatre.

Herniography can demonstrate effectively posterior wall lesions that are not apparent clinically (Ekberg 1981; Ekberg *et al.* 1988). However, herniography is not the easiest investigation to perform, nor is it the safest (Ekberg 1983).

Dynamic ultrasound is effective in the detection of posterior inguinal wall deficiencies in asymptomatic male athletes (Orchard *et al.* 1998) and it shows promise as a non-invasive and safe diagnostic tool in athletes suspected of having a sports hernia.

Bone scan, CT and MRI are often negative (Lacroix *et al.* 1998), although the bone scan may show non-specific increased uptake at the groin (Taylor *et al.* 1991). All of these investigations can be used to exclude various differential diagnoses.

Treatment

If examination and investigation fail to demonstrate any abnormality, then a period of conservative treatment may be tried. However, if there is strong clinical suspicion of a sports hernia and the athlete is anxious to return to sport quickly, early surgery may be appropriate.

Conservative treatment includes rest, NSAIDs and muscle stretching and strengthening exercises.

It will resolve symptoms in only a small number of cases.

If conservative treatment fails and there is a good history of hernia-type pain, herniorrhaphy is indicated. This usually allows a diagnosis to be made, with definitive treatment and cure of the problem. Operative results are good, and the athlete should be able to return to full activity within 5–12 weeks of surgery (Taylor *et al.* 1991; Williams & Foster 1995).

Prevention

The authors are not aware of any studies that address prevention of this injury. Attention should be directed at improving poor pelvic or hip flexibility, addressing malalignment issues such as pelvic imbalance and leg length discrepancy and correcting any muscle weakness around the pelvis. Those athletes at risk such as soccer, rugby and ice-hockey players should be assessed in the preseason period for any of the above problems as part of their preparticipation examination.

Whether these measures help, or not, is unproven.

Conclusion

With the present emphasis on year-round endurance training, overuse injuries are becoming more frequent. Training errors are the commonest aetiological factor. Inadequate strength and flexibility, biomechanical factors, playing surface and equipment are other important influences.

As we gain a better understanding of these factors, prevention will be the key element in offering suitable training programmes for the high-performance athlete.

References

Acevedo, J.L. & Beskin, J.L. (1998) Complications of plantar fascia rupture associated with corticosteroid injection. *Foot and Ankle International* 19, 91–97.

Anderson, D.L., Taunton, J.E. & Davidson, R.G. (1992) Surgical management of chronic Achilles tendinitis. *Clinical Journal of Sports Medicine* 2, 38–42.

Archambault, J.M., Wiley, J.P. & Bray, R.C. (1995) Exercise loading of tendons and the development of overuse injuries. *Sports Medicine* 20, 77–89.

Arroll, B., Ellis-Pegler, E., Edwards, A. & Sutliffe, G. (1997) Patellofemoral pain syndrome: a critical review of the clinical trials on nonoperative therapy. *American Journal of Sports Medicine* 25, 207–212.

Astrom, M. & Westlin, N. (1994a) Blood flow in the human Achilles tendon assessed by laser Doppler flowmetry. *Journal of Orthopaedic Research* 12, 246–252.

Astrom, M. & Westlin, N. (1994b) Blood flow in chronic Achilles tendinopathy. *Clinical Orthopaedics and Related Research* 308, 166–172.

Baquie, P. & Brukner, P. (1997) Injuries presenting to an Australian sports medicine centre: a 12-month study. *Clinical Journal of Sports Medicine* 7, 28–31.

Bates, B.T., Osternig, L.R., Mason, B. & James L.S. (1979) Foot orthotic devices to modify selected aspects of lower extremity mechanics. *American Journal of Sports Medicine* 7, 338–342.

Batt, M.E., Tanji, J.L. & Skattum, N. (1996) Plantar fasciitis: a prospective randomized clinical trial of the tension night splint. *Clinical Journal of Sports Medicine* 6, 158–162.

Bennell, K.L. & Crossley, K. (1996) Musculoskeletal injuries in track and field: incidence, distribution and risk factors. *Australian Journal of Science and Medicine in Sport* 28, 69–75.

Bennell, K.L., Malcolm, S., Thomas, S.A., Wark, J.D. & Brukner, P.D. (1996a) The incidence and distribution of stress fractures in competitive track and field athletes. *American Journal of Sports Medicine* 24, 211–217.

Bennell, K.L., Malcolm, S.A., Thomas, S.A. *et al.* (1996b) Risk factors for stress fractures in track and field athletes. A twelve month prospective study. *American Journal of Sports Medicine* 24, 810–818.

Blazina, M.E., Kerlan, R.K., Jobe, F.W., Carter, V.S. & Carlson, G.J. (1973) Jumper's knee. *Orthopedic Clinics of North America* 4, 665–678.

Bodne, D., Quinn, S.F., Murray, W.T. *et al.* (1988) Magnetic resonance images of chronic patellar tendinitis. *Skeletal Radiology* 17, 24–28.

Bradshaw, C. & McCrory, P. (1997) Obturator nerve entrapment. *Clinical Journal of Sports Medicine* 7, 217–219.

Briner, W.W. Jr & Kacmar, L. (1997) Common injuries in volleyball. Mechanisms of injury, prevention and rehabilitation. *Sports Medicine* 24, 65–71.

Brubaker, C.E. & James, S.L. (1974) Injuries to runners. *Journal of Sports Medicine* 2, 189–198.

Brukner, P. & Bennell, K. (1997) Stress fractures in female athletes. *Sports Medicine* 24, 419–429.

Brukner, P., Bradshaw, C., Khan, M.K., White, S. & Crossley, K. (1996) Stress fractures: a review of 180 cases. *Clinical Journal of Sports Medicine* 6, 85–89.

Cardinal, E., Chhem, R.K., Beauregard, C.G., Curkin, B.R. & Petellier, M. (1997) Plantar fasciitis: sonographic evaluation. *Radiology* 201, 257–259.

Chandler, T.J. & Kibler, W.B. (1993) A biomechanical approach to the prevention, treatment, and rehabilitation of plantar fasciitis. *Sports Medicine* 15, 344–352.

Clancy, W. (1982) Tendinitis and plantar fasciitis in runners. In: Drez, D. & D'Ambrosia, R.D. (eds) *Prevention and Treatment of Running Injuries*, pp. 77–87. Slack Publishers, Thorofare.

Clancy, W.G. (1990) Tendon trauma and overuse injuries. In: Leadbetter, W.B., Buckwalter, J.A. & Gordon, S.L. (eds) *Sports-Induced Inflammation: Clinical and Basic Science Concepts*, pp. 609–618. American Academy of Orthopedic Surgeons, Park Ridge, IL.

Clement, D.B. (1975) Tibial stress syndrome in athletes. *American Journal of Sports Medicine* **2**, 81–85.

Clement, D.B. (1987) Stress fractures of the foot and ankle. *Medicine and Science in Sports and Exercise* **23**, 56–70.

Clement, D.B., Taunton, J.E., Smart, G.W. & McNicol, K. (1981) A survey of overuse running injuries. *Physician and Sportsmedicine* **9**, 47–58.

Clement, D.B., Taunton, J.E. & Smart, G.W. (1984) Achilles tendinitis and peritendinitis: etiology and treatment. *American Journal of Sports Medicine* **12**, 179–184.

Clement, D.B., Ammann, W., Taunton, J.E. *et al.* (1993) Exercise-induced stress injuries to the femur. *International Journal of Sports Medicine* **14**, 347–352.

Congeni, J., McCulloch, J. & Swanson, K. (1997) Lumbar spondylolysis. A study of natural progression in athletes. *American Journal of Sports Medicine* **25**, 248–253.

Cook, J.L., Khan, K.M., Harcourt, P.R., Grant, M., Young, D.A. & Bonar, S. (1997) A cross sectional study of 100 athletes with jumper's knee managed conservatively and surgically. *British Journal of Sports Medicine* **31**, 332–336.

Coventry, M.B. & Mitchell, W.C. (1961) Osteitis pubis: observations based on a study of 45 patients. *Journal of the American Medical Association* **178**, 898–905.

Curwin, S. & Stanish, W. (1984) *Tendinitis: its Etiology and Treatment*. Collamore Press, Lexington, Massachusetts.

Cyriax, J.H. (1980) Clinical applications of massage. In: Rogoff, I.B. (ed.) *Manipulation, Traction and Massage*, pp. 152–169. Williams & Williams, Baltimore.

DiMarcangelo, M.T. & Yu, T.C. (1997) Diagnostic imaging of heel pain and plantar fasciitis. *Clinics in Podiatric Medicine and Surgery* **14**, 281–301.

Dorman, P. (1971) A report of 140 hamstring injuries. *Australian Journal of Sports Medicine* **4**, 30–36.

Doxey, G.E. (1987) Assessing quadriceps femoris muscle bulk with girth measurements in subjects with patellofemoral pain. *Journal of Orthopaedic and Sports Physical Therapy* **9**, 5.

Eckstrand, J. & Gillquist, J. (1983) Soccer injuries and their mechanisms: a prospective study. *Medicine and Science in Sports and Exercise* **15**, 267–270.

Ekberg, O. (1981) Inguinal herniography in adults: technique, normal anatomy, and diagnostic criteria for hernias. *Radiology* **138**, 31–36.

Ekberg, O. (1983) Complications after herniography in adults. *American Journal of Roentgenology* **140**, 491–495.

Ekberg, O., Persson, N.H., Abrahamsson,

P.-A. *et al.* (1988) Longstanding groin pain in athletes. *Sports Medicine* **6**, 56–61.

Engstrom, B., Forssblad, M., Johansson, C. & Tomkvist, H. (1990) Does a knee injury indefinitely sideline an élite soccer player. *American Journal of Sports Medicine* **18**, 101–105.

Ferretti, A. (1986) Epidemiology of jumper's knee. *Sports Medicine* **3**, 289–295.

Ferretti, A., Puddu, G., Mariani, P.P. *et al.* (1984) Jumper's knee: an epidemiological study of volleyball players. *Physician and Sportsmedicine* **12**, 97–103.

Frankel, V.H. (1978) Editorial comment. *American Journal of Sports Medicine* **6**, 396.

Fredericson, M. (1996) Common injuries in runners. *Sports Medicine* **21**, 49–72.

Fricker, P.A. (1997) Management of groin pain in athletes. *British Journal of Sports Medicine* **31**, 97–101.

Fricker, P.A., Taunton, J.E. & Ammann, W. (1991) Osteitis pubis in athletes: infection, inflammation or injury? *Sports Medicine* **12**, 266–279.

Garrett, W.E. Jr (1996) Muscle strain injuries. *American Journal of Sports Medicine* **24** (Suppl.), S2–S8.

Gillespie, H.S. & George, E.A. (1969) Results of surgical repair of spontaneous rupture of the Achilles tendon. *Journal of Trauma* **9**, 247–249.

Gilmore, O.J.A. (1992) Gilmore's groin. *Sportsmedicine and Soft Tissue Trauma* **3**.

Gordon, G.A. (1991) Stress reactions in connective tissues: a molecular hypothesis. *Medical Hypotheses* **36**, 289–294.

Gudas, C.L. (1980) Patterns of lower extremity injury in 224 runners. *Comprehensive Therapy* **6**, 50–59.

Gudeman, S.D., Eiscle, S.A., Heidt, R.S. Jr, Colosimo, A.J. & Stronpe, A.L. (1997) Iontophoresis of 0.4% dexamethasone for plantar fasciitis. *American Journal of Sports Medicine* **25**, 312–316.

Hackney, R.G. (1993) The sports hernia: a cause of chronic groin pain. *British Journal of Sports Medicine* **27**, 58–62.

Harrington, T., Crichton, K.J. & Anderson, I.F. (1993) Overuse ballet injury of the base of the second metatarsal. *American Journal of Sports Medicine* **21**, 591–598.

Hastad, K., Larsson, L.-G. & Lindholm, A. (1959) Clearance of radioisosodium after local deposit in the Achilles tendon. *Acta Chirurgica Scandinavica* **116**, 251–255.

Holt, A.M., Keene, J.S., Graf, B.K. & Helwig, D.C. (1995) Treatment of osteitis pubis in athletes. Results of corticosteroid injections. *American Journal of Sports Medicine* **23**, 601–606.

Hoppenfeld, S. (1976) *Physical Examination of the Spine and Extremities*, p. 218. Apple-

ton & Lange, Norwalk, Connecticut.

James, S.L., Bates, B.T. & Osternig, L.R. (1978) Injuries to runners. *American Journal of Sports Medicine* **6**, 40–50.

Jarvinen, M., Jozsa, L., Kannus, P., Jarvinen, T.L., Kvist, M. & Leadbetter, W. (1997) Histopathological findings in chronic tendon disorders. *Scandinavian Journal of Medicine and Science in Sports* **7**, 86–95.

Johnson, A.W., Weiss, C.B. & Wheeler, D.L. (1994) Stress fractures of the femoral shaft in athletes—more common than expected. A new clinical test. *American Journal of Sports Medicine* **22**, 248–256.

Johnson, L.C. (1963) Morphologic analysis in pathology in bone biodynamics. In: Frost, H.M. (ed.) *Bone Dynamics*, pp. 535–549. Little, Brown, Boston.

Karlsson, J., Sward, L., Kalebo, P. & Thomee, R. (1994) Chronic groin injuries in athletes: recommendations for treatment and rehabilitation. *Sports Medicine* **17**, 141–148.

Karpos, P.A.G., Spindler, K.P., Pierce, M.A. & Shull, H.J. Jr (1995) Osteomyelitis of the pubic symphysis in athletes: a case report and literature review. *Medicine and Science in Sports and Exercise* **27**, 473–478.

Kibler, W.B. & Chandler, T.J. (1994) Sport-specific conditioning. *American Journal of Sports Medicine* **22**, 424–432.

Kibler, W.B., Goldberg, C. & Chandler, T.J. (1991) Functional biomechanical deficits in running athletes with plantar fasciitis. *American Journal of Sports Medicine* **19**, 66–71.

Kilmartin, T.E. & Wallace, W.A. (1994) The scientific basis for the use of biomechanical foot orthoses in the treatment of lower limb sports injuries: a review of the literature. *British Journal of Sports Medicine* **28**, 180–184.

Klingman, R.E., Liaos, S.M. & Hardin, K.M. (1997) The effect of subtalar joint posting on patellar glide position in subjects with excessive rearfoot pronation. *Journal of Orthopaedic and Sports Physical Therapy* **25**, 185–191.

Knight, A.T.C. (1990) Cold as a modifier of sports-induced inflammation. In: Leadbetter, W.B., Buckwalter, J.A. & Gordon, S.L. (eds) *Sports-Induced Inflammation: Clinical and Basic Science Concepts*, pp. 463–478. American Academy of Orthopedic Surgeons, Park Ridge, Illinois.

Krissoff, W.B. & Ferris, W.D. (1979) Runner's injuries. *Physician and Sportsmedicine* **7**, 55–64.

Krivickas, L.S. (1997) Anatomical factors associated with overuse injuries. *Sports Medicine* **24**, 132–146.

Kujala, U.M., Osterman, K., Kvist, M.,

Aalto, T. & Friberg, O. (1986) Factors predisposing to patellar chondropathy and patellar apicitis in athletes. *International Orthopaedics* 10, 195–200.

Kujala, U.M., Orava, S. & Jarvinen, M. (1997) Hamstring injuries: current trends in treatment and prevention. *Sports Medicine* 23, 397–404.

Kvist, M. (1994) Achilles tendon injuries in athletes. *Sports Medicine* 18, 173–201.

Lacroix, V.J., Kinnear, D.G., Mulder, D.S. & Brown, R.A. (1998) Lower abdominal pain syndrome in national hockey league players: a report of 11 cases. *Clinical Journal of Sports Medicine* 8, 55–59.

Lagergren, C. & Lindholm, A. (1959) Vascular distribution in the Achilles tendon: an angiographic and microangiographic study. *Acta Chirurgica Scandinavica* 116, 491–495.

Leach, R., Jones, R. & Silva, T. (1987) Rupture of the plantar fascia in athletes. *Journal of Bone and Joint Surgery [American]* 60, 537–539.

Leadbetter, W.B. (1993) Tendon overuse injuries: diagnosis and treatment. In: Renstrøm, P.A.F.H. (ed.) *Sports Injuries: Basic Principles of Prevention and Care*, p. 457. Blackwell Scientific Publications, Oxford.

Lian, O., Engebretson, L., Ovrebo, R.V. & Bahr, R. (1996) Characteristics of the leg extensors in male volleyball players with jumper's knee. *American Journal of Sports Medicine* 24, 380–384.

Lindholm, A. & Arner, O. (1959) Subcutaneous rupture of the Achilles tendon: a study of 92 cases. *Acta Chirurgica Scandinavica* Suppl. 239, 1–51.

Lutter, L.D. (1981) Cavus foot in runners. *Foot and Ankle* 1, 225–228.

Macintyre, J.G., Taunton, J.E. & Clement, D.B. (1991) Running injuries: a clinical study of 4,173 cases. *Clinical Journal of Sports Medicine* 1, 81–89.

Mafulli, N., Regine, R., Angelillo, M., Capasso, G. & Filice, S. (1987) Ultrasound diagnosis of Achilles tendon pathology in runners. *British Journal of Sports Medicine* 21, 168–172.

Mair, S.D., Seaber, A.V., Glisson, R.R., Garrett, W.E. Jr (1996) The role of fatigue in susceptibility to acute muscle strain injury. *American Journal of Sports Medicine* 24, 137–143.

Malycha, P. & Lovell, G. (1992) Inguinal surgery in athletes with chronic groin pain: the sportsman's hernia. *Australian and New Zealand Journal of Surgery* 62, 123–125.

Martin, A.D. & McCulloch, R.G. (1987) Bone dynamics: stress, strain and fracture. *Journal of Sports Sciences* 5, 155–163.

Matheson, G.O., Clement, D.B. & McKenzie, D.C. (1987) Stress fractures in athletes. *American Journal of Sports Medicine* 15, 46–58.

Micheli, L.J. & Wood, R. (1995) Back pain in young athletes. Significant differences from adults in causes and patterns. *Archives of Pediatric and Adolescent Medicine* 149, 15–18.

Morberg, P., Jerre, R., Sward, L. & Karlsson, J. (1997) Long-term results after surgical treatment of partial Achilles tendon ruptures. *Scandinavian Journal of Medicine and Science in Sports* 7, 299–303.

Newell, S.G. & Miller, S.J. (1977) Conservative treatment of plantar fascial strain. *Physician and Sportsmedicine* 5 (11), 68–73.

Niesen-Vertommen, S.L., Taunton, J.E., Clement, D.B. *et al.* (1992) The effect of eccentric versus concentric exercise in the management of Achilles tendonitis. *Clinical Journal of Sports Medicine* 2, 109–113.

Nikolau, P.K., Macdonald, B.L., Glisson, R.R., Seaber, A.V., Garrett, W.E. Jr (1987) Biomechanical and histological evaluation of muscle after controlled strain injury. *American Journal of Sports Medicine* 15, 9–14.

Obremsky, W.T., Seaber, A.V., Ribbeck, B.M. & Garrett, W.E. Jr (1994) Biomechanical and histological assessment of a controlled muscle strain injury treated with piroxicam. *American Journal of Sports Medicine* 22, 558–561.

Orchard, J., Marsden, J., Lord, S. & Garlick, D. (1997) Preseason hamstring muscle weakness associated with hamstring muscle injury in Australian footballers. *American Journal of Sports Medicine* 25, 81–85.

Orchard, J.W., Read, J.W., Neophyton, J. & Garlick, D. (1998) Groin pain associated with ultrasound finding of inguinal canal posterior wall deficiency in Australian rules footballers. *British Journal of Sports Medicine* 32, 134–139.

Puddu, G., Ippolito, E. & Postacchini, F. (1976) A classification of Achilles tendon disease. *American Journal of Sports Medicine* 4, 145–150.

Puranen, J. & Orava, S. (1988) The hamstring syndrome: a new diagnosis of gluteal sciatic pain. *American Journal of Sports Medicine* 16, 517–521.

Ralston, E.L. & Schmidt, E.R. (1971) Repair of the ruptured Achilles tendon. *Journal of Trauma* 11, 15–21.

Reeder, M.T., Dick, B.H., Atkins, J.K., Pribis, A.B. & Martinez, J.M. (1996) Stress fractures. Current concepts of diagnosis and treatment. *Sports Medicine* 22, 198–212.

Renstrom, P. & Peterson, L. (1980) Groin injuries in athletes. *British Journal of Sports Medicine* 14, 30–36.

Roels, J., Martens, M., Mulier, J.C. & Burssens, A. (1978) Patellar tendinitis (jumper's knee) *American Journal of Sports Medicine* 6, 362–368.

Schepsis, A.A., Wagner, C. & Leach, R.E. (1994) Surgical management of Achilles tendon overuse injuries: a long-term follow up study. *American Journal of Sports Medicine* 22, 611–619.

Scully, T.J. & Besterman, G. (1982) Stress fracture: a preventable training injury. *Military Medicine* 147, 285–287.

Shields, C., Stein, S.R., Perez Tueffer, A. *et al.* (1976) Achilles tendon problems increase—round table discussion. *Physician and Sportsmedicine* 4, 43–56.

Shin, A.Y., Morin, W.D., Gorman, J.D., Jones, S.B. & Lapinsky, A.S. (1996) The superiority of magnetic resonance imaging in differentiating the cause of hip pain in endurance athletes. *American Journal of Sports Medicine* 24, 168–176.

Simonet, W.T., Saylor, H.L. III & Sim, L. (1995) Abdominal wall muscle tears in hockey players. *International Journal of Sports Medicine* 16, 126–128.

Slocum, K.A., Gorman, J.D., Puckett, M.L., & Jones, S.B. (1997) Resolution of abnormal MR signal intensity in patients with stress fractures of the femoral neck. *American Journal of Roentgenology* 168, 1295–1299.

Smart, G.W., Taunton, J.E. & Clement, D.B. (1980) Achilles tendon disorders in runners—a review. *Medicine and Science in Sports and Exercise* 12, 231–243.

Smith, A.D., Stroud, L. & McQueen, C. (1991) Flexibility and anterior knee pain in adolescent figure skaters. *Journal of Paediatric Orthopaedics* 11, 77–82.

Smith, L.S., Clarke, T.E. & Hamill, C.L. (1986) The effects of soft and semi-rigid orthoses upon rearfoot movement in running. *Journal of the American Podiatric Medical Association* 76, 227–233.

Smodlaka, V.N. (1980) Groin pain in soccer players. *Physician and Sportsmedicine* 8 (8), 57–61.

Swenson, E.J. Jr, Dehaven, K.E., Sebastianelli, W.J., Hanks, G., Kallnak, A. & Lynch, J.M. (1997) The effect of a pneumatic leg brace on return to play in athletes with tibial stress fractures. *American Journal of Sports Medicine* 25, 322–328.

Taunton, J.E., Clement, D.B. & Webber, D. (1981) Lower extremity stress fractures in athletes. *Physician and Sportsmedicine* 9, 77–86.

Taunton, J.E., Clement, D.B. & McNicol, K. (1982) Plantar fasciitis in runners. *Cana-*

dian Journal of Sports Medicine **7**, 41–44.

Taylor, D.C., Meyers, W.C., Moylan, J.A., Lohnes, J., Bassett, F.H. & Garrett W.E. Jr (1991) Abdominal musculature abnormalities as a cause of groin pain in athletes. *American Journal of Sports Medicine* **19**, 239–242.

Tudor, G.R., Finlay, D., Allen, M.J. & Belton I. (1997) The role of bone scintigraphy and plain radiography in intractable plantar fasciitis. *Nuclear Medicine Communications* **18**, 853–856.

Upton, P.A., Noakes, T.D. & Juritz, J.M. (1996) Thermal pants may reduce the risk of recurrent hamstring injuries in rugby players. *British Journal of Sports Medicine* **30**, 57–60.

Waterston, S.W., Mafulli, N. & Ewan, S.W.B. (1997) Subcutaneous rupture of the Achilles tendon: basic science and some aspects of clinical practice. *British Journal of Sports Medicine* **31**, 285–298.

Watkins, J. & Green, B.N. (1992) Volleyball injuries: a survey of injuries of Scottish national league male players. *British Journal of Sports Medicine* **26**, 135–137.

Watson, A.W. (1996) Sports injuries in school Gaelic football: a study over one season. *Irish Journal of Medical Science* **165**, 12–16.

Williams, J.G.P. (1978) Limitation of hip joint movement as a factor in traumatic osteitis pubis. *British Journal of Sports Medicine* **27**, 76–79.

Williams, P. & Foster, M.E. (1995) 'Gilmore's groin'—or is it? *British Journal of Sports Medicine* **29**, 206–208.

Wilson, A.M. & Goodship, A.E. (1994) Exercise-induced hyperthermia as a possible mechanism for tendon degeneration. *Journal of Biomechanics* **27**, 899–905.

Zamora, A.J. & Marini, J.F. (1988) Tendon and myo-tendinous junction in an overloaded skeletal muscle of the rat. *Anatomy and Embryology* **179**, 89–96.

Zernicke, R., McNitt-Gray, J., Otis, J. *et al.* (1993) Stress fracture assessment among collegiate women runners. International Society of Biomechanics, XIVth Congress, 1506–1507.

Chapter 53

Countering Inflammation

HINNAK NORTHOFF AND ALOIS BERG

Inflammation in the setting of sports medicine usually occurs as a highly undesirable phenomenon (Berg *et al.* 1992; Northoff *et al.* 1994). It accompanies acute injuries of all degrees of severity and affects all kinds of tissue; it also develops as a consequence of overuse in tendons, fasciae, joints and muscles. When considering inflammation, it is appropriate to begin with the role that inflammation plays in the first place in satisfying the overall aim of the body of maintaining or re-establishing homeostasis after it has been challenged by infection or injury. In this context, injury should be used in a very broad sense, to include subtle, camouflaged forms such as overuse or overstrain.

The role of inflammation

Although inflammation has a high potential for causing damage beyond the primary insult, it is of fundamental importance to keep in mind that inflammation, or at least certain aspects of it, is intimately associated with vital functions of tissue defence. With all the havoc that inflammation can cause, it should never be viewed as a fault of nature, or as an unnecessary, unpleasant side-effect which should simply be eradicated. The pain caused or aggravated by inflammation is a serious and meaningful signal of nature, and it is intended to force the body to keep itself, or at least the affected part, at rest. Patients with defective pain recognition are very prone to all kinds of injuries. In the same way, effective pain killing can be medically counterproductive if it leads to further strain on top of the primary injury (Stanley & Weaver 1998).

Apart from the symptom of pain and its protective role, inflammation is an integral part of any healing process (Berg *et al.* 1992; Northoff *et al.* 1994; Northoff *et al.* 1995). The mediators that cause inflammation all have important functions themselves, either in the healing process itself, or in offering an effective defence against invading microbes once an injury has breached the skin or mucosal barrier (Fig. 53.1). All of these factors are also present in sterile or internal wounds in the absence of any visible defects in the outer barriers of the body. Any injury leads to a complicated sequence of events, driven by a cascade of soluble mediators and by expression of receptors and adhesion molecules. These processes are designed to stop bleeding, keep out invading microorganisms, remove debris, induce controlled growth of the different tissues to form a scar, and restore normal function. The first wave of mediators is liberated by injured cells of epithelial, endothelial, fibroblastic or muscular origin, and by platelets. Besides activated complement and coagulation factors, they comprise a number of growth factors (EGF, FGF, IGF, FGFβ, PDGF), together with interleukin-6 (IL-6), eicosanoids and members of the IL-8 family which function as chemokines (Bennett & Schultz 1993; Lowry 1993). The latter provoke a wave of neutrophil immigration into the affected tissues. Somewhat later, macrophages follow, called in by chemoattractants which are generated for example by PDGF-stimulated smooth muscle cells from the vessel walls. Macrophages themselves deliver a number of cytokines which work as growth factors or activate polymorph neutrophils (PMN) and lymphocytes.

800

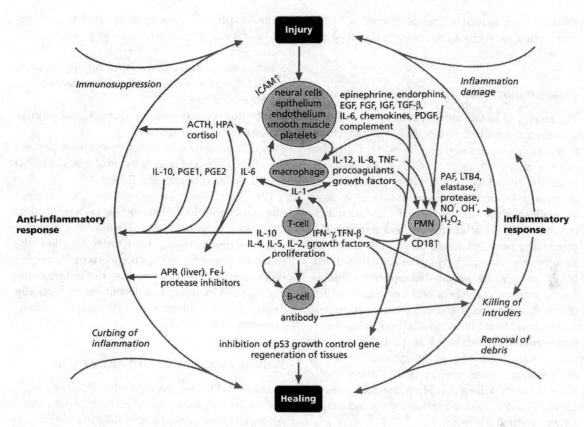

Fig. 53.1 Some factors involved in healing and inflammation (adapted from Northoff *et al.* 1995).

IL-1, tumour necrosis factor-α (TNF-α), IL-6 and IL-12 are some of these monokines. Lymphocytes finally follow to the scene, contributing their own shower of cytokines. Some of these cytokines, such as interferon-γ (IFN-γ), are essential for the activation of local macrophages and immigrating monocytes. They can also grossly enhance the action of other cytokines. This is particularly true for IFN-γ, which is not toxic in itself, but massively enhances the action of TNF in *in vivo* experiments. TNF is a notorious killer molecule and thus a very effective weapon in the body's defences. But, like all lethal weapons, it can also be dangerous for the host (Ferrante *et al.* 1992).

Injury alone is sufficient to cause inflammation, but inflammation is dramatically enhanced by bacterial products. Some of these, like endotoxin, a cell wall constituent of Gram-negative bacteria, cause major alarm reactions in macrophages at pg·ml^{-1} or low ng·ml^{-1} concentrations.

The neutrophils, which are the first type of leucocytes to enter the site of injury and inflammation, produce little or no cytokines in themselves. They are designed to perform phagocytosis, to kill microorganisms, and then to die. Together with bacteria or remnants of them, they form the main constituent of pus. Neutrophils possess an array of highly toxic substances which are normally stored in their granules, but are released upon stimulation with TNF or other cytokines. Cytotoxic macrophages and natural or specific killer lymphocytes all dispose of their own arsenal of attack molecules, including oxygen radicals (Favier 1997). This arsenal of deadly weapons is indispensable for an effective fight against microbial intruders. In the next section, we focus on the damage that they can cause to the host.

Inflammatory damage and its regulation

The arsenal of agents used by cells of the immune system comprises hydrolyses, elastase, collagenase, pore-forming molecules and a host of reactive oxygen species like NO, O_2^-, H_2O_2 and the extremely toxic OH radical. These substances are designed to kill microorganisms, but once they have been released, they are also toxic for the surrounding host cells. The attack molecules are induced by proinflammatory cytokines, particularly TNF and IL-8, by eicosanoids, by platelet-activating factor (PAF), and also by activated complement components, immune complexes and bacterial products (Baggiolini *et al.* 1994). TNF can induce neutrophils and eosinophils to kill endothelial cells. It has strong procoagulatory effects which are probably meant to confine intruders to their site of entrance. However, the proinflammatory mediators and attack molecules, besides killing invading microorganisms, cause cell death, vascular leakage, pain and coagulation (Northoff *et al.* 1995).

Inflammatory damage is essentially oxidative damage, and it can substantially exacerbate the primary injury (Jenkins 1993; Northoff *et al.* 1994; Sen *et al.* 1994). Its potency can be illustrated by the reperfusion damage of the heart that follows occlusion of a coronary artery. Reperfusion of the ischaemic tissue leads to a considerable enlargement of the damaged area. Adult respiratory distress syndrome (ARDS) is another condition in which radicals from invading phagocytes play a pivotal and fatal role (Donnelli *et al.* 1994). Systemic overexpression of TNF, leading to massive induction of oxygen radicals, also plays an essential role in causing the septic shock syndrome. Injection of TNF can induce all of the symptoms of sepsis. Inflammatory damage is thus a risk that is automatically associated with an effective immune response.

In the normal healing process, inflammation and associated damage are effectively balanced by several anti-inflammatory factors and mechanisms (Northoff *et al.* 1995). To these belong:

1 the induction of heat shock proteins, which act as radical scavengers and help with repair mechanisms;

2 induction of acute phase proteins in the liver, which help to reduce radical formation and work as protease inhibitors;

3 induction of receptor antagonists and soluble receptors (IL-1ra; sIL-2r); and

4 regulation of proinflammatory cytokine production. This is effected mainly by prostaglandins (PG) of the E series, cortisone and IL-10.

The overall effect of anti-inflammatory regulation can be decidedly immunosuppressive. Just as inflammation itself, the anti-inflammatory response must be finely balanced, in order to allow the tissue to proceed towards homeostasis. Excessive immunosuppression in response to the inflammation induced by injury or infection can be clinically deleterious, and indeed is one of the major problems in septic shock.

Role of eicosanoids and nitric oxide

Eicosanoids like the prostaglandins PGE_1 and PGE_2 and the leukotrienes (LT) deserve further attention. Although they have some inhibitory effects on inflammatory cells, particularly lymphocytes, and therefore play some regulatory, anti-inflammatory role, their overall spectrum of effects is decidedly proinflammatory (König *et al.* 1997a). They are the main transmitters delivering the pain signal to the local nerve endings. Their elimination by drugs causes prompt pain relief, but also shuts down the neural reflexes which take part in the normal inflammatory sequence (Leadbetter 1995; Stanley & Weaver 1998).

Prostaglandins and LT both stem from membrane phospholipids which are broken down to yield arachidonic acid (AA) as soon as they become accessible to phospholipase A_2 (PLA) through the activation or damage of cells (Adam 1992; König *et al.* 1997a; Stanley & Weaver 1998). This happens not only in activated macrophages, but also in many different types of somatic cells and tissues. Arachidonic acid is then processed into the prostaglandin-2 series by cyclooxygenase (COX), or into LT_4 by 5-lipoxygenase (5LG). Animal fat is the body's main source of AA, and the normal western diet contains more AA than is physiologically required. Anything which reduces the amount of available AA (particularly a reduced intake of meat) or interferes with the activity of PLA decreases both PG_2 and LT_4 and therefore has an anti-inflammatory effect (Adam 1992; König *et al.* 1997a). A major increase in the intake of essential fatty acids such as eicosapentaenoic acid (EPA, fish oil), α-linoleic acid (linseed oil) or γ-linoleic acid (GLA, evening primrose oil) shifts metabolism away from PG_2 into the PG_1 and PG_3 series, which act in part as antagonists of PG_2 metabolites (König *et al.* 1997a). Inhibition of COX by non-steroidal anti-inflammatory drugs (NSAIDs) shuts down the PG pathway (Parker 1986, 1987).

NSAIDs can have other, non-PG-related anti-inflammatory effects. Some are potent pain killers independently of PG. Moreover, some NSAIDs will inhibit both the COX and 5LG pathways (Leadbetter 1995; Stanley & Weaver 1998).

Besides the induction of pain and inflammation, PG have some critical protective functions for gastric mucosa and kidney tissue. This is why prolonged blockade of PGs can have adverse side-effects on these organs. COX comes in two versions: the constitutive one (COX1) and an inducible one (COX2). COX1 is largely responsible for protective and COX2 for inflammatory and pain-related effects (Stanley & Weaver 1998). Selective inhibition of COX2 with a sparing of COX1 has been an important target of the pharmaceutical industry for a number of years. At best, partially selective drugs have been developed (nabumetone, etodolac), and their clinical relevance has not yet been proven. Truly selective COX2 inhibitors are in experimental use, and some (e.g. celebrex) have now reached the US market (Taylor 1998). If they realize their promise, they will totally revolutionize the world of pharmaceutical pain killing.

Another mediator which is increased in wounded and inflamed tissues deserves mention: nitric oxide (NO) (Schaffer *et al.* 1997). NO radicals are part of the cytotoxic arsenal, but NO is also involved in blood pressure regulation and it may play an important role in the healing process (Schaffer *et al.* 1996). Research in this area is still in its early stages, but it is known that collagen synthesis is hampered by too little NO, whereas cellular proliferation suffers from overexpression of NO. As with COX, there are inducible and constitutive forms of NO synthase (iNOS, cNOS) and a mediator (NO) which need to be carefully regulated to achieve an appropriate balance of destructive and protective effects.

Causes of exercise-induced tissue injury

Given the increasing number of people who engage in some type of sport in their leisure time, and the increased training intensity and load needed to meet today's standards of competitive physical performance, the number of sports injuries has increased substantially over the last decade. Some 50–70% of all sports participants at some time sustain a sport-related injury (Renström & Johnson 1985; Brody 1987; Berg *et al.* 1989; Korkia *et al.* 1994; Ashbury 1995; Fallon 1996; Biundo *et al.* 1997; Fulcher *et al.* 1998).

In addition to the growing number of traumatic injuries, there is an increased incidence of overuse syndromes at the musculotendinous junction, both in leisure-time and competitive athletes. Special attention should be directed to the indirect type of sport injury, because clinical experience seems to indicate that it can be prevented by correcting extrinsic factors such as training mode, equipment, nutritional behaviour, and by physical and pharmacological pretreatment. However, neither the aetiology nor the possible effects of behavioural adjustments are proven by convincing prospective studies (Renström & Johnson 1985; Biundo *et al.* 1997; Fulcher *et al.* 1998).

Overuse leading to clinical syndromes and tissue injuries has been defined as a level of repetitive microtrauma sufficient to overwhelm the tissue's ability to adapt (Leadbetter 1995; Stanley & Weaver 1998). Tissue disturbances develop at the microscopic and/or molecular level as a result of extensive stress on the musculotendinous unit, particularly from repetitive bouts of combined eccentric and concentric exercise. Overload can occur at any point of the musculotendinous unit: within the muscle fibres themselves, at the musculotendinous junction, in the tendon or at the attachment of muscle or tendon to bone. Depending on the anatomical unit that has been disturbed, the overuse syndrome appears to the athlete as a muscle strain (delayed onset), muscular soreness, tendinitis, tendosynovitis or bursitis.

Even if prospective studies are lacking, we (and probably most practitioners) are strongly convinced from our experience that indirect, non-traumatic injuries are often related to training levels and training errors. Injuries are most common in athletes starting a training programme in combination with an excessive mileage (Renström & Johnson 1985; Brody 1987). Although the mechanism and the location of the overuse syndrome may differ in relation to the type of sports activity (Berg & Haralambie 1978), a local and a systemic inflammatory response can be observed immediately after the stressful episode (Fielding *et al.* 1993; Bruunsgaard *et al.* 1997; Weinstock *et al.* 1997). When the inflammatory response is essential to recovery and healing, it may be difficult to decide whether the inflammatory reaction should be therapeutically weakened or not. However, factors influencing, preventing or diminishing exercise-induced tissue injury and its corresponding inflammatory response should be taken into account more frequently.

With regard to countering exercise-induced inflammation, the first step in management should be the prevention of tissue injury by energetic, mechanical or structural overload (Renström & Johnson 1985; Brody 1987; Berg *et al.* 1989). However, the individual reaction to physical loading varies widely, and the extent of muscular

and systemic responses to exercise stress seems to be influenced by various cofactors (Fig. 53.2).

Factors influencing tissue injury and the inflammatory reaction

Training form and training status

For most practitioners, there is no doubt that incorrect training methods and a poor level of training significantly increase the incidence of overuse problems. Among external factors, improper training techniques or incorrect use of equipment are often mentioned as trigger mechanisms for overuse syndromes (Renström & Johnson 1985; Brody 1987; Berg *et al.* 1989; Korkia *et al.* 1994; Archambault *et al.* 1995; Almekinders & Temple 1998). It is thought that a combination of extrinsic factors such as excessive training intensity and duration, repetitive loading stress at an excessive force or elongation level, anatomical predisposition (inflexibility, weakness or malposition), strength deficits and muscular imbalance is responsible for common exercise injuries. As stated above, the correct answer to the aetiology of overuse syndromes remains to be established, because the majority of studies of physical activity and the incidence of sport-induced tissue injuries are retrospective in type, and have not been confirmed by controlled investigations. In addition, the relation-

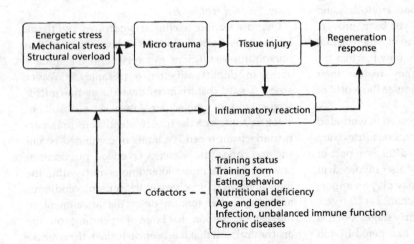

Fig. 53.2 Factors influencing exercise-induced overuse injuries.

ship between the extrinsic factors discussed and the theoretical pathways of the corresponding inflammatory response are not sufficiently documented. Some studies have indicated a correlation between running mileage and sport injuries, but on the other hand, there is an increased risk of injuries in persons who start their physical activity from a very low level. Serological findings indicating an increased level of muscular stress following endurance exercise have been reported in running novices (Noakes & Carter 1982). Adaptation to training decreases both the muscular and the inflammatory response to a given exercise load (Berg & Haralambie 1978; Noakes & Carter 1982).

Our own data on a homogeneous group of regional endurance athletes ($n = 100$) demonstrate that only a small proportion of athletes (about 15%) show moderately elevated resting IL-6 serum concentrations ($\geq 1.5\,pg\cdot ml^{-1}$) during the course of normal training (samples collected at 8.00 a.m. with no competitive event during the preceding 7 days) (Wagner et al. 1996). Nevertheless, there was a direct correlation between the training load (expressed as training hours per week) and the morning serum IL-6 levels in our athlete group. There was also an increased incidence of IL-6 concentrations of $>1.5\,pg\cdot ml^{-1}$ in athletes who were training for more than $15\,h\cdot week^{-1}$.

Special attention should be paid to the type of muscular exercise undertaken. In sports like cycling, which involve largely concentric work, the muscular stress reaction is significantly less than in other endurance sports with an appreciable percentage of eccentric loading (Berg & Haralambie 1978; Renström & Johnson 1985; Korkia et al. 1994). Thus, some authors have theorized that sports injuries and accompanying inflammation are particularly fostered by eccentric contractions of the muscle–tendon unit.

Age and gender

Age and gender are among the better documented factors supposedly playing an aetiological role in sports injuries and inflammation (Kannus et al. 1989; Ross & Woodward 1994; Almekinders & Temple 1998). The regulation of muscular and systemic stress significantly deteriorates with ageing, and the incidence of sports injuries in athletes increases with age, peaking between 30 and 50 years of age. The underlying mechanism for this, however, is unclear. Elderly athletes are predominantly male, well-educated, health conscious and of good cardiovascular fitness. Apparently, the majority of them are endurance sportsmen, differing substantially in their sports habits from their younger colleagues. This could be one reason why they have significantly more overuse injuries. There is no study indicating that the corresponding inflammatory response may be amplified with age. However, it is a reasonable assumption that elderly athletes have a more degenerative basis for their sports injuries. This may be accompanied by a chronic inflammatory response. A repeated inflammatory response may cause unwanted and non-specific (fibrous/collagenous) healing processes in elderly athletes. It has yet to be examined whether the countering of inflammation would be beneficial in this context.

The hypothesis that individual regulation of the inflammatory response may play a role in the incidence of overuse injuries is supported by new data about gender and neurogenic variables in tendon biology and repetitive motion disorders (Hart et al. 1998). Traditionally, overuse injuries have been discussed as primarily a consequence of tissue fatigue, with a subsequent inflammatory response. In the case of tendons, no investigation has ever found conventional signs of inflammation in the tendon itself. The inflammatory response seems to be confined to surrounding tissues.

Factors which can initiate the inflammatory process, such as vasoactive substances, PG, neurotransmitters and neurogenic substances, are influenced by sex hormones and gender-related factors (Hart et al. 1998). These findings are in good agreement with observations that females have a higher incidence of overuse or repetitive motion injuries in the workplace (Ross & Woodward 1994; Ashbury 1995). In addition, syndromes which are accompanied by fluctuations or disturbances of sex hormones during the menstrual cycle, e.g. secondary amenorrhoea and premenstrual syndrome, are related to sports injuries (Lloyd et al. 1986). Therefore, it must be assumed that there is a sex-related cellular and molecular component to the development of overuse injuries (Hart *et al.* 1998). More understanding of this neurogenic mechanism is needed before a specific rather than an empirical treatment of sex-related overuse injuries can be adopted.

Nutritional aspects

As already mentioned in the section on prostaglandins, some nutrients may play an important role in regulating inflammatory processes, including those caused by intensive physical exercise. To this group of nutrients belong vitamin E, selenium (Se) and several polyunsaturated fatty acids (PUFAs) (Ursini & Bindoli 1987; Dekkers *et al.* 1996; Halliwell 1996; König *et al.* 1997a,b; Berg *et al.* 1998). These nutrients are involved in inflammatory regulation by direct and indirect mechanisms, influencing the structure of blood cells and muscle cell membranes, the metabolism of eicosanoids and the functional capacity and action of cortisol. Other nutrients, such as Zn, Cu and Mn, are involved in the regulation of antioxidative stress (Dekkers *et al.* 1996; König *et al.* 1998), but there are as yet no sufficient data to show that the acute inflammatory response after exhaustive physical exercise can be modulated by products or special diets containing substantial amounts of these trace elements.

VITAMIN E

Intensive physical activity, particularly of the aerobic type, can cause an increased production of reactive oxygen species (ROS) (Jenkins 1993; Sen *et al.* 1994; Berg *et al.* 1998). Sources for the formation of free radicals include the working muscles (mitochondrial oxygen consumption, xanthine oxidation) and several processes that accompany muscular activities (e.g. acidosis, PG stimulation, the phagocytic oxidative burst, intracellular calcium accumulation, iron release and increased exposure to environmental sources such as ozone). Since vitamin E can reduce lipid peroxidation, it is assumed that this vitamin may protect against free radical damage and exercise-induced inflammation. Although several studies indicate correlations

between exhaustive aerobic exercise and oxidative stress, no direct cause and effect relationship has yet been established. Our own recently published data (Berg *et al.* 1998) indicate that neither the exercise-induced peroxidation rate, expressed by diene production, nor the muscular cell damage, expressed by an increase in serum creatine kinase activity, is related to the individual plasma vitamin E concentration. Our tests were based on a homogeneous group of endurance athletes. In contrast, athletes in the same experimental group who showed high plasma vitamin E levels had a decreased exercise-induced inflammatory response as indicated by a significantly smaller increase in serum IL-6 (Berg *et al.* 1998). However, it is important to notice that vitamin E mildly inhibits 5LG, thereby reducing the biosynthesis of LTA_4, LTB_4 and LTC_4. This biochemical effect of vitamin E may explain the possible benefit from pharmacological doses of vitamin E (a dose of 400 IU vitamin E or more per day), given as a dietary supplement in patients with osteoarthritis (Scherak *et al.* 1990).

SELENIUM

As an essential component of the enzyme glutathione peroxidase, the trace element selenium (Se) is involved in the regulation and breakdown of hydroperoxides (Tiran 1997). Thus, Se may play a significant role in the prevention of free radical damage and oxidative stress, even in situations of muscular stress and exhaustive exercise (Ursini & Bindoli 1987). Se has a similar action to vitamin E, and indeed, vitamin E deficiency synergistically augments symptoms of Se deficiency. Muscular discomfort and/or weakness are documented after continuous periods of Se-free diets (e.g. parenteral feeding) (Tiran 1997). In conditions of Se deficiency (for example, in patients undergoing haemodialysis), significant limitations of cellular antioxidative properties can be observed. Controlled studies concerning the impact of Se supplementation on lipid peroxidation in athletes are not yet available. However, there is growing evidence that the local application of Se (as Na selenite) significantly decreases symptoms of arthralgia, tendinitis and bursitis in general and sports medicine practice

(Al-Bazaz 1995). The therapeutic effects of local Se application have been attributed to a combination of anti-inflammatory, immunomodulating and radical-catching properties (Tiran 1997).

POLYUNSATURATED FATTY ACIDS

PUFAs are essential components of cellular membranes and structures; they significantly influence the plasticity and rigidity of muscle and blood cells, both of which are stressed by exhaustive aerobic exercise (König et al. 1997a). In addition, essential fatty acids, particularly EPA and GLA, can weaken the inflammatory response to physical stress by modulating the eicosanoid pathway (see above). Available results document that both muscular and systemic inflammatory stress can be influenced in apparently healthy individuals, including endurance athletes, by modulating the composition and quality of dietary fat (König et al. 1997a). The practical implication is that in contrast to the usual dietary aim (lowering total fat intake to 30–35% of total energy intake), athletes should pay greater attention to the intake of essential fatty acids. When more than 60% of the fat energy intake is derived from meat, the distribution of ω-6 to ω-3 PUFAs, as well as the content of AA probably becomes unfavourable for the tolerance of muscular and systemic stress (Adam 1992). Since PUFAs are known to influence (i) the structure of red blood cell and muscle cell membranes (creatine kinase, myoglobin) and (ii) the inflammatory response (IL-6, C reactive protein (CRP)) to training and physical exercise, athletes may profit from an increased intake of EPA and/or GLA products, as well as from low AA diets (König et al. 1997a).

Prevention and treatment of inflammation and tissue injuries

The primary basis for the prevention of exercise-induced injuries is the correction of extrinsic factors, such as overuse, training errors, use of inadequate equipment and dietary inadequacies. Excessive repetitive movement, leading to overload of specific musculotendinous groups, carries a risk of muscular injury. Training methods, training load and

intensity all have to be adjusted to ensure the individual health and training status of the athlete. Body conditioning programmes should be an obligatory component of all sports practice, but particularly in the case of elderly athletes and untrained beginners (Renström & Johnson 1985; Brody 1987; Fulcher et al. 1998; Hart et al. 1998).

Once inflammation and overuse syndromes are manifest, corrections of behavioural factors and relative rest of the respective area are the first lines of treatment and a precondition for further therapeutic steps. This seems true for both acute and chronic overuse injuries; however, the absolute necessity of relative rest has not been proven scientifically. Absolute rest is required in syndromes that are accompanied by wounds and tears, unless the defect has been surgically corrected. Lack of compliance in such cases leads to inadequate healing, with unnecessary enlargement of fibrous or collagenous scar tissue. Rest and compression bandages can also help to reduce swelling, particularly when the inflamed part can be put into an elevated position.

Non-pharmaceutical treatment

Although little scientific proof is available, application of ice and cryotherapy are widely considered as effective measures for curbing inflammation when treating soft tissue injuries (Almekinders 1993; Almekinders & Temple 1998). Ice is also a potent pain killer. Application of ice, preferably within the first seconds and minutes after an inflammatory stimulus, can reduce subsequent inflammatory damage (Swenson et al. 1996). The efficacy of ice therapy is probably attributable not simply to a reduction in swelling and pain; ice also reduces the secretory activity of the inflammatory cells. Once the first round of inflammatory mediators has been produced, ice may still be effective, but not to the same extent as in the first minutes after injury. Ice is also effective in chronic inflammatory syndromes. The fact that cryotherapy is not only a pain killer but also interferes deeply with the metabolic mediators of inflammation can be seen from the fact that repetitive local ice application causes similar topical side-effects to local cortisone application, particularly atrophy of the skin.

Pharmaceutical treatment

When inflammation and pain are prominent symptoms of the acute or chronic exercise injury, most physicians use pharmacological remedies to achieve relief. The medical benefit of such treatment mainly remains dubious, but it usually makes the patient 'feel better' (Almekinders & Almekinders 1994). Common forms of therapy include oral aspirin or other NSAIDs, topical application of NSAIDs and local injection of corticosteroids. Several excellent reviews are available (Leadbetter 1995; Almekinders & Temple 1998; Stanley & Weaver 1998).

Oral aspirin is still widely used despite the development of many alternative drugs. Diclofenac, piroxicam and naproxen are some of the more frequently used alternative remedies (Leadbetter 1995; Stanley & Weaver 1998). Their efficacy in terms of relieving pain and anti-inflammatory symptoms has been documented in various controlled and prospective studies (Almekinders & Temple 1998). Their efficacy in terms of pain relief seems generally accepted, but improvements in the healing process cannot be expected from such drugs. In contrast, it has been discussed whether the anti-inflammatory effects of NSAIDs may actually delay healing, for example in minor stretch injuries. The situation may differ in conditions where inflammatory damage is a very prominent component of the overall tissue injury. In addition to rheumatic conditions, this is probably also the case in delayed-onset muscle soreness (DOMS).

Leukotriene inhibitors have also been discussed as a possible treatment for tissue injuries (Stanley & Weaver 1998). Leukotriene inhibitors increase the efficacy of NSAIDs in an experimental model of rheumatoid arthritis, but we do not know of any study yet performed in the context of exercise-induced injuries.

Oral NSAIDs should generally be prescribed with care, since side-effects are not uncommon, and can be disastrous in individual patients. Gastrointestinal complications are the most frequent and well-known side-effects (Stanley & Weaver 1998), but renal complications have also been documented (Farquhar & Kenney 1997). Several case studies have linked acute renal failure to the use of NSAIDs in the context of exercise and related heat stress and dehydration (Farquhar & Kenney 1997). Long-term use of NSAIDs can contribute to chronic renal failure, independently of any sport involvement. Gastrointestinal problems can also be fatal. Chronic gastrointestinal ulceration and fatal ulcer-related complications are commonly associated with NSAID therapy. Of the many different NSAIDs which have been prescribed to date, none is free of such side-effects. Truly specific COX2 inhibitors may change the situation substantially in the very near future (Taylor 1998) (see 'Role of eicosanoids and nitric oxide' above).

The risk of gastrointestinal toxicity can be diminished by complementary prescription of protective drugs like misoprostol, a PGE_1 analogue, or omeprazole, a proton pump inhibitor (Stanley & Weaver 1998). Topical application of NSAIDs provides an alternative way of avoiding critical systemic side-effects. Effective levels of NSAIDs are found in muscle and connective tissues after local application of such drugs, whereas systemic concentrations remain less than 10% of those measured after oral NSAID therapy (Dominikus *et al.* 1996).

Corticosteroids are potent anti-inflammatory drugs. Multiple mechanisms underlie their anti-inflammatory action, ranging from inhibition of phospholipase, inhibition of cytokine and chemokine expression to stabilization of membranes (Leadbetter 1995). Interference with the cytokine cascade has indirect effects on other proinflammatory systems like PGs. Since the cytokine cascade is intimately involved in the healing sequence, it is not surprising that cortisone can severely impair wound healing. This is also the major drawback limiting the use of corticosteroids in inflammatory conditions.

Local, peritendinous infiltration of cortisol has been advocated for the treatment of chronic tendon injuries. Nevertheless, caution is warranted, and a strict limitation must be placed on the number of injections and the duration of treatment (Almekinders & Temple 1998; Stanley & Weaver

1998). There is a substantial danger of tendon rupture associated with local injection of corticosteroids. Existing literature weighing the benefits and side-effects of local steroid injection in sport injuries is inconsistent, and is characterized by a lack of long-term prospective studies.

References

Adam, O. (1992) Immediate and long range effects of the uptake of increased amounts of arachidonic acid. *Clinical Investigation* 70, 721–727.

Al-Bazaz, S. (1995) Schmerzminderung bei Arthralgien verschiedener Genese durch intraartikuläre Selengaben. *Orthopedische Praxis* 31, 710–714.

Almekinders, L.C. (1993) Anti-inflammatory treatment of muscular injuries in sports. *Sports Medicine* 15, 139–145.

Almekinders, L.C. & Almekinders, S.V. (1994) Outcome in the treatment of chronic overuse sports injuries: a retrospective study. *Journal of Orthopedic and Sports Physical Therapy* 19, 157–161.

Almekinders, L.C. & Temple, J.D. (1998) Etiology, diagnosis, and treatment of tendonitis: an analysis of the literature. *Medicine and Science in Sports and Exercise* 30, 1183–1190.

Archambault, J.M., Wiley, J.P. & Bray, R.C. (1995) Exercise loading of tendons and the development of overuse injuries. A review of current literature. *Sports Medicine* 20, 77–89.

Ashbury, F.D. (1995) Occupational repetitive strain injuries and gender in Ontario, 1986–1991. *Journal of Occupational and Environmental Medicine* 37, 479–485.

Baggiolini, M., Moser. B. & Clark-Lewis, I. (1994) Interleukin-8 and related chemotactic cytokines. *Chest* 105, 95–98.

Bennett, N.T. & Schultz, G.S. (1993) Growth factors and wound healing: Part II. Role in normal and chronic wound healing. *American Journal of Surgery* 166, 74–81.

Berg, A. & Haralambie, G. (1978) Changes in serum creatine kinase and hexose phosphate isomerase with exercise duration. *European Journal of Applied Physiology* 39, 191–201.

Berg, A., Jakob, E. & Keul, J. (1989) 'Exercise Myopathie'—metabolische Ätiologie und die Konsequenzen für den Sportarzt. *Therapiewoche* 39, 1852–1857.

Berg, A., Northoff, H. & Keul, J. (1992) Immunologie und Sport. *Internist* 33, 169–178.

Berg, A., König, D., Grathwohl, D., Frey, I. & Keul, J. (1998) Antioxidantien im Leistungssport. Was ist Gesichert? *Deutsch Zeitschrift für Sportmedizin* 49 (Suppl.1), 86–92.

Biundo, J.J. Jr, Mipro, R.C. Jr & Fahey, P. (1997) Sports-related and other soft-tissue injuries, tendinitis, bursitis and occupation-related syndromes. *Current Opinion in Rheumatology* 9, 151–154.

Brody, D.M. (1987) Running injuries—prevention and management. *Clinical Symposia* 39, 1–36.

Bruunsgaard, H., Galbo, H., Halkjaer-Kristensen, J., Johansen, T.L., MacLean, D.A. & Pedersen, B.K. (1997) Exercise-induced increase in serum interleukin-6 in humans is related to muscle damage. *Journal of Physiology (London)* 499, 833–841.

Dekkers, C., Doornen, L.J.P.V. & Kemper, H.C.G. (1996) The role of antioxidant vitamins and enzymes in the prevention of exercise-induced muscle damage. *Sports Medicine* 21, 213–238.

Dominikus, M., Nicolakis, M. & Kotz, R. (1996) Comparison of tissue and plasma levels of ibuprofen after oral and topical administration. *Arzneimittelforschung* 46, 1138–1143.

Donnelli, S.C., Strieter, R.M., Kunkel, S.L. et al. (1994) Chemotactic cytokines in the established adult respiratory distress syndrome and at-risk patients. *Chest* 105, 98–105.

Fallon, K.E. (1996) Musculoskeletal injuries in the ultramarathon: the 1990 Westfield Sydney to Melbourne run. *British Journal of Sports Medicine* 30, 319–323.

Farquhar, B. & Kenney, W.L. (1997) Anti-inflammatory drugs, kidney function, and exercise. *Sports Science Exchange* 11, 1–5.

Favier, A. (1997) Le stress oxydant: intérêt de sa mise en évidence en biologie médicale et problèmes posés par le choix d'un marqueur. *Annales de Biologie Clinique (Paris)* 55, 9–16.

Ferrante, A., Kowanko, I.C. & Bates, E.J. (1992) Mechanisms of host tissue damage by cytokine-activated neutrophils. *Immunology Series* 57, 499–521.

Fielding, R.A., Manfredi, T.J., Ding, W., Fiatarone, M.A., Evans, W.J. & Cannon, J.G. (1993) Acute phase response in exercise. III. Neutrophil and IL-1 beta accumulation in skeletal muscle. *American Journal of Physiology* 265, R166–R172.

Fulcher, S.M., Kiefhaber, T.R. & Stern, P.J. (1998) Upper-extremity tendinitis and overuse syndromes in the athlete. *Clinical Journal of Sports Medicine* 17, 433–448.

Halliwell, B. (1996) Oxidative stress, nutrition and health. Experimental strategies for optimization of nutritional antioxidant intake in humans. *Free Radical Research* 25, 57–74.

Hart, D.A., Archambault, J.M., Kydd, A., Reno, C., Frank, C.B. & Herzog, W. (1998) Gender and neurogenic variables in tendon biology and repetitive motion disorders. *Clinical Orthopedics* 351, 44–56.

Jenkins, R.R. (1993) Exercise, oxidative stress, and antioxidants: a review. *International Journal of Sport Nutrition* 3, 356–375.

Kannus, P., Niittymaki, S., Jarvinen, M. & Lehto, M. (1989) Sports injuries in elderly athletes: a three-year prospective, controlled study. *Age and Ageing* 18, 263–270.

König, D., Berg, A., Weinstock, C., Keul, J. & Northoff, H. (1997a) Essential fatty acids, immune function, and exercise. *Exercise Immunology Review* 3, 1–31.

König, D., Keul, J., Northoff, H. & Berg, A. (1997b) Rationales für eine gezielte Nährstoffauswahl aus sportmedizinischer und sportorthopädischer Sicht. *Orthopäde* 26, 942–950.

König, D., Weinstock, C., Keul, J., Northoff, H. & Berg, A. (1998) Zinc, iron, and magnesium status in athletes—influence on the regulation of exercise-induced stress and immune function. *Exercise Immunology Review* 4, 2–21.

Korkia, P.K., Tunstall-Pedoe, D.S. & Maffulli, N. (1994) An epidemiological investigation of training and injury patterns in British triathletes. *British Journal of Sports Medicine* 28, 191–196.

Leadbetter, W.B. (1995) Anti-inflammatory therapy in sports injury. The role of non-steroidal drugs and corticosteroid injection. *Clinical Journal of Sports Medicine* 14, 353–410.

Lloyd, T., Triantafyllou, S.J., Baker, E.R. et al. (1986) Women athletes with menstrual irregularity have increased musculoskeletal injuries. *Medicine and Science in Sports and Exercise* **18**, 374–379.

Lowry, S.F. (1993) Cytokine mediators of immunity and inflammation. *Archives of Surgery* **128**, 1235–1241.

Noakes, T.D. & Carter, J.W. (1982) The responses of plasma biochemical parameters to a 56-km race in novice and experienced ultra-marathon runners. *European Journal of Applied Physiology* **49**, 179–186.

Northoff, H., Weinstock, C. & Berg, A. (1994) The cytokine response to strenuous exercise. *International Journal of Sports Medicine* **15** (Suppl. 3), S167–S171.

Northoff, H., Enkel, S. & Weinstock, C. (1995) Exercise, injury, and immune function. *Exercise Immunology Review* **1**, 1–25.

Parker, C.W. (1986) Leukotrienes and prostaglandins in the immune system (review). *Advances in Prostaglandin, Thromboxane and Leukotriene Research* **16**, 113–134.

Parker, C.W. (1987) Lipid mediators produced through the lipoxygenase pathway. *Annual Reviews of Immunology* **5**, 65–84.

Renström, P. & Johnson, R.J. (1985) Overuse injuries in sports. A review. *Sports Medicine* **2**, 316–333.

Ross, J. & Woodward, A. (1994) Risk factors for injury during basic military training. Is there a social element to injury pathogenesis? *Journal of Occupational Medicine* **36**, 1120–1126.

Schaffer, M.R., Tantry, U., Gross, S.S., Wasserburg, H.L. & Barbul, A. (1996) Nitric oxide regulates wound healing. *Journal of Surgical Research* **63**, 237–240.

Schaffer, M.R., Tantry, U., Wesep, R.A.V. & Barbul, A. (1997) Nitric oxide metabolism in wounds. *Journal of Surgical Research* **71**, 25–31.

Scherak, O., Kolarz, G., Schödl, C. & Blankenhorn, G. (1990) Hochdosierte Vitamin-E-Therapie bei Patienten mit aktivierter Arthrose. *Zeitschrift für Rheumatologie* **49**, 369–373.

Sen, C.K., Atalay, M. & Hanninen, O. (1994) Exercise-induced oxidative stress: glutathione supplementation and deficiency. *Journal of Applied Physiology* **77**, 2177–2187.

Stanley, K.L. & Weaver, J.E. (1998) Pharmacologic management of pain and inflammation in athletes. *Clinical Journal of Sports Medicine* **17**, 375–392.

Swenson, C., Sward, L. & Karlsson, J. (1996) Cryotherapy in sports medicine. *Scandinavian Journal of Medicine and Science in Sports* **6**, 193–200.

Taylor, C. (1998) The great pain debate. *TIME* **152**, 47.

Tiran, B. (1997) Selen—ein essentielles Spurenelement. *Wiener Klinische Wochenschrift* **109**, 3–6.

Ursini, F. & Bindoli, A. (1987) The role of selenium peroxidases in the protection against oxidative damage of membranes. *Chemistry and Physics of Lipids* **44**, 255–276.

Wagner, J.D., Zhang, L., Williams, J.K. *et al.* (1996) Esterified estrogens with and without methyltestosterone decrease arterial LDL metabolism in cynomolgus monkeys. *Arteriosclerosis, Thrombosis and Vascular Biology* **16**, 1473–1480.

Weinstock, C., Konig, D., Harnischmacher, R., Keul, J., Berg, A. & Northoff, H. (1997) Effect of exhaustive exercise stress on the cytokine response. *Medicine and Science in Sports and Exercise* **29**, 345–354.

PART 8

SPECIFIC ISSUES IN INDIVIDUAL AND TEAM SPORTS

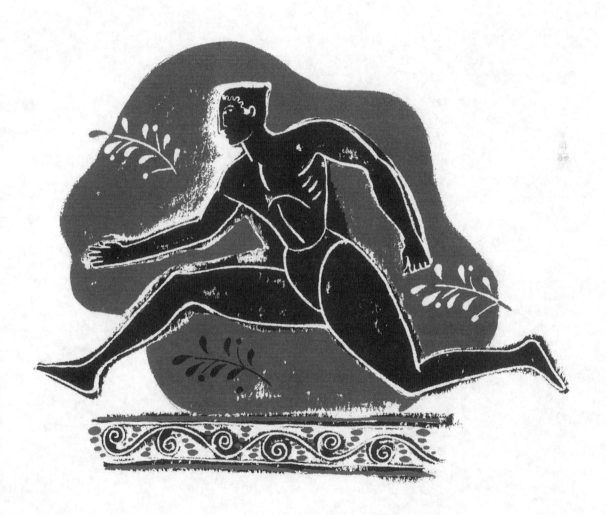

Chapter 54

Energetics of Running

PIETRO E. DI PRAMPERO

The energetics of running, and indeed of many other forms of locomotion on land and in water, can be appropriately described, provided that their energy costs are known. This cost, which will here be given the symbol C_r, is defined as the amount of energy required to transport the runner over one unit of distance: C_r is therefore conceptually identical to the notion of 'petrol consumption per 100 km' for a car. In the case of a vehicle, determination of the fuel consumed over a given distance is made trivial by the presence of the tank. In the human body, however, no well-defined 'tank(s)' can be identified, so that C_r can only be determined indirectly, from the amount of O_2 consumed. As a first approximation, the energy equivalent of O_2 amounts to 20.9 kJ·l^{-1} (5.0 kcal·l^{-1})* so that C_r can be expressed in $1O_2$·km^{-1}, kcal·km^{-1} or kJ·km^{-1}, the choice being essentially a matter of convenience, even if, according to SI units, C_r ought to be expressed in kJ·km^{-1} or in J·m^{-1}. So, C_r is generally obtained from the ratio of the steady-state O_2 consumption above resting to the running speed (Fig.

54.1). It goes without saying that it is often convenient to express C_r per kg of transported mass.

The energy cost of running

During treadmill running, C_r is independent of speed (Fig. 54.2); for level running it amounts, on average, to 3.8 kJ·kg^{-1}·km^{-1} (di Prampero 1986). When running uphill, C_r increases approximately linearly with the incline, to reach about 8 kJ·kg^{-1}·km^{-1} at a slope of +20%. For downhill running, C_r decreases to attain a minimum of about 3 kJ·kg^{-1}·km^{-1} at a slope of −10%; for steeper slopes it increases again to about 3.5 kJ·kg^{-1}·km^{-1} for a slope of −20% (Margaria 1938).

The interindividual variability in C_r is rather small, amounting to ±8% (s.d.) (di Prampero 1986). Even so, this variability can be responsible for substantial differences in performance times (see section on 'Long-distance running' below); it is therefore not surprising that the underlying reasons have been thoroughly investigated. These will not be reviewed here; nevertheless the results of some studies devoted to the effects on C_r of: (i) training (Bourdin et al. 1993; Morgan et al. 1995; Lake & Cavanagh 1996); (ii) sex (Bunc & Heller 1989; Padilla et al. 1992; Bourdin et al. 1993; Helgerund 1994); (iii) age (MacDougall et al. 1983); and (iv) body mass (Padilla et al. 1992; Bourdin et al. 1993; Helgerund 1994) are briefly summarized below. There is far from a consensus as to the effects of training on C_r. However, a retrospective analysis of seven publications over a 20-year period showed that, on average, élite runners were more economical than the less

*The energy equivalent of O_2 depends on the respiratory quotient, i.e. on the ratio of metabolic CO_2 output to O_2 consumption (RQ = $\dot{V}_{CO_2}/\dot{V}_{O_2}$). RQ depends on the type of fuel and varies from 1.00 for pure carbohydrates to 0.71 for pure lipids, the corresponding energy equivalent of O_2 ranging from 21.13 kJ·l^{-1} (5.05 kcal·l^{-1}) for RQ = 1.00, to 19.62 kJ·l^{-1} (4.68 kcal·l^{-1}) for RQ = 0.71. The value used throughout this chapter (20.9 kJ·l^{-1} or 5.00 kcal·l^{-1}) applies for RQ = 0.96, as can be expected during heavy aerobic exercise. It is based on the additional assumption that, during exercise, the net oxidation of proteins is not increased substantially above the value at rest.

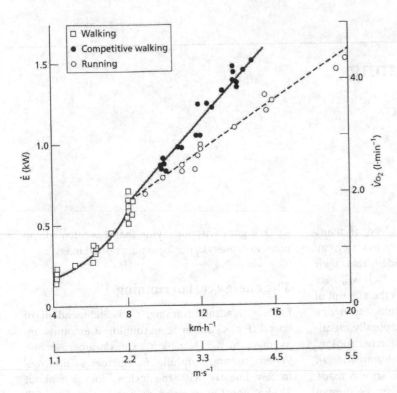

Fig. 54.1 Metabolic energy expenditure in excess of resting ($\dot{E}$, kW, left; $1O_2 \cdot min^{-1}$, right) in one subject as a function of the speed (km·h⁻¹ or m·s⁻¹) during walking (filled squares, w), competitive walking (filled dots, w*) or running (open dots, r) on a treadmill.

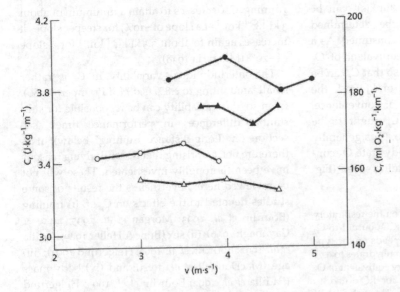

Fig. 54.2 Energy cost of running (C_r, J·kg⁻¹·m⁻¹, left; mlO_2·kg⁻¹·m⁻¹, right) as a function of treadmill speed (v, m·s⁻¹) in four representative subjects. From di Prampero (1986).

talented ones and trained subjects had a lower C_r than untrained controls (Morgan *et al.* 1995). The within-group variability was high in all groups, and there was a substantial overlap of minimum and maximum C_r values. When C_r is expressed per kg body mass, it is the same in men and women (Bunc & Heller 1989). Some studies, however, show that C_r per kg body mass is smaller the larger the body mass (Padilla *et al.* 1992; Bourdin *et al.* 1993; Helgerund 1994) (see section on 'Performance and body size' below), so that, strictly speaking C_r is the same in men and women only for the same body mass. In children, C_r is larger than in adults; according to MacDougall *et al.* (1983), it amounts on average to 5.05, 4.66, 4.26 and 4.08 (kJ·kg^{-1}·km^{-1}) in children of 7–9, 10–12, 13–14 and 15–16 years of age, respectively, as compared with an average value of 3.8 kJ·kg^{-1}·km^{-1} in adults. The data of MacDougall *et al.* show that in children C_r is essentially independent of speed, and the coefficient of variation of C_r amounts to about 16%, twice that observed in adults.

When running in the field, C_r is larger than observed on the treadmill (C_{rtr}):

$$C_r = C_{rtr} + k' \cdot v^2$$

where k' is a constant and v (m·s^{-1}) is the air speed. For normal running conditions ($P_B \approx 760$ mmHg, T $\approx$ 20°C), k' = 0.40 J·s^2·m^{-3} and per m^2 of body surface area, i.e. about 0.01 J·s^2·m^{-3} and per kg body mass (see Table 54.1). Since C_{rtr} is constant, amounting to about 3.8 kJ·kg^{-1}·km^{-1} for level running (see above), it can be calculated that the energy expended against the wind is ≤ 8% for speeds ≤ 20 km·h^{-1}. For larger speeds it increases substantially, to reach 32% at maximal absolute running speeds of about 40 km·h^{-1}.

Long-distance running

The metabolic power ($\dot{E}_r$) required to run at any given speed v is set by the product of C_r and speed:

$$\dot{E}_r = C_r v = C_r d / t_p \tag{1}$$

where d is the distance covered in the performance time t_p. If C_r and v are expressed in SI units (J·m^{-1} and m·s^{-1}), $\dot{E}_r$ is expressed in W, or, if C_r is expressed in mlO$_2$·kg^{-1}·m^{-1} and v in m·min^{-1}, $\dot{E}_r$ is in ml O$_2$·kg^{-1}·min^{-1}, the traditional units in which metabolic power has been expressed. Rearranging Equation 1, it becomes apparent that the maximal speed is set by the ratio of the maximal metabolic power of the runner ($\dot{E}_{max}$) to his/her C_r at that speed:

$$v_{max} = \dot{E}_{max} / C_r \tag{2}$$

Table 54.1 The constant (k') relating the energy expended against the wind to the square of air speed, together with the energy cost of treadmill running in excess of resting (C_{rtr}) ± 1 s.d. and the overall cost of running in excess of resting (including air resistance, for a 70-kg, 1.75-m runner (body surface area (BSA) = 1.85 m^2)).

k'	C_{rtr} ± s.d.	Overall cost
J·s^2·m^{-3} (per m^2 BSA)	J·kg^{-1}·m^{-1}	J·m^{-1} (for 70 kg, 1.75 m)
0.40	3.80 ± 0.30	265 + 0.74v^2

The constant k' is expressed per m^2 of BSA, at 760 mmHg barometric pressure and 20 °C ambient temperature; v is the air velocity in m·s^{-1}.

In aerobic conditions, $\dot{E}_{max}$ is proportional to the subject's maximal O$_2$ intake, so that Equation 2 becomes:

$$v_{end} = F \dot{V}_{O_{2max}} / C_r \tag{3}$$

where v_{end} is the endurance speed and F is the fraction of $\dot{V}_{O_{2max}}$ that can be maintained throughout the run. In Equation 3, $\dot{V}_{O_{2max}}$ and C_r must be expressed in the same units (see footnote on p. 813).

The validity of Equation 3 was investigated in 36 male amateur runners who performed the marathon (42.195 km) or the semimarathon (21 km). In these subjects, $\dot{V}_{O_{2max}}$ and C_r (at a speed equal to the average they had actually maintained during the event) were determined 1–2 weeks after competition. F was then estimated from published data, on the basis of individual performance time and v_{end} calculated from Equation 3. The results showed that v_{end} was linearly correlated to the actual average speed during competition ($r^2 = 0.72$) and did not differ significantly from it (Fig. 54.3 & Table 54.2) (di Prampero *et al.* 1986).

The data reported in Fig. 54.3 showed that v_{end} was slightly greater than the actual speed of performance, the more so the larger the speed. A fraction of this difference was due to underestimation of the denominator of Equation 3 (C_r). Indeed, the value of C_r utilized to calculate v_{end} was determined 1–2 weeks after competition, during a brief experimental session of 15–20 min duration. So, the calculated value was that applicable to a non-fatigued subject. If C_r increased as the runners became fatigued in the

Table 54.2 Ratios of the actual average speed over competition (v_{comp}) to the speed predicted from Equation 3 (v_{end}) for semimarathoners (1/2 M), marathoners (M) and all subjects combined (All). Number of subjects (n) is also indicated. The three columns report the ratios obtained: (i) when $v_{end}(1)$ is calculated assuming C_r as measured on the treadmill (see Table 54.1); (ii) when $v_{end}(2)$ is calculated correcting C_r for the average wind resistance (see Table 54.1); and (iii) when $v_{end}(3)$ is calculated correcting C_r for the average wind resistance and for the fatigue incurred throughout competition (see section on 'Long-distance running'). Data from di Prampero *et al.* (1986) and Brückner *et al.* (1991).

	n	$v_{comp} \cdot v_{end}(1)^{-1}$	$v_{comp} \cdot v_{end}(2)^{-1}$	$v_{comp} \cdot v_{end}(3)^{-1}$
M	12	0.948 ± 0.082	0.974 ± 0.084	0.999 ± 0.085
1/2 M	24	0.946 ± 0.067	0.980 ± 0.070	1.005 ± 0.073
All	36	0.947 ± 0.076	0.978 ± 0.079	1.003 ± 0.083

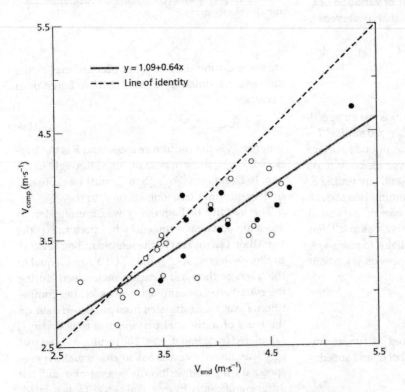

Fig. 54.3 Actual average speed during the marathon (filled dots) or semimarathon (open dots) (v_{comp}, m·s⁻¹) is plotted as a function of the speed predicted from Equation 3 (v_{end}, m·s⁻¹). Straight line is described by: $y = 1.09 + 0.64x$ ($r^2 = 0.72$). The line of identity is also shown. From di Prampero *et al.* (1986).

course of an actual race, then the 'true' value of C_r used in the calculation should have been larger than that determined in non-fatigued conditions, thus yielding a smaller value of v_{end}, presumably closer to the actual speed. This possibility was investigated in 10 amateur long-distance runners who ran twice, at 15–30-day intervals, distances of 15, 32 and 42.195 km. The experiments were completed on a 400-m indoor track, and the subjects were asked to run at a constant speed, 3% slower than their best individual contemporary performance over the marathon. The speed was checked at regular intervals throughout the experiment. During the initial and final 5–7 min, the subjects ran on a treadmill at the same speed at which they were supposed to run, or at which they were actually running. Thus, for each runner, C_r was determined in non-fatigued conditions and after covering 15, 32 and 42.195 km. The results showed that, in comparison with non-fatigued conditions, C_r was unchanged up to 15 km.

For greater distances C_r increased, on average by about 0.12% per km distance (Brückner *et al.* 1991). On these bases, therefore, v_{end} was recalculated for the runners mentioned above, assuming that in this group also, C_r increased with distance by the same amount. The values of v_{end} thus calculated were essentially equal to the actual speed of performance (see Table 54.2). It can be concluded that the value of C_r to use in Equation 3 to obtain a correct estimate of v_{end} must take into account the slight but significant increase of C_r that takes place over race distances longer than about 15 km.

The increase of C_r with distance was astonishingly small, at least in the trained amateur long-distance runners in whom it was determined: indeed, at the end of the marathon, C_r had increased on average by only about 4%. This is small, particularly if compared to the apparent qualitative deterioration of running 'style' in fatigued subjects. However, the change is substantial in terms of performance. It can easily be calculated that a 4% increase in C_r is accompanied by an equal increase in the performance time, i.e. slightly more than 5 min for world-class marathon performances. This is particularly relevant, since the increase of C_r with the distance varies markedly from one subject to the other, the extremes ranging from 0.06% to 0.19% per km. This large variability so far remains unexplained; it shows, however, that if a long-distance runner is to achieve world-class performance, in addition to being characterized by a high $\dot{V}_{O_2max}$ and a low C_r, she/he must also be a 'non-augmenter' of C_r over the event.

As mentioned above, F in Equation 3 is the fraction of $\dot{V}_{O_2max}$ that can be maintained throughout the run. It is rather difficult to measure. In the study reported above, F was estimated on the basis of individual performance times, since the data of Saltin (1973) showed that the fraction of $\dot{V}_{O_2max}$ used by trained subjects decreased linearly with the duration of runs to exhaustion (t_e, s) as described by di Prampero (1981):

$$F = 0.94 - 1.67 \cdot 10^{-5} t_e \tag{4}$$

This equation applies only for $F \leq 0.9$, since for $F > 0.94$ Equation 4 yields negative values for t_e, a nonsensical result.

More recently, Péronnet and Thibault (1989) have shown that, for performance times shorter than 7 min, $F = 1.0$, whereas for longer performance times, F decreases with the natural logarithm of the performance time (t_e, s):

$$F = 1.00 \qquad \text{(for } 45\,s < t_e < 420\,s\text{)}$$

$$F = 1.00 - 0.0568 \ln (t_e/420) \quad \text{(for } t_e > 420\,s\text{)} \tag{5}$$

Equation 3 shows unequivocally that the performance time depends critically not only on $\dot{V}_{O_2max}$ and C_r but also on F. A precise assessment of individual values of F, even if rather tedious experimentally, appears of crucial importance when evaluating the athletic capabilities of long-distance runners.

In conclusion, Equation 3 is a faithful description of the energetic bottleneck that determines endurance performance. In practice, once individual values of $\dot{V}_{O_2max}$, F and C_r of a given runner are known, Equation 3 can be utilized to predict his or her performance. Alternatively, the same information allows the training strategy of a given runner to be individually tailored, so that it is directed towards improving the weakest of the three quantities that determine performance.

Performance and body size

In the preceding paragraphs, it has been implicitly assumed that the three variables that set v_{end}: $\dot{V}_{O_2max}$, C_r and F (Equation 3), are independent of the subject's body mass. Many studies have shown, however, that in the animal kingdom the maximal oxygen intake and the energy cost of locomotion (be it on land, in water or in the air) increase with the animal's body mass raised to an exponent < 1.0. The few paragraphs that follow are therefore devoted to a brief analysis of the relationship between body mass and performance in mammals, and more specifically in humans. The analysis will be limited to performance times allowing the animal to exercise at 100% $\dot{V}_{O_2max}$. So, as a first approximation, it can be assumed that, of the three variables at stake, $F = 1.0$ is constant, whereas $\dot{V}_{O_2max}$ and C_r depend on the animal's body mass (M):

$$F = 1.0 M^0 \tag{6}$$

$$\dot{V}O_{2max} = aM^{\alpha} \qquad (7)$$

$$C_r = bM^{\beta} \qquad (8)$$

where a, b are the appropriate constants and α, β the corresponding exponents. Thus, as from Equation 3:

$$v_{end} = aM^{\alpha}(bM^{\beta})^{-1} \qquad (9)$$

or, setting $c = ab^{-1}$ and $\gamma = \alpha - \beta$:

$$v_{end} = cM^{\gamma} \qquad (10)$$

Taylor et al. (1980) observed that in mammals ranging in mass from 0.6 to 260 kg, $\dot{V}O_{2max}$ (W) increased with the animal's mass (M, kg) as described by the equation:

$$\dot{V}O_{2max} = 34.9 M^{0.85} \qquad (11)$$

It was also observed that over a similar body mass range, C_r (J·m^{-1}) increased to a lesser extent:

$$C_r = 10.7 M^{0.60} \qquad (12)$$

for quadrupedal running (Taylor 1977; McMahon & Bonner 1983) and:

$$C_r = 11.5 M^{0.76} \qquad (13)$$

for bipedal running (Taylor 1977).

Equations 10–13 allow one to calculate that the maximal running speeds at $\dot{V}O_{2max}$ depend on the animal's mass, as described by:

$$v@ \dot{V}O_{2max} = 3.26 M^{0.25} \qquad (14)$$

for quadrupeds and:

$$v@ \dot{V}O_{2max} = 3.03 M^{0.09} \qquad (15)$$

for bipeds. So, whereas for quadrupeds the speed attained at $\dot{V}O_{2max}$ (Equation 14) should increase substantially with the animal's mass (from 6.9 m·s^{-1} for a 20-kg dog to 15.4 m·s^{-1} for a 500-kg horse), for bipedal running, the maximal aerobic speed as predicted from Equation 15 is very nearly independent of speed, increasing only from 4 m·s^{-1} for 20 kg to 5.3 m·s^{-1} for 500 kg body mass.

The maximal aerobic speed, as from Equation 15, amounts to 4.4 m·s^{-1} (16.0 km·h^{-1}) for a 70-kg biped, not far from the values that can be expected in trained humans. In humans, however, analysis of the relationship between $\dot{V}O_{2max}$ or C_r, and hence of maximal aerobic speed, on the one side, and body mass, on the other, is fraught with difficulties because of (i) the large variability of $\dot{V}O_{2max}$ among subjects and (ii) the limited range of body mass. Nevertheless, Åstrand and Rodahl (1986; from data provided by O. Vaage & L. Hermansen) showed that, in a group of élite male Norwegian athletes, as a first approximation $\dot{V}O_{2max}$ (W) increased with the body mass (kg), as described by:

$$\dot{V}O_{2max} = 100 M^{0.67} \qquad (16)$$

The 0.67 exponent reported by Åstrand and Rodahl is close to that obtained by von Døbeln (1956) for the relationship between $\dot{V}O_{2max}$, predicted from the Åstrand nomogram, and fat-free body mass (an exponent of 0.71).

The relationship between C_r and body mass in running humans has been investigated by several authors (Williams et al. 1987; Berg et al. 1991; Padilla et al. 1992; Bourdin et al. 1993). On the whole, the results indicate that C_r increases with body mass raised to an exponent < 1.0. Indeed, the data collected by Lacour and coworkers (Padilla et al. 1992; Bourdin et al. 1993) in a group of boys and girls and men and women with body masses ranging from about 25 to about 80 kg (10–30 years of age) showed that the relationship between C_r (J·m^{-1}) and body mass (M, kg) could be approximated by the following equation:

$$C_r = 12.5 M^{0.7} \qquad (17)$$

This equation should be taken with a pinch of salt: (i) because of the variability of C_r for a given body mass, and (ii) because the body mass differences in the subjects investigated were due to a combination of sex, age and body structure, furthermore (iii) Ferretti et al. (1991) and Minetti et al. (1994) reported lower C_r values (per kg body mass) in pygmies, as compared to Caucasians, thus flatly contradicting Equation 17. In the case of Minetti et al. (1994), C_r was on average 12.7% lower in pygmies, as compared to Caucasians, instead of 9% larger, as predicted from Equation 17 for the corresponding average body masses (pygmies, 51.6 kg; Caucasians, 69.2 kg). The different running economy of pygmies and Caucasians was attributed by the authors to as yet unexplained differences in the mechanics of running between the two population groups.

The above reported data and considerations show that the relationship between C_r and M in running humans, as well as its underlying causes, deserves further scrutiny. Even so, Equation 17 is fairly close to the analogous equation for running bipeds (Equation 13), in terms of both constants (12.5 versus 11.5) and exponents (0.70 versus 0.76). Assuming therefore that Equation 17 is indeed an appropriate description of the dependence of C_r on body mass, the maximal aerobic speed in élite human athletes is given by the ratio of Equations 16 to 17:

$$v@\ \dot{V}O_{2max} = 8.00\,M^{-0.03} \tag{18}$$

If this is so, the maximal aerobic speed in humans is essentially independent of the subject's body mass, amounting to about $7\,\text{m·s}^{-1}$ ($25\,\text{km·h}^{-1}$) for a 70-kg runner. This may appear a little high, even if it refers to the élite athletes from whom the relationship between $\dot{V}O_{2max}$ and M was obtained (see above). It should be noted, however, that (i) it refers to the speed that can be maintained at $\dot{V}O_{2max}$, i.e. for at most 7–10 min, and (ii) $\dot{V}O_{2max}$ in Equation 16 includes the resting metabolism so that, when this last item is subtracted, the speed predicted by Equation 18 is reduced by about 1–$1.5\,\text{km·h}^{-1}$.

Finally, it should be pointed out that expressing $\dot{V}O_{2max}$ and C_r per unit of body mass, each raised to a given exponent, may be appropriate when comparing subjects of different body size and hence understanding the underlying physiological determinants (Helgerund 1994). However, Equations 9 and 10 show that, in order to compare the individual speeds of different subjects, both $\dot{V}O_{2max}$ and C_r should be expressed per unit body mass raised to the same exponent. If this is not the case, the resulting speed (v_{end} in Equation 10) is expressed per unit body mass raised to the residual exponent ($\gamma = \alpha - \beta \neq 0$), a rather unusual way of expressing athletic performances. For practical athletic purposes, the most reasonable choice is to normalize both $\dot{V}O_{2max}$ and C_r per unit body mass ($M^{1.0}$).

Middle-distance running

The preceding discussion was devoted to running speeds at or below $\dot{V}O_{2max}$. Over short times (and distances), the maximal metabolic power can exceed $\dot{V}O_{2max}$ by a substantial amount, thanks to exploitation of the anaerobic energy stores. Under these conditions, the amount by which the maximal metabolic power exceeds the subject's $\dot{V}O_{2max}$ depends on the duration of the effort, being large for short efforts and decreasing progressively as the duration of effort is increased. The next few paragraphs provide a brief discussion of factors that determine performance when a substantial fraction of the overall maximal metabolic power is derived from anaerobic sources.

As pointed out above (Equation 1), in this case the metabolic power ($\dot{E}_r$) required to proceed at any given speed v is determined by the product of C_r and the speed:

$$\dot{E}_r = C_r v = C_r d/t_p \tag{1}$$

Since C_r is constant (or increases slightly with speed) for any given distance, $\dot{E}_r$ is larger the shorter t_p. Thus, the shortest time (fastest speed) over a given distance will be achieved when $\dot{E}_r$ is equal to the maximal metabolic power of the subject ($\dot{E}_{max}$).

Many studies have shown that $\dot{E}_{max}$ is a decreasing function of the duration of exercise to exhaustion (exhaustion time, t_e). According to Wilkie (1980):

$$\dot{E}_{max} = \text{AnS}\,t_e^{-1} + [\dot{V}O_{2max} - \dot{V}O_{2max}\,(1 - e^{-t_e/\tau})\,\tau\,t_e^{-1}] \tag{19}$$

where AnS is the amount of energy derived from complete exploitation of the anaerobic sources (maximal lactic acid formation and maximal phosphocreatine breakdown) and where AnS and $\dot{V}O_{2max}$ are expressed in the same units. The third term of Equation 19 takes into account the fact that, at the onset of exercise, $\dot{V}O_{2max}$ is not reached instantaneously, but with a time constant τ; this term represents the aerobic power loss due to the O_2 deficit incurred at the onset of exercise and averaged throughout the time to exhaustion t_e. As a consequence, the actual aerobic power, averaged throughout exercise, is given by the term in square brackets. Equation 19 shows that the contribution of anaerobic stores to $\dot{E}_{max}$ becomes progressively smaller, and that of aerobic sources progressively larger, with increasing t_e. The example that follows illustrates this point. For an élite athlete, $\dot{V}O_{2max}$ above resting and AnS can be assumed to be 25.8 W·kg^{-1} and 1.42 kJ·kg^{-1} (74 ml·kg^{-1}·min^{-1} and 68.0 ml·kg^{-1} in O_2 equivalents) (di Prampero 1981). Assuming $\tau = 24$ s (Binzoni *et al.* 1992), $\dot{E}_{max}$ amounts to 39.2 W·kg^{-1} for $t_e = 60$ s, and to 26.7 W·kg^{-1} for $t_e = 15$ min. Equation 19 shows that the corresponding anaerobic contributions decrease from 23.7 W·kg^{-1} (60.5%) for $t_e = 60$ s to 0.67 W·kg^{-1} (2.5%) for $t_e = 15$ min. It necessarily follows that the remaining fractions, representing the average aerobic power, increase from 39.5% to 97.5%. Strictly speaking, Equation 19 applies for $45 s \leq t_e \leq 7$ min, i.e. over a time range sufficient for full utilization of AnS, but within which $\dot{V}O_{2max}$ can be fully maintained throughout exercise (see Equation 5). Equation 5 shows, however, that from 7 to 15 min, F decreases only from 1.00 to 0.96, so that the validity of the equation can be extended up to 15 min, if one is prepared to accept an error $\leq 4\%$.

The preceding discussions and calculations show that if τ, $\dot{V}O_{2max}$ and AnS are known, $\dot{E}_{max}$ can be described analytically as a function of t_e by means of Equation 19. On the other side, if C_r is known, $\dot{E}_r$ can be described analytically as a function of t_p, over any given distance d, by means of Equation 1. Furthermore, it can be assumed that the best performance time, over a given distance and for a given runner, is the time value for which exhaustion and performance coincide ($t_e = t_p$). If this is so, the best performance time (for any given runner and distance) can be obtained (graphically or by numerical iteration) as the time value for which $\dot{E}_{max}$ (Equation 19) and $\dot{E}_r$ (Equation 1) become equal. A graphical example of this approach is reported in Fig. 54.4 for an élite athlete whose characteristics are assumed to be as follows: $\dot{V}O_{2max}$ above resting = 25.8 W·kg^{-1} (74 ml O_2·kg^{-1}·min^{-1}), AnS = 1.42 kJ·kg^{-1} (68.0 ml O_2·kg^{-1}), $C_r = 3.78$ J·kg^{-1}·m^{-1} (0.180 ml O_2·kg^{-1}·m^{-1}), $\tau = 24$ s. For times shorter than that at which the two functions $\dot{E}_r$ and $\dot{E}_{max}$ cross, $\dot{E}_r$ is greater than $\dot{E}_{max}$; these times will therefore be unattainable by the runner in question. For greater times, the opposite is true: $\dot{E}_{max}$ is larger than $\dot{E}_r$, so the runner could have run faster. Hence the best performance time for any given runner and distance is indeed the time value where the two functions $\dot{E}_r$ and $\dot{E}_{max}$ cross.

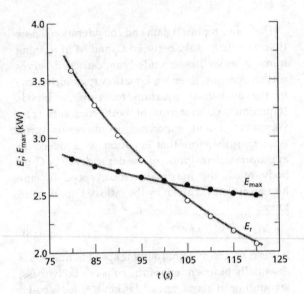

Fig. 54.4 The metabolic power ($\dot{E}_r$) required to cover 800 m from a stationary start in the time reported on the abscissa is indicated by open dots. The filled dots indicate the maximal power ($\dot{E}_{max}$) sustainable for the time reported on the abscissae. The time at which the two functions cross (98.7 s) is the individual best performance time. Data refer to a hypothetical top-class athlete: $\dot{V}O_{2max}$ in excess of resting = 25.8 W·kg^{-1} (74 ml O_2·kg^{-1}·min^{-1}), AnS = 1.42 kJ·kg^{-1} (68.0 ml O_2·kg^{-1}), $C_r = 3.78$ J·kg^{-1}·m^{-1}. Metabolic power is expressed in kW, time in s. See text for details.

The validity of this approach was investigated in 16 runners of intermediate level competing over middle distances (0.8–5.0 km). Their $\dot{V}O_{2max}$ was measured during an incremental running test. C_r during constant speed track running (3.7–6.0 m·s^{-1}) was subsequently determined from the ratio of steady-state oxygen consumption above resting (corrected for blood lactate accumulation) to speed, and AnS was assumed from published data. Assuming further that $\tau = 24$ s (Binzoni *et al.* 1992), this made it possible to calculate time values equating the left sides of Equations 1 and 19, for distances from 0.8 to 5.0 km, as described above. These times were then compared to the actual best times obtained by the same subjects during contemporary competitions over the same distances (di Prampero *et al.* 1993).

C_r amounted on average to 3.72 J·kg^{-1}·m^{-1} (±0.24,

Table 54.3 Average ratios (±1 s.d.) between actual best performance times (t_{act}) and theoretical times (t_{theor}) over the corresponding distances are reported for medium-class and élite athletes. From di Prampero *et al.* (1993). Theoretical times for élite athletes were calculated from data reported by Lacour *et al.* (1990). Values significantly different from 1.00 ($p < 0.05$) are indicated by *; n = number of observations.

| Distance (km) | Medium level | | Élite | |
	n	$t_{act} \cdot t_{theor}^{-1}$	n	$t_{act} \cdot t_{theor}^{-1}$
0.8	12	1.16 ± 0.093*	13	1.075 ± 0.033*
1.0	8	1.065 ± 0.091		
1.5	11	1.038 ± 0.064	24	1.016 ± 0.025
3.0	7	1.026 ± 0.066	18	1.015 ± 0.027
5.0	3	1.025 ± 0.022	18	1.016 ± 0.024
Overall mean	41	1.078 ± 0.095*	73	1.026 ± 0.0042*

s.d.; n = 58). For distances between 1 and 5 km, theoretical times were on average, 4.1% shorter (±6.8%, s.d.; n = 29), but not significantly different, than actual best times. For the shortest distance (0.8 km), however, theoretical times were significantly shorter than actual best times, the average difference amounting to 16% (±9.3%, s.d.; n = 12) (diPrampero *et al.* 1993) (Table 54.3). The above approach was also applied to similar data obtained by Lacour *et al.* (1990) on French élite middle-distance runners. In this case, the agreement between theoretical and actual best times was even better: for distances between 1.0 and 5.0 km, the theoretical times were 1.6% shorter (±2.5%, s.d.; n = 60), but not significantly different from actual best times. Again, for the shortest distance (0.8 km), theoretical times were significantly shorter than actual best times, the average difference amounting to 7.5% (±3.3%, s.d.; n = 13) (Table 54.3). For both groups of subjects, the theoretical performance times are plotted in Fig. 54.5 as a function of the actual individual contemporary records over the same distance.

The data reported above show that the agreement between fact and theory for distances of between 1.0 and 5.0 km is rather good. It is likely that the agreement would have been better if, in addition to $\dot{V}O_{2max}$ and C_r, AnS had also been individually determined, rather than estimated from the literature. For shorter distances, however, the model yields theoretical performance times that are shorter than

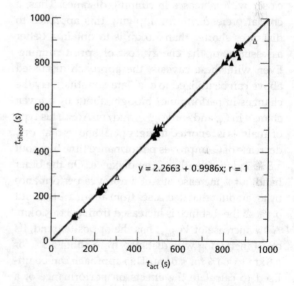

Fig. 54.5 Theoretical best performance times (t_{theor}) for two groups of athletes (medium level, open triangles; élite, filled triangles) are plotted as a function of contemporary actual best performance times (t_{act}). From di Prampero *et al.* (1993).

actual times, and hence speeds that are greater. This is presumably due to the fact that, in both sets of calculations, C_r was determined during constant speed running. Therefore, before inserting it into Equation 1, C_r was corrected for the energy spent to accelerate the body from a stationary start to the final running speed. This was done by calculating the kinetic energy (E_k) per kg body mass and per unit of distance ($(d/t_p)^2/d$) and dividing this quantity by the efficiency of running (η): $E_k = (d/t_p)^2 (d\eta)^{-1}$. Since the recovery of elastic energy is negligible in the initial acceleration phase, η was assumed to be 0.25, i.e. close to the value observed when running uphill on very steep slopes (Margaria 1938). E_k was then added to the value of C_r as obtained during constant speed running: it amounted to about 10% of C_r for the shortest distance and highest speed (0.8 km), but decreased for longer distances and smaller speeds, attaining a value of about 1% for 5.0 km. Any possible error in calculating E_k is bound to affect the theoretical times to a larger extent over shorter distances. Indeed, it was observed that the agreement between theoretical and actual times became progressively closer with increases in running distance. Thus, a crucial prerequisite for applying this approach to distances shorter than 1.0 km is to obtain a better assessment of the energy cost of sprint running. Even with these caveats, the approach discussed above can be utilized to evaluate quantitatively the changes in performance brought about by a given change in C_r, and/or $\dot{V}O_{2max}$, and/or AnS. This type of analysis is reported in Fig. 54.6. It shows that a 5% decrease of C_r improves performance time by about 3.8%, independently of the distance. On the other hand, a 5% increase of AnS improves performance by an amount that decreases from about 2% to about 0.3% as the distance is increased from 0.8 to 5.0 km. A 5% increase of $\dot{V}O_{2max}$ has the opposite trend, its effect increasing with distance, from about 2.8% for 0.8 km to 3.9% for 5.0 km. This approach can be utilized to calculate the effects on performance of a change in any of the variables included in the model, or any combination thereof. Individualized use of the model may aid in the selection of a more successful training strategy for any given runner. In conclusion, the approach explained here seems to provide an appropriate description of the energetics of best performances in running. The model has also been applied recently to track cycling over distances of 1.0–10.0 km, with equally good results (Capelli *et al.* 1998).

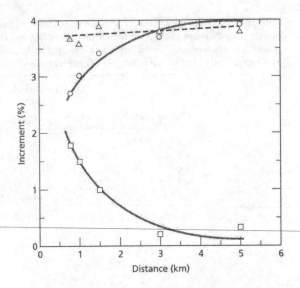

Fig. 54.6 Percentage increase of performance (decrease of performance time) over the indicated distances (km) when $\dot{V}O_{2max}$ (open dots) or AnS (open squares) are increased by 5%, or when C_r (open triangles) is decreased by 5%. The reference values are those applicable for an élite athlete: $\dot{V}O_{2max}$ in excess of resting = 25.8 W·kg^{-1} (74 ml O$_2$·kg^{-1}·min^{-1}), AnS = 1.42 kJ·kg^{-1} (68.0 ml O$_2$·kg^{-1}), C_r = 3.78 J·kg^{-1}·m^{-1} (0.180 ml O$_2$·kg^{-1}·m^{-1}). See text for details. From di Prampero (1997).

Conclusions

The agreement between theoretical estimates and actual running performances is remarkably good. The precision of estimates depends essentially on the accuracy with which we can assess individual values for the energy cost of running, maximal anaerobic capacity, maximal aerobic power and the fraction of this last variable which can be sustained throughout the required effort. This seems sound proof that our knowledge of the energetics of muscular exercise, on the one hand, and of running, on the other, is quite satisfactory.

Theoretical estimates, based on the energetics of running, have practical value in sports physiology and also help to clarify the basic mechanisms underlying human motion.

References

Åstrand, P.O. & Rodahl, K. (1986) *Textbook of Work Physiology*, pp. 391–411. McGraw-Hill, New York.

Berg, U., Sjödin, B., Forsberg, A. & Svedenhag, J. (1991) The relationship between body mass and oxygen uptake during running in humans. *Medicine and Science in Sports and Exercise* **23**, 205–211.

Binzoni, T., Ferretti, G., Schenker, K. & Cerretelli, P. (1992) Phosphocreatine hydrolysis by ^{31}P-NMR at the onset of constant-load exercise in humans. *Journal of Applied Physiology* **73**, 1644–1649.

Bourdin, M., Pastene, J., Germain, M. & Lacour, J.R. (1993) Influence of training, sex, age and body mass on the energy cost of running. *European Journal of Applied Physiology* **66**, 439–444.

Brückner, J.C., Atchou, G., Capelli, C. *et al.* (1991) The energy cost of running increases with the distance covered. *European Journal of Applied Physiology* **62**, 385–389.

Bunc, V. & Heller, J. (1989) Energy cost of running in similarly trained men and women. *European Journal of Applied Physiology* **59**, 178–183.

Capelli, C., Schena, F., Zamparo, P., Dal Monte, A., Faina, M. & di Prampero, P.E. (1998) Energetics of best performances in track cycling. *Medicine and Science in Sports and Exercise* **30**, 614–624.

Døbeln, W., von (1956) Maximal oxygen uptake, body size and total haemoglobin in normal man. *Acta Physiologica Scandinavica* **38**, 193–199.

Ferretti, G., Atchou, G., Grassi, B., Marconi, C. & Cerretelli, P. (1991) Energetics of locomotion in African Pygmies. *European Journal of Applied Physiology* **62**, 7–10.

Helgerund, J. (1994) Maximal oxygen uptake, anaerobic threshold and running economy in women and men with similar performances level in marathons. *European Journal of Applied Physiology* **68**, 155–161.

Lacour, J.R., Padilla-Magunacelaya, S., Barthélémy, J.C. & Dormois, D. (1990) The energetics of middle distance running. *European Journal of Applied Physiology* **60**, 38–43.

Lake, M.J. & Cavanagh, P.R. (1996) Six weeks of training does not change running mechanics or improve running economy. *Medicine and Science in Sports and Exercise* **28**, 860–869.

MacDougall, J.D., Roche, P.D., Bar-Or, O. & Moroz, J.R. (1983) Maximal aerobic capacity of Canadian schoolchildren: predictions based on age related oxygen cost of running. *International Journal of Sports Medicine* **4**, 194–198.

McMahon, T.A. & Bonner, J.T. (1983) *On Size and Life*, pp. 151–165. Scientific American Library, W.H. Freeman, New York.

Margaria, R. (1938) Sulla fisiologia epecialmente sul consumo energetico della marcia e della corsa a varia velocità e inclinazione del terreno. *Atti della Accademia Nazionale dei Lincei* **7**, 299–368.

Minetti, A.E., Saibene, F., Ardigò, L.P., Atchou, G., Schena, F. & Ferretti, G. (1994) Pygmy locomotion. *European Journal of Applied Physiology* **68**, 285–290.

Morgan, D.W., Bransford, D.R., Costill, D.L., Daniels, J.T., Howley, E.T. & Krahenbuhl, G.S. (1995) Variation in the aerobic demand of running among trained and untrained subjects. *Medicine and Science in Sports and Exercise* **27**, 404–409.

Padilla, S., Bourdin, M., Barthélémy, J.-C. & Lacour, J.R. (1992) Physiological correlates of middle-distance running performance. A comparative study between males and females. *European Journal of Applied Physiology* **65**, 561–566.

Péronnet, F. & Thibault, G. (1989) Mathematical analysis of running performance and world running records. *Journal of Applied Physiology* **67**, 453–465.

di Prampero, P.E. (1981) Energetics of muscular exercise. *Reviews of Physiology, Biochemistry and Pharmacology* **89**, 143–222.

di Prampero, P.E. (1986) The energy cost of human locomotion on land and in water. *International Journal of Sports Medicine* **7**, 55–72.

di Prampero, P.E. (1997) Energetica della corsa. *Medicina dello Sport* **50**, 1–8.

di Prampero, P.E., Atchou, G., Brueckner, J.-C. & Moia, C. (1986) The energetics of endurance running. *European Journal of Applied Physiology* **55**, 259–266.

di Prampero, P.E., Capelli, C., Pagliaro, P. *et al.* (1993) Energetics of best performances in middle distance running. *Journal of Applied Physiology* **74**, 2318–2324.

Saltin, B. (1973) Oxygen transport by the circulatory system during exercise in man. In: Keul, J. (ed.) *Limiting Factors of Physical Performance*, pp. 235–252. Georg Thieme, Stuttgart.

Taylor, C.R. (1977) The energetics of terrestrial locomotion and body size in vertebrates. In: Pedley, T.J. (ed.) *Scale Effects in Animal Locomotion*, pp. 127–141. Academic Press, London.

Taylor, C.R., Maloiy, G.M.O., Weibel, E.R. *et al.* (1980) Design of the mammalian respiratory system. III. Scaling maximum aerobic capacity to body mass: wild and domestic mammals. *Respiration Physiology* **44**, 25–37.

Wilkie, D.R. (1980) Equations describing power input by humans as a function of duration of exercise. In: Cerretelli, P. & Whipp, B.J. (eds) *Exercise Bioenergetics and Gas Exchange*, pp. 75–80. Elsevier, Amsterdam.

Williams, K.R., Cavanagh, P.R. & Ziff, Z.L. (1987) Biomechanical studies of élite female distance runners. *International Journal of Sports Medicine* **8**, 107–118.

Chapter 55

Swimming as an Endurance Sport

LENNART GULLSTRAND

Introduction

Swimming is in many ways a peculiar sport. From a physiological point of view, one of the most striking aspects of competitive swimming is that it is dominated by anaerobic events (Table 55.1; Houston 1978; Maglischo 1982; Troup 1984), although practices for most distances are still dominated by aerobic workouts. This is supported by the fact that 10 out of a total of 13 events for both sexes in international competitions are swum over distances taking less than about 2 min. When all 4 × 100-m and 4 × 200-m relays are included, the number of anaerobic events is increased even further.

During 1986, the 50-m freestyle event was added to the international programme for both men and women. By analogy with track and field, this event is similar in duration to the running distance of 200 m. Even more 50-m distances are now included in international competitions. That swimming training is dominated by aerobic exercises can be seen by the high maximal oxygen intake values measured for swimmers (Holmér 1979). In a review table that includes participants in other sports, we find female and male swimmers with values of 3.5 and 5.5 $l \cdot min^{-1}$, respectively, in the top third of athletes from endurance sports such as long-distance running, cross-country skiing and orienteering. Similar figures have been measured repeatedly for Swedish national team swimmers since the early 1960s (Åstrand & Rodahl 1986). Nevertheless records in different distances and strokes are continuously broken. Increased strength and refined technique (swimming economy) are prob-

ably the most reasonable factors to explain this development.

Comparison of maximal oxygen intake values expressed in $ml \cdot kg^{-1} \cdot min^{-1}$ is not justified in this sport because the static lifting force of buoyancy influences the body's performance. Extra body fat has only a minor negative effect on performance in water when compared with dry land.

A superficial analysis of the training performed by élite swimmers allows us to understand why they have a large aerobic power. It is usual to swim between eight and 12 workouts per week, covering a distance of 4000–12 000 m (60–120 min) per workout. Large muscle groups are thereby involved, stressing the cardiopulmonary system to adapt. Strangely enough, the character of the conditioning programme is similar for long periods, regardless of the distance for which athletes are training.

It is unrealistic to draw up a training plan for most swimmers competing over 50, 100 and 200 m based on a physiological competition profile, as in Table 55.1. A 100-m or 200-m swimmer cannot, for example, withstand workouts in which 80–90% of training is at an anaerobic intensity, especially since 65% of this training is calculated to be of a lactic acid nature, with the remaining part being aerobic. Nevertheless, there has been a certain change in the design of training programmes over the past 10 years. More and more anaerobic sessions are seen in a 100-m swimmer's training, as well as more frequent periods of both active and passive rest (Gullstrand 1985, 1986a,b).

One of the reasons for the continued dominance

824

Table 55.1 Relative contribution of anaerobic and aerobic metabolism in international swim distances.

Race distance (m)	Approximate time* (min:s)	ATP–PCr (alactic) (%)			HLa (lactic) (%)			Total (%)			Aerobic metabolism (%)		
		M	T	H	M	T	H	M	T	H	M	T	H
50	0:23	78	98	—	20	2	—	98	100	—	2	—	—
100	0:50	25	80	—	65	15	—	90	95	80	10	5	20
200	1:50	10	30	—	65	65	—	75	95	60	25	5	40
400	3:50	7	20	—	40	55	—	47	75	40	53	25	60
800	7:50	5	—	—	30	—	—	35	—	17	65	—	83
1500	15:00	3	10	—	20	20	—	23	30	10	77	70	90

*Male élite swimmers.

ATP, adenosine triphosphate; PCr, phosphocreatine; HLa, lactic acid; M, Maglischo (1982); T, Troup (1984); H, Houston (1978).

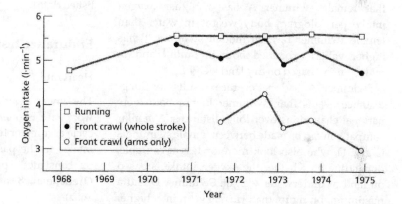

Fig. 55.1 Oxygen intake during maximal swimming and running for world and Olympic medal swimmer Gunnar Larsson over a period of 8 years. From Åstrand and Rodahl (1986).

of aerobic training is probably that swimming is very much an 'arm and upper body sport'. All leg-dependent athletes on land have special training for the lower extremities, plus the daily stimulation of walking and standing.

A swimmer who is not actually swimming receives virtually no training of the upper body, and especially not of the 'proper' arm muscles that are required for swimming. Perhaps this is one of the reasons for the distance and time a swimmer must cover in order to be successful, regardless of whether he or she is preparing for short- or long-distance performance. Swimmers could reduce their workout time as compared to runners if they could swim to and from school, their place of employment or a training session. In such a fantasy

situation, the 100-m swimmer would probably perform better with training based on the competitive profile mentioned above.

The fact that the arms and upper body must be well trained locally can be deduced from longitudinal oxygen intake measurements made on the Olympic champion Gunnar Larsson from 1970 to 1975 (Fig. 55.1). The top values in swimming performance were recorded when he was a double gold medal winner at the 1972 Olympics. Between major competitions, his maximal oxygen intake was reduced when swimming, but it remained unchanged for running. The conclusion which can be drawn is that treadmill testing does not mirror swimming performance.

It was mentioned above that the maximal oxygen

intake of swimmers should not be expressed in $ml \cdot kg^{-1} \cdot min^{-1}$. Litres per minute provides a better measure of swimming ability, but the evaluation remains incomplete when expressing endurance in swimming.

A better way to explain an athlete's physiological ability is probably to express the oxygen intake in $l \cdot min^{-1}$ per kg *body weight in water* because this is the environment in which the athlete is performing. Hydrostatic weight is measured with the swimmer completely submerged after a maximal exhalation. This way of expressing swimming endurance includes some of the swimmer's sinking force, which has a crucial impact on the water resistance the swimmer must overcome to attain certain swim speeds.

Using this method, we can see from Table 55.2 that female swimmer A has a higher oxygen intake per kilogram body weight in water than female swimmer B, even though swimmer B has higher values expressed both in $l \cdot min^{-1}$ and in $ml \cdot kg^{-1} \cdot min^{-1}$ based on dry land weight.

Swimmer A had better race results for long-distance events than swimmer B, but both were national champions over long distances. A similar comparison can be made between female swimmers C and D, who also look more or less favourable, depending on whether the oxygen intake is based on land or underwater weight. Swimmer D had a maximum of more than $12 \, ml \cdot kg^{-1} \cdot min^{-1}$ higher than C on dry land, but C had a higher oxygen intake when weight in water was used in the calculation. However, these women competed over distances of 100 and 200 m, where maximal aerobic power plays only a minor role. The swimmers thus had similar competitive times.

Other findings further illustrate the problem of correlating high oxygen intake values with swimming endurance. Earlier longitudinal studies on top swimmers had shown that they could beat national records for 400-m distances during championships, despite approximately 15% lower maximal oxygen intake values when compared with their corresponding measurements during the preseason months (Gullstrand & Holmér 1983). Less remarkably, the maximal oxygen intake values for 100- and 200-m swimmers usually decline at the time of championships when they are compared with figures for periods of hard training. The dominance of anaerobic energy delivery over these distances could explain the decline (L. Gullstrand, unpublished data).

Endurance testing in swimming

Heart rate

The linear relationship between heart rate and work rate is one of the cornerstones of Åstrand's cycle ergometer test for predicting maximal oxygen intake. In the past, this correlation has been used to construct sport-specific tests in swimming (Treffene 1978) and in other sports (Conconi *et al.* 1982).

The heart rate (oxygen intake)/performance line is shifted rightwards as endurance capacity improves. This means, for example, that given swim speeds can be performed at a lower heart rate. The

Table 55.2 Comparison of maximal oxygen intake calculated using dry land weight and hydrostatic weight in female subjects A–D. The measurements were made in a swimming flume. From Gullstrand (1988).

Race distance (m)	Subject	$\dot{V}O_{2max}$ ($l \cdot min^{-1}$)	Mass (kg)	Test value ($ml \cdot kg^{-1} \cdot min^{-1}$)	Hydrostatic weight (kg)	Test value in water ($l \cdot kg^{-1} \cdot min^{-1}$)
400, 800 & 1500	A	2.8	57.3	48.9	1.3	2.2
	B	3.6	61.8	58.3	2.9	1.2
100 & 200	C	2.8	74.3	37.7	2.2	1.3
	D	3.4	67.6	50.3	3.0	1.1

linear part of the lactate–performance curve undergoes a similar rightward shift.

Conconi's test identifies a so-called heart rate deflection point (HR_d), where the heart rate no longer increases linearly with work rate, but does so at a reduced rate (Chapter 22).

Approximately 700 tests on Swedish national and other national team swimmers have indicated that, when swimming, the HR_d point does not coincide with the start of the rise in blood lactate concentration in the stepwise manner that Conconi has imputed to runners. In a 10×100-m increased swim-speed test with simultaneous measurements of heart rate and blood lactates, the HR_d occurred at higher speeds than the increase in lactate concentrations. Figure 55.2 shows an example of one world-class swimmer where the HR_d correlates better with what other investigators have called maximal lactate steady state, at a blood lactate concentration of about $4\,\mathrm{mmol\cdot l^{-1}}$.

This finding, together with the linear relationship

of heart rate to performance, could be useful when evaluating and monitoring endurance training in swimmers.

The same figure shows that the maximal heart rate was about 10 beats lower when training was dominated by extensive aerobic exercise, as compared to a 3-week period when speed and anaerobic training was completed. Similar fluctuations are seen in other highly trained subjects.

Oxygen consumption

Measurement of peak oxygen consumption can be one method of evaluating prolonged endurance in swimming. But, as mentioned earlier, the correlation with swimming performance is not always clear. By making additional measurements of O_2 consumption at one or two relatively high submaximal standardized speeds one can obtain valuable information about an athlete's swimming economy. The smaller the percentage of $\dot{V}O_{2max}$ that is used at high submaximal speeds, the better the economy. This is of importance in longitudinal studies and when analysing swimming performance on an individual basis.

However, this measure includes a variety of components such as hydrostatic weight (reflecting body composition), breathing pattern, streamlining, propulsion by the arms and legs and overall technique. After controlling for at least some of these components, swimming economy may be very informative.

Equipment for measuring the oxygen intake of swimmers is expensive and complicated to handle. In general, such devices (including a swimming flume or a mobile measurement platform over a 25- or 50-m pool) are only available in research institutes and major testing centres and then must be operated by skilled personnel.

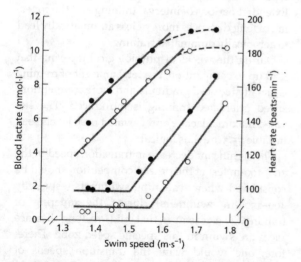

Fig. 55.2 Blood lactate and heart rate values at 8–10 × 100-m freestyle for one world-class 200-m swimmer. Values shown as open circles are from an extensive and aerobically dominated period of training. Black circles denote values obtained after a 3-week period of increased training for speed and anaerobic qualities with less distance training. The dashed lines indicate heart rates beyond the deflection point (see text). From Gullstrand (1988).

Blood lactate

In recent years the use of lactate tests in swimming has become very popular world-wide. Different kinds of lactate–performance curves and threshold tests based on 'micro' blood samples have been constructed after various swim performances. The aims of these tests are to evaluate training, to predict race results and to detect talent.

Such methods are particularly applicable to swimming, because the pool offers relatively constant conditions over time, and swimming is a 'cyclic sport', with maintenance of an even pace as one of the most important objectives during both races and training.

Mader's two-point test is one of the most well-known threshold tests (Mader *et al.* 1976). However, it has been criticized because it uses a fixed $4 \, mmol \cdot l^{-1}$ point to describe the aerobic–anaerobic threshold and define the optimal training load. Heck *et al.* (1985) and colleagues have pointed out that this threshold is individual and can occur either below or above $4 \, mmol \cdot l^{-1}$ (see Stegmann *et al.* 1983; Olbrecht *et al.* 1985).

The aerobic–anaerobic threshold is defined as the maximal power at which there is a balance between the production and elimination of lactate (Chapter 22). It has also been termed the maximal lactate steady state (Heck *et al.* 1985). From 1977 to 1982, Swedish national swimmers were frequently evaluated with a battery of tests. The first year included the two-point test described by Mader *et al.* (1976). But certain problems in this approach led to the adoption of more training-related tests (L. Gullstrand, unpublished results). One hundred metres were swum from eight to 10 times at progressively increased effort, starting at a low speed and ending with a maximal effort. With this test design, the time reduction per repetition of the 100-m swim was about 2 s. Microsamples of blood were taken from the earlobe after each 100 m. The resulting lactate–performance curve covers lactate levels during aerobically dominated metabolism, the individual aerobic–anaerobic transition and lactate levels during anaerobically dominated metabolism (Fig. 55.2). All parts of the curve are of interest for evaluation and training, as swim training is traditionally carried out over the entire 'metabolic scale'. A standardized treatment of the lactate–performance curve (Fig. 55.2) allows comparison of the base lactate level, the speed at the aerobic–anaerobic transition, and the increase in (and maximal) lactate concentration at different periods during training. The true maximal anaerobic metabolism can prob-

ably be determined only after maximal effort races during important competitions, or during simulated races where the swimmers are highly motivated (L. Gullstrand, unpublished results). Measurement of maximal anaerobic power is probably impossible, because the actual energy demand cannot be predicted.

The lactate–performance profile shows typical variations, depending on whether tests are conducted during hard training or in direct connection with championships (Table 55.3). The Swedish national team swimmers from whom data were derived had differing specializations with regard to both distance and technique. However, very rarely did anyone break the general pattern by showing a lower base level, a higher transition speed or a lower maximal lactate concentration when hard training periods were compared with tests connected with important races.

Lower base levels of lactate at aerobically dominated speeds and a lower maximal lactate value after the final 10th 100-m repetition during hard training could reflect metabolic adaptation to the type of training which has been conducted. Extended periods of interval training and the covering of long distances more or less automatically lead to aerobically dominated training.

During the weeks of physiological tapering that lead up to competition, the total amount of training is usually reduced gradually and more competition-speed orientated training is introduced. The elevated maximal lactate and elevated base levels seen in Table 55.3 are thus logical.

The significant decrease in transition speed in the 10×100-m test at the time of competition should be considered when evaluating swimmers (especially 400–1500-m swimmers) during the tapering of training. The reason is that mid- to long-distance races are swum in this specific speed zone. Therefore, one would want the transition speeds of 400–1500-m swimmers to increase, and definitely not to decline. The same probably applies to 200-m swimmers.

Critical swim speed

Coaches are always looking for valid, fast feedback

Table 55.3 Comparison of mean values from four well-defined parts of the lactate–performance curve obtained during extensive training and at the time of competition. Values are from 8 to 10 × 100-m freestyle stroke (see also Fig. 55.2). From Gullstrand (1988).

	Base level (mmol·l^{-1})	Transition speed (m·s^{-1})	Slope ($y = a + bx$)	HLa$_{max}$ (mmol·l^{-1})
Men ($n = 11$)				
Preparation training	1.3	1.550	39.8	7.3
Competition	1.7	1.532	44.6	9.2
p value	0.01	n.s.	n.s.	0.01
Women ($n = 11$)				
Preparation training	1.2	1.425	51.1	7.0
Competition	1.7	1.402	50.8	8.7
p value	0.001	0.01	n.s.	0.05

HLa$_{max}$, maximal blood lactate concentration; n.s., not significant.

and easy field handling methods, which are possible to use in their own training environment.

For several years heart rate and blood lactate devices have to some extent met these needs, and such methods have become valuable tools in evaluating and monitoring swim training. Reliable lactate analysers are still not cheap enough to allow each club or élite coach to possess one for frequent measurements. Costs of reagents and maintenance, handling of the analyser and evaluation of results still make coaches interested in yet more accessible methods.

During recent years a variety of non-invasive tests have been suggested. One of the most interesting is the method of critical swim speed (CSS), described by Wakayoshi et al. (1992) and frequently evaluated in the scientific literature (Wright & Smith 1994; Toussaint et al. 1998). This method is claimed to be a sensitive method of quantifying training status over time (Maclaren & Coulson 1999). In brief, maximal swims of 50-, 100-, 200- and 400-m distances are performed with push-off starts. Time is recorded, and the CSS is calculated as the slope of a regression line relating distance against time.

CSS as well as other non-invasive methods based on time/distance recording have been compared to blood lactate tests. For further information, see Matsunami et al. (1999).

Consequently there now are a variety of methods for evaluating swim performance, mostly reflecting endurance capacity.

Correlation of swim test and competitive performance

In a typical endurance sport, the triathlon, the Olympic version includes a 1500-m swim. To evaluate the endurance capacity of eight national team triathletes, lactate thresholds were established from an incremental 10 × 100-m freestyle swim in a 25-m pool, and peak oxygen intake measurements were made in a swimming flume. Results from these analyses were correlated with competitive 1500-m swim times in a lake.

The threshold velocity (m·s^{-1}) and the peak oxygen intake (l·min^{-1}) correlated significantly ($p < 0.05$) with water swimming speed ($r = 0.92$ and 0.79, respectively). The overall swim velocity was 5% slower in free water swimming than the individual threshold speed in the pool. The difference can be explained by factors such as orienteering problems, the lack of speed increasing and microrest push-offs during free water swimming (Gullstrand 1997).

In this case, the results from field and laboratory tests correlated significantly with swimming performance during competition, as well as with each other. In such a case, one could talk about a *golden triangle* of laboratory and field test and performance in competition and training. These relationships are relatively easy to establish in indoor and outdoor pool swimming, when compared to many other sports. The normal environment for training and competition is well standardized in most pools; water and air temperatures are also consistent and the distance is usually 25 or 50 m.

Specific methods of endurance training

Without doubt, the most frequently practised method of swim training is the interval approach. To develop aerobic power and capacity, extended series of laps are often performed with relatively short resting intervals of 10–30 s. The total distance covered in a series can range from 1000 to 5000 m or more, usually divided into distances of from 50 to 800 m. The series can be 'straight', which means that the same distance is repeated throughout, or it can consist of mixed distances.

The rest periods between laps and swim strokes are also varied. Every coach and swimmer have their own preference, and their inventive capacity is enormous. Often the top athlete group comprises 15–20 swimmers using a very limited pool space. The swimmers are thus usually organized to swim in a 'loop' in the lanes. In such situations, the straight series are the easiest, for both swimmers and coaches to control, with regard to speed, heart rate and rest intervals.

Long-distance swimming of 2000–3000 m, or the maximal distance covered over a given time of 20–50 min, are less frequently used. Such series are mostly swum with the whole stroke, to create the greatest possible load on the cardiovascular system (see more about endurance training at the end of this chapter).

A study of top-level swimmers by Huber *et al.* (1978) revealed a less than expected discrepancy in heart rate between series of whole stroke, pulling and kicking (170, 160 and 150 beats·min^{-1}, respectively). The differences were even less among regional swimmers (175, 175 and 170 beats·min^{-1}). These findings indicate that the muscle mass engaged during kicking and pulling is large enough to result in a good central stimulation of the cardiovascular system for less trained swimmers.

Risks in endurance training

Several risks are involved in the intensive training regarded as necessary for top-level swimmers to attain a high level of swimming endurance. One is that a major portion of the training does not correspond well with the metabolic profile of competition, as described in Table 55.1.

Endurance training is frequently executed at too high an intensity. This results in substantial lactate accumulation, which in top-level swimming often leads to overtraining. The swimmer feels very weak, and cannot reproduce normal training speeds. It can take days or even weeks of easy swimming or rest to recover to 'normal' capacity (Chapter 34).

Madsen (1982/1983) emphasized the need for controlled-intensity training in order to obtain the desired effect. The method of control that he recommended was frequent measurement of blood lactate concentration.

Too low a training intensity is often the result of extensive workouts that stimulate primarily aerobic metabolism. One reason for an inadequate intensity is that stored glycogen is only partially replenished between training sessions (Costill 1985). Fat then becomes the dominant energy source during training. Poor training results, and tiredness during the third day of a two-workouts-per-day training camp is a classical consequence of emptied or partially emptied glycogen stores.

This theory is supported by a lower base lactate level in the lactate–performance curve. Values of RQ (respiratory quotient) for a given submaximal oxygen intake are also lower during endurance training than during periods of competition. Some of these negative metabolic effects can be eliminated by a more effective scheduling of training. Good nutrition must also be emphasized; according to several investigations, athletic nutrition can be greatly improved.

Trappe *et al.* (1997) showed recently that during a 5-day training camp, five national team and world-ranked female swimmers had a negative energy balance of –47%! The swimmers trained for 5–6 h per day, and the double labelled water method was used to measure energy output. There are good reasons to believe that if male swimmers had been included, an even larger negative balance would have been discovered.

Another risk associated with extensive low-speed training is found at the neuromuscular level. During low-speed training, swimming movements are accomplished at a low limb speed. Several investigators have shown that such low-speed training gives good results for the limb speed at which practice has occurred, but transfer of the training effect to higher limb speeds is doubtful. On the other hand, high-speed movements give good training effects for both high and low speeds of movements (Lesmes et al. 1978).

Most other researchers agree with these findings, but some narrow the conditioning effect of fast-movement training to fast limb movements (Caiosso et al. 1981; Kanehisa & Miyashita 1983). The stroke frequency of a good 100-m freestyle swimmer who repeats 100-m training swims at a speed of 60–70 s corresponds to 30–38 arm cycles per minute (one cycle comprising one left and one right arm stroke). At maximal swim speeds (50 s over a 100-m distance), the frequency of the same swimmer will be roughly 66 cycles per minute (Craig et al. 1979). The difference between training and race movement speeds is approximately 50%. Because much endurance training for good male 100-m swimmers today is swum at speeds of 60–70 s, it can be concluded that there is a substantial difference between the movement speed in training and in competitions.

One way of solving both metabolic and neuromuscular problems is to adopt 15:15 training; this is based on a large number of repetitions of 15-s exercise at race pace plus 15-s rest. The first study of this approach was performed on runners (Christensen et al. 1960). In recent years, the same design has been used for good swimmers (Gullstrand & Lawrence 1987) and for national team rowers (Gullstrand 1996). Figure 55.3 shows the acute effect on blood lactate levels and heart rate during and after 40 × 25-m freestyle swims at an average speed corresponding to the race pace for 100 m. The relatively low lactate level (3 mmol·l^{-1}) and the high mean heart rate (179 beats·min^{-1}) indicate a low level of anaerobic metabolism and a high aerobic loading. After a 100-m maximal swim, the same subjects had a mean lactate concentration of 7.1 mmol·l^{-1} and a heart rate of 191 beats·min^{-1}. The 40 × 25-m freestyle swim with a 15:15 design thus resulted in values that were 43% of maximal lactate and 93% of maximal heart rate.

In a similar study, national team rowers were exercised on a Gjessing rowing ergometer. Oxygen intake measurements were also included. The 40 × 15:15 results were compared to $\dot{V}O_{2max}$ as determined by a continuously incremental rowing test (to exhaustion). The results showed that the intermittent exercise demanded 89, 78 and 32% of maximal heart rate, oxygen intake and blood lactate, respectively.

In conclusion, both studies of typical endurance sports show the advantage of 'short, intermittent training': swimming and rowing a substantial volume at race pace; the attainment of a high aerobic load; and training periods with a low level of anaerobic lactic stress.

Tapering and endurance

It is not yet fully understood how the tapering phase affects factors related to swimming endurance. The problem seems to be how to become rested and 'superadapted' for competition without losing endurance quality during tapering. Few investigations of this question have yet been completed, although the physiological changes that develop in well-trained endurance athletes after the cessation of training have been described (Houston et al. 1979; Costill et al. 1985).

Endurance is reduced more quickly than maximal oxygen intake with detraining and inactivity. The reason is the reduction of oxidative enzyme activity. This activity is reduced by 50% after a week of inactivity (Henriksson & Reitman 1977). Houston et al. (1979) studied a group of highly trained runners after a training interruption of 15 days. They noted a 4% decrease in maximal oxygen intake, a 24% reduction of SDH (succinate dehydrogenase) activity, and a 25% reduction in endurance during a 15–18-min run. Costill et al. (1985) studied the

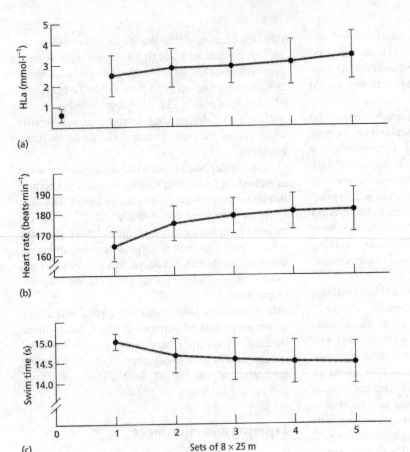

Fig. 55.3 Mean values of (a) blood lactate (HLa), (b) heart rate and (c) swim time for five sets of 8 × 25-m swim efforts at 100-m race pace (*n* = 9). From Gullstrand and Lawrence (1987).

phosphorylase and phosphofructokinase activity of top-level swimmers during a 4-week period when training had ceased, but they did not find any significant change in these variables. This last investigation was carried out after a tapering and competition phase, and it can be hypothesized that the swimmers had already started to reduce their enzyme activity during tapering. They probably also competed with a reduced endurance capacity. These swimmers had trained for 5 months, with 6 days of training per week and an average swimming distance of 10 900 m per day.

In another study, eight female national team swimmers were followed over a 6-week tapering period (L. Gullstrand, unpublished data). Maximal oxygen intake was significantly (*p* < 0.05) reduced, from 3.5 to 3.2 l·min⁻¹, during the 6-week period.

Lactate–performance testing was conducted

every week, using an 8–10 × 100-m protocol. Aerobic–anaerobic transition speeds were significantly reduced, by an average of 2.4 s on 100 m, from 3 weeks before to 1 day after the championships. These results indicate that the traditional tapering pattern reduced performances in both types of endurance test.

The female swimmers had specialized for 100- and 200-m distances, and as a group they performed well at the meet. A reduced endurance is not particularly important at these distances. On the other hand, the swimming times might have been better, given larger maximal oxygen intake and lactate threshold values.

Conclusion

Endurance training is very important in top-level

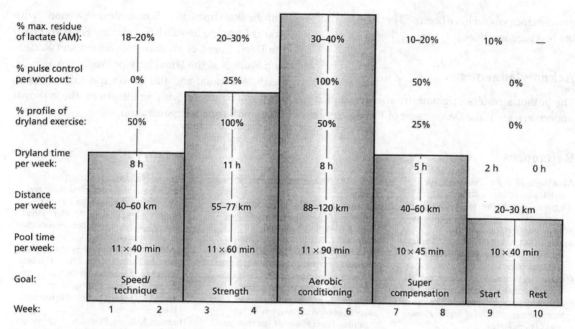

% max. residue of lactate (AM):	18–20%	20–30%	30–40%	10–20%	10%	—
% pulse control per workout:	0%	25%	100%	50%	0%	
% profile of dryland exercise:	50%	100%	50%	25%	0%	
Dryland time per week:	8 h	11 h	8 h	5 h	2 h	0 h
Distance per week:	40–60 km	55–77 km	88–120 km	40–60 km	20–30 km	
Pool time per week:	11 × 40 min	11 × 60 min	11 × 90 min	10 × 45 min	10 × 40 min	
Goal:	Speed/ technique	Strength	Aerobic conditioning	Super compensation	Start	Rest
Week:	1 2	3 4	5 6	7 8	9	10

Fig. 55.4 Coach Koshkin's basic training pattern for 1500-m swimmer Salnikov and other Soviet top swimmers. The pattern is repeated five times a year in 10-week cycles. From Koshkin (1984).

swimming, over both short and long distances. In fact, many world-class short-distance swimmers were highly ranked when competing over 400–1500-m distances at a younger age. Whether this reflects a necessary and natural development of better performance over shorter distances or a failure to identify sprinting talent is unclear.

The trend over the past years has been to adapt swim training more closely to the physiological profile of the intended competitive distance. This should not be regarded as a way of reducing the training necessary to become a top-level swimmer, but rather as a trial of more effective approaches to training.

The effectiveness of swim training can be enhanced by use of sophisticated test methods such as measurements of blood lactate concentrations, although reliance should not be placed on any one test method. Several physiological qualities need to be considered, and a battery of relevant tests is desirable.

For endurance, oxygen intake or heart rate mea-

surements will be suitable for evaluation of the central capacity, while lactate–performance tests will provide more information about the peripheral capacity.

Föhrenbach et al. (1984) divided the lactate–performance test into five intensity zones, attributing to each zone a major training effect. Absaliamow (1984) constructed a table showing lactate and heart rate values for each training zone. This way of classifying training has major advantages for the understanding, monitoring and evaluation of swim training. Nevertheless, it is important to understand that these recommendations must be adapted for the individual swimmer.

A coach from the former Soviet Union (Koshkin 1984) demonstrated how frequent heart rate and lactate measurement was a part of Vladimir Salnikov's training programme (Fig. 55.4). During one period, all training was controlled by heart rate. As a world record holder for the longest distance in swimming (1500 m), Salnikov may be seen as one of the leading representatives of endurance training in swimming. However, we do not know whether his performance would have been still better if his train-ing had been modified.

Acknowledgements

The author's results originate from investigations undertaken at: (i) the Department of Physiology III, Karolinska Institute, Stockholm, Sweden with grants from the Swedish Swimming Federation; (ii) the Department of Human Movement and Recreation Studies at the University of Western Australia, Perth, Australia; and (iii) Bosön Institute of Sport, Lidingö, Sweden, with grants from the national Olympic Support Organization.

References

Absaliamow, T. (1984) Controlling the training of top level swimmers. In: Cramer, J.L. (ed.) *How to Develop Olympic Level Swimmers*, pp. 14–21. International Sport Media, Finland.

Åstrand, P.-O. & Rodahl, K. (1986) *Textbook of Work Physiology*, 3rd edn. McGraw-Hill, New York.

Caiosso, V.J., Perrine, J.J. & Edgerton, W.R. (1981) Training induced alterations of the *in-vivo* force–velocity relationships of human muscle. *Journal of Applied Physiology* 51 (3), 750–754.

Christensen, E.H., Hedman, R. & Saltin, B. (1960) Intermittent and continuous running. *Acta Physiologica Scandinavica* 50, 269–286.

Conconi, F., Ferrari, M., Liglio, P., Drogetti, P. & Codeca, L. (1982) Determination of the anaerobic threshold by a non-invasive field test in runners. *Journal of Applied Physiology* 52 (4), 869–873.

Costill, D.L. (1985) Carbohydrate nutrition before, during and after exercise. *Federation Proceedings* 44, 364–368.

Costill, D.L., Fink, W.J., Hargreaves, M., King, D.S., Tomas, R. & Fielding, R. (1985) Metabolic characteristics of skeletal muscle during detraining from competitive swimming. *Medicine and Science in Sports and Exercise* 17, 339–343.

Craig, A.B., Boomer, W.L. & Gibbons, J.F. (1979) Use of stroke and velocity relationships during training for competitive swimming. In: Terauds, J. & Beddingfield, E.W. (eds) *Swimming III*, pp. 263–272. University Park Press, Baltimore.

Föhrenbach, R., Liesen. H., Mader, A., Heck, H., Vellage, E. & Hollmann, W. (1984) Wettkampf und Trainings-teuerung von Marathonläuferinnen und -läufern mittels leistungsdiagnostischer Felduntersuchungen. (Competition and training monitoring of female and male marathon runners by means of performance diagnostic field tests.) In: Heck, H., Hess. G. & Mader, A. (eds) *Comparative Study of Different Lactate Threshold Concepts*. Special issue. *Deutsche Zeitschrift für Sportmedizin*, Vol. 36, Nos 1 and 2.

Gullstrand, L. (1985) Soviet swimming: analysis, planning and research. *Simsport* 1, 36–37 (in Swedish).

Gullstrand, L. (1986a) Periodization in training swimmers. In: Quinlan, P. (ed.) *Swim 86 Yearbook*, pp. 45–48. Australian Swimming Incorporated and Swimming Coaches Association, Mt Gravatt.

Gullstrand, L. (1986b) Physiological aspects of tapering swimmers. In: Quinlan, P. (ed.) *Swim 86 Yearbook*, pp. 39–43. Australian Swimming Incorpo-rated and Swimming Coaches Associa-tion, Mt Gravatt.

Gullstrand, L. (1988) Swimming. In: Forsberg, A. & Saltin, B. (eds) *Konditionsträn-ing*, pp. 280–291. Idrottens Forskningsråd, Sveriges Riksidrottsför-bund (in Swedish).

Gullstrand, L. (1996) Physiological responses to short-duration high-intensity intermittent rowing. *Canadian Journal of Applied Physiology* 21, 197–208.

Gullstrand, L. (1997) Laboratory and com-petition measurements in élite level triathlon, with special reference to swim-ming. In: Daniel, K., Hoffmann, U. & Klauck, J. (eds) *Kölner Schwimmsport-tage*, pp. 150–154. Sport Fahnemann, Brockenem.

Gullstrand, L. & Holmér, I. (1983) Physio-logical characteristics of champion swimmers during a five year follow-up period. In: Hollander, P. & de Groot, G. (eds) *Biomechanics and Medicine in Swim-ming*, pp. 258–262. Human Kinetics, Champaign, IL.

Gullstrand, L. & Lawrence, S. (1987) Heart rate and blood lactate response to short intermittent work at race pace in highly trained swimmers. *Australian Journal of Science and Medicine in Sport* 19 (1), 10–14.

Heck, H., Mader, A., Hess, G., Mucke, S., Muller. P. & Hollmann, W. (1985) Justifi-cation of the 4-mmol/l lactate threshold. *International Journal of Sports Medicine* 6, 117–130.

Henriksson, J. & Reitman, S. (1977) Time course of changes in human skeletal muscle succinate dehydrogenase and cytochrome oxidase activities and maximal oxygen uptake with physical activity and inactivity. *Acta Physiologica Scandinavica* 99, 91–97.

Holmér, I. (1979) Physiology of swimming man. In: Hutton, R.S. & Miller, D.I. (eds) *Exercise and Sport Sciences Reviews* 7, pp. 87–123. American College of Sports Medicine Series, The Franklin Institute Press.

Houston, M.E. (1978) Metabolic responses to exercise with special reference to training and competition in swimming. In: Eriksson, B. & Furberg, B. (eds) *Swimming Medicine IV*, pp. 207–232. Univer-sity Park Press, Baltimore.

Houston, M.E., Bentzen, H. & Larsen, H. (1979) Interrelationships between skele-tal muscle adaptations and performance as studied by detraining and retraining. *Acta Physiologica Scandinavica* 105, 163–170.

Huber, G., Keul, J., Kindermann, W. & Stocklasa, L. (1978) Herzfrequenzen, Lactatspiegel, und pH-Wert bei ver-schiedenen Trainingsformen im Kraulswimmen. (Heart rate, lactate level and pH value at different training regimes in front crawl swimming.) *Deutsche Zeitschrifte für Sportmedizin* 10, 282–291.

Kanehisa, H. & Miyashita, M. (1983) Speci-ficity of velocity in strength training. *European Journal of Applied Physiology* 52, 104–106.

Koshkin, I. (1984) The training program that developed Salnikov. In: Cramer, J.L. (ed.) *How to Develop Olympic Level Swim-mers*, pp. 107–116. International Sport Media, Finland.

Lesmes, G.R., Costill, D.L., Coyle, E.F. & Frick, W.J. (1978) Muscle strength and power changes during maximal isomet-ric training. *Medicine and Science in Sports and Exercise* 10 (4), 266–269.

Maclaren, D.P.M. & Coulson, M. (1999) Critical swim speed can be used to deter-mine changes in training status. In:

Keskinen, K.L., Komi, P.V. & Hollander, A.P. (eds) *Biomechanics and Medicine in Swimming VIII*, pp. 232–272. Gummerus Printing, Jyväskylä, Finland.

Mader, A., Heck, H. & Hollmann, W. (1976) Evaluation of lactic acid anaerobic energy contribution by determination of post lactic acid concentration of capillary blood in middle distance runners and swimmers. In: Landry, F. & Orban, W. (eds) *Exercise Physiology*, pp. 187–199. Symposia Specialists Incorporated, Florida.

Madsen, Ö. (1982/83) Aerobic training: not so fast there. *Swimming Technique* **19** (53), 17–19.

Maglischo, E. (1982) *Swimming Faster*. Mayfield Publishing Company, Palo Alto, CA.

Matsunami, M., Taguchi, M., Taimura, A. *et al.* (1999) Comparison of swimming speed and exercise intensity during non-invasive and invasive test in competitive swimming. In: Keskinen, K.L., Komi, P.V. & Hollander, A.P. (eds) *Biomechanics*

and Medicine in Swimming VIII, pp. 239–244. Gummerus Printing, Jyväskylä, Finland.

Olbrecht, J., Madsen, Ö., Liesen, H. & Hollmann, W. (1985) Relationship between swimming velocity and lactic acid concentration during continuous and intermittent training exercises. *International Journal of Sports Medicine* **6**, 74–77.

Stegmann, H., Weiler, B. & Kindermann, W. (1983) Vergleich verschiedener anaerober Schwellenkonzepte bei Sportarten. (Comparison of different anaerobic threshold concepts for athletes representing various sports events.) In: Heck, H., Hollmann, W., Liesen, H. & Rost, R. (eds) *Sport, Leistung und Gesundheit*, pp. 163–167. Deutsche Ärzte-Verlag, Cologne.

Toussaint, H.M., Wakayoshi, K., Hollander, A.P. & Ogita, F. (1998) Simulated front crawl swimming performance related to critical speed and critical power. *Medicine and Science in Sports and Exercise* **30**, 144–151.

Trappe, T.A., Gastadelli, A., Jozsi, A.C., Troup, J.P. & Wolfe, R.R. (1997) Energy expenditure of swimmers during high volume training. *Medicine and Science in Sports and Exercise* **29**, 950–954.

Treffene, R. (1978) Swimming performance test. A method of training and performance time selection. *Australian Journal of Sports Medicine* **10** (2), 33–38.

Troup, J. (1984) Energy systems and training considerations. *Journal of Swimming Research* **1**, 13–16.

Wakayoshi, K., Ikuta, K., Yoshida, T. *et al.* (1992) Determination and validity of critical velocity as an index of swimming performance in the competitive swimmer. *European Journal of Applied Physiology* **64**, 153–157.

Wright, B. & Smith, D.J. (1994) A protocol for the determination of critical speed as an index of swimming endurance performance. In: Miyashita, M., Mutoh, Y. & Richardson, A.B. (eds) *Medicine and Science in Aquatic Sports*, pp. 55–59. Karger, Basel.

Chapter 56

Rowing

NIELS H. SECHER

Introduction

Rowing combines intense dynamic exercise with a need for development of a large force during each stroke. Accordingly, the circulation has to adapt not only to a large cardiac output, but also to the increase in blood pressure at the 'catch'. These demands are reflected in the hearts of rowers, which show large internal diameters and wall thicknesses (Pelliccia *et al.* 1991); even in advanced age, rowers maintain superior systolic function (Gustafsson *et al.* 1996). At the same time, the way in which rowers apply simultaneous pressure of the right and left legs against the stretcher may be unique to human motion, pointing to the neurophysiological problems involved in coordination for this sport (Secher 1983). In contrast to many other sports, rowing is associated with few injuries. The main problems are concerned with extreme fatigue, although chronic low back pain may also be a problem for some rowers, besides more trivial blisters. For reviews of the biomechanics and physiology of rowing see Secher (1983, 1990), Hagerman (1984), Körner and Schwanitz (1985), Steinacker (1987), Steinacker and Secher (1993) and Shephard (1998).

Rowing competitions

Competitions are divided into two distinct, yet related, disciplines: sweep rowing and sculling. In sweep boats, each rower uses a single oar approximately 4 m long, whereas in sculling each uses two smaller (approximately 3-m) sculls on each side of the boat. Both types of boat are rowed by pulling the

oar at a cadence of between 34 and 38 strokes·min^{-1}, with the competitor's back towards the direction of the course. In contrast to traditional rowing boats, as well as to the first racing shells, the stroke is made more efficient by the use of a sliding seat, thereby adding leg extension to the work performed with the upper body and arms. In sweep rowing, the boats may include two, four or eight rowers. Pairs and fours are rowed both with and without a coxswain, but a coxswain is always present in the eights (Table 56.1). Sculls are rowed without a coxswain and encompass boats for one, two or four competitors. The minimum body mass of the coxswain is 50 kg for male and 40 kg for female events.

Regattas

Race rowing started on the River Thames in England, with the 'Doggett's Coat and Badge' race for professional watermen (1715) and the Oxford and Cambridge Boat Race (1829) and the Henley Regatta (1839) for 'gentlemen'. Championships have been arranged by the Féderation Internationale des Sociétés d'Aviron (FISA) since 1893. Rowing first appeared on the Olympic programme in 1900. FISA championships for women were added in 1954. Unofficial lightweight championships (maximum body mass 72.5 kg; mean body mass 70 kg) were introduced in 1974 and made 'official' in 1985. Lightweight championships for women (maximum body mass 59 kg; mean body mass 57 kg) were added in 1985, after an unofficial regatta had been held in 1984, and the distance

Table 56.1 Minimum boat weight allowed in Féderation Internationale des Sociétés d'Aviron (FISA) championships, and the FISA competitions arranged for men and women including lightweight competitors.

	Boat type*							
	4+	2×	2−	1×	2+	4−	4×	8+
Boat weight (kg)	51	27	27	14	32	50	52	96
Men	•	•	•	•	•	•	•	•
Male lightweights		•	•	•	•		•	•
Women		•	•	•	•		•	•
Female lightweights		•			•		•	

*Digits indicate number of rowers; +/− denotes the presence or absence of a coxswain; × indicates scull boats. •, current events.

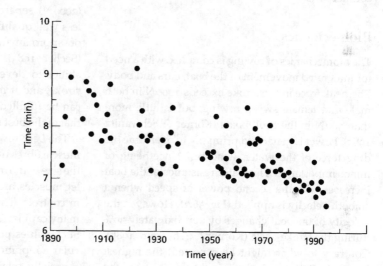

Fig. 56.1 Results obtained by FISA regatta winning single scull over 2000 m from 1893 to 1995.

rowed by women was increased to the 2000 m rowed by men. Weighing takes place about 2 h before a regatta, and the normal body mass of the lightweight rower is usually above the one 'allowed' in the race.

Improvement of results

Since the first FISA regatta took place, the mean result for the 2000-m distance has improved by about 0.7 s (range 0.6–0.9 s) per year (Fig. 56.1). It is possible to detect a similar 0.6 s (range 0.2–2.1 s) per year improvement in the results for the women over the 1000-m course. The improvement in rowing performance reflects the composite effect of an increase in size of the general population and changes in the training and selection of rowers; contributions have also been made by technical modifications in the construction of boats and oars, as well as the effort to standardize racing courses. The introduction of 'big blades' (1992) made a significant contribution. Currently, FISA has also standardized the weights of boats to the values presented in Table 56.1.

Duration of competitions

The median results in recent FISA regattas indicate a race duration of 6.5 min (6.6 min for lightweight competitors). For women, the times are 7.1 min, 10% longer than for men competing in similar events.

The difference between the two types of women's races is somewhat larger than in the men's (12%), suggesting that the 'cut' separating lightweight women and men is different. However, for both men and women the highest body mass allowed in lightweight events is about 75% of the average body mass of the rowers in the open classes, 94 and 79 kg, respectively. Values indicate a difference between results obtained in lightweight events of 2.5% for men and 5% for women, supporting the need for a division of races into weight categories, but also indicating that the quality of the lightweight women's races does not yet meet that of their male counterparts.

Biomechanics

The biomechanics of rowing is complex, with a need for integrated movement of the boat, oars and body. The peak force in the stroke exceeds 1000 N in both male and female sweep rowing, but is little more than 500 N in the scull boats (Körner & Schwanitz 1985). Power is generated primarily to overcome the drag force of the water, wind resistance being of minor importance. The water resistance of the boat increases with the second power of speed when a smooth velocity is applied (Fig. 56.2). However, the velocity of the boat changes by approximately 30% during the stroke cycle (Körner & Schwanitz 1985). Contrary to what might be expected, the highest boat velocity is reached when the oar is out of the water and the heavy bodies of the rowers are

moving in the opposite direction to that of the shell. Similarly, during the stroke, the movement of the bodies in the direction of the boat decreases the propagation of the shell. Only when the total system is taken into consideration, including rowers, shell and oars, is the highest velocity reached at the end of the stroke.

Muscle strength

Rowers are large and strong individuals, but their ability as rowers is not related in any simple way to their muscle strength. Only when measured in a simulated rowing position does muscle strength (2000 N) separate the best rowers from groups of less well qualified rowers with a 'rowing strength' of approximately 1800 and 1600 N, respectively (Secher 1983). Nevertheless, rowing requires an ability to develop a large peak force during the stroke, and it may be argued that this requirement can be fulfilled only if rowing strength is close to that of the best rowers.

The best rowers tend to have many slow-twitch muscle fibres (Körner & Schwanitz 1985). Moreover, the size of the muscle fibres of rowers is large: for the leg muscles, an average of 3970 μm^2 versus 3330 μm^2 in controls. The muscle fibres of rowers also have many capillaries per fibre: 7.3 versus 3.1 in controls. Such values point to the importance of local muscular adaptations in rowing. This consideration is especially relevant when training on the water is impossible and indoor training must be undertaken.

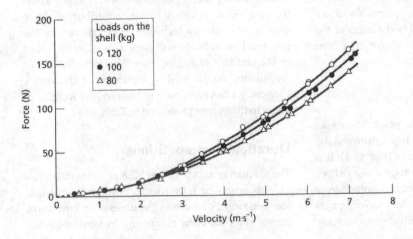

Fig. 56.2 Drag force applied to a single scull at different velocities. Three loads on the shell are presented: 120 kg, 100 kg and 80 kg. From Balukow (1964).

The use of rowing ergometers and tank rowing is recommended, and indeed the former has become a discipline of its own, with unofficial national and world championships.

Aerobic metabolism

An increase in ideal boat resistance to the second power of boat velocity suggests that the metabolism of rowers should increase with the third power of boat velocity (Secher 1983), although in practice a lower power has been reported (Fig. 56.3), possibly reflecting a significant contribution from movement of the rower on the sliding seat. At the present speed

of competitive rowing, the metabolic cost of rowing may be calculated as $6.7 \, l \cdot min^{-1}$ for men ($5.9 \, l \cdot min^{-1}$ for male lightweight competitors), $5.3 \, l \cdot min^{-1}$ for women and $4.9 \, l \cdot min^{-1}$ for lightweight female competitors. These high metabolic rates are reflected in the metabolic capacity of rowers as expressed by their maximal oxygen intakes, average values being $6.1 \, l \cdot min^{-1}$ for men ($5.1 \, l \cdot min^{-1}$ for lightweight men) and $4.3 \, l \cdot min^{-1}$ for women (Secher 1990). Moreover, a direct relationship has been demonstrated between the results obtained in a FISA championship and the crew's average maximal oxygen intake (Fig. 56.4). In fact, an almost perfect relationship ($r = 0.99$) can be demonstrated when the

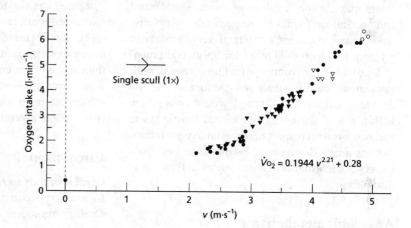

Fig. 56.3 Oxygen intake during rowing a single scull for two oarsmen. Values indicated with an open circle were not included in the regression. $\dot{V}O_2 = 0.1944 \, v^{2.21} + 0.28$.

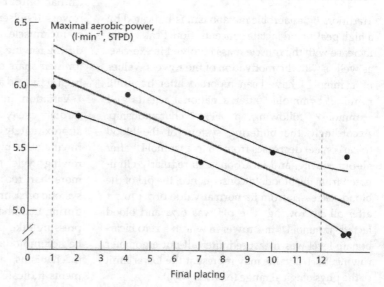

Fig. 56.4 Regression line between average maximal oxygen intake of a crew and its placing in a FISA championship regatta (1971). The 95% confidence limits are also shown. From Secher (1983).

metabolic capacity of the crew is balanced with boat resistance and compared with the results obtained in FISA regattas (Secher 1983).

When rowing, the results are correlated to the maximal oxygen intake of rowers expressed in $l \cdot min^{-1}$ (Fig. 56.4) rather than $ml \cdot kg^{-1} \cdot min^{-1}$ (Secher 1983). On the other hand, if maximal oxygen intake values are to be compared between subjects, the dimensions of the athlete should be taken into consideration, and a unit based on body surface area (or $kg^{-2/3}$) may be applied. When expressed in terms neutral to body dimensions, the rowers' maximal oxygen intakes are only approximately $300 \, ml \cdot kg^{-2/3} \cdot min^{-1}$ for men and $250 \, ml \cdot kg^{-2/3} \cdot min^{-1}$ for women, whereas the best runners, cyclists and skiers may approach values of $370 \, ml \cdot kg^{-2/3} \cdot min^{-1}$ and $270 \, ml \cdot kg^{-2/3} \cdot min^{-1}$, respectively. Applying these figures to rowers, a maximal oxygen intake of $7.5 \, l \cdot min^{-1}$ for men ($6.2 \, l \cdot min^{-1}$ for lightweight men) and $5.0 \, l \cdot min^{-1}$ for women would be obtained, with associated improvements of performance. The data also indicate that although women rowers are within 10% of the best international female skiers and runners with respect to maximal oxygen intake, there is a 20% discrepancy between the best male rowers and international élite athletes in these other disciplines.

Anaerobic metabolism

Traditionally, anaerobic metabolism is indicated by a high peak blood lactate concentration. Peak values increase with the muscle mass involved in exercise, as well as with the motivation of the rowers. Values of $11 \, mmol \cdot l^{-1}$ have been reported after treadmill running, $15 \, mmol \cdot l^{-1}$ after a national regatta and $17 \, mmol \cdot l^{-1}$ following a FISA championship. Accordingly, the buffering system of the blood (bicarbonate) decreases from 26 to $13 \, mmol \cdot l^{-1}$ after all-out rowing, and bicarbonate is regularly eliminated from the blood. In consequence, the pH of the blood decreases from its normal value of 7.4 to 7.1 after all-out rowing. The pH was 6.74 and blood lactate $32 \, mmol \cdot l^{-1}$ in a rower in whom a zero bicarbonate level was measured after all-out ergometer rowing. Such a value may represent the lower limit of the physiological range (Nielsen 1999).

These values give little indication of the amount of anaerobic metabolism. For that purpose the 'oxygen deficit' can be calculated. The oxygen deficit is that part of metabolism that is not covered by oxygen intake during exercise (Chapter 22). In rowers, the reported oxygen deficit of $88–97 \, ml \cdot kg^{-1}$ is substantially larger than in runners. The anaerobic contribution to metabolism varies between 21% and 30%. Rowers also have the highest plasma catecholamine values measured during exercise, 35 and $120 \, nmol \cdot l^{-1}$ for adrenaline and noradrenaline, respectively. These high plasma catecholamine values may explain the persistent mobilization and activation of immunocompetent cells during rowing (Nielsen *et al.* 1996; Chapter 50).

Interest has also focused on the 'anaerobic threshold' or the work rate that elicits a blood lactate concentration of $4 \, mmol \cdot l^{-1}$ (Chapter 22). This work rate increases with training, and it seems to depend on the muscle fibre composition of the rower; those with many slow-twitch fibres are able to exercise at a high intensity for any given blood lactate level (Körner & Schwanitz 1985).

Circulation

Cardiac output showed values of only $13–17 \, l \cdot min^{-1}$ in ordinary rowing (Liljestrand & Lindhard 1920). During ergometer rowing with a sliding seat, the cardiac output is about $30 \, l \cdot min^{-1}$ for lightweight rowers (Nielsen *et al.* 1999). The involvement of many muscle groups presents a special problem during rowing. Different groups of muscle compete for their share of cardiac output when they have all been activated at maximal intensity (Secher 1983).

Variation in blood pressure is related to the cardiac cycle, resulting in a pulse pressure of approximately 45 mmHg (6 kPa) at rest. During rowing, the blood pressure also varies with the rowing cycle, giving rise to a 'pulse pressure' of more than 100 mmHg (13 kPa). In consequence, the systolic pressure may approach 200 mmHg (27 kPa) during maximal rowing. The fluctuations in blood pressure take place at a rate much faster than can be accommodated by the cerebral autoregulatory mechanisms, and transcranial Doppler measurements indicate that flow to the brain fluctuates in close parallel with blood pressure during rowing (Fig. 56.5). The heart rate has been determined repetitively during rowing and is currently used to guide training intensity, often with the aim of keeping effort close to the intensity that elicits a blood lactate value of $4 \, mmol \cdot l^{-1}$.

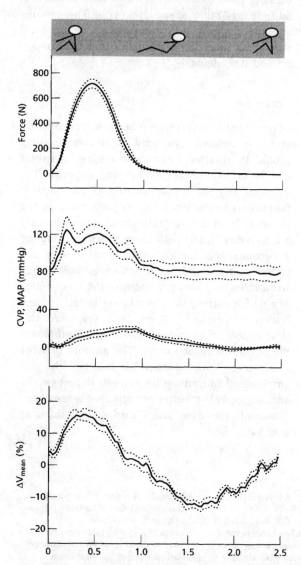

Fig. 56.5 Averaged results of rowing force, mean arterial pressure (MAP), central venous pressure (CVP) and middle cerebral artery mean flow velocity (V_{mean}) during ergometer rowing. From Pott *et al.* (1997).

Ventilation

As during other types of exercise, the respiratory minute volume increases linearly with oxygen intake until approximately 80% of the rower's maximal oxygen intake is reached. At higher work rates, the increase in ventilation becomes steeper, with a peak recorded value of $243 \, l \cdot min^{-1}$ (Secher 1983). The vital capacity of rowers is also large; the male mean is $6.8 \, l$, and a peak value of $9.1 \, l$ has been measured.

The high ventilation rate during intense rowing induces a marked increase in alveolar oxygen pressure. Yet the large cardiac output elicited during maximal exercise makes oxygen saturation of haemoglobin difficult, especially when exercise involves large muscle groups. Thus, although there is no decrease in haemoglobin saturation during maximal arm exercise, during 'all-out' rowing a reduction of 8% or more takes place regularly. It may be speculated that during rowing, the decrease in haemoglobin saturation is due to the decrease of the blood pH, but arterial oxygen tension also decreases from a resting value of $105 \, mmHg$ ($14 \, kPa$) to $83 \, mmHg$ ($11 \, kPa$). This finding points to a limitation in oxygen transport across the alveolar membrane. Indeed, an inspired oxygen fraction of 0.30, compared to the normal atmosphere of 0.21 oxygen, restores haemoglobin saturation even during maximal exercise, with a corresponding increase in maximal oxygen intake (Nielsen *et al.* 1999). Arterial desaturation is reflected in the brain during all-out rowing, cerebral oxygenation decreasing to an extent (approximately 15%; Fig. 56.6) that is seen otherwise only during fainting (Madsen & Secher 1999).

Altitude training

With the difficulty of increasing maximal oxygen intake in well-trained athletes, altitude training has remained popular among some rowers and is carried out immediately before the FISA championship in any given year. Early studies, involving mainly untrained subjects, showed a dramatic increase in maximal oxygen intake following altitude training. But such an effect has been more difficult to demonstrate in well-trained individuals,

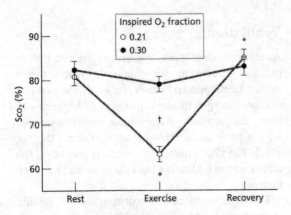

Fig. 56.6 Cerebral oxygenation (Sco_2) in ambient air, with an inspired O_2 fraction of 0.21 and 0.30: at rest, during a 6-min maximal ergometer row; and into the recovery from exercise. * different from control, $p < 0.05$; † different from the trial with O_2 supplementation, $p < 0.05$. Modified from Nielsen *et al.* (1999).

and in athletes it has sometimes been difficult to maintain even the prealtitude maximal oxygen intake (Secher 1990). The problems with altitude training are related both to the foreign environment and to the reduced tolerance of training while at altitude. Both difficulties can be taken care of by using an 'altitude chamber'. In this manner, athletes can sleep at simulated altitude, while training is performed outside the chamber in the normal sea-level environment. The stimulating effect of hypoxia on the blood-forming organs may thus be combined with normal training. However, even after weeks of sleeping in such a chamber, it is difficult to see any effect either on the haemoglobin content of newly formed red cells (the reticulocytes) or on blood volume.

Equally, no increase in performance on a rowing ergometer has been demonstrated following altitude training. In a controlled study, the same increase in maximal oxygen intake was noted when training at altitude and at sea-level (Levine *et al.* 1992). However, in the group that trained at sea-level, endurance at sea-level increased more (68%) than at altitude (46%). Conversely, in the altitude training group, endurance was more enhanced at altitude (73%) than at sea-level (43%). These results strongly suggest that competitions at sea-level should be preceded by training that is also performed at sea-level.

Training

Given the strong correlation between performance and the metabolic capacity of rowers, training should be directed towards increasing anaerobic and especially aerobic power and capacity. The maximal oxygen intake of rowers increases in proportion to the work that is performed during training, from 400 to 700 h·year^{-1} (approximately 1.1–2.2 h·day^{-1}), but with more prolonged training it becomes increasingly difficult to develop any further increase (Körner & Schwanitz 1985). High work rates may serve to increase the work intensity which corresponds to a blood lactate concentration of 4 mmol·l^{-1}. It has been suggested that this variable offers the best physiological estimate of the performance of rowers. The amount of work rather than work intensity has traditionally been emphasized in training for rowing. Recent experience suggests that better performance is associated also with the time spent during high-intensity exercise.

References

Balukow, C.N. (1964) Hydrodynamische Charakteristik der Sport-Ruderboote (German translation). *Katera I Yachti* **3**, 187–191.

Gustafsson, F., Ali, S., Hanel, B., Toft, J.C. & Secher, N.H. (1996) The heart of the senior oarsman: an echocardiographic evaluation. *Medicine and Science in Sports and Exercise* **28**, 1045–1048.

Hagerman, F.C. (1984) Applied physiology of rowing. *Sports Medicine* **1**, 303–326.

Körner, T. & Schwanitz, P. (1985) *Rudern*. Sportsverlag Berlin, Berlin.

Levine, B.D., Friedman, D.B., Engfred, K. *et al.* (1992) The effect of normoxic or hypobaric hypoxic endurance training on the hypoxic ventilatory response. *Medicine and Science in Sports and Exercise* **24**, 769–775.

Liljestrand, G. & Lindhard, J. (1920) Zur Physiologie des Ruderns. *Skandinavische Archives für Physiologie* **39**, 215–235.

Madsen, P.L. & Secher, N.H. (1999) Near-infrared oxymetry of the brain. *Progress in Neurobiology* **56**, 1–20.

Nielsen, H.B. (1999) pH after competitive rowing: the lower physiological range? *Acta Physiologica Scandinavica* **165**, 113–114.

Nielsen, H.B., Secher, N.H., Christensen, N.J. & Pedersen, B.K. (1996) Lymphocytes and NK cell activity during repeated bouts of exercise. *American*

Journal of Physiology 271, R222–R227.

Nielsen, H.B., Boushel, R., Madsen, P. & Secher, N.H. (1999) Cerebral desaturation during exercise reversed by O_2 supplementation. American Journal of Physiology 277, H1045–H1052.

Pelliccia, A., Maron, B.J., Spataro, A., Proschan, M.A. & Spirito, P. (1991) The upper limit of cardiac hypertrophy in highly trained elite athletes. New England Journal of Medicine 324, 295–301.

Pott, F., Knudsen, L., Nowak, M., Nielsen, H.B., Hanel, B. & Secher, N.H. (1997) Middle cerebral artery blood velocity during rowing. Acta Physiologica Scandinavica 160, 251–255.

Secher, N.H. (1983) The physiology of rowing. Journal of Sports Sciences 1, 23–53.

Secher, N.H. (1990) Rowing. In: Reilly, T., Secher, N.H., Snell, P. & Williams, C. (eds) Physiology of Sports, pp. 259–285. E. & F.N. Spon, London.

Shephard, R.J. (1998) The biology and medicine of rowing. Journal of Sports Sciences 16, 603–620.

Steinacker, J.M. (1987) Rudern. Springer-Verlag, Berlin.

Steinacker, J.M. & Secher, N.H. (eds) (1993) Advances in physiology and biomechanics of rowing. International Journal of Sports Medicine 14, S1–S46.

Chapter 57

Cross-Country Ski Racing

ULF BERGH AND ARTUR FORSBERG

Introduction

Cross-country skiing has been practised for at least 4000 years, most of the time for basic transportation. Nowadays, activities such as recreational touring and racing are the more common reasons for such skiing. As a result, skiing equipment has become more specialized and the level of performance has increased. This chapter focuses on cross-country ski racing, particularly performance at a very advanced level. The data presented are mostly taken from the literature but some of the authors' as yet unpublished results are included.

Skiing competitions

Cross-country skiing competitions for adults are performed over distances ranging from 5 to 90 km. In the world championships, the Olympic games and the World Cup, the distances for individual races range from 5 to 30 km for females, and from 10 to 50 km for males. Relay races consist of 4 × 5-km and 4 × 10-km events for females and males, respectively. The duration of these races is, at present, approximately 12–90 min for females and 22–140 min for males. In individual events, competitors usually start at 30-s intervals. However, since 1992, the Olympic games and the world championships have included a competition consisting of a classic race and a freestyle race, performed on two consecutive days. The event starts with an ordinary race (classic). The following day there is a 'pursuit race' (freestyle); the start is arranged based on the competitors' time intervals obtained on the first day, and

the first to finish is the winner. The distances are 5 km and 10 km for women, while men race for 10 km and 15 km. In relay races, all teams start at the same time.

Occasionally, 'mass starts' are used in individual events. These races are usually quite long (60–90 km), and the courses are flatter. A number of these are part of the so-called 'worldloppet', which is a long distance equivalent to the World Cup.

As in most sports, the results in cross-country skiing have improved over the decades (Fig. 57.1). This is due to better equipment, better preparation of courses and greater physical capacity of the skiers. There are considerable variations in this overall trend within relatively narrow timespans (a few years), probably resulting from differences in factors such as snow conditions and altitude. The results have improved more in cross-country skiing than in some other endurance events (Fig. 57.2). This is probably due to the fact that there has been room for considerable improvement in at least four areas of cross-country skiing: courses, equipment, skiing technique and physical capacity of the skiers, whereas in other sports major contributions to a better performance have been possible in only one or two of these areas.

According to the rules, a racing course should contain uphill, downhill and flat terrain in equal proportions. Usually, more than half of the racing time is spent skiing uphill, and 10–15% skiing downhill (Frost et al. 1984). Consequently, one would expect the major part of the time differences between skiers to occur during the uphill parts of the course. This has been confirmed by timing the

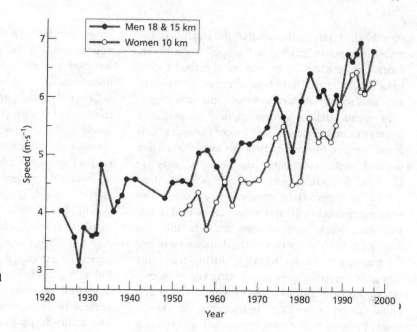

Fig. 57.1 Average speeds in world championships and Olympic games in men's shortest individual event (18 km up to 1948 and thereafter 15 km) and the longest event (50 km).

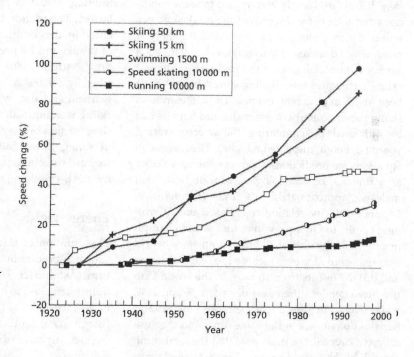

Fig. 57.2 Relative improvement of the results (men) in some endurance sports, calculated according to the expression $100 \cdot (v_i - v_0) \cdot v_0^{-1}$, where v_i is the speed in a given year and v_0 is the speed at the earliest of the displayed competitions. For cross-country skiing, the calculations are based on the winning results in Olympic games and world championships. Values are presented as averages for each decade. For the other events, the world records are used to indicate performance.

participants in various races (Frost *et al.* 1984). However, if one compensates for differences in duration between uphill and downhill skiing the data become conflicting. Thus, there are data indicating that (compared with the winner) the fraction

of the total time difference for a specific part of the course is directly proportional to the fraction of total racing time spent in this section of the course (Frost *et al.* 1984). In contrast, a study based on four events in the 1989 World Championships (A. Forsberg, unpublished data) indicates that the fraction of the time differences occurring in the uphill segments is much greater than its fraction of the total racing time. Similar results have been obtained by Welde in 1991 and 1997 (B. Welde, personal communication).

In events such as swimming and running, the average velocity is lower over longer distances. This is mainly due to the fact that the available power declines with increasing duration of exercise (Åstrand & Rodahl 1986). Hence, such a pattern would be expected in cross-country skiing. The winning results in Olympic games and world championships from 1978 to 1985 indicate that the average velocity decreases as the distance increases for males, but not for females. During this time, classic skiing techniques (see 'Racing styles' below) were used over all distances. However, the anticipated distance–velocity relationship in cross-country skiing is obscured by the fact that courses may differ considerably with regard to snow conditions and total climb. Moreover, the total climb per unit of distance tends to be greatest in the shortest races, which decreases the average velocity for such events. Additionally, since the mid-1980s different skiing techniques (see 'Racing styles' below) have been used in different events. The difference in skiing performance between males and females can be estimated by comparing the average racing speed (U. Bergh, unpublished data). The regression equations for prediction of average racing velocity as a function of chronological time indicate that males ski approximately 14% faster than females. Distance–velocity relationships based on: (i) winning results in Olympic games and world championships; (ii) the fastest Olympic games or world championship race ever recorded for each distance; and (iii) the results from 10 races in the World Cup produced gender differences of 13%, 14% and 15%, respectively. In these competitions males and females do not race at the same time, and they use different courses; the rules state that the total climb should be less for females. These factors make the comparison more difficult, with a tendency to underestimate the difference between genders. In the Wasa Race (90 km), where men and women have been racing on the same day, on the same course, since 1981, the difference in average speed is approximately 16% (Ekblom & Bergh 1994). These figures tend to be somewhat higher than those reported for other endurance events (Åstrand & Rodahl 1986).

Generally, the performance in events such as cross-country skiing is strongly influenced by forces acting in the forward direction and forces acting in the opposite direction. The former are limited by the rate of energy yield (motor power) of the skier (and in downhill segments the force of gravity) and the capability to utilize this energy in the forward direction (technical skill). The skier has to expend power to: (i) overcome the friction between the ski and the snow; (ii) overcome air resistance; (iii) elevate the centre of gravity during each stride and in uphill skiing; and (iv) accelerate the body's centre of mass (translational kinetic energy) and the mass of various body segments (rotational kinetic energy). The ability to produce power can be increased by training, but it is strongly influenced by genetic factors. The friction between ski and snow is influenced by the condition of the snow surface, waxing of the ski and by pressure distribution characteristics (Ekström 1980). Air resistance can be diminished by the design and material of the skier's outer garment and also by the skier's body position. The skiing technique aims at directing the largest possible fraction of the available metabolic power (and in skiing down hills the force of gravity) in a forward direction, parallel to the track, while minimizing the resisting forces.

Energy yield

The duration of ski races is such that the energy source is predominantly (85–99%) aerobic metabolism (Åstrand & Rodahl 1986). Oxygen intake is quite often close to its maximum in uphill segments of the race, judging from observed heart rate values (Bergh 1982; Saltin 1997), and measurements of oxygen uptake during racing-like conditions (Mygind et al. 1994). Even higher demands have been reported. Norman et al. (1989) filmed skiers during the 1988 Olympics and calculated their power outputs. In short (<20 s) uphill segments the demand corresponded to $110-120 \, ml \cdot kg^{-1} \cdot min^{-1}$. Skiing can induce a higher oxygen intake than uphill running (Strömme *et al.* 1977). For these reasons, a very high maximal oxygen intake is likely to be a prerequisite for success in international cross-country ski racing (see Fig. 7.2). The anaerobic energy-yielding system may be taxed substantially during racing conditions, judging from the blood lactate levels obtained at the finish of races (Åstrand *et al.* 1963; U. Bergh, unpublished data), and during a simulated 14-km competition where blood samples were obtained every 2.75 km (Mygind *et al.* 1994). That study also demonstrated that the blood lactate concentration rises to almost 10 mmol·l^{-1} during the first couple of kilometres, and it increases slightly further (a few mmol·l^{-1}) during the rest of the race. Based on lactate uptake data, Saltin (1997) has estimated the quantitative aspects; and he postulated that approximately 10% of the total energy may come from anaerobic sources during a 15-km race, and up to 20% in a 5-km race. On the other hand, in order to oxidize the lactate produced when delivering these amounts of anaerobic energy, the oxygen uptake needs to be higher than that observed during races. This discrepancy becomes even greater if the muscle is using fuels other than lactate, thus leaving less oxygen for lactate oxidation and less room for lactate production. Such calculations indicate an anaerobic contribution of about half the figures mentioned above. Hence, even if the anaerobic energy yield is greater than previously believed, the anaerobic capacity is probably of minor importance for cross-country skiing performance, especially in longer events, and its influence can be decisive only if the differences in other functions are small.

The main substrates for muscular activity are fat and carbohydrates. The latter are stored as glycogen in the skeletal muscles and in the liver. If the racing time exceeds 1 h, there is a risk of emptying carbohydrate stores, in which case the tempo will drop dramatically. This is not infrequent in races of 50 km or longer, where minutes may be lost within a few kilometres. Glycogen cannot be moved from one muscle to another; therefore, some muscles may become depleted of glycogen, while others are far from empty. Carbohydrates can be supplied to the skier during a race. These carbohydrates primarily serve the very important purpose of maintaining an adequate blood glucose concentration; but they may also decrease the rate of glycogen degradation, although to a limited extent (see Chapter 29). Hence, the vast majority of the glycogen needed during a race must be stored in the body of the skier before the start of the race.

Racing styles

At present, skiing competitions are classified into two styles: classic skiing (Fig. 57.3a,b) and freestyle (Fig. 57.3c). In classic skiing three main techniques are used: diagonal (Fig. 57.3a), double pole and kick/double pole (Fig. 57.3b). In the freestyle events, skating is by far the most frequently used technique; classic skiing is hardly used at all, except for double poling. Skating is nowadays performed almost exclusively as double skate (V-skate). The one leg skate (marathon skate) is used only as a means of changing direction. The double skate is performed in different ways, depending on prevailing conditions, the main difference being the timing between arms and legs. Generally, if the resistance to propagation is low (e.g. good glide, slightly downhill), the number of arm cycles per leg cycle is lower ('low gear') than in less favourable conditions (uphill, harsh snow); the extreme situation is skating without using the poles ('overdrive').

Skating is approximately 10% faster than classic skiing (Stray-Gundersen & Ryschon 1987). The question is: why? There are a number of possible explanations: (i) the attainable aerobic power is higher in skating than in classic skiing; (ii) for a given metabolic rate, skating develops a greater power in the forward direction; and (iii) the forces resisting the forward progression are lower in skating. Comparison of the diagonal technique and the V-skate in nine male international calibre skiers during maximal uphill skiing did not reveal any significant difference in oxygen intake between techniques (Table 57.1). In contrast, with six female national calibre skiers, the diagonal technique produced significantly higher values than the V-skate (Table 57.1). Hence, these observations do not indicate that the superiority of skating is due to a higher aerobic power. On the other hand, there are indications that higher oxygen intake values can be

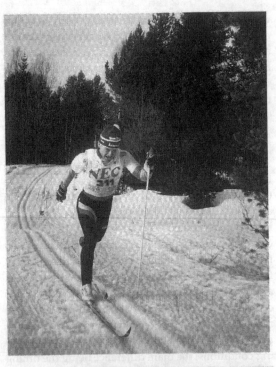

(a)

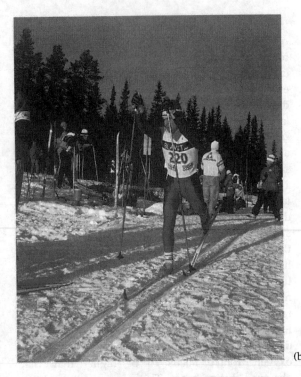

(b)

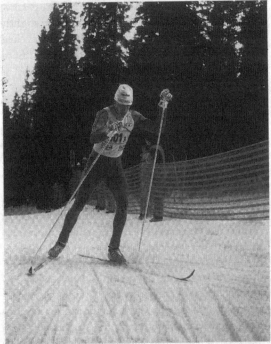

(c)

Fig. 57.3 (a) Diagonal technique; (b) kick double/pole technique; (c) V-skate (double skate) technique.

Table 57.1 Oxygen uptake and heart rate during approximately 3 min of maximal uphill skiing preceded by at least 30 min of warm-up skiing. The male skiers were all of international calibre; most of the females were not, although all of them belonged to the Swedish national team. From Forsberg *et al.* (1988) and unpublished data.

	Diagonal		Skate	
	Mean	s.d.	Mean	s.d.
Males (n = 9)				
Oxygen intake (l·min⁻¹)	5.65	0.61	5.59	0.60
Heart rate (beats·min⁻¹)	177	8	177	8
Females (n = 6)				
Oxygen intake (l·min⁻¹)	3.41	0.18	3.27	0.27
Heart rate (beats·min⁻¹)	178	5	179	4

attained in skating compared with the kick double pole technique (Nilsson & Löfstedt 1984). However, the latter technique is used mainly on flat terrain, where the oxygen intake is not usually taxed to its maximum (Bergh 1982). It is therefore not possible to state whether the attainable oxygen intake over an entire race will be higher in skating compared with classic skiing. At racing pace, blood lactate concentration and heart rate tend to be higher in skating than in classic skiing (Mygind *et al.* 1994).

For a given velocity, skating has been reported to be metabolically approximately 10% less costly than classic skiing (Zupan *et al.* 1988). The same trend was found by Saibene *et al.* (1989), but double poling seems to be even less costly than skating (Hoffman & Clifford 1990). Skating also produces a higher velocity than classic skiing at a given blood lactate concentration (Nilsson & Löfstedt 1984), which further supports the theory that skating is less costly than other cross-country skiing techniques. Hence, one probable explanation why skating is faster than classic skiing is that the metabolic rate for a given skiing velocity is lower in skating than in classic skiing; for a given aerobic power, skating produces a higher speed. The question is again: why? There are several possibilities: (i) resisting forces (air resistance and friction between the ski and the snow) are less; (ii) less work is performed against gravity; (iii) increases in kinetic energy are smaller; and (iv) there is a better transformation of energy between body segments. There are no data on the air resistance for different racing styles. However, the body position is a crucial factor, and when conditions allow the

skier to skate without using poles, the skating technique may allow a more crouched posture, as in speed skating. In addition, skating can be performed without kick waxes and that reduces the frictional force. The glide becomes better, which is an advantage in almost all parts of a racing track; it may also contribute to a lowering of air resistance, by reducing the trend to slowing on flats after downhill segments, thus allowing the skier to stay longer in a crouched position. Another possible difference between classic and skating techniques is that the work performed against gravity within a given step cycle may be lower in skating, since the vertical displacement of the centre of gravity, as well as the frequency of cycles, appears to be less than in classic skiing. The velocity changes during the step cycle are much smaller in skating (Frederick 1992), which helps to reduce the power requirement.

On the other hand, if the course is very soft, the V-skate may be more costly than both the kick/double pole technique and the marathon-skate (Nilsson & Löfstedt 1984). This may be due to the fact that the skis are tilted during skating, so that the edges cut rather deeply into the snow during both planting and the thrust. Among classic techniques, the kick/double pole technique has been found to demand either less oxygen than the diagonal technique (Westergren & Nylander 1977; U. Bergh, unpublished data) or more (MacDougall *et al.* 1979). The latter result is not compatible with the fact that the kick/double pole technique is the predominant one adopted on flats during classic skiing, at least among élite skiers.

Skiing techniques differ with regard to the velocity attained over a distance of 90 m (Nilsson & Löfstedt 1984). The V-skate is significantly faster (9%) than the kick/double pole technique, which in turn tends to be slower than the marathon skate (3%).

The general opinion is that the use of double poling techniques has increased during recent decades. This probably results from a better preparation of courses and better skis and waxes; these factors increase speed, making the use of the diagonal technique too costly. In turn, this has put more emphasis on upper body strength and endurance (see 'Training' below).

Characteristics of élite cross-country skiers

Top skiers can vary considerably in body mass (Table 57.2). World-class male skiers during the 1970s and early 1980s differed from each other by approximately 30 kg (Bergh 1987). Thus, the influence of body size appears to be no greater than the differences in quality (the variation in capacity for a given body size). This contrasts with the situation in many other sports, even endurance events, e.g. rowing (Secher 1983). Cross-country skiers tend to be heavier than long-distance runners (Bergh et al. 1978), but lighter than rowers (Secher 1983).

Maximal oxygen intake is extremely high, both in absolute volume and relative to body mass (Åstrand 1955; Saltin & Åstrand 1967; Hanson 1973; Bergh et al. 1978; Ingjer 1991) (Table 57.3). World-class skiers have a significantly higher maximal oxygen intake than less successful skiers (Bergh 1987; Ingjer 1991). Among world-class skiers, the greatest variation appears when expressing the values in $l \cdot min^{-1}$, whereas the unit $ml \cdot kg^{-2/3} \cdot min^{-1}$ produces the smallest interindividual variation (Bergh 1987; Ingjer 1991). Without an oxygen intake of at least 350 $ml \cdot kg^{-2/3} \cdot min^{-1}$ for males and 290 $ml \cdot kg^{-2/3} \cdot min^{-1}$ for females, the probability of winning gold medals in individual events in the Olympic games or world championships seems to be quite low (Bergh 1987). This is supported by data on Swedish and Norwegian male medallists in individual events (Table 57.3). The medallists in the junior world championships had lower values for maximal oxygen intake (Table 57.3), and none of them had won a medal in a world championship or the Olympic games while they were of junior age. Also, the fraction of maximal oxygen intake that the skier can attain during upper body exercise is higher among élite skiers when compared with less experienced skiers (Dittmer et al. 1980; Sharkey & Heidel 1981), and it has been reported as increasing over the last few decades (Saltin 1997).

When using maximal oxygen intake to characterize cross-country skiers, it seems appropriate to compensate for differences in body mass by expressing values as $ml \cdot kg^{-2/3} \cdot min^{-1}$ rather than as $ml \cdot kg^{-1} \cdot min^{-1}$ (Bergh 1987; Ingjer 1991). This reflects the fact that the power cost of skiing increases less than in direct proportion to body mass (Bergh 1987;

Table 57.2 Age, height, body mass and body mass index (body mass·height^{-2}) of international-calibre cross-country skiers during the mid-1990s.

	Age (years)	Height (m)	Body mass (kg)	Body mass index (kg·m^{-2})
Males				
Mean	30	1.81	74	22.7
Standard deviation	5	0.05	7	1.2
Extreme values	22–44	1.69–1.90	58–84	20.3–23.8
Females				
Mean	31	1.69	58	20.1
Standard deviation	5	0.05	7	1.4
Extreme values	22–39	1.62–1.75	45–68	17.1–22.2

Table 57.3 Body mass and maximal oxygen intake of Swedish male individual events medallists in Olympic Games or World Championships and in Junior World Championships.

	Body mass (kg)	Maximal oxygen intake		
		$l \cdot min^{-1}$	$ml \cdot kg^{-1} \cdot min^{-1}$	$ml \cdot kg^{-2/3} \cdot min^{-1}$
1960s* (n = 4)	68 ± 3	5.56 ± 0.2	82.0 ± 2.27	335 ± 9
1970s* (n = 4)	72 ± 7	6.14 ± 0.4	84.9 ± 6.44	353 ± 20
1980s† (n = 4)	73 ± 5	6.33 ± 0.5	87.2 ± 1.61	363 ± 14
1990s (n = 5)‡	78 ± 4	6.95 ± 0.4	88.8 ± 2.95	388 ± 14
Juniors (n = 5)				
1979–1998	70 ± 3	5.53 ± 0.2	78.7 ± 2.56	324 ± 8

n denotes the number of subjects.

* Maximal oxygen uptake was measured during uphill running on a treadmill.

† Maximal oxygen uptake was measured during uphill skiing which produces approximately 3% higher values compared with uphill running (Strömme *et al.* 1977).

‡ Norwegian and Swedish skiers. Data on Norwegian skiers courtesy of Frank Ingjer.

Bergh & Forsberg 1992), i.e. if two skiers differ in body mass by 20%, the difference in power expense during skiing is less than 20%.

The oxygen cost of skiing at any given speed is lower in élite than in non-élite cross-country skiers (Harkins 1978), indicating that élite skiers are technically superior. In contrast, another study comparing skiers of national calibre with recreational skiers did not confirm this finding (MacDougall *et al.* 1979). The latter study indicated considerable interindividual differences within the group of élite skiers, in line with data on subjects whose skiing capability ranged from being close to national level down to recreational level (Wehlin *et al.* 1970). In contrast, a much lower interindividual variation was found among skiers of international calibre (Åstrand *et al.* 1963). Variation seems to be less at the international level, which is logical since individuals with unfavourable qualities will not reach this high level of performance.

Muscle fibres in the leg muscles of élite skiers appear to be predominantly slow-twitch fibres, although again the interindividual variation is considerable (Rusko 1976; Bergh *et al.* 1978; Mygind 1995). A predominance of slow-twitch fibres is logical for several reasons: (i) in both arm and leg muscles, slow-twitch fibres display a more complete glycogen depletion than fast-twitch fibres (Tesch *et al.* 1978) during cross-country skiing, indicating that the demands of this sport involve slow-twitch more than fast-twitch fibres; (ii) metabolism during cross-country skiing is predominantly aerobic, and slow-twitch fibres have a high oxidative capacity; (iii) the number of capillaries per fibre is higher in slow-twitch fibres, which enhances oxygen transport; and (iv) slow-twitch fibres consume less glycogen for a given energy output (see Chapter 9).

Results from recent decades show that it is possible for both male and female skiers to be successful in all the present combinations of racing style and racing distance. It is very unusual that skiers are successful in only one style or distance. Thus, there is no clear trend for skiers to specialize either for distance or for style. One reason is that the metabolism is predominantly aerobic in all races. Moreover, for a given racing style, the technique is very much the same regardless of distance. However, a group of skiers who are very successful in the so-called 'worldloppet' ('flat' courses 2–5 h in duration) do not reach nearly the same standard in normal skiing competitions. Possible differences from ordinary races, apart from the above-mentioned factors, are the extensive use of double poling, and the mass start procedure. The former makes the capacity for upper body exercise more important, and the latter makes the performance during the last few hundred metres of the race much more decisive.

Predicting performance from physiological variables

Table 57.4 displays the correlation coefficients between a number of variables and different performance criteria. As expected, no single variable fully explains observed inter-individual differences in skiing performance. Moreover, skiing performance as measured by the outcome of races varies even within a period of a few days. Comparing the results from two races during the world championships tends to give a correlation coefficient of around 0.85, the average difference in rank being approximately four places (U. Bergh, unpublished data). Hence, the chances of predicting the outcome of a ski race correctly from physiological data are small. However, some characteristics show a considerable covariation with skiing performance. Maximal oxygen intake is one of these, and the skiing velocity at a given fraction of maximal oxygen intake is another, although oxygen intake at a given speed displays less covariation with skiing performance. Mygind et al. (1991) found that a combination of peak oxygen intake data from treadmill running and data obtained during exercise on a ski ergometer (upper body exercise) correlated better with skiing performance than either of these variables used separately. In running, maximal oxygen intake explained 61% of the variation in marathon performance, and the fraction of maximal oxygen intake utilized during treadmill running at a given speed explained 88% of the variation, whereas oxygen intake at a given running velocity accounted for 55% of the variation (Sjödin & Svedenhag 1985). Corresponding figures for the performance in 5000-m events were 35%, 88% and 53%, respectively (Sjödin & Schele 1982). The discrepancy between running and skiing is probably explained by the fact that the subjects used only one skiing style during measurements of oxygen intake, whereas additional styles were used during the race. Hence, in the skiing experiments the measured oxygen intake reflected only one aspect of the skiers' technical skill, whereas in

running a single measurement is likely to be more representative of the oxygen cost in competition, because the intraindividual variation of style during a race is much less than in skiing. In order to establish valid figures for individual differences in the oxygen cost of skiing under racing conditions, one would need to make measurements for all of the actual combinations of skiing techniques and terrain, preferably at racing speed. Moreover, one must know for what fraction of the total racing time the skier uses each of the different techniques. Hence, available data on the correlation between performance and the oxygen cost of skiing are hardly representative of the influence of technical skill on skiing performance.

Among variables other than physiological characteristics, the amount of cross-country skiing training seems to be a valuable predictor of performance, since it explains the vast majority (90%) of the interindividual variation in performance (Holm et al. 1976). A much lower figure (31%) was found for ski racing experience (Niinimaa et al. 1978).

Training

Cross-country skiing is characterized by repeated contractions of a number of muscles over extended periods. Sometimes the active muscle mass is large enough to tax the cardiopulmonary system maximally, while in other instances the active muscle groups are small. For small muscle groups, the attainable oxygen intake can vary substantially without any change in the maximal oxygen intake (Holmér 1974; Clausen 1976), and performance may also vary considerably for a given maximal oxygen intake (Holmér 1974; Clausen 1976). Hence, there is a need for both a high maximal oxygen intake and a high aerobic power of the individual muscles engaged in the various skiing styles. These qualities can be improved considerably by training. Furthermore, it is important not to empty the glycogen stores in muscles that are active during the race. Endurance training, where intensities below maximal aerobic power are maintained for hours, causes adaptations in the muscles that increase fat metabolism, sparing glycogen (see Chapters 7 & 9). The ability to convert the available energy into a

Table 57.4 Correlation between cross-country skiing performance and different variables.

Performance criterion	No. of subjects	Maximal oxygen intake§	Oxygen intake at given speed§	% of maximal oxygen intake at given speed	Muscle fibre composition (% slow-twitch fibres)	Muscle strength (Nm·kg⁻¹)	Racing experience (years)	Racing success in the previous race	Training*	Reference
Rank†	4	1.00								Åstrand (1955)
Rank†	5	0.40	0.23	0.3						Åstrand et al. (1963)
Rank†	6	0.89								Bergh (1982)
Speed	3	0.98								Bergh (1982)
Speed (medium)	11	0.72	0.16	0.75						Wehlin et al. (1970)
Speed (high)	11			0.86						Wehlin et al. (1970)
Speed	11	0.89			0.26					Holm et al. (1976)
Speed	11					0.35			0.93	Holm et al. (1976)
Rank††	6	0.03								Forsberg (unpublished)
Rank	11	0.70								Forsberg (unpublished)
Racing success	10	0.40					0.56			Forsberg (unpublished)
Rank	50							0.87		Bergh (unpublished)

* Kilometres of skiing during the year of the race.
† Position to finish. Spearman's rank correlation coefficient is used.
‡ Women.
§ ml·kg⁻¹·min⁻¹.

forward motion of the body, i.e. the individual's skiing skill, is likely to be important, although the correlation between racing performance and the oxygen cost of skiing is not very impressive (Table 57.4). Another potentially important quality is the ability to choose the most effective racing style with regard to prevailing conditions. This is especially difficult in events with individual starting times, since there is then limited feedback as to what style is the most effective. Consequently, training should include exercises that: (i) induce a high cardiovascular load to increase maximal oxygen intake; (ii) involve all muscles that are used during competitive skiing, in order to increase the attainable oxygen intake in skiing styles that only involve relatively small muscle groups, and to increase the capacity to spare glycogen; and (iii) improve technical skill in order to increase skiing velocity at a given metabolic rate. The attainable oxygen intake is of similar magnitude in running and in roller-skiing (Bergh 1982). Ski-walking (walking up a fairly steep hill using poles to imitate uphill skiing) and cross-country skiing produce slightly higher values compared with running in subjects who have trained for cross-country skiing (Hermansen 1973; Strömme et al. 1977). One advantage of roller-skiing training compared with running is that the upper body is also engaged in a manner similar to that of actual skiing (Petterson et al. 1977). It is important that the muscles participating in poling have a good endurance, since this movement contributes substantially to most racing styles (Petterson et al. 1977; Ekström 1980). Another reason is that double poling, the most efficient of all racing styles, cannot be used extensively unless the skier can attain a high aerobic power during upper body exercise. Training can substantially increase peak oxygen intake and performance during upper body exercise (~10%) within a couple of months even in well-trained skiers (Mygind et al. 1991). Moreover, a high aerobic power in the muscles of the upper body facilitates the attainment of maximal oxygen intake during combined arm and leg exercise (Bergh et al. 1976).

One disadvantage of roller-skiing might be that the skis can roll quite fast without much effort from the skier. Thus, the load on the oxygen-transporting system may be insufficient, since the skiers do not seem to compensate fully for a decreased rolling resistance by increasing their speed, either on flat or uphill terrain (Forsberg & Karlsson 1987). Therefore, skiers whose off-snow training consists predominantly of roller-skiing should not always use fast roller-skis.

Skiing technique should be learned by skiing, because exercises such as roller-skiing and ski-walking do not require identical patterns of motion (Petterson et al. 1977). Training in skiing technique has a greater priority among youngsters, because it seems harder for adults to achieve the necessary coordination and youngsters cannot tolerate the same quantities of endurance and strength training.

The top skiers of today train so much and so hard that only a well-trained body can endure this. Since the body needs time to adapt to high levels of physical stress, it takes several years of increased training volume and intensity before the necessary level is attained (Table 57.5). This partly explains why junior skiers rarely compete successfully in Olympic games and world championships, and why the average age of international-calibre skiers is almost 30 years (see Table 57.2). The body adapts not only to increases in training, but also to decreases. Therefore, the increments in training should be fairly gentle, and long breaks in training should be avoided, unless the individual's medical status dictates otherwise.

The content of training varies both between and within groups. There are, however, three main activities: cross-country running, roller-skiing and cross-country skiing. In the off-snow season, roller-skiing

Table 57.5 Approximate amount of training ($h \cdot year^{-1}$) for cross-country skiers in different age groups. Exercises such as warm-up and stretching are not included in these figures, which are representative of the present (1998) situation in Sweden.

	Age (years)	Males	Females
Adults	>20	650–750	500–700
Juniors	16–20	400–550	300–550
Youth	12–15	250–350	250–350

accounts for 50–70% of the time devoted to endurance training. The intensity of this training varies because skiers most often train on hilly terrain, where it is hard to maintain a constant work rate. Skiers tend to exercise at a higher metabolic rate uphill than on flat terrain, during both running and roller-skiing (Forsberg & Karlsson 1987). There are also seasonal variations. After the competitive season, high intensities should be avoided, especially at the beginning of the off-snow season (when there is a risk of overuse injuries; see Chapter 34). High-intensity training is performed just before the competitive season, whereas the greatest amounts of training are carried out after the beginning of the on-snow season. The intensity is usually such that the blood lactate concentration is increased, but it rarely approaches the levels attained immediately after skiing competitions (Bergh 1982).

The aforementioned increased use of poling techniques has changed the pattern of training. More time is now devoted to training the upper body. Thus, the trend seems to be that skiers are increasing their upper body strength and endurance, allowing them to use more poling and less leg exercise. In turn, skiers can use less kick wax and put more emphasis on the glide. This trend is particularly pronounced in long-distance races, where the courses are flatter.

Heat balance

Cross-country skiing is frequently performed in comparatively cold weather, and a substantial body heat loss as well as cold injuries may be expected.

The temperature of a body tissue is the result of the balance between the sum of the heat production plus heat gain on the one hand and the heat loss on the other (Chapter 17). For the body as a whole, the metabolic heat production during ski racing is usually greater than the heat loss due to convection, conduction and radiation, and therefore the skier must sweat to maintain the heat balance of the body. In spite of this, certain parts of the body, e.g. nose, ears and feet, can become quite cold, and sometimes even suffer cold injuries. This may seem paradoxical, but it is explained by the fact that the local heat loss can be greater than the sum of the local heat production and heat gained via the warm blood. The rate of local heat loss is high, because the velocity of the wind is added to the velocity of the skiers. Furthermore, the convective and evaporative heat losses are considerably elevated for body parts facing the wind. To reduce these problems, competitions should not be held at temperatures below –20 °C. However, there are risks of cold injuries even at temperatures above these limits, especially in strong winds and/or if the course contains long downhill segments. Another problem is that the skier inhales thousands of litres of cold, dry air, which may cause irritation of the respiratory tract (see also Chapter 17). The skier sweats during racing. The volume of sweat may, at least in longer races, amount to 4% of body mass (Holm *et al.* 1976) and may exceed that which can be tolerated without a reduction in performance capability. Consequently, there is a need for fluid replenishment during cross-country ski racing over longer distances.

References

Åstrand, P.-O. (1955) New records in human power. *Nature* 176, 922–923.

Åstrand, P.-O., Hallbäck, I., Hedman, R. & Saltin, B. (1963) Blood lactates after prolonged severe exercise. *Journal of Applied Physiology* 18, 619–622.

Åstrand, P.-O. & Rodahl, K. (1986) *Textbook of Work Physiology*, 3rd edn. McGraw-Hill, New York.

Bergh, U. (1982) *Physiology of Cross-Country Ski Racing*. Human Kinetics, Champaign, IL.

Bergh, U. (1987) The influence of body

mass in cross-country skiing. *Medicine and Science in Sports and Exercise* 19, 324–331.

Bergh, U. & Forsberg, A. (1992) Influence of body mass on cross-country ski racing performance. *Medicine and Science in Sports and Exercise* 24, 1033–1039.

Bergh, U., Kanstrup, I.-L. & Ekblom, B. (1976) Maximal oxygen uptake during exercise with various combinations of arm and leg exercise. *Journal of Applied Physiology* 41, 191–196.

Bergh, U., Thorstensson, A., Sjödin, B.,

Hultén, B., Piehl, K. & Karlsson, J. (1978) Maximal oxygen uptake and muscle fiber types in trained and untrained humans. *Medicine and Science in Sports* 10, 151–154.

Clausen, J.P. (1976) Circulatory adjustments to dynamic exercise and effect of physical training in normal subjects and in patients with coronary disease. *Progress in Cardiovascular Diseases* 18, 459–495.

Dittmer, S., Schantz, P. & Forsberg, A. (1980) Betydelsen av grennära styr-

keträning för längdåkare. (The importance of sports-specific strength training
for cross-country skiers.) *Svensk Skidsport*, October, **9**, 21–23.

Ekblom, B. & Bergh, U. (1994) Physiology
and nutrition for cross-country skiing.
In: Lamb, D.R., Knuttgen, H.G. &
Murray, R. (eds) *Perspectives in Exercise
Science and Sports Medicine. Vol. 7 Physiol-
ogy and Nutrition for Competitive Sports*.
Cooper Publishing, Carmel, IN.

Ekström, H. (1980) *Biomechanical research
applied to skiing: a developmental study and
an investigation of cross-country skiing,
alpine skiing and knee ligaments*.
Linköping Studies in Science and Technology, Dissertation no. 53. University of
Linköping, Sweden.

Forsberg, A. & Karlsson, E. (1987) Rullar
det för lätt? (Are roller-skis too fast for
aerobic training?) *Svensk Skidsport* **7**,
48–50.

Forsberg, A., Palmgren, L.-E. & Karlsson,
E. (1988) 'Konditionsträna båda stilarna'.
(Use both classic and skating techniques
in aerobic training.) *Svensk Skidsport* **10**,
44–46.

Frederick, E.C. (1992) Mechanical constraints in Nordic ski performance. *Medicine and Science in Sports and Exercise* **24**,
1010–1014.

Frost, P., Gabrielsson, L. & Jalderyd, G.
(1984) *Kapacitetsanalys av svenska damju-
niorer*. (Analysis of racing capacity in
Swedish junior female cross-country
skiers.) Physical Education Student
Thesis. Report 1984: 16, Gymnastik–och
idrottshögskolan, Stockholm, Sweden.

Hanson, J. (1973) Maximal exercise performance in members of the US Nordic ski
team. *Journal of Applied Physiology* **35**,
592–595.

Harkins, K.J. (1978) Metabolic cost comparison of cross-country skiing between
élite and non élite. *Canadian Journal of
Sports Sciences* **3**, 186 (abstract).

Hermansen, L. (1973) Oxygen transport
during exercise in human subjects. *Acta
Physiologica Scandinavica* Suppl. 399.

Hoffman, M.D. & Clifford, P.S. (1990) Physiological response to different cross
country skiing techniques on level
terrain. *Medicine and Science in Sports and
Exercise* **22**, 841–848.

Holm, I., Sjödin, B., Nilsson, J., Tesch, P. &
Forsberg, A. (1976) Muskelfunktionens
förändring under Vasaloppet. (Changes
in muscle functions during long distance
skiing, Vasaloppet.) *Svensk Skidsport* **8**,
27–30.

Holmér, I. (1974) Physiology of swimming
man. *Acta Physiologica Scandinavica*
Suppl. 407.

Ingjer, F. (1991) Maximal oxygen uptake as
a predictor of performance ability in
women and men élite cross-country
skiers. *Scandinavian Journal of Medicine
and Science in Sports* **1**, 25–30.

MacDougall, J.D., Hughson, R., Sutton, J.R.
& Moron, J.R. (1979) The energy cost of
cross-country skiing among élite competitors. *Medicine and Science in Sports* **11**,
270–273.

Mygind, E. (1995) Fibre characteristics and
enzyme levels of arm and leg muscles in
élite cross-country skiers. *Scandinavian
Journal of Medicine and Science in Sports* **5**,
76–80.

Mygind, E., Larsson, B. & Klausen, T.
(1991) Evaluation of a specific test in
cross-country skiing. *Journal of Sports Sciences* **9**, 249–257.

Mygind, E., Andersen, L.B. & Rasmussen,
B. (1994) Blood lactate and respiratory
variables in élite cross-country skiing at
racing speeds. *Scandinavian Journal of
Medicine and Science in Sports* **4**, 243–
251.

Niinimaa, V., Dyon, M. & Shepard, R.J.
(1978) Performance and efficiency of
intercollegiate cross-country skiers. *Medicine and Science in Sports* **10**, 91–93.

Nilsson, C. & Löfstedt, M. (1984) *Effek-
tivitetsanalys av några av skidorienterin-
gens olika åksätt*. (Analyses of different
cross-country skiing-techniques in ski-
orienteering.) Physical education
student thesis, Report 1984: 19,
Gymnastik-och Idrottshögskolan,
Stockholm, Sweden.

Norman, R.W., Ounpuu, S., Fraser, M. &
Mitchell, R. (1989) Mechanical power
outputs and estimated metabolic rates of
Nordic skiers during Olympic competition. *International Journal of Sport Biomechanics* **3**, 359–369.

Petterson, L.-G., Skogsberg, L. &
Zackrisson, U. (1977) Muskelaktivitet
under olika träningsformer för
längdåkning på skidor. (EMG activity
during cross-country skiing.) Physical
education student thesis, College of
Physical Education, Stockholm.

Rusko, H. (1976) *Physical performance characteristics in Finnish athletes*. Studies in
Sports, Physical Education and Health
no. 8, University of Jyväkylä, Jyväkylä.

Saibene, F., Cortili, G., Roi, G. &
Colombini, A. (1989) The energy cost of
level cross-country skiing and the effect

of friction of the ski. *European Journal of
Applied Physiology* **58**, 791–795.

Saltin, B. (1997) The physiology of competitive C.C. skiing across a four decade
perspective: with a note on training
induced adaptations and the role of
training at medium altitude. In: Müller,
E., Schameder, H., Kornexl, E. &
Raschner, C. (eds) *Science and Skiing*, pp.
435–469. E. & F. N. Spon, London.

Saltin, B. & Åstrand, P.-O. (1967) Maximal
oxygen uptake in athletes. *Journal of
Applied Physiology* **23**, 353–358.

Secher, N.H. (1983) The physiology of
rowing. *Journal of Sports Sciences* **1**, 23–53.

Sharkey, B.J. & Heidel, B. (1981) Physiological test of cross-country skiers. *Journal of
United States Ski Coaches Association* **5**,
1–6.

Sjödin, B. & Schele, R. (1982) Oxygen cost
of treadmill running in long distance
runners. In: Komi, P. (ed.) *Exercise and
Sport Biology*, pp. 61–67. Human
Kinetics, Champaign, IL.

Sjödin, B. & Svedenhag, J. (1985) Applied
physiology of marathon running. *Sports
Medicine* **2**, 83–99.

Stray-Gundersen, J. & Ryschon, T. (1987)
Economy of skating versus classic roller-
skiing. *Medicine and Science in Sports and
Exercise* **19**, 46 (abstract).

Strömme, S.B., Ingjer, F. & Meen, H.D.
(1977) Assessment of maximal aerobic
power in specifically trained athletes.
Journal of Applied Physiology **42**, 833–
837.

Tesch, P., Forsberg, A. & Karlsson, J. (1978)
Selective muscle glycogen depletion
during cross-country skiing. *Journal of
United States Ski Coaches Association* **2**,
12–17.

Wehlin, S., Agnevik, G., Sjödin, B. & Saltin,
B. (1970) Fysiologiska undersökningar
under Engelbrektsloppet. (Physiological
studies during the Engelbrekt ski race.)
Svensk Idrott **15–16**, 1–6.

Westergren, T.-G. & Nylander, P. (1977)
Spannhårdhetens inverkan på start-och
glidfriktion samt på energikravet vid
olika åkstätt. (Influence of camber stiffness on starting and gliding friction and
on energy cost for different skiing techniques.) Physical education student
thesis. Gymnastik-och Idrottshögskolan,
Stockholm, Sweden.

Zupan, M.F., Shepard, T.A. & Eisenman,
P.A. (1988) Physiological responses to
nordic tracking and skating in élite
cross-country skiers. *Medicine and Science
in Sports and Exercise* **20**, 81 (abstract).

Chapter 58

Cycling

GEORG NEUMANN

Cycling events

Cycling comprises several disciplines (Table 58.1). Besides classic road and track events, mountain-biking has become an attractive sport for many. To an increasing extent, cycling has become part of combination sports such as the triathlon, biathlon and winter triathlon. In the triathlon, cycling follows swimming and running comes at the end. In the biathlon, competitors run first, cycling follows and the athletes run again at the end. In the winter triathlon the first segment is running, cycling follows (mostly mountain-biking) and in the final segment the athletes are cross-country skiing.

Both men and women take part in cycling. Different types of bicycle are used for the various events. The bicycle used for road cycling weighs about 9 kg. The bicycle frame is made from a special light metal or carbon fibre. New frames are continually being developed for the bicycle, and the spokes have become an object of investigation too. In mild winds, carbon disk wheels are advantageous compared with spoked wheels. Combinations of disk and spoked wheels are also possible.

In track cycling, a lighter bicycle (about 6 kg) without brakes or gear-change is used. Braking is carried out by using the incline of the track. Cycling tracks are between 170 and 400 m in length. They are covered with cement or wood. As a consequence of high traffic density, off-road cycling has become more popular, and mountain-biking represents a real alternative in leisure-time sport.

Competitive cycling speed increases by 0.5–1% annually. The reasons include technical improve-ments in the bicycle, but also an enhancement of athletic performance preparation and conditioning. Among the aspects of physical conditioning, aerobic endurance in particular must be increased. An example of the dynamic development of strength endurance ability in cycling is provided by the preparation of Chris Boardman (UK) for his 4000-m world record in 1996 (Fig. 58.1). After his participa-tion in the Tour de France and in the individual time trial for the 1996 Olympic Games, he raced to a fan-tastic world record of 4 min 11.1 s in the 4000-m indi-vidual pursuit during the World Championship in September 1996.

Factors influencing cycling speed

Cycling speed does not always indicate the athlete's performance potential; speed is influenced by several components of resistance:
- air resistance;
- slope resistance;
- rolling resistance; and
- frictional forces.

Air resistance (Fig. 58.2) has the greatest influence. Energy consumption is significantly reduced by drafting. When riding in second or third position, approximately 30% of energy is saved relative to the lead cyclist. In a large group of cyclists, up to 50% of energy can be saved. This fact is currently intro-duced into tactical considerations for stage races. The athlete who aims at winning the race overall is relieved by other members of his or her team. He or she drafts wherever possible, thus saving strength for riding hills, for the time trial or for the final spurt

Table 58.1 Cycling events.

Event	Short-term endurance (1–2 min)	Medium-term endurance (2–10 min)	Long-term endurance			
			I (10–35 min)	II (35–90 min)	III (90–360 min)	VI (>360 min)
Track cycling	1000 m	Sprint (11–25 s and 2-min preload) 4000-m pursuit cycling (individual) 4000-m pursuit cycling (team) 3000-m pursuit cycling (women, individual)				
Road cycling			30–50-km criterion, time trial	100-km team competitions 80–180-km individual competitions	>200-km competitions	
Biathlon			30–50 km			
Triathlon (Olympic distance)			40 km	180-km Ironman (men and women)	540 km (ultratriathlon/ triple triathlon)	
Tourism			20–50 km	50–120 km		
Cross-country race (off-road cycling)		2–5 km (downhill)	5–20 km	30–50 km	50–70 km	

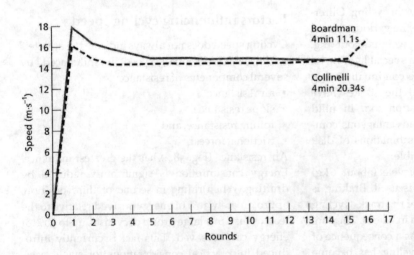

Fig. 58.1 4000-m individual pursuit. Speeds developed by Chris Boardman during world record in 1996.

of the stage. Cycling as part of a group is the most efficient way of saving energy. With increasing cycling speed, the energy expenditure needed to overcome air resistance increases as the square of the cycling speed. To overcome all of the resistance factors mentioned above, the total force must increase as the third power of speed. Air resistance is significantly influenced by the riding position.

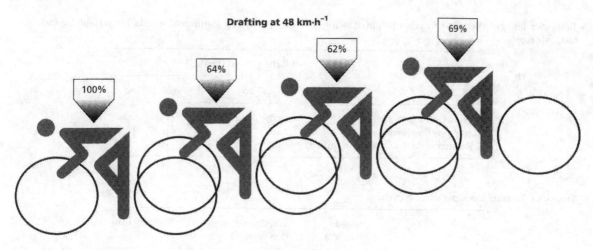

Fig. 58.2 Energy expenditure in drafting position in cycling.

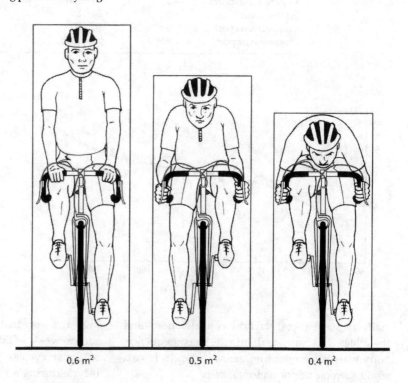

Fig. 58.3 Surface area presented to air resistance in different cycling positions.

0.6 m²   0.5 m²   0.4 m²

The wind impact area can be reduced from 0.6 m² in the upright position to 0.4 m² in a flat-back body position (Fig. 58.3). In certain situations, body mass may also have an influence on cycling performance. Athletes with a low body mass (less than 65 kg) have an advantage when riding uphill (Table 58.2). On the other hand cyclists with a body mass above 75 kg have an advantage on a flat course, because air resistance has to be overcome with great strength (Table 58.2). A comprehensive study of élite time trials found that heavier athletes tended to have faster times (Swain 1994). Small cyclists must do everything they can to optimize their aerodynamics.

When cycling in a group of several athletes (espe-

Table 58.2 Energy expenditures in the upright or racing position when riding at different speeds. From Hagberg and McCoyle (1996).

	Riding speed (km·h⁻¹)				
	10	20	30	40	50
Upright position (watts)	23.6	79.4	199.1	415.0	759.3
Racing position (watts)	22.6	70.8	170.2	346.8	625.7
% Reduction (watts or power required)	4	11	15	17	18

Table 58.3 Training loads per week in cycling.

Sport	Speed (km·h⁻¹)	Training volume (km·week⁻¹)	Training load (h)
Leisure-time sport	<20	60–120	3–6
Fitness sport	25	150–300	6–12
Competition sport	27	400–600	15–25
Professional sport	30	700–1000	25–35

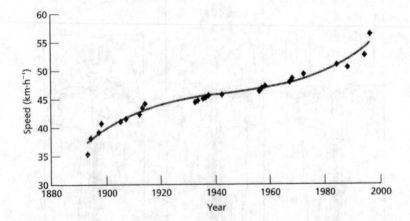

Fig. 58.4 Development of the 1-h world record in cycling.

cially in stage races), tactical considerations and the athlete's experience dominate. In consequence, body mass has a minor influence if cyclists have a similar aerobic performance capacity.

Training load in cycling

Cycling is a typical endurance-based sport, with one of the highest number of annual training hours. In this respect, cyclists are now being overtaken by triathlonists. Professional cyclists train over 700–1000 kilometres a week. For preventive train-ing, 10% of that distance is enough, i.e. 60–120 km·week⁻¹ (Table 58.3). Top international professional cyclists train about 35 000 km on their bicycle during a year, spending more than 30 h per week in training. Successful professional cyclists use races with several stages to prepare for even tougher races (such as the Tour de France). Since an increasing number of cyclists aim at reaching the international level, the performance density is increasing. For example in the 1-h world record (Fig. 58.4), the first record in 1883 was registered with a speed of 35.3 km·h⁻¹. Today, this speed is

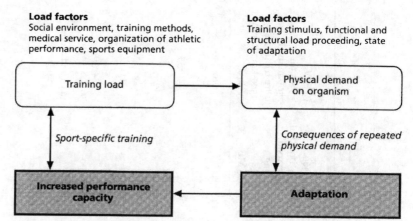

Fig. 58.5 Relationship between training load and adaptation of the organism. Adaptation should be evaluated by means of laboratory and field tests and the training programme corrected according to the data measured.

quite normal for group training. The 1996 1-h World Record was set by Boardman (United Kingdom) with a speed of 56.4 km·h⁻¹.

Physiology of cycling training

To achieve top-level athletic performance in cycling, 8 ± 2 years of training are required. The age for top-class results in cycling is about 25 ± 2 years (s.d.). With appropriate social and financial motivation, top results are possible for about 10 years (Fig. 58.5).

In this period, the necessary adaptations of the cardiovascular system, metabolism and specific muscular strength have to be achieved. Technical and tactical abilities are acquired and stabilized by participation in competitions.

The temporal duration of competition determines the training plan. Distinction is drawn between short-term endurance, medium-term endurance and long-term endurance events (Table 58.4).

Demands on functional systems in short-term and medium-term endurance events

THE MOTOR SYSTEM

Short-term endurance exercise lasts between 1 and 2 min, and medium-term endurance exercise lasts between 2 and 10 min. In 1000- and 4000-m track cycling, a high level of activation of the central nervous system is required. In track cycling, there is a predominant recruitment of fast-twitch fibres (FTF). Among track cyclists, sprinters have the highest proportion of FTF (from 35 to 65%). Intensive training programmes change the metabolic qualities and substrates of the FTF. Special strength training leads to hypertrophy of muscle fibres, especially the FTF (Table 58.5). Hypertrophy of these muscle fibres is a consequence of different training contents.

ENERGETIC BASIS OF PERFORMANCE

For short-term endurance performance in track cycling, mainly local energy stores are used. In particular, adenosine triphosphate (ATP), phosphocreatine (PC) and glycogen are required to accelerate a bicycle from a standstill (Fig. 58.6). Because start and finish follow each other within a few seconds, energy can be supplied only via alactic and glycolytic mechanisms. In competitions of 1–5-min duration, 30–50% of the energy is supplied from anaerobic sources. The values are similar to those obtained by Åstrand and Rodahl (1986) and Medbø and Tabata (1989). In efforts that last longer than 1 min, aerobic energy supply processes are dominant.

The training-induced adaptation of enzyme capacity differs significantly between track and road cyclists (Table 58.6).

The high proportion of anaerobic activity in the track competitor is indicated by the lactate concentration, although the extent of anaerobic

Table 58.4 Performance structure, cycling events.

Measured value	STE 35s–2min 1000-m track, sprint	MTE >2min–10min 3000-m female, 4000-m male (individual and team pursuit) Keirin, MB-downhill	LTE I >10min–30min Hill climb, point race	LTE II >30min–90min 30–60-m time trial, 40-km triathlon, 30–50-km MB	LTE III >90min–360min 60–80-km time trial, 80–250-km road, 180-km long triathlon, 55–70-km MB	LTE IV >360min 250-km road, ultra triathlon, <500-km ultra road cycling
Heart rate (beats·min⁻¹)	185–205	190–210	180–195	175–190	140–180	110–150
Oxygen intake (% $\dot{V}o_{2max}$)	95–100	97–100	90–95	80–95	60–85	40–55
Energy exchange						
% Aerobic	50	80	85	95	98	99
% Anaerobic	50	20	15	5	2	(1)
Energy consumption†						
kJ·min⁻¹	230–250	170–190	90–120	84–105	50–84	34–50
kJ (total)	250–290	630–960	1170–2760	3140–7450	7540–41400	36000–50200 (24h and more)
Lactate (mmol·l⁻¹)	14–15	16–22	12–14	8–12	1.5–4	1.0–2.0
Free fatty acids (mmol·l⁻¹)	0.50*	0.50*	0.80	0.90–1.0	1.2–2.0	1.5–3.0
Urea (mmol·l⁻¹)	6	6	7	7–9	8–10	9–15
Cortisol (nmol·l⁻¹)	200–400*	200–400*	200–450	400–800	500–900	600–1200

* Stress lipolysis (adrenaline); † dependent on speed and body mass; MB, mountain-bike; STE, short-term endurance; MTE, medium-term endurance; LTE, long-term endurance.

Table 58.5 $\dot{V}_{O_{2max}}$, proportion and cross-sectional area of fibres in vastus lateralis muscle of national (former East German) élite cyclists.

Sport	No. of cyclists	$\dot{V}_{O_{2max}}$ (ml·min⁻¹·kg⁻¹)	Fibre type (%)			Cross-sectional area (μm²)	
			I (STF)	II (FTF)	Ia (FTG)	STF	FTF
Sprinters	5	64.0	65	35	30	9000	13500
1000-m track	5	66.0	72	28	25	8500	12000
4000-m track	10	76.0	78	22	22	8000	10000
Road cyclists	20	78.0	80	20	20	7000	8000

STF, slow-twitch fibre; FTF, fast-twitch fibre; FTG, fast-twitch glycolytic fibre.

Table 58.6 Enzyme activity of vastus lateralis muscle in national élite cyclists in former East Germany.

Enzyme activity (μmol·g⁻¹ wet muscle)	Road cyclists ($n = 19$)	Track cyclists ($n = 12$)	P
Glycogen synthetase	7.62 ± 1.38	4.1 ± 2.1	0.002
Phosphoglycerate kinase	174 ± 48	274.2 ± 60	0.001
Pyruvate kinase	103.2 ± 21.6	450.0 ± 48.0	0.001
Lactate dehydrogenase	229.2 ± 72.0	390.0 ± 114.0	0.001
Citrate synthetase	43.0 ± 11.3	29.3 ± 10.1	0.005

Values are mean ± s.d.

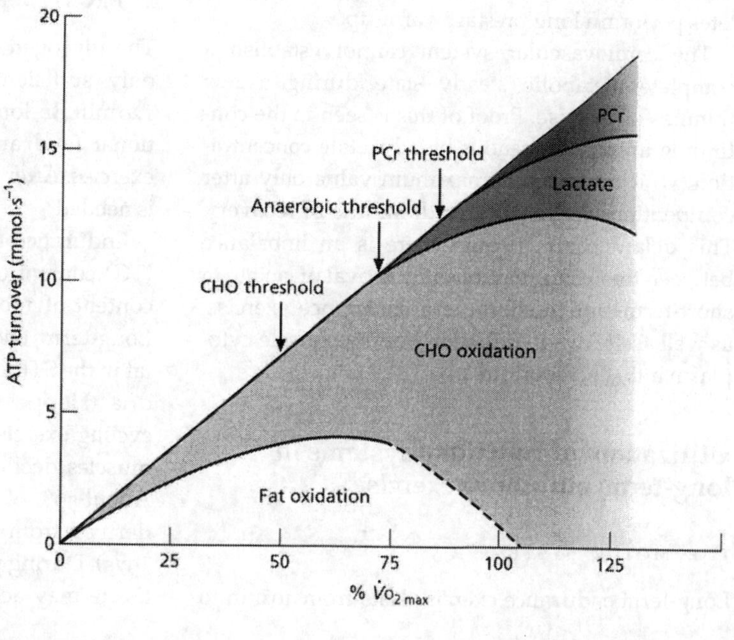

Fig. 58.6 Metabolic thresholds (carbohydrate (CHO), aerobic–anaerobic and phosphocreatine (PCr)) related to adenosine triphosphate (ATP) turnover (Sahlin 1986).

metabolism cannot be quantified exactly. In competitions of between 1000 and 4000 m, blood lactate concentrations reach 18–22 mmol·l^{-1}. In track cycling performance, the energy exchange per unit time is also high. Due to their intensive training, track cyclists have a higher anaerobic power than road cyclists, as may be concluded from the higher activity of the anaerobic enzymes in muscles (Table 58.6). In 1000-m time trials, anaerobic metabolism provides about 230 kJ·min^{-1} of energy, and in 4000-m team pursuit events it yields about 170 kJ·min^{-1}. The high degree of central nervous system activation required in heavy track cycling efforts results in a substantial release of catecholamines. The elevated levels of adrenaline (epinephrine) and noradrenaline (norepinephrine) induce glycolysis, lipolysis and proteolysis. The resulting increase in free fatty acids (FFA) and amino acids is of no use to metabolism in short-term endurance workouts.

CARDIOVASCULAR BASIS OF PERFORMANCE

In short- and medium-term endurance performances, the cardiovascular system is maximally activated. Maximal heart rates range between 185 and 210 beats·min^{-1}. The maximal oxygen intake can be fully utilized only after a latency of 40–60 s. In order to raise the metabolism to a higher level, athletes perform a long prestart warm-up.

The cardiovascular system cannot establish a complete metabolic steady state during a few minutes of exercise. Proof of this is seen in the continuing increase in venous blood lactate concentration, which reaches its maximum value only after competition, in the 5th to 15th minute of recovery. This delay occurs because there is an imbalance between the accumulation and removal of lactate in short-term and medium-term endurance exercise, as well as delays in diffusion from the muscle cytoplasm into the blood stream.

Utilization of functional systems in long-term endurance exercise

THE MOTOR SYSTEM

Long-term endurance exercise lasts from 10 min to several hours (see Table 58.4). Due to very different motor, energy and psychic demands, long-term endurance exercise is subdivided based on duration. The following categories are described (Neumann *et al.* 1998): long-term endurance I (10–30 min), long-term endurance II (30–90 min), long-term endurance III (90–360 min) and long-term endurance IV (>360 min). Over all of these events, the potential power of the muscles depends particularly on fatigue-resistant slow-twitch fibres (STF). Successful road cyclists have a high proportion of STF (70–95%). To sustain bicycle exercise for several hours, a motor stereotype is required. This stereotype is developed by prolonged training and is characterized by the dominant recruitment of STF. A stable motor stereotype considerably restricts motor readjustments. The motor variability only increases if FTF are again included in the motor programme by short-term exercise bouts. If cycling training is combined with training to augment explosive power or to maintain and enhance strength, the STF will hypertrophy, increasing cross-sectional area to about 7000–8000 μm^2. Endurance training improves the blood supply of the muscles, because capillarization is increased.

ENERGETIC BASIS OF PERFORMANCE

The glycogen stores in the muscles and liver are only sufficient for intensive efforts lasting 90–120 min. In long-term endurance III exercise, additional food and fluid intake is necessary during exercise. After 1 h, an intake of 40–50 g carbohydrate is needed.

Endurance training increases the triacylglycerol (TG) content of the muscles in road cyclists. A TG content of 100–350 g serves as a stable fat reserve. Long-term endurance-trained athletes store more fat in the STF, in droplets located near the mitochondria (Hoppeler 1986). After 3 days of prolonged cycling exercise (4.5 h·day^{-1}), the TG content of the muscles declines significantly (Brouns *et al.* 1989). About 50% of the FFA oxidized during exercise are derived from local energy stores (Paul & Holmes 1975). During prolonged exercise, FFA from adipose tissue may account for up to 60% of total energy

Table 58.7 Urea, free fatty acids (FFA) and betahydroxybutyrate (BHB) after cycling competitions.

Distance (km)	No. of cyclists	Speed (km·h^{-1})	Urea (mmol·l^{-1})	FFA (mmol·l^{-1})	BHB (μmol·l^{-1})
40*	12	40	7.0 ± 2.2	0.70 ± 0.12	50 ± 20
100	12	37	7.8 ± 1.3	1.00 ± 0.25	210 ± 30
210	6	32	9.8 ± 2.0	1.25 ± 0.29	450 ± 80
300	6	27	8.8 ± 1.4	1.50 ± 0.30	—
540	9	20	11.0 ± 3.0	1.72 ± 0.60	640 ± 520

*Time trial.

needs (Hultman & Sjöholm 1983). Fat metabolism spares muscle glycogen.

In cycling training lasting several hours, the availability of carbohydrates is always limited. At first the muscle breaks down amino acids for hepatic gluconeogenesis (Wahren *et al.* 1971). Knowing that 1 g of amino acid yields an average of 0.65 g of glucose (Poortmans 1988), protein catabolism could account for more than 10% of energy requirements during prolonged exercise, when muscle glycogen is low (Lemon & Mullin 1980). A serum urea concentration of about 7 mmol·l^{-1} reveals elevated protein catabolism. The longer the duration of exercise, the greater the increase in serum urea (Table 58.7). The concentration of ketone bodies also rises, because the decreased availability of carbohydrate augments fat metabolism (see Table 58.7).

THE CARDIOVASCULAR SYSTEM

In cycling exercise of several hours' duration, the heart rate lies between 140 and 170 beats·min^{-1}. The increase in core temperature caused by the active muscles is of great importance with regard to the increase in heart rate. Due to increasing dehydration, the transport of heat to the body surface is impeded. During dehydration, the blood volume is reduced proportionally less than the loss of body water. The wind protects the body from overheating during cycling. With increasing muscle fatigue, the heart rate rises further. In long-term endurance exercise, only about 70% of $\dot{V}O_{2max}$ is utilized. This means, in road cycling, that an athlete with a body mass of 72 kg and a $\dot{V}O_{2max}$ of 78 ml·kg^{-1}·min^{-1} will

utilize approximately 54 ml oxygen·kg^{-1}·min^{-1} at a speed of 37 km·h^{-1}.

Assessment of functional capacity

Laboratory tests

The most important device for laboratory testing of a cyclist is the cycle ergometer. In most laboratories, the test exercise starts at a power output between 90 and 120 W. It is then increased by steps of 30–50 W. Individual steps may last for 2–5 min. One test widely used in Germany is described in Fig. 58.7; it may be performed as an incremental test. Important data recorded during the test include heart rate, oxygen intake, pulmonary ventilation and blood lactate concentration.

Significant parameters for the assessment of performance capacity include the $\dot{V}O_{2max}$, the work rate at a lactate concentration of 2 mmol·l^{-1} and the percentage of $\dot{V}O_{2max}$ developed at a lactate concentration of 2 mmol·l^{-1}.

MAXIMAL OXYGEN INTAKE

Élite cyclists achieve a $\dot{V}O_{2max}$ of 75–80 ml·kg^{-1}·min^{-1}, but several years of performance-oriented training are necessary to achieve such high values. A hereditary predisposition to excellence in endurance-based sports also has considerable influence. Depending on the content of the training programme, the $\dot{V}O_{2max}$ may vary by 8–12 ml·kg^{-1}·min^{-1} over the training year. Only in an ideal case does a cyclist achieve his or her individual

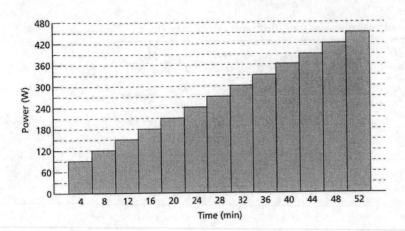

Fig. 58.7 An incremental ergometer test for cyclists.

best $\dot{V}_{O_{2max}}$ value at the time of a world championship. If the proportion of intensive training at the aerobic–anaerobic transition is increased, the $\dot{V}_{O_{2max}}$ will drop again (Fig. 58.8).

One reliable indicator is the power output (W) that can be sustained at a lactate concentration of $2\,mmol\cdot l^{-1}$ (PL2). Former calculations, based on concentrations of 3 or $4\,mmol\cdot l^{-1}$ (PL3 or PL4), are too high for road cycling. The determination of PL2 allows a better differentiation of aerobic power than the use of $\dot{V}_{O_{2max}}$ alone (Neumann & Schüler 1994). The PL2 is representative of the economy in endurance or strength-endurance training. With an increase in aerobic capacity, the lactate–performance graph (aerobic–anaerobic threshold) shifts to the right (Fig. 58.9).

Determination of the maximum lactate concentration at the end of effort gives information on the ability to mobilize anaerobic metabolism.

Although track cyclists reach blood lactate values of 10–$14\,mmol\cdot l^{-1}$ in laboratory tests, road cyclists reach values of only 6–$10\,mmol\cdot l^{-1}$ lactate. In road cyclists, training reduces the level of anaerobic enzymes (see Table 58.6).

The endurance training of cyclists is performed at about 70–80% of $\dot{V}_{O_{2max}}$, or a blood lactate concentration of less than $2\,mmol\cdot l^{-1}$.

Field tests

An incremental test may be performed under field conditions. Distances may vary between 3 and 5 km.

The velocities set may increase from 70%, 80%, 85% and 90% up to 100% of individual maximal performance. Between these steps a break of 2 min is required to measure the blood lactate concentration. Lactate is measured 1 min after each bout of effort. As in all progressive tests, four stages are considered a minimum, and five stages are a desirable optimum.

FOLLOW-UP DURING THE TRAINING PROCESS

To evaluate the optimal intensity and volume of exercise, fitness level and the degree of recovery, such parameters as heart rate, lactate, serum urea and creatine kinase (CK) are suggested.

TRAINING INTENSITY

Depending on the type of event, adaptation to cycling is facilitated by performing training in a combination of aerobic, aerobic–anaerobic and anaerobic metabolic states. The data necessary to control the intensity of exercise are listed in Table 58.8. The heart rate, in particular, is an appropriate parameter for individual differentiation of intensity during aerobic exercise (lactate $<2\,mmol\cdot l^{-1}$). The dominant part of training is performed at the level of basic endurance (see Table 58.8); 70–80% of training (for professionals $30\,000$–$35\,000\,km\cdot year^{-1}$) is performed at this aerobic level.

The heart rate is a reliable parameter to control

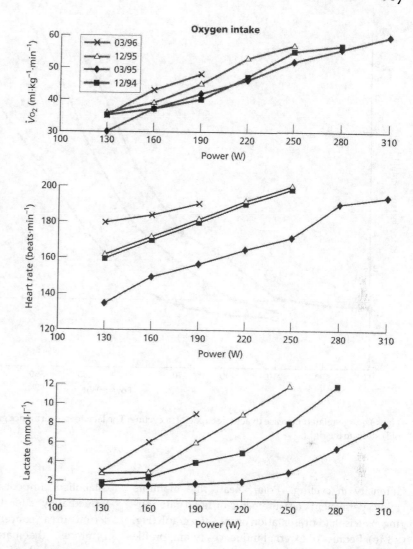

Fig. 58.8 Longitudinal study of a female cyclist showing $\dot{V}O_2$, heart rate and performance at the aerobic–anaerobic transition.

Table 58.8 Follow-up of élite cyclists during the training process.

	Basic endurance	Basic endurance and intensity	Intensity	Short-term endurance intervals
Distance	100–250 km	60–100 km	30–50 km	200–1000 m
Speed (km·h⁻¹)	27–32	33–37	37–40	42–50
Pedal frequency (pedalling rate·min⁻¹)	80–100	95–105	100–120	110–120
Energy exchange *Measurement of actual adaptation in field tests*	Aerobic	Aerobic–anaerobic	Aerobic–anaerobic	Alactacid–lactacid
Lactate (mmol·l⁻¹)	1–2	2–3	4–7	>7
Heart rate (beats·min⁻¹)	110–140	130–160	150–190	180–200

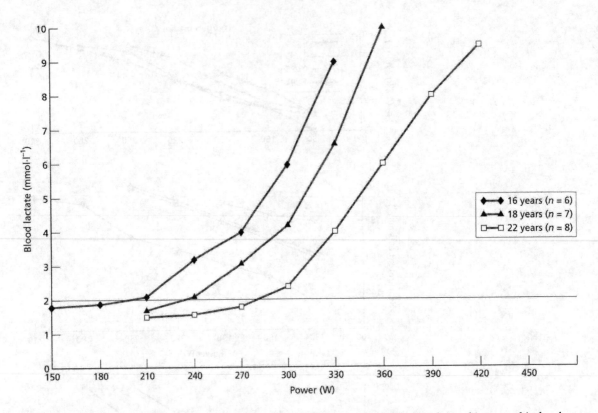

Fig. 58.9 Age-related increase in aerobic capacity in cycling. The lactate–performance graph (aerobic–anaerobic threshold) shifts to the right.

intensity in cycling. 'Polar' heart rate monitors allow permanent measurements of heart rate during exercise and presentation of data as a graph (Fig. 58.10). Because of external influences (wind, profile of the road course, road surface) speed gives an uncertain indication of the intensity of exertion during cycling.

PROTEIN CATABOLISM

Measurements of serum urea can indicate an elevated protein metabolism. Depending on the individual's fitness level and the duration of exercise, the concentration of serum urea is increased at subsequent rest. Training may induce resting serum urea levels of 6–8 mmol·l^{-1}. If the resting serum urea reaches 10 mmol·l^{-1} on two successive days, there is a danger the athlete is overreaching and the training volume must be reduced. A high rate of protein

catabolism impedes the process of adaptation. Immediately after long-term endurance exercise, serum urea concentration may rise by up to 15 mmol·l^{-1} (haematocrit 0.43); see Table 58.7. A recovery period of approximately 15 h causes a decline in serum urea of 2–3 mmol·l^{-1}. A good method to evaluate the intensity of cycling, especially the effect of heavy training, is to measure the activity of CK. Heavy-interval training can push CK levels to 3–10 μmol·s^{-1}·l^{-1}. If the level of CK exeeds 10–15 μmol·s^{-1}·l^{-1}, the rate of exercise must be reduced or the recovery period prolonged.

THE INFLUENCE OF RECOVERY

Replenishment of energy stores, especially the glycogen in muscle and liver, is of central significance in cycling training and competition. In prolonged daily training on the road (>180 km) or in

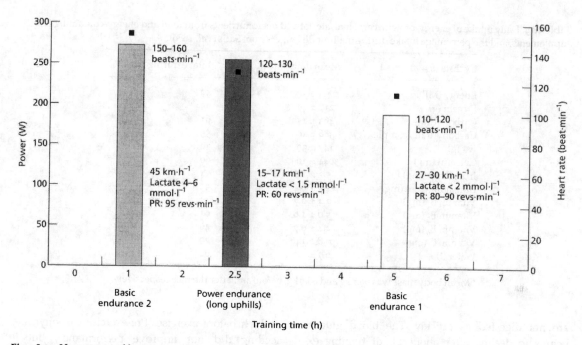

Fig. 58.10 Heart rate and lactate in endurance training of cycling capability. PR, pedalling rate.

tour races, the glycogen stores cannot be replenished within 24 h if the athlete remains on a normal diet. For cyclists the percentage of carbohydrate in their food should be 55–60%, the share of fat 20–25% and of protein 15–18%. Chronic consumption of a high carbohydrate diet facilitates a greater training capacity, whereas chronic consumption of a moderate carbohydrate diet may produce suboptimal cycling training and performance capabilities (Costill & Miller 1980; Costill *et al.* 1981; Sherman *et al.* 1989, 1991; Coyle 1991; Wright *et al.* 1991; Lugo *et al.* 1993).

It is reasonable for cyclists to consume a diet that contains 8–10 g carbohydrate·kg body mass^{-1}·day^{-1}.

Because liver stores are limited (100–120 g), the blood glucose concentration will decline, and fatigue will occur without carbohydrate supplementation.

Significant glycogen sparing, as well as supercompensation within 24 h of recovery, was observed after consumption of a high maltodextrin/low fructose beverage (Brouns *et al.* 1989). If catabolism predominates, body mass will decrease. Saris *et al.* (1989) found a beverage energy intake of 25–

26 MJ·day^{-1} (5900–6200 kcal·day^{-1}) during the Tour de France. The highest energy intake was 32.7 MJ·day^{-1} (7780 kcal·day^{-1}). The energy intake while cycling was 40–50% of total daily intake during the event.

If environmental temperatures are high, the athlete's fluid requirements may reach 10 l·day^{-1}, with 6 l being ingested during a race. Road cycling has high requirements of both energy and fluid compared with other sports. If the energy consumption during normal training does not surpass 20 MJ·day^{-1} (about 4800 kcal·day^{-1}), recovery may be ensured by consumption of a high carbohydrate diet. Any higher energy consumption requires an additional intake of glucose concentrates, glucose fluids, vitamins and minerals (Table 58.9). One-third of carbohydrate requirements may be met from carbohydrate-rich liquids. The polysaccharides prevent stomach disorders or diarrhoea during exercise. The amount of carbohydrate needed during cycling is 40–60 g of glucose for each hour of exercise. In practice, cyclists consume both liquid and solid forms of carbohydrate during cycling. Carbohydrates that are ingested without fluid

Table 58.9 Daily intake of energy, protein, carbohydrate, fat and micronutrients from food and energy-containing food supplements, and the percentage intake during the Tour de France (from Saris *et al.* 1989).

Cyclists ($n = 5$)	Mean daily intake ($\pm$ s.d.)	Intake during race (%)
Energy (MJ)	24.3 ± 5.3	49
Protein (g)	217 ± 47	35
Carbohydrate, simple (g)	463 ± 159	61
Carbohydrate, complex (g)	386 ± 100	55
Fat (g)	147 ± 39	39
Calcium (mg)	3044 ± 1000	60
Iron, haem (mg)	5.3 ± 1.6	1
Iron, non-haem (mg)	24.9 ± 9.4	55
Vitamin B_1 (mg)	2.4 ± 0.7	44
Vitamin B_2 (mg)	5.0 ± 1.6	61
Vitamin B_6 (mg)	2.4 ± 0.7	46
Vitamin C (mg)	158 ± 146	29
Water (l)	6.7 ± 2.0	61

*Mean body mass was 69.2 kg and 68.9 kg, before and after the race respectively.

are not digested as quickly. The blood glucose begins to decline after about 2 h of training exercise. Carbohydrate ingestion must begin before there is a significant decline in the body's carbohydrate reserves. If only 20 g of glucose·h^{-1} are taken, a marked gluconeogenesis and ketogenesis may develop and hypoglycaemic reactions may occur.

The majority of published studies have reported that pre-exercise carbohydrate feeding improves cycling performance capabilities (Gleeson *et al.* 1986; Neuffer *et al.* 1987; Sherman *et al.* 1989, 1991; Wright *et al.* 1991). Between 2 and 5 g of liquid carbohydrate·kg body mass^{-1} was consumed between 1 and 4 h before exercise. Pre-exercise carbohydrate feeding did not improve performance, but it increased the rate of carbohydrate oxidation and impeded the mobilization of FFA (Essig *et al.* 1980; Sasaki *et al.* 1987; Sherman 1991).

In the postexercise recovery phase, carbohydrate ingestion (1–1.5 g·kg body mass^{-1}) stimulates glycogen synthesis. When carbohydrate is consumed immediately after exercise and at 2-h intervals thereafter, the rate of muscle glycogen synthesis is 6 mmol·kg^{-1}·h^{-1} (Blom *et al.* 1987; Ivy *et al.* 1988a, b; Reed *et al.* 1989). Carbohydrate ingestion should begin immediately after glycogen-depleting endurance exercise.

References

Åstrand, P.-O. & Rodahl, K. (1986) *Textbook of Work Physiology*. McGraw-Hill Book Company, New York.

Blom, P.C.S., Hostmark, A.T., Vaage, O., Kardel, K.R. & Maehlum, S. (1987) Effect of different postexercise sugar diets on the rate of glycogen synthesis. *Medicine and Science in Sports and Exercise* **19**, 491–496.

Brouns, F., Saris, W.H.M., Beckes, E. *et al.* (1989) Metabolic changes induced by sustained exhaustive cycling and diet manipulation. *International Journal of Sports Medicine* **10**, S49–S62.

Costill, D.L. & Miller, J.M. (1980) Nutrition for endurance sport: carbohydrate and fluid balance. *International Journal of Sports Medicine* **1**, 2–14.

Costill, D.L., Sherman, W.M., Fink, W.J., Maresh, C., Whitten, M. & Miller, J.M. (1981) The role of dietary carbohydrates in muscle glycogen resynthesis after strenuous running. *American Journal of Clinical Nutrition* **34**, 1831–1836.

Coyle, E.F. (1991) Timing and method of increased carbohydrate intake to cope with heavy training, competition and recovery. *Journal of Sports Science* **9** (Suppl.), 29–52.

Essig, D., Costill, D.L. & van Handel, P.J. (1980) Effects of caffeine ingestion on utilization of muscle glycogen and lipid during leg ergometer cycling. *International Journal of Sports Medicine* **1**, 86–90.

Gleeson, M., Maughan, R.J. & Greenhaff, P.L. (1986) Comparison of the effects of preexercise feedings of glucose, glycerol and placebo on endurance and fuel homeostasis in man. *European Journal of Applied Physiology* **55**, 65–76.

Hagberg, J. & McCole, S. (1996) Energy expenditure during cycling. In: Burke, E.R. (ed.) *High-Tech Cycling*, pp. 167–184. Human Kinetics, Champaign, IL.

Hoppeler, H. (1986) Exercise-induced

ultrastructural changes in skeletal muscle. *International Journal of Sports Medicine* 7, 187–204.

Hultman, E. & Sjöholm, H. (1983) Substrate availability. In: Knuttgen, H., Vogel, J.A. & Poortmans, J. (eds) *Biochemistry of Exercise*, pp. 63–75. Human Kinetics, Champaign, IL.

Ivy, J.L., Katz, A.L., Cutler, C.L., Sherman, W.M. & Coyle, E.F. (1988a) Muscle glycogen synthesis after exercise: effect to time of carbohydrate ingestion. *Journal of Applied Physiology* 64, 1480–1485.

Ivy, J.L., Lee, M.C., Brozinick, J.T. & Reed, M.J. (1988b) Muscle glycogen storage after different amounts of carbohydrate ingestion. *Journal of Applied Physiology* 65, 2018–2023.

Lemon, P.W.R. & Mullin, J. (1980) Effect of initial muscle glycogen levels on protein catabolism during exercise. *Journal of Applied Physiology* 48, 624–629.

Lugo, M.J., Sherman, W.M., Wimer, G.S. & Garleb, K. (1993) Metabolic responses when different forms of carbohydrate energy are consumed during cycling. *International Journal of Sport Nutrition* 3, 398–407.

Medbø, J.I. & Tabata, I. (1989) Relative importance of aerobic and anaerobic energy release during short-lasting exhaustive bicycle exercise. *Journal of Applied Physiology* 67, 1881–1886.

Neuffer, P.D., Costill, D.L., Flynn, M.G., Kirwan, J.P., Mitchell, J.B. & Houmard, J. (1987) Improvements in exercise performance: effects of carbohydrate feedings and diet. *Journal of Applied Physiology* 63, 983–988.

Neumann, G. & Schüler, K.-P. (1994) *Sportmedizinische Funktionsdiagnostik.* J.A. Barth, Leipzig.

Neumann, G., Pfützner, A. & Berbalk, A. (1998) *Optimales Ausdauertraining.* Meyer & Meyer, Aachen.

Paul, P. & Holmes, W.L. (1975) Free fatty acid and glucose metabolism during increased energy expenditure and after training. *Medicine and Science in Sports and Exercise* 7, 176–184.

Poortmans, J.R. (1988) Protein metabolism. In: Poortmans, J.R. (ed.) *Principles of Exercise Biochemistry.* Med Sport Sci, Vol. 27, pp. 164–193. Karger, Basel.

Reed, M.J., Brozinick, J.T., Lee, M.C. & Ivy, J.L. (1989) Muscle glycogen storage post-exercise: Effect of mode of carbohydrate administration. *Journal of Applied Physiology* 66, 720–726.

Sahlin, K. (1986) Metabolic changes limiting muscle performance. In: Saltin, B. (ed) *Biochemistry of Exercise VI*, pp. 232–343. Human Kinetics, Champaign, IL.

Saris, W.H.M., van Erp-Baart, M.A., Brouns, F., Westerterp, K.R. & ten Hoor, F. (1989) Study on food uptake and energy expenditure during extreme sustained exercise: the Tour de France. *International Journal of Sports Medicine* 10, S25–S31.

Sasaki, H., Maeda, J., Usui, S. & Ishiko, T. (1987) Effect of sucrose and caffeine
ingestion on performance of prolonged strenuous running. *International Journal of Sports Medicine* 8, 261–265.

Sherman, W.M. (1991) Carbohydrate feedings before and after exercise. In: Lamb, D.R. & Williams, M.H. (eds) *Perspectives in Exercise Science and Sports Medicine: Ergogenics*, pp. 1–34. Brown & Benchmark, Indianapolis.

Sherman, W.M., Brodowicz, G., Wright, D.A., Allen, W.K., Simonsen, J.C. & Dernbach, A.R. (1989) Effects of 4-hour preexercise carbohydrate feedings on cycling performance. *Medicine and Science in Sports and Exercise* 21, 598–604.

Sherman, W.M., Peden, M.C. & Wright, D.A. (1991) Carbohydrate feedings 1 hour before exercise improve cycling performance. *American Journal of Clinical Nutrition* 54, 866–870.

Swain, D.P. (1994) The influence of body mass in endurance bicycling. *Medicine and Science in Sports and Exercise* 26, 58–63.

Wahren, J., Ahlborg, G., Fehling, P. & Jorfeld, L. (1971) Glucose metabolism during exercise in man. In: Pernow, B. & Saltin, B. (eds) *Muscle Metabolism during Exercise*, pp. 179–203. Plenum Press, New York.

Wright, D.A., Sherman, W.M. & Dernbach, A.R. (1991) Carbohydrate feedings before, during, or in combination improve endurance performance. *Journal of Applied Physiology* 71, 1082–1088.

Chapter 59

The Triathlon

GORDON G. SLEIVERT

A triathlon event requires the uninterrupted and sequential completion of swimming, cycling and running events. There are two major classifications of triathlon: the 'Olympic' distance and the ultra-endurance or 'Ironman' triathlon. The Olympic triathlon usually comprises a 1.5-km swim, a 40-km cycle and 10-km run, whereas the Ironman triathlon requires competitors to complete nearly 4 km of swimming, about 180 km of cycling and (usually) 42.2 km of running (a full marathon). Completion times are generally in the range of 2–4 h for the short-course event and 8–14 h for ultra-endurance triathlons. This chapter reviews the demands of training and competition for these two classifications of triathlon and discusses the factors that impact on or are related to triathlon performance.

Demands of the triathlon

The demands of the triathlon differ from other endurance events, because of the sequential performance of three different modes of exercise, using different muscle groups and differing amounts of muscle mass in different postures and markedly different environments. Although each phase of the triathlon relies on aerobic rephosphorylation of ATP, the percentage of $\dot{V}O_{2max}$ that can be sustained and the challenge of maintaining cardiovascular and thermoregulatory homeostasis while exercising at a maximal sustainable pace differ between exercise modes. These differences are accentuated in the triathlon, because of the sequential nature of the swim–cycle–run event.

Thermoregulation

Kreider et al. (1988a) were the first to investigate the thermoregulatory responses to triathlon competition. They studied nine male triathletes who performed a simulated short-course triathlon, comparing their physiological responses to a control cycle and run. The water temperature was maintained at 23°C, and the air temperature during the cycling and run segments was maintained at 29°C. Postswim, the core temperature averaged 37.8°C; values continued to rise throughout the triathlon cycle, and rose more steeply during the run, to average approximately 39.6°C by the end of the triathlon. In the light of this final core temperature, it is not surprising that five out of the nine triathletes who were studied experienced heat complications. It therefore appears that thermoregulatory homeostasis can be a major challenge for competing triathletes. The run phase probably provides the biggest heat challenge, since a large muscle mass is actively producing heat, and the convective and conductive cooling, available in cycling and swimming, respectively, are much reduced.

Although water is an excellent heat sink, many triathletes wear a wetsuit to increase their buoyancy and decrease hydrodynamic drag (Toussaint et al. 1989). This may improve swimming performance (Parsons & Day 1986), but it also has the potential to impair performance in subsequent triathlon segments, since the insulative effects of neoprene potentiate exercise-induced hyperthermia. Several studies have examined whether a wetsuit adversely affects thermal homeostasis. Trappe et al. (1995)

studied the thermoregulatory responses of nine competitive triathletes and/or swimmers who were swimming at water temperatures of 20.1, 22.7 and 25.6°C with and without full-body 3–4-mm-thick wetsuits. The subjects swam for 30 min, had a 3-min transition and then rode a cycle ergometer for 15 min. There were large individual variations in the core temperature response. On average, the core temperature rose similarly whether or not a wetsuit was worn at all three water temperatures. The wetsuit maintained skin temperature of the trunk 3–4°C warmer than when the subjects were in the swimsuit condition, and at the two cooler water temperatures several swimmers demonstrated a drop in core temperature when wearing only a swimsuit. This drop was attenuated or prevented when wearing a wetsuit. At the warm water temperature of 25.6°C, the wetsuit did not cause greater hyperthermia than a swimsuit alone. In fact, the core temperature rose to a greater extent in the swimsuit versus the wetsuit condition. This is a surprising finding; the researchers suggested that it could be due to a large peripheral vasoconstrictor response in the swimsuit condition, decreasing the core to skin temperature gradient to a greater extent than when a wetsuit was worn. This would impair heat loss and accelerate the rise in core temperature.

Cycling in an air temperature of 21°C after the swim caused a transient drop in body temperature; this is probably explained by warm blood being circulated through a cold periphery (Webb 1986). Thus, the swim essentially acts as a precooling manoeuvre, and precooling has previously been shown to enhance endurance performance (Lee & Haymes 1995; Booth *et al.* 1997). It is possible that the thermoregulatory advantages of cooling down during a swim confer transient benefits later, in the other segments of the triathlon, and the swimsuit condition might achieve a greater precooling effect. Alternatively, the performance gains from using a wetsuit may be more worthwhile, since the swimmers covered a 188-m greater distance (a 9.8% improvement) and also had longer stroke distances when wearing a wetsuit versus a swimsuit.

Another recent study by the same research group has more completely examined the influence of a wetsuit on body heat storage during the triathlon.

Kerr *et al.* (1998) studied five well-trained male triathletes who randomly completed two simulated triathlons (comprising a 30-min swim, a 40-km cycle ride and a 10-km run). The only difference between the two triathlons was that in one subjects wore a 3–4-mm-thick neoprene wetsuit that covered the torso and legs during the swim. The water temperature averaged 25.4°C; environmental conditions for the cycle and run were hot, and maintained at 31.9 ± 0.1°C and 65% relative humidity. Although the skin temperature was warmer during the wetsuit swim, by 15 min into the cycling segment there were no differences between the swimsuit and wetsuit conditions in skin, core or mean body temperatures. Therefore, even in relatively warm water and a hot air environment, a wetsuit worn during swimming does not compromise thermoregulation in the latter phases of the triathlon. However, the swims undertaken in this study were controlled to occur at identical paces and the metabolic cost of swimming in the wetsuit appeared to be less than when wearing the swimsuit. It is likely that, in actual competition, the triathlete would swim faster in the wetsuit condition and therefore more heat would be stored. This distinction could be particularly relevant for triathletes with higher body fat percentages who do not dissipate heat easily. Individual differences in body composition must be considered when deciding whether to wear a wetsuit or not.

Dehydration

Kreider *et al.* (1988a) monitored dehydration and fluid consumption during a simulated triathlon. Subjects ingested 56% and 72% more water during triathlon cycling and running, respectively, than in control runs or cycles. Despite the greater water intake, the triathletes had dehydrated by 3% of body mass at the end of the triathlon and a half of this dehydration occurred during the running segment of the event. Consequently, stroke volume decreased and heart rate increased during both the cycling and running segments to a significantly greater extent than was seen during control cycling and running. However, the cardiac output was significantly lower than control only during the triathlon cycle. This could reflect the lower mean cycling power output that occurred in the triathlon. Similar information was reported by Farber *et al.* (1991), who studied an Ironman triathlon event over 2 years; they observed that dehydration occurred progressively throughout the event, despite allowing competitors free access to food and fluid. The swim occurred in a water temperature of 21–22°C and dehydration averaged 0.9% of pretriathlon body mass by the end of the 2.4-mile (3.85-km) swim. The land temperature was between 19 and 26°C and the relative humidity was between 50 and 96%. Triathletes dehydrated by a further 0.6% of body mass over the 112-mile (180-km) cycling segment and by yet another 2.1% of body mass during the 42.5-km run. By the end of the triathlon, the competitors had lost a total of 3.6% of body mass. These patterns of dehydration reflect the difficulty of hydrating the competitor adequately during all phases of the event. Little hydration probably occurs during the swim, whereas cycling may be the easiest phase in which to consume fluid. The rate of dehydration was greatest during the running phase, reflecting the whole-body nature of this exercise mode driving sweat rate; moreover, triathletes perhaps find it difficult to consume adequate volumes of fluid when running, due to the gastric discomfort that may be associated with impact exercise and a full stomach. When triathlons are held in hotter climates, the extent of dehydration would probably be markedly greater and the consequences of dehydration more severe.

Conversely, there have been documented cases of triathletes consuming too much fluid during a race, and becoming hyponatraemic (see Chapter 40). Most recently, Speedy *et al.* (1999) reported the results of a large prospective study that examined changes in body mass and plasma sodium concentrations in those completing the Ironman race. They found that 18% (58) of race finishers were clinically hyponatraemic (serum sodium < 135 mmol·l^{-1}), but only 31% were symptomatic and sought medical care. A small percentage of the hyponatraemic athletes had severe hyponatraemia (serum sodium < 130 mmol·l^{-1}). Three-quarters of these individuals either maintained or gained body mass over the triathlon, suggesting that a primary aetiology of hyponatraemia may be an excessive fluid consump-

tion, rather than a large salt loss through excessive sweating. This prospective study also reported that female triathletes were at a higher risk of hyponatraemia, possibly because they sweat less and are more likely to maintain body mass during the race.

Acute effects of sequential exercise

The sequential completion of swimming, cycling and running stages presents the triathlete with unique demands when compared to endurance specialist sports. For example, many triathletes experience difficulty in the early stages of the run after the cycle–run transition, but the reason for this is unknown. Quigley and Richards (1996) studied 11 competitive biathletes and triathletes in order to determine whether previous exercise disrupted running mechanics; they found that running mechanics were unchanged after either previous running or cycling. This finding was replicated in a more recent study of seven male competitive triathletes who performed a 10-km run either with or without 40 km of previous cycling (Hue *et al.* 1998). One study has, however, reported greater forward trunk lean and decreases in stride length (7%) after previous swimming and cycling. These biomechanical changes were attributed primarily to local muscle fatigue, but no single kinematic variable could account fully for the decrease in running economy observed in the triathlon run compared to the control run (Hausswirth *et al.* 1997). These studies suggest therefore that the feeling of awkwardness experienced in running immediately after cycling may be due to changes in a combination of motor control, physiological and biomechanical factors. For example, triathletes entrain their breathing rate to the rhythm of exercise, and this has a small effect on ventilatory efficiency (Bonsignore *et al.* 1998). Since cycling cadence generally occurs at 1.5–2.0 Hz and running cadence is slower at 1.0–1.25 Hz, the entrainment of breathing and ventilatory efficiency may be disrupted in the early stages of a run after cycling. It is possible that with regular transition training (BRICK training), which involves two or more modes within a single session, triathletes may develop strategies to entrain their breathing quickly with stride rate, and ventilatory efficiency may be improved. This remains to be confirmed.

Economy may change throughout the course of an event. Kreider *et al.* (1988a) observed that compared to a control run, triathlon running at an identical pace was performed at a higher core temperature, with a significantly lower stroke volume and mean arterial pressure. The triathlon run required a significantly larger oxygen consumption, ventilation and heart rate, a finding replicated in several recent studies (Guezennec *et al.* 1996; Hausswirth *et al.* 1996, 1997; Hue *et al.* 1998). Besides biomechanical factors, other changes known to occur over the course of a triathlon have been suggested as decreasing the economy of running after previous cycling and swimming. Possibilities include progressive muscle damage, glycogen depletion and a resulting increase in fat metabolism, and thermal stress and dehydration leading to increased cardiac and ventilatory work (Kreider *et al.* 1988a; Farber *et al.* 1991; Guezennec *et al.* 1996; Hausswirth *et al.* 1996, 1997). With these problems in mind, it has been suggested that detrimental changes in economy can be minimized by proper pacing strategies, utilizing a progressively increasing intensity of effort as the race progresses (Kreider *et al.* 1988b; O'Toole & Douglas 1995).

De Vito *et al.* (1995) examined the impact of residual fatigue from one exercise mode on the performance of another by measuring the treadmill $\dot{V}O_{2max}$ in a rested state and after completion of the first two segments of a triathlon (1.5 km swimming, 32 km cycling). They found that the $\dot{V}O_{2max}$ decreased from 69 to 64 ml·kg^{-1}·min^{-1}. The oxygen consumption at the running ventilatory threshold (V_T) was also a smaller percentage of $\dot{V}O_{2max}$ (74.3 versus 84.6%) after completion of the partial triathlon, indicating that the ability to sustain a high percentage of $\dot{V}O_{2max}$ in running is impaired after completing the swimming and cycling sections of a triathlon. In addition, the heart rate at the V_T was lower after previous exercise, which has implications for setting training and competition pace. Regular exposure to sequential exercise in training as a means of simulating the physiological responses experienced in a triathlon may be important in this respect.

Triathlon training

The triathlete must train regularly in the three exercise modes of swimming, cycling and running. The reported volumes and intensities of training in each mode are diverse, depending upon the competitive level of the triathlete and the type of triathlon for which training is being undertaken.

Training and performance

An early study of 65 Olympic distance triathletes showed strong systematic relationships between training practices and triathlon performance (Zinkgraf *et al.* 1986). These triathletes averaged 4–5 workouts in each exercise mode per week, and the specificity of their training was evident, since the training distance for each exercise mode was correlated most strongly with performance in the matching phase of the triathlon. Additionally, the fastest triathletes of the sample studied had completed the greatest number of triathlons, trained for more months prior to the race, had longer single workouts and engaged in higher training volumes.

O'Toole (1989) was one of the first to report on training practices of Ironman triathletes. She reported data on 323 Hawaii Ironman participants. In general, these triathletes prepared themselves seriously for at least 8 months before the event, training approximately 21 h·week^{-1}. Swim training took place on average 3.5 h·week^{-1}, bicycle training 12 h·week^{-1} and run training about 6 h·week^{-1}. Swimming was spread over 3–5 days·week^{-1}, cycling 4–5 days·week^{-1} and running 4–6 days·week^{-1}. This necessitated multiple workouts each day. Approximately 46% of the swim training was interval based, whereas 80% of the cycle and run training was continuous in nature. When relating training practices to finishing times, it appeared that bicycle and run training volumes were most important to a fast finish time, and that 11 km of swimming, 320 km of cycling and 65 km of running per week were the minimum volumes required for any triathlete to finish in a faster time than 10.5 h.

Hendy and Boyer (1995) used a questionnaire to collect information on training behaviour from 203

Ironman competitors and 421 competitors in an Olympic distance triathlon. As previously reported, the training behaviour was diverse, but those competitors training for the Ironman had greater average training volumes (10, 290, 57 km·week^{-1}) than the Olympic distance competitors (8, 198, 48 km·week^{-1}) in swimming, cycling and running, respectively. In contrast to the previous studies that had observed training volume to be most strongly correlated with triathlon performance, Hendy and Boyer (1995) reported that training intensity in the same exercise mode was the best predictor of swimming and running performance for both Olympic and Ironman triathlons, reinforcing the importance of training specificity. Cycling performance over either the Olympic or the Ironman distance could not be predicted very well from training data. The researchers suggested that this could be because cycling is the longest of the triathlon stages, and it offers a longer time for external factors to influence performance. Alternatively, the quality of the bicycle can have a large impact on performance, and now that drafting is allowed during the cycling stage, this will further attenuate the strength of any relationship between cycling training and triathlon cycle performance.

Training and injuries

It seems logical that with the high training volumes reported for triathletes, susceptibility to overuse injuries would be high. O'Toole et al. (1989b) reported training and injury statistics in a group of 95 Ironman competitors. There was wide variability in triathlete training practices, but on average the sample trained 210, 684 and 350 min·week^{-1} in swimming, cycling and running, respectively, spending 3–5 days·week^{-1} in each exercise mode. A massive 90.3% of these competitors had had at least one injury during the previous year. The most common site of injury was the back, although many triathletes (72%) reported multiple injury sites that included the lower limbs. Surprisingly, no training variables were related to injury.

Ireland and Micheli (1987) reported on the training practices and injury patterns of 168 recreational and competitive triathletes who had previously completed a mean of six triathlons. These triathletes trained an average of 17 h·week^{-1}, but the range was large (5–60 h). Similar to the findings of O'Toole (1989), most training time was spent on the bicycle (7.5 h·week^{-1}, 44%), followed by running (6 h·week^{-1}, 35%) and swimming (3.5 h·week^{-1}, 21%). At least 66% of the triathletes studied had sustained at least one injury; the lower extremity was involved in 85% of these injuries, most of which were due to overuse. Running training accounted for the bulk of the overuse injuries (78%), but no training variables were related to either the occurrence or the number of injuries. A more recent study of 155 British triathletes whose normal competitive distance ranged from a sprint to a full Ironman event reported relatively low training volumes for sprint triathletes of 7 h·week^{-1}, the corresponding figures for an 8-week period being 10 h·week^{-1} for half and full Ironman competitors (Korkia et al. 1994). For both the sprint and the ultra-endurance competitors, about half the training time was spent cycling, with the remaining training time split equally between running and swimming. Thirty-seven per cent of the sample sustained an injury over the 8 weeks of training that were studied, with 41% of injuries being diagnosed as overuse and 86% of the injuries occurring in the lower limb. Sixty-five per cent of the injuries occurred while running. Similar to previous studies, however, there was no association between the extent of training practices and injury. Several other studies have shown weak associations between training practices and injury.

Williams et al. (1988) surveyed 332 triathletes competing in a variety of events ranging from Olympic to Ironman distance triathlons. The mean training volumes were 7, 157 and 47 km·week^{-1} in swimming, cycling and running exercise modes, respectively. Fifty per cent of this sample reported injuries, and 20% of these injuries were of sufficient severity to cause cessation of training or withdrawal from an event. The principal sites of injury were the knee (22%), lower back (17%) and foot or ankle (14%). The majority of injuries were thought to arise from run training (53%), although there was no significant correlation between the run training volume and the likelihood of injury. Significant but weak correlations were obtained between the weekly training distances in cycling and the number of injuries, and between the number of years involved in triathlons and the number of injuries. Taken together, these training variables only accounted for 4% of the variance in occurrence of injuries. Manninen and Kallinen (1996) surveyed 92 Japanese triathletes retrospectively. This sample trained on average 14.6 h·week^{-1}, spending 29, 38 and 33% of their triathlon training time in swimming, cycling and running, respectively; the majority (79%) of their training was performed at or below the anaerobic threshold. Seventy-two per cent of the triathletes sustained at least one training-related musculoskeletal injury in the previous year, with most of the injuries occurring in the lower limbs, primarily the knees. Similar to previous studies, running was the most common perceived cause of the lower limb injury. Thirty-two per cent of the triathletes surveyed had also experienced lower back pain in the previous year, and there was some indication that the average weekly training load was associated with the incidence of lower back pain. Neither cycling position nor the use of triathlon aerobars was associated with back pain, but nevertheless the authors suggested that cycling may cause most of the lower back pain in triathletes, since there was an almost significant difference in average weekly cycling time ($P = 0.065$) between those triathletes with and those free of lower back pain. This agrees with the findings of Williams et al. (1988) that a high cycling volume may relate to injury risk.

Vleck and Garbutt (1998) studied the training and injury characteristics of 12 élite, 17 developmental and 87 male British club triathletes, using a 5-year retrospective questionnaire. The élite (15.6 h) and developmental (13.1 h) triathletes trained more hours per week than the club-level triathletes (5.3 h). For example, the élite group spent 5.6, 6.3 and 3.7 h·week^{-1} swimming, cycling and running, respectively, compared to the 2.3, 4.4 and 2.4 h·week^{-1} average time that the club triathletes spent in training in the same exercise modes. Despite differences in training behaviour, the prevalence of injuries did not differ between ability groups. Between 56 and 75% of the triathletes suffered an overuse injury over the time studied, and the number of injured sites ranged from 1.9 to 2.9, with lower extremity injuries accounting for 43–48% of the total number of overuse injuries. The most common sites of injury were the knees and lower back, although multiple sites of injury were common. Additionally, each group identified run training as responsible for the greatest fraction of injuries. When the groups were combined, the number of overuse injuries sustained was significantly related to a variety of indices of training volume and intensity. Injuries in one discipline, for example running, were correlated not only with the training volume in that discipline but also with the training volume in other disciplines. As Vleck and Garbutt (1998) suggest, this may reflect simply that those with high training volumes in one mode are likely to have high training volumes in other modes, or it may indicate that the recovery interval between disciplines is an important injury risk factor.

It can be concluded from these studies that the high volume of training required to excel in the triathlon predisposes these athletes to overuse injuries. In particular, lower limb injuries appear to be related to run training volume and back injuries may be related to cycle training volume. However, the interaction effect of training in three exercise modes on the incidence of injuries is not well understood, since training variables do not generally relate strongly to injury. As first suggested by Williams et al. (1988), it may not be training volume per se that leads to injury in triathletes, but rather rapid increases in training volume. Further prospective studies of this issue are required.

Characteristics of triathletes and their relationship to performance

Physical characteristics

Élite male triathletes (O'Toole et al. 1987; Horrell 1989; Travill et al. 1994; Bunc et al. 1996; Vallier et al. 1996; Hoogeveen & Schep 1997; Vleck & Garbutt 1998) are similar in height to specialist cyclists (Burke et al. 1977; Neumann 1992; Coyle et al. 1988), but tend to be taller than specialist runners (Pollack 1977; Conley & Krahenbuhl 1980; Tittel & Wutsherk 1992) and shorter than specialist distance swimmers

(Holmér *et al.* 1974; Tittel & Wutsherk 1992; Travill *et al.* 1994) (Fig. 59.1a). There seems to be little difference in height between Ironman and Olympic triathlon competitors. Female Ironman triathletes (O'Toole *et al.* 1987) tend to be taller than their Olympic triathlete counterparts (Leake & Carter 1991; Laurenson *et al.* 1993); both groups of triathletes are taller than élite female endurance runners (Wilmore & Brown 1974; Tittel & Wutsherk 1992), but similar in height to élite cyclists (Åstrand & Rodahl 1986; Neumann 1992) and swimmers (Tittel & Wutsherk 1992; Travill *et al.* 1994) (Fig. 59.1b).

Taller triathletes may have an advantage over shorter triathletes, since longer limbs offer greater leverage. Long limbs allow a greater running stride and a longer swimming stroke, with lower stride and stroke frequencies for a given velocity. Longer stride lengths are more economical than a high stride frequency, as demonstrated by oxygen uptake and blood lactate measurements (Tittel & Wutsherk 1992). Conversely, an excessive height may be a disadvantage. Increased height is associated with an increased body surface area, and the greater the surface area, the greater resistance opposing movement of the athlete (Neumann 1992; Tittel & Wutsherk 1992). Air resistance is the major component

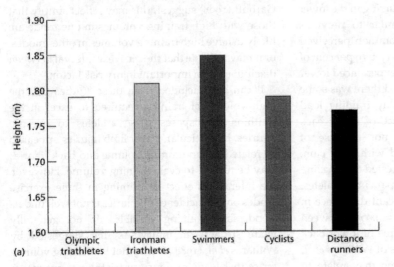

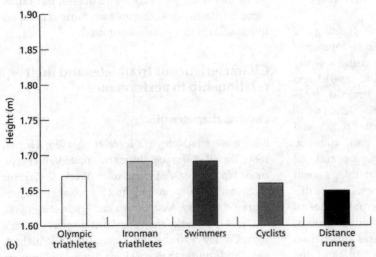

Fig. 59.1 Weighted mean height values for male (a) and female (b) élite Olympic and Ironman triathletes compared to that of élite 1500/800-m swimmers, road cyclists and distance runners. Mean height values for each population were generated by taking a mean of the means weighted against the sample size of athletes used in each study referenced in the text, using the equation: $X = \hat{A}pi\,(ni.xi)/N$ where: X is the mean of the means, $\hat{A}pi$ is the sum of sample size weighted means, ni is the sample number in each study, xi is the mean value for each study and N is the sum of ni for all studies.

of resistance to movement during level cycling (Neumann 1992; Chapter 58), and it is also a significant form of resistance during running (Åstrand & Rodahl 1986).

Élite male triathletes (O'Toole *et al.* 1987; Horrell 1989; Travill *et al.* 1994; Bunc *et al.* 1996; Vallier *et al.* 1996; Hoogeveen & Schep 1997; Vleck & Garbutt 1998) have a similar body mass to élite cyclists (Burke *et al.* 1977; Coyle *et al.* 1988; Neumann 1992), but weigh less than swimmers (Holmér *et al.* 1974; Tittel & Wutsherk 1992; Travill *et al.* 1994) and more than runners (Pollack 1977; Conley & Krahenbuhl 1980; Tittel & Wutsherk 1992) (Fig. 59.2a). Surpris-

ingly, élite ultra-endurance male triathletes have a larger body mass than their Olympic distance counterparts. Similar patterns are evident in female triathletes (Fig. 59.2b), with the élite Ironman females (O'Toole *et al.* 1987) weighing more than their Olympic triathlete counterparts (Leake & Carter 1991; Laurenson *et al.* 1993), cyclists (Åstrand & Rodahl 1986; Neumann 1992) and runners (Wilmore & Brown 1974; Tittel & Wutsherk 1992), but having similar weights to élite swimmers (Tittel & Wutsherk 1992; Travill *et al.* 1994).

The body composition may influence performance in swimming, cycling and running differen-

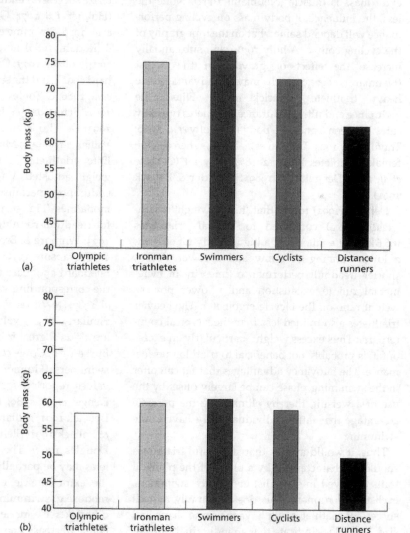

Fig. 59.2 Weighted mean mass values for male (a) and female (b) élite and average (all triathletes) endurance and ultra-endurance triathletes compared to that of élite 1500/800-m swimmers, road cyclists and distance runners. Weighted mean values were generated as detailed in Fig. 59.1.

tially. In swimming, extra body fat may improve buoyancy, thus helping to reduce hydrodynamic drag (Gullstrand 1992; Chapter 55). In contrast to swimming, where hydrodynamic drag is the greatest force to overcome (Gullstrand 1992; Tittel & Wutsherk 1992), gravity is the major force to overcome during running. As a result, excess weight is detrimental to running performance (Deitrick 1991; Houtkooper & Going 1994). However, excess weight may not be detrimental to weight-supported cycling. In cyclists, the increase of frontal surface area with an increase in body mass is offset by an increased absolute power output, as long as the extra mass is muscle (Neumann 1992). None the less, the influence of body mass on cycling performance will depend somewhat on the topography of the cycling course. A hilly route will substantially increase the effect of gravity on the cyclist (Neumann 1992), which may disadvantage the heavy triathlete (Deitrick 1991). Élite male endurance and ultra-endurance triathletes typically carry between 6 and 11% body fat (Holly et al. 1986; Travill et al. 1994; De Vito et al. 1995), whereas élite female triathletes have 12–18% body fat (O'Toole et al. 1987; Dengel et al. 1989; Schneider & Pollack 1991).

Deitrick (1991) found that 'heavy-weight' triathletes (90.9 kg) compared to 'typical' triathletes (66.6 kg) were taller, had a higher body fat content, a lower running economy and a lower $\dot{V}O_{2max}$, shorter treadmill performance times in an incremental run to exhaustion and a lower power/weight ratio on the bicycle ergometer. The heavier triathletes also trained less than their typical counterparts. Thus excess weight, particularly an excess of fat, is probably not beneficial to triathlon performance. The buoyancy advantages that fat can offer in the swimming phase can be largely offset by the use of a wetsuit, thereby eliminating the possible advantage that fatter individuals may have while swimming.

Thus, it would appear that successful triathletes should be characterized by a blend of the physical traits observed in specialist endurance swimmers, cyclists and runners. This does not imply that all successful triathletes will have the same shape and size, but it does indicate that an individual's physical attributes can help to predict in which exercise mode a triathlete is most likely to be successful, or in which mode they have the potential to improve. Similarly, triathletes with different physical attributes may excel on one type of course (e.g. flat) but not be suited to another (e.g. hills), or they may excel in one exercise mode at the expense of the other two.

Physiological characteristics

AEROBIC POWER ($\dot{V}O_{2max}$)

High levels of aerobic power generally characterize successful endurance specialists in swimming (Holmér et al. 1974; Gullstrand 1992), cycling (Burke et al. 1977; Strömme et al. 1977; Burke 1980; Åstrand & Rodahl 1986) and running (Wilmore & Brown 1974; Pollack 1977; Davies & Thompson 1979; Shephard 1992), and the same is true for triathletes (Holly et al. 1986; O'Toole et al. 1987; Millard-Stafford et al. 1991; Schneider & Pollack 1991; Laurenson et al. 1993; De Vito et al. 1995; O'Toole & Douglas 1995; Vallier et al. 1996; Miura et al. 1997; Kerr et al. 1998). Élite triathletes generally have slightly lower weight-adjusted $\dot{V}O_{2max}$ values than single-sport endurance specialists in their respective exercise modalities (Fig. 59.3a–c). The mean $\dot{V}O_{2max}$ values for treadmill running in élite runners (Costill et al. 1973; Wilmore & Brown 1974; Pollack 1977; Davies & Thompson 1979; Conley & Krahenbuhl 1980; Shephard 1992) are on average 8–23% higher than the corresponding values for triathletes (O'Toole et al. 1987; De Vito et al. 1995; O'Toole & Douglas 1995). Similarly, $\dot{V}O_{2max}$ values in élite single-sport athletes are 15–23% greater in cyclists (Strömme et al. 1977; Burke 1980; Coyle et al. 1988) and 18–20% greater in swimmers (Holmér et al. 1974) than most of the values reported for triathletes (Holly et al. 1986; Dengel et al. 1989; Douglas 1989; Toussaint 1990; Deitrick 1991; Millard-Stafford et al. 1991; Schneider & Pollack 1991; Sleivert & Wenger 1993; O'Toole & Douglas 1995). The lower $\dot{V}O_{2max}$ values in triathletes may be partially attributable to the carrying of the extra muscle mass required in one exercise mode, e.g. swimming, which is not required in the other exercise modes, e.g. cycling or running. This could decrease the $\dot{V}O_{2max}$ in any given mode of

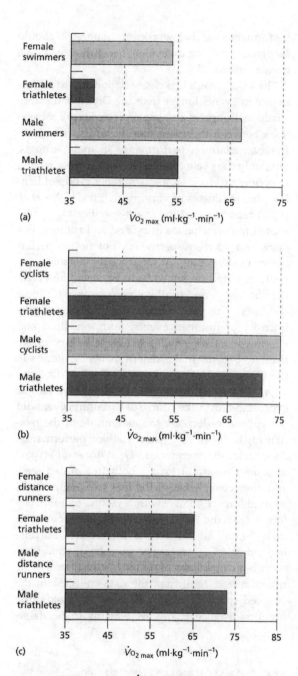

(a) $\dot{V}_{O_2 max}$ (ml·kg^{-1}·min^{-1})

(b) $\dot{V}_{O_2 max}$ (ml·kg^{-1}·min^{-1})

(c) $\dot{V}_{O_2 max}$ (ml·kg^{-1}·min^{-1})

Fig. 59.3 Weighted mean $\dot{V}_{O_2 max}$ values for élite male and female Olympic and Ironman triathletes compared to (a) élite distance swimmers, (b) élite road cyclists and (c) élite distance runners. Weighted mean values were generated as detailed in Fig. 59.1.

exercise. That $\dot{V}_{O_2 max}$ values are lower in triathlete than in endurance specialists may also be due to differences in training volumes, since the triathlete necessarily spreads training between three exercise modes (O'Toole *et al.* 1989a). The greater $\dot{V}_{O_2 max}$ values generally obtained by single-sport specialists reinforce the concept of a specificity of training response. Some studies, however, have shown $\dot{V}_{O_2 max}$ improvements in both cycling and running after training in only one exercise mode, with the magnitude of $\dot{V}_{O_2 max}$ improvements being largest for the exercise mode adopted during training (Boutcher *et al.* 1989; Hoffman *et al.* 1993). Conversely, the addition of 6 weeks of increased cycling training resulted in an increase of running performance of similar magnitude to that achieved by the addition of extra run training in well-trained male distance runners (Flynn *et al.* 1998). It therefore appears that training in one exercise mode may cross over and influence performance in another exercise mode, even in well-trained athletes, although the bulk of evidence still suggests that specificity of training should remain a central premise in any triathlete training programme.

Relatively few data exist, but it appears that élite triathletes have greater $\dot{V}_{O_2 max}$ values than subélite and recreational triathletes. For example, treadmill $\dot{V}_{O_2 max}$ values of 70–85 ml·kg^{-1}·min^{-1} have been reported for élite male triathletes (Holly *et al.* 1986; O'Toole *et al.* 1987; De Vito *et al.* 1995; O'Toole & Douglas 1995), whereas lower-level triathletes have $\dot{V}_{O_2 max}$ values of between 55 and 67 ml·kg^{-1}·min^{-1} (Zinkgraf *et al.* 1986; Kreider *et al.* 1988b; Douglas 1989; Delistraty *et al.* 1990; Sleivert & Wenger 1993; Miura *et al.* 1997; Rowbottom *et al.* 1997; Zhou *et al.* 1997). Similarly, élite and recreational female triathletes have treadmill $\dot{V}_{O_2 max}$ values of between 54 and 73 ml·kg^{-1}·min^{-1} (Schneider & Pollack 1991; Laurenson *et al.* 1993) and 44–65 ml·kg^{-1}·min^{-1} (Laurenson *et al.* 1993; Sleivert & Wenger 1993; Bunc *et al.* 1996), respectively. These results suggest a relationship between $\dot{V}_{O_2 max}$ and triathlon performance.

When triathletes of mixed abilities compete in short-course triathlons, swimming, cycling and running performances have been reported to be related to event-specific $\dot{V}_{O_2 max}$ in some cases. For example, in a mixed gender sample, Butts *et al.*

(1991) found the swim time to correlate with the absolute ($l \cdot min^{-1}$) tethered swimming $\dot{V}O_{2max}$ ($r = -0.49$), the cycling time to correlate with both the absolute ($r = -0.57$) and the relative ($ml \cdot kg^{-1} \cdot min^{-1}$) $\dot{V}O_{2max}$ ($r = -0.78$), and the running time to correlate with the relative $\dot{V}O_{2max}$ ($r = -0.84$). These relationships must be interpreted with care, since a mixed gender sample may have elevated these correlations by increasing the range of both $\dot{V}O_{2max}$ and performance scores. Sleivert and Wenger (1993) reported gender-specific correlations. They found that the swimming time was related to the relative tethered swim $\dot{V}O_{2max}$ in both females ($r = -0.93$) and males ($r = -0.48$), but the cycling time was not related to the cycle $\dot{V}O_{2max}$ in either gender, and the running time was related to the treadmill $\dot{V}O_{2max}$ in females ($r = -0.88$) but not in males. The small sample of females in this study ($n = 7$) exhibited greater variance in abilities than the males ($n = 18$), which is likely to have inflated the observed correlations for the female sample. Another recent study of a very heterogeneous sample of triathletes (e.g. running $\dot{V}O_{2max}$ values ranging from 54 to 82 $ml \cdot kg^{-1} \cdot min^{-1}$) reported significant correlations between the run time in an Olympic distance triathlon and the relative treadmill $\dot{V}O_{2max}$ ($r = -0.73$); however, there was no relationship between the cycling $\dot{V}O_{2max}$ and the cycling performance, despite the fact that the absolute cycling $\dot{V}O_{2max}$ was correlated with the overall triathlon time ($r = -0.72$) (Zhou et al. 1997). In a more homogeneous group of 17 male competitive triathletes, Miura et al. (1997) reported that the exercise mode-specific $\dot{V}O_{2max}$ was significantly related to performance in swimming ($r = -0.65$), cycling ($r = -0.82$) and running ($r = -0.73$) phases of an Olympic distance triathlon; moreover, each $\dot{V}O_{2max}$ measure was correlated with the overall triathlon completion time ($r = -0.62$ to -0.89). In recreational triathletes of low average fitness, Loftin et al. (1988) reported significant relationships between cycling and running $\dot{V}O_{2max}$ and cycling and running performance in the triathlon ($r = -0.56$ and -0.58, respectively), but no relationship between the arm crank $\dot{V}O_{2max}$ and swimming performance. It therefore appears that $\dot{V}O_{2max}$ is important to performance over the Olympic distance, but the relationship is moderate and often not statistically significant. In triathletes of mixed abilities, the $\dot{V}O_{2max}$ is a valid predictor of

performance, and lower-level triathletes should emphasize training to develop this attribute in each exercise mode.

The $\dot{V}O_{2max}$ has a less clear relationship to performance in events longer than the Olympic distance triathlon. Dengel et al. (1989) reported weak correlations between the event-specific $\dot{V}O_{2max}$ and half-Ironman triathlon performance in male subjects, with only the cycle ergometer $\dot{V}O_{2max}$ being related to cycling time ($r = -0.70$). In another group of half-Ironman triathletes of varying abilities, Kohrt et al. (1987) reported that the event-specific $\dot{V}O_{2max}$ was related to performance in cycling and running ($r = -0.68$ and -0.78, respectively), but not to performance in swimming. At the Ironman distance, one study reported no relationship between the event-specific $\dot{V}O_{2max}$ and triathlon performance (O'Toole et al. 1987). This may be because of the lower relative intensity of Ironman events; nutrition, fluid and electrolyte balance and psychological factors are likely to become major determinants of success in these ultra-endurance events (O'Toole & Douglas 1995). One study observed that cumulative fatigue experienced over the course of a triathlon event did not appear to decrease the magnitude of the relationship between $\dot{V}O_{2max}$ and triathlon performance. As previously mentioned, De Vito et al. (1995) measured treadmill $\dot{V}O_{2max}$ both in a rested state and after completion of the first two segments of a triathlon (1.5-km swim, 32-km bike). They found that the $\dot{V}O_{2max}$ decreased from 69 to 64 $ml \cdot kg^{-1} \cdot min^{-1}$ at the second assessment. Surprisingly, the $\dot{V}O_{2max}$ measured from basal conditions was a better predictor of running performance in the triathlon ($r = -0.86$) than the data collected in the fatigued state ($r = -0.77$). Whether this holds true for ultradistance triathlons remains to be determined.

FRACTIONAL UTILIZATION OF $\dot{V}O_{2max}$

Performance in the triathlon has been significantly related to the ability of the triathlete to exercise at a low percentage of $\dot{V}O_{2max}$ for any given submaximal work rate (Dengel et al. 1989). This ability is influenced by a combination of factors, including aerobic power, economy of movement and anaerobic threshold (An_T).

The ability to exercise at a high fraction of $\dot{V}O_{2max}$ is largely influenced by An_T, expressed as either ventilatory threshold (V_T) or lactate threshold (L_T). A non-linear increase in either respiratory minute ventilation or blood lactate concentration when plotted against $\dot{V}O_2$ or velocity is commonly used to determine A_{nT} (Thoden 1991; Chapter 22). Endurance time at an exercise intensity above A_{nT} is reduced due to metabolic acidosis and accelerated glycogen depletion (MacDougall et al. 1977). Therefore, the successful endurance athlete is often characterized by an ability to perform high amounts of work at or just below A_{nT} (Costill et al. 1973; Tanaka et al. 1984).

In Olympic triathletes, V_T has been reported at 72–75% of swimming $\dot{V}O_{2max}$, 63–85% of cycling $\dot{V}O_{2max}$ and 74–91% of running $\dot{V}O_{2max}$ (Schneider & Pollack 1991; Sleivert & Wenger 1993; De Vito et al. 1995; Bunc et al. 1996; Zhou et al. 1997). Likewise, L_T has occurred at 72–88% of cycling $\dot{V}O_{2max}$ and 80–85% of treadmill $\dot{V}O_{2max}$ (Kohrt et al. 1989). These percentages are similar to or slightly lower than those reported in endurance specialists (Withers et al. 1981; Sjodin et al. 1985; Simon et al. 1986). It has been suggested that the amount of muscle mass involved in a movement partially determines the percentage of $\dot{V}O_{2max}$ at which A_{nT} occurs. This may be because the average metabolic rate per unit of contracting muscle is greater in exercise modes where less muscle mass is recruited (Koyal et al. 1976; Schneider & Pollack 1991). The training history may alter this relationship.

Kohrt et al. (1989) reported that over the course of a triathlon season, the cycling L_T increased by 6%, and the running L_T by 10%, without improvements in $\dot{V}O_{2max}$. Similarly, Rowbottom et al. (1997) reported that over 9 months of training, the running velocity at L_T in a group of well-trained male triathletes improved from 15.6 to 16.6 km·h⁻¹, with no change in $\dot{V}O_{2max}$. Withers et al. (1981) found cyclists could use larger fractions of $\dot{V}O_{2max}$ than runners when tested on a cycle ergometer, whereas runners had a higher fractional utilization on a treadmill. Hoffman et al. (1993) reported that with run training, V_T improved on the treadmill but not the cycle ergometer; however, cycle ergometer training improved V_T in both cycling and treadmill running. Others also have reported improvements of L_T in

cycling through run training (Boutcher et al. 1989). The data therefore indicate that training may improve V_T and L_T measures specifically, allowing triathletes to compete at higher percentages of $\dot{V}O_{2max}$; the findings also provide some support for the benefits of cross-training.

Sleivert and Wenger (1993) reported that the running velocity at V_T was related to the run time in both females ($r = -0.88$) and males ($r = -0.73$), and the resistance pulled at V_T during tethered swimming was related to the swimming time ($r = -0.81$) for females in a short-course triathlon. The overall triathlon time was related to the velocity at the running V_T in both genders ($r = -0.78$). The sample of recreational triathletes used in this study was heterogeneous in terms of performance ability, particularly in the female triathletes, and this may have inflated the magnitude of the correlations. Nevertheless, V_T measures have also been related to performance in a small group ($n = 6$) of well-trained male triathletes (De Vito et al. 1995).

In the study of De Vito et al. (1995), the $\dot{V}O_2$ at the running V_T was measured both starting from resting conditions and after completion of a partial triathlon (1.5 km of swimming, 32 km of cycling). After completion of the partial triathlon, the V_T occurred at a lower percentage of $\dot{V}O_{2max}$ (74.3 versus 84.6%), demonstrating that the ability to sustain a high percentage of $\dot{V}O_{2max}$ in running is impaired after the swimming and cycling sections of a triathlon. In addition, the heart rate at V_T was lower after previous exercise, a finding which has implications for setting training and competition pace. De Vito's group also found that $\dot{V}O_2$ at the running V_T was related to running performance in an Olympic triathlon ($r = -0.79$), and this relationship was even stronger when V_T was tested after completion of the partial triathlon ($r = -0.85$). The L_T has also been related to performance in running and cycling during a half-Ironman event ($r = -0.73$ and -0.72, respectively) (Kohrt et al. 1989). Zhou et al. (1997) have similarly reported that the work rate at V_T for both cycling ($r = -0.79$) and running ($r = -0.68$) was significantly correlated to the overall Olympic triathlon performance; the work rate at the cycling V_T was not related to cycling performance, but the speed at the running V_T was correlated with running performance in the triathlon ($r = -0.85$). Thus, the ability to perform high rates of work at or below V_T or L_T, and to minimize muscle acidosis, are probably important determinants of success in short-course triathlons. The one study that has reported no relationship between V_T and triathlon performance examined a homogeneous group of triathletes who were competing in a long-course triathlon (O'Toole et al. 1988). It may be that other factors, such as energy reserves, fluid and electrolyte balance and economy of movement are more important in ultra-endurance triathlons (O'Toole & Douglas 1995).

ECONOMY OF MOVEMENT

Economy has been defined by numerous researchers as the oxygen cost of exercising at a standard, predetermined velocity (Daniels et al. 1977; Farrell et al. 1979; Morgan et al. 1995). An economic triathlete uses less oxygen than her or his less economic peers at a standard velocity, and theoretically such an individual is able to move faster or to conserve energy for the later stages of an event. Economy has been shown to account for the large variation in 10-km race performance times of highly experienced runners with similar $\dot{V}O_{2max}$ values (Conley & Krahenbuhl 1980). Other studies have shown significant relationships between economy and cycling (Coyle et al. 1988) and swimming (Montpetit et al. 1988) performance.

Economy is important to performance in triathletes. Laurenson et al. (1993) reported that élite female triathletes were significantly more economical than club-level triathletes during treadmill running at 15 km·h⁻¹ (respective oxygen costs of 51.2 versus 53.8 ml·kg⁻¹·min⁻¹). The élite females also exercised at a lower percentage of their $\dot{V}O_{2max}$ (78.2 versus 89.2%) and had lower lactate and heart rate values at submaximal running velocities. The percentage of $\dot{V}O_{2max}$ at 15 km·h⁻¹ was a significant predictor of Olympic-distance triathlon performance. Dengel et al. (1989) also reported that the $\dot{V}O_2$ values at submaximal speeds of running, cycling and swimming were strong predictors of corresponding performance times in a half-Ironman triathlon, the strongest predictors being the ability to use a low

percentage of $\dot{V}O_{2max}$ at a given submaximal work rate in each exercise mode ($r = 0.91, 0.78$ and 0.87 for swimming, cycling and running performance times, respectively). O'Toole et al. (1989a) also reported that the percentage of $\dot{V}O_{2max}$ used during submaximal cycling was significantly related to the cycle finish time in an Ironman-distance triathlon. Most recently, Miura et al. (1997) measured the economy of 17 competitive male triathletes during a simulated triathlon comprising flume swimming, cycle ergometry and treadmill running (60% $\dot{V}O_{2max}$ in each exercise mode, for fixed durations of 30, 75 and 45 min, respectively). The economy index (% $\dot{V}O_{2max}$) was taken during the last minute of each stage, since it is known that the oxygen cost will drift higher during prolonged exercise, as demonstrated in numerous triathlon studies (Kreider et al. 1988a; Guezennec et al. 1996; Hausswirth et al. 1996, 1997; Hue et al. 1998). This study found significant relationships between the percentage of $\dot{V}O_{2max}$ used during the swimming ($r = 0.55$), cycling ($r = 0.61$) and running ($r = 0.55$) stages and performance in the corresponding phases of an Olympic triathlon. The swimming economy was not related to the overall triathlon performance, but the cycling and running economies were reasonable predictors of triathlon performance ($r = 0.60$ and 0.77, respectively). The index of economy used in this study reflects the ability to maintain a stable percentage of $\dot{V}O_{2max}$ over the course of a triathlon; therefore, it probably reflects the degree of cardiovascular and thermal stability that the triathletes were able to maintain. This might explain the lack of correlation between economy in swimming, the first event of the triathlon, and overall performance. The fact that the relationship between economy and overall performance strengthened on moving from cycling to the running mode, the latter phases of the triathlon, lends some support to the importance of minimizing cardiovascular drift during sequential endurance exercise.

Although the economy of movement in swimming did not predict overall triathlon performance in the study of Miura et al. (1997), it may still be an important determinant of success in the swimming phase of the triathlon, where a large emphasis is placed on technique. Toussaint (1990) compared propulsion efficiency (the energy used to overcome drag/total energy used) between élite swim specialists and élite triathletes. At an equal power output, the two groups did not differ in gross efficiency, stroke frequency or work per stroke, but the élite swimmers covered a greater distance per stroke (1.23 versus 0.92 m) and had a greater mean swimming velocity (1.17 versus 0.95 m·s^{-1}). The élite swimmers used a higher proportion of their power output to overcome drag, and expended less power in moving the water backwards. The overall mean propulsion efficiency for swimmers was 61%, but it was only 44% for the triathletes. It was concluded that the triathletes should focus their attention on improving swimming technique, rather than on improving their ability to generate power. The distance covered per stroke may be a simple criterion that triathletes can use to evaluate their swimming skill.

A number of extrinsic factors may influence exercise economy. The use of a wetsuit in the swimming section can reduce drag by up to 14% (Toussaint et al. 1989). Cycling economy can be affected by factors such as seat position, crank length, body position and shoe–pedal interface (Cavanagh & Kram 1985; Gregor & Wheeler 1994). A triathlete's cycling performance is also affected by the quality of the bicycle, including the design of its wheels, tyres and handlebars (Faria 1992).

Conclusions

The triathlon significantly challenges human capacity for thermoregulatory and cardiovascular homeostasis. This is particularly evident in the latter stages of the event, when hyperthermia, dehydration, a reduced $\dot{V}O_{2max}$ and a poor economy of movement are all observed. Successful triathletes are able to minimize homeostatic disturbances over the course of the event, probably largely as a result of high volumes of training in swimming, cycling and running. Unfortunately, these necessarily large volumes of training predispose the triathlete to overuse injuries, with the knees and lower back being the most common sites of injury. Triathletes develop physical and physiological characteristics that are a blend of those seen in endurance swimming, cycling and running specialists, largely through specific training, but probably partially through cross-training. Élite triathletes have high $\dot{V}O_{2max}$ values in swimming, cycling and running, and are able to exercise at high fractions of $\dot{V}O_{2max}$ in each exercise mode, due to well-developed anaerobic thresholds and economy of movement. More research is required on acute interaction effects arising from sequential exercise in swimming, cycling and running, and there is also need for further information on the influence of different training interventions on triathlon performance.

References

Åstrand, P.-O. & Rodahl, K. (1986) Textbook of Work Physiology: Physiological Bases of Exercise, 3rd edn. McGraw-Hill, New York.

Bonsignore, M.R., Morici, G., Abate, P., Romano, S. & Bonsignore, G. (1998) Ventilation and entrainment of breathing during cycling and running in triathletes. Medicine and Science in Sports and Exercise 30, 239–245.

Booth, J., Marino, F. & Ward, J.J. (1997) Improved running performance in hot humid conditions following whole body precooling. Medicine and Science in Sports and Exercise 29, 943–949.

Boutcher, S.H., Seip, R.L., Hetzler, R.K., Pierce, E.F., Snead, D. & Weltman, A. (1989) The effects of specificity of training on rating of perceived exertion at the lactate threshold. European Journal of Applied Physiology 59, 365–369.

Bunc, V., Heller, J., Horcic, J. & Novotny, J. (1996) Physiological profile of best Czech male and female young triathletes. Journal of Sports Medicine and Physical Fitness 36, 265–270.

Burke, E.R. (1980) Physiological characteristics of competitive cyclists. The Physician and Sports Medicine 8, 79–84.

Burke, E.R., Cerney, F., Costill, D. & Fink, W. (1977) Characteristics of skeletal muscle in competitive cyclists. Medicine and Science in Sports and Exercise 9, 109–112.

Butts, N.K., Henry, B.A. & McLean, D. (1991) Correlations between $\dot{V}O_{2max}$ and performance times of recreational triathletes. Journal of Sports Medicine and Physical Fitness 31, 339–344.

Cavanagh, P.R. & Kram, R. (1985) Mechanical and muscular factors affecting the efficiency of human movement. Medicine and Science in Sports and Exercise 17, 326–331.

Conley, D.L. & Krahenbuhl, G.S. (1980) Running economy and distance running performance of highly trained athletes. Medicine and Science in Sports and Exercise 12, 357–360.

Costill, D.L., Thomason, H. & Roberts, E. (1973) Fractional utilisation of aerobic capacity during distance running. Medicine and Science in Sports and Exercise 5, 248–252.

Coyle, E.F., Coggan, A.R., Hoper, M.K. & Walters, T.J. (1988) Determinants of endurance in well trained cyclists. Journal of Applied Physiology 64, 2622–2630.

Daniels, J., Krahenbuhl, G., Foster, C., Gilbert, J. & Daniels, S. (1977) Aerobic responses of female distance runners to submaximal and maximal exercise. *Annals of the New York Academy of Sciences* 301, 726–733.

Davies, C.T.M. & Thompson, M.W. (1979) Aerobic performance of female marathon and male ultramarathon athletes. *European Journal of Applied Physiology* 41, 233–245.

Deitrick, R.W. (1991) Physiological responses of typical versus heavy weight triathletes to treadmill and bicycle exercise. *Journal of Sports Medicine and Physical Fitness* 31, 367–375.

Delistraty, D.A., Noble, B.J. & Wilkinson, J.G. (1990) Treadmill and swim bench ergometry in triathletes, runners and swimmers. *Journal of Applied Sports Science Research* 4, 31–36.

Dengel, D.R., Flynn, M.G., Costill, D.L. & Kirwan, J.P. (1989) Determinants of success during triathlon competition. *Research Quarterly in Exercise and Sport* 60, 234–238.

De Vito, G., Bernardi, M., Sproiero, E. & Figura, F. (1995) Decrease in endurance performance during Olympic triathlon. *International Journal of Sports Medicine* 16, 24–28.

Douglas, P.S. (1989) Cardiac considerations in the triathlete. *Medicine and Science in Sports and Exercise* 21, S214–S218.

Farber, H.W., Schaefer, E.J., Franey, R., Grimaldi, R. & Hill, N.S. (1991) The endurance triathlon: metabolic changes after each event and during recovery. *Medicine and Science in Sports and Exercise* 23, 959–965.

Faria, I.E. (1992) Energy expenditure, aerodynamics and medical problems in cycling. *Sports Medicine* 14, 43–63.

Farrell, P.A., Wilmore, J.H., Coyle, E.F., Billing, J.E. & Costill, D.L. (1979) Plasma lactate accumulation and distance running performance. *Medicine and Science in Sports and Exercise* 11, 338–344.

Flynn, M.G., Carroll, K.K., Hall, H.H., Bushman, B.A., Brolinson, P.G. & Weideman, C.A. (1998) Cross training: indices of training stress and performance. *Medicine and Science in Sports and Exercise* 30, 294–300.

Gregor, R.J. & Wheeler, J.B. (1994) Biomechanical factors associated with shoe/pedal interfaces. Implications for injury. *Sports Medicine* 17, 117–131.

Guezennec, C.Y., Vallier, J.M., Bigard, A.X. & Durey, A. (1996) Increase in energy cost of running at the end of a triathlon. *European Journal of Applied Physiology* 73, 440–445.

Gullstrand, L. (1992) Swimming as an endurance sport. In: Shephard, R.J. & Åstrand, P.-O. (eds) *Endurance in Sport*, 1st edn, pp. 531–541. Blackwell Science, Oxford.

Hausswirth, C., Bigard, A.X., Berthelot, M., Thomadis, M. & Guezennec, C.Y. (1996) Variability in energy cost of running at the end of a triathlon and a marathon. *International Journal of Sports Medicine* 17, 572–579.

Hausswirth, C., Bigard, A.X. & Guezennec, C.Y. (1997) Relationships between running mechanics and energy cost of running at the end of a triathlon and a marathon. *International Journal of Sports Medicine* 18, 330–339.

Hendy, H. & Boyer, B.J. (1995) Specificity in the relationship between training and performance in triathlons. *Perceptual and Motor Skills* 81, 1231–1240.

Hoffman, J.J., Loy, S.F., Shapiro, B.I. et al. (1993) Specificity effects of run versus cycle training on ventilatory threshold. *European Journal of Applied Physiology* 67, 43–47.

Holly, R.G., Barnard, R.J., Rosenthal, M., Applegate, E. & Pritikin, N. (1986) Triathlete characterisation and response to prolonged strenuous competition. *Medicine and Science in Sports and Exercise* 18, 123–127.

Holmér, I., Lundin, A. & Eriksson, B.O. (1974) Maximal oxygen uptake in swimming and running by élite swimmers. *Journal of Applied Physiology* 36, 711–714.

Hoogeveen, A.R. & Schep, G. (1997) The plasma lactate response to exercise and endurance performance: relationships in élite triathletes. *International Journal of Sports Medicine* 18, 526–530.

Horrell, S.A. (1989) *An investigation into the physiological responses of triathletes during running and cycling*. Masters dissertation, University of Otago.

Houtkooper, L.B. & Going, S.B. (1994) Body composition: how should it be measured? Does it affect sport performance? *Gatorade Sports Science Exchange* 7 (5).

Hue, O., Le Gallais, D., Chollet, D., Boussana, A. & Préfaut, C. (1998) The influence of prior cycling on biomechanical and cardiorespiratory response profiles during running in triathletes. *European Journal of Applied Physiology* 77, 98–105.

Ireland, M.L. & Micheli, L.J. (1987) Triathletes: biographic data, training, and injury patterns. *Annals of Sports Medicine* 3, 117–120.

Kerr, C.G., Trappe, T.A., Starling, R.D. & Trappe, S.W. (1998) Hyperthermia during Olympic triathlon: influence of

body heat storage during the swimming stage. *Medicine and Science in Sports and Exercise* 30, 99–104.

Kohrt, W.M., Morgan, D.W., Bates, B. & Skinner, J.S. (1987) Physiological responses of triathletes to maximal swimming, cycling and running. *Medicine and Science in Sports and Exercise* 19, 51–55.

Kohrt, W.M., O'Conner, J.S. & Skinner, J.S. (1989) Longitudinal assessment of responses by triathletes to swimming, cycling and running. *Medicine and Science in Sports and Exercise* 21, 569–575.

Korkia, P.K., Tunstall-Pedoe, D.S. & Maffulli, N. (1994) An epidemiological investigation of training and injury patterns in British triathletes. *British Journal of Sports Medicine* 28, 191–196.

Koyal, S.N., Whipp, B.J., Huntsman, D., Bray, G.A. & Wasserman, K. (1976) Ventilatory responses to the metabolic acidosis of treadmill and cycle ergometry. *Journal of Applied Physiology* 40, 864–867.

Kreider, R.B., Boone, T., Thompson, W.R., Burkes, S. & Cortes, C.W. (1988a) Cardiovascular and thermal responses of triathlon performance. *Medicine and Science in Sports and Exercise* 20, 385–390.

Kreider, R.B., Cundiff, D.E., Hammett, J.B., Cortes, C.W. & Williams, K.W. (1988b) Effects of cycling on running performance in triathletes. *Annals of Sports Medicine* 3, 220–225.

Laurenson, N.M., Fulcher, K.Y. & Korkia, P. (1993) Physiological characteristics of élite and club-level female triathletes during running. *International Journal of Sports Medicine* 14, 455–459.

Leake, C.N. & Carter, J.E.L. (1991) Comparison of body composition and somatotype of trained female triathletes. *Journal of Sports Sciences* 9, 125–135.

Lee, D.T. & Haymes, E.M. (1995) Exercise duration and thermoregulatory responses after whole body precooling. *Journal of Applied Physiology* 79, 1971–1976.

Loftin, M., Warren, B.L., Zingraf, S., Brandon, J.E., Skudlt, A. & Scully, B. (1988) Peak physiological function and performance of recreational triathletes. *Journal of Sports Medicine and Physical Fitness* 28, 330–335.

MacDougall, J.D., Ward, G.R., Sale, D.G. & Sutton, J.R. (1977) Biochemical adaptation of human skeletal muscle to heavy resistance training and immobilisation. *Journal of Applied Physiology* 43, 700–703.

Manninen, J.S.O. & Kallinen, M. (1996) Low back pain and overuse injuries in a group of Japanese triathletes. *British Journal of Sports Medicine* 30, 134–139.

Millard-Stafford, M., Sparling, P.B., Rosskopf, L.B. & DiCarlo, L.J. (1991) Differences in peak physiological responses during running, cycling and swimming. *Journal of Applied Sport Science Research* **5**, 213–218.

Miura, H., Kitawaga, K. & Ishiko, T. (1997) Economy during a simulated laboratory test triathlon is highly related to Olympic distance triathlon. *International Journal of Sports Medicine* **18**, 276–280.

Montpetit, R.R., Smith, H. & Boie, G. (1988) Swimming economy: how to standardise the data to compare swimming proficiency. *Journal of Swimming Research* **4**, 5–8.

Morgan, D.W., Bransford, D.R., Costill, D.L., Daniels, J.T., Howley, E.T. & Krahenbuhl, G.S. (1995) Variation in the aerobic demand of running among trained and untrained subjects. *Medicine and Science in Sports and Exercise* **27**, 404–409.

Neumann, G. (1992) Cycling. In: Shephard, R.J. & Åstrand, P.-O. (eds) *Endurance in Sport*, 1st edn, pp. 582–596. Blackwell Science, Oxford.

O'Toole, M.L. (1989) Training for ultraendurance triathlons. *Medicine and Science in Sports and Exercise* **21**, S209–S213.

O'Toole, M.L. & Douglas. P.S. (1995) Applied physiology of triathlon. *Sports Medicine* **19**, 251–267.

O'Toole, M.L., Hiller, W.D.B., Crosby, L.O. & Douglas, P.S. (1987) The ultraendurance triathlete: a physiologic profile. *Medicine and Science in Sports and Exercise* **19**, 45–50.

O'Toole, M.L., Douglas, P.S. & Hiller, W.D.B. (1988) The relation of exercise test variables to bike performance times during the Hawaii Ironman triathlon. *Medicine and Science in Sports and Exercise* **20**, S50.

O'Toole, M.L., Douglas, P.S. & Hiller, W.D.B. (1989a) Lactate, oxygen uptake and cycling performance in triathletes. *International Journal of Sports Medicine* **10**, 413–418.

O'Toole, M.L., Hiller, W.D.B., Smith, R.A. & Sisk, T.D. (1989b) Overuse injuries in ultraendurance triathletes. *American Journal of Sports Medicine* **17**, 514–518.

Parsons, L. & Day, S.J. (1986) Do wet suits affect swimming speed? *British Journal of Sports Medicine* **20**, 129–131.

Pollack, M.L. (1977) Characteristics of élite class distance runners. *Annals of the New York Academy of Sciences* **301**, 278–282.

Quigley, E.J. & Richards, J.G. (1996) The effects of cycling on running mechanics. *Journal of Applied Biomechanics* **12**, 470–479.

Rowbottom, D.G., Keast, D., Garcia-Webb, P. & Morton, A. (1997) Training adaptation and biological changes among well-trained male triathletes. *Medicine and Science in Sports and Exercise* **29**, 1233–1239.

Schneider, D.A. & Pollack, J. (1991) Ventilatory threshold and maximal oxygen uptake during cycling and running in female triathletes. *International Journal of Sports Medicine* **12**, 379–383.

Shephard, R.J. (1992) Maximal oxygen intake. In: Shephard, R.J. & Åstrand, P.-O. (eds) *Endurance in Sport*, pp. 192–200. Blackwell Scientific Publications, Oxford.

Simon, J., Young, J.L., Blood, D.K., Sega, K.R., Case, R.B. & Gutin, B. (1986) Plasma lactate and ventilatory thresholds in trained and untrained cyclists. *Journal of Applied Physiology* **60**, 777–781.

Sjodin, B., Jacobs, I. & Svendenhag, J. (1985) Changes in the onset of blood lactate accumulation (OBLA) and muscle enzymes after training at OBLA. *European Journal of Applied Physiology* **49**, 45–57.

Sleivert, G.S. & Wenger, H.A. (1993) Physiological predictors of short-course triathlon performance. *Medicine and Science in Sports and Exercise* **25**, 871–876.

Speedy, D.B., Noakes, T.D., Rogers, I.R. et al. (1999) Hyponatremia in ultradistance triathletes. *Medicine and Science in Sports and Exercise* **31**, 809–815.

Strömme, S.B., Ingjer, F. & Meen, H.D. (1977) Assessment of maximal aerobic power in specifically trained athletes. *Journal of Applied Physiology* **42**, 833–837.

Tanaka, K., Matsuura, Y., Matsuzaka, A. et al. (1984) A longitudinal assessment of anaerobic threshold and distance-running performance. *Medicine and Science in Sports and Exercise* **16**, 278–282.

Thoden, J. (1991) Testing aerobic power. In: MacDougall, J.D., Wenger, H.A. & Green, H.J. (eds) *Physiological Testing of the Élite Athlete*, pp. 107–173. Human Kinetics, Champaign, IL.

Tittel, K. & Wutsherk, H. (1992) Anatomical and anthropometric fundamentals of endurance. In: Shephard, R.J. & Åstrand, P.-O. (eds) *Endurance in Sport*, 1st edn, pp. 35–45. Blackwell Science, Oxford.

Toussaint, H.M. (1990) Difference in propelling efficiency between competitive and triathlon swimmers. *Medicine and Science in Sports and Exercise* **22**, 409–415.

Toussaint, H.M., Bruinunk, L., De Coster, R. et al. (1989) Effect of triathlon wet suit on drag during swimming. *Medicine and Science in Sports and Exercise* **21**, 325–328.

Trappe, T.A., Starling, R.D., Jozsi, A.C. et al. (1995) Thermal responses to swimming in three water temperatures: influence of a wet suit. *Medicine and Science in Sports and Exercise* **27**, 1014–1021.

Travill, A.L., Carter, J.E.L. & Dolan, K.P. (1994) Anthropometric characteristics of élite male triathletes. In: Bell, F.I. & Van Gyn, G.H. (eds) *Proceedings of the 10th Commonwealth and International Scientific Congress. 'Access to Active Living'*, pp. 340–343. University of Victoria, Canada.

Vallier, J.M., Chateau, C.Y. & Guezennec, C.Y. (1996) Effects of physical training in a hypobaric chamber on the physical performance of competitive triathletes. *European Journal of Applied Physiology* **73**, 471–478.

Vleck, V.E. & Garbutt, G. (1998) Injury and training characteristics of male élite, development squad, and club triathletes. *International Journal of Sports Medicine* **19**, 38–42.

Webb, P. (1986) Afterdrop of body temperature during rewarming: an alternative explanation. *Journal of Applied Physiology* **60**, 385–390.

Williams, M.M., Hawley, J.A., Black, R., Freke, M. & Simms, K. (1988) Injuries amongst competitive triathletes. *New Zealand Journal of Sports Medicine* **March**, 2–6.

Wilmore, J.H. & Brown, C.H. (1974) Physiological profiles of woman distance runners. *Medicine and Science in Sports and Exercise* **6**, 178–181.

Withers, R.T., Sherman, W.M., Miller, J.M. et al. (1981) Specificity of the anaerobic threshold in endurance trained cyclists and runners. *European Journal of Applied Physiology* **47**, 93–104.

Zhou, S., Robson, S.J., King, M.J. & Davie, A.J. (1997) Correlations between short-course triathlon performance and physiological variables determined in laboratory cycle and treadmill tests. *Journal of Sports Medicine and Physical Fitness* **37**, 122–130.

Zinkgraf, S.A., Jones, C.J., Warren, B. & Krebs, S.A. (1986) An empirical investigation of triathlon performance. *Journal of Sports Medicine and Physical Fitness* **26**, 350–356.

Chapter 60

Canoeing

ANTONIO DAL MONTE, PIERO FACCINI AND GIOVANNI MIRRI

Introduction

Canoeing was invented out of necessity, but has since become a popular form of sport and pleasure activity. Canoes were the first objects built for travelling on rivers and lakes. Three characteristics differentiate the canoe from most other types of watercraft:

1 the participant(s), seated or on their knees, look in the direction in which they are heading;

2 the propelling element is a paddle without a fixed support on the boat, held freely in the hands of the paddler; and

3 the canoe is a craft with a pointed stem and stern. These particular characteristics permit a great mobility and manageability. Some small rowing boats built by canoe makers in Canada have also adopted this design.

A report written by some Russian hunters indicates that around 1745, Europeans already knew about the use of this particular type of boat by Inuits from Greenland. About 100 years later, the Scot John McGregor designed and built a canoe similar to the kayak. Even if he was founder of the sport, he always preferred to stress the recreational aspect of canoeing rather than competitive racing.

In 1866 he founded the first canoe club which, in 1873, became the Royal Canoe Club. In April 1867, the first canoe race was held on the River Thames, over a distance of 1.6 km (1 mile). By 1900, the kayak had been adopted by the majority of European countries. The first treatise on paddling dates back to this year. It was written by the Norwegian Nansen. The pioneer period ended in 1936, at the Olympic Games in Berlin, when canoeing became an Olympic speciality. At present, the sport is regulated by the ICF (International Canoe Federation) and by various national federations. Canoeing has developed as a sport with two main specializations: speed canoeing (in calm water) and whitewater canoeing (in rough water). Other specialities include polo canoeing, sail canoeing and marathon canoeing.

Contestants in speed canoeing follow parallel courses in calm water. The classic races cover distances of 500 and 1000 m. The following types of craft are used: kayaks (K1, K2, K4, according to the number of crew members) and Canadian canoes (C1, C2) (Fig. 60.1).

Whitewater canoeing (an Olympic speciality from 1992) involves slalom events on a river with falls, on which has been installed a race course with obligatory 'gates' (doors) to be passed by either stem or stern. The craft used are the kayak (K1) and the Canadian canoe (C1, C2); the latter has a different design to the high-speed canoe; whitewater canoes are less rapid, but more stable.

The materials from which paddles and canoes are made, and their shapes, have evolved over time. The paddles, in particular, have undergone a dramatic change, from wood to synthetic material such as kevlar and carbon, and from a flat blade to the most recent wing-shaped type.

Biomechanics

Kayak technique

The following description is valid both for speed

Kayak 1

Kayak 2

Kayak 4

Canoe 1

Canoe 2

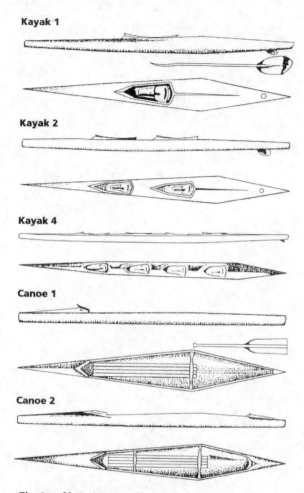

Fig. 60.1 Various types of kayak and Canadian canoe.

canoeing in calm water with any number of crew members, and for whitewater canoeing in rough water. To make the technique more easily understood, four fundamental phases can be distinguished.

1 *Position of attack*, or beginning of the paddling cycle. The trunk is in a position of maximum rotation; the attacking shoulder is stretched forward, and the corresponding arm is extended and horizontal. The active shoulder moves backward behind the head; the arm and the forearm are flexed at about 90°. The pelvis rotates forwards on the attack side and the corresponding leg flexes at around 130°.

2 *Passage in the water*. The first phase is dominated by pushing of the leg corresponding to the traction

and opposing rotation of the trunk, so that the traction arm, remaining extended, receives and transmits to the paddle the power resulting from the above-mentioned thrust. In the second phase, the rotation of the trunk and the thrust of the leg continue, while the rotation of the traction arm begins until the forearm reaches a minimum angle of 90°. The active arm completes the extension at the same time.

3 *Extraction*. After passage through the water, made with a rapid outward rotation of the traction arm, the extraction phase begins. This is also called the return phase.

4 *Aerophase*. In this phase, the paddle cycle ends and the next one begins. As in extraction, the aerophase is made by the traction arm, which completes the outward rotation. The rotation and upward movement permit the paddle to achieve the semirotation necessary to change sides.

Canadian technique

Here again we can distinguish four phases in the paddling cycle.

1 *Position of attack*. Both arms are extended: the trunk is in a position of maximum rotation and flexion; and the forward leg maintains the angle of the basic position. The angle formed between the paddle and the water surface in the phase of attack is about 65°.

2 *Phase of traction*. From the position of attack, while maintaining extension of the arms, an opposing rotation and extension of the trunk is effected until returning to the basic position. The active arm makes a downward pressure on the paddle, trying to keep this pressure perpendicular. The uppermost arm, by moving the wrist, makes the paddle rotate outwards until the extraction phase.

3 *Phase of extraction*. In this phase, the extracting fist is at the level of the hip and the semiflexed arm moves rapidly outwards.

4 *Aerophase*. In this phase, the athlete passes from the basic position to the position of attack, keeping the arms extended and achieving a torsion of the body, with the trunk flexed.

Figure 60.2 shows the forces applied during the paddling cycle as registered by means of a

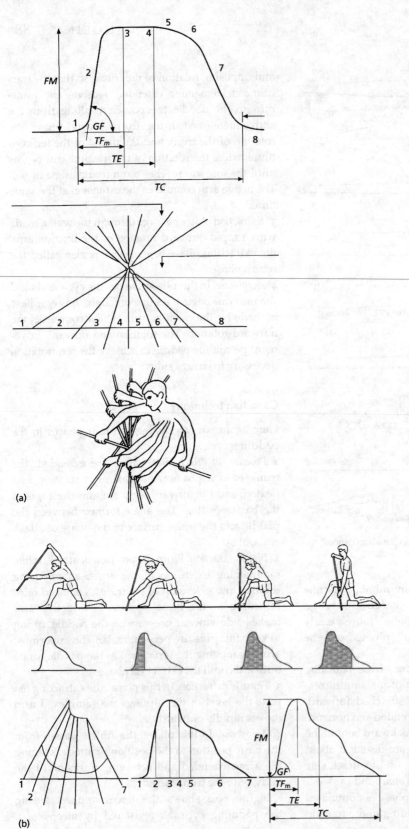

Fig. 60.2 (a) Force exerted during kayak paddling, as registered with a dynamometric paddle. (b) Force developed during Canadian canoe paddling, as registered with a dynamometric paddle. *FM*, maximal force; *GF*, angle of force; *TC*, paddling time; *TE*, effective time; *TFm*, time to reach maximal force.

dynamometric paddle (Perri *et al.* 1990) both in the kayak canoe (Fig. 60.2a) and in the Canadian canoe (Fig. 60.2b).

Anthropometry

Height

Hirata (1977) has demonstrated from a study of Olympic winners that the ideal paddler is generally 0.02–0.08 m taller than the average person. He has also shown that there is a height difference of about 0.03–0.05 m between the best kayakers and the best canoeists, the former being the taller.

Body mass

According to Sidney and Shephard (1973), junior competitors are relatively light. On the other hand, senior competitors carry a substantial excess mass (an average of 5.8 kg in men and 9.5 kg in women). This influences their performance. The correlation between lean body mass and overall ability is 0.72. In support of this view, Hirata (1977) showed that the gold medal winners in the Montreal Olympics were 3–10 kg heavier than the average contestant.

Muscle fibres

Canoeists have an unusual body composition; the deltoid muscles contain 63% slow-twitch fibres, as compared with 44% in a student population (Gollnick *et al.* 1972; Tesch & Karlsson 1985). The 'ideal' composition would be 50%, 65% and 70% of slow-twitch fibres for distances of 500, 1000 and 10 000 m, respectively (Shephard 1987).

Muscle force

Canoeists show large peak isometric forces for hand-grip, elbow flexion and knee extension. The coefficients of correlation between such measurements and overall performance are, however, quite low: 0.58 for knee extension, 0.29 for hand-grip and 0.11 for elbow flexion (Sidney & Shephard 1973). However, some researchers have not found particularly high values in the muscular regions of the trunk, especially in extension. In this region the peak muscle force is only 29% higher than in untrained students (Cermak *et al.* 1975).

We studied force–velocity curves for the upper limbs, using an isokinetic ergometer at an angular velocity similar to that of the stroke frequency during competition. The canoeists reached their maximum power at about 70 r.p.m. (Table 60.1). Studies completed by Armand (1983) and Vandewalle *et al.* (1983) have demonstrated that the force–velocity relationship plotted with data obtained on an arm ergometer gives higher figures for canoeists than for athletes practising other sport disciplines (Table 60.2).

Anaerobic metabolism

The literature gives conflicting data as far as blood lactate is concerned, with results perhaps depending on the type of test and ergometer used and on the motivation of the subjects. Cermak *et al.* (1975) observed peak blood lactate concentrations as high as $18.4\,mmol\cdot l^{-1}$ in men and $16.8\,mmol\cdot l^{-1}$ in women canoeists. Tesch and Lindberg (1984) reported values of $5\,mmol\cdot l^{-1}$ (males) and $6\,mmol\cdot l^{-1}$ (females). Dal Monte (1983) observed a final concentration of $14\,mmol\cdot l^{-1}$ in a test that simulated

Table 60.1 Average isokinetic data: the canoeists reached their maximum power at about 70 strokes·min⁻¹.

	Maximum velocity (r.p.m.)	Maximum force (N)	Maximum power (W)	No. of subjects
Junior kayak (male)	70	514	705	4
Senior kayak (male)	70	674	928	7
Senior kayak (female)	70	393	471	5

Table 60.2 Force–velocity relationship for various types of athlete, using an arm ergometer.

Reference	Sport	Maximum velocity (r.p.m.)	Maximum force (N)	Maximum power (W)
Vandewalle	Canoe/kayak			
et al. (1983)	men	243	165	948
	women	218	103	549
	Handball (men)	230	134	768
	Boxing (men)	240	124	768
	Tennis (men)	237	112	662
	Sedentary (men)	222	104	578
Armand	Senior kayak (male)	226	122	1045
(1983)	Junior kayak (male)	216	171	698
	Senior canoe (male)	233	147	916
	Junior canoe (male)	213	180	642
	Senior canoe/kayak (female)	211	187	583
	Junior canoe/kayak (female)	193	222	413

Table 60.3 'Fractionated' laboratory test, simulating the distances covered by Olympic kayak canoes in 500- and 1000-m races.

Time of work (4 min)	Mechanical work (kJ)	Mechanical power (W)	Oxygen intake during test (l·min^{-1})	Blood lactate mmol·l^{-1}*	mmol·l^{-1}†
Total test (0–4 min)	94.10	392	15.03		
I min (0–1 min)	26.26	437	1.82	6.70	6.70
II min (1–2 min)	21.80	363	4.36	8.00	1.3
III min (2–3 min)	—	366	4.40	8.12	0.12
IV min (3–4 min)	—	401	4.45	8.44	0.32

*Lactate concentration: difference between maximal blood lactate value and resting value.
†Difference between peak blood lactate concentration and peak value the minute before.

competition. In a laboratory test simulating the duration and energy outputs anticipated in races over 500 and 1000 m in speed-racing kayak canoes and a kayak ergometer ('Modest' kayak ergometer), Colli *et al.* (1990) obtained blood lactate measurements of 12.7 mmol·l^{-1} and 11.7 mmol·l^{-1}, respectively.

Table 60.3 presents laboratory data in tests simulating these same distances. Notice that the blood lactate concentration reached a high level after the first minute and then maintained a constant value for the rest of the test. We may conclude that there is no accumulation of blood lactate even if the metabolic intensity far exceeds the anaerobic threshold and is close to $\dot{V}O_{2max}$. This indicates that the measurement of blood lactate concentration alone could give misleading information about anaerobic glycolytic activity. In 500- and 1000-m competitions of highly specialized athletes, we obtained values of 16.0 (s.d. ± 0.70) mmol·l^{-1} and 13.5 (s.d. ± 0.47) mmol·l^{-1}, respectively (Colli *et al.* 1990).

Heller *et al.* (1984) compared test data on two groups of top-level canoeists. The first group ($n = 14$) were evaluated on the cycle ergometer and subsequently on the paddle ergometer, and the second group ($n = 10$) were tested on the treadmill and paddle ergometer. Respective lactate values of 8.6 mmol·l^{-1} and 8.8 mmol·l^{-1} were not significantly different for the first group; values for the second group were 13.2 and 12.5 mmol·l^{-1} ($P < 0.1$). These figures suggest that notable muscular and metabolic adjustments occur in canoeists, so that when using the specific ergometer, and thereby activating a relatively small muscular mass, the lactate value remains similar to that obtained on the treadmill or cycle ergometer.

We have also carried out studies on whitewater canoeists, both during slalom performance and during specific tests, in order to study their maximal lactate capacity (D'Angelo et al. 1987). The 'figure of eight' distance (Fig. 60.3) had to be completed as many times as possible in 1 min, and the distance covered was calculated according to the landmarks between the two gates. When that slalom had ended, we found a mean blood lactate concentration of 7.0 (s.d. ± 0.51) mmol·l^{-1}, whereas during specific tests in water we found a maximum of 13.2 (s.d. ± 1.11) mmol·l^{-1}. Field studies on Canadian canoeists have indicated values similar to those for kayakers. The only trend to a difference was between the two racing distances, i.e. 500 and 1000 m, with respective blood lactate values of 14.9 (s.d. ± 0.78) mmol·l^{-1} and 13.0 (s.d. ± 0.95) mmol·l^{-1}

(not significantly different) (Colli et al. 1990, personal communication).

When the anaerobic capacity was evaluated by measurement of oxygen deficit, we (Faina et al. 1997) found a positive ($r = 0.55$), but not statistically significant, correlation between the time limit at the minimum exercise intensity capable of inducing the maximal oxygen intake ($I\dot{V}O_{2max}$) and the accumulation oxygen deficit (AOD). These data suggest that, in kayakers, during an effort at the $I\dot{V}O_{2max}$, which is close to the intensity adopted in actual competition, endurance seems to be influenced heavily by the anaerobic capacity.

Anaerobic threshold

Cerretelli et al. (1979) and Tesch and Lindberg (1984) have noted a high anaerobic threshold in paddlers. Possible factors include rapid oxygen kinetics at the onset of exercise, a high capillary density in the shoulder muscles, and a high oxidative power (Gollnick et al. 1972) or a low lactate dehydrogenase activity.

Bunc et al. (1981) examined anaerobic thresholds, using various ergometric tests. They found that when paddlers were tested on the treadmill, they had a threshold at 79% of $\dot{V}O_{2max}$, whereas the value on the kayak ergometer was around 86% of $\dot{V}O_{2max}$ (Tesch et al. 1976). Colli et al. (1990) measured the

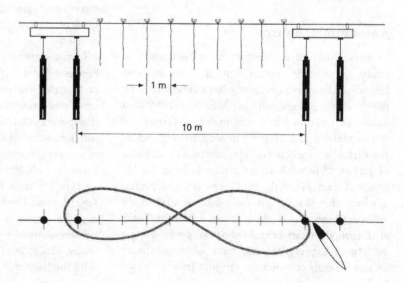

Fig. 60.3 Specific test for white-water canoeing: plan of the course.

Table 60.4 Power at 4-mM blood lactate concentration measured on the kayak ergometer in the five fastest Italian paddlers.

	Power (W)	$\%\dot{V}O_{2max}$	Heart rate (beats·min^{-1})	No. of subjects
500-m kayak (male)	268	79	178	1
1000-m kayak (male)	356	86	179	1
500-m kayak (female)	225	88	181	1
500-m canoe (male)	260	77.5	180	1
1000-m canoe (male)	299	87.3	177	1

anaerobic threshold by an incremental test on the kayak ergometer (the power at a blood lactate concentration of 4 mM); values for the best Italian canoeists, divided according to their specialities, are shown in Table 60.4. When Dal Monte's kayak ergometer was used on members of the Italian national kayak team, an anaerobic threshold 82% (s.d. ± 6.3%) of $\dot{V}O_{2max}$ was obtained (Paselli *et al.* 1986).

The heart rate at the anaerobic threshold also reaches high values. During an incremental test on the treadmill, with a constant slope of 5% and speed increments of 1 km·h^{-1}·min^{-1}, Bunc *et al.* (1981) found a heart rate of 177 beats·min^{-1} in top Hungarian male canoeists who had a maximum heart rate averaging 192 beats·min^{-1}. Corresponding values for women were 182 and 195 beats·min^{-1}, respectively.

Aerobic metabolism

Various tests and ergometers have been used to study the aerobic metabolism of canoeists and kayakers. Data have frequently been obtained using the treadmill. Sidney and Shephard (1973) reported values of 3.8 l·min^{-1} in junior males, 4–5 l·min^{-1} in senior males and 2.8 l·min^{-1} in women whitewater paddlers. Vaccaro *et al.* (1984) recorded a mean value of 4.7 l·min^{-1} in whitewater canoeists from the US national team. Horvath and Finney (1969) reported a mean of 3.8 l·min^{-1} in male contestants. Many authors (Cermak *et al.* 1975; Vrijens *et al.* 1975; Tesch *et al.* 1976; Dransart 1977; Rusko *et al.* 1978), using a variety of leg ergometers, have obtained mean values for male competitors ranging from 5.3 to 5.6

l·min^{-1}. Data referring to winners are larger: Tesch and Lindberg (1984) reported a $\dot{V}O_{2max}$ of 4.9 l·min^{-1} in Swedish junior males, 5.0 l·min^{-1} in senior males and 5.4 l·min^{-1} in a male world-champion. Dransart (1977) presented exceptional data, 5.6 l·min^{-1} (85 ml·kg^{-1}·min^{-1}) in a French male competitor.

However, the canoeist provides a classic example of a fundamental feature of living beings: adaptability. The athlete continuously modifies her or his morphofunctional characteristics in relation to the specific requirements of the sport. The canoeist develops the upper part of the body, thus opposing the evolutionary law which privileges the upright position of humans and thus the usual morphofunctional difference between upper and lower limbs. Therefore, in order to obtain valid and specific information on the functional qualities of a canoeist as well as on his or her training status, ergometers that can simulate paddling should be used. If such apparatus is not available, an upper limb ergometer can be used.

In canoeists and kayakers, the difference in $\dot{V}O_{2max}$ between a test carried out with the lower limbs and one carried out with a specific ergometer is very small (the same is not true for athletes in other sport disciplines). Dal Monte and Leonardi (1975) found a difference (in ml·kg^{-1}·min^{-1}) of only 7.3% in favour of the results obtained by the cycle ergometer test. Likewise, Heller *et al.* (1983) obtained a value of 4.45 l·min^{-1} with the cycle ergometer versus 4.16 l·min^{-1} with the kayak ergometer. Differences are slightly larger if comparison is made with the results of treadmill tests: in the above-mentioned study, Heller *et al.* obtained a value of 4.87 l·min^{-1} with the treadmill, compared with 4.01 l·min^{-1} with the kayak ergometer. It is generally agreed that when sedentary people exercise on an upper limb ergometer, they reach only about 70% of the maximal oxygen intake attained during running, but canoeists attain much higher values on a specific ergometer (Table 60.5).

Faina *et al.* (1988, personal communication) tested eight good-level kayakers and found a $\dot{V}O_{2max}$ of 54.4 ml·kg^{-1}·min^{-1} on the kayak ergometer and of 53.3 ml·kg^{-1}·min^{-1} on the cycle ergometer. In contrast, a group of eight cyclists showed a $\dot{V}O_{2max}$ of 68.7 ml·kg^{-1}·min^{-1} on a cycle ergometer and of 46.8 ml·kg^{-1}·min^{-1} on an upper limb ergometer. Dal Monte (1975) noted that a highly specialized athlete was even able to reach a higher $\dot{V}O_{2max}$ on a kayak ergometer than on a cycle ergometer. However, this last observation is not universally true; in fact, this is not the case with medium-level athletes or young athletes (Colli *et al.* 1990).

The efficiency of paddling seems to be quite an important limiting factor too. In a laboratory simulation of speed-canoe races over distances of 1000 m and 300 m, and in non-specific tests, Colli *et al.* (1990) found that the amount of energy released aerobically ($\dot{V}O_2$) and anaerobically (lactate) was the same, both in high-level Olympic canoeists and in national-level canoeists, but the mechanical power produced was higher in the high-level competitors (Tables 60.6–60.8). These data could indicate that the latter group developed more specific coordinative,

Table 60.5 Percentage of leg $\dot{V}O_{2max}$ developed by paddlers. From Shephard (1987).

Reference	% leg $\dot{V}O_{2max}$
Vrijens *et al.* (1975)	
Paddlers	89
Controls	81
Cermak *et al.* (1975)	
Male paddlers	95
Female paddlers	100
Dransart (1977)	77
Tesch & Lindberg (1984)	
Paddlers	87
Vaccaro *et al.* (1984)	89

Table 60.7 Comparison between top-level and good-level athletes in two kayak ergometer tests simulating distances of 1000 and 300 m.

	Top level	Good level	P
1000 m			
W·kg^{-1}	3.66 ± 19	3.37 ± 0.34	0.05
J·paddle^{-1}·kg^{-1}	2.129 ± 3.6	2.016 ± 0.12	0.05
r.p.m.	102.7 ± 3.6	100 ± 1.0	n.s.
300 m			
W·kg^{-1}	5.01 ± 0.24	4.62 ± 0.57	0.05
J·paddle^{-1}·kg^{-1}	2.360 ± 0.15	2.310 ± 0.10	n.s.
r.p.m.	127.0 ± 7	119 ± 10	0.05

Values are mean ± s.d.; n.s., not significant; r.p.m., revolutions per min.

Table 60.6 Comparison between top-level and good-level athletes using non-specific tests. The performance of top-level athletes in running, traction and pushing with weights did not differ from that of good-level athletes.

	Top level	Good level	P	Student's *t* test
Swimming 100 m (s)	77 ± 8	90 ± 15	0.05	2.22
Swimming 300 m (s)	284 ± 38	327 ± 56	0.05	1.82
Running 1200 m (s)	247 ± 27	231 ± 8	n.s.	1.51
Tractions on bench (rep·50 kg^{-1}·60 s^{-1})	40.4 ± 5	40.4 ± 6.8	n.s.	0.02
Push on bench (rep·50 kg^{-1}·60 s^{-1})	34.6 ± 9.8	33.6 ± 4.8	n.s.	0.24
Tractions on bar (rep·60 s^{-1})	43.8 ± 6.8	47.1 ± 12	n.s.	0.69

Values are mean ± s.d.; n.s., not significant; rep, repetitions.

technical and muscular adaptations that can be detected either by means of specific tests that reproduce the race situation or on the field.

Cardiovascular system

Echocardiography has produced some interesting data on the heart volumes and ventricular mass of canoeists and kayakers. Values are similar to those of athletes who practice middle-distance running events (Table 60.9). Similar results are obtained when data are related to body surface area (Fig. 60.4) (Pelliccia et al. 1991).

Sidney and Shephard (1973) noted that the resting heart rate of their sample of whitewater canoeists was relatively high: they reported values of 71 beats·min⁻¹ in young male competitors.

The systolic blood pressure is relatively high in this class of athletes, around 135 mmHg. Armand (1983) attributes this to a high stroke volume and to a blockage of the peripheral circulation by the thoracic ribcage during paddling. The lung volumes are not particularly remarkable and within the average range for body size. However, Sidney and Shephard (1973) found a relatively high correlation between lung volumes and performance (0.64 for the absolute vital capacity and 0.69 for the percentage according to age and height standards).

Table 60.8 Comparison between metabolic parameters in top-level and good-level athletes during kayak ergometer tests simulating the distance of 1000 m (duration 4 min). The only statistically significant difference is in mechanical efficiency.

	Top level	Good level	P
Oxygen consumption (ml·kg⁻¹)			
0–1 min	21 ± 3	21 ± 4	n.s.
1–2 min	52 ± 4	51 ± 4	n.s.
2–3 min	54 ± 3	53 ± 4	n.s.
3–4 min	53 ± 3	53.5 ± 5	n.s.
Efficiency (%)	14.6 ± 0.74	13.4 ± 0.51	0.005

Values are mean ± s.d.; n.s., not significant.

Conclusions

The aforementioned differences in level of

Table 60.9 Left ventricular end-diastolic volume and left ventricular mass (mean value ± s.d.) in aerobic sports. From Pelliccia et al. (1991).

	Left ventricular end-diastolic volume (ml)	Left ventricular mass (g)
Males		
Cross-country skiing	167 ± 14	314 ± 46
Walking	121 ± 6	255 ± 20
Marathon	162 ± 16	332 ± 42
Long-distance running	151 ± 22	258 ± 12
Middle-distance running	163 ± 8	336 ± 28
Canoeing	162 ± 14	388 ± 52
Rowing	168 ± 23	365 ± 55
Cycling	164 ± 30	355 ± 80
Control	118 ± 22	197 ± 36
Females		
Cross-country skiing	111 ± 16	213 ± 31
Marathon	122 ± 30	228 ± 19
Long-distance running	104 ± 10	183 ± 18
Middle-distance running	115 ± 10	227 ± 22
Cycling	121 ± 12	251 ± 19

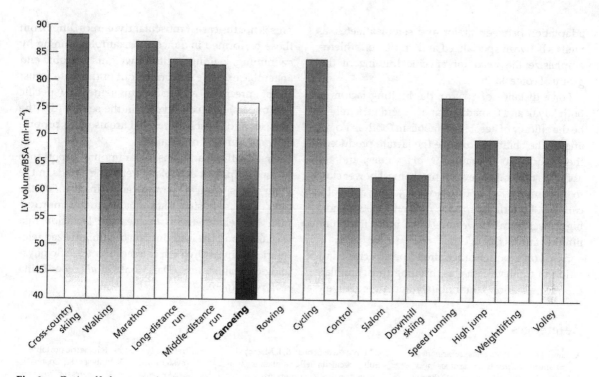

Fig. 60.4 Ratio of left ventricular (LV) volume to body surface area (BSA) in male athletes (aerobic and anaerobic sports).

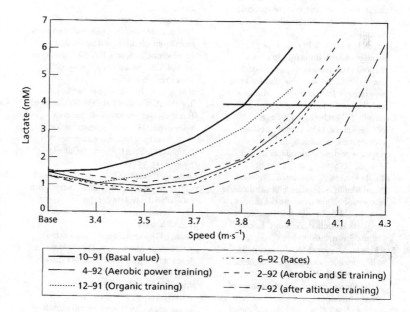

Fig. 60.5 Training monitoring of kayaking. The figure shows the results of six tests completed by a top-level Italian kayaker before the Olympic Games of Barcelona 1992. The tests were established to detect the lactate/velocity curve and were carried out in the field. The last test was carried out after a period of residence at an altitude training camp.

— 10–91 (Basal value)   ····· 6–92 (Races)

— 4–92 (Aerobic power training)   – – – 2–92 (Aerobic and SE training)

········ 12–91 (Organic training)   — — 7–92 (after altitude training) adaptation between junior and senior athletes, as well as between specialized and 'top-level' athletes, emphasize the need for specific training of this group of contestants.

For a distance of 1000m, the limiting factors in both kayak and Canadian canoes seem generally to be the efficacy of aerobic metabolism (both as $\dot{V}O_{2max}$ and as the ability to oxidize the lactate produced), the capacity to tolerate low pH values, and the ability to maintain a level of mechanical power close to maximum. For a distance of 500m, anaerobic capacity, buffering capacity, oxygen kinetics and a high mechanical power are even more important limiting factors than $\dot{V}O_{2max}$.

Based on experience acquired from specific adaptation in top-level athletes, training must simulate the race situation continuously and progressively.

This is not the case if muscular dynamics differ from those performed in a race, for example, training by swimming, jogging or lifting weights. Aerobic and anaerobic exercise performed out of the water must adopt precisely simulated movements (specific ergometers) that can involve in the same order the muscles and muscle fibres that are used for propulsion and removal of lactate.

On the other hand, it is of paramount importance to use equipment capable of detecting trends in the main physiological parameters directly 'in the field'. This is possible today, thanks to the improvement of field methods to measure lactacidaemia (Fig. 60.5) and the introduction of miniaturized telemetric equipment which can monitor specific physiological parameters (Dal Monte *et al.* 1989; Faina *et al.* 1992, 1996).

References

Armand, J.C. (1983) *Surveillance médicale de l'entrainement d'une équipe de canoe kayak de haut niveau de performance.* MD thesis, Université de Paris Ouest.

Bunc, V., Leso, J., Heller, J., Novak, J., Strejkova, B. & Novotnj, V. (1981) Anaerobic threshold by specific and non-specific load. *Lekar a TV—Physician and Physical Education* 3, 35–37.

Cermak, J., Kuta, I. & Parizkova, J. (1975) Some predispositions for top performance in speed canoeing and their changes during the whole year training programme. *Journal of Sports Medicine and Physical Fitness* 15, 243–251.

Cerretelli, P., Pendergast, D., Paganelli, W.C. & Rennie, D.W. (1979) Effects of specific muscle training on $\dot{V}O_2$ on response and early blood lactate. *Journal of Applied Physiology* 47, 761–769.

Colli, R., Faccini, P., Schermi, C., Introini, E. & Dal Monte, A. (1990) Della valutazione funzionale all'allenamento del canoista. (Functional evaluation and training of canoeists.) Scuola dello Sport. *Rivista di Cultura Sportiva* 18, 26–37.

Dal Monte, A. (1975) Metodologia della valutazione funzionale specifica negli atleti praticanti attività sportive di media e lunga durata. (Methodology of specific functional evaluation of long and middle distance athletes.) *Medicina dello Sport* 28, 323–353.

Dal Monte, A. (1983) *La Valutazione Funzionale dell'Atleta.* (*The Functional Evaluation of Athletes.*) Ed. Sansoni, Florence.

Dal Monte, A. & Leonardi, L.M. (1975) Sulla specificità della valutazione funzionale negli atleti: esperienze sui canoisti. (The specificity of functional evaluation of athletes: data on canoeists.) *Medicina dello Sport* 28, 213–219.

Dal Monte, A. & Leonardi, L.M. (1976) Functional evaluation of kayak paddlers from biomechanical and physiological viewpoints. In: Komi, P. (ed.) *Biomechanics*, Vol. VB., pp. 258–267. University Park Press, Baltimore.

Dal Monte, A., Faina, M., Leonardi, L.M., Todaro, A., Guidi, G. & Petrelli, G. (1989) Il massimo consumo di ossigeno in telemetria. (Maximal oxygen intake measured by telemetric equipment). Scuola dello Sport. *Rivista di Cultura Sportiva* 15, 35–44.

D'Angelo, R., Coan, G., Mazzanti, L., Perli, C.P. & Trompetto, M. (1987) Costruzione ed analisi dei test da campo. (Planning and evaluation of field tests.) *Canoa Ricerca* 2, 9–14.

Dransart, G. (1977) *Contribution à la connaissance du canoe kayak.* Thesis, National Institute of Sport and Physical Education, Paris.

Faina, M., Marini, C., Sardella, F. *et al.* (1992) La scienza ed il controllo dell'allenamento. (Sport science and monitoring of training.) Scuola dello Sport. *Rivista di Cultura Sportiva* 26, 7–14.

Faina, M., Pistelli, R., Franzoso, G., Petrelli, G. & Dal Monte, A. (1996) Validity and

reliability of a new telemetric portable system with CO_2 analyser (K4 Cosmed). In: *Proceedings of 1st Congress of European College of Sports Science (ECSS)*, Nice, p. 572.

Faina, M., Billat, V., Squadrone, R., De Angelis, M., Koralstein, J.P. & Dal Monte, A. (1997) Anaerobic contribution to the time to exhaustion at the minimal exercise intensity at which maximal oxygen uptake occurs in élite cyclists, kayakists and swimmers. *European Journal of Applied Physiology* 76, 13–20.

Gollnick, P.D., Armstrong, R.B., Saubert, I.V.C.W., Piehl, K. & Saltin, B. (1972) Enzyme activity and fiber composition in skeletal muscle of trained and untrained men. *Journal of Applied Physiology* 33, 312–319.

Heller, J., Bunc, V. & Kuta, M. (1983) *Functional predisposition for top canoe and kayak performance*, p. 15 (abstract). International Congress on Sport and Health, Maastricht.

Heller, J., Bunc, V., Novak, J. & Kuta, I. (1984) A comparison of bicycle, paddling and treadmill spiroergometry in top paddlers. In: Lollgen, H. & Mellerowicz, H. (eds) *Progress in Ergometry: Quality Control and Test Criteria*, pp. 236–241. Springer, Berlin.

Hirata, K. (1977) *Selection of Olympic Champions*, Vols 1 & 2. Karger Publishers, Basel.

Horvath, S.M. & Finney, B.R. (1969) Paddling experiments and the question of Polynesian voyaging. *American Anthropology* **71**, 271–276.

Paselli, L., Dal Monte, A., Faccini, P. & Faina, M. (1986) Fosfati e prestazione fisiche. (Phosphates and performance.) *Canoa Ricerca* **1**, 3–11.

Pelliccia, A., Maron, B.J., Spataro, A., Proschan, M.A. & Spirito, P. (1991) The upper limit of physiologic cardiac hypertrophy in highly trained elite athletes. *New England Journal of Medicine* **324**, 295–301.

Perri, O., Dal Santo, A., Haszik, E. & Toth, A. (1990) La tecnica di pagaiata in kayak e canadese. (Paddling technique in kayaking and canoeing.) *Canoa Ricerca* **5**, 5–15.

Rusko, H., Havu, M. & Karvinen, E. (1978) Aerobic performance capacity in athletes. *European Journal of Applied Physiology* **38**, 151–159.

Shephard, R.J. (1987) Science and medicine of canoeing and kayaking. *Sports Medicine* **4**, 19–33.

Sidney, K.H. & Shephard, R.J. (1973) Physiological characteristics and performance of the whitewater paddler. *European Journal of Applied Physiology* **32**, 55–70.

Tesch, P. & Karlsson, J. (1985) Muscle fiber type and size in trained and untrained muscles of elite athletes. *Journal of Applied Physiology* **59**, 1716–1720.

Tesch, P. & Lindberg, S. (1984) Blood lactate accumulation during arm exercise in world class kayak paddlers and strength-trained athletes. *European Journal of Applied Physiology* **52**, 441–445.

Tesch, P., Piehl, K., Wilson, G. & Karlson, J.

(1976) Physiological investigations of Swedish élite canoe competitors. *Medicine and Science in Sports* **8**, 214–218.

Vaccaro, P., Clarke, D.H., Morris, A.F. & Gray, P.R. (1984) Physiological characteristics of the world champion whitewater slalom team. In: Bachl, N., Prokop, L. & Suckert, R. (eds) *Current Topics in Sports Medicine*, pp. 637–647. Urban & Schwarzenberg, Vienna.

Vandewalle, H., Pers, G. & Monod, H. (1983) Relation force–vitesse lors d'exercises cycliques realisés avec les membres supérieurs. *Motricité Humaine* **2**, 22–25.

Vrijens, J., Hoestra, P., Bouckaert, J. & Van Vytvanck, P. (1975) Effects of training on maximal work capacity and haemodynamics response during arm and leg exercise in a group of paddlers. *European Journal of Applied Physiology* **36**, 113–119.

Chapter 61

Endurance Aspects of Soccer and Other Field Games

THOMAS REILLY

Introduction

Field games impose different physiological demands on participants than do individual sports such as running, cycling and swimming, where activity is continuous. Exercise in field games is intermittent, brief recovery periods or pauses intervening between exercise bouts. The intensity and duration of activity vary in an irregular manner. In all field games there is an underlying reliance on aerobic metabolic processes, but the energy provided for the critical actions of match-play may be largely anaerobic. It is nevertheless imprudent to generalize to all field games, despite their common characteristics, since each of the sports has unique aspects.

Pitch dimensions vary among games, the largest being for Australian Rules and the Gaelic games (football and hurling), and field hockey having relatively the smallest area for play. The number of players allowed on the field at one time (and the freedom to substitute players) also differs among games. Within those football codes in which use of the hand is permitted, exchange of players is relatively rigid for the rugby games and more fluid for American football. In association football (soccer), use of the hand is prohibited, whereas use of the foot is illegal in hockey, the goalkeeper being excepted in both cases. The professional games (Rugby Union, Rugby League, American football, soccer) are more systematized than are the amateur games (field hockey, Australian Rules, lacrosse and the Gaelic games codes) in terms of training and remuneration of players. There are also mini-football versions of the football games, e.g. seven-a-side for outdoor

play and four- or five-a-side for indoor soccer. The 'Rugby-Sevens' form of Rugby Union had its first world championships in 1993 and was introduced to the Commonwealth Games in Malaysia in 1998. A hybrid version of Australian Rules and Gaelic football, 'Compromise Rules', combines these two codes, so that teams from each subdiscipline can compete against one another.

The theme of this chapter is endurance in the context of the major field games. Emphasis is placed first on soccer. It is the leading sport world-wide and has attracted more attention from researchers than any of the other games. The rugby codes are then considered together, followed by the national codes. Special attention is given to field hockey; the other stick-and-ball games (hurling and lacrosse) are evaluated together.

For each of the sports discussed, the demands of the game are covered initially. The intensity of exercise and physiological responses to match-play are reviewed. Of the many factors influencing performance in the game, those related to endurance are identified. The fitness characteristics of players provide insights into how individual capabilities match the games' demands. Consideration is also given to training and the problems of preparing for competition in the different games.

The physiological demands of association football (soccer)

Activity profiles

The physiological demands of soccer are indicated

by the exercise intensities at which players perform their many activities during match-play. This exercise pattern has implications for the fitness of players and for the designing of appropriate training regimens. The training and competitive schedules of players and their habitual activities determine their daily energy expenditures and hence their nutritional requirements. There are repercussions also for injury prevention and proper rehabilitation following soft tissue injuries.

The exercise intensity during competitive soccer can be gauged by the overall distance covered. This index represents a global measure of energy expended, encompassing all the discrete movements of an individual player over a whole game. Activities can be classified according to type (action), intensity (quality), duration (distance) and frequency. Juxtaposing the activity profile on a time base allows average exercise-to-rest ratios to be calculated. These ratios may be used in physiological studies that model the demands of soccer, and they also help in the design of soccer players' training programmes. Information from these profiles can be augmented by monitoring physiological responses during actual or simulated play.

Motion analysis has been conducted on national league players; the various methods of recording

activities were reviewed by Reilly (1994). The most comprehensive system employed to date utilizes six cameras from vantage points high in the stands. Linked to a computer, such monitors enable the intensity of effort to be documented for an entire team during the game. Whatever method is adopted must comply with quality control specifications of validity and reliability.

A summary of the overall activity patterns reported in the literature (Table 61.1) indicates that outfield players cover a distance of 8–12 km during a match, movement being more or less continuous. The overall distance covered during a game masks frequent changes in activities; each player completes about 1000 different activities in a typical game, representing a change in either the level or the type of activity every 6 s. Alterations in the pace and direction of movement also incorporate game skills and the tracking of opponents' movements.

The distance covered by outfield players during a match consists of 25% walking, 37% jogging, 20% submaximal cruising, 11% sprinting and 7% moving backwards (Reilly 1997a). Within these broad categories are included sideways and diagonal movements. These proportions (Fig. 61.1) are representative of contemporary play in the European top leagues, in international tournaments

Table 61.1 Mean distance covered per soccer game according to various sources. Original sources are in Reilly (1994) and Rienzi et al. (1998).

Source and year	n	Distance covered (m)	Method
Czechoslovakia (1967)	1	11 500	Undisclosed
Sweden (1970)	10	10 200	Cine-film
Sweden (1973)	9	10 900	Cine-film
England (1974)	40	4834	Hand notation
England (1976)	40	8680	Tape-recorder
Finland (1980)	7	7100	TV cameras (two)
Japan (1981)	–	9971	Trigonometry
Australia (1982)	20	11 527	Video
Sweden (1986)	10	9800	Hand notation
Japan (1988)	2	9845	Trigonometry (two cameras)
Belgium (1988)	7	10 245	Cine-film
Denmark (1991)	14	10 800	Video (24 cameras)
Japan (1991)	50	11 529	Trigonometry
Uruguay (1998)	17	8638	Video

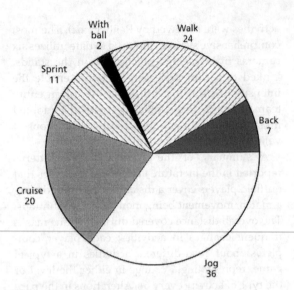

Fig. 61.1 Proportion of various categories of activity during soccer match-play (from Reilly 1996).

and at top-level matches in Japan (Ogushi *et al.* 1993).

Cruising (striding) and sprinting can be combined to represent high-intensity activity in soccer. The ratio of low-intensity to high-intensity exercise is then about 2.2:1 in terms of distance covered, but is about 7:1 in terms of time. This proportion denotes a predominantly aerobic outlay of energy. Each outfield player has a short rest pause, averaging only 3 s every 2 min; rest breaks are longer and occur more frequently at lower levels of play, where players are more reluctant to run to support a colleague in possession of the ball. Less than 2% of the total distance covered by top players is with possession of the ball. Actions are mainly 'off the ball', running to contest possession, supporting team mates, counter running by a marking player, jumping for the ball, tackling an opponent, or playing the ball with one touch only.

Whilst the majority of activity during a top-level game is submaximal, high-intensity efforts are extremely important. Players generally have to run with effort (cruise) or sprint every 30 s, but on average sprint all-out only once every 90 s. The timing of these anaerobic efforts, whether in posses-

sion of the ball or without, is crucial, since their success may determine the outcome of the game.

Factors affecting intensity of effort

The team configuration in contemporary top-level soccer is relatively flexible; nevertheless, the intensity of effort is influenced by a player's positional role. The greatest distances are covered by midfield players, who act as links between defence and attack (see Reilly 1996). Among English league players, the full-backs have shown the greatest versatility (Fig. 61.2). Although they cover more overall distance than the centre-backs, they sprint less. The greatest distances covered in sprinting are by strikers and midfield players. The greatest overall distance covered is found in players who undertake more running at low speeds. This profile denotes an aerobic type of activity for midfield players in particular. A more anaerobic profile is displayed by the centre-back, sweeper or libero. The pace of walking is slower in centre-backs than for any other outfield position (Reilly & Thomas 1976). Centre-backs and strikers jump more frequently than full-backs or midfield players. However, the frequency of once every 5–6 min indicates that jump endurance may not be particularly important in soccer.

The goalkeeper covers about 4 km during a match (Reilly & Thomas 1976). Time spent standing still is much greater than for outfield players. Their activity profile emphasizes anaerobic efforts of brief duration, when the goalkeeper is directly involved in play. The goalkeeper is engaged in play more than any outfield player; nevertheless, this involvement has been reduced by the rule introduced in 1992, which prevents back-passes from defenders. This rule has had only a marginal effect on the activities of outfield players. The endurance training requirements for playing outfield are not necessary for the goalkeeper.

The ability to exercise at a high power output depends on the maximal aerobic power ($\dot{V}o_{2max}$), but the upper limit at which continuous exercise can be maintained is influenced by the so-called 'anaerobic threshold' and a high fractional utilization of $\dot{V}o_{2max}$. Soccer play calls for an oxygen intake of

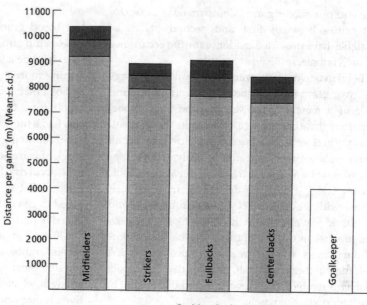

Fig. 61.2 Distance covered per game according to positional roles (from Reilly & Thomas 1976).

roughly 75% $\dot{V}_{O_{2max}}$ (Bangsbø 1994a,b), a value which is close to the 'anaerobic threshold' of top soccer players. The $\dot{V}_{O_{2max}}$ of English league players is correlated significantly with the distance covered in a game, underlining the need for aerobic fitness, particularly in midfield players (Reilly 1994). The $\dot{V}_{O_{2max}}$ also influences the number of sprints that players attempt (Smaros 1980). Bangsbø and Lindquist (1992) showed that the distance covered during a game was correlated with performance in a continuous 2.16-km field test, and also with the $\dot{V}_{O_{2max}}$ and the $\dot{V}_{O_2}$ corresponding to a blood lactate level of 3mM. It seems the intensity of effort in soccer matches depends on physiological indications of aerobic fitness as found in endurance athletes.

The style of play may influence a player's energy expenditures. Emphasis on retaining possession of the ball, controlling the pace of the game and delaying attacking moves until opportunities to penetrate defensive line-ups are presented underlines the dependence on speed and timing of movement in such critical phases of the game. Conversely, the direct method of play, as used by the Ireland team in the 1990 World Cup and later by Norway in 1994

and 1998, raises the overall pace of the game. The main elements are fast transfer of the ball from defence to attack to create scoring chances, use of long passes rather than a sequence of short passes, exploitation of defensive errors, harrying opponents into mistakes when they possess the ball, and alternating midfield players to support the strikers when they are on the offensive (Reilly 1996). This style of play has an equalizing effect on the energy expenditure of outfield players, since they are expected to exercise at a high intensity 'off the ball' and throughout all the playing zones of the field. A similar levelling of aerobic fitness demands applies to the 'total football' style, exhibited first by the Netherlands national side in the 1970s and characteristic of current top European club sides. The pace of play in international matches within South America is more rhythmic than in Europe; as a result players cover about 1 km less during a game (Rienzi *et al.* 1998).

Fatigue

Fatigue is defined as a decline in performance and is manifest as a deterioration in power output towards the end of a soccer game. Comparisons of exercise intensities between first and second halves of matches have provided evidence for the occurrence of such fatigue.

Belgian university players were found on average to cover 444 m more in the first than in the second half of a match. Likewise, Bangsbø *et al.* (1991) reported that the distance covered in the first half was 5% greater than in the second. However, not all players show such a decrement. Reilly and Thomas (1976) noted an inverse relation between aerobic power ($\dot{V}_{O_{2max}}$) and the decrement in work rate. Those with the higher $\dot{V}_{O_{2max}}$ values, midfield and full-back players, were the least likely to show fatigue. In contrast, all of the centre-backs and 86% of the strikers covered greater distances in the first half than in the second half. It seems that the impact of a high aerobic fitness level is especially evident in the later parts of a match.

The amount of glycogen stored in the leg muscles prematch appears to be an important determinant of resistance to fatigue. Swedish club players with a low glycogen content in the vastus lateralis muscle covered 25% less overall distance than the other players (Saltin 1973). A more marked effect was noted for running speed; those with low muscle glycogen stores prematch covered 50% of the total distance walking and 15% at top speed compared to 27% walking and 24% sprinting for players who started with high muscle glycogen concentrations. Attention to diet and a tapering of training are recommended in the immediate build-up for competition. Benefits would be most evident when drawn matches are extended into 30 min extra time, in 'cup' matches or in the professional 'J' League in Japan, for example.

Whilst goals may be scored at any time, an above-average proportion are scored towards the end of a game. In the 1998 World Cup finals, a higher than average scoring rate was evident for the final 15 min of play. This cannot be explained simply by a fall in power output of players, since this should be balanced out between the two opposing teams. Deteriorations of performance among defenders may give an advantage to attackers towards the end of a game. Alternatively, the late scores may be linked with 'mental fatigue', lapses in concentration as a consequence of sustained physical effort and/or a low blood glucose level leading to tactical errors and opening up goal-scoring chances. The phenomenon may be a factor inherent in the game, play becoming more urgent and adventurous towards the end of a match despite a fall in the players' physical capabilities. Goals scored in the 1998 World Cup also had a higher than expected incidence in the first 3 min following half-time: whether this is related to a lack of warm-up or a lapse similar to that assumed to be occurring late in the game is unknown. Clearly, a team that is physiologically and tactically prepared to last 90 min of intense play is likely to be an effective unit.

Gleeson *et al.* (1998) investigated the effects of endurance exercise, designed to simulate the physiological demands of match-play, on leg strength, electromechanical delay and knee laxity. Even though peak torque was preserved following the activity, the authors considered that the risk of ligamentous damage may be increased by a concomitant impairment of electromechanical delay and anterior tibiofemoral displacement.

Environmental conditions can impose a limit on the exercise intensity that is maintained throughout a soccer game, and/or hasten the onset of fatigue during a match. Major soccer tournaments are often held in hot conditions with ambient temperatures around 30°C. The intensity of effort is adversely affected when such conditions are combined with high humidity. Performance is influenced both by the rise in core temperature and by dehydration, and sweat production is ineffective in dissipating body heat when the relative humidity approaches 100%. During 90 min of continuous exercise, cognitive function, akin to the kind of decision-making required during match-play, is better maintained when fluid is supplied intermittently than in a control condition (Reilly & Lewis 1985). Adequate hydration pre-exercise and during intermissions is important when players have to play in the heat. The opportunity to acclimatize to heat prior to competing in tournaments in hot climates is an essential element of preparing for such events. Acclimatization may be achieved in training camps, a good physiological adaptation being realized within 10–14 days of initial exposure to hot weather. Alternatively, regular repeated exposures to heat in an environmental chamber are partially effective.

The major consequence of playing in cold conditions is likely to be an increased liability to injury. Icy pitches that lack facilities for underground heating promote risk. Muscle performance deteriorates as muscle temperature falls below optimum; a good warm-up prior to playing in cold weather and the use of appropriate sportswear (more than one layer) to maintain core body temperature and avoid the deterioration in performance synonymous with fatigue are important. Injury is more likely to occur if the warm-up routine is inappropriate (Reilly & Stirling 1993). Therefore, prematch exercises should engage the muscle groups employed during the game, particularly in executing soccer skills.

Physiological responses to match-play

The relative metabolic loading during soccer play can be calculated, given direct measurements for both energy expenditure during competition and $\dot{V}_{O_{2max}}$. Analysis of expired air collected in Douglas bags has indicated energy expenditure rates of $22–44\,kJ\cdot min^{-1}$ and $32.2\,kJ\cdot min^{-1}$ in two studies (see Reilly 1996). These values are probably underestimates, due to the restrictions placed on players by the apparatus and also the low skill levels of the subjects investigated. Seliger (1968a,b) reported values of $54.8\,kJ\cdot min^{-1}$ for energy expenditure and $76\,l\cdot min^{-1}$ for minute ventilation in Czech players. The $\dot{V}_{O_2}$ of $35.5\,ml\cdot kg^{-1}\cdot min^{-1}$ agrees with figures of $35–38$ and $29–30\,ml\cdot kg^{-1}\cdot min^{-1}$ for Japanese players (Kawakami et al. 1992). An alternative research strategy is to measure the heart rate during match-play and to juxtapose the observations on heart rate–$\dot{V}_{O_2}$ regression lines determined during running on a treadmill. The heart rate itself is a useful indicator of the overall physiological strain.

The circulatory strain is relatively high and does not fluctuate greatly during a game. The heart rate is about 77% of the heart rate range (maximal minus resting heart rate) for 66% of the playing time (Rohde & Espersen 1988). For a large part of the remaining time, the heart rate exceeds this level.

The heart rate during soccer varies with the exercise intensity and so may differ between playing positions and between the first and second half of a game. Van Gool et al. (1988) reported mean figures of 155 beats·min^{-1} for a centre-back and a full-back, 170 beats·min^{-1} for a midfield player and 168 and 171 beats·min^{-1} for two forwards. These values were closely related to the distances covered by the corresponding players in a match. Mean values for a Belgian university team were 169 beats·min^{-1} in the first half and 165 beats·min^{-1} in the second half of a friendly match (Van Gool et al. 1988). Again, the physiological responses reflected a drop in energy expenditures during the second half. These trends have been confirmed in matches played by English university teams (Florida-James & Reilly 1995).

Several studies have employed heart rate to estimate the relative metabolic loading during match-play. Generally, the exercise intensity during soccer is about 75% of $\dot{V}_{O_{2max}}$ and heart rate averages 170 beats·min^{-1}. Use of heart rate regressions may overestimate the real $\dot{V}_{O_2}$, but the error is generally small (Bangsbø 1994a).

Progressively higher blood lactate levels during matches have been observed on progressing from the fourth to the top division in the Swedish league (Ekblom 1986). Higher blood lactate levels were associated with person-to-person marking roles when compared with zone coverage responsibility (Gerisch et al. 1988). Peak values above 12 mM were frequently observed in higher league players (Ekblom 1986). Physical activity cannot be sustained continuously under such conditions which reflect the intermittent consequences of anaerobic metabolism during competition. Whilst other studies of blood lactate concentration have yielded values of 4–6 mM during play (Table 61.2), such measures are determined by the activity just prior to blood sam-

Table 61.2 Mean (± s.d.) blood lactate concentrations (mM) during soccer.

1st half	2nd half	Reference
5.1 ± 1.6	3.9 ± 1.6	Rohde & Espersen (1988)
5.6 ± 2.0	4.7 ± 2.2	Gerisch et al. (1988)
4.9	3.7	Bangsbø et al. (1991)
4.4 ± 1.2	4.5 ± 2.1	Florida-James & Reilly (1995)

pling. Consequently, higher values are noted at half-time compared to the end of the match.

Muscle glycogen appears to be the most important substrate for the exercising muscles during soccer play. Glucose taken up from the blood and lipids mobilized from triglyceride stores become important towards the end of a game. The metabolic responses closely resemble those of endurance runners, for whom the sparing of muscle glycogen stores is important to overall performance.

Physiology of game-related activities

The total distance covered in a game underrepresents the energy expended, because it does not take account of the extra demands of game skills and match events. These demands include frequent accelerations and decelerations, angular runs, changes of direction, jumps to contest possession, tackles, avoidance of tackles and other multiple aspects of involvement in play. There have been attempts to quantify the additional physiological demands of game skills over and above the physiological cost of locomotion.

Reilly and Ball (1984) examined physiological responses to dribbling a soccer ball at four different speeds, each for 5 min. A rebound box on the front of a treadmill returned the ball to the player's feet after each touch. The simulation allowed precise control over the player's activity while expired air, blood lactate and perceived exertion were measured. The energy cost of dribbling, with one touch of the ball every 2–3 full stride cycles, increased linearly with running speed. The added cost of dribbling averaged $5.2 \, \text{kJ·min}^{-1}$ (Fig. 61.3).

When dribbling the ball, the player's stride rate increases and the stride length shortens compared with normal running at the same speed; these changes add to the energy cost. Changing stride length from that freely chosen by the individual increases the $\dot{V}O_2$ for a given speed (Cavanagh & Williams 1992). The energy cost is further accentuated by changing stride irregularly, or feigning lateral movements whilst possessing the ball in order to outwit an opponent. Stride length must be reduced when dribbling in order to control the ball properly and propel it forward with the right amount of force. The energy cost is also increased by the muscle activity required to kick the ball and the action of synergistic and stabilizing muscles to maintain balance while the ball is being kicked.

Blood lactate levels and perceived exertion are elevated as a consequence of dribbling the ball, lactate increasing disproportionately at high speeds (Fig. 61.3). Reilly and Ball (1984) estimated that the lactate inflection point occurred at a speed of

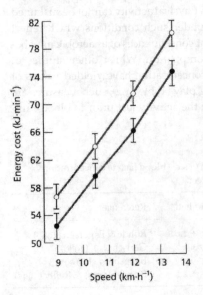

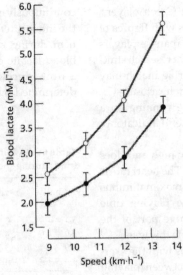

Fig. 61.3 The added physiological cost of dribbling a soccer ball at four different speeds (from Reilly & Ball 1984).

10.7 km·h^{-1} for dribbling but not until 11.7 km·h^{-1} in normal running. The metabolic strain of fast dribbling is underestimated unless the additional anaerobic loading is considered.

Moving backwards or sideways can account for 16% of the distance covered by players. The percentage is highest in defenders who often must back up quickly under high forward kicks from the opposition's half, or move sideways when jostling for position before making a tackle. The added physiological costs of unorthodox movements have been examined by getting nine soccer players to run on a treadmill at three different speeds whilst running normally, running backwards and running sideways (Reilly & Bowen 1984). The extra energy cost of the unorthodox movements increased disproportionately with the speed of movement. There was no difference in energy expenditure or perceived exertion between running backwards or sideways (Table 61.3). Improving muscular efficiency during these unorthodox modes of movement should benefit the player's performance.

Fitness measures

As the capability for a high energy expenditure is important in soccer, top players tend to have a high level of aerobic fitness. The significance of aerobic fitness was demonstrated by Apor (1988); the mean $\dot{V}O_{2max}$ of top Hungarian teams was inversely related to their position in the league. Wisloff et al. (1998) confirmed the relationship between maximal aerobic power ($\dot{V}O_{2max}$) and performance in the Norwegian soccer league. The mean $\dot{V}O_{2max}$ of 29 players was 63.7 ml·kg^{-1}·min^{-1}: the authors concluded that the $\dot{V}O_{2max}$ should be scaled by a factor of 0.75 when evaluating aerobic power of soccer players, to allow for the influence of body size. Whilst the $\dot{V}O_{2max}$ does not necessarily limit performance in soccer, the high values observed in élite players underline the aerobic contribution to play. This point is further emphasized by the physiological characteristics of muscle samples taken from soccer players.

Oxidative enzyme activities in leg muscle biopsies of Danish players taken at the time of full training were characteristic of endurance-trained athletes (Bangsbø & Mizuno 1988). Findings in Finnish and Japanese players were similar. Smaros (1980) reported that glycogen depletion occurred mainly in slow-twitch muscle fibres, reflecting the aerobic regimens of match-play. The fibre type distribution tends to be mixed, and exhibits a wide range within a team (see Bangsbø 1994b).

Training and habitual activities

The dimensions of the training programme—intensity, frequency, duration and mode of exercise—are manipulated by the trainer. The stimuli therefore depend on how the training regimens are organized. A fundamental principle is that training should be specific to game requirements. The training classification shown in Fig. 61.4 depicts the proportionate allocation of time adopted traditionally in English league soccer (Reilly 1979).

The training intensity as reflected by the mean heart rate is indicated in Table 61.4. Players are prepared to endure higher physiological stresses when engaged in actual matches. Field-based drills without the ball are relatively unreliable, so activity patterns from the game should be incorporated into training regimens where possible.

There is a need for balance among the integral components of a training programme. Preseason regimens usually emphasize aerobic training stimuli, which may interfere with the development

Table 61.3 Mean (±s.d.) for energy expended and ratings of exertion at three speeds and three directional modes of motion ($n = 9$). From Reilly and Bowen (1984).

Speed (km·h^{-1})	Direction of motion		
	Forwards	Backwards	Sideways
	Energy expended (kJ·min^{-1})		
5	37.0 ± 2.6	44.8 ± 6.1	46.6 ± 3.2
7	42.3 ± 1.7	53.4 ± 3.5	56.3 ± 6.1
9	50.6 ± 4.9	71.4 ± 7.0	71.0 ± 7.5
	Perceived exertion (Borg units)		
5	6.7 ± 0.1	8.6 ± 2.0	8.7 ± 2.0
7	8.0 ± 1.4	11.2 ± 2.9	11.3 ± 3.2
9	10.2 ± 2.1	14.0 ± 2.0	13.8 ± 2.5

Table 61.4 Heart rates (± s.d.) and estimated energy expenditure during various components of soccer training. From Reilly (1990).

	Heart rate (beats·min^{-1})	Energy expended (kJ·min^{-1})
Warm-up	120 ± 2	38.9
Flexibility	112 ± 3	31.4
Running	144 ± 4	58.6
Circuit and weight training	125 ± 4	43.1
Skills practice	128 ± 5	45.2
Drills	137 ± 4	53.6
Games	157 ± 7	68.6
Recovery periods	102 ± 3	22.6

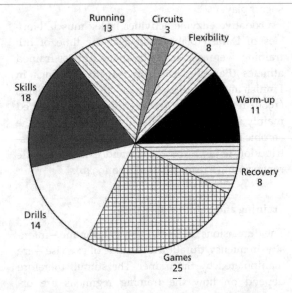

Fig. 61.4 Distribution of time in training according to its components.

of muscle strength (Reilly & Thomas 1977). During the competitive season, the aerobic fitness tends to remain stable. Muscle strength is depressed at the start of the playing season, and at this time, players may be more vulnerable to injury. Players with greater muscle strength at the start of a season are more likely to remain injury free throughout the season (Reilly & Thomas 1980).

Typically, soccer players compete each weekend. This schedule permits a gradual build-up to a peak training load in midweek, and a tapering off in preparation for match-play (Fig. 61.5). This pattern

of conditioning safeguards the player against overtraining and a reduction of prematch muscle glycogen levels (Reilly & Thomas 1979). This regimen cannot be employed when players have a hectic competitive schedule, including extra matches midweek. Under such circumstances, only certain components of physiological training can be included between matches and the matches themselves provide the major physiological stimuli. Emphasis should be placed on accelerating recovery following each game so that players are prepared fully for the subsequent game. Priorities are warmdown after the game, restoration of fluid and energy losses soon afterwards and appropriate modification of training on the next day.

Variations in energy expenditure over the week have implications for the way footballers organize their diets. The dietary practices of soccer players tend to be imperfect, in terms of both overall energy intake and the distribution of macronutrients (Piearce 1993). Recommendations for soccer players are 10–12% protein, 25% fat and 65–70% carbohydrate, compared to respective percentages of 12, 42 and 46 in the normal population. Manipulating the nutritional intake of players enhances both performance in training (Miles *et al.* 1992) and resynthesis of muscle glycogen following competition (see Reilly 1990).

Top soccer teams experience phases during the season when recovery between successive matches is short, for instance when cup and league matches are played in the same week. The high frequency of full-scale competitive engagements may compro-

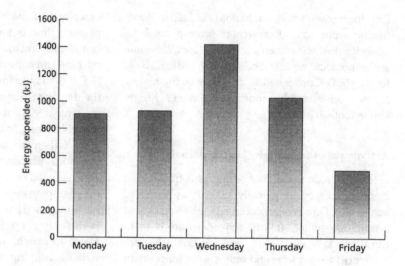

Fig. 61.5 Distribution of average energy expended in training within a professional soccer team according to the day of the week (from Reilly & Thomas 1979).

mise the immune system. The immune system may be depressed following strenuous exercise, but usually returns to resting values within 20 h. Rebelo *et al.* (1998) failed to provide evidence of any immune system impairment in soccer players during a season of intense training and competition. Nevertheless, following matches during the high-frequency phase of the competitive season, players should take steps to restore fluids and energy following a match and to speed recovery before the next engagement.

The physiology of rugby football

Historical introduction

Rugby Union had been nurtured in the grammar schools of England. The Union split off from the professional game of Rugby League in 1895 (following the breakaway of the Northern Union 2 years earlier), with league players coming mainly from a working-class background in northern England. The divide was complete until 1995, when Rugby Union became professional. Rugby Union is played in more countries than is Rugby League. The first World Cup competition was held in Australia and New Zealand in 1987; subsequent championships were located in Great Britain and France (1991), South Africa (1995) and Wales (1999). New Zealand, Australia, South Africa and Australia again were

victorious in the first four tournaments, the inauguration of which marked the escalation of scientific approaches towards preparing teams. The demands of Rugby League and Rugby Union have been reviewed elsewhere (Brewer & Davis 1995; Reilly 1997b). The focus here is primarily on Rugby Union, with observations on endurance aspects of Rugby League where appropriate. The physiological demands are outlined first; then fitness and training aspects of the game are considered.

Many factors determine the physiological load on individual players. Each positional role in rugby football has its unique demands, and there is less homogeneity among these roles than in soccer. The type and frequency of training also vary with the level of play. Game performance relies on tactical awareness, interplay of individuals in tactical moves, competence of players in catching, passing, kicking and tackling, and skills specific to playing position. Rugby Union and Rugby League both require an amalgam of fast reactions, speed, agility, muscular strength and anaerobic and aerobic power, although combined in a complex manner. Nevertheless, an attempt can be made to assess rugby games from a physiological perspective and to match this assessment of physiological responses to match-play with fitness profiles of the players.

The increase in women's participation in football games is reflected in the growing popularity of women's Rugby Union football. The first World

Cup for women's national teams was held in Wales during April 1991. Researchers have given little attention to the women's game, except for some anthropometric reports (Sedlock *et al.* 1988; Kirby & Reilly 1993). Consequently, this part of the review focuses on research reported for men's Rugby Union football.

Activity patterns in Rugby Union football

A Rugby Union game lasts 80 min plus time added by the referee, but it typically has only 25–30 min of actual play. On average, it contains 140 sequences of action. Altogether, 32% of sequences are 0–5 s in duration, 24% are 5–10 s, 29% 10–20 s, 10% are sequences 20–30 s long and only 5% are longer than 30 s. These figures imply an emphasis on anaerobic metabolism during the intense periods of play (56% < 10-s duration) (see Reilly 1997b). The total distance covered in a match may be divided according to the different exercise intensities demanded by discrete activities and it can be complemented by establishing ratios of exercise to rest durations.

The overall distance covered in amateur Rugby Union is 5.5 km for forwards and 3.8 km for backs, with values ranging to a maximum of 9.6 km (Reid & Williams 1974). These distances are relatively modest compared with élite soccer play, even after allowing for the 10 min shorter duration of Rugby Union play. Morton (1978) reported that Rugby Union play comprised 37% walking, 29% jogging and 34% striding/sprinting. Contemporary top-class play emphasizes support of the player with the ball, or seeking to regain it, and this has increased the energy expenditure required of the backs. Australian centre-backs and half-backs (5530 m) and wingers and full-backs (5750 m) covered more ground than props and locks (4400 m) and back-row (4080 m) players over 70 min of under-19 matches (Deutsch *et al.* 1998). Rugby Union players spend more time in 'game-related activities' than players in other football codes, with scrums, rucks and mauls engaging groups of forwards together for protracted periods. About 85% of players' time is spent in low-intensity activity (Docherty *et al.* 1988). Players have to resume formations in order for play to continue following a quick switch of play to the other half of the field. The remaining 15% of the player's time is taken up by intense exercise, 6% being related to running and 9% to tackling, pushing and competing for the ball.

The demands imposed by the game differ from the demands players impose on themselves. Consequently, McLean (1992), in his analysis of the 'Five-Nations Championship', concentrated on the game (when the ball was in play) rather than on individual players' energy expenditures. The analysis was based on video recordings of all matches in the championship. On average, the ball was in play for 29 min each game. The exercise/rest ratio ranged from 1:1 to 1:1.9. These ratios were consistent from match to match, and were later employed in prescribing training and designing field-based tests (McLean 1993). In 63% of cases, the rest exceeded in length the preceding sequence of play; in 37% of cases the rest was shorter than the exercise bout it followed. The exercise periods were mainly in the range 11–25 s, the overall average being 19 s.

The time during five matches at the 1987 Rugby World Cup was divided between 25 min (31%) of play and 55 min (69%) of stoppages. The mean time for single actions was 7.3 s for forwards and 6.5 s for three-quarters; time for stoppages averaged 33 s. During any one match, there were 181 pieces of action, 96 stoppages and 30 scrummages. Altogether, 70% of playing sequences were 4–10 s in duration and 75% of stoppages lasted between 5 and 40 s. Recovery from periods of fast intense play was often incomplete (Menchenelli *et al.* 1992a). Special endurance capabilities were recommended to speed recovery after intense passages of play.

Docherty *et al.* (1988) reported a mean (±s.d.) blood lactate of 2.8 (± 1.6) mM in players at the end of Canadian university matches, reflecting the moderate intensity of exercise at this standard. McLean (1993) tested players in top Scottish clubs, repeated measurements being made during natural breaks in the game (injuries, penalty kicks and so on). Values ranged from 5.8 to 9.8 mM, indicating that competitive rugby can entail appreciable lactate production. Roughly similar values (range 6–12 mM) were reported for top Italian and Argentinian sides (Menchenelli *et al.* 1992b). Values in the blood considerably underestimate concentrations in the active muscles (Chapters 3 and 22). Deutsch *et al.* (1998) showed that the mean blood lactate (4.8–7.2 mM) did not differ between positional roles: they concluded that there was a need for 'lactate tolerance' training to improve hydrogen ion buffering and facilitate lactate removal following high-intensity efforts. Further, the distances covered (4.2–5.6 km in 70 min) and the intermittent nature of match-play indicated a need for sound aerobic conditioning to minimize fatigue in both backs and forwards.

The energy expenditure in competitive rugby was first evaluated by Yamaoka (1965), who calculated an 11-fold average increase of metabolism. Forwards expended more energy (2510–3350 kJ) than backs (1840–2930 kJ). Assuming an average $\dot{V}_{O_2max}$ of 4.5 l·min^{-1}, this expenditure would correspond to an energy expenditure about 52% of $\dot{V}_{O_2max}$. The exercise intensity in contemporary professional Rugby Union may be greater than these findings (particularly among the backs), owing to the faster current pace of play, but it is still below the intensity in soccer (estimated 75% $\dot{V}_{O_2max}$).

Muscle glycogen stores are not exhausted at the end of a rugby match, confirming that the overall energy expenditure is low compared to that observed in soccer. Carbohydrate loading increases carbohydrate utilization during play, but it does not offer the ergogenic benefits seen in endurance athletes. Nevertheless, carbohydrate loading may be advantageous during tournaments, when a number of matches have to be played within a short time. Many teams in the late 1990s have used creatine loading regimens to prepare their players for competition. Whilst creatine loading has proved beneficial in reloading creatine phosphate stores within muscle, its value lies chiefly in preventing a decline in performance during a sequence of high-intensity sprints. Its ergogenic effects in a game context are unproven.

Factors affecting work rate

As the traditional European Rugby Union season spans the winter months, matches may frequently take place in temperatures that are too cold for thermal comfort. Warm-up is especially important in cold conditions, in order to raise body temperature for the more strenuous activities to follow, either in training or in competition. Players attribute about 18% of injuries to inadequate warm-up. To reduce injury risk, the warm-up regimen should include flexibility exercises with actions similar to those employed in the game (Reilly & Stirling 1993). Reilly & Hardiker (1981) reported a greater incidence of injury shortly after half-time than at other points in the game. This was attributed to players getting cold while standing outdoors during the half-time break.

Environmental temperatures during the competitive Rugby Union season are generally much warmer in the southern than in the northern hemisphere. Rugby matches—in Australia and the Southern African countries, in particular—may be played in conditions that precipitate heat stress. Players competing in air temperatures of 24–25 °C had rectal temperatures of 39.4 °C at the end of a game (Doncaster 1972). Temperatures were elevated equally in backs and forwards, but the forwards sweated more, being larger in body size. Rehydration at half-time should follow guidelines designed for soccer players (Maughan & Leiper 1994). More attention should also be given to the fabric of team clothing in conditions where hyperthermia is a risk.

Altitude challenges the oxygen transport system due to the reduction in alveolar oxygen tension. This is likely to affect aerobic performance, $\dot{V}_{O_2max}$ declining by 15% at an altitude of 2280 m (Åstrand & Rodahl 1986). Teams competing in South Africa in the 1995 Rugby Union World Championships had to consider altitude training as a part of their preparation. The physiological adaptations to sojourns at altitude, notably increased red blood cell production stimulated by renal secretion of erythropoietin, have also been employed in attempts to improve aerobic performance at sea-level. Whilst altitude training has been used by some endurance athletes since the early 1970s, its systematic use in Rugby Union has been limited largely to French teams (Bishon 1993).

During the 1995 World Cup tournament, the South African team applied patches to the bridge of the nose with the aims of decreasing nasal resistance and increasing respiratory minute volume ($\dot{V}_E$). The practice was adopted by British players in the subsequent Five-Nations Championship and it spread also to soccer, Rugby League and Gaelic football players. Whilst such patches may have marginal benefits when playing at altitude, they have no physiological justification when players are competing at sea-level. Similarly, the benefit of the provision of pure oxygen to speed recovery in Rugby Union or Rugby League, as in American football, is unsupported by any evidence (Winter *et al.* 1989).

Fitness characteristics of players

ANTHROPOMETRY

Physical characteristics vary widely among rugby players, depending on the positional role, the level of play and the range of skills required by the game. As styles of play are altered to maintain or gain a competitive edge over opponents, so too may the players chosen to implement the game plan vary in their physical characteristics.

The most striking comparison of the anthropometric characteristics of Rugby Union players is between backs and forwards. On average the forwards are 0.2 m taller. The shape and body composition of both Rugby Union and Rugby League players favour strength and muscular power rather than endurance capability.

Body mass is an important factor in Rugby Union, particularly in tackling or breaking tackles. It also bestows an advantage in scrummaging, since forwards find it hard to shove a heavy opposing pack backwards. It is preferable to have this weight as lean body mass rather than as adipose tissue since the latter would constitute an extra load for the muscles to lift repeatedly against gravity in locomotion and in jumping. Forwards can enhance mobility by trimming adipose tissue levels; this indirectly improves their endurance capabilities. The heaviest of the Rugby Union club players studied by Rigg and Reilly (1988) were the second-row forwards (101 ± 7 kg); the lightest were the half-backs, with 24 kg less body mass. Wing-backs were traditionally light, their major requirement being sprinting ability. A recent trend has seen the use of three-quarter line players large in body size and so able to contribute to the other aspects of the game that demand a high power output. Nevertheless, the need to recover quickly from short-term efforts and to reproduce high-intensity bouts after only a brief pause requires a high anaerobic endurance capability.

MUSCLE STRENGTH AND ENDURANCE

Muscle strength is employed in a host of activities during Rugby Union match-play, especially in view of the contact nature of the sport. This feature is even more evident in Rugby League. Muscle strength is required of forwards in all aspects of scrummaging in Rugby Union; force is applied isometrically in the first instance, and is coordinated in a sustained team push. It is also required in rucks and mauls, in ripping the ball from opponents and by all players in tackling and breaking tackles. In many of these contexts, muscle endurance is also required. In view of the many ways in which forces are exerted during a game, muscle strength has been measured by various methods.

Tests of 'muscular fitness' have incorporated both strength and endurance factors. Performance in press-ups (either the number completed at a set rhythm before exhaustion, or the number achieved in a given time) discriminated between first-class and second-class Rugby Union club players; among forwards, values were best in front-row players (Rigg & Reilly 1988). The 'push-ups' used in assessing the US national squad players (Maud 1983) consisted of extending the elbows, with the hands leaving the ground and being clapped together, the criterion being the number of 'clap' push-ups achieved in 45 s. The backs (35 ± 6.8) were better performers than the forwards (31.7 ± 8.1). This superiority was evident also in sit-ups and squat thrusts over the same time frame of 45 s.

Carlson *et al.* (1994) used a motor performance test battery along with kinanthropometric variables to 'profile' US national rugby players. The performance variables that best distinguished between backs and forwards were the repeated jump in place (as many as possible in 45 s), push-ups and vertical jump. These variables contributed 76% to correct classification, the backs having the better performances on all tests.

Laboratory and performance tests have measured anaerobic endurance in terms of jumping ability, power output on a treadmill and on a cycle ergometer, repeated short sprints, shuttle runs and maximal accumulated oxygen deficit (MAOD). The ability to sustain maximal power output has been measured in 'anaerobic capacity' tests. Maud (1983) measured power output by means of a 40-s cycle ergometer test, reporting higher anaerobic power and anaerobic capacity in the forwards than in the backs. Rigg and Reilly (1988) observed a similar trend in measurements of peak power and mean power over 30 s. The absolute power output was higher in the forwards than in the backs, but this apparent superiority was reversed when data were corrected for body mass.

Cheetham *et al.* (1988) measured the power output of Rugby Union forwards during a 30-s test on a non-motorized treadmill. Results were compared with those previously observed for backs. The forwards performed worse than the backs, mainly due to a greater fatigue in the forwards during the test. The forwards with the highest peak power outputs also fatigued most and had the largest elevations in blood lactate concentrations.

The MAOD test was used by Holmyard and Hazeldine (1993) as a measure of anaerobic capacity. Values improved systematically during the 1990 Five-Nations Championship, but had dropped by September prior to a build-up for the 1991 World Championships. At the start of the next home nations international competition, performance was significantly better in the backs compared to the forwards. Mean values of $70 \, ml \cdot kg^{-1}$ were still below the target of $78 \, ml \cdot kg^{-1}$ set for a 'good' level of anaerobic endurance fitness, $88 \, ml \cdot kg^{-1}$ being the target for an élite standard.

Muscle fibre characteristics provide information about the dominance of aerobic and anaerobic predispositions. A predominance of slow-twitch fibres is characteristic of endurance athletes. Jardine *et al.* (1988) reported that university rugby players had 55% fast-twitch fibres in the vastus lateralis muscle, similar to middle-distance runners. This proportion is indicative of the mixture of metabolic attributes associated with competitive Rugby Union play. Rugby League players are likely to have more fast-

twitch fibres and place even greater emphasis on speed and strength training than Rugby Union teams.

FIELD TESTS

Distances of 15 m and 30 m have been employed in field tests for rugby players, on the basis that these represent typical all-out efforts during a game. A sequence of sprint tests with brief recovery periods (6–30 s) may be employed to measure the ability to repeat all-out sprints. The ability to continue reproducing such sprints places rugby in an endurance context.

McLean (1992) developed a shuttle run test, the task being to maintain shuttle running at 85% $\dot{V}O_{2max}$. The recovery period of 30 s was determined according to average exercise/rest ratios in the game. Backs in the national Scottish team could maintain the required velocity for 9 shuttles on average, performances by the forwards being as low as 5 shuttles at various times during the season.

The 20-m shuttle run has been adopted as a field test to estimate $\dot{V}O_{2max}$. A number of players can be tested simultaneously and the test incorporates some agility in turning that is related to the rugby games. Observations on players using this test are included in the results for $\dot{V}O_{2max}$ to be considered later.

McLean (1993) designed a functional field test for use with the Scotland national Rugby Union team. It included slalom runs across a football field over a well-marked course. Fifteen points were marked by flags, round or past which the player ran. Games skills were incorporated, including passing the ball, driving a tackle dummy over 2 m backwards, diving to win the ball on the ground and so on. The test took about 30 s for forwards to perform, the backs being about 2 s faster.

Whilst field tests have face validity, they have to be interpreted cautiously. Results are difficult to express in physiological terms once skills have been added to the demands of locomotion. There may also be influences from environmental conditions and ground surface conditions. Crucially, results depend entirely on the motivation of players to produce maximal efforts.

AEROBIC MEASURES

Maximal oxygen intake values have been reported for various Rugby Union teams (see Table 61.5). Values generally increase with the standard of play. They are higher for backs than for forwards, even though the latter cover more distance in the game. Maximal oxygen intake may not be so important in a game which makes proportionately more demands on the anaerobic system, but it can provide the basis for sustained and repeated anaerobic efforts and recovery from them. Consequently, $\dot{V}_{O_{2max}}$ values tend to be well below the standards accepted for top soccer players, the exception being the Italian players studied by Menchenelli *et al.* (1992b).

The 'anaerobic threshold' (Chapter 22) may be determined as a breakpoint in the linear relationship between running velocity and $\dot{V}_E$ or blood lactate. Alternatively, the exercise intensity corresponding to a fixed lactate concentration (such as 4 mM) may be used as a reference. Douge (1988) reported that the running speed corresponding to the 'anaerobic threshold' was lower in Rugby Union players than in Australian Rules or soccer players. In the latter group, the breakpoint is usually observed at about 75% $\dot{V}_{O_{2max}}$.

The average ($\pm$ s.d.) maximal heart rates of US Rugby Union club players were 182 ($\pm$9) beats·min^{-1} and 189 beats·min^{-1} for forwards and backs, respectively, both groups being within the normal population range (Maud 1983). The corresponding $\dot{V}_{Emax}$ values were 174.6 ($\pm$25.6) l·min^{-1} and 176.1 ($\pm$16.0) l·min^{-1}. Values for university players of 110 ($\pm$16.6) l·min^{-1} (Williams *et al.* 1973) were closer to normal population values, reflecting the smaller body size of university players compared to their club counterparts. The poor endurance-run performances of these players compared to professional soccer players suggest that aerobic fitness was neglected in their training.

The university forwards studied by Jardine *et al.* (1988) demonstrated higher $\dot{V}_{Emax}$ values than the backs (133.1 $\pm$ 13.8 and 110.8 $\pm$ 21.6 l·min^{-1}, respectively). This difference could be due to the greater body size of the forwards (body height 1.88 $\pm$ 0.08 m, body mass 98.0 $\pm$ 8.7 kg) compared to the latter (1.81 $\pm$ 0.05 and 75.4 $\pm$ 5.8, respectively). The maximal heart rates of these players (188 $\pm$ 7 and 193 $\pm$ 5 for forwards and backs, respectively) were close to those of US club players. These figures highlight the unexceptional nature of the heart rate response to maximal exercise in rugby players.

Table 61.5 Mean values for maximal oxygen intake ($\dot{V}_{O_{2max}}$) of Rugby Union players reported in the literature.

Source	Level of play	$\dot{V}_{O_{2max}}$ (ml·kg^{-1}·min^{-1})	n
Williams *et al.* (1973)	University College forwards	46.3	
Maud (1983)	US club backs	59.5	
	US club forwards	54.1	
Ueno *et al.* (1988)	Japan college half-backs	55.8 ($\pm$6.7)	17
	Japan college three-quarters	54.5 ($\pm$6.4)	38
	Japan college forwards	54.7 ($\pm$7.2)	44
* Holmyard & Hazeldine (1993)	England squad	58.4 ($\pm$3.3)	18
Menchenelli *et al.* (1992b)	Italy club players	61.9 ($\pm$7.1)	18
* McLean (1993)	Scotland squad	52.0	23
Tong & Mayes (1995)	Wales squad: backs	59.1 ($\pm$2.8)	18
	Wales squad: forwards	54.3 ($\pm$3.1)	21
Mayes & Nuttall (1995)	Wales squad: seniors	55.6 ($\pm$3.8)	37
	Wales squad: under-14s	55.2 ($\pm$4.5)	42
Jardine *et al.* (1988)	South Africa university backs	55.8 ($\pm$4.1)	14
	South Africa university forwards	52.0 ($\pm$4.8)	15

*Indicates value estimated from shuttle run test.

TRAINING AND LIFESTYLE

Rugby Union was traditionally a sport where a scientific approach towards training was eschewed and the lifestyle of players was rarely such as to enhance athletic performance. Rugby League players, on the other hand, have a longer history of systematic training for competitive play. Even since introduction of the Rugby Union World Cup, the fitness levels of international players demonstrate seasonal variations. Players alternate systematic training with pronounced detraining in the off-season. Rugby players have traditionally been negligent with regard to diet and nutrition. Nine rugby players were among the group whose dietary habits were studied by Piearce (1993). Protein intake was above the guidelines recommended for athletes and alcohol intake was above the maximum amount (5% of total energy intake) recommended for the general population. Many players did not consume any carbohydrate in the first 2 h following exercise, a factor which would delay their recovery.

Alcohol consumption was traditionally embedded in the postmatch socializing of Rugby Union players. Many players also drank alcohol on the night before playing. O'Brien (1992) reported a 'hangover' effect of alcohol. Players consumed their normal quota on a typical night out and were tested at noon the next day, following a 6-h sleep and a standard breakfast. Whilst anaerobic performance was unaffected, there was an 11.4% decrement in aerobic performance. Clearly, players need to be educated about the adverse effects of drinking the night before playing.

Rugby Union demands mobility, agility, muscular strength and muscular power. These vary with positional role and the level of competition. Anthropometric characteristics are more variable between playing positions than between competitive level, and such characteristics may determine the specialization of players in particular roles. Rugby League players tend to be more homogeneous, since scrums and line-outs form only a minor part of the game and the intermissions between exercise bouts are invariably short. Anaerobic parameters play a more dominant role in game-related performance in both rugby codes than in soccer. Nevertheless, aerobic capacities provide relevant background fitness status and help sustain work rates to the end of matches. A systematic approach to training and competing has been adopted within Rugby Union in recent years, in turn altering the attitudes and lifestyles of players at an élite level. Those aspiring to play at the highest level in either rugby code must now adopt a scientific approach to training and preparing for competition.

American football

Background to the game

American football is the largest spectator sport in the US and its major spectacle, the Super Bowl, is watched live on TV worldwide. Games consist of four quarters. Although each lasts only 15 min of actual play, the game itself may be spread over 3–4 h. The frequent interchange of offensive and defensive line-ups on the field of play as possession of the ball changes hands means that players are only intermittently involved directly in play. When play is in progress, the action is intense. Consequently, the game makes high and prolonged demands on speed, anaerobic power and muscular strength rather than on aerobic power.

Each team has a 45-man squad, consisting of three quarter-backs, five running backs, four wide receivers, two tight ends, eight offensive linemen, seven defensive linemen, seven linebackers, four defensive backs, one kicker and one punter, plus three others. The offence contains linemen (tackles, guards and ends) and centres; the defence has secondary lines (safety, guards), linebackers (outside, middle) and linemen (ends and tackles). A typical 3–4–4 defensive unit will have a tackle and two ends, four linebackers and four defensive backs.

As the game is a physical contact sport, tackling and blocking are important skills. The game is unique among the football codes in the amount of protective clothing worn by players. The clothing should not interfere with running, execution of other game skills or heat loss when playing in hot conditions.

Demands of the game

Periods of play (usually < 30 s) are generally intense before players gain respite at each 'down' or change of possession. As players regularly have intervals off the field of play, they are not required to make multiple repeated sprints, as in soccer or Australian Rules football. Nevertheless, they must maintain attention for the entire game, since at any time they could be called into action.

The main demands seem to be on alactic anaerobic power, with some demands on anaerobic power and capacity. It is unlikely that blood lactate reaches very high levels, or that there is pronounced hypoxia within the active muscles. The current use of oxygen for recovery when players reach the sideline is unnecessary and has little to recommend it (Winter *et al.* 1989). Demands placed on aerobic metabolism are relatively light, the average rate of energy expenditure being 37.7 kJ (9 kcal)·min^{-1} (Brooks & Fahey 1984).

Characteristics of players

American footballers on average tend to be taller and leaner than participants in the other football codes. The contemporary game at top level calls for larger players than in the previous generation, and the physiques predispose towards muscular strength and power output rather than endurance. An excess of adipose tissue predisposes against endurance as well as mobility in sprinting.

Studies on US college players (Burke *et al.* 1980) show a mean body fat of 13% for 20 backs and 21.8% for 33 linemen. Defensive backs have less body fat than offensive, 7.3 and 11.5%, respectively. In four separate studies (reviewed by Reilly 1990), comparative mean values were 6.7–11.5% for defensive backs and 11.5–13.8% for offensive backs. The defensive backs rely more on agility and speed of movement, whilst the extra weight helps the offensive backs to maintain momentum after impacts. The overall values are lower than in normal populations of comparable age, but are higher than values reported for endurance athletes.

Professional footballers have below-average vital capacities, the mean being 94.3% of values predicted from a standard nomogram. Wilmore and Haskell (1972) found no consistent relationship between height or body mass and vital capacity or total lung volume. Vital capacity values for defensive backs (83% of predicted vital capacity) were especially poor. These results contrast with an earlier study of 16 collegiate footballers (Novak *et al.* 1969), where players were smaller, but averaged a 1-l larger vital capacity than the professionals.

The average maximal heart rate of the professional American footballers studied by Wilmore and Haskell (1972) was 185 beats·min^{-1}. Values varied from 179 (offensive backs and receivers) to 198 beats·min^{-1} in defensive backs. The $\dot{V}_{\text{Emax}}$ values similarly varied from an average of 149.3 for three linebackers to 189.6 l·min^{-1} for four offensive linemen and tight ends.

The $\dot{V}_{\text{O}_2\text{max}}$ values of American footballers are quite modest, average values being highest in defensive backs (54.5 ml·kg^{-1}·min^{-1}) and lowest in defensive linemen (43.5 ml·kg^{-1}·min^{-1}). Since defensive linemen carry a greater proportion of body mass as fat than other players, expressing $\dot{V}_{\text{O}_2\text{max}}$ per kg lean body mass brought values for the defensive linemen closer to those for defensive and offensive backs and wide receivers (Wilmore & Haskell 1972). Nevertheless, figures were still well below those observed for linebackers and offensive linemen. Although the defensive backs had the largest aerobic power, their values were below expectations in endurance sports, reflecting the pronounced anaerobic metabolic load in playing the game. This was corroborated by Gettman *et al.* (1987), whose professional players had an average $\dot{V}_{\text{O}_2\text{max}}$ of 49.2 ml·kg^{-1}·min^{-1}. A strenuous 14-week conditioning programme improved this value by only 6%.

Training

Training for American football emphasizes the development of strength and muscle power, in accordance with the demands of the game. Consequently, the vast majority of teams are well equipped with weight-training facilities, including isokinetic and multistation apparatus. Free weights are still widely used in training specific muscle groups, and many coaches prefer such training to aerobic, circuit weight-training. Specific dynamic practices include use of tackle dummies, where game skills can be improved against fabricated resistance.

Despite being recommended to continue fitness training in the off-season, many players return to preseason practices overweight. Frequently, they lack the stamina for long training sessions at this time. In the past, the use of sweat-suits in a mis-guided attempt to shed unwanted weight quickly led to fatalities from hyperthermia. The footballer clad in the usual protective clothing and exercising in the heat has difficulty in evaporating sweat. This can cause a dangerous elevation of body tempera-ture and slow dehydration of the player. Use of a mesh jersey allows more effective evaporative and convective cooling of the body. Aerobic fitness also helps thermal homeostasis. The risks of heat injury are now recognized by trainers and a high priority is given to replacement of body fluids during practices.

Australian Rules and Gaelic football

Introduction to the games

Australian Rules matches are held in a large oval field, with 18 players on each team. The game con-sists of four quarters, each of 25-min duration. The ball is moved quickly from end to end with the purpose of scoring, thereby promoting a flowing style of game. Six points are awarded when the ball crosses between two central uprights, and one point if it goes between the two side uprights. As the game is continually in motion, all players need good running ability, agility in avoiding tackles, catching and kicking skills and tactical sense.

The Gaelic football field is approximately 40 m longer than a soccer pitch, with 15 players on each side. Goalposts at each end have a crossbar, a goal (equal to 3 points) being scored beneath it, and a point if the ball crosses above the bar and between the posts. The ball is round like a soccer ball, in con-trast to the oval shape of the Australian Rules ball. Apart from the shape of the ball and the scoring system, the two games are close relatives, having many skills in common. These include high catch-

ing, long-distance kicking for accuracy, passing and moving the ball downfield. Players from the two codes quickly adapt to the 'Compromise Rules' game which has been played at international level (Ireland versus Australia) since the 1960s.

Gaelic football consists of two 30-min halves. Time is increased to 70 min in intercounty champi-onship games. The normal energy reserves of the body should sustain intense match-play more easily in this than in the Australian Rules game, because of its shorter duration. The extent to which glycogen stores are deployed in competition depends on the work-rate profiles and patterns of activity in each of these football codes.

Demands of the games

The movement patterns of Australian Rules players are in general similar to those observed in soccer. Players cover over 10 km per game (27% walking, 53% jogging and 20% striding or sprinting); 30% of sprints are <5 m, 27% are between 5 and 10 m, 21% 10–20 m, 11% 20–30 m, 6% 30–40 m and only 5% are >40 m. Players sprint more than 40 m only a few times per game.

The activity profiles differ according to position. The rover, ruckman and centreline players have to cope with sustained efforts whilst the half-back flanker and backpocket player have comparatively short bursts of activity. The distance covered in a game by a half-back flanker was 77% that of a rover (Pyke & Smith 1975), roughly the difference between the work rate of a centre-back and a mid-field player in soccer.

As in Australian Rules, Gaelic footballers need to accelerate to receive or intercept a pass, or leap to catch a high ball. The ball is seldom out of play for long, so players have few respites during a match. The toe-to-hand method of travelling with the ball means that many forwards cover more distance in possession than do Australian Rules or soccer players. Nevertheless, the distance covered in pos-session of the ball is a mere 2% of the overall dis-tance covered in a Gaelic football match and only 4 min is occupied with high-intensity activity likely to place demands on anaerobic metabolism (Keane et al. 1993).

The overall distance covered in intercounty Gaelic football was calculated to be 8594 (±s.d. = 1056) m (Keane *et al.* 1993). Walking and jogging accounted for two-thirds of the total distance. The greatest distances were covered by centrefield players (9131 ± 977m), followed by backs (8523 ± 1175m) and forwards (8490 ± 673m). Gaelic footballers demonstrate higher average speeds of movement (133 m·min^{-1}) than those reported for Australian soccer players (124 m·min^{-1}: Withers *et al.* 1982) and Australian Rules players (106 m·min^{-1}: Douge 1988). The shorter durations of Gaelic football matches mean that fatigue due to depleted muscle glycogen stores is unlikely.

The energy expenditures of the Gaelic football goalkeeper are relatively light, but physiological demands are well distributed among the other players. These consist of three full-backs, three half-backs, two midfield players, three half-forwards and three full forwards. In the Australian Rules game the highest work rate is accomplished by the 'rovers'. McKenna *et al.* (1988) reported that walking took 44% of rovers' match time, jogging 40%, high-intensity runs 5% and game-related activity 2.5%, and for less than 9% of the time were they stationary. The mean duration of a high-intensity run was 2.7 (± 0.7) s, the maximum being 10.4 s, and one such run occurred every 73 s on average.

The overall physiological strain on players in these two football codes is represented by the irregular superimposition of changes of pace and anaerobic efforts on a background of light to moderate aerobic activity. The activity patterns denote a call on aerobic metabolism and on intramuscular phosphagens. Anaerobic breakdown of glycogen is implicated in the longer sprints. Pohl *et al.* (1981) observed that the anion gap increased and blood bicarbonate levels decreased during Australian Rules football, changes compatible with a mild metabolic acidosis.

An Australian Rules football game is likely to reduce muscle glycogen stores to low levels. The activity patterns and distance covered are broadly similar to those of soccer players, whose thigh muscle glycogen depots are nearly depleted by full-time (Saltin 1973). On the day following a match, the peak values for $\dot{V}O_2$ and $\dot{V}_E$ are below normal

(McKenna *et al.* 1988), an observation compatible with reduced muscle glycogen. A diet rich in carbohydrate is thus recommended to aid recovery from exercise-related decrements in aerobic power.

Indices of cardiorespiratory strain during Australian Rules matches confirm a relatively high aerobic load. The mean heart rate during play (161 beats·min^{-1}) is comparable to observations on soccer players (Douge 1988). The heart rates of club Gaelic footballers have been measured as 157 ± 10 and 164 ± 10 beats·min^{-1} for first and second halves, respectively. Blood lactates measured at the end of each half are 4.3 ± 1.0 and 3.4 ± 1.6mM, respectively (Florida-James & Reilly 1995). The overall relative loading is estimated at 72% $\dot{V}O_{2max}$. 'Rovers' in Australian Rules seem to have higher heart rates than other players during games. Pyke and Smith (1975) reported values of between 170 and 185 beats·min^{-1} (mean 178 beats·min^{-1}); it is unlikely that in any Gaelic football outfield player operates at this high level.

Characteristics of players

Australian Rules players tend to be large. Mean height and body mass were 1.83 m and 80 kg, respectively (see review by Douge 1988), with ranges of 1.76–1.93 m for height and 79–93 kg for body mass. Interindividual variability was attributed to the demands of specific positional roles. Tallness is an advantage in contesting aerial possession of the ball and catching is an important skill in the game. Not surprisingly, there is a gradation in body size with the level of competition, top professional players being the tallest and heaviest, players in amateur clubs being the smallest and lightest and those in low-level professional clubs having intermediate values.

The sprinting performance of Australian Rules players compares poorly with that of top American football players. Pyke and Smith (1975) reported 40-yard (36.6-m) times averaging 5.25 s for Perth (Western Australia) players. The corresponding time for Dallas Cowboy professionals was 0.35 s faster, although they were 23 kg heavier than the Australian Rules players. This reflects the emphasis on anaerobic power in the American game, compared with the more aerobic nature of the Australian code.

The inference of a moderately high aerobic demand in the Australian Rules game is supported by observations on $\dot{V}_{O_{2max}}$. The $64\,ml\cdot kg^{-1}\cdot min^{-1}$ average for élite players (Douge 1988) is much higher than corresponding values for rugby and American football. Most positional roles demand a high aerobic power, the 'rovers' having the highest aerobic requirements.

The $\dot{V}_{O_{2max}}$ of Gaelic footballers depends on the level of competition. University players had average values of $47\,ml\cdot kg^{-1}\cdot min^{-1}$ (Kirgan & Reilly 1993), whilst a more successful club team had values of $52.6\,(\pm\,4)\,ml\cdot kg^{-1}\cdot min^{-1}$. Successful county teams had mean values of 56 (Keane et al. 1997) and $58.6\,ml\cdot kg^{-1}\cdot min^{-1}$ (Watson 1995; Reilly & Doran, 1999) as they prepared for the All-Ireland finals. Outfield players tended to be homogeneous with respect to $\dot{V}_{O_{2max}}$.

Similar inferences can be made from the data on the physical working capacity of Gaelic footballers. Watson (1977) found that power output at a heart rate of 170 beats$\cdot min^{-1}$ (PWC_{170}) was higher in successful than in less successful county teams, even when data were adjusted for the larger body size of the successful players. Values were highest close to provincial or All-Ireland championship finals, suggesting the impact of training for such events.

Training

The training among top sides is much more systematic for Australian Rules than for Gaelic football. It usually involves 4–5 sessions a week, with 1–2 rest days. Besides, players engage in one and sometimes two matches per week.

The traditional conditioning programme emphasized aerobic exercise. Jones and Laussen (1988) introduced a more comprehensive programme which incorporated strength training. Running drills were also designed to resemble activity patterns in the game. The programme adopted by the Fitzroy FC team also utilized a game skill combat-running circuit: this was intended to develop the agility and acceleration related to competitive play. The conditioning drills included, for example,

blocks of short sprints, repeated every 20 s with 2-min rests between sets.

During the playing season, the training load tends to be distributed unevenly over the week. The most arduous sessions are on Tuesday evening: from then on, training is tapered in preparation for Saturday's competition. Training is resumed on Sunday, but tends to be light in order to recover from the effects of the previous day's contest. This cyclical organization resembles soccer practices, ensuring that players start their match physiologically recovered from training sessions during the week.

Gaelic football is still an amateur game, and this is reflected in training programmes. Highly organized training is concentrated mainly in the championship season, May to September. League and friendly matches provide the main training stimulus in the remainder of the year. Teams eliminated in the first round of championship matches may not attain high fitness standards. Watson (1977) found the highest PWC_{170} among players preparing for provincial and All-Ireland finals. The same trend was reported for All-Ireland champions in the mid-1990s (Keane et al. 1997).

Field hockey

Historical background

The game of field hockey is thought to have evolved from prehistoric human's delight in stick-and-ball games. Its origins as a semiorganized activity have been traced to Asia, about 2000 BC. A form of the game was played by the Egyptians 4000 years ago, and later by Ancient Greeks. The Romans developed the game, passing it on to the European nations that they conquered. Thus, German (Kolbe), Dutch (het kolven—a forerunner of ice hockey) and French (hocquet—meaning shepherd's crook) versions evolved. The true ancestor of field hockey is thought to be Irish hurling, the original Gaelic term 'iomán' meaning a vigorous forward drive (see Reilly & Borrie 1992).

Field hockey is played on a pitch 90 m long and 55 m wide. Teams are composed of 11 players, including a goalkeeper. Unlike other stick-and-ball games (hurling, lacrosse, bandy and shinty), the ball is played with the stick on the ground and the use of the hand in catching is prohibited. A match is played over two 35-min halves, with a 5–10-min interval. The game requires a wide repertoire of skills and physical and psychomotor attributes. Two areas of technical development have affected physiological requirements: the hockey stick and the playing surface.

Field hockey is similar to most field-invasive games, with one unique feature. The rules governing use of the stick and its design preclude any left-handed sticks, since the player may use only the flat side of the stick. The easiest position from which to exercise game skills is with the ball out to the right of the body. The effectiveness of this body–ball position determines the pattern of play when two opposing players confront each other. An attacker will try to take the ball around the left side of the defender, the defender's weakest tackling area, whereas the defender tries to force the attacker to pass down his/her right side, the strongest tackling area. Playing right-sided dictates that the right wing is the main channel of attack.

Hockey therefore has an in-built asymmetry in terms of individual and team play. This should raise the physiological demands, as players must pay attention to body position in relation to both ball and opponent. Maintenance of correct positioning increases the work rate when playing, and in particular when defending.

Energy expenditures in field hockey

Fox (1984) included hockey with lacrosse and soccer among sports with a 30% aerobic, 70% anaerobic contribution to energy expenditure. Sharkey (1986) classified the game as bordering on the aerobic side (40% anaerobic, 60% aerobic), grouping it with sports of mixed demands that included canoeing, kayaking, lacrosse, motocross and mountaineering. The contemporary game is aerobically more demanding than previously, with frequent though brief anaerobic efforts superimposed on aerobic metabolism.

The exercise intensity in hockey can be gauged from motion analysis. Male players at the 1973 World Cup were active for 20.6 min (30% of match time) and in that time covered 5.61 km, implying an exercise to rest ratio of 2:5 (Wein 1981). Defenders covered less (5.14 km) and midfield players more (6.36 km) ground. The player covering the greatest distance (on the New Zealand team) had a value of 8.82 km.

A task analysis of players' actions suggested differences among outfield players, at least with the conventional game. Overall, hockey players were reported to 'make more light than strenuous movements', 69% compared with 31%. Centre-forwards made the highest number of strenuous movements (36%), whilst defenders and 'halves' functioned with 70% of light movements. The 'heavy' movements call for great muscular effort in hitting the ball strongly, whereas light movements encompass push passing for precision and dribbling (Wein 1981). Of all the activity on the ball, 61% lasted between 0.5 and 2.0 s, only 5% lasting more than 7 s. Clearly, much of the activity of players involves motion 'off the ball'.

Energy expenditure estimates approaching 50 kJ·min^{-1} in field hockey have categorized the men's game as 'heavy exercise' (Reilly 1981). Boyle et al. (1994) reported mean heart rates of 155 beats·min^{-1} in international players, which yielded an energy expenditure estimation higher than this value. The greatest energy expenditure was among central midfield players, the lowest in the left corner forward. In the women's game, the most strenuous position, centre-midfield, has an associated energy expenditure of approximately 35 kJ·min^{-1} (Skubic & Hodgkins 1967). The figures are based on predictions rather than direct measurements, due to difficulties in monitoring during play. Direct measurements of Indian soldiers during recreational play yielded a value of 36.4 kJ·min^{-1} (8.7 kcal·min^{-1}) (Malhotra et al. 1962). The energy expenditure is probably higher in competitive match-play.

Reilly and Seaton (1990) measured energy expenditure, heart rate and perceived exertion in hockey players dribbling a ball on a treadmill at speeds of 8 and 10 km·h^{-1}. Dribbling increased energy expenditure by 15–16 kJ·min^{-1} above that observed in normal running. The heart rate was elevated by 23 beats·min^{-1}, whilst perceived exertion increased from 'very light' and 'light' to 'somewhat hard' and 'hard' at the two speeds examined. The greater additional energy cost in field hockey compared to dribbling in soccer (Reilly & Ball 1984) reflects postural factors and arm and shoulder exercise when using the hockey stick. The physiological costs of accelerating, decelerating and changing the direction of motion add to energetic requirements. As with soccer, the physiological cost of hockey play is underestimated if prediction of $\dot{V}O_2$ and hence energy expenditure is based solely on the distance covered during a game.

The playing surface can influence physical and physiological strain. The effective duration of a hockey match played on grass at the second World Cup in Amsterdam was only 53% of the total game time (Wein 1981). Interruptions lasted 8.7s on average, and were about twice as numerous as in soccer at a comparable standard. There were 230 stoppages per match in the 1975 Pre-Olympic Tournament at Montreal. These averaged one every 18s. Adoption of synthetic surfaces at the 1976 Olympic Games and subsequent international tournaments increased playing times and decreased the number of interruptions. This trend was enhanced by rule changes in 1981–2 which speeded up the game and kept the ball in play for longer than before.

Playing characteristics are more consistent on synthetic surfaces than on grass. The ball also travels over the surface at a faster pace. Both factors have changed the style of play and affected physiological requirements (Malhotra et al. 1983). Both anaerobic and aerobic demands on players are likely to have increased.

It is easier to execute individual skills on a synthetic surface, thereby retaining possession of the ball under pressure. The speed of ball movement and higher individual skills have increased emphasis on a team's ability to play as a cohesive unit. Teams now adhere more closely to the concept of 'total' hockey, players being able to interchange positions during a game without disrupting team balance. Players thus cover greater distances within a game and must have the aerobic fitness to do so.

Malhotra et al. (1983) studied physiological demands using a Kofranyi–Michaelis meter during a field hockey game. Physiological responses were greater on an artificial pitch compared to grass, mean $\dot{V}_E$ being 56.8 versus 46.6 l·min^{-1} and mean $\dot{V}O_2$ 2.26 versus 1.91 l·min^{-1}. The $\dot{V}O_2$ values correspond to energy expenditures of 46.5 kJ·min^{-1} (11.1 kcal·min^{-1}) and 39.3 kJ·min^{-1} (9.4 kcal·min^{-1}) for artificial and grass pitches, respectively. The higher physiological stress on the synthetic pitch was due to faster play and higher running speeds. However, the game was a six-a-side match, played on half a normal-sized pitch, and so is not representative of normal field hockey matches.

Positional role

The evolution of playing formations within hockey initially followed the same pattern as in soccer. The classical 2:3:5 formation dominated tactical thinking until the mid-1960s, when a sweeper system was introduced in West Germany (Wein 1981). In the mid-1980s, the formations became more varied and dynamic, the most popular systems being 1:3:3:3, 1:3:2:4 and 4:2:4 (Whitaker 1986). Synthetic playing surfaces also altered styles of play, and players now interchange positions frequently during a game.

Ready and van der Merwe (1986) examined positional differences in the Canadian Olympic women's squad. Players were classified as defenders, midfield and strikers, corresponding to the backs, halves and forwards of Indian and Australian researchers. It was thought that the Canadian training programme and system of play would even out the fitness demands of outfield positions, but forwards had the highest $\dot{V}O_{2max}$ (Fig. 61.6), midfield players had the greatest anaerobic capacity as measured in a treadmill run test, and defenders had the lowest peak lactate level and $\dot{V}O_{2max}$.

A fitness evaluation of 24 English female hockey players (Reilly & Bretherton 1986) failed to separate players according to positional roles. This applied to kinanthropometric measures, muscular strength and power, aerobic fitness and field tests. However, goalkeepers tended to be high in anaerobic power measures and poor to moderate in aerobic fitness indices.

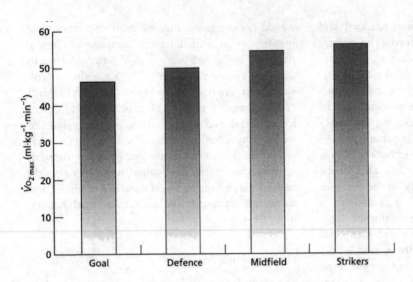

Fig. 61.6 Maximum oxygen intake in Canadian female hockey players according to positional role (from Ready & van der Merwe 1986).

Fitness profiles: women's field hockey

MUSCLE PERFORMANCE

Female field hockey players show a high anaerobic power output relative to other games players (Reilly & Secher 1990). Their mean performance on the stair run (955 W) is similar to netball players (953 W) and superior to endurance athletes—orienteers and cross-country skiers. When adjusted for body mass, the performance of the field hockey players was 3.7 W·kg^{-1} greater than that of netball players. A high anaerobic power output facilitates changes of pace and direction during a game. Anaerobic power discriminates successfully between élite and county-level players (Reilly & Bretherton 1986). Élite players are also superior to county players in a range of muscular fitness measures.

Principal components analysis of data on 24 female hockey players identified components of anaerobic power and dribbling speed which were significantly correlated ($r = 0.694$). The 'dribbling speed' component incorporated a 50-yard (45.5-m) sprint and a 60-yard (54.6-m) run over a 'T'-shaped course whilst dribbling a hockey ball around skittles (Reilly & Bretherton 1986). 'Dribbling speed' discriminated between levels of play, indicating the importance of this skill in field hockey. The relation with run time suggests that sprinting ability contributes to fast dribbling.

Reilly and Bretherton (1986) evaluated English élite female players. Their first test was a 2-min 'T' run over a 60-yard (54.5-m) course, dribbling a leather ball around skittles. Sports that engage large muscle groups for 1 min or more may tax $\dot{V}_{O_{2max}}$, so this test implies a high aerobic loading (Åstrand & Rodahl 1986). Use of reversed sticks is excluded, and the best of three trials is recorded. Performance is significantly correlated with both aerobic ($r = 0.48$) and anaerobic ($r = 0.60$) power, and it differentiates between élite and county-level players.

AEROBIC FACTORS

The mean $\dot{V}_{O_{2max}}$ of élite female field hockey squads (Table 61.6) ranges from 45 to 59 ml·kg^{-1}·min^{-1} (Reilly & Secher 1990). This is comparable to values for lacrosse players, but lower than for cross-country skiers and orienteers.

Élite English squad players had predicted $\dot{V}_{O_{2max}}$ mean values of 46 ± 9 ml·kg^{-1}·min^{-1}, distinguishing them from county players who had mean values of 41 ± 6 ml·kg^{-1}·min^{-1} (Reilly & Bretherton 1986). American (Zeldis *et al.* 1978) international players demonstrated mean values of 52 ml·kg^{-1}·min^{-1}, rising to 57 ml·kg^{-1}·min^{-1} before the 1996 Olympic Games (Sparling *et al.* 1998).

Table 61.6 Mean $\dot{V}_{O_{2max}}$ of top female and male field hockey players: only figures obtained in a treadmill test are included (from Reilly & Borrie 1992; Boyle *et al.* 1994; Sparling *et al.* 1998).

Level of play	n	$\dot{V}_{O_{2max}}$ (ml·kg^{-1}·min^{-1})
Females		
College (US)	10	42.9
Provincial (Australia)	6	50.1
College and national (US)	10	51.7
County (England)	12	52.2
National (Wales)	10	54.5
National (US)	12	57.1
National (Canada)	16	59.3
Males		
Provincial (Australia)	9	64.1
Provincial and national (Australia)	14	60.7
National (UK)	20	62.2
National (West Germany)	5	63.5
National (Ireland)	9	61.8
National Senior B and Junior (Spain)	26	59.7

There is a large genetic component to $\dot{V}_{O_{2max}}$, and improvement with training is normally only about 25–30% (Åstrand & Rodahl 1986). Nevertheless, such an effect could contribute to the spread of values reported for top players, reflecting the phase of the competitive season and training status. In the year leading up to the Los Angeles Olympics, the $\dot{V}_{O_{2max}}$ of the Canadian Olympic team increased from 52.7 ± 6.0 to 55.7 ± 4.5 and finally to 59.3 ± 4.1 ml·kg^{-1}·min^{-1} just before the tournament (Reilly & van der Merwe, 1986). Higher values during peak training periods may be attributable in part to a loss of fat mass during training. In the year's build-up to the Los Angeles games, the average body fat content of players decreased from 18.9 to 15.7% of body mass. This alone would account for 25% of the reported increases in $\dot{V}_{O_{2max}}$.

Typically, intensifying the training programme of field hockey players entails superimposing specific drills on the normal regimen. The mean $\dot{V}_{O_{2max}}$ of Welsh international players was 54 ml·kg^{-1}·min^{-1} in the early stages of planning for an intercontinental tournament (Reilly *et al.* 1985). The squad had a good background of match-play, endurance and general fitness training in the 2 months prior to initial measurements (3 months before the tourna-

ment). From then on, the training programme was designed to maintain aerobic fitness, but also introduced elements of sprint training. In the month of the competition, the $\dot{V}_{O_{2max}}$, $\dot{V}_{Emax}$, % body fat, ventilatory threshold and anaerobic capacity were all unaltered, whereas flexibility and sprinting speed were significantly enhanced. It was concluded that flexibility and anaerobic power could be improved prior to major tournaments without detrimental effects on aerobic fitness.

Cheetham and Williams (1987) noted similar findings in English county players. Six weeks of high-intensity training included four or five training sessions per week (two fast runs of 5–9 km, two interval sessions of repeated 30–300-m runs and at least one circuit training session), in addition to normal hockey commitments of one or two skill/tactical sessions and one or two matches per week. The improvement in $\dot{V}_{O_{2max}}$ was small, from 50.1 ± 4.1 to 52.2 ± 3.7 ml·kg^{-1}·min^{-1}. These values compared with 43.9 ± 2.5 and 44.9 ± 2.7 ml·kg^{-1}·min^{-1} for club players who were measured at the same times but did not undertake supplementary training. Aerobic rather than anaerobic factors best distinguished between the two levels of play. Peak blood lactate levels measured 5 min after a 30-s all-out treadmill sprint were similar for the county and club players (15.4 ± 2.2 and 14.9 ± 1.7 mM, respectively).

The predominance of aerobic over anaerobic factors in female field hockey players is further suggested by muscle biopsy studies. Prince *et al.* (1977) reported that female college players possessed a significantly higher proportion of fast oxidative glycolytic (Type IIb) and slow oxidative (Type I) skeletal muscle fibres than controls. Whether this trend was due to endowment or training could not be established.

Pulmonary and cardiac function data have been reported for female field hockey players. The vital capacity was 17.6 and 16% greater than normal values matched for age, gender and body size in élite and county squads, respectively (Reilly & Bretherton 1986). Corresponding values for 1-s forced expiratory volume ($FEV_{1.0}$) were 14 and 13% above expected. The $\dot{V}_{Emax}$ of the Canadian national squad (Ready & van der Merwe 1986) peaked just prior to the Olympic tournament at 96.4 ± 10.7 l·min^{-1}. The corresponding maximal heart rates were 195 ± 9 beats·min^{-1}. The mean $\dot{V}_{Emax}$ of the Welsh national team (Reilly *et al.* 1985) was 100.3 ± 19.2 l·min^{-1}. The maximal heart rate of English players (combined élite and county) was 192 ± 7 beats·min^{-1}, close to general population values (Reilly & Bretherton 1986).

The 'ventilatory threshold' of Welsh international players was $76.8 \pm 6.6\%$ of $\dot{V}_{O_2max}$ (Reilly *et al.* 1985). This indicates a good training status, comparing favourably with values expected in good distance runners.

The power output corresponding to a heart rate of 170 beats·min^{-1} has traditionally been used as a measure of aerobic capability. Values in the English élite squad members averaged 2.3 W·kg^{-1}, compared to 2.0 W·kg^{-1} for county players (Reilly & Bretherton 1986). Mean PWC_{170} values were about 24% greater in the élite squad than in sedentary females (Davies & Daggett 1977). The average for Welsh international players was 2.87 W·kg^{-1}, recorded after a good background of match-play and fitness training. It seems that aerobic fitness influences the standard of play in female field

hockey players and so aerobic training should form an essential part of preparation for competition.

Fitness profiles: men's field hockey

Reviewing competitors at the 1964 Olympic Games in Tokyo, Hirata (1966) concluded that the physique of male field hockey players was almost the same as that of soccer players. The age of peak performance for ball players was 24–27 years, soccer success being accomplished earliest and hockey latest.

Training programmes for Olympic competitors have improved considerably in the intervening three decades, but field hockey is still largely an amateur game; social pressures rather than ageing determine the duration of top players' careers and the fitness levels they reach and maintain.

AEROBIC FACTORS

The average $\dot{V}_{O_2max}$ of teams reviewed by Reilly and Secher (1990) ranged from 48 to 65 ml·kg^{-1}·min^{-1}. The lowest figure was a step-test value for the Argentinian team obtained at the Olympic village in Mexico in 1968 (Di Prampero *et al.* 1970). The figure for top German players (Rost 1987) was estimated from a graphical presentation of results (Table 61.6); findings were comparable with top German tennis players and middle-distance runners, and exceeded values for handball players and ice hockey specialists. It seems that values in excess of 60 ml·kg^{-1}·min^{-1} are required in top field hockey players, much as in professional soccer players (Reilly 1996).

The heart size of field hockey players approximated that found in soccer players, and exceeded that noted in ice hockey and handball (Rost 1987). Greater heart dimensions were observed in decathletes, who might be expected to have much more arduous training programmes.

The $\dot{V}_{Emax}$ of the Senior B and Junior Internationals in Spain averaged 148.4 ± 10.9 l·min^{-1} (Drobnic *et al.* 1989). These values compare favourably with observations on professional soccer players (Reilly 1996).

Apart from a high aerobic power, field hockey requires a capability to accelerate and decelerate quickly; this is more critical to performance than maximal speed. In an analysis of state-level Australian sportsmen hockey players had a mean relative leg power which compared favourably with state footballers (Withers *et al.* 1977).

Training

Data on the most appropriate training regimens for field hockey are sparse. The significant aerobic contribution to energy expenditure is evident in the $\dot{V}o_{2max}$ of both male and female players (Withers *et al.* 1977; Reilly & Bretherton 1986; Rost 1987; Reilly 1990). Training must therefore develop aerobic power. The increased speed of movement demanded by synthetic surfaces suggests that the majority of aerobic training needs to be done over shorter distances (5–9 km) at high pace, or using interval sessions with high-intensity repetitions.

Élite hockey players must also possess significant anaerobic power. The game requires frequent acceleration, deceleration and turning movements. A high peak power output from the leg is therefore important to the physiological profile of the élite player. No specific data are available on the effectiveness of sprint training, but it is likely that regimens successfully utilized by soccer players will benefit field hockey players (Reilly & Borrie 1992). Short (30-m) sprints with maximally explosive starts and an exercise/rest ratio of 1:5 improve sprinting speed in male soccer players (Apor 1988).

Daily energy expenditure

The severity of the training programme in top-level performers is reflected in daily energy expenditures. Grafe (1971) considered an intake of 23 MJ (5600 kcal) daily was adequate for male field hockey players. A similar intake was advised for basketball and handball specialists. In view of the relatively moderate training regimens of players at the time, these figures may have overestimated the real requirements.

More recent figures give an actual energy intake of $181\,kJ\cdot kg^{-1}\cdot day^{-1}$ for élite male field hockey players. For a 75-kg individual, this amounts to 13.6 MJ (3250 kcal), below the figure for soccer players ($192\,kJ\cdot kg^{-1}\cdot day^{-1}$). Values for female players were $145\,kJ\cdot kg^{-1}\cdot day^{-1}$ or 8.7 MJ (2080 kcal) for a 60-kg individual (Erp-Baart *et al.* 1989), marginally above the figure for handball players ($142\,kJ\cdot kg^{-1}\cdot day^{-1}$). These values were derived from 4- to 7-day food diaries, an approach that often underestimates energy requirements (Westerterp & Saris 1991).

The activity profiles during play do not suggest the likelihood of muscle glycogen depletion. Consequently, glycogen loading is not essential, but it may have some value in serial competitions or after prolonged training sessions. In these instances, a high carbohydrate diet guards against starting subsequent matches with inadequate glycogen reserves. Carbohydrate supplementation has reduced fatigue during intense training of US national players (Kneider *et al.* 1995).

The US women's team trained 3–4 h a day, 6 days each week in preparation for the 1996 Olympics (Sparling *et al.* 1998). The percentage body fat was 16–17%; bone mineral density was 13% above age-related and weight-matched norms. The elevated bone density and nutritional profile contrast with reports of premature bone loss, stress fractures and eating disorders in élite female endurance runners.

Physical strain

Skill requirements and postural stress are superimposed on the energy expenditures demanded by the game and its pattern of play. This is accentuated when players dribble the ball or move in a semi-crouched posture. Spinal flexion is ergonomically unsound for fast locomotion, and it may predispose to back injury. Cannon and James (1984) reported that 8% of patients referred to a back-pain clinic for athletes over a 4-year period were field hockey players. A survey of local male clubs in the Merseyside region showed that 53% of respondents had experienced low back pain (Reilly & Seaton 1990).

Compressive loading of the intervertebral discs during play and practices causes players to lose height. Water is extruded from the disc when the compressive load exceeds the interstitial osmotic pressure. The result is a decrease in total body length which can be demonstrated by high-resolution stadiometry (Troup *et al.* 1985). Dribbling a hockey ball on a motor-driven treadmill for 7 min at a speed of 8.5 km·h^{-1} induced a shrinkage of 0.4 mm·min^{-1} (Reilly & Seaton 1990), about four times that observed in running and almost twice that found in circuit weight training (Leatt *et al.* 1986). Training of back strength and flexibility (Garbutt *et al.* 1990) may reduce the risk of back injury in field hockey players. Procedures for unloading the spine, notably gravity inversion and Fowler's posture, adopted before and after exercise or during intermissions, may also help (Leatt *et al.* 1985).

Hurling and lacrosse

Introduction

Hurling is the national game in Ireland; the pitch has the same dimensions as for Gaelic football. The female version of the game (camogie) has similar rules to the men's game. Teams are 15-a-side. Positional roles are relatively rigid, and marking of players is usually adopted. Traditional hurling sticks are made of ash, but in recent years synthetic versions of the 'camán' have been accepted. Typically, a long puck of the ball could propel it over 100 m, and it is usual for players to score directly with a shot 70 m from goal.

The implement used in lacrosse is very different from the camán, allowing the player to catch and cradle the ball. The game originated among North American Indians and has traditionally been popular among females. It has a wider following than hurling (or the Scottish version known as shinty), particularly in Canada, the US and the UK.

There are 10 players per side in lacrosse. The pitch is 100 m shorter than in hurling. Matches are 60 min in duration.

Demands of the games

The physiological demands of hurling probably resemble those of Gaelic football. The play may change quickly from end to end, in view of the large distances the ball can be hit. Players cover distance with the ball by carrying it or tapping it with the base of the hurling stick, but they are tracked by markers. The game demands a substantial amount of upper body effort as well as leg exercise associated with contesting possession and playing the leather ball or sliotar. There is a small but not appreciable effect of carrying the camán, entailing an elevation in heart rate of 3 beats·min^{-1} (Fenton 1996).

The pattern of play in lacrosse is broadly similar to that in hurling. Lacrosse players have more freedom to roam, since fewer players are on the pitch. Good running abilities are important for play. As in other field games, the majority of the total distance travelled is taken up with movement away from play, in order to become available for a pass or afford an outlet for a player under pressure whilst in possession.

The camán is responsible for the majority of injuries in shinty (the Scottish form of hurling). The whole body is vulnerable (MacLean 1989). In hurling and camogie injuries are largely to the hand and to the face (Crowley & Condon 1989). Eye injuries have been highlighted in lacrosse (Livingston & Forbes 1996). Protective measures are clearly important in all stick-and-ball games.

Fitness

In both sports, players require a good aerobic fitness to withstand the endurance demands of competitive matches. Fitness programmes should incorporate anaerobic components, in view of the need for repeated short sprints. There is also considerable shoulder-blocking body contact, especially in the men's games. Neither sport is on the Olympic games calendar, but both provide a convenient reference for comparisons with field hockey; hurling, in particular, also bears comparisons with Gaelic football.

The $\dot{V}O_{2max}$ of 10 intercounty hurlers was measured at 56.8 ($\pm$ 5.0) ml·kg^{-1}·min^{-1} (Fenton 1996). Watson (1977) studied fitness over a competitive season of hurling. The training programmes of successful players increased physical capabilities

(PWC$_{170}$). It was concluded that endurance contributes to performance in both Gaelic football and hurling.

Conclusions

Field games incorporate bouts of high-intensity exercise superimposed on lower-intensity aerobic activity. Methods of quantifying physiological loading include motion analysis, estimated $\dot{V}_{O_2}$, heart rate and blood lactate measurements. The highest relative loading among football games is in soccer (about 75% $\dot{V}_{O_{2max}}$), followed by Australian Rules, Gaelic football, Rugby Union and Rugby League. American football emphasizes muscle strength and anaerobic power, with aerobic factors providing only part of general conditioning. The physiological demands are reflected in fitness measures and are accentuated by environmental stressors such as heat and altitude.

A considerable amount of data now describes the physiological characteristics of field hockey players of both genders. Such profiles need to be interpreted with caution, as competitive level, stage of season, player position and other factors should be considered.

In contrast there have been relatively few attempts to measure directly the physiological demands of match-play in field hockey, hurling, shinty or lacrosse. Nevertheless, inferences have been made from model games and motion analyses. Information about conditioning has been gathered from fundamental research on training and its physiological effects, and from training studies on football players. Information on environmental stressors must as yet be borrowed from exercise physiology literature (or studies of soccer players) and applied to the specific context of these stick-and-ball games, especially when play takes place in hot conditions.

References

Apor, P. (1988) Successful formulae for fitness training. In: Reilly, T., Lees, A., Davids, K. & Murphy, W. (eds) *Science and Football*, pp. 95–107. E. & F. N. Spon, London.

Åstrand, P.-O. & Rodahl, K. (eds) (1986) *Textbook of Work Physiology*. McGraw-Hill, New York.

Bangsbø, J. (1994a) The physiology of soccer—with special reference to intense intermittent exercise. *Acta Physiologica Scandinavica* 151 (Suppl.), 619.

Bangsbø, J. (1994b) Energy demands in competitive soccer. *Journal of Sports Sciences* 12, S5–S12.

Bangsbø, J. & Lindquist, F. (1992) Comparison of various exercise tests with endurance performance during soccer in professional players. *International Journal of Sports Medicine* 13, 125–132.

Bangsbø, J. & Mizuno, M. (1988) Morphological and metabolic alterations in soccer players with detraining and retraining and their relation to performance. In: Reilly, T., Lees, A., Davids K. & Murphy, W. (eds) *Science and Football*, pp. 1124–1135. E. & F. N. Spon, London.

Bangsbø, J., Norregaard, L. & Thorso, F. (1991) Activity profile of professional soccer. *Canadian Journal of Sport Sciences* 16, 110–116.

Bishon, M. (1993) Mean altitude training to prepare for altitude and sea level events. The Font–Romeau experience. In: *Proceedings of the International Symposium on 'the Altitude Factor in Athletic Performance'*, pp. 116–141. British Olympic Association, London.

Boyle, P., Mahoney, C.A. & Walker, W.F.M. (1994) The competitive demands of élite male field hockey. *Journal of Sports Medicine and Physical Fitness* 34, 235–241.

Brewer, J. & Davis, J. (1995) Applied physiology of Rugby League. *Sports Medicine* 13, 129–135.

Brooks, G.A. & Fahey, T.D. (1984) *Exercise Physiology: Human Bioenergetics and its Applications*. John Wiley, New York.

Burke, E.J., Winslow, E. & Straub, W.V. (1980) Measures of body composition and performance in major College football players. *Journal of Sports Medicine and Physical Fitness* 20, 173–180.

Cannon, S.R. & James, S.E. (1984) Back pain in athletes. *British Journal of Sports Medicine* 18, 159–164.

Carlson, B.R., Carter, J.E.L., Patterson, P., Petti, K., Orfanos, S.M. & Noffal, G.J. (1994) Physique and motor performance characteristics of US national rugby players. *Journal of Sports Sciences* 12, 403–412.

Cavanagh, P.R. & Williams, K.R. (1992) The effect of stride length variations on oxygen uptake during distance running. *Medicine and Science in Sports and Exercise* 14, 30–35.

Cheetham, M.E. & Williams, C. (1987) High intensity training & treadmill sprint performance. *British Journal of Sports Medicine* 21, 14–17.

Cheetham, M.E., Hazeldine, R.J., Robinson, A. & Williams, C. (1988) Power output in Rugby forwards during maximal treadmill sprinting. In: Reilly, T., Lees, A., Davids, K. & Murphy, W.J. (eds) *Science and Football*, pp. 206–210. E. & F. N. Spon, London.

Crowley, P.J. & Condon K.C. (1989) Analysis of hurling and camogie injuries. *British Journal of Sports Medicine* 23, 183–185.

Davies, B. & Daggett, A. (1977) Responses of adult women to programmed exercise. *British Journal of Sports Medicine* 11, 122–126.

Deutsch, M.U., Maw, G.J., Jenkins, D. & Reaburn, P. (1998) Heart rate, blood lactate and kinematic data of élite colts (under-19) rugby union players during competition. *Journal of Sports Sciences* 15, 561–570.

Di Prampero, P.E., Pinera Limas, F. & Sassi,

G. (1970) Maximal muscular power, aerobic and anaerobic in 116 athletes performing at the XIXth Olympic Games in Mexico. *Ergonomics* 13, 665–674.

Docherty, D., Wenger, W.A. & Neary, P. (1988) Time–motion analysis related to the physiological demands of Rugby. *Journal of Human Movement Studies* 14, 269–277.

Doncaster, C.P. (1972) Body temperature after rugby. *South African Medical Journal* 4C, 1872–1874.

Douge, B. (1988) Football: the common threads between the games. In: Reilly, T., Lees, A., Davids, K. & Murphy, W.J. (eds) *Science and Football*, pp. 3–19. E. & F. N. Spon, London.

Drobnic, F., Galiles, P.A., Pons, V., Riera, J. & Rodriguez, F.A. (1989) The breath frequency as a limiting factor for the ventilation of maximal effort in different sports. In: *Proceedings of the First IOC Congress on Sports Science, Colorado Springs*, pp. 122–123.

Ekblom, B. (1986) Applied physiology of soccer. *Sports Medicine* 3, 50–60.

Erp-Baart, A.M.J., van Saris, W.H.M., Binkhorst, R.A., Vos, J.A. & Elvers, J.W.H. (1989) Nationwide survey on nutritional habits in élite athletes. Part 1: Energy, carbohydrate, protein and fat intake. *International Journal of Sports Medicine* 10, S17–S21.

Fenton, C. (1996) A comparison in hurling of the physiological cost between carrying and not carrying a hurley. *Journal of Sports Sciences* 14, 81–82.

Florida-James, G. & Reilly, T. (1995) The physiological demands of Gaelic football. *British Journal of Sports Medicine* 23, 41–45.

Fox, E.L. (1984) *Sports Physiology*. Saunders, Philadelphia.

Garbutt, G., Boocock, M.G., Reilly, T. & Troup, J.D.G. (1990) An evaluation of warm-up procedures using spinal shrinkage. In: Lovesey, E.J. (ed.) *Contemporary Ergonomics 1990*, pp. 305–309. Taylor & Francis, London.

Gerisch, G., Rutemöller, E. & Weber, K. (1988) Sports medical measurements of performance in soccer. In: Reilly, T., Lees, A., Davids, K. & Murphy, W. (eds) *Science and Football*, pp. 60–67. E. & F. N. Spon, London.

Gettman, L.R., Storer, T.W. & Ward, R.D. (1987) Fitness changes in professional football players. *Physician and Sportsmedicine* 15 (9), 92–101.

Gleeson, N.P., Reilly, T., Mercer, T.H., Rakawaki, S. & Rees, D. (1998) Influence of endurance activity on key neuromus-cular and musculoskeletal performance. *Medicine and Science in Sports and Exercise* 30, 596–608.

Grafe, H.H. (1971) Nutrition. In: Larson, L.A. (ed.) *Encyclopaedia of Sports Sciences and Medicine*, pp. 1126–1130. Collier MacMillan, London.

Hirata, K.I. (1966) Physique and age of Tokyo Olympic champions. *Journal of Sports Medicine and Physical Fitness* 17, 207–222.

Holmyard, D.J. & Hazeldine, R.J. (1993) Seasonal variations in the anthropometric and physiological characteristics of international Rugby Union players. In: Reilly, T., Clarys, J. & Stibbe, A. (eds) *Science and Football II*, pp. 21–26. E. & F. N. Spon, London.

Jardine, M.A., Wiggins, T.M., Myburgh, K.H. & Noakes, T.D. (1988) Physiological characteristics of rugby players including muscle glycogen content and muscle fibre composition. *South African Medical Journal* 73, 529–532.

Jones, C.J. & Laussen, S. (1988) A periodised conditioning programme for Australian Rules football. In: Reilly, T., Lees, A., Davids, K. & Murphy, W. (eds) *Science and Football*, pp. 125–133. E. & F. N. Spon, London.

Kawakami, Y., Nazaki, D., Matsuo, A. & Fukinaga, T. (1992) Reliability of measurement of oxygen uptake by a portable telemetric system. *European Journal of Applied Physiology* 65, 409–414.

Keane, S., Reilly, T. & Hughes, M. (1993) Analysis of work rates in Gaelic football. *Australian Journal of Science and Medicine in Sport* 25, 100–102.

Keane, S., Reilly, T. & Borrie, A. (1997) A comparison of fitness characteristics of élite and non-élite Gaelic football players. In: Reilly, T., Bangsbø, J. & Hughes, M. (eds) *Science and Football III*, pp. 3–6. E. & F. N. Spon, London.

Kirby, W.J. & Reilly, T. (1993) Anthropometric and fitness profiles of élite female Rugby Union players. In: Reilly, T., Clarys, J. & Stibbe, A. (eds) *Science and Football II*, pp. 27–30. E. & F. N. Spon, London.

Kirgan, B. & Reilly, T. (1993) A fitness evaluation of Gaelic football players. In: Reilly, T., Clarys, J. & Stibbe, A. (eds) *Science and Football II*, pp. 59–61. E. & F. N. Spon, London.

Kneider, R.B., Hull, D., Horton, G., Downes, M., Smith, S. & Anders, B. (1995) Effects of carbohydrate supplementation during intense training on dietary sufferers, physiological status and performance. *International Journal of Sports Nutrition* 5, 115–135.

Leatt, P., Reilly, T. & Troup, J.D.G. (1985) Spinal loading during weight-training and running. *British Journal of Sports Medicine* 20, 119–124.

Leatt, P., Reilly, T. & Troup, J.D.G. (1986) Unloading the spine. In: Oborne, D. (ed.) *Contemporary Ergonomics*, pp. 227–232. Taylor & Francis, London.

Livingston, L.A. & Forbes, S.L. (1996) Eye injuries in women's lacrosse: strict rule enforcement and mandatory eyewear required. *Journal of Trauma—Injury, Infection and Critical Care* 40, 144–145.

McKenna, M.J., Sandstrom, E.R. & Chennalls, M.H.D. (1988) The effects of training and match-play upon maximal aerobic performance: a case study. In: Reilly, T., Lees, A., Davids, K. & Murphy, W.J. (eds) *Science and Football*, pp. 87–92. E. & F. N. Spon, London.

McLean, D.A. (1992) Analysis of the physical demands of international Rugby Union. *Journal of Sports Sciences* 13, 13–14.

McLean, D.A. (1993) Field testing in Rugby Union football. In: MacLeod, D.A., Maughan, R.J., Williams, C., Madely, C.R., Sharp, J.C.M. & Nutton, R.W. (eds) *Intermittent High-Intensity Exercise: Preparation, Stresses and Damage Limitation*, pp. 79–84. E. & F. N. Spon, London.

MacLean, J.G.B. (1989) A survey of injuries in the Highlands during 1987–88. *British Journal of Sports Medicine* 23, 179–182.

Malhotra, M.S., Ramaswamy, S.S. & Ray, S.V. (1962) Influence of body weight on energy expenditure. *Journal of Applied Physiology* 17, 433–435.

Malhotra, M.S., Ghosh, A.K. & Khanna, G.L. (1983) Physical and physiological stresses of playing hockey on grassy and Astroturf fields. *Society for National Institutes of Sport Journal* 6, 13–20.

Maud, P.J. (1983) Physiological and anthropometric parameters that describe a Rugby Union team. *British Journal of Sports Medicine* 17, 16–23.

Maughan, R.J. & Leiper, J.B. (1994) Fluid replacement requirements in soccer. *Journal of Sports Sciences* 12, S29–S34.

Mayes, R. & Nuttall, F.E. (1995) A comparison of the physiological characteristics of senior and under 21 élite rugby union players. *Journal of Sports Sciences* 13, 13–14.

Menchenelli, C., Morandini, C. & De Angelis, M.A. (1992a) A functional model of rugby: determination of the characteristics of sports performance. *Journal of Sports Sciences* 10, 196–197.

Menchenelli, C., Morandini, C. & Gardini, F. (1992b) A function model of rugby players: drawing up a physiological profile. *Journal of Sports Sciences* **10**, 152–153.

Miles, A., MacLaren, D. & Reilly, T. (1992) The efficacy of a new energy drink: a training study. *Communication to Olympic Scientific Congress*, 14–19 July (Benalmadena, Spain).

Morton, A.R. (1978) Applying physiological principles to rugby training. *Sports Coach* **2**, 4–9.

Novak, L.P., Hyatt, R.E. & Alexander, J.R. (1969) Body composition and physiologic function of athletes. *Journal of the American Medical Association* **205**, 764–770.

O'Brien, C. (1992) The hangover effect of alcohol on aerobic and anaerobic performance of a rugby population. *Journal of Sports Sciences* **10**, 139.

Ogushi, T., Ohashi, J., Nagahama, H., Isokawa, M. & Suzuki, S. (1993) Work intensity during soccer match-play (a case study). In: Reilly, T., Clarys, J. & Stibbe, A. *Science and Football II*, pp. 121–123. E. & F. N. Spon, London.

Piearce, L. (1993) Dietary habits of football. In: MacLeod, D.A.D., Maughan, R.J., Williams, C., Madeley, C.R., Sharp, J.C.M. & Nutton, R.W. (eds) *Intermittent High-Intensity Exercise: Preparation, Stresses and Damage Limitation*, pp. 159–173. E. & F. N. Spon, London.

Pohl, A.P., O'Halloran, M.W. & Pannall, P.R. (1981) Biochemical and physiological changes in football players. *Medical Journal of Australia* **1**, 467–470.

Prince, F.P., Hikida, R. & Hagerman, F.C. (1977) Muscle fibre types in women athletes and non athletes. *Pflügers Archives* **371**, 161–165.

Pyke, F. & Smith, R. (1975) *Football: the Scientific Way*. University of Western Australia, Nedlands.

Ready, A.E. & van der Merwe, M. (1986) Physiological monitoring of the 1984 Canadian women's Olympic field hockey team. *Australian Journal of Science and Medicine in Sport* **18** (3), 13–18.

Rebelo, A.N., Candelus, J.R., Freya, M.M. *et al.* (1998) The impact of soccer training on the immune system. *Journal of Sports Medicine and Physical Fitness* **38**, 258–261.

Reid, R.H. & Williams, C. (1974) A concept of fitness and its measurement in relation to Rugby football. *British Journal of Sports Medicine* **8**, 96–99.

Reilly, T. (1979) *What Research Tells the Coach About Soccer*. AAHPERD, Washington.

Reilly, T. (1981) *Sports Fitness and Sports Injuries*. Faber & Faber, London.

Reilly, T. (1990) Football. In: Reilly, T., Secher, N., Snell, P. & Williams, C. (eds) *Physiology of Sports*, pp. 372–425. E. & F. N. Spon, London.

Reilly, T. (1994) Motion characteristics. In: Ekblom, B. (ed.) *Football (Soccer)*, pp. 31–42. Blackwell Science, Oxford.

Reilly, T. (1996) *Science and Soccer*. E. & F. N. Spon, London.

Reilly, T. (1997a) Energetics of high-intensity exercise (soccer) with particular reference to fatigue. *Journal of Sports Sciences* **15**, 257–263.

Reilly, T. (1997b) The physiology of Rugby Union football. *Biology of Sport* **14**, 83–101.

Reilly, T. & Ball, D. (1984) The net physiological cost of dribbling a soccer ball. *Research Quarterly for Exercise and Sport* **55**, 267–271.

Reilly, T. & Borrie, A. (1992) Physiology applied to field hockey. *Sports Medicine* **14**, 10–26.

Reilly, T. & Bowen, T. (1984) Exertional cost of changes in directional modes of running. *Perceptual and Motor Skills* **58**, 49–50.

Reilly, T. & Bretherton, S. (1986) Multivariate analysis of fitness in female field hockey players. In: Day, J.A.P. (ed.) *Perspectives in Kinanthropometry*, pp. 135–142. Human Kinetics, Champaign, IL.

Reilly, T. & Doran, D. (1999) Kinanthropometric and performance profiles of élite Gaelic footballers. *Journal of Sports Sciences* **17**, 922 (Abstract).

Reilly, T. & Hardiker, R. (1981) Somatotype and injuries in adult student Rugby Union football. *Journal of Sports Medicine and Physical Fitness* **21**, 186–191.

Reilly, T. & Lewis, W. (1985) Effects of carbohydrate loading on mental functions during sustained physical work. In: Brown, I.D., Goldsmith, R., Coombes, K. & Sinclair, M. (eds) *Ergonomics International 85*, pp. 700–702. Taylor & Francis, London.

Reilly, T. & Seaton, A. (1990) Physiological strain unique to field hockey. *Journal of Sports Medicine and Physical Fitness* **30**, 142–146.

Reilly, T. & Secher, N. (1990) Physiology of sports: an overview. In: Reilly, T., Secher, N., Snell, P. & Williams, C. (eds) *Physiology of Sports*, pp. 465–485. E. & F. N. Spon, London.

Reilly, T. & Stirling, A. (1993) Flexibility, warm-up and injuries in mature games players. In: Duquet, W. & Day, J.A.P. (eds) *Kinanthropometry IV*, pp. 119–123. E. & F. N. Spon, London.

Reilly, T. & Thomas, V. (1976) A motion analysis of work-rate in different positional roles in professional football match-play. *Journal of Human Movement Studies* **2**, 87–97.

Reilly, T. & Thomas, V. (1977) Effect of a programme of pre-season training on the fitness of soccer players. *Journal of Sports Medicine and Physical Fitness* **17**, 401–412.

Reilly, T. & Thomas, V. (1979) Estimated energy expenditures of professional association footballers. *Ergonomics* **22**, 541–548.

Reilly, T. & Thomas, V. (1980) The stability of fitness factors over a season of professional soccer as indicated by serial factor analyses. In: Ostyn, M., Beunen, G. & Simons, J. (eds) *Kinanthropometry II*, pp. 245–257. University Park Press, Baltimore.

Reilly, T., Parry-Billings, M. & Ellis, A. (1985) Changes in fitness profiles of international female hockey players during the competitive season. *Journal of Sports Sciences* **3**, 210.

Rienzi, E., Mazza, J.C., Carter, J.E.L. & Reilly, T. (1998) *Footbolista Sudamericano de Élite: Morfologia, Analisis del Juego y Performance*. Biosystem Servicio Educativo, Rosario.

Rigg, P. & Reilly, T. (1988) A fitness profile and anthropometric analysis of first and second class Rugby Union players. In: Reilly, T., Lees, A., Davids, K. & Murphy, W.J. (eds) *Science and Football*, pp. 194–200. E. & F. N. Spon, London.

Rohde, H.C. & Espersen, T. (1988) Work intensity during soccer training and match-play. In: Reilly, T., Lees, A., Davids, K. & Murphy, W. (eds) *Science and Football*, pp. 68–75. E. & F. N. Spon, London.

Rost, R. (1987) *Athletics and the Heart Year Book*. Medical Publishers, Chicago.

Saltin, B. (1973) Metabolic fundamentals in exercise. *Medicine and Science in Sports and Exercise* **5**, 137–146.

Sedlock, D.A., Fitzgerald, P.I. & Knowlton, R.G. (1988) Body composition and performance of collegiate women rugby players. *Research Quarterly for Exercise and Sports* **59**, 78–82.

Seliger, V. (1968a) Heart rate on an index of physical load in exercise. *Scripta Medica* **41**, 231–240. Medical Faculty, Brno University, Czechoslovakia.

Seliger, V. (1968b) Energy metabolism in selected physical exercises. *Internationale Zeitschrift für Angewandte Physiologie* **25**, 104–120.

Sharkey, B. (1986) *Coaches' guide to Sport Physiology*. Human Kinetics, Champaign, IL.

Skubic, V. & Hodgkins, J. (1967) Relative strenuousness of selected sports as performed by women. *Research Quarterly* 38, 305–313.

Smaros, G. (1980) Energy usage during football match. In: Vecchiet, L. (ed.) *Proceedings of the 1st International Congress on Sports Medicine Applied to Football*, Vol 11, pp. 795–801. D. Guanello, Rome.

Sparling, P.B., Snow, T.K., Rosskopf, L.B., O'Donnell, P.M., Freedson, P.S. & Byrnes, W.C. (1998) Bone mineral density of the United States Olympic women's field hockey team. *British Journal of Sports Medicine* 32, 315–318.

Tong, R.J. & Mayes, R. (1995) The effect of pre-season training on the physiological characteristics of international Rugby Union players. *Journal of Sports Sciences* 13, 507.

Troup, J.D.G., Reilly, T., Eklund, J.A.E. & Leatt, P. (1985) Changes in stature with spinal loading and their relation to perception of exertion or discomfort. *Stress Medicine* 1, 303–307.

Ueno, Y., Watai, E. & Ishii, K. (1988) Aerobic and anaerobic performance of Rugby football players. In: Reilly, T., Lees, A., Davids, K. & Murphy, W.J. (eds) *Science and Football II*, pp. 201–205. E. & F. N. Spon, London.

Van Gool, D., Van Gervess, D. & Boutmans, T. (1988) The physiological load imposed on soccer players during real match-play. In: Reilly, T., Lees, A., Davids, K. & Murphy, W. (eds) *Science and Football*, pp. 51–59. E. & F. N. Spon, London.

Watson, A.W.S. (1977) A study of the physical working capacity of Gaelic footballers and hurlers. *British Journal of Sports Medicine* 11, 133–137.

Watson, A.W.S. (1995) Physical and fitness characteristics of successful Gaelic footballers. *British Journal of Sports Medicine* 29, 229–231.

Wein, H. (1981) *The Advance Science of Hockey*. Pelham Books, London.

Westerterp, K.R. & Saris, W.H.M. (1991) Limits of energy turnover in relation to physical peformance, achievement of energy balance on a daily basis. *Journal of Sports Sciences* 9 (Suppl. 1), 1–15.

Whitaker, D. (1986) *Coaching Hockey*. Crowood Press, Marlborough.

Williams, C., Reid, R.M. & Coutts, R. (1973) Observations on the aerobic power of University Rugby players and professional soccer players. *British Journal of Sports Medicine* 7, 390–391.

Wilmore, J.H. & Haskell, W.L. (1972) Body composition and endurance capacity of professional football players. *Journal of Applied Physiology* 33, S64–S67.

Winter, F.D., Snell, P.G. & Stray-Gunderson, J. (1989) Effects of 100% oxygen on performance of professional soccer players. *Journal of the American Medical Association* 262, 227–229.

Wisloff, U., Helgerud, J. & Hoff, J. (1998) Strength and endurance of élite soccer players. *Medicine and Science in Sports and Exercise* 30, 462–467.

Withers, R.T., Roberts, R.G.D. & Davies, G.J. (1977) The maximum aerobic power, anaerobic power and body composition of South Australian male representatives in athletics, basketball, field hockey and soccer. *Journal of Sports Medicine and Physical Fitness* 17, 391–400.

Withers, R.T., Maricic, Z., Wesilewski, S. & Kelly, L. (1982) Match analysis of Australian professional soccer players. *Journal of Human Movement Studies* 8, 159–176.

Yamaoka, S. (1965) Studies on energy metabolism. *Research Journal of Physical Education (Taiikugaku Kenkyu)* 9, 28–40.

Zeldis, S.M., Morganroth, J. & Rubler, S. (1978) Cardiac hypertrophy in respect to dynamic conditioning in female athletes. *Journal of Applied Physiology* 44, 849–852.

Chapter 62

Mountaineering

ROBERT B. SCHOENE AND THOMAS F. HORNBEIN

Introduction

Mountaineering encompasses a broad range of physical activities, from the intense muscular conditioning and gymnastic agility of the rock climber to the durability and endurance of the high-altitude mountaineer. Common to all forms of mountaineering, from fast and difficult short ascents of artificial or real rock walls to remote ascents in unexplored regions, is the element of verticality, i.e. high-angle terrain where error or unforeseen events can result in death. Therefore, common to all forms of mountain climbing are such elements as difficulty, a variable quantum of risk and the need for skill, knowledge and judgement.

Aside from the elements of risk and uncertainty, the physical demands upon the human body are analogous to those of other sports, such as gymnastics, skiing and endurance running. The unique element of mountain venture derives from the decrease in barometric pressure and the partial pressure of inspired oxygen. For example, at the summit of Mount Everest, the barometric pressure is but one-third of that at sea-level. The resulting hypoxia impedes performance and places special demands on the human body with regard to strength, endurance and nutrition. Certain illnesses caused by hypoxia may at times be fatal.

In this chapter we will limit our discussion to the effects of high altitude upon human performance. We shall review the physiological adaptations to hypoxia, discuss the limits to maximum exercise at extreme altitude, define endurance in this environment, and consider attributes that are conducive to

better performance at high altitude. Additionally, we shall briefly discuss nutritional requirements and make suggestions for training.

The environment

Although the high-altitude environment includes other environmental stresses such as cold and exposure to intense ultraviolet radiation which may have an impact on elements of performance such as muscle fatigue, dehydration, malnutrition and mental fatigue, the decreasing barometric pressure with increasing altitude is the unique problem for the high-altitude mountaineer (Table 62.1). Because of a variety of physiological adaptations, oxygen delivery to the tissues is remarkably well maintained in spite of the decreased partial pressure of oxygen (Po_2) in the inspired air (Fig. 62.1). Adaptation minimizes the magnitude of steps in the oxygen cascade, helping to maintain an adequate delivery of oxygen to the mitochondria. Without any adaptation, a sudden exposure to severe hypoxia can result in a loss of consciousness and even death.

Adaptation

The body adjusts to hypoxia with changes in ventilation, gas exchange from the alveoli to the blood, haemoglobin affinity for oxygen, red blood cell mass and transfer of oxygen from the capillaries to the mitochondria (Schoene & Hornbein 1988). The most important recipients of oxygen are the exercising muscle and the central nervous system.

Table 62.1 Mean ± s.d. of values for resting ventilation and arterial blood gases in seven subjects, measured during a simulated 40-day ascent of Mount Everest, in a chamber (Operation Everest II). Modified from Goldberg and Schoene (1992).

Altitude		Barometric pressure (Torr)	Partial pressure of inspired oxygen (Torr)	Pulmonary ventilation (l·min⁻¹)	pH	Partial pressure of carbon dioxide (Torr)	Partial pressure of oxygen (Torr)	Oxygen saturation (%)
Feet	Metres							
0	0	760	150	11.0 ± 1.0	7.43 ± 0.04	33.9 ± 3.5	99.3 ± 9.3	97.6 ± 0.1
15 000	4570	429	80	14.6 ± 2.7	7.46 ± 0.02	25.0 ± 2.2	52.4 ± 4.0	84.8 ± 4.0
20 000	6100	347	63	20.9 ± 6.3	7.50 ± 0.04	20.0 ± 2.8	41.1 ± 3.3	75.2 ± 6.0
26 500	8080	282	49	36.6 ± 7.9	7.53 ± 0.03	12.5 ± 1.1	36.6 ± 2.2	67.8 ± 5.0
29 029	8840	240	43	42.3 ± 7.7	7.56 ± 0.03	11.2 ± 2.1	30.3 ± 2.1	58.0 ± 4.5

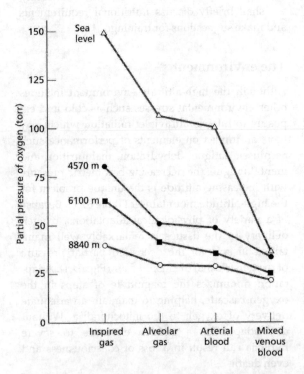

Fig. 62.1 The cascade of oxygen partial pressures at four different altitudes.

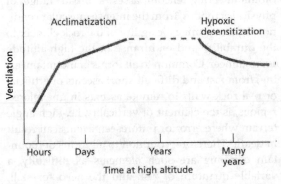

Fig. 62.2 Course of ventilatory response to acclimatization to high altitude at different durations of exposure, from hours to a lifetime. From Weil (1986), with permission.

Ventilation

With the initial exposure to high altitude, breathing increases (Weil 1986). The hyperventilation (relative to sea-level) is initiated by the peripheral chemoreceptors, notably the carotid body (Lahiri *et al.* 1981), although there is much inter-individual variability in the magnitude of this response. Much of the increased ventilation occurs within the first few days after ascent, but a steady level of ventilation at a particular altitude may not develop for several weeks. Many years of residence at high altitude can result in a decrease of ventilation (Fig. 62.2) (Weil 1986). Hyperventilation results in a decrease in alveolar $P\text{co}_2$ and an increase in alveolar $P\text{o}_2$ which is reflected by an increased arterial $P\text{o}_2$ and oxygen content of arterial blood (West *et al.* 1983b). Ventilatory acclimatization is associated with renal bicarbonate excretion in compensation for the respiratory alkalosis. However, compensation is never complete, and there is a persistent respiratory alkalaemia.

Pulmonary function

Upon initial ascent, lung compliance, vital capacity and air flow decrease and gas trapping increases (Coates *et al.* 1979; Jaeger *et al.* 1979; Gautier *et al.* 1982). These changes are attributed to an increase in interstitial lung water, which normally resolves within the first day or two at altitude. Lifelong residence at high altitude results in an increase of lung volume and diffusion capacity, documented in high-altitude natives of the Andes and Himalayas (Remmers & Mithoefer 1969; Frisancho *et al.* 1973; Vincent *et al.* 1978).

Gas exchange

Alveolar hypoxia results in an increase in pulmonary arterial pressure, which at rest improves perfusion of non-dependent regions of the lung. Prolonged stay at high altitude can result in severe pulmonary hypertension, leading to chronic mountain sickness (Monge's disease), characterized by pulmonary hypertension, polycythaemia, mental slowing and cor pulmonale (Monge 1928; Winslow & Monge 1987).

Diffusion

Transfer of oxygen from the air to the blood is decreased because of the lower driving pressure of oxygen in alveolar gas (Fig. 62.3) (West & Wagner 1980). This limitation to oxygen transfer from the air to the blood is accentuated during exercise, when a higher cardiac output results in a shorter transit time for red blood cells across the pulmonary capillaries and a briefer opportunity for end-capillary Po_2 to approach that in the alveoli (Fig. 62.3). The arterial oxygen desaturation that occurs with exercise at high altitude can be quite profound (Fig. 62.4) (West *et al.* 1983a).

Blood

Two adaptations of oxygen transport occur at high

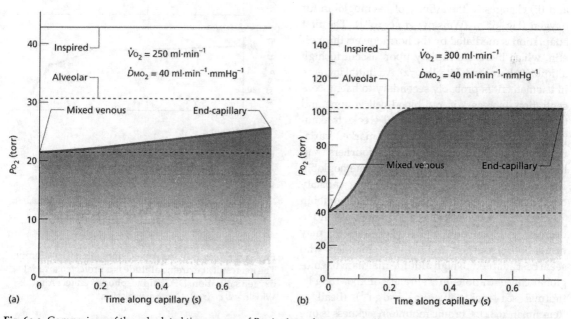

Fig. 62.3 Comparison of the calculated time course of Po_2 in the pulmonary capillary of a climber at rest on the summit of Mount Everest (P_B 250 torr, PIO_2 43 torr) (a) to sea-level values (P_B 760 torr, PIO_2 150 torr) (b). From West and Wagner (1980), with permission. $\dot{D}MO_2$, membrane diffusion capacity for oxygen, P_B, barometric pressure; PIO_2, inspired partial pressure of oxygen.

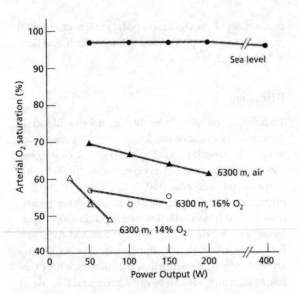

Fig. 62.4 Arterial oxygen saturation (%) does not decrease with exercise at sea-level but drops progressively more rapidly with higher levels of exercise at greater altitudes. From West *et al.* (1983a), with permission.

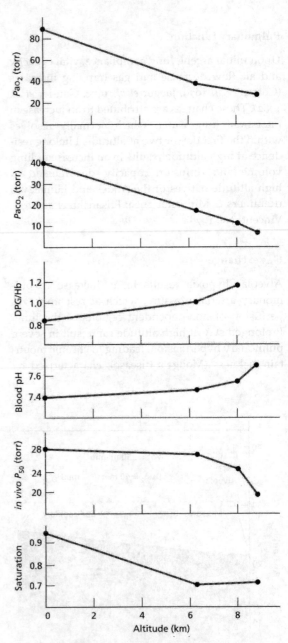

Fig. 62.5 Effectors of oxygen–haemoglobin (Hb) affinity. The net result at extreme altitude is a protected arterial oxygen saturation. DPG, diphosphoglycerate. From Winslow *et al.* (1984), with permission.

altitude: (i) an increase in red blood cell production; and (ii) changes in the affinity of haemoglobin for oxygen (Fig. 62.5) (Winslow *et al.* 1984). The first adaptation is mediated by the hormone erythropoietin, which increases rapidly upon ascent to high altitude (Abbrecht & Littell 1972). An initial increase in haematocrit is probably secondary to haemoconcentration. Increases in red blood cell volume and total blood volume require several weeks to complete (Sanchez *et al.* 1970). There is marked variability in this response in both sojourners and high-altitude natives. An increase in haemoglobin concentration increases oxygen-carrying capacity but, if the increase is too great (haemoglobin $>190\,g\cdot l^{-1}$), blood viscosity also increases and a decrease in blood flow and oxygen delivery may result. Both sojourners and native highlanders who seem best adapted to high altitude maintain haemoglobin concentrations in the range of $160–180\,g\cdot l^{-1}$ (normal sea-level value $130–150\,g\cdot l^{-1}$) (Beall & Reischman 1984). Chronic mountain sickness is one example of the adverse consequence of a surfeit of red blood cell production (Winslow & Monge 1987).

The affinity of haemoglobin for oxygen influences

both loading of oxygen at the lung and unloading at the tissues. At moderate altitudes a rightward shift of the oxyhaemoglobin dissociation curve enhances unloading of oxygen to the tissue (Aste-Salazar & Hurtado 1944; Moore & Brewer 1981). Although the arterial Po_2 is high enough to minimize the effect of the shift on arterial oxygen saturation, at very high altitudes (where alveolar Po_2 is much less), a left-shifted curve might better optimize intake of oxygen at the lungs (Fig. 62.5) (Winslow et al. 1984). Some animals who live at or birds that fly at very high altitude have left-shifted oxyhaemoglobin dissociation curves (Swan 1970; Faraci et al. 1984), and the marked respiratory alkalosis noted in humans at extreme altitude also results in a leftward shift of the curve (Winslow et al. 1984).

Tissue adaptation

Adaptation at the cellular level is less well understood. Some studies suggest that several weeks' exposure to high altitude results in increases in capillary and mitochondrial density, as well as a decrease in cell size, all of which would decrease the

radial diffusion distance for oxygen from the capillaries to the mitochondria (Ou & Tenney 1970; Tenney & Ou 1970; Banchero 1975). There is controversy about what occurs to oxidative enzymes upon ascent to high altitudes (Hochachka et al. 1982; Green et al. 1989), but the sum total of all these mentioned changes is presumably beneficial to oxidative metabolism.

Limitation to exercise

Although little is known about endurance performance at high altitude, a great deal is known about maximal aerobic power. Maximal oxygen intake ($\dot{V}o_{2max}$) decreases with increasing altitude (West et al. 1983a; Reeves et al. 1987; Cymerman et al. 1989). Studies both in the field and in a high-altitude chamber have shown that at the summit of Mount Everest (barometric pressure of approximately 250 torr), $\dot{V}o_{2max}$ is about 20% of the sea-level value (Fig. 62.6) (West et al. 1983a; Cymerman et al. 1989). Interestingly, even though individuals may start with different values of $\dot{V}o_{2max}$ at sea-level, those who have been studied have similar values when exercis-

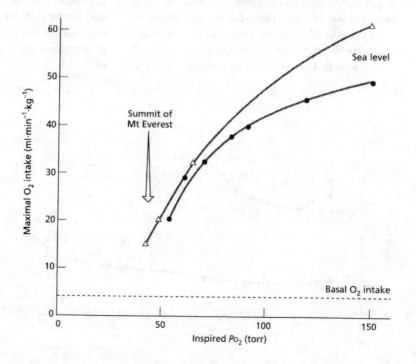

Fig. 62.6 Maximal oxygen intake ($\dot{V}o_{2max}$) against inspired Po_2. There is a predictable decrease in $\dot{V}o_{2max}$ at high altitudes. From West et al. (1983a). △, 1981 expedition; •, from Pugh et al. (1964).

ing at a barometric pressure equivalent to that at the summit of Mount Everest.

The cause of the decrease in exercise performance is probably multifactorial, including impaired diffusion of oxygen from air to blood in the lungs and consequently a lesser availability of oxygen to the exercising muscles and brain (Gale *et al.* 1985; Torre-Bueno *et al.* 1985; Wagner *et al.* 1986, 1987). At very high altitude, diffusion of oxygen to the tissues may also be compromised by the low Po_2.

The ventilatory response to exercise at high altitude is a marked increase in ventilation. This helps maintain arterial oxygen saturation (Fig. 62.7) (Schoene 1984), but is not sufficient to reverse the diffusion limitation and the subsequent desaturation of arterial blood. In the high-altitude sojourner, a greater ventilatory response results in less arterial oxygen desaturation (Schoene *et al.* 1984), whereas in high-altitude natives who have a more blunted ventilatory response, desaturation is minimized in part by an increased surface area for oxygen transfer (diffusion capacity) (Dempsey *et al.* 1971).

For a given work rate, cardiac output is, for the most part, similar at high altitude to that at sea-level (Reeves *et al.* 1987). After exposure of several weeks or longer at moderate to extreme altitude, maximal heart rate is decreased (West *et al.* 1983a). Inhalation of oxygen results in an increase in maximum heart rate and in maximal aerobic power, although values remain well below those at sea-level. The mechanism for the lower maximal heart rate is not understood.

Limits to short bouts of intense exercise may reflect a failure of oxygen delivery to the brain rather than muscle. Hypoxia may impair central nervous system function. Numerous accounts exist of climbers at these heights who, upon further exertion, hallucinate, have narrowed or blurred vision, or come close to losing consciousness. Several studies have shown neurobehavioural dysfunction after return from extreme altitude (Cavaletti *et al.* 1987; Hornbein *et al.* 1989; Regard *et al.* 1989). This is particularly notable in individuals with a more vigorous ventilatory response to hypoxia, an attribute that correlates with a better physical performance while at high altitude (Hornbein *et al.* 1989). The authors speculate that the greater ventilatory response results in more profound hypocapnia and cerebral vasoconstriction, and consequently a larger decrease in oxygen delivery to the brain.

Endurance performance at high altitude

For high-altitude mountaineering, endurance is defined not in hours, but in days, weeks or months. Therefore, data taken from brief, maximal exercise may not predict performance at high altitude. Much information on the effect of high altitude on athletic performance was obtained in the 1960s, at the time of the Mexico City Olympics (altitude 2300 m). For

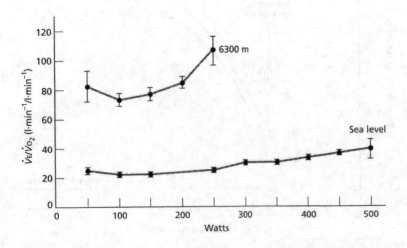

Fig. 62.7 The ventilatory response expressed as the ventilatory equivalent ($\dot{V}_E/\dot{V}o_2$) in subjects at sea-level (P_B 755 torr) and at 6300 m (P_B 350 torr), demonstrating that the ventilatory response for a given metabolic rate is almost four times the sea-level value. From Schoene (1984).

events lasting for more than 2 min, some period of acclimatization is necessary for optimal performance. Most studies looked at $\dot{V}o_{2max}$ or performance time over measured distances (Dill *et al.* 1966; Buskirk *et al.* 1967; Grover *et al.* 1967), but improvement in submaximal exercise performance rather than intense exercise to exhaustion is more pertinent to high-altitude climbing (Maher *et al.* 1974). Here little objective information exists. As any high-altitude mountaineer can relate, at altitudes up to 5000 m, performance improves with time. One study suggested that endurance time at 75% of $\dot{V}o_{2max}$ was greater at day 12 than at day 2 of exposure at 4300 m (Maher *et al.* 1974). This improvement was associated with decreased blood lactate concentrations, suggesting that improved exercise capacity resulted from better tissue oxygenation. No similar longitudinal studies have been performed above 6000 m.

Based on anecdotes, an altitude of 5500 m, where the barometric pressure is half that at sea-level, appears to represent the limit of permanent human habitation. Above that altitude, performance deteriorates after the initial period of acclimatization. It has become fashionable during expeditions to extreme altitude to acclimatize at moderate altitude with occasional short forays to extreme altitude, before making a final rapid ascent. This approach may optimize the adaptive processes while minimizing the deleterious effects of extreme altitude.

Training

Although aerobic fitness is generally associated with greater speed of travel and thus safety in the mountains, it is not clear whether maximal aerobic power correlates with performance at extreme altitude. Aerobic training at low altitude or intermediate altitude is still the most beneficial way of enhancing performance at high altitude. Gains may be achieved by optimization of ventilation, haematological response, cardiovascular fitness and peripheral tissue adaptation, the benefits of which are common to both low- and high-altitude performance. Of these adaptations, those of the blood and tissues may be particularly important. At low alti-

tude, a modest increase in haemoglobin concentration is associated with improved endurance performance (Buick *et al.* 1980). One might presume that the high-altitude sojourner would gain similar benefits. All of these adaptations occur spontaneously over days to weeks at high altitude. In order to optimize performance, the mountaineer should ascend at a comfortable pace that will allow adaptation to take place, while minimizing the possibility of incurring altitude illness.

Controversy has existed regarding the benefit of high-altitude training for low-altitude events. Anecdotal evidence suggested that living and training at moderate altitude, for the aforementioned reasons, conveyed benefit for the competitor in aerobic events at low altitude, but no good data were available to substantiate that claim until recently. Levine and Stray-Gundersen (1997) tested accomplished runners in four well-controlled situations. One group lived and trained at low (1250 m) altitude, one lived and trained high (2500 m), another lived high and trained low, while a fourth lived low and trained high. The group that lived high and trained low had the greatest improvement in maximal oxygen intake, sustainable time of maximal power output (Figs 62.8 & 62.9) and 5000-m run time. The improvement was attributed in part to the increase in haemoglobin and ability to maintain high-intensity workouts at the lower altitude which was not possible if training occurred at the higher altitude. The investigators found, however, that there was individual variation in the erythropoietic response such that not everyone responded to high-altitude training, and only enough data were available to substantiate the claim in men.

The élite climber

Unlike most sports in which élite performers have many common characteristics, the élite mountaineer cannot be so simply described. Several researchers have studied some physiological markers of mountaineers who have climbed on one or more occasions to 8000 m or higher (Schoene 1982; Masuyama *et al.* 1986; Oelz *et al.* 1986). Factors such as hypoxic ventilatory responses, aerobic power, strength, muscle fibre type and bio-

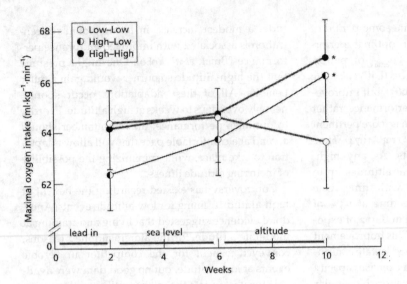

Fig. 62.8 Maximal oxygen uptake at baseline after sea-level training in Dallas (sea-level) and after altitude training camp or sea-level control (altitude). *$P < 0.05$ compared with previous time point for a given group.

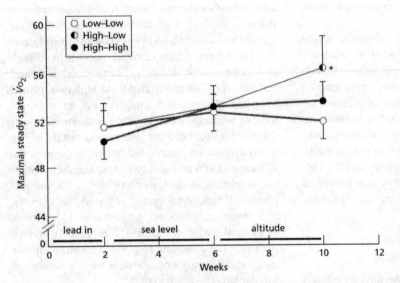

Fig. 62.9 Oxygen uptake ($\dot{V}o_2$) at maximal steady state, determined from ventilatory threshold, at baseline, after sea-level training in Dallas (sea-level), and after altitude training camp or sea-level control (altitude). Group characteristics and figure symbols are defined as in Fig. 62.8. *$P < 0.05$ compared with previous time point.

mechanics were investigated, to see whether any of these characteristics predicted climbing performance at extreme altitude (Oelz *et al.* 1986). Most, but not all, of the climbers had high $\dot{V}o_{2max}$ values (>60 ml·kg^{-1}·min^{-1}). On the other hand, one of the world's best climbers had a $\dot{V}o_{2max}$ that was only moderately greater than the normal expected value (48 ml·kg^{-1}·min^{-1}). Previously, a very high $\dot{V}o_{2max}$ was thought to be a requisite for the Himalayan climber. Perhaps the efficient climber may be able to climb for prolonged periods at a high percentage of

their $\dot{V}o_{2max}$, in a manner similar to long-distance runners. The absolute value of $\dot{V}o_{2max}$ at sea-level may not be a relevant predictor of performance at extreme altitude, because the factors limiting $\dot{V}o_{2max}$ at sea-level (primarily cardiovascular) are not those that limit performance at extreme altitude — diffusion limitation at either the lung and/or the peripheral tissues becomes the critical factor.

A number of studies have found that many successful climbers to extreme altitude have moderate to high ventilatory responses (HVR) to hypoxia

(Schoene 1982; Masuyama *et al.* 1986; Oelz *et al.* 1986) and exercise (Oelz *et al.* 1986). A greater alveolar ventilation ensures a higher alveolar P_{O_2} and subsequently minimizes the arterial oxygen desaturation during exercise (Schoene *et al.* 1984). This characteristic is probably only important for those who go to extreme altitudes, where a slight increase in ventilation can make a substantial difference in oxygen saturation. On the other hand, some individuals with blunted HVR and ventilation upon ascent appear to be more prone to mild and severe altitude illness (Hackett *et al.* 1982, 1988). A higher breathing response may, therefore, be a helpful but not essential attribute of the high-altitude climber.

These studies have not found any characteristic common to all élite climbers. What may be more important are some of the less tangible traits without which no mountain can be climbed. A strong psychological drive, tenacity, patience, team work, knowledge, skill, judgement and joy in the activity are all prerequisites that are difficult to define by objective data.

Nutrition

Although many of the physiological responses to high altitude are well described, another key element to success or failure with prolonged stay at high altitude is nutrition. The well-described shift in food preference from fats and carbohydrates to primarily carbohydrates as one ascends may reflect the body's needs. A unique factor found in high-altitude climbers is malabsorption in both the small and large intestines (Boyer & Blume 1984). This has been documented at altitudes above 6000 m. Carbo-hydrates are probably better absorbed than other fuels; thus, to optimize performance, carbohydrates should be ingested to the point of tolerance to ensure adequate blood glucose, muscle glycogen and free fatty acid and triglyceride stores. Although weight loss is generally the rule in individuals climbing at high altitude for weeks or more, there is an individual variability in this response which may reflect the difference in preferences and tolerance for food (Boyer & Blume 1984).

Both field and high-altitude chamber studies have documented a decrease in muscle mass, while fat stores (although decreased from sea-level) are still present (Boyer & Blume 1984; Green *et al.* 1989). These findings reflect muscle catabolism, which suggests utilization of gluconeogenesis to maintain blood glucose and muscle glycogen. Interestingly, studies even at extreme altitude show adequate muscle glycogen stores (Green *et al.* 1989).

Summary

Physiological adaptations to high altitude optimize aerobic power in an environment characterized by a diminished oxygen supply. Although these adaptations improve aerobic capacity during a stay at moderate altitude, sea-level capacities are never fully restored. Even less information is known about endurance performance for the high-altitude mountaineer during prolonged exposure to altitude. Much anecdotal evidence suggests that, at moderate altitude, continual activity and adequate nutrition are the key elements in sustaining endurance and performance. At extreme altitude much more individual variability may exist based on psychological rather than physiological characteristics.

References

Abbrecht, P.H. & Littell, J.K. (1972) Plasma erythropoietin in men and mice during acclimatization to different altitudes. *Journal of Applied Physiology* 32, 34–58.

Aste-Salazar, H. & Hurtado, A. (1944) The affinity of hemoglobin for oxygen at sea level and high altitude. *American Journal of Physiology* 142, 733–743.

Banchero, N. (1975) Capillary density of skeletal muscle in dogs exposed to simu-lated altitude. *Proceedings of the Society for Experimental Biology and Medicine* 148, 435–439.

Beall, C.M. & Reischman, A.B. (1984) Hemoglobin levels in the Himalayan high altitude population. *American Journal of Physical Anthropology* 63, 301–306.

Boyer, S.J. & Blume, F.D. (1984) Weight loss and changes in body composition at high altitude. *Journal of Applied Physiology* 57, 1580–1585.

Buick, F.J., Gledhill, N., Froese, A.B., Sprite, L. & Meyers, E.C. (1980) Effect of induced erythrocythemia on aerobic work capacities. *Journal of Applied Physiology* 48, 636–642.

Buskirk, E.R., Collias, J., Akers, R.F., Prokop, E.K. & Reategui, E.P. (1967) Maximal performance at altitude and on return from altitude in conditioned runners. *Journal of Applied Physiology* **23**, 259–266.

Cavaletti, G., Moroni, R., Garavaglia, P. & Tredici, G. (1987) Brain damage after high altitude climbs without oxygen. *Lancet* **i**, 101.

Coates, G., Gray, G., Mansell, A. *et al.* (1979) Changes in lung volume, lung density, and distribution of ventilation during hypobaric decompression. *Journal of Applied Physiology* **46**, 752–755.

Cymerman, A., Reeves, J.T., Sutton, J.R. *et al.* (1989) Operation Everest II: maximal oxygen uptake at extreme altitude. *Journal of Applied Physiology* **66**, 2446–2453.

Dempsey, J.A., Reddun, W.G., Birnbaum, M.L. *et al.* (1971) Effects of acute through life-long hypoxic exposure in exercise pulmonary gas exchange. *Respiration Physiology* **13**, 62–89.

Dill, D.B., Myrhe, L.G., Phillips, E.E. Jr & Brown, D.K. (1966) Work capacity in acute exposure to altitude. *Journal of Applied Physiology* **21**, 1168–1176.

Faraci, F.M., Kilgore, D.L. Jr & Feddle, M.R. (1984) Oxygen delivery to the heart and brain during hypoxia: Peking duck versus bar-headed goose. *American Journal of Physiology* **247**, R69–R75.

Frisancho, A.R., Velasquez, T. & Sanches, J. (1973) Influence of developmental adaptation on lung function at high altitude. *Human Biology* **45**, 583–594.

Gale, G.E., Torre-Bueno, J.R., Moon, R.E., Saltzman, H.A. & Wagner, P.D. (1985) Ventilation–perfusion inequality in normal humans during exercise at sea level in simulated altitude. *Journal of Applied Physiology* **58**, 978–988.

Gautier, H., Peslin, R., Grassino, A. *et al.* (1982) Mechanical properties of the lungs during acclimatization to altitude. *Journal of Applied Physiology* **52**, 1407–1415.

Goldberg S. & Schoene, R.B. (1992) Mountain sickness and other disorders at high altitude. In: Aghabadian, R.V. (ed.) *Emergency Medicine*. Little Brown & Company, Boston.

Green, H.J., Sutton, J.R., Young, P., Cymerman, A. & Houston, C.S. (1989) Operation Everest II: muscle energetics during maximal exhaustive exercise. *Journal of Applied Physiology* **66**, 142–150.

Grover, R.F., Reeves, J.T., Grover, E.B. & Leathers, J.E. (1967) Muscular exercise in young men native to 3100 meters altitude. *Journal of Applied Physiology* **22**, 555–564.

Hackett, P.H., Rennie, D., Hofmeister, S.E., Grover, R.F., Grover, E.B. & Reeves, J.T.

(1982) Fluid retention and relative hyperventilation in acute mountain sickness. *Respiration* **43**, 321–329.

Hackett, P.H., Roach, R.C., Schoene, R.B., Harrison, G.L. & Mills, W.R. Jr. (1988) Abnormal control of ventilation in high altitude pulmonary edema. *Journal of Applied Physiology* **64**, 1268–1272.

Hochachka, K.W., Stanley, C., Merkt, J. & Sumar-Kalinowski, J. (1982) Metabolic meaning of elevated levels of oxidative enzymes of high altitude adapted animals: an interpretive hypothesis. *Respiration Physiology* **52**, 303–313.

Hornbein, T.F., Townes, B.D., Schoene, R.B., Sutton, J.R. & Houston, C.S. (1989) The cost to the central nervous system of climbing to extremely high altitude. *New England Journal of Medicine* **321**, 1714–1719.

Jaeger, J.J., Sylvester, J.T., Cymerman, A., Berberich, J.J., Denniston, J.C. & Maher, J.T. (1979) Evidence for increased intrathoracic fluid volume in man at high altitude. *Journal of Applied Physiology* **47**, 670–676.

Lahiri, S., Edelman, N.H., Cherniack, N.S. & Fishman, A.P. (1981) Role of carotid chemoreflex in respiratory acclimatization to hypoxia in goat and sheep. *Respiration Physiology* **46**, 367–382.

Levine, B.D. & Stray-Gundersen, J. (1997) 'Living high–training low': effect of moderate-altitude acclimatization with low-altitude training on performance. *Journal of Applied Physiology* **83**, 102–112.

Maher, J.T., Jones, L.G. & Hartley, L.H. (1974) Effects of high altitude exposure on submaximal endurance capacity of men. *Journal of Applied Physiology* **37**, 895–898.

Masuyama, S., Kimura, H., Sugita, T. *et al.* (1986) Control of ventilation in extreme altitude climbers. *Journal of Applied Physiology* **61**, 500–506.

Monge, M.C. (1928) La enfermadad de los Andes. Sindromes eritremicos. *Ann. Fac. Med* (Univ. San Marcos, Lima) **11**, 1–16.

Moore, L.G. & Brewer, G.J. (1981) Beneficial effect of rightward hemoglobin-oxygen dissociation curve shift for short-term high altitude adaptations. *Journal of Laboratory and Clinical Medicine* **98**, 145–154.

Oelz, O., Howard, H., di Prampero, E. *et al.* (1986) Physiological profile of world-class high altitude climbers. *Journal of Applied Physiology* **60**, 1734–1742.

Ou, L.C. & Tenney, S.M. (1970) Properties of mitochondria from hearts of cattle acclimatized to high altitude. *Respiration Physiology* **8**, 151–159.

Pugh, L.G. (1964) Cardiac output in muscular exercise at 5800 m (19000 feet). *Journal of Applied Physiology* **19**, 441–450.

Reeves, J.T., Groves, B.M., Sutton, J.R. *et al.* (1987) Operation Everest II: preservation of cardiac function at extreme altitude. *Journal of Applied Physiology* **63**, 531–539.

Regard, M., Oelz, O., Brugger, P. & Landis, T. (1989) Persistent cognitive impairment in climbers after repeated exposure to extreme altitude. *Neurology* **39**, 210–213.

Remmers, J.E. & Mithoefer, J.C. (1969) The carbon monoxide diffusing capacity in permanent residents at high altitude. *Respiration Physiology* **6**, 233–244.

Sanchez, C., Merino, C. & Figallo, M. (1970) Simultaneous measurement of plasma volume and cell mass in polycythemia of high altitude. *Journal of Applied Physiology* **28**, 775–778.

Schoene, R.B. (1982) The control of ventilation in climbers to extreme altitude. *Journal of Applied Physiology* **53**, 886–890.

Schoene, R.B. (1984) Hypoxic ventilatory response in exercise ventilation at sea level and high altitude. In: West, J.B. & Lahiri, S. (eds) *Man at High Altitude*, pp. 19–30. American Physiologic Society Clinical Physiology Series. Waverly Press, Baltimore.

Schoene, R.B. & Hornbein, T.F. (1988) Respiratory adaptation to high altitude. In: Murray, J.F. & Nadel, J.A. (eds) *Textbook of Respiratory Medicine*, pp. 196–220. W.B. Saunders, Baltimore.

Schoene, R.B., Lahiri, S., Hackett, P.H. *et al.* (1984) Relationship of hypoxic ventilatory response to exercise performance on Mt. Everest. *Journal of Applied Physiology* **56**, 1478–1483.

Swan, L.W. (1970) Goose of the Himalaya. *Natural History* **79**, 68–75.

Tenney, S.M. & Ou, L.C. (1970) Physiological evidence for increased tissue capillarity in rats acclimatized to high altitude. *Respiration Physiology* **8**, 137–150.

Torre-Bueno, J.R., Wagner, P.D., Saltzman, H.A., Gale, G.E. & Moon, R.E. (1985) Diffusion limitation in normal subjects during exercise at sea level in simulated altitude. *Journal of Applied Physiology* **58**, 989–995.

Vincent, J., Hellot, M.F., Vargas, E., Gautier, H., Pasquis, P. & Lefrancois, R. (1978) Pulmonary gas exchange, diffusing capacity in natives and newcomers at high altitude. *Respiration Physiology* **34**, 219–231.

Wagner, P.D., Gale, G.E., Moon, R.E., Torre-Bueno, J.R., Stolp, B.W. & Saltzman, H.A. (1986) Pulmonary gas exchange in humans exercising at sea level in simulated altitude. *Journal of Applied Physiology* **61**, 280–287.

Wagner, P.D., Sutton, J.R., Reeves, J.T., Cymerman, A., Groves, B.M. & Malconiun, N.K. (1987) Operation Everest II: pulmonary gas exchange during a simulated ascent of Mt. Everest. *Journal of Applied Physiology* **63**, 2348–2359.

Weil, J.V. (1986) Ventilatory control at high altitude. In: Fishman, A.P., Cherniack, N.S., Widdicome, J.G. & Gieger, S.R. (eds) *Handbook of Physiology. The Respira-*

tory System, Section 3, Vol. II, *Control of Breathing*, Part 1, pp. 730–737. American Physiologic Society, Bethesda, MD.

West, J.B. & Wagner, P.D. (1980) Predicted gas exchange on the summit of Mt. Everest. *Respiration Physiology* **42**, 1–16.

West, J.B., Boyer, S.J., Graber, D.J. *et al.* (1983a) Maximal exercise at extreme altitudes on Mt. Everest. *Journal of Applied Physiology* **55**, 688–702.

West, J.B., Hackett, P.H., Maret, K.H. *et al.* (1983b) Pulmonary gas exchange on the summit of Mt. Everest. *Journal of Applied Physiology* **55**, 678–687.

Winslow, R.M. & Monge, C.C. (1987) *Hypoxia, Polycythemia, and Chronic Mountain Sickness.* Johns Hopkins University Press, Baltimore.

Winslow, R.M., Samaja, M. & West, J.B. (1984) Red cell function at extreme altitude on Mt. Everest. *Journal of Applied Physiology* **56**, 109–116.

Chapter 63

The Physiology of Human-Powered Flight

ETHAN R. NADEL AND STEVEN R. BUSSOLARI

Introduction

Humans have always been fascinated with the concept of flight, yet throughout history the actuality of flight has been relegated to winged animals or assigned to the realm of myth. Only in very recent times has an understanding of the requirements of flight and the development of strong and light structures enabled flight to be accomplished under human power alone.

The first record of human-powered flight was from the ancient Greek civilizations. As first reported by Homer around the 8th–7th century BC, a Mycenean craftsman and inventor named Daedalus fashioned wings from feathers and wax and flew under his own power from a hillside cleft in King Minos' Labyrinth, in which he was imprisoned, across the Aegean Sea to his freedom. According to later versions of the myth, Daedalus flew with his son, Icarus, who, ignoring his father's advice, flew too close to the sun and fell to his death when the heat of the sun melted his wings.

Drela and Langford (1985) have charted the progress of human-powered flight since the time of Daedalus. They noted that only within the past 30 years or so has human-powered flight progressed beyond the realm of extended glides from a catapult take-off. This was undoubtedly because the early human-powered aircraft required more power to maintain steady flight than the pilot could produce. Progress in the realm of human-powered flight was stimulated by the challenge of competition for monetary prizes established by the British industrialist Henry Kremer in 1959. The first Kremer prize,

awarded for flying a human-powered aircraft around a 1-mile (1609-m), figure-of-eight course under human power alone, was claimed in 1977 by Bryan Allen, flying the Paul MacCready-designed *Gossamer Condor*. The second Kremer prize of £100 000 went to the same team, when Bryan Allen pedalled the *Gossamer Albatross* across a 37-km strait of the English Channel in 1979. This was indeed an endurance event; the flight time was nearly 3 h. In 1988, *Daedalus*, designed by a team of engineers from the Massachusetts Institute of Technology, flew under human power from the north coast of Crete to the island of Santorini, a distance of 119 km, in just under 4 h.

Aeroplane aerodynamics

To understand the reasons why human-powered flight has become possible only in recent times, it is important to appreciate the basics of aeroplane aerodynamics (for an expanded discussion see Shevell 1983). Four forces—lift, weight, thrust and drag—are the determinants for flight. As an aircraft moves through the air, the shape of its wing imparts differential velocities to the air passing over its upper and lower surfaces, creating a higher pressure beneath the wing and a lower pressure above the wing. This results in a net upward force called lift. In level flight, lift is balanced by the downward force of gravity, the aircraft weight. A horizontal thrust force is furnished by the propeller which is driven by the aircraft engine. In level, unaccelerated flight, thrust balances the total horizontal resistive force, drag, which is produced by a combination of the movement of air past the exposed surfaces of the aircraft (form and parasite drag) and the disturbance of the air caused by the wing as it produces lift (induced drag).

The power required for flight is the product of thrust and velocity, or, in level flight, drag and velocity. Since form and parasite drag increase roughly as the square of the velocity, the power (force × velocity) required to overcome these components of drag will increase as the cube of velocity. Thus, doubling the airspeed of a given aircraft would require roughly an eight-fold increase in the power applied by the engine (the human engine in the case of a human-powered aircraft). A more exact relationship between power required and aircraft design parameters may be obtained by consideration of the equations that describe the production of lift and induced drag:

$$\text{power} = [2/\rho S]^{1/2} W^{3/2} C_D / C_L^{3/2}$$

where ρ is the air density, S is the wing area, W is the total weight of the aircraft including payload (in a human-powered aircraft, the pilot is a significant fraction of W), and C_D and C_L are coefficients of drag and lift that depend on the aircraft shape. The above equation confirms that it is important for the aircraft designer to minimize weight and drag, while maintaining a high lift and a large wing area to keep the required power low.

Design strategies

Over the years, human-powered aircraft designers have attempted to solve the problem of reducing the power requirement to that which a human could be expected to maintain by adopting several strategies. One strategy was to design a very light structure with a large wing area by using external wire bracing. Compensation for the high parasite drag of the wire bracing was achieved by keeping the design airspeed (velocity) low to minimize its contribution to the power required. The success of the *Gossamer* human-powered aircraft was the result of this design strategy. The disadvantage of this type of aircraft is its low speed, which requires its pilot to remain aloft for a long time in order to cover a given distance. The development of strong, lightweight graphite–epoxy and other composite materials allowed designers to eliminate the external wire bracing, while maintaining a large wing area with little weight penalty. The *Daedalus* aircraft (Fig. 63.1), with its 34.1-m semicantilever wingspan, is an example of this design strategy.

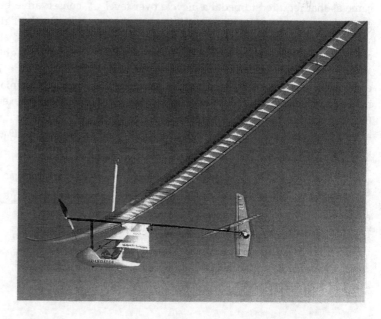

Fig. 63.1 The *Daedalus* undergoing flight-testing at Edwards Air Force Base in California. In April 1988, K. Kanallopoulos flew the *Daedalus* between the Greek islands of Crete and Santorini, a distance of 119 km, in just under 4 h. The distance and duration are the current world records for human-powered flight. Photo courtesy of the Daedalus Project, Massachusetts Institute of Technology.

Table 63.1 Characteristics of the 25 final pilot candidates.

Parameter	Mean ± s.d. value
Maximal oxygen intake (semirecumbent position) (ml oxygen·min^{-1}·kg^{-1})	69.2 ± 5.2
Maximal mechanical power output (W·kg^{-1})	5.25 ± 0.53
70% maximal power output (W·kg^{-1})	3.54 ± 0.36
Mechanical efficiency (%)	24.1 ± 3.7

Power requirements for flight

The outcome of aerodynamic and materials innovations led to the design of a low-power, moderate-speed aircraft that could be flown for extended periods. Preliminary calculations and measurements, derived largely from tow tests of the aircraft, showed that the mechanical power requirement to fly the *Daedalus* was about 3.0–3.5 W·kg^{-1} pilot weight at the design speed of 24 km·h^{-1}. Assuming the pilot's ability to convert 24% of the potential energy of stored fuels to mechanical work in the muscle machinery (Åstrand & Rodahl 1986), the pilot must maintain a fuel conversion rate of nearly 15 W·kg^{-1}, requiring an oxygen intake of about 45 ml oxygen·min^{-1}·kg^{-1}, to generate mechanical power at 3.5 W·kg^{-1}. This metabolic cost is approximately the same as that required to pedal a bicycle over level ground at a speed of 37 km·h^{-1} (Whitt & Wilson 1982). Based upon knowledge of performance characteristics, the metabolic cost of flying the *Gossamer Albatross* at its design speed of 18 km·h^{-1} has been estimated to be 20% higher, a remarkable output to maintain throughout the English Channel crossing. (Note: a human-powered aircraft is flown like any aircraft; the pilot adds power to gain altitude and decreases power to descend. Because the human-powered aircraft flies within 6 m of the surface, the loss of altitude due to a reduction in power for more than a few seconds will cause the aircraft to land, or worse.)

As human-powered aircraft designers have refined their designs and used lighter and stronger materials, the power requirements for flight have come into the realm of the possible for more than just the élite endurance athlete. It is notable that the *Daedalus* pilot team of five athletes was selected from more than 300 initial applicants (Nadel & Bussolari 1988). The maximal mechanical power production of the 25 athletes who were invited for objective testing was 5.25 W·kg^{-1} (Table 63.1). The 70% maximum power, which most fit people should be able to sustain aerobically for extended periods, was therefore 3.54 W·kg^{-1}, higher than the most conservative estimate of power required to maintain steady flight in the *Daedalus*. The ability to generate power at this rate is the critical factor for extended flight. Factors that can limit prolonged flight include hyperthermia, dehydration and/or hypoglycaemia, the same factors that can limit other endurance exercise bouts (for a discussion of the strategies to limit the development of these factors during the *Daedalus* flight, see Nadel & Bussolari 1988).

References

Åstrand, P.-O. & Rodahl, K. (1986) *Textbook of Work Physiology*. McGraw-Hill, New York.

Drela, M. & Langford, J.S. (1985) Human-powered flight. *Scientific American* **253**, 144–151.

Nadel, E.R. & Bussolari, S.R. (1988) The Daedalus project: physiological problems and solutions. *Scientific American* **76**, 351–360.

Shevell, R.S. (1983) *Fundamentals of Flight*. Prentice Hall, New Jersey.

Whitt, F.R. & Wilson, D.G. (1982) *Bicycling Science*. MIT Press, Cambridge, Massachusetts.

Chapter 64

Endurance in Other Sports

PER-OLOF ÅSTRAND

Individual sport events with demands for endurance during training and competition have been discussed in preceding chapters. *Orienteering* was mentioned only in passing, but it is certainly an endurance sport because it involves long distances of cross-country running (the 'ideal' time is about 1 h 30 min for men and about 1 h for women). Armed with a compass and a map, the competitor must find his or her way to checkpoints in the terrain (see Creagh & Reilly 1997). Many countries have annual meetings with up to 5 days of competitions. In Sweden, more than 20 000 people participate, with classes from beginners up to élite, and age groups from children up to master athletes. The endurance training for orienteering follows the same principles as those discussed in Chapters 28 and 57. Orienteering is also a popular sport when performed on skis.

Many other events are time consuming with regard to both training sessions and competition time. However, physical activity during competition is often not continuous but intermittent, i.e. short bursts of vigorous exercise are followed by rest or low-intensity activity. The physiology of this type of exercise was briefly discussed in Chapter 2. A few examples of such events are given below.

Several studies on *soccer* have been carried out (see Ekblom 1986; Chapter 61). On average the players cover about 10 km during the 90-min game, and it has been estimated that top-class performers in British premier-division teams walk and run 13.5 km in total (see Ekblom 1986). Soccer involves high-intensity, intermittent exercise although the total number of tackles in a game per player is only some 15–20, with 10–15 headings of the ball. Even so, the heart rate is often high and close to the player's maximum. Ekblom estimated that the average oxygen intake during the game could be about 80% of the maximum. The maximal aerobic power of players in good national teams seems to be around 65–67 ml·kg^{-1}·min^{-1}, with individual values exceeding 70 ml·kg^{-1}·min^{-1}. Peak blood lactate concentrations above 12 mmol·l^{-1} have frequently been measured. It is evident that soccer players must devote time to endurance training. In the recent world championships many games were extended by 2×15-min periods. (See also Ekblom 1994.)

Other games involving high-intensity, non-continuous, intermittent exercise are European handball, basketball, volleyball, netball, field hockey, ice hockey and water polo.

A high maximal aerobic power can lower the demand on anaerobic energy yield. The importance of myoglobin oxygen stores was discussed in Chapter 2 (see Fig. 2.1). However, training does not seem to increase the myoglobin concentration in human skeletal muscle. One aspect of the importance of separate endurance training for players is the fact that training sessions often last for 2–2.5 h.

A similar situation arises in racquet sports. A *tennis* match can last for 4 h or more, sometimes in a hot environment. In *table tennis*, the three sets may take from 20 to 30 min. In the Swedish national team, which included world champions, the maximal oxygen intake averaged 65 ml·kg^{-1}·min^{-1}. The mean oxygen intake during games was about 70% of the maximum. During major tournaments a player must often play several matches per day.

Fencing is another event with many matches per day; this complicates food and water intake. A competition often lasts for 2 days, and the fencers are usually active for 10–12h on each day of competition. Six members of the Swedish national épée team have been studied. Altogether, the fencers won 13 gold, one silver and four bronze medals in world championships and Olympic games. The mean maximal oxygen intake was $5.2 \, l \cdot min^{-1}$, $67.3 \, ml \cdot kg^{-1} \cdot min^{-1}$ (Nyström *et al.* 1990). Endurance training is considered an important part of their training. The muscle mass was significantly larger in their 'forward leg' than in the contralateral leg, although the fibre composition was similar.

This list could be much longer. The conclusion is that the training of aerobic power has importance for all athletes, not least because habitual physical activity is essential for optimal function. In addition, there is the health aspect. Many studies have shown convincingly that training of the oxygen transport system can significantly reduce the morbidity and mortality from cardiovascular disease (for references see US Department of Health and Human Services 1996; Åstrand 1997; Chapter 51).

References

Åstrand, P.-O. (1997) Why exercise? *Advances in Exercise and Sports Physiology* **3** (2), 45–54.

Creagh, U. & Reilly, T. (1997) Physiological and biomechanical aspects of orienteering. *Sports Medicine* **24** (6), 409–418.

Ekblom, B. (1986) Applied physiology of soccer. *Sports Medicine* **3**, 50–60.

Ekblom, B. (1994) *Football (Soccer)*. Blackwell Scientific Publications, Oxford.

Nyström, J., Lindwall, O., Ceci, R., Harmenberg, J., Svedenhag, J. & Ekblom, B. (1990) Physiological and morphological characteristics of world class fencers. *International Journal of Sports Medicine* **11**, 136–139.

US Department of Health and Human Services (1996) *Physical Activity and Health: A Report of the Surgeon General*. Superintendent of Documents, P.O. Box 371954, PA 15250-7954, S/N 017-023-00196-5, USA.

Index

Page numbers in bold refer to tables; page numbers in *italics* refer to figures. This index is in letter-to-letter order whereby spaces and hyphens between words in main entries are ignored in alphabetization. 'Training' refers to endurance training unless otherwise noted. Likewise, all athletes and performance levels relate to endurance athletes and endurance performance.

abortion, spontaneous 536–537
accessory respiratory muscles 54
accidents 33
    see also injury, sports
acclimatization 614
    cold stress 294
    heat 265, 288, 288–289
    high altitude 12, 296, 614, 617–619,
        932, 937
    muscle blood flow 111
    soccer in hot environment 904–
        905
accumulated oxygen deficit (AOD)
    canoeists 893
    rugby players 913
acetazolamide 321, 622
acetyl coenzyme A (CoA) 757
Achilles tendinosis 462, 469
Achilles tendon 777
    blood supply 777
    chronic tears 783
    pain 780
    rupture 779
        complete 780–781, 783
        partial 780, 783
    tightness 786
Achilles tendon overuse injuries
    777–783
    aetiology 778–779
    anatomy 777
    classification 777–778
    diagnosis 780
    differential diagnosis 781
    investigations 781
    pathogenesis 779–780
    prevention 783

treatment 781–783
acid–base balance 320–322
    high altitude 616–617
    measurements 320–321
    modifications 321–322
    pregnancy 532
acid–base imbalance
    acute mountain sickness 621
    respiratory acidosis 321
    respiratory alkalosis 321, 532
    see also metabolic acidosis
acrophase 640
actin
    eccentric exercise effect 166–167
    F-actin/G-actin 164
    monomers 164
    myosin interactions 159–160
action potentials
    changes in fatigue 29, 30
    failure in repetitive activity 174
    sarcolemma and T tubules 171
activities of daily living (ADL) 566,
    753
actomyosin
    failure 158
    interactions 159–160
    see also actin; myosin
acute mountain sickness 296, 618,
    620–621
acute phase proteins 802
adaptation(s) 501
    adverse 528
        see also overtraining
    ATP regeneration 178
    autonomic nervous system 596,
        708
    biochemical, to high-intensity
        exercise 180
    Ca^{2+}-ATPase 177
    canoeists 894
    cardiac 70–71, *71*, 520
    chronic, excitation–contraction
        coupling 176
    circulatory 12
    cycling 866
    cytoskeletal system 179–180
    ECG changes 677
    enzymes *see* enzymes

'first in, last out pattern' 122
high resistance training 168
membrane excitability 177
mitochondria *see* mitochondria
mountaineering 931, 935
muscle *see* muscle, adaptation
neurones 136
overuse injury prevention 766
pulmonary system 59, 61–64
regression after discontinuation of
    training 130
respiratory muscle training (RMT)
    62–64
respiratory system 59, 61–64
sensorimotor systems 144
signalling systems 177
skiing 852, 854
tissue, mountaineering 935
to training 97, 501
    ATP regeneration 178
    in women *see* women
ventricular function 75
see also plasticity
adductor injuries 791, 792–793
adductor longus, injuries 792
adenosine 96
adenosine diphosphate (ADP) 21,
    331
adenosine monophosphate (AMP)
    21
adenosine triphosphatase (ATPase)
    see ATPase
adenosine triphosphate (ATP) 21,
    330–331
    intermittent exercise 10–11
    muscle blood flow control 96
    regeneration 178, 334
        energy requirement 31
    structure 331, *332*
    synthesis 179, 271, 330–331
        fatty acid degradation 336–337
        glycolysis 333, 334–336
        phosphocreatine 334
        sites 177
    triathlon 872
    utilization 84, *179*
adipose tissue 329
    blood flow 107

adipose tissue (*continued*)
　fat mobilization 28
　in pregnancy 534
　triglycerides 201
　see also fat, body
adolescents
　anthropometric characteristics
　　41–42, *42*
　athletic success prediction 41
　cardiovascular screening *see*
　　cardiovascular screening
　growth spurts 397, *398*
　height increase 397, *398*
　injuries 462, 466–468
　marathon running 399
　maximal oxygen intake ($\dot{V}O_{2max}$)
　　512
　　age-related changes 45, 47
　　body size relationship 45, *45*, *46*
　　endurance training effect 509
　menstrual cycle 514, 720
　overuse injuries 462
　scaling factors, submaximal $\dot{V}O_2$
　　48, *49*
　talent identification and
　　development 400
　training 509
　see also children
adrenaline (epinephrine) 184, 185
　muscle sensitivity, training effect
　　130
　overtraining marker 494
　response to endurance exercise
　　184, 185
　secretion increased by caffeine 441
　use prohibition 653
adrenergic blocking agents 549
　alpha-blockers 567
　beta-blockers 567, 569
adrenergic receptors 184, 634
adrenocorticotrophic hormone
　　(ACTH) 185–187
　actions 493
　decreased, overtraining marker
　　493
　E-endorphin correlation 188–189
　response to exercise 185–186
　training effect 186–187
adult respiratory distress syndrome
　　(ARDS) 802
aerobic activities 866, *867*
　injuries in elderly 558, 559
　see also aerobic exercise training
aerobic–anaerobic threshold 318
　cycling 866, *867*
　economy of movement and 247
　swimmers 828
　see also anaerobic threshold
aerobic capacity 311, 318
　alcohol effects 447
　cycling 857, *868*
　definition 301

smoking effect 445
　see also anaerobic threshold
aerobic conditioning 533–534
aerobic exercise training
　benefits 458
　children *see* children
　diffusive oxygen flux 90–91
　muscle blood flow 90–91
　pregnancy 533–534, 537
　women 518–519
aerobic fitness 767
　guidelines for elderly 554, 555
　hot environment 289–290
　maximal oxygen intake as marker
　　507
　soccer 907
　see also maximal oxygen intake
　　($\dot{V}O_{2max}$)
aerobic metabolism
　canoeing 894–896
　continuous exercise 13
　glycolysis *see* glycolysis
　hockey 922–924, *924*
　isokinetic ergometer 278
　rowing 839–840
　skeletal muscle 84
　skiing 846
　swimming 824, *825*
　training in women 521
　transition to anaerobic 311, 315
　　see also anaerobic metabolism;
　　　anaerobic threshold
aerobic power
　age-related decline 714
　body fat relationship 350
　elderly 552–555
　as input to perception of effort 377
　maximal *see* maximal oxygen
　　intake ($\dot{V}O_{2max}$)
　measurement 271, 272
　peak, disabled persons 566
　post-myocardial infarction 566
　pregnancy 533
　rate of loss with age 753
　swimmers 824
　triathletes 880–882, *881*
　see also oxygen intake
aerodynamic drag 253, 279
aerodynamics 252–253, 279
aeroplane aerodynamics 942–943
A-frame stands 609
afterload 34
age, chronological *vs* biological
　　397–398, 513
age-related changes *38–40*, 548–551
　Achilles tendon overuse injuries
　　778
　aldosterone 550
　baroreceptor reflex function 549
　blood pressure 549
　body composition 555, *556*
　bone loss 551

cardiac function 548, 550
cardiovascular disease risk 701
catecholamine response to exercise
　185
circadian rhythm control 640
endurance athletes *38–40*
endurance preparation 397–401
flexibility loss 558, 756
hepatic function 550
hyperthermic exercise effect on
　vasoconstriction 112
injuries associated 466–468
jet lag response 641–642
maximal oxygen intake ($\dot{V}O_{2max}$)
　45, 47, 713–714, 753, *756*
musculoskeletal changes 550–
　551
peak height velocity (PHV) 397,
　398
performance at and prediction of
　success 399
physical limitations 547
physiological/pathological
　changes 547–551
rating of perceived effort 390
renal function 549–550
renin–angiotensin–aldosterone
　550
stress fracture 768
temperature intolerance 548
tissue injury and inflammation
　805–806
vasoconstrictor responses 107
see also elderly
air–liquid partition coefficient 23
air pollutants 628–638
　carbon monoxide 297, 635–636
　ozone *see* ozone
　performance reduced 629–630
　primary 297
　respiratory discomfort 628
　secondary 297–298, *298*
　sulphur dioxide 297, 634–635
air pollution 53
　episodes 298
　high altitude 298, 615
air quality 297–298
　assessment 298
air resistance
　cycling 857, *859*, 860
　energy costs 252
　high altitude 252–253, 614–615
　shielding from 254
　skiing 846
　triathlon 878–879
air travel 639
　sedative use with 646–647
　see also jet lag
airway
　hyperresponsiveness to ozone
　　632
　inflammation 632

ozone pollution effect 632
resistance 53, 632
alcohol 445–448
  adverse effects 447
  catabolism 446
  consumption 760
    rugby football 915
    social 447
  content of drinks 445–446
  effects on CNS 446
  as energy source 446
  misuse 447–448
  oxidation 328
  physiological effects 446
  warning before mass participation
    events 661
aldosterone 190
  elderly 550
  high altitudes 616
alertness, maintenance after jet lag
    646, 647
alkalosis
  input to perception of effort 376
  respiratory 321, 532
allelic variations 234
allergies, medical screening before
    competition 653
allometric equations 44, 45
allometry 44
alpha-adrenergic receptor blockers
    567
Δ-motoneurones 137, 139
altitude
  acclimatization see acclimatization
  high see high altitude
  moderate
    acute effects 616–617
    diet 618
  training see high altitude, training
altitude chamber, rowing training
    842
alveolar–capillary surface area 53
alveolar hyperventilation 55
alveolar macrophage 737
alveolar oxygen pressure
  high altitude 616
  rowers 841
alveolar to arterial partial pressure
    gradient (A–aD_{O_2}) 55
alveolar ventilation ($\dot{V}_A$) 52
alveoli, oxygen transport from 23
amantadine hydrochloride 581
amenorrhoea
  adolescents 514
  bone (density) loss 361, 718, 719
  causative hypotheses 723–725
  characterization 720–723
  consequences 718–719
  eumenorrhoeic athletes
    comparison 720
  factors associated 721–723
  ovarian function and hormone

changes 720–721
  secondary 410, 514
  sports injuries and 805
  stress fractures 466
American Academy of Orthopedic
    Surgeons 479–480
American College of Sports Medicine
    (ACSM)
  exercise for
    cardiorespiratory/muscular
    fitness 554
  exercise prescription for elderly
    557
  heat stress 287
American football/footballers
    915–917
  background and principles 915
  characteristics of players 916
  dehydration 917
  heart rate 916
  jet lag effect 643–644
  maximal oxygen intake 916
  protective equipment 478, 479
  rule and injuries 464
  training 916–917
American Heart Association
    667–668, 668, 672, 715
Americans with Disability Act (ADA)
    565
amino acids
  branched-chain see branched-chain
    amino acids (BCAAs)
  changes in fatigue 33
  essential 329
  ingestion 201, 203–204
  supplements 201, 204–205
  synthesis 329
5-aminolevulinic acid 133
amphetamine 439–440, 657
  derivatives 439
  effects and dosages 440
amputations, lower extremity
    576–577
amyotrophic lateral sclerosis
    582–583
anabolic–androgenic steroids (AAS)
    443, 443–444
  abuse 657
  adverse effects 444
  effect on bone mass 358
  mechanisms of action 444
anaemia 424–425
  erythropoietin treatment 428
  haemoglobin levels 424
  iron deficiency 415
  'sports' 190, 424–425
anaerobic capacity 318
anaerobic conditions, aerobic training
    session with 12
anaerobic events, swimming 824
anaerobic metabolism 311–328,
    410–411

American footballers 916
canoeing 891–893
concepts 311–312
congestive heart failure 91
cycling 866
glycolysis 328, 331, 335
  maximal power 334, 336
hockey 922
inefficiency 312
intermittent exercise 10
interval exercise 11
isokinetic ergometer 278
lactate accumulation limitation
    312
markers of competitive
    performance 312
middle-distance running and
    819–820
pace training effect 519
rowing 840
skiing 847
swimming 824, 825
training influence 312
transition to 311, 315
anaerobic threshold (lactate
    threshold) 13–14, 315, 318–320
  altitude acclimatization 618
  canoeing 893–894
  carboxyhaemoglobin effect 635
  concept 318
  cycling 863, 866, 867
  definition 315
  economy of movement and 247
  endurance performance and
    403–404
  exercise below 27
  first/second breakpoints 318–320
  as marker for training intensity
    381, 382, 389–390
  measurement methods 320
  overtraining marker 489, 490, 491,
    492
  pace training in women 519, 521
  perception of effort 381, 382
  performance and 524–525
  pregnancy 533
  rating of perceived effort 389–390
  rowers 840
  rugby football 914
  running, training effect 407–408,
    408
  running velocity (V_{La4}) and
    403–404
  soccer 902–903
  swimmers 828
  training at speed corresponding
    404
  triathlon 883
  ventilation curves and 318
  ventilatory threshold relationship
    54
  women 521–522, 524

anaerobic threshold (*continued*)
  see also aerobic capacity
anaesthetics, local injection 657–658
analysis of covariance (ANCOVA) 44
anaphylactic reactions, dextran
      infusions 432
androgenic steroids 443–444
aneurysms 568–569, 577
  aortic 568
  circle of Willis 712
  exercise/training guidelines 569
angina pectoris 548, 695
angiotensin II 190
angiotensin-converting enzyme
      (ACE) gene 234–235
  I/D polymorphism 235
angiotensin-converting enzyme
      (ACE) inhibitors 567
ankle
  braces for stabilization 480, 480
  dorsiflexion 779
  injury 476
  taping 481
  venous pressure 97
ankle drop protocol 788
anorexia nervosa 723
anovulation 720
anterior cruciate ligament injuries
      465, 471, 472, 473
  injury prevention 476, 477
anterior tibial muscle, chronic
      stimulation effect 118, 120
anthropometry 37–38
  biological age 397
  body composition assessment 349
  canoeing 891
  characteristics of athletes 38–40,
      38–41
  child and adolescent athletes
      41–42, 42
  Heath–Carter protocol 38
  heat loss and cold stress 292–293
  physiological/biomechanical
      considerations 43
  rugby football 912
  somatotype 37–38, 232, 233
  see also body size; height; physique
anticholinergic drugs 584
anticoagulants 568
anticonvulsants 578, 583
antidepressants 570, 582
antidiarrhoeals 660
antidiuretic hormone (ADH) 190,
      432, 447
antihypertensive agents 572, 578
anti-inflammatory agents 808–809
  see also non-steroidal anti-
      inflammatory drugs (NSAIDs)
anti-inflammatory cytokines 738, 802
anti-inflammatory effects 802, 803
antioxidants 417
anxiety 214

benefits of exercise 759
fatigue association 33
input to perception of effort 382
performance relationship 215, 456
precompetition 214–215, 456
aorta
  aneurysms 568
  enlargement 568
  rigidity, elderly 549
  rupture 670
aortic valve stenosis 670
appetite, diminished in overtraining
      496
arachidonic acid (AA) 802
arctic trips 663–664
area equipment 463–464
arousal 216, 760
arrhythmias see cardiac arrhythmias
arterial oxygen saturation see oxygen;
      oxygen transport
arterial pressure see blood pressure
arteries
  occlusion, muscle blood flow
      reduction 91
  rigidity, elderly 549
arteriovenous oxygen difference 103,
      104, 224
  age-related changes 548
  elderly 552
arthritis 575
  rheumatoid 575, 752
  see also osteoarthritis
arthropathies, Achilles tendon
      injuries 779
articular cartilage see cartilage
aspirin 808
association–dissociation factors
      216–217, 454
  input to perception of effort 383,
      388
  pain and discomfort management
      456
association football see soccer
asthma 53, 298
  benefits of exercise 750
  exacerbation by exercise 634
  exercise training effects 569
  ozone effect 629, 632
  sulphur dioxide effect 634
  training recommendations 570
atherosclerosis 77, 566, 568
  benefits of exercise 695
  stroke due to 696
  sudden death due to 712
atherosclerotic plaque 691
'athlete's heart' (concept) see heart
athleticism, personality impact
      211–212
Athletic Motivation Inventory (AMI)
      368
atmosphere, high altitude 296, 615,
      931

ATP see adenosine triphosphate
      (ATP)
ATPase
  muscle cells 170
  myofibrillar see myofibrillar
      ATPase
  myosin 160, 164
atrial natriuretic factor/peptide
      (ANF; ANP) 190, 683
  during and after exercise 685, 685
atrioventricular accessory pathway
      79
atropine sulphate 632
attentional focus, input to perception
      of effort 381
'augmenters,' input to perception of
      effort 382–383
Australian Rules football 917–919
  maximal oxygen intake 919
autonomic nervous system
  adaptation induced by training
      596, 708
  circulation control 103
  failure, blood pressure changes
      105
awareness of effort 374, 388
axotomy 149

back pain
  gestational 536
  stress fractures 771
  triathletes 877
badminton, rules and injury
      prevention 464
banned substances 439, 439, 657
  blood doping 427, 657
  drugs used for bronchospasm 653
  ephedrine 443
  erythropoietin 430, 657
  reasons for use 439
barometric pressure 294–295
baroreceptors 113
baroreflex 112–113
  blood pressure control 112–113,
      113
  elderly 549
  sensitivity in exercise 112, 113
base, excess 321
baseball, rules and injury prevention
      464
basketball, left ventricle dimensions
      76
Bassler hypothesis 77
baths, heatstroke management 610
Bayes theorem 715
B cells 495, 732
Becker muscular dystrophy 580
benzodiazepines 646
Bergström needle biopsy 342, 343
beta-agonists 634
beta-blockers 567, 569
beta-endorphin see E-endorphin

betamethasone, cerebral oedema 621–622
bicarbonate 26
  buffering action 321
  cerebral fluid, high altitude 617, 619
  doping 26, 322
  measurement and normal level 321
  metabolic acidosis 321
biceps femoris 789
bicycle, types 857
biochemical markers, of overtraining 491–492
biochemical tests, muscle metabolism 338–341
bioelectric impedance analysis 349, 685
biological age 397–398
  chronological vs 397–398, 513
  training effect in children 513
biological factors, endurance performance 21
bioluminescence assays 340
biomechanical constraints 245–258
  drag forces 252, 253
  economy of movement relationship 250–251
  fluid resistance and 252–253
  mechanical power and economy 246, 246–248
  performance vs controlled conditions 245
  stride length and speed 250–251
  see also mechanical power
biomechanics
  Achilles tendon overuse injuries 778
  anthropometry 43
  canoeing 888–891
  orthotics (shoe) 482
  rowing 838
  stress fracture prevention 773–774
biophosphates 576
biopsy, muscle 118, 338, 342–343
biopsy needles 342, 343
bladder
  catheterization 606
  spinal cord injuries and 579
blindness 586
blood
  pH 321
  redistribution during exercise 684
  removal and re-infusion 427
  solubility factors for gases 23, 23, 24–25
  storage, glycerol cell-freezing technique 426
blood doping 425, 657, 682
  blood viscosity changes 425–426, 427
  detection 427–428

erythropoietin 428–431, 657
  maximal oxygen intake 425
  time course of RBC changes 427
blood flow 103–117
  adipose tissue 107
  blood pressure and vascular resistance 104–105, 105
  cerebral 107
  cutaneous see cutaneous blood flow
  to legs in runners 34
  maternal 535
  oxygen consumption relationship 103, 104
  pooling below heart level 263, 264
  redistribution 103, 104
    blood pressure maintenance 104–105
    reduced cardiac output 106
  restriction in excess muscle contraction 31, 32
  skeletal muscle see muscle blood flow
  uterine 107
blood glucose see glucose
blood–muscle oxygen exchange capacity 89
blood packing see blood doping
blood pressure
  autonomic failure 105
  baroreflex control 112–113, 113
  blood flow and vascular resistance relations 104–105, 105
  canoeists 896
  control 689
  elderly 549
  endurance exercise benefits 689–691
    dose–response 691
    exercise types 691
    intensity threshold 689
  maintenance 104–105
  measurement 305–306
  myocardial work rate 711
  preliminary screening before competition 654
  raised 689–691
    incidence 690
    in isometric/isotonic exercise 751
    response to endurance exercise 751, 751
    see also hypertension
  rowing 840, 841
  systolic see systolic blood pressure
  unconscious patient 603
  women and effect of training 520
blood samples, doping detection 427–428
blood transfusions
  autologous 426, 428, 657

erythrocythaemia induction 426
  risks associated 657
blood viscosity
  agents reducing 568
  increased 425–426
    adverse effects 429
    altitude acclimatization 618, 934
    erythropoietin use 429
blood volume 682
  central 683
    after exercise 685, 685–686
    fall in 'heat exhaustion' 594
    increase during exercise 683
    prolonged standing effect 684
  changes 427
  decreased, hot environment 263, 264
  estimation 431
  increased 70–71, 431–432, 432–434, 683
    see also volume loading
  pregnancy 531–532, 534
  regulation 683
  role in oxygen transport 431–435
  see also plasma volume
body awareness 759
body build 4
body clock see circadian rhythm
body composition 346–365
  assessment 346–349
    criterion methods 346–349
    errors 348
    field methods 349
  definition 346
  elderly 555, 556
  endurance athletes 351–362
    bone mass/density 350, 355–361
    extreme leanness, problems 361–362
    fat-free mass 350, 354–355
    female 351
    male 352
    percentage fat 351–354
  genetic influences 232–234
  menstrual disorder mechanism 724
  models 346
    multiple-component 346, 348–349
    three-component 348, 349
    two-component 43, 346, 347–348
  performance 349–350
  role of specific genes 238
  triathlon 879–880
  young athletes 353–354
body mass
  amenorrhoea vs eumenorrhoea 721
  Australian Rules football 918
  calculations 347
  canoeists 891
  children and adolescents 41, 42

body mass (*continued*)
  cycling 859
  distribution (male and female) *41*
  economy relationship 250
  excess 43
  fat *see* fat, body
  fat-free (FFM) *see* fat-free mass
    (FFM)
  genetic influences 233–234
  maximal oxygen intake relation
    45, 405, 817
  monitoring during intensive
    training 654–655
  rugby players 912
  scaling 44, 48, 49
  skiers 850, *850*
  smokers 757
  for specific sports 38–40
  triathlon 878, 879, *879*
  see also fat, body
body mass index (BMI)
  genetic influences 233–234
  maximum oxygen intake
    measurement 307
  obesity 574
body shape, athletes 757
body size 38–40, 346
  assessment 37–38
  consequences for performance 43,
    48–50, *49*
  economy of movement and 250
  'ideal' values 37
  individual variability 42–43
  performance in cold conditions
    292–293
  physiological/biomechanical
    considerations 43
  runners 39, 40, 42, 43
  running performance and 817–819
  scaling *see* scaling
  submaximal energy cost of
    locomotion 47–48, *48*
  $\dot{V}O_{2max}$ relationship 45, 45–47,
    48–49, 817
    children and adolescents 45, *45*,
    46
  $\dot{V}O_{2submax}$ relationship 47–48, *48*,
    49
  see also anthropometry
body surface area
  left ventricular volume ratio *897*
  thermoregulation and 43
  volume relationship 44
body temperature *see* temperature,
    body
bone
  age 397
  density *see* bone mineral density
  exercise effect 356, 358, 361
  force applied 768
  loss
    amenorrhoea 718, 719

elderly 551
  women 415
mass
  anabolic steroids effect 358
  endurance athletes 355–361
  injuries in women and 466
  performance and 350
  see also bone mineral density
microtrauma 399
mineral content (BMC), gender and
    355, 356, 357, 359–361
remodelling 768
spinal cord injuries 579
stress
  fractures due to 768
  training in children 513
bone mineral density
  benefit of exercise 752–753
  benefits of training children 512
  endurance athletes 350, 355–361
  heritability 358
  influences/factors affecting 752,
    754–755
  oligomenorrhoea/amenorrhoea
    361
  performance and 350
  women 361, 415
  see also bone, mass
bone scans 772, 787
  stress fractures 771, 772
boredom 33
Borg's scale 374, 376, 384, *384*, 389
boundary layer (air) 27
bowel maintenance programme 579
braces
  ankle stabilization 480, *480*
  elbow 480
  injury prevention 479–481
  knee 480
  patellar stabilizing 776, 785
bradycardia, fetal 535
brain
  blood sugar decrease effect 28
  see also entries beginning cerebral
branched-chain amino acids
    (BCAAs) 204
  mountaineers 618
  oxidation 499
  performance improvement 419,
    655
  transport to brain 205
  tryptophan relationship 499
breakfast, pre-competition 198–199
breast cancer, risk reduction 758
breast milk, lactic acid 539
breath-by-breath equipment 283, *284*
breathing
  excessive work during prolonged
    exercise 56
  increase at high altitude 932
  input to perception of effort 376,
    381

mechanics during exercise 53–54
  ozone-induced alterations 629, 632
  pregnancy-induced changes 532
  rate 53, 54, 64
  respiratory muscle training effect
    64
  work *58*, 60
  see also ventilation ($\dot{V}_E$)
breathlessness *see* dyspnoea
'bright light,' jet lag management
    647–648, *648*
bronchial C fibres 633
bronchitis, chronic 750
bronchoconstriction, pollutants
    causing 629, 634
bronchodilators 571, 632
bronchospasm, exercise-induced 653
Brozek formula 347, 349
buffering capacity 321
  altitude acclimatization 617–618
  intramuscular 320
bundle branch block 617
burnout *see* overtraining
bursae 777

Ca^{2+}-ATPase 170, *170*
  chronic adaptation effect 177
  content in muscle fibres 85, *85*,
    172–173
  function 172
  sarcoplasmic reticulum 172–173
cadence, stride length and speed
    250–251
Caesarean section 539
caffeine 201, 440–442
  content of drinks/products 441
  dosages 441–442
  effects and mechanisms 441
  ergogenic benefit 201–202, 657
  health risks 442
calcaneal spur 787
calcitonin 576
calcium/calcium ions
  cycling and free calcium levels
    175, *176*
  in fatigue 29–30, 170–171
  intake, children 514
  muscle contraction 28, 29–30
  post-tetanic potentiation 163
  release, prolonged exercise effect
    176
  sarcoplasmic reticulum 169–170
  supplements 415, 753
  troponin complex action 164
calcium channel blockers 567
calcium ion (pCa)–force relationship
    164, *165*, 166
  chronic adaptation effect 168
calcium release channel 170, 173
  repetitive activity and 175
  T tubule interface 173–174
calf muscle pump 596

calisthenics 560
calories 5
camán 926
camogie 926
Canadian technique, canoeing 889,
    889–891, 890
cancer, benefits of exercise 758–759
canoeing 888–899
    accumulation oxygen deficit
        (AOD) 893
    adaptations 894
    aerobic metabolism 894–896
        kayakers vs canoeists 894–895
    anaerobic metabolism 891–893
    anaerobic threshold 893–894
    anthropometry 891
    biomechanics 888–891
    blood lactate levels 891–892, 894
    blood pressure 896
    Canadian technique 889, 889–891,
        890
    cardiovascular system 896
    equipment 888
    ergometers 274, 274, 275, 276
    force exerted during paddling 889,
        890
    heart rate 894
    historical aspects 888
    isokinetic data 891, 891
    kayak technique 888–889, 889, 890
        isokinetic data 891, 892
        metabolic/cardiac parameters
            281
        monitoring 897
    left ventricular mass 896, 897
    muscle fibre type 891
    muscle force 891
    paddling efficiency 895
    speed canoeing 888
    watercraft types 888
    whitewater canoeing 888, 889, 893
capillarization, muscle, training effect
    122, 127–129, 128, 130, 169
capillary bed, gas exchange 23
capillary density 13, 520
capillary electrophoresis (CE) 340
carbohydrate(s) 197–207
    availability, and perception of
        effort 379, 387
    classification 199
    cyclists 869, 870
    energy per gram 329
    energy source 27, 198, 847
    food containing 199, 413
    high-CHO diet 197, 411–412, 757
        before/during exercise 420
        effect on glycogen stores 418
        jet lag management 646
    ingestion 197–201, 410–411
        amino acids with 201
        children 514
        cyclists 869, 870, 870

effect on glycogen stores 417
    during exercise 200
    glycogen resynthesis rate 412,
        412
    immediately pre-exercise 200
    post-exercise 200–201, 870
    precompetition meals 198–199
    prior to exercise 198–200, 870
    timing during exercise 200
    women athletes 205–206, 525
loading regimens 198
    rugby football 911
    women 525
low-CHO diet 418
metabolism 27, 198
    alcohol effects 447
    pregnancy-induced changes 531
    training in women 521
    oxidation (aerobic glycolysis)
        329–330, 334, 336
    requirements 410, 411–412
    restriction, hypoglycaemia with
        606
    sources 412
    sports drinks see carbohydrate
        beverages
    stores 197–198, 411
        elevated and detrimental aspects
            198
    'supercompensation' 198
    supplementation 741
        immune benefits 740
    synthesis 329, 329
    threshold, cycling 863
    utilization rate 411–412
carbohydrate beverages 200, 201,
    742
    benefits on immune system 731,
        740–741, 741
    see also sports drinks
carbon cycle 329, 329
carbon dioxide
    adverse effects 24
    arterial partial pressure 52
    blood solubility factor 24–25
    conductance 24, 24–25, 25
    output
        as input to perception of effort
            377
        pregnancy 534
    partial pressure (ambient air) 24
    retention/accumulation 31, 321
    total flux 24
    transport 24
    underwater athletes 24, 31
carbonic anhydrase inhibitors 621
carbon monoxide
    air pollution 297, 635–636
    binding to haemoglobin 635, 684
    diffusing capacity see pulmonary
        diffusing capacity (DLco)
    exposure, causes 635

high altitude interaction 615
carboxyhaemoglobin 635, 636
cardiac arrest/events 306, 601
    mass participation events 663
    reduced risk by exercise 696
    risk at high altitude 622
    see also myocardial infarction;
        sudden cardiac death
cardiac arrhythmias 653, 654
    fetal bradycardia 535
    sudden death 670, 712
    tachycardia 320, 594
    ventricular fibrillation 306, 696
cardiac disease see cardiovascular
        disease
cardiac failure 58, 604
    congestive see congestive heart
        failure
    detection methods 709
cardiac fatigue 69, 80
cardiac hypertrophy 708
    benefits 713–714
    biochemical and cellular changes
        75
    endurance sports effect 76–77,
        708–709
    haemodynamic basis 70–71, 708
    health impact 714
    historical aspects 68, 708
    investigation methods 709
    molecular triggers 71
    myocardial ischaemia and 710–711
    pathological 71–75, 78, 709
        indicators 710
    physiological 71–75, 709, 711, 713
        pathological vs 68, 71–75, 73,
            709, 710
        types of sport and 76, 76–77
    septal 710, 712
    stimulus causing 70
    wall stress 71, 72
    wall thickness 709
cardiac output 34
    central limitation of effort 34
    distribution 58
    elderly 548, 552
    genetic influence 228–229
    high altitude 617, 936
    hot environment 112
    increased 70, 682
    pregnancy 531–532
    reduced, blood flow redistribution
        106
    rowers 840
    triathlon 873
cardiac reserve, children 513
cardiac transplantation 106
cardiomegaly, physiological 70,
    70–71
    see also cardiac hypertrophy
cardiomyopathy 73
    dilated 75, 670

cardiomyopathy (*continued*)
  hypertrophic *see* hypertrophic
    cardiomyopathy (HCM)
  overdiagnosis, danger 708, 709,
    713
cardiorespiratory fitness 701
  ACSM recommendations 554
cardiorespiratory function
  age-related decline 714
  hockey 924
  screening before competition 653
cardiothoracic ratio 708
cardiovascular abnormalities,
    sudden death and 668–671
cardiovascular benefits, of exercise
    688–707
  blood lipids and lipoproteins
    698–699
  blood pressure 689–691
  confounding factors in studies
    688–689
  coronary heart disease prevention
    691–696
  exercise recommendations *see*
    exercise
  glucose intolerance 699
  insulin sensitivity 699
  obesity 698
  research methodological issues
    688–689
  stroke risk reduction 696–698
cardiovascular consequences
  of exercise in children 508
  of respiratory muscle work 57–58
  women and effect of training 520
cardiovascular disease 566–571,
    688
  age-related risk 701
  epidemiology, exercise link
    691–696, 693, 694
  exercise testing 306
  reduction by exercise 458
  skeletal muscle blood flow and
    91–92
  see also cardiovascular system;
    coronary heart disease
cardiovascular drift 54, 109, 109–110
cardiovascular fitness 776, 781
cardiovascular resistance, oxygen
    transport 24
cardiovascular risks, of exercise 671,
    708–717
  see also cardiac hypertrophy;
    sudden cardiac death
cardiovascular screening 667–681
  abnormalities/disorders 668–671
  American Heart Association
    guidelines 667–668, 668, 672,
    715
  cost-efficiency 671, 676, 715
  definitions and background
    667–668

efficacy/limitations of non-
    invasive tests 675–677
  ethical considerations 671
  examiners 673, 674
  expectations of strategies 674–675
  impact and limitations 675, 715
  importance 714–715
  legal considerations 672
  limitations in use 673, 715
  methods/diagnostic testing 676
  obstacles 671
  practice in US 672–673
  purpose 667
  questionnaires 673, 673, 674
  race and gender aspects 677–678
cardiovascular system
  alcohol effects 446
  canoeing 896
  cycling 864, 865
  genetic aspects 228–229
  pregnancy 531–532
  see also cardiovascular disease
carnitine 336, 416
carotid body 932
cartilage
  benefit of exercise 751–752
  degeneration with age 551
catecholamines 184
  cardiac hypertrophy 70
  effect of strenuous exercise 184,
    185, 440, 682
  glycogenolysis stimulation 185
  input to perception of effort 379
  myocardial response, in elderly
    548
  overtraining marker 494
  release in exercise 184, 185, 864
  sudden cardiac death due to 79–80
  see also adrenaline; noradrenaline
catheterization
  bladder 606
  muscle metabolism analysis
    341–342
Cattell sixteen personality factor
    questionnaire (16PF) 368, 370
cavus feet 469
CD25 (IL-2R), overtraining marker
    495
cell trafficking, cortisol effect 735
central fatigue *see* fatigue
central limitations, of effort 34–35,
    301, 304
  see also fatigue, central
central nervous system (CNS)
  alcohol effect 446
  thermoregulatory centre 262
central venous pressure
  exercise in hot environment 263
  rowers 840–841, 841
cerebral blood flow 22, 107, 759
  velocity, rowers 840–841, 841
cerebral fatigue 28–29, 29

cerebral hypoxia 623
cerebral oedema 598–599, 606
  acute mountain sickness 621–622
  treatment 621–622
cerebral oxygenation, rowers 841,
    842
cerebral palsy 583–584
Cerebral Palsy–International Sport
    and Recreation Association
    (CP-ISRA) 3 583
cerebral perfusion 759
cerebral vascular accident (CVA)
    577
  see also stroke
cervical spine injuries 464
cervix, incompetent 539
C fibres, bronchial 633
channel swimmers, body
    temperature 266, 600
chemiluminescence, enhanced 338
chemokines, inflammation 800
chemoreceptors 54, 932
chest disease, carbon dioxide
    conductance 25
childbirth, training after 539
childhood, 'disappearance' 515
children 507
  aerobic trainability 507–512
    implications 511–512
    mechanisms 509–511
    reduced response to training
      509–510
  anthropometric characteristics
    41–42, 42
  athletes 507
  athletic success prediction 41
  biological age 397–398, 398
  burnout 515
  carbohydrate intake 514
  early maturers 398–399
  early specialization in sports
    398–399
  energy expenditure 510
  growth 397
  growth spurts 397, 398, 399
  heart rate 510
  heart size and cardiac reserve 513
  height development 397–398, 398
  injuries 466–468
  late maturers 398
  maximal oxygen intake ($\dot{V}_{O_{2max}}$)
    45, 47, 227, 507–509, 508,
    511
    body size relationship 45, 45, 46
  musculoskeletal system 513
  nutrient deficiencies 513
  nutrition 513–514
  oxygen intake variations 509
  participation in sport 507
  performance trainability 512
  physical activity levels 510
  psychosocial variables 514–515

scaling factors, submaximal $\dot{V}_{O_2}$
   48, 49
selection of wrong sport 398–399
sexual maturation 514
soccer, early selection 399
stroke volume 510, 511, 513
talent identification and
   development 400
tennis, early selection 399
thermoregulation 514
training 399, 507–516, 512
   benefits and risks 512–515
   effect on growth 41–42, 513
weight 514
cholesterol, reduction by exercise
   698–699, 757
chondromalacia 473
chondromalacia patellae see
   patellofemoral pain syndrome
   (PFPS)
chronic fatigue syndrome 499, 660,
   742
   plasma glutamine 500, 500
chronic pulmonary disease (CPD)
   569–570
chronic stimulation, electrical see
   electrical stimulation
chronological age 397–398, 513
cigarette smoke, composition 445
cigarette smoking see smoking
ciprofloxacin 660
circadian rhythm 639–641
   adjustment 644–645
      bright light and exercise
         647–649, 648
      improving 645–649
      maintaining alertness 646, 647
      meal timing/composition 646
      melatonin 647
      process 645–646
      schedule to facilitate 645–646
      sedatives 646–647
   control 639
   desynchronization see jet lag
   exercise 640
   factors affecting 640
   intensity of exercise 641
   phase delay and advance 645
   rectal temperature 640, 645
   signals controlling 644–645
   ventilation ($\dot{V}_E$) 640, 641
circle of Willis, aneurysms 712
circulation
   control 103
   coronary see coronary circulation
   gastrointestinal 105
   maximal aerobic power and 13
   pregnancy 531–532, 537, 538
   problems, fatigue development
      31–32
   rowers 836, 840–841
   splanchnic see splanchnic

circulation
circulatory discomfort, in heat stress
   265
circulatory failure 32, 594
cisternae, terminal 172
citrate synthase 119
citric acid (Krebs) cycle 25, 332, 333,
   337
   branched-chain amino acids 205
   enzymes 119, 120
   increased in altitude
      acclimatization 618
claudication, intermittent 91, 568
clothing
   cold stress 291, 294
   economy of movement and 253
   hot environments 290–291
   mass participation events 663
   soccer 905
   wind chill reduction 291
clumsiness 29, 32
cognitive disorders 584–586
cognitive factors 216–217
cognitive strategies 453, 456
   input to perception of effort 383
cold environment 259–267, 291–292
   exercise in 265–266
   shivering 260
   soccer 905
cold injuries 465
   prevention 481
   risks during competition 291–292
   skiers 855
cold stress 265–266, 291–294
   acclimatization 294
   assessment 291–292
   clothing 291, 294
   determinants 291–292
   hydration 294
   performance factors 292–294
   poor air quality and 298
cold tolerance 293, 294
cold water 292
collagen disorders 779
collapse 607
   conditions causing 601, 601
   diagnosis 598
   exercise-associated see exercise-
      associated collapse (EAC)
   management 601–607
      in conscious patient 606–607
      diagnostic information required
         603
      diagnostic steps 602–604
      flowchart 611
      initial 601–602
      protocols 604–606, 606–607
      in unconsciousness 604–606
   postexercise see exercise-associated
      collapse (EAC)
   rates 601, 602
   rectal temperature 663

risk reduction by prerace planning
   608–609
severity assessment 602, 602
vasomotor 594
see also hypoglycaemia;
   unconsciousness
colonic cancer, reduction 758
coma 603
common colds 742
communication system, prerace
   planning 609
compartment syndrome, hamstring
   791
competition
   anxiety before 214–215, 456
   carbohydrate meal 198–199
   cold injury risks 291–292
   diet 417–419
   high altitude, strategies 296–297
   hot environment, strategies
      288–291
   international see international
      competition
   medical supervision during
      659–660
   mental preparation 453–454, 456
   return to after childbirth 539
Competitive Reflections 456
complement, in inflammation 800
computed tomography (CT), stress
   fractures 771, 772
concanavalin-A, overtraining marker
   495
concentric actions 475
Concept II rowing ergometer 275,
   275
conchotome technique 342–343
Conconi principle 320
Conconi test 13, 320, 827
conditioning, endurance 4, 402–408
   hamstring injury prevention 791
   oxygen intake 405
   physiological factors 402–405
   safe limits in pregnancy 536–538
   training considerations 405–408
   see also training
conductance, definition 22
conductance analysis 22
conductance theory 22–28
   carbon dioxide 24, 24–25
   heat 26, 26–27
   lactate 25, 25–26
   metabolites 27–28
   oxygen 22–24
confectionery 412
confounding factors, benefits of
   exercise 688–689
congestive heart failure 580
   anaerobic metabolism 91
   muscle blood flow reduction 91
   vasodilatation impairment 91, 92
continuous exercise 12–14, 15

contractile proteins 159–164
  failure 158–159
  types 161
convection, heat 260
cooling-down 474–475
  elderly athletes 557
coordination
  failure, fatigue 29
  training for injury prevention
    476
core temperature *see* temperature,
  body
coronary anomalies, congenital
  669–670, 676, 712
coronary arteries, intramural
  (tunnelled) 670
coronary circulation 696
  impairment 653
coronary heart disease 691
  anabolic–androgenic steroid
    increasing 444
  benefits of exercise 691–696
    epidemiological features
      692–693
    mechanisms 695
    risk assessments 692, 692–694,
      693, 694
  benefits of training children 512
  ECG and diagnosis 549
  elderly 548–549
  ephedrine effect 443
  lower extremity amputees 577
  marathon runners 77
  risk factors 548, 551
    reduction by exercise 695
  sudden cardiac death 670
  see also cardiovascular disease;
    myocardial infarction
cor pulmonale 569
corpus luteum 719
corticosteroids
  anti-inflammatory actions 808
  injections 658, 809
    adverse effects 477
    contraindication 782, 783
corticotrophin-releasing hormone
  (CRH) 185
cortisol 185–187
  consequences of elevation 186
  elevated levels in amenorrhoea
    723, 725
  input to perception of effort 380
  local infiltration 808–809
  neutrophil/lymphocyte count
    changes 735
  overtraining marker 492, 493, 656
  response to exercise 186
  testosterone ratio 493, 656
  training effect 186–187
COSMED telemeter 304
C-protein *160*
creatine 416

loading 201, 911
  muscle stores 416
  supplements 416–417
creatine kinase (CK) 236
  adaptation to chronic stimulation
    121
  overtraining marker 491
creatine kinase, skeletal muscle-
    specific (CKMM)
  fatigue resistance and 236
  gene 236–237
  maximal oxygen intake linkage
    236
creatine phosphate 21, 416
critical power 317, 318
  see also anaerobic threshold
cromolyn sodium 634
cross-country running, rating of
    perceived effort 390
cross-reinnervation 144–145
cruciate ligament injury *see* anterior
    cruciate ligament injuries
crutches 790
cryotherapy 807
cutaneous blood flow 26, 103–117,
    107–109, 263
  alcohol effect 447
  body temperature relationship
    107–108, *108*
  exercise in hot environment 263
  muscle blood flow competition
    108–109, 110, 263
  role in cardiovascular drift *109*,
    109–110
  thermoregulation 596
  threshold temperature for
    vasodilatation 108
  vasoconstriction 108–109
cyanmethaemoglobin assay 424,
    738–739
cybex strength testing 790
cycle ergometer/ergometry 274,
    865–866
  cerebral palsy 583–584
  diabetics 573
  disabled persons 565
  incremental test 866
  maximal oxygen intake
    measurement 11–12, 304,
      865–866
  overtraining 489
  wetsuit effect 873
cycling and cyclists 857–871
  adaptations 866
  aerobic–anaerobic transition 866,
    867
  aerobic capacity 857, *868*
  aerodynamic clothing/equipment
    253
  age, body size and physique *38*
  air resistance 254, 857, *859*, 860
  anaerobic metabolism 866

bicycle variables affecting
    economy 252
blood glucose 869, 870
blood lactate 861, 864, 866, *869*
body fat 352
body mass effect 859
body surface area *859*, 860
cadence and economy 251
caffeine intake effect 442, 657
cardiovascular system 864, 865
catecholamine release 864
circadian rhythm control 640
cross-country races 858
dehydration 865
diet 869–870, *870*
drafting 857–858, *859*
economy of movement 245, 524,
    885
energetics 861–864, 864–865
energy consumption 857–858
energy costs 517, *859*
  per unit of body mass 250
energy sources 864, 865
environmental conditions 869
events 857, 858
external/internal locus of control
    383
fatigue mechanism 34, 869
fluid ingestion 597
fluid requirements 869
functional capacity assessment
    865–870
glycogen loading 655
gravity effect 614
heart rate 865, *867*, 869
heat loss 873
immune system changes 732
ketone bodies 865
laboratory *see* cycle
    ergometer/ergometry
left ventricle dimensions 76
long-term, physiology 864–865
lower extremity amputees 577
maltodextrin/low fructose
    beverage 869
maximal oxygen intake 863, *867*
medium-term, physiology
    861–864
metabolic data 282
metabolic rate 409
metabolic thresholds *863*
motor system 861, 864
muscle enzymes 863
muscle fibres 861, 864
  area 863
  recruitment patterns 127
ozone effect 630, 631
pedalling rates 251
perceived effort application 385
performance structure 862
power output 866
pregnancy 537

protein catabolism 865, 868
recovery, diet and 868–869
respiratory muscle training effect
  61
road 858
rolling resistance 252
short-term events, physiology
  861–864
sitting positions 858–859, *859*, *860*
speeds 857, *858*
  factors influencing 857–860
  wind resistance 279, *280*
sudden cardiac death 711
tactics 857, 860
track 857, 858
training
  follow-up 866, 867
  intensity 866–868
  physiology 861
  rating of perceived effort 390
  for world record *860*, 860–861
  years required 861
training load 860, 860–861, *861*
triacylglycerol content of muscles
  864
triathlons 873, 874, 885
wind speed/direction effect 253
  in wind tunnel 279, *279*
work components 246, *246*
cyclooxygenase 802
cyclooxygenase inhibitors 633, 803
  COX2 inhibitors 803, 808
cystic fibrosis 61, 570–571
cytochrome c oxidase 119
cytochromes 337
cytokines
  anti-inflammatory 738, 802
  ex vivo production reduced 739
  increased by prolonged exercise
    738–739, *739*
  inflammation process 802, 808
  pro-inflammatory 738–739, 802
cytoskeletal system, muscle cells
  177–178
  adaptations 179–180
  disruption by eccentric exercise
    167

Daedalus 942, *943*, *944*
dancers, amenorrhoea 724
dead space ventilation 53
deafness 585–586
deceleration, work 6
decompression chamber 620
deep vein thrombosis, in air travel
  639
degenerative changes, elderly 468
dehydration
  air travel 639
  American football 917
  cold environments 294
  cyclists 865

due to fluid restriction 591–592
elderly, susceptibility 550
during exercise 200
  wartime studies 595
exercise-associated collapse 607
fatigue due to 419
heart rate increase 14
heat cramps association 592–593
heat exhaustion 593, 607
heatstroke and 596
hot environment 290
impaired performance in 597, 598
physiological changes 597
pre-exercise 595
role in heat illnesses 591–592,
  597–599
triathlon 873–874
unconsciousness 605
delayed hypersensitivity 738, *738*
delayed-onset muscle soreness
  (DOMS) 808
densitometry 347
depression 214
  benefits of exercise 759
detraining 147
dexamethasone, plantar fasciitis 787
dextran 432
dextran infusion 432, 434
  blood volume increase 432
dextroamphetamine 439
diabetes mellitus 572–574
  benefits of exercise 757–758
  complications 758
  effects of exercise training 573, 699
  endurance training
    recommendations 573–574
  gestational 534, 572–573
  injury predisposition 473
  reduced risk with exercise 699,
    757–758
  type I (insulin-dependent; juvenile-
    onset) 572, 758
  type II (non-insulin dependent;
    adult-onset) 572, 758
    lower extremity amputees 577
    obesity reduction 574
    prevention 573
dialysis 571, 572
diaphragm, shortening 63
diaphragmatic fatigue 54, 56–57, *57*,
  61
diarrhoea, traveller's 659
diastasis recti 536, 539
diastolic blood pressure, elderly
  549
diastolic function 75
  training-induced changes 70
diclofenac 808
diet
  acute mountain sickness
    prevention 621
  benefits of exercise 760

carbohydrate ingestion *see*
  carbohydrate(s)
for competition 417–419
cyclists 869–870, *870*
  recovery 868–869
at high altitude 618
high-carbohydrate *see*
  carbohydrate(s)
high-fat 202, 412, 413, 757
high-fat, low carbohydrate
  412–413
high-fibre 203, 204
infection prevention 742
injury prevention 477
luteinizing hormone pulsatility
  726
meal timing/composition, jet lag
  646
pre-competition 418
pre-exercise 418
prerace advice to athletes 609
rugby football 915
soccer players 908
training 409–417
  energy substrates 409–413
  micronutrients 414–415
  protein intake 413–414
  supplements 415–417
vegetarian 203, 415
see also nutrition; *individual
  nutrients*
dietary fibre, high 203, 204
dietary supplements *see* nutritional
  supplements
dihydropyridine receptors (DHPR)
  170, 176
dimensionality theory 44
diphenoxylate 660
2,3-diphosphoglycerate 618
disabilities
  classification 567
  definition 565
  see also individual disabilities
disability, persons with 565–587
  endurance training principle 565
  importance of training 566
discomfort, cognitive control
  strategies 456
disease, classification 567
dissociation 216, 454
  see also association–dissociation
    factors
diuresis, caffeine effect 442
diuretics 606
  effect on exercise training 567, 570
diurnal rhythm *see* circadian rhythm
dopamine
  reduced 584
  role in central fatigue 419
dopaminergics 584
doping 657–658
  bicarbonate 26, 322

doping (*continued*)
  blood *see* blood doping
  erythropoietin *see* erythropoietin
  hormones 191, 194, 657
  international competition 657–658
  see also banned substances
dorsal root ganglion 151–152
  neurones 142–144, 151
  succinate dehydrogenase activity
    151–152
dorsospinocerebellar neurones 138
Douglas bags 305, 905
Down's syndrome 585
drafting, cycling 857–858, 859
drag forces 252, 253
drinking stations 658, 661
drinks 200
  caffeine content 441
  composition during exercise 420
  glycerol-containing 419–420
  sodium addition 420, 421
  see also carbohydrate beverages;
    sports drinks
drugs 438
  ergogenic *see* ergogenic drugs
  injury prevention 477
  for medical facilities at races 610,
    611
  prohibited 657
    bronchospasm treatment 653
    see also banned substances
  social (recreational) 438, 439,
    444–448
dual-energy X-ray absorptiometry
  (DXA) 349
Duchenne muscular dystrophy 580
duration of exercise/training
  ACSM recommendations 554
  elderly 552
  input to perception of effort 380,
    386, 388, 389
    application 385–386
  metabolic changes 125–127
  muscle metabolism 125–127
  periodization and 527
  pregnancy 538
dye dilution technique 341
dynamic stretching 476
dyspnoea 548–549
  development 750
  reduction in performance
    enhancement 64
  respiratory muscle
    loading/unloading 58, 63

ear guards 479
East Germany, swimming medals
  400, 400
eating, grazing pattern 412
eating disorders 362, 514, 723
eccentric exercise 475
  effect on cytoskeletal system 178

effect on myofibrillar proteins
  166–167
  muscle strain injuries 788
  triceps surae 781–782
echocardiography 69
  abnormalities detectable 676
  hypertrophic cardiomyopathy
    675, 709
  M-mode 74, 74
  prescreening of competitors 675,
    676, 715
  two-dimensional 677, 709
  use and misuse 709–710
ecological physiology 44
economy index, triathlons 884
economy of movement 245–258, 402
  biomechanical measures and
    250–251
  body size relationship 250
  cycling 245, 524, 885
  equipment relationship 251–252,
    253
  external resistance forces 252–254
  footwear 248, 251–252
  kinematic/kinetic measures 251
  lower limb flexibility 249
  mechanical power relationship
    246–248
  optimization 254
  performance relationship 245, 524
    exceptions 245
  running *see* running
  skiing 251
  small improvement with large
    benefits 245–246
  stretch–shortening cycle 248–250
  technique affecting 251
  triathletes 875, 884–885
  utilization of maximal aerobic
    capacity 402–403
  variations 246
  women 521, 524
ecstasy 439
ectomorphy 37–38, 41, 42
education
  Achilles tendon injury prevention
    782
  health 477
  prerace planning 608
  stress fracture prevention 773
effective temperature (ET*) 288
efficiency *see* economy of movement
efficiency ratio 247
effort awareness 374, 388
Ehlers–Danlos syndrome 779
eicosanoids 802
  role in inflammation 802–803
eicosapentaenoic acid 803
ejection fraction 709
elbow
  braces 480
  pads 479, 479

tennis 463, 480
elderly 547–564
  ACSM recommendations for
    exercise 554
  activity level 547
  baroreceptor reflex function 549
  blood pressure 549
  body composition 555, 556
  cardiac function 548
  cardiac hypertrophy benefits
    713–714
  cerebral performance
    improvement 759
  chronic disease 547
  cool-down exercises 557
  coronary artery disease 548–549
  dyspnoea 750
  eccentric exercise not
    recommended 475
  electrocardiography (ECG) 549
  endurance training effects 552–555
  exercise prescription 555–560
    guidelines 555–559
    to prevent disease 551
  falls 576
  frail, exercise programme 756
  graded exercise testing 548–549
  hepatic function 550
  hyperkalaemia 550
  injuries associated 468, 558, 558,
    805
  intensity of training 558
  maximal oxygen intake ($\dot{V}O_{2max}$)
    552–555, 553
  medical examination, clearance for
    exercise 477, 551, 551–552
  muscular strength training 555
  musculoskeletal changes 550–551
  physical activity levels 753
  physiological/pathological
    changes 547–551
  prolongation of independence
    753–756
  renal function 549–550
  renin–angiotensin–aldosterone
    system 550
  strength training 559–560
  sudden deaths 670
  tennis 468
  warm-up exercises 557
electrical impedance 349, 685
electrical stimulation, chronic
  effects on muscle 118, 120–122, 121
  enzyme changes 118, 119
electrocardiography (ECG) 69
  cardiovascular screening for
    training 672, 677
  changes due to training
    adaptations 677
  elderly 549
  electrode placement 305
  exercise test 305

high altitude 617
hypertrophic cardiomyopathy 677
long QT syndrome 677
ST depression 549
electroencephalography (EEG) 646
electrolyte analysers 610
electrolytes
    administration, exercise-associated
        collapse 607
    balance, women during training
        525–526
    heat cramps and 593
    loss during sweating 419
    replacement 420–421, 421
    see also potassium; sodium
electromyography (EMG) 141, 174
electrophoresis, erythropoietin
    determination 430–431
élite athletes 239
    anxiety 214, 215
    body composition 351, 352
    cognitive factors 216, 217
    genetic markers 234
    infections 732
    maximal oxygen intake ($\dot{V}O_{2max}$)
        402
    mental skills 452
    mountaineering 937–939
    overtraining 487
    performance determinants 271,
        272
    pulmonary blood–gas barrier
        impairment 53
    skiing 850–852
    veteran, injuries 468
emergency departments, mass
        participation events 661
emergency evacuation see evacuation
        of athletes
emergency transport, prerace
        planning 609
emotional risks, training of children
        512, 514–515
endergonic reactions 330
endocrine response
    high altitude 616
    see also hormones
endometrium, oestrogen and
        progesterone effect 719
endomorphy 37, 41, 42
β-endorphin 188–189, 749
    ACTH release correlation 186,
        188–189
    euphoric sensations 189, 749
    input to perception of effort 379
    response to exercise 188–189
    secretion ('runner's high') 749, 759
endotenon 777
endothelium-dependent
        vasodilatation 96–97
    congestive heart failure 92
endotoxin 801

endurance
    definition 7–8, 37
    perceived effort relationship 385
endurance activities 9–16
    categories 653
endurance conditioning see
        conditioning, endurance
endurance factors 184–207
endurance time 12–13
energetics
    cycling 861–864, 864–865
    running see running
energy
    ATP resynthesis 31, 331
    balance
        negative see below
        women 525
    chemical 5, 21
    consumption (internal) 6
    costs (C_r) 813
        air resistance 252
        competitive walking 282
        cycling 857–858
        fluid resistance 252–253
        reducing see economy of
            movement
        rowing 839
        running see running
    elastic 248, 249
    expenditure
        activities of daily living (ADL)
            753
        children 510
        cycling 517, 859
        hockey 920–921, 925
        international competitions 655
        leisure, optimal 747
        resting 6
        rugby football 911
        running 517, 815
        'running and walking' 814
        skiing 846–847
        soccer see soccer
        in training 410
        weight maintenance 700
        women 517–518
    'free' 21
    intake 410, 414
        amenorrhoeic vs eumenorrhoeic
            athletes 721
        cyclists 869, 870, 870
        runners 410, 410
        women athletes 202, 205, 410
    kinetic 6, 97
    low availability
        consequences 725
        menstrual disorder mechanism
            724, 725
    metabolism
        elderly 550–551
        pathways 331–334, 332, 333
    for muscle cells 158, 329, 330–331

negative balance
    decreased bone density due to
        752
    swimmers 830–831
    origins 329
    potential 5
    protein oxidation 414
    relationship to work 6
    release 330, 331, 411
        anaerobic glycolysis 335
    replenishment, cyclists 868–869
    requirement for women 517
        luteinizing hormone pulsatility
            725, 726
    requirements during exercise 410,
        411
    reserves 22
    resting expenditure 6
    sources 329, 410–413
        alcohol 446
        carbohydrate 27, 198, 847
        for cycling 864, 865
        fat see fat
        for skiing 846–847
        see also glycogen
    stores 5, 330
    submaximal costs of locomotion
        47–48, 48
    supply and demand, skeletal
        muscle 84, 85–86, 98
    utilization by muscle 330–331
'energy drain', amenorrhoea in
        dancers 724
English Channel swimmers,
        hypothermia 266, 600
enhanced chemiluminescence (ECL)
        338
environmental conditions
    conditions for event cancellation
        662
    contribution to competitive success
        4
    cycling 869
    injuries associated 465
    mass participation events 662, 663
    potential hazards 658
    rugby football 911
    soccer 904–905
environmental extremes
    assessment 287–300
    stressor interactions 298
    see also cold environment; high
        altitude; hot environment
enzyme immunosorbent assay
        (ELISA) 340
enzymes 330
    adaptation 120–121, 122–124
        citric acid cycle enzymes 120
    adaptations, training-induced
        mechanisms 131–133
    chronic electrical muscle
        stimulation effect 118, 119

enzymes (*continued*)
 endurance training effects
  122–124, *124*
  aerobic enzymes 27, *314*
 lifespan 131
 in mitochondria 332
 muscle metabolism 118
  genetic determinants 231, *232*
 overtraining effect 656
 reactions catalysed by 330
 synthesis rate 131
 vastus lateralis muscle, cyclists
  863
ephedrine 442–443
 side-effects 443
epic expeditions 653
epinephrine *see* adrenaline
  (epinephrine)
epiphyseal plate (growth plate)
  injuries 399
 children 513
epitenon 777
equipment
 arena 463–464
 canoeing 888
 economy of movement and
  251–252, *253*
 medical facility at race finish
  609–611, *610*
 poor, injuries due to 463
 preventive 478–482
  braces 479–481
  shoes 481–482
  tape 481
 protective *478*, 478–479
ergogenic aids 438
 alcohol 446
 caffeine 442
 creatine 416–417
 Macrodex™ 434
ergogenic drugs 438, 439–444
 reasons for use 439
 see also banned substances
ergometer pools 276–277
ergometers
 canoeing 274, *274*, 275
 Concept II rowing *275*, *275*
 cycle *see* cycle
  ergometer/ergometry
 Gjessing–Nilsen 275, *275*, *276*, 831
 isokinetic 277–278, *278*, 891
 lower extremity amputees 577
 for maximum oxygen intake
  ($\dot{V}o_{2max}$) 304, 865–866
 rowing 275, 275–276, *276*
 skiing *276*, 277
 stroke and head injury patients
  578
 types 274–279
 wheelchair athletes 278, *278*
ergometry 273–274
 definition 273–274

muscular dystrophy 580
erythrocytes *see* red blood cells
erythrocythaemia 425–428
 induction methods 425, *426*
 input to perception of effort 376
erythrocytosis, autosomal dominant
  235
erythropoiesis
 altitude training in women
  526–527
 increased by anabolic–androgenic
  steroids 444
 signs 682
erythropoietin (EPO) 190, 236
 abuse 190
 actions 190
 anaemia treatment 428
 blood doping method 428–431,
  657
 dangers of use 429
 effect on training on serum levels
  429–430
 gene 235–236, 428
 improved aerobic power 428
 recombinant 428, 429
  anabolic–androgenic steroids
   effect 444
  detection 430–431
  renal failure therapy 572
  sudden cardiac death 711
 role 428
 serum level determination 430
 synthesis 428
 urine levels 430
erythropoietin receptor (EPOR) gene
  236
Escherichia coli
 diarrhoea due to 659
 phagocytosis 735, *736*
ethics, cardiovascular screening 671
ethnic aspects
 blood pressure and exercise effect
  689–690
 cardiovascular screening 677–678
 sudden death *678*
ethyl alcohol *see* alcohol
eumenorrhoeic athletes,
  characterization 720–723
evacuation of athletes 609, 664
 wilderness trips 664
evaporation 260–261
examination, medical
 cardiovascular 672, *673*
  impact and limitations *675*
  see also cardiovascular screening
 pregnancy 536–537
 before sports for injury prevention
  477
excess post-exercise oxygen
  consumption (EPOC) 574
excitation–contraction coupling *see*
  muscle

exercise
 benefits 547, 551, 688–707
  see also cardiovascular benefits
 bronchospasm 653
 circadian rhythm 640
 deaths related to 712
  see also sudden cardiac death;
   sudden deaths
 definition 3
 duration *see* duration of
   exercise/training
 effect on heart 68, 688
 elderly *see* elderly
 health benefits *see* health benefits
 infection reduction 732
 intensity *see* intensity of
   exercise/training
 intermittent *see* intermittent
   exercise
 jet lag management 647–649
 lack 688
 leisure-time
  coronary heart disease risk 692,
   692–694, *693*, *694*
  high blood pressure incidence
   690
  reduced risk/mortality of stroke
   697
 lipids and lipoproteins 698–699
 medical clearance for in elderly
  551, 551–552
 in peripheral vascular disease 91
 programme for frail elderly 756
 recommendations
  cardiovascular health 699–700,
   700–701
  by health organizations 700–701
 stress, menstrual disorder
  mechanism 723, 724–725
 types and injury relationship 805
 whilst unwell, recommendations
  742–743
 year 2000 goals in US 701
exercise-associated collapse (EAC)
  594, 595
 diagnosis 607
 management 606–607
exercise-induced arterial hypoxaemia
  (EIAH) 55–56, 62
exercise machines, lower extremity
  amputees 577
exercise rehabilitation, chronic
  pulmonary disease 570, 750
exercise testing
 contraindications 306, *306*, 551
 ECG 305
 elderly 548–549, 551
 graded *see* graded exercise testing
  (GXT)
 precautions 306, *306*
exergonic reactions 330
expiratory flow limitation (EFL) 56

expiratory flow rates 53, 59
external oblique aponeurosis 795
external resistance forces 252–254
extrasarcomeric proteins 178
extroversion 382, 640
   circadian rhythm 640
   exercise intensity relationship 382
eye, injury prevention 478–479
eye-protecting devices 478–479
Eysenck Personality Inventory (EPI)
   382

face masks 464
   protective 478, 478, 479
facioscapulohumeral dystrophy
   (FSHD) 580
falls, elderly 576
fasting, short-term 413
fast-twitch muscle fibres see muscle
   fibre types
fat 197–207, 201
   avoidance by athletes 202
   energy per gram 329
   as energy source 329, 519, 847
   high-fat diet 202, 412, 413, 757
   increased utilization after training
      60
   inflammation and 807
   ingestion/intake 201–202
   metabolism 27, 521
      pregnancy-induced changes 531
   mobilization 28, 201–202
   oxidation 410–411
   requirements 412
   stores 197
   see also lipids
fat, body
   adverse effects of accumulation
      757
   aerobic power relationship 350
   American footballers 916
   critical level and amenorrhoea
      aetiology 724
   density relationship 347
   endurance athletes 351–354
   excessive 349–350
   gender influences 293
   genetic influences 233–234
   increasing prior to prolonged
      exercise 655
   intra-abdominal in elderly 555
   mass 43, 346
      assessment 347
      performance and 349–350
      two-component model and 346,
         347
   men, by sport type 354
   percentage
      determination 347, 349
      endurance athletes 351–354
   reduction in diabetics after exercise
      573

tissue insulation in cold water
   immersion 292–293, 293
women 353, 410, 525
young athletes 353–354
fat-free mass (FFM) 43, 346
   assessment 347
   calculation 347, 348
   constituents 346, 348
   elderly 560
   endurance athletes 354–355
   gender differences 354–355, 355
   genetic influences 233
   interindividual variations 347–348
   performance and 350
   resistance training effect 555
   two-component model and 346,
      347
fatigue 22, 28–33, 418–419
   accident risk 33
   acute after training session 501
   anxiety association 33
   branched-chain amino acids role
      205
   causes 28, 259, 336
   central causes 28, 205
      dopamine role 419
      nutrition and 418–419
      overtraining 499
      susceptibility 33
   central vs peripheral limitations
      34–35
   cerebral 28–29, 29
   clumsiness 29, 32
   cumulative chronic 32
   cyclists 34, 869
   definition 259, 903
   dehydration causing 419
   diaphragmatic 54, 56–57, 57, 61
   excitation–contraction coupling
      174
   failure of drive mechanisms 28–30
   failure of power supply 31
   glycogen reserves and 31, 411
   heart rate 259
   high-frequency 174
   homeostasis failure 31–32, 95
   hormonal 32
   hot environment 419
   hyperthermia relationship 111
   hypoglycaemia as cause 336
   hypothermia susceptibility 294
   immune system deterioration 32,
      33
   inappropriate calcium level 29–30,
      170–171
   injuries 461
   interindividual differences 33–34
   intermittent exercise protocol 11
   internal temperature and 111, 419
   marathon runners 31
   masked by amphetamine 440
   medical aspects 33

mental, goals in soccer 904
metabolic 120, 158, 166, 178–180
   avoidance 166
   cause (theory) 205
   protective role 166
metabolic acidosis 95
mitochondrial damage 33
muscle see muscle
myocardium 110
myofibrillar function 165–167
neural component 29, 29
neuromuscular 146, 153
neurotransmitters involved 419
non-metabolic 178–180
perceptions 33
peripheral cause, onset speed
   33–34
perseverance aspect 453
physiological 28–32
projected 32–33
psychological 32–33, 453
resistance 180
   adaptations in myofibrillar
      system 167–168
   enzyme activities 146
   low CKMM activity 236
   Na^+/K^+ pump role 177
   soccer 904
   training effect 168–169
respiratory muscles see respiratory
   muscles
soccer see soccer
time to, acclimatization effect 111
travel 639
triathlons 874, 875
warm environment 419
fatigue fractures 33
fat pad atrophy 788
fatty acid-binding protein (FABPPM)
   334
fatty acids
   degradation, ATP production
      336–337
   energy metabolism 333, 334, 337
   essential 803, 807
   free see free fatty acids (FFA)
   long-chain 202
   metabolism 337
   oxidation 332, 336–337
      chronic stimulation effect 119,
         119, 120
   polyunsaturated (PUFAs) 807
   short-chain 202
   transport across mitochondria 334,
      336
   transport to muscle 31
Fédération Internationale des
   Sociétés d'Aviron (FISA) 836,
   837, 839
feedback, body 216, 217
   perceived effort 375, 386–387, 388
feed-forward mechanisms 54

femur, stress fracture 768, 769, 770
fencing 946
fenoterol, prohibition 653
fetus
    bradycardia 535
    growth, endurance exercise effect
        535
    heart rate 534–535, 535, 538
    obstetric outcomes 536
    response to maternal exercise 534,
        534–535
    stress 538
fibrinolysis 696
fibula, stress fracture 768, 770
Fick principle/equation 103, 510
Fick's first law 89
field games
    physiological demands 900
    pitch dimensions 900
    types 900
    see also rugby football; soccer
field hockey see hockey
field independent input, to
        perception of effort 383
field sports 900–930
first-aid helpers 609, 660
first-aid stations
    mass participation events 662, 663
    positions 609
fish oil 803
fitness 3–4
    ACSM recommendations for
        exercise 554
    aerobic/anaerobic 767
        see also aerobic fitness
    athletic 767
    basic level for injury prevention
        473–474
    blood pressure control 689
    cardiorespiratory 554
    cardiovascular 776, 781
    hurling and lacrosse 926–927
    rugby football 912–915
    soccer 907
    sport-specific 767
Five-Nations Championship 910
flexibility
    age-related loss 756
    elderly 558
    injuries due to 470–471
    stretch–shortening cycle and
        249–250
    training 471
        ACSM recommendations 554
        elderly 558
        to prevent injury 475–476
flight see air travel; human-powered
        flight; spaceflight
flow–volume loop 53, 56
fluid
    absorption 599
    accumulation 598–599

advice before international
        competitions 659
balance, women during training
        525
ingestion
    during exercise 597
    marathon running 592
    mass participation events 661
loss
    diarrhoea 659
    see also dehydration
overload in prolonged exercise
        598–599
    diagnosis 604
    management 606
    see also hyponatraemia
replacement 420–421, 421
    see also hydration
requirements 419–421
    cyclists 869
    before exercise 419–420
    postexercise 420–421
resistance 246, 246
    work to overcome 252–253
restriction during exercise 591
retention 598
    pathogenic mechanisms 599
    see also drinks; genetic
        determinants; water
fluid-regulating hormones 190
fluorescein isothiocyanate (FITC)
        175
fluorometric pyridine nucleotide
        method 338, 339
follicle-stimulating hormone (FSH)
        719
foods
    advice before international
        competitions 659
    glycaemic index 199, 199–200
    see also diet; nutrition
food supplements see nutritional
        supplements
foot
    care 477–478
    dorsiflexion 779
football
    American see American
        football/footballers
    association see soccer
    Australian Rules 917–919
    Gaelic 917–919
    rugby see rugby football
footwear
    Achilles tendon injury prevention
        778–779
    cushioning effect on energy costs
        252
    economy of movement and 248,
        251–252
    energy storage and economy of
        movement 248

heel (shoe) 778–779
heel lifts 782
ideal 481–482
injury prevention 481–482,
        778–779
mass participation events 663
motion control 779
plantar fasciitis 786
running 248, 481
stress fracture prevention 774
force 5, 768
    aeroplane aerodynamics 942–943
    drag, rowing 838, 838
forced expiratory volume in 1 s
        (FEV$_1$) 629
forced vital capacity (FVC) 629
force–velocity curves, canoeists 891,
        892
fractures
    fatigue 33
    Jones' 771
    risk after menstrual disorders
        718
    stress see stress fractures
    tibial, anterior cortical 770
    vertebral 576
Frank–Starling mechanism 520, 548,
        683
free fatty acids (FFA)
    availability, input to perception of
        effort 379, 387
    degradation 336–337
    intravenous administration 655
    metabolism, caffeine effect 441
    mobilization 201
free radicals
    damage to muscle 417
    Na$^+$/K$^+$ pump susceptibility 175
    reactive oxygen species 801, 802,
        806
frostbite 291, 654
fructose, uptake by liver 199
fruit, carbohydrate content 199, 200
fuel reserves, catecholamine effect
        185
functional field test, rugby 913

Gaelic football 917–919
gait
    analysis 780, 787
    kinetic chain 471–472
gamma (γ)-motoneurones 137–138
gas exchange 52–53
    capillary bed 23
    maternal–fetal 532
    mountaineering 933
    prolonged exercise 52
    training effect 59
gastric emptying 420
gastrocnemius muscle 777, 788
gastrointestinal circulation 105
gel electrophoresis 341

GENATHLETE Study 235, 236, 237, 239
gender differences
  aerobic trainability of children 509
  blood pressure and effect of exercise 690
  body fat 293, 353, 354
  bone mineral density/content 355, 356, 357, 359–361
  cardiovascular screening 677–678
  fat-free mass 354–355, 355
  heart size 75–76
  jet lag 642
  maximal aerobic power, adolescents 397, 398
  nutritional needs 205–206
  performance 523
  rating of perceived effort 390
  skiing distance–velocity relationships 846
  stress fracture 767, 768
  tissue injury and inflammation 805–806
  see also women
genes
  amplification in motor units 142
  candidate for endurance performance 237, 239
  contribution to competitive success 4
genetic determinants 21, 223–242
  bone density 358
  cardiovascular 228–229
  maximal oxygen intake 224–228
    familial resemblance assessment 224–225, 225
    heritability 225–227
    maternal effects 227
    response to training 227–228
  molecular markers 234–238
  muscle 229–232
  muscle blood flow control 97
  physique and body composition 232–234
  quantitative studies 224–234
  research directions 238–239
  skiing performance 846
genetic markers, performance phenotypes 234–238
genu varum 468
Gestalt rating 384, 748
gestational diabetes 534, 572–573
Gjessing–Nilsen ergometers 275, 275, 276, 831
glandular fever 660
glaucoma 586
glomerular filtration rate (GFR) 549–550
glucagon 189–190
glucocorticoids 570
  see also corticosteroids

gluconeogenesis 31, 198, 313, 329, 336
glucose
  advice before international competitions 659
  blood
    amenorrhoea vs eumenorrhoea 721
    cerebral decrease in fatigue 28–29
    cyclists 869, 870
    improved control by exercise 573
    pregnancy-induced changes 531
  insulin secretion stimulation 189
  intake 27–28
  intolerance, benefits of exercise 699
  preliminary screening before competition 654
  reduction by endurance exercise 758
  regulation 336, 654
  replacement 606
  solutions, ingestion/absorption rate 27–28
  sources during exercise 198
  supplements 27–28, 29, 387
  synthesis 31
glucose analysers 610
glucose–electrolyte solutions, mass participation events 662
glucose/polymer solutions 27–28
glutamine 33, 204
  chronic fatigue syndrome 500, 500
  depletion 417, 740
  overtraining marker 491–492, 492, 492, 496, 500
  role in immune system 496
  supplements 204, 740
gluteus medius, weakness 776
glycaemic index 199–200
  foods 199, 413, 418
glycerol, hyperhydration 419–420
glycerol cell-freezing technique 426
glycerol-containing drinks 419–420
glycogen 328
  breakdown 411
  depletion 411, 418
    Gaelic football 918
    hypoglycaemia 606
    overtraining marker 491
    oxidative enzyme relationship 131
    rate 27
    specific muscles 847
    swimming training 830
    ultra-long distance events 313
  glycolysis 333, 334–335
  loading 655, 925
  muscle stores 198, 336, 411, 417
    amphetamines effect 440

Australian Rules football 918
    diet to increase 417–418
    rugby football 911
    soccer 904, 906
    type of carbohydrate diets 417, 418
  replenishment after exercise 655
    cyclists 870
    jogging effect 519
  reserves
    fatigue development 31, 411
    utilization rate 27
    women 521
  resynthesis rates 412, 412
  sources, skiing 847
  storage 200, 314, 864
  structure 335
glycogenolysis 185, 328
  see also glycolysis
glycogen phosphorylase, regulation 185
glycolysis 328, 333, 334–336
  aerobic 334, 335, 336
  anaerobic 328, 331, 334, 335
  energy release 335, 411
  maximal power from 334, 336
  muscle 334–336
  pathway 331
  reactions 333, 334–335
  terminology 328
glycolytic enzymes 126
  chronic stimulation effect 118, 119, 119, 121
  inhibition by hydrogen ions and lactate 312
  muscle cell content 127
  training effect 127–129
goals
  outcome/performance/process 455
  setting 216, 455–456
  training 518
gonadotrophin-releasing hormone (GnRH) 719, 720–721, 723
gonadotrophins 188
Gossamer human-powered craft 942, 943
graded exercise testing (GXT)
  disabled persons 565
  elderly 548–549
granulocytes 735, 737
gravitational unloading syndrome (GUS) 144
gravity
  at high altitudes 614
  neuromotor responses 144, 151
  potential energy stores 5
  reduced (spaceflight), effects 144, 146, 149, 151
groin
  mass 792
  pain 791–792

growth
  submaximal energy costs of
      running 48, *48*
  training in childhood effect 41–42,
      513
growth factors, inflammation 800
growth hormone 187–188
  actions/effects 187
  response to training 187–188, 511
growth retardation, intrauterine 539
growth spurts 397, *398*, 399
  flexibility exercises after 475
  injury predisposition 466
  muscle strength imbalance 466
gunshot wounds 577
gymnasts
  growth and training effect 513
  injuries 467, *467*, 513
  stress fractures 771

haematocrit 424
  determination 427
  improvement in women 526
  increase with erythropoietin use
      429
  optimal 425
haematoma, hamstring injury 789,
    790
haemoconcentration 191, 618
haemodilution, from volume
    expanders 433
haemodynamic overloading 70
haemoglobin 423–437
  altitude acclimatization 617, 934
  blood volume changes and 427,
      431
  carbon monoxide binding 635, 684
  control of levels 429
  erythrocythaemia and 425–428
    see also erythrocythaemia
  maximizing before competitions
      655–656
  oxygen affinity, high altitude 934,
      934
  oxygen-carrying capacity 423
  oxygen transport 423–431
  structure 423
  see also anaemia
haemoglobin A 423
haemopoiesis
  increase, altitude acclimatization
      618
  suppression after return to sea-
      level 620
  see also erythropoiesis
Haglund's deformity 470, 781
hamstring 789
hamstring compartment syndrome
    791
hamstring injuries 789–791
  avulsion 790
  strains 470

treatment 790–791
hand grip, strength after spinal cord
    injuries 579
'handicapping,' allometric scaling for
    50
Hanin's individual zone of optimal
    functioning (IZOF) 456
'hardiness,' coping with training 498
Hawthorne effect 216
head
  injury 577–578, *578*
  protective equipment 478, *478*
healing, after tissue injury 802
health, perceived 748–749, *749*
  consequences of changes 749–750
health benefits, of exercise 699,
    747–765
  cardiovascular *see* cardiovascular
      benefits
  humoral disorders 756–758
  immune function 732, 759
  independence prolongation
      753–756
  lifestyle 760–761
  metabolic 756–758
  musculoskeletal 750–753
  neoplasms 758–759
  psychological function 759–760
  respiratory function 750
  in specific diseases 747, 748
health promotion 458
hearing aids 585
hearing difficulties 585–586
heart
  conduction abnormalities 79, 710
  failure *see* cardiac failure
  function, elderly 548
  malformations 668
  murmurs 674
  rhythm abnormalities 653
    see also cardiac arrhythmias
  size
    effect of training of children 513
    enlargement 70–71
    genetic influence 229, 710
    hockey players 924
    see also cardiac hypertrophy
  training effect *see* heart, athlete's
  transplantation 106
heart, athlete's 68–83, 75–76
  characteristics 71–75
  concept relating to 708–709
  diagnostic advances 69
  gender issues 75–76
  historical aspects 68–69
  hypertrophy *see* cardiac
      hypertrophy
  natural selection and 710
  shape 73
  sudden death *see* sudden cardiac
      death
  systolic and diastolic functions 70

ventricular performance 69–70
  see also ventricular remodelling
heart rate
  age-associated decline 548
  American footballers 916
  anaerobic threshold measure
      (Conconi test) 13, 320, 827
  body temperature relationship
      109, 110
  canoeists 894
  children 510
  cycling 865, 867, 869
  deflection point 827
  elderly 555, 557, 560
  environmental factors effect 14
  factors affecting 280–281
  in fatigue definition 259
  fetal 534, 535, 538
  hockey 924
  increase 107
  input to perception of effort 376,
      385
  intensity of endurance training
      14
  interval exercise 11, *11*
  marathon runners 385
  measurement 14
  myocardial work rate 711
  overtraining marker 490
  pace training in women 519
  peak 14, 490
  power output relationship 13, 320
  pregnancy 533, 537, *538*
  reserve 14, 555, 557, 560
  rugby football 914
  skiing 849
  soccer 905, 908
  swimming 826–827, *827*
  training recommendation 14
  in unconscious patient 603
  women during sustained distance
      training 518
heat
  acclimatization 265, 285, 288,
      288–289
  conductance 26, *26*–27, 260
    water immersion 27, 292
  convection 260
  dissipation 26, 27
  environmental *see* hot environment
  flux 27
  generation 7, 26, 108, 260
  injury
    children 514
    prevention 481, *481*
  intolerance by elderly 548
  loss 260, 419
    cold conditions 291
    importance 108
    mechanisms 107–108, 260–261,
        419
    predictions 292

reduction in mass participation events 663
skiing 855
triathlon 873
response to exercise by children 514
storage 260
tolerance 289
transfer 260, 261, 262, 290
during exercise 263
water immersion 261
wetsuit effect 872, 873
heat cramps 592–593
heat exhaustion (syncope) 593–596, 607
Heath–Carter anthropometric protocol 38
heat illnesses 591–599, 663
heat prostration (exhaustion) 593–596, 607
heat retainers 481
heat-shock proteins 802
heat strain 593, 595, 597
heat stress 263–265, 287–288
see also hot environment
heat stress index (HSI) 288
heatstroke 288, 592, 596–597
amphetamine interactions 657
body temperature 595
diagnosis 603
emergency treatment 601
management 604–605, 610
mortality 605
physiological changes 604
predisposing factors 596
heel pain 786
height
canoeists 891
increase in boys 397, 398
peak height velocity (PHV) 397, 398
triathletes 877–878, 878
see also body size; stature
helmets, aerodynamic 253
Henry's law 423
hepatic blood flow, exercise in hot environments 264–265
hepatic function, elderly 550
hepatitis B, protection against 659
hepatitis C, protection against 659
heritability 224
maximal oxygen intake 225–227, 226, 865
see also genetic determinants
HERITAGE family study 227, 228, 228, 233, 234, 237
hernia, sports 794–796
herniography 795
herniorrhaphy 796
hexokinase (HK) 120
high altitude 294–297, 614–627, 931

acclimatization 12, 296, 614, 617–619, 932
acid–base balance 616–617
acute effects (moderate altitude) 616–617
air density reduction 296, 615
air quality deterioration 298, 615
air resistance decrease 252–253
assessment 294–295
cardiac output 617, 936
competing above 3000m 619
competitive strategies 296–297
disorders associated 620–623
endocrine response 616
endurance performance 936–937
heat conductance 27
hyperventilation 321, 932
hypoxia 55, 58, 616, 933, 936
lung volume 933
maximum oxygen intake ($\dot{V}o_{2max}$) 55, 295, 295–296
medical conditions at 614, 622–623
muscle oxidative capacity 133
oxygen partial pressure reduced 295, 295, 615–616, 931
performance relationship 295–296, 296
physical environment 614–616
polycythaemia 619
pulmonary arterial pressure 617, 933
pulmonary oedema 296, 622
risks of competitions at 614
training 12, 296–297, 321–322
for low-altitude events 937
rowing 841–842
rugby football 911
women 526–527
see also mountaineering
high-altitude training camps 619–620
high-density lipoprotein (HDL) 566, 698
increased by exercise 698, 700, 701, 757
high intensity training see training
high-performance liquid chromatography (HPLC) 339–340
high ventilatory response 938–939
hip
examination 784
injuries 770
loss of rotatory function 473
rotation abnormality 792, 793
'hitting the wall' 27, 216, 313
dissociation methods linked 216–217
HIV infection 657, 659
hockey 919–926
cardiorespiratory system 924
demands of specific positions 920

dribbling, and demands of 920–921
energy expenditure 920–921, 925
exercise intensity 920
fitness profiles 922–924
men 924–926
women 921, 922–924
heart rate 924
historical background 919–920
maximal oxygen intake 922, 922–923, 923, 924–925
muscle performance 922
physical strain 925–926
playing surfaces 921
positional role 921
rules/principles 920
training 923, 925, 926
ventilatory threshold 924
homeostasis failure 31–32
signs 28
homocystinuria 779
hormonal fatigue 32
hormone replacement therapy (HRT) 576
hormones 184–207
abuse 194
adolescents, training 511
doping 191, 194, 657
exercise-induced changes 192–193
fluid-regulating 190
markers of overtraining 492–494
measurements 191
Na^+/K^+ pump regulation by 176–177
peptide, doping 657
pregnancy-induced changes 531
prolonged events 313
response to training 191, 511
sympathoadrenal 184–185
variables affecting 191
horseradish peroxidase 139
hospitals
admission in heatstroke 605
liaison for mass participation events 661
warning in prerace planning 609
hot environment 259–267, 287–291
aerobic fitness 289–290
caffeine effect 442
cardiac output 112
casualty number prediction 608
circulatory homeostasis failure 32
clothing 290–291
competitive strategies 288–291
exercise–heat acclimatization 285, 288, 288–289
exercise in 262–265, 287–291
fatigue 419
fluid and electrolyte loss 419
fluid intake 597
heart rate increase 14
'heat exhaustion' pathogenesis 594

hot environment (*continued*)
  heat stress assessment 287–288
  hydration levels 290
  intolerance by elderly 548
  mineral depletion 656
  muscle blood flow 111, 112
  soccer 904–905
  temperature regulation influence
    110, 290
  training in women 526
  see also heat stress
human-powered flight 942–944
  aeroplane aerodynamics 942–943
  characteristics of pilots 944
  design strategies 943
  factors limiting prolonged flight
    944
  historical aspects 942
  power requirements 943, 944
humidity, soccer 904
hunger, exercise and 726
hurling 926–927
  demands 926
  fitness 926–927
  maximal oxygen intake 926–927
hydration 290, 294
  rugby footballers 911
hydride ions 334, 335, 337
hydrogen ions
  accumulation
    decreased by respiratory muscle
      training 64
    in fatigue 29–30
    muscle 312
    repetitive activity 166
  effect on lactate transport 26
  high-intensity exercise 95
  muscle blood flow control 95
  pregnancy 533
3-hydroxyacyl CoA dehydrogenase
  (HAD) 119, 119
5-hydroxytryptamine *see* serotonin
hygiene 477–478
hyperbaric chamber 621
hypercapnia, as input to perception
  of effort 377
hypercarbia 620
hypercortisolism 186–187
hyperextension, injury risk factor
  467, 467
hyperglycaemia 572
hyperhydration 290, 419–420
hyperinsulinaemia 699
hyperkalaemia 550
hyperlipidaemia 698
hypermobility 471
hyperoxia, in perception of effort 376
hyperpnoea, exercise 53, 54, 56
hyperpronation, compensatory 468,
  469
hyperreactivity, in perception of
  effort 382

hyperreflexia, amyotrophic lateral
  sclerosis 582
hypersensitivity, delayed 738, *738*
hypertension
  benefits of endurance exercise 688
  elderly 550
  risk factor for disease 689
  risk factor for stroke 578
  screening 671
  systolic 549
  see also blood pressure
hyperthermia 26, 591–613, 659
  American footballers 917
  cooling procedure 604
  fatigue relationship 111
  malignant 597, 605
  in triathlon 872
  visceral vasoconstriction 111–112
hypertrophic cardiomyopathy
  (HCM) 71–72, 79, 654
  athlete's heart *vs* 72, 74
  detection 674, 675
  diagnostic criteria 713
  ECG screening 677
  false-negative screening 677
  gene mutations 669, 713
  overdiagnosis 708, 709, 713
  pathology 669
  as post-mortem finding 711, 712
  race and gender aspects 677
  screening by genetic testing
    675–676
  sudden cardiac death 78, 712–713
hypertrophy, cardiac *see* cardiac
  hypertrophy
hyperventilation 54, 312
  altitude acclimatization 617, 932
  compensatory 55
  exercise-induced 54
  high altitude 321, 932
hypervolaemia 70–71, 431–432
  see also blood volume; volume
    loading
hypnosis, fatigue and 28, 29
hypocapnia, high altitude 616
hypoestrogenaemia 514
hypoglycaemia
  cause of fatigue 336
  coma 603
  detection 602
  effects 313–314
  management 606
  precautions against 573–574
  preliminary screening before
    competition 654
  reactive 418
hypoglycaemic agents, oral 573
hypoglycaemic crisis 654, 758
hypogonadism 188
hypohydration *see* dehydration
hyponatraemia
  diagnosis 603

emergency treatment 601, 602
of exercise 598–599, 599
management 605–606
mass participation events 662
triathletes 874
hypotension 579
postural *see* postural hypotension
hypothalamic dysfunction,
  overtraining 493
hypothalamic–pituitary–adrenal axis
  186, 740
hypothalamic–pituitary–ovarian
  (HPO) axis 719, 720
  amenorrhoeic *vs* eumenorrhoeic
    athletes 720–721, 721
  causative hypothesis for
    amenorrhoea 724
hypothalamus 262, 639
hypothermia 261, 266, 591–613, 659
  cold exposure 291
  consequences 600
  high altitude 615
  management 605, 610
  predisposing factors 600
  during running 599–600
  susceptibility in fatigue 294
  water immersion 266
hypovolaemia 263, 264
hypoxaemia, arterial, exercise-
  induced (AIAH) 55–56, 62
hypoxia
  adjustment in mountaineers 931
  aerobic training session combined
    12
  cerebral 623
  diaphragmatic fatigue 56
  high altitude 55, 58, 616, 933, 936
  input to perception of effort 376
  oxygen dissociation curve 616

ice, inflammation management 807
'iceberg profile' (mood states) 212,
  212, 213
  personality 370
ice-cold water, hyperthermia therapy
  604, 610
ice hockey 464
  protective equipment 478, 478
ilioinguinal neuralgia 792
iliopsoas bursitis 792
iliotibial band friction syndrome 462,
  469
imagery, mental 215
immobilization, adverse effects 474
immune system 731–746
  benefits of regular exercise 732,
    759
  deterioration in fatigue 32, 33
  endurance exercise adverse effects
    731, 735–740
    countermeasures 740–742
    implications 734–745

'open window' theory 731,
    735–740
  policy recommendations
    742–743
  see also immunosuppression
impairment by overtraining 656,
    731–732
marker of overtraining 494–496
monitoring before competition 654
non-athletes vs endurance athletes
    731–733
soccer players 908–909
immunity
  adaptive 732
  innate 732–734
immunoblotting 338
immunoglobulin, overtraining
    marker 495–496, 656
immunoglobulin A 735–736
  decreased after prolonged exercise
    735–736
  nasal 735–736
  overtraining marker 495–496
  salivary, reduced in athletes 734,
    735–737
immunomodulators 740
immunoradiometric assay 430
immunosuppression, exercise-
    induced 735–740, 759
  countermeasures 740–742, 741
immunosuppressive agents 575
impact force
  protective equipment role 479, 479
  shoes to prevent 481
  sports surface 462
impact injuries, chronic 468
'impaired competitor' policy 609
impedance, electrical 349, 685
inactivity, physical and injuries 474,
    779
independence, prolongation 753–756
'indifference point' 684
'individual zones of optimal
    functioning' (IZOF) 214–215,
    456
infections
  benefits of regular exercise 732,
    759
  fatality rates 712, 732
  IgA levels as risk marker 734–735
  overtraining association 494, 712,
    732, 742, 749–750
  prolonged exertion linked
    731–732, 734, 742, 759
    prevention recommendations
    742
  tropical, prevention 658
infectious mononucleosis 660
infertility, female athletes 718
inflammation 800–810
  age and gender effect 805–806
  chronic 807

damage due to 802
  initiation 800, 801, 805
  nutritional influences 806–807
  overuse injuries 800, 804
  polyunsaturated fatty acids
    affecting 807
  prevention and treatment 807–809
    non-pharmaceutical 807
    pharmaceutical 808–809
  process/reaction 800, 801, 804–807
  prolonged exercise causing 735
  regulation 802, 805, 806
  role 800–802
  training form and status affecting
    804–805
inflammatory mediators 738–739,
    800
influenza, vaccination 742
inguinal hernia 794
injury, sports 458, 749, 803
  acute 460, 461
  aetiological factors/mechanisms
    460–461
    arena equipment 463–464
    environmental conditions 465
    extrinsic factors 461–465, 462
    ineffective rules 464
    intrinsic factors see below
    poor equipment 463
    sports surface adjustment
    462–463
    training errors 462, 462, 766–
    767
  age relationship 805
  chronic impact injuries 468
  elderly 468, 558, 558–559
  epidemiology 460
  exercise type relationship 805
  fatigue 461
  impact 461
  intrinsic factors causing 465–473
  mass participation events 660
  mechanisms, education on 477
  overuse see overuse
    injuries/syndromes
  previous and reinjury 472–473
  reinjury risk 470
  repeated overload 461
  running mileage link 805
  sites, triathlons 876–877
  skiing 463
  societal costs 458
  surveillance system 460–461
  tennis 463
  tissue inflammation see
    inflammation; tissue injury
  triathlon 876–877
  women 465–466
injury prevention 458–465
  cold environment 481
  cooling-down 474–475
  general methods 473–475

at individual and group level
    458–459
  inflammation and tissue injury 807
  load and speed decrease 461
  in obesity 574
  preparation for sports 478
  preventive equipment see
    equipment
  preventive training 475–478
    coordination and proprioceptive
    476
    diet and drugs 477
    education 477
    flexibility 475–476
    hygiene 477–478
    medical examination 477
    muscle training 475
    sport-specific 476–477
  primary 459
  risk factor identification 459
  secondary and tertiary 459
  sequence 459, 459–460, 460
  slow progression 475
  at societal level 459
  tactics 458–460, 459
  warm-up 458, 474
inspiratory capacity, decreased 629
inspiratory flow rates, training effect
    59
insulin 189–190, 572
  amenorrhoeic vs eumenorrhoeic
    athletes 721, 723
  basal levels in athletes 189
  decreased secretion 189, 572
  hypoglycaemic crisis 654
  pregnancy 531
  receptor density 699
  resistance 572
  secretion 189, 531
  sensitivity
    improved by exercise 573, 699
    of muscle 132–133
  therapy 573
insulin-like growth factor (IGF) 71,
    187, 723
insulin-like growth factor-binding
    protein I (IGFBP-I) 721, 723
insulin receptor substrate-1 337
intellectual performance 759
intensity of exercise/training
  ACSM recommendations 554
  anaerobic threshold as marker
    389–390
  children 508
  circadian rhythm 641
  disabled persons 565
  effect on blood pressure 689
  elderly 552, 557, 558
  high-density lipoprotein increase
    701
  hockey 920
  importance in training 125–127

intensity of exercise (*continued*)
  input to perception of effort 381,
    382, 386
  maximal oxygen intake 406
  metabolic effects 125–127
  periodization and 527
  personality relationship 382
  pregnancy 537–538
  rating of perceived effort 390
  soccer 907
interactional theory, personality
    assessment 370
interferon-γ, inflammation 801
interleukin-1 (IL-1) 741
interleukin-2 (IL-2), receptor (CD25)
    495
interleukin-6 (IL-6) 739, 800, 805
intermittent claudication 91, 568
intermittent exercise 9–11, 14–15
international competition 653–660
  cardiovascular screening 714–715
  doping 657–658
  immediate preparation 658–659
  medical supervision during
    659–660
  nutrition 654–656
  overtraining 656–657
  preliminary medical screening
    653–654
  preliminary site visit 658
  preparation 654–658
International Conference on
    Overtraining in Sport 486
International Olympic Committee
  banned substances *see* banned
    substances
  standards for medical/athletic
    facilities 658
interval training 11–12, 15
  aerobic 518
  continuous *vs* 391
  elderly 559
  lactate data role 314
  swimming 830
  women 518–519
interventricular septum, thickness
    710
intervertebral disc, loading in hockey
    players 925–926
intestinal ischaemia 112
intracellular signalling, muscle
    337–338
intracerebral haemorrhage 696
intramuscular pressure, arterial
    supply reduction 31, 32
intrasarcomeric system 178
intravascular fluids, decrease in hot
    environment 263, 264
intravenous fluids, hyponatraemia
    misdiagnosis 606
introversion 382, 640
inverted U-hypothesis 214

iontophoresis 787
ion transport, in muscle cells 169
iron
  altitude acclimatization 618
  deficiency 424–425
  intake recommendation 425
  losses 425
  supplements/therapy 415, 656
ischaemia–reperfusion injury,
    Achilles tendon 779
isokinetic ergometer 277–278, 278,
    891
isokinetic training 475
isoleucine, supplements 204
isometric exercise 475
isoprenaline, prohibition 653
Italy, preparticipation screening 672,
    675, 676

jet lag 639, 641–642
  age and gender differences
    641–642
  effects on performance 642–644,
    643, 644
  management *see* circadian rhythm
  symptoms 641, 647
jogging
  injuries in elderly 558–559
  lactate removal 519
joint
  instability 471, 472
  laxity, injury predisposition 471
  malalignments 468–469
  mobility and flexibility training
    475
Jones' fracture 771
joules 5
jumper's knee *see* patellar tendinitis
jumping
  fat mass and performance 349
  patellar tendinitis 784
  repeated overload 461
  stress fractures 768, 771
  stretch–shortening cycle
    contribution 249

K2 COSMED 281
K4b² metabolimeter 282, 283, 284
K4RQ metabolimeter 281, 282, 282,
    283
kayak canoeing *see* canoeing
kayak ergometer 274, 274, 892, 895
ketoacidosis 572
ketoacids 328
ketone bodies, cycling 865
kinematic measures 251
kinetic chain 471–472
kinetic measures 251
knee
  braces 480
  examination 775, 784
  imaging 776

injuries 766
  pain 775, 783
  referred pain 775
  sprains 463
  unstable 480
knee-bend, stretch–shortening cycle
    248
knee ligament, instability 471, 472
Krebs cycle *see* citric acid (Krebs)
    cycle
kyphosis 576

lacrosse 926–927
  demands 926
  fitness 926–927
  maximal oxygen intake 926–927
lactate 314–318
  accumulation 311, 318, 319
    adverse effects 312
    benefits of limitation 312
    decrease by respiratory muscle
      training 63–64
    effect on standard bicarbonate
      321
    factors influencing 312
    as input to perception of effort
      377, 387
    mechanisms 316–317
    in muscle 25, 312
    muscle endurance and 312–313
    patterns during exercise
      315–316
    practical applications 317–318
    see also anaerobic threshold
  blood levels
    accumulation 318, 319
    Australian Rules football 918
    canoeists 891–892, 894
    cycling 861, 864, 866, 869
    factors affecting 316, 317
    during hyperthermic exercise
      111
    implications of data 314
    increase during exercise 111, 316
    maximal oxygen intake
      correlation 313
    maximum levels 25, 311
    measurement 315
    overtraining marker 490, 491
    patterns during exercise
      315–316
    power output relationship 316,
      316
    rowers 840
    rugby football 910–911
    skiing 847
    soccer 905, 905–906, 906–907
    swimming 827, 827–828
    training 318
  buffering, high altitude 616
  conductance from muscles 25,
    25–26

curve, shift 404
implications of data on 314
input to perception of effort 377, 378, 387
intermittent exercise 9, 10, 11
intramuscular levels 316, 335
marathon running 11
maximal steady state 828
measurement methods 314–315
metabolism 25, 317, 335
post-exercise 316
production 335, 377, 387, 521
rating of perceived effort and 498, 498
removal 12, 317, 335
 continuous jogging 519
 gentle exercise after intense exercise 335
 increasing 656
running 312
salivary 315
threshold see anaerobic threshold
tolerance, rugby football 911
transport from muscle to blood 25–26
turning point see anaerobic threshold
ventilation relationship 60
lactate dehydrogenase (LDH) 119
lactation, exercise and 539
lactic acidosis, hyperventilation 54
Laplace, law 71, 711
lateral retinacular release 776–777
lateral retinaculum 774, 775
leanness, extreme, problems 361–362
lean soft tissue (LST), calculation 348
left anterior descending coronary artery 670, 895
left main coronary artery, anomalous 669–670, 676
left ventricle
 dimensions 71, 72, 72
  endurance sports 76–77
  hypertrophic cardiomyopathy 78
  for specific sports 76
  strength training 76, 77
  training effect 76
 ejection time 520
 end-diastolic diameter 710
 end-diastolic volume 683
  canoeists 896
  increased 70–71
 gender-related differences 75–76
 hypertrophy 71, 708
  detection 69
  patterns and haemodynamics 73
  physiological vs pathological 73, 74
  women 76
mass
 ACE gene alleles and 235

canoeists 896
 women 520
 mass index (LVMI) 72
 structure, genetic influence 229
 volume 72–75, 520
  ratio to body surface area 897
  training-induced changes 69
 wall stress/tension 71, 72
 wall thickness 72–75, 709, 710
leg
 length discrepancy 469–470, 769, 775
 raises 776
 stiffness, measures 248
 see also limb blood flow
legal aspects, cardiovascular screening 672
leptin, diurnal rhythm 721, 723
leucine, supplements 204
leucocyte count, overtraining 494–495
leukotrienes 802, 806
 inhibitors 808
life expectancy 68
 cross-country skiers 760, 760, 761
 effect of exercise 747
 endurance athletes 714
 quality-adjusted 714, 748
lifestyle 438
 benefits of regular exercise 760–761
 benefits of training children 512
 effect on biological age 398
 healthy, importance 478
 rugby football 915
ligaments, benefit of exercise 751–752
light exposure, jet lag management 647–649, 648
limb blood flow
 effect of respiratory muscle work 58–59
 'steal effect' of respiratory muscles 57–58, 63
lipids
 blood, benefits of exercise 698–699, 757
 peroxidation, reduction 806–807
 see also fat
lipogenesis 329
lipolytic enzymes 699, 757
lipoprotein(a) 698
lipoproteins, benefits of exercise 698–699
little leaguer's elbow 467
liver
 carbohydrate stores 198
 function, elderly 550
 ischaemia 112
locomotion, energy costs 47–48, 48
locus of control, input to perception of effort 383

longevity, exercise benefit 747
long QT syndrome 670, 677
loperamide 660
low back pain see back pain
low-density lipoprotein (LDL) 698
lower extremity amputees 576–577
lower limb, flexibility 249
lower motor neurones, degeneration 582
Lown–Ganong–Levine syndrome 79
lumbar spine, hyperextension 771
lung
 anatomical dead space 53
 minute volume 22
 size 684
 vital capacity 750
 volume
  canoeists 896
  high altitude 933
  static, effect of training 59–60
 see also entries beginning pulmonary
lung disease 566–571
 chronic 569–570, 750
  exercise rehabilitation 570, 750
 obstructive 750
lung fluid movements 682–687
 exercise-induced changes 683–684, 684
 see also blood volume
lung function 684
 mountaineering 933
 ozone effect 629, 629
 training effect 59–60
luteinizing hormone (LH)
 amenorrhoeic vs eumenorrhoeic athletes 722
 pulsatile secretion 719, 722, 725
  low energy availability disrupting 725, 726
lymphatic drainage 53
lymphocyte(s) 740
 mitogen-induced proliferation 732, 738
 overtraining marker 495
 reduced counts due to cortisol 735, 736
 see also B cells; T cells

McArdle's disease 54, 319
macrocycles 527
Macrodex™ 432, 434
macronutrients 197–207
macrophage 737, 800
 alveolar 737
Mader's two-point test 828
magnesium
 deficiency, sudden death 79
 intravenous therapy 607
magnetic resonance imaging (MRI)
 cardiac 69, 676
  use and misuse 709–710
 plantar fasciitis 787

magnetic resonance imaging
    (*continued*)
    stress fractures 770, 772
major histocompatibility complex
    (MHC), class II antigens 739
malabsorption, high altitude 939
maladaptations, of overtraining 528
malalignments 468–469, 769
malaria 658
malpractice liability 672
maltodextrin/low fructose beverage
    869
marathon runners
    carbohydrate fluid ingestion
        740–741
    children and teenagers 399
    coronary heart disease and 77
    dissociation methods 216
    fatigue 31
    fluid ingestion rules 592
    fluid restriction 591–592
    hypothermia 600
    immune system and infection
        reduction 732
    injuries associated with
        environment 465
    lactate levels 11
    maximal oxygen intake 13
    mood state profiles 212, 212
    perceived effort application
        385–386
    psychological response 213
    serum erythropoietin 429–430
    see also running
marathons
    first-aiders 660
    speeds 815, 816, 816
    see also mass participation events;
        ultra-long distance events
Marfan's syndrome 568–569, 670,
    673, 675
    Achilles tendon injuries 779
massage, deep friction 782
mass participation events 653
    application forms and waiver
        clauses 661
    casualty types 660
    clothing and equipment 663
    conditions for cancellation 662
    detailed planning 661–662
    immediate preparation 662
    initial preparation 660–661
    medical supervision 660–663
    participants' information sheets
        661
    plan of treatment 663
    route planning 661
    withdrawal from 662
    see also marathons
Masters athletes
    high altitude 623
    infection reduction 732

injury prevention 468
medical condition screening 654
smoking cessation 760
maximal accumulated oxygen deficit
    (MAOD), rugby 913
maximal aerobic power 13, 259, 301
    see also maximal oxygen intake
maximal isometric force 161
maximal oxygen intake ($\dot{V}_{O_{2max}}$) 22,
    224, 301–310
    age-related changes 45, 47, 107,
        713–714, 753, 756
    alcohol effect 447
    American footballers 916
    Australian Rules football 919
    benefits of exercise 714, 750
    blood doping to increase 425
    blood lactate correlation 313
    blood volume effect 431–432
    body mass relationship 405
    body size and *see* body size
    carboxyhaemoglobin effect 635,
        636
    cardiovascular responses 12, 12
    children 227, 303, 507, 508
        endurance training effect 509,
            511
    criteria 301–303
    cross-country skiers 400
    cycling 863, 867
    definition 301
    determinants 224
    disabled persons 566
    elderly athletes 552–555, 553
    élite athletes 402
    endurance performance
        relationship 402
    factors affecting 309
    fatigue development 31
    Gaelic football 919
    gender differences in adolescents
        397, 398
    genetic aspects *see* genetic
        determinants
    heritability 225–227, 226, 865
    high altitude effects 55, 295, 295,
        295–296, 617
    hockey 922, 922–923, 923, 924–925
    hot/cold environment effect 259
    hurling and lacrosse 926–927
    input to perception of effort 377
    intensity of endurance training 14
    interindividual differences 309
    intermittent exercise 9
    interval exercise 11–12
    marathon runners 13, 402, 404–405
    measurement 271
        ancillary equipment 305
        blood pressure during 305
        cardiac arrest and 306
        central limitation of effort 301,
            304

conditions for 303
contraindications 306
cycle ergometer 304, 865–866
ergometer choice 304
factors adversely affecting 303
field tests 307, 309
halting, indications 306
preparations 303
principle 301, 302
reproducibility 309
result interpretations 309
safety precautions 306–307
standard errors 307
submaximal tests 307
uses 309
mountaineers 935, 935–936, 938
muscle 87
muscle specific creatine kinase link
    236
overtraining effect 309, 489
ozone effect 631–632
plasma volume expansion effect
    433
pregnancy 533
pre-/post-pubertal differences 510
prolonged exercise 52
respiratory muscle training and 61
rowers 840
rugby 914, 914
running 403, 405, 815, 852
    speed correlations 308
significance 301
skiing *see* skiing
soccer 902–903, 905, 907
swimming *see* swimming
training effects 14, 406
    running 406, 406
    women 522, 524
triathletes 880–882, 881
    fractional utilization 882–884
utilization and economy of
    movement 402–403
values by specific sports 302, 945,
    946
wheelchair athletes 34
women 519–520, 522–524
meal, timing and composition 646
measurement of endurance
    factors 271–272, 272
    laboratory and field 273–286
    sport-specific 273–286
mechanical constraints *see*
    biomechanical constraints
mechanical efficiency 6–7
mechanical power 246–248
    economy and 247–248
    measures 247
    reduction, benefits 247
medial collateral ligament, training
    effect 752
medial tibial stress syndrome 462
medical examination *see* examination

medical facility organization 607–611
  collapse prevention by prerace planning 608–609
  first-aid stations positions 609
  flowchart for management 611
  layout 609, 610
  for mass participation events 662
  medications needed 610, 611
  planning/equiping at race finish 609–611, 610
  prerace 607–608
  rate of admission to 601
  triage 603, 604
medical history, in cardiovascular screening 674, 675
medical records 658–659
medical screening
  hypertension 671
  international competition 653–654
  see also cardiovascular screening
medical surveillance 653–666
  international competition 653–660
  mass participation events 660–663
  wilderness expeditions 663–664
  see also international competition; mass participation events
medications, for medical facilities at races 610, 611
melatonin 639, 647
  levels and temperature effect 640, 647
  secretion 642, 647
  supplements 647
membrane permeability, increased in fatigue 33
memory loss, cerebral hypoxia 623
men (athletes)
  age, body size and physique 38–39
  body composition 352
  body fat, by sport type 354
  body mass distribution 41
  bone mineral density 355, 356, 359
  exercise, benefit on cardiovascular disease 693, 693
  fat-free mass 354–355, 355
  hockey 924–926
  reproductive disorders 723
menarche, average age 399, 514, 720
menstrual cycle
  changes in eumenorrhoeic athletes 720–721
  follicular phase 719
  jet lag severity 642
  length and regularity variations 719–720
  luteal phase shortening 718, 719
  regulation 719–720
  sports injuries relationship 466, 805
menstrual disorders/irregularities 718

adolescents 514, 720
  clinical consequences 718–719
  effect on bone mineral density 361
  hypotheses relating to 723–725
  induction experiments 725
  injuries and 466, 805
  jet lag 642
  prospective experiments 725–727
mental coping strategies 454
mental health model 211–212
mental imagery 215
mental preparation
  for competition 453–454
  to optimize preparation 456
  warm-up exercises 474
mental retardation 584–585
  definition 584
mental skills
  development 455–456
  goal setting 216, 455–456
  used by élite athletes 452
mental strategy training program 388, 454
mental tension, adverse reactions 478
mental training 454–455
meromyosin 160
mesocycles 527
mesomorphy 37, 41, 42, 232
metabolic acidosis 321
  fatigue mechanism 95
  high-intensity exercise 95
  input to perception of effort 378
metabolic control hypothesis 94–95
metabolic disease 571–575, 756–758
metabolic efficiency, perceived effort relationship 378
metabolic power (E_r), long-distance running 815
metabolic rate 409
  input to perception of effort 377
metabolism 118–136
  alcohol effects 446
  heat generation 26
  input to perception of effort 376–378, 391
  muscle see muscle metabolism
  total body 328
metabolites
  conductance 27–28
  muscle blood flow control 94–95
  muscle fatigue 95
metatarsal, stress fractures 771
metatarsal heads 779
metatarsal shafts 770
methacholine 632
methamphetamine (speed) 439
methylene-dioxymethamphetamine (ecstasy) 439
methylxanthines 570
micro-Åstrup apparatus 320
microdialysis technique 343–344

microgravity environment 144
micronutrients 414–415
microstatellites, erythropoietin receptor gene 236
Minnesota Multiphasic Personality Inventory (MMPI) 368
minute ventilation $(\dot{V}_E)$ 53–54, 54
  decreased after training 60, 64
  ozone effect 630, 631
  rowers 841
minute volume 22
'miserable malalignment syndrome' 469
misoprostol 808
mitochondria
  adaptation 123, 167, 935
  damage in fatigue 33
  density in motoneurones 138, 138
  density in muscles after training 13
  high altitudes 935
  intermyofibrillar pool 124
  pools in skeletal muscle 124
  subsarcolemmal pool 124
  transport chain 22
mitochondrial DNA (mtDNA) 237–238
mitochondrial enzymes 87, 332
  increase by training 90
mitogen-activated protein kinases (MAPK) 338
mitogen-induced lymphocyte proliferation 732, 738
mitral regurgitation 710
mitral stenosis 106
mitral valve prolapse 670
mixing-chamber metabolimeter 281
modified discomfort index (MDI) 287
Monge's disease (chronic mountain sickness) 621, 933
monoamine oxidase type B (MAO-B) inhibitors 584
monocytes 735
mood
  disturbances, training association 213
  positive effect of exercise 749, 759
  'profile of mood states' see Profile of Mood States (POMS)
motivation 374
  body temperature effect 419
  decreased, overtraining marker 496
  goal setting 455–456
  maintenance, psychological aspects 453
  poor, in fatigue 33
motoneurones 136–157
  adaptive response 152–153

motoneurones (*continued*)
  changes with training/detraining
      147
  firing frequency 140
  functions and conduction
      velocities 137
  heteronymous 138
  mitochondria density 138, *138*
  modulation of myosin isoforms
      144–145
  muscle fatiguability and 140–142
  muscle fibre type relationship
      139–140, 152
  nucleus and myonuclei
      relationship 142
  overloading effect 147–149
  oxidative enzymes 140
  properties 137–140, 152
  reduced loading effect 149
  spaceflight effect 149, 150–151
  spinal cord 149–151
  succinate dehydrogenase *148*,
      148–149
motor development 759
motor pools 137–140, *139*, 147
motor system, cycling 861, 864
motor units
  fatigue and 140–142, 146
      mechanism 29, *30*
  firing frequencies 140
  gene amplification in 142
  plasticity 146, 147
  properties and metabolism
      137–140
  recruitment 136–137, 140, 153
  training and detraining effects 147
mountain-biking 857
mountaineering 614, 931–941
  acclimatization *932*, 937
  adaptation 931
  blood changes 933–935
  diet 618
  élite climbers 937–939
  environment 931–936
  gas exchange 933
  limitation to exercise 935–936
  maximal oxygen intake *935*,
      935–936, *938*
  nutritional aspects 939
  oxygen partial pressure and 615
  oxygen transport 933
  pulmonary function 933
  respiratory alkalosis treatment 321
  risks 931
  tissue adaptation 935
  training 937–939
  ventilation *932*, 932
  ventilatory response *936*, 936,
      938–939
mountain expeditions 663–664
mountain sickness
  acute 296, 618, 620–621

chronic 621, 933
  prevention 621
mouthpieces, protective 479
movement
  economy of *see* economy of
      movement
  mechanics 245
  velocity, aerobic energy
      relationship 517
mucociliary clearance, reduced 737
multiple sclerosis 581
muscle 158–183, *159–169*
  action potential *see* action
      potentials
  active transport of ions 169
  adaptation 122–124, 167–169,
      178–179, *179*, 475
      chronically stimulated 167–168
      genetic aspects 231–232
      metabolism 120–121, 130–131
      skiing 852, 854
      to stress 475
  agonist/antagonist imbalance
      470
  area, adaptation to training 179
  atrophy, fatigue 146
  biopsy 118, 338, 342–343
  blood flow *see* muscle blood flow
  capillarization 122, 127–129, *128*,
      130, 169
  catabolism, high altitude 939
  chronically stimulated 167–168
  conditioning programme, elderly
      559
  contractile characteristics 130
  contraction 158
      forces 93
      frequency and muscle pump
          effect 97
      increased after warm-up 474
      initiation 28
      maximal velocity 161
      maximum voluntary 93
      myosin heavy/light chain
          isoforms 162–163
      pH effect and perceived effort
          378
      post-tetanic potentiation 163
      sliding filament theory 159
      training effect 168
  contraction–relaxation cycle 93
  cramps 593, 607
  creatine stores 416
  cross-bridges 160–161
      cycling 161, 164
      inhibition in fatigue 29–30
      maximal isometric force 161
  denervation 581, 582
  design and structure 84–91
  discomfort, exercise during heat
      stress 265
  disruptive injury 789

elasticity and need for warm-up
      474
endurance 312–314
  definition 312–313
  training effects 314, 526
  women 526
energy supply and demand 84,
      85–86, 98
excitation–contraction coupling
      169–177, *170*
  adaptation to endurance training
      178–179
  caffeine effect 441
  chronic adaptation effect
      176–177
  failure 176
  repetitive activity 174–176
  sarcolemma and T tubules
      171–172
  sarcoplasmic reticulum 172–173
  T tubule–sarcoplasmic reticulum
      Ca^{2+} 173–174
fatigue 33, 57
  fibre types and 86–87
  input to perception of effort 379
  metabolites involved 95
  motor unit plasticity 146
  motor units and 140–142
  substrate availability aspect 379,
      411
  triathletes 874
force 121, 891
force sharing 180
function in prolonged events 313
glycogen stores *see* glycogen
growth hormone effect 511
heterogeneity 86
hypertrophy 314, 413
injury 470, 792
  overuse 788–789
  prevention by warm-up 474
insulin sensitivity 132–133
isometric contraction 248
lesions, in fatigue 33
mass
  elderly 550, 560
  perceived effort application 386
mechanical properties, training
      effect 169
membrane 169
metabolism *see* muscle metabolism
mitochondria pools 124
myofibrillar proteins and protein
      isoforms 161
nuclei, changes 123–124
overloaded 147–149
oxidative enzyme content 124, 125
oxygen consumption 103, 260
oxygen transport 682
peak blood flow 23
perfusion 97
potassium release 95

recruitment *see* muscle fibre types
regulatory proteins 164–165
response to training, genetic
    aspects 231–232
sensitivity to epinephrine after
    training 130
strain 788, 789
strength
    benefit of exercise 750–751
    improvement 314, 471
    rowing 838–839
    rugby football 912–913
strength imbalance 470
    growth spurts and 466
    injuries 470
    renal failure 571
strength training
    elderly 555
    women 526
stretch, failure 789
temperature, warm-up exercise
    474
training, injury prevention 475
triacylglycerol content in cyclists
    864
vascular resistance 104–105, *105*
volume, oxygen consumption
    303
weakness 178, 179–180, 470, 751
    muscular dystrophy 580
'wisdom' 140
muscle blood flow 26, 84–102, *93*, 263
    capacity (Q_{cap}) 87, *87*, 87–88, *88*
    cardiovascular disease and 91–
        92
    chronic electrical stimulation effect
        121–122
    forearm 97
    hot environments and 111, 263,
        264
    hyperthermic exercise effect
        111–112
    impedance by maximum voluntary
        contraction 93
    implications for endurance sport
        97
    increase to active muscle 93–94
    injury prevention 474
    input to perception of effort 379
    limiting conditions 91–92
    oxidative enzymatic capacity
        relationship 87–89
    oxygen delivery 93
    redistribution effect 104
    regulation 93–98, *94*, *99*
        endothelium-dependent 96–97
        metabolic 94–95
        muscle pump control 93, 97–98
        myogenic control 96
        nitric oxide role 97
    resistance 93–94
    response to exercise 92, *92*–93

skin blood flow competition
    108–109, 110, 263
steady-state 92–93
temperature regulation effect 111
training effect 90–91
muscle-building programmes,
    middle-aged 750–751
muscle cells 159–169, 331–332
    cytoskeletal system 177–178
    see also myofibrillar system
muscle fibre types 85, *85*–86
    adaptation 167–169
    Ca^{2+}-ATPase content 172–173
    calcium ion (pCa)–force
        relationship 164, *165*
    calcium-release channels 173
    canoeists 891
    continuous exercise 13
    cycling 861
    detraining effects 147
    distribution 86–87, 229–231
        men/women 162
    elderly 550
    energy supply and demand 85–86
    fast-twitch 162
        adaptations 167
        cycling 861
        endurance training effect 126
        fatigue 29, 379
        force–velocity characteristics
            163, *163*
        motoneurones 140
        recruitment 318–319
        types IIA and IIB 128, 161
    fast-twitch glycolytic (FG) 85, *85*
        endurance training effect
            128–129
        functions 86
    fast-twitch oxidative glycolytic
        (FOG) 85, *85*, 86
    force–velocity characteristics 163,
        163
    functional properties 85, *85*–86
    functions of specific types 86
    genetic aspects 229–232
    hydrogen ion release 95
    innervation 137–138
    input to perception of effort 379
    modification by endurance
        training 13
    motoneurone relationship
        139–140, 152
    Na^+/K^+ ATPase content and
        isoforms 171, *171*–172
    neural modulation 144–145
    plasticity 136
    recruitment patterns 86, 93, 127
        effects 126–127
        fatigue and 86–87
        training effect 126
        women 521
    rowers 838

rugby players 913
sarcoplasmic reticulum
    characteristics 172–173, *173*
size, endurance training effect 129
skiing 851
slow-twitch (type I) 85, *85*, 86, 162
    endurance training effect 126,
        128–129
    enzymes 126
    fatigue 379
    genetic influence 230–231, *231*
    long-distance cycling 864
    marathon runners 13
    motoneurones 140
    rowers 838
    skiing 13, 851
    in specific sports 7
    succinate dehydrogenase *148*,
        148–149
    training effect 127–129, *128*–129,
        147, 168
    type determination 127
muscle filaments, thick and thin 159,
    159, *160*
muscle metabolism 328–345
    ATP production (from) 334–337
    capacity determination 118–119,
        337
    citric acid cycle 337
    endurance training effects
        122–124, 328
        duration of exercise 125–127
        enzyme changes 122–124
        intensity of exercise 125–127
    energy utilization 330–331
    enzyme-catalysed reactions 330
    enzymes 118
        adaptation 120–121
        profile, genetic influence 231,
            232
        rate-limiting 337
    genetic aspects 231
    impairment in amenorrhoea 719
    intracellular signalling 337–338
    maximal adaptability 120–122
    metabolic pathways 118, 328–330,
        331–334
    methods of study 338–344, *339*
    oxidation–reduction 334
    oxidative enzyme(s) 124, *125*
    oxidative enzyme capacity 85, *85*,
        123
        high altitude 133
        overloading and 147–149
        oxygen exchange capacity linked
            89–90
        training effect 90, 122–124, *123*
    principles 329–330
    rate variations 328
    regulation 328
    training-induced adaptation,
        significance 130–131

muscle pump model 93, 97–98
muscle spindles, innervation 137–138
muscular dystrophy 580–581
muscular fitness
  ACSM recommendations 554
  rugby football 912
musculoskeletal system
  adaptation to stress 475
  benefits of exercise 750–753
  changes in elderly 550–551
  children 513
  injuries in elderly 558–559
  medical screening before competition 653
  problems, screening before competition 654
musculotendinous injuries 470
musculotendinous junction, overload 803
music, input to perception of effort 381
M wave 177
mycolytic therapy 571
myocardial capillary development 711
myocardial contractility 34
  training-induced changes 70, 520
myocardial function, increased 695
myocardial hypertrophy 708
  see also cardiac hypertrophy
myocardial infarction 566–568
  endurance exercise after 688
  exercise training effect 566
  recommendations for training 567–568
  risk at high altitude 622
  risk factors 307
  risk reduced by endurance exercise 694
myocardial ischaemia 566
  cardiac hypertrophy and 710–711
  fatal 712
  high altitudes and 615
  transient 78
myocardial oxygen demand, reduced by exercise 695, 696
myocardial perfusion 711
myocardial work rate 711
myocarditis 656, 670, 670, 750
myocardium
  electrical stability increased by exercise 695
  fatigue 110
  response to catecholamines 548
myocyte, stretch 71, 78
myofibrillar ATPase 127, 170
  assay 340
  failure in repetitive activity 174
myofibrillar proteins
  isoform patterns 129, 166
  plasticity 168

types 161
  see also myosin
myofibrillar system 159–169, 331–332
  chronic adaptations 167–169
  composition 167–169
  contractile proteins 159–164
    see also myosin
  function 165–167
  regulatory proteins 164–165
    see also tropomyosin; troponin
  repetitive activity 165–167
myofibrils, structure 159, 159
myoglobin 9, 618, 945
myonuclei 142, 142
myosin 159, 160
  actin interactions 159–160
  ATPase 160, 164
  eccentric exercise effect 166–167
  filaments 159, 159
  force generation 160–161
  heavy chains 145, 160
    adaptation effect 167
    effects on contractile properties 162–163
    fast-twitch/slow-twitch muscles 162
    isoforms 161, 161–162
    submaximal exercise and 166
    tropomyosin isoform association 165
  isoforms, neural modulation 144–145, 147
  light chains 160
    adaptation effect 167
    effect on force–velocity characteristics 163
    effects on contractile properties 162–163
    heterogeneity 162
    phosphorylation 162, 163
  structure 160

Na^+/K^+ pump 169, 170
  chronic low-frequency stimulation effect 176, 177
  content/isoforms in muscle fibres 171, 171–172
  free radical susceptibility 175
  hormonal regulation 176–177
  increase in skeletal muscle 95
  muscle fibre membrane content 171–172
  role in muscle contraction 177
  sarcolemma and T tubules 169, 171–172
  structure 171
  training effect 176, 179
naproxen 808
nasal patches 911
natural killer (NK) cells 33, 732–733
  activity measurement 732–733

decreased by prolonged exercise 656, 737, 737, 759
  enhancement by exercise 732–733, 734
  as overtraining marker 495, 656
navicular stress fractures 768, 770–771
nedocromil 571
neoplasms
  benefits of exercise 758–759
  risk associated with athletes 758
neoprene, for triathletes 872, 873
neoprene sleeves 481
nerve conduction 29
net efficiency value, definition 6
neuralgia, ilioinguinal 792
neural modulation, myosin isoforms 144–145
neuroendocrine system 184
neuromuscular aspects, in perception of effort 378
neuromuscular disease/conditions 471, 577–578
neuromuscular fatigue 146, 153
neuromuscular junction, physiology of fatigue 29
neurones
  adaptations 136
  dorsal root ganglion 142–144, 151
  dorsospinocerebellar 138
  ionic balance 137
  pseudounipolar 151
  size, succinate dehydrogenase activity and 142, 143
  ventral horn 149–151
  see also motoneurones; sensory neurones
neurosis 382
neurotransmitters 144
neutrophils
  cortisol-induced changes 735, 736
  inflammation 800, 801
  overtraining marker 495–496
  prolonged exercise-induced changes 735, 736
  role 733
  suppressed activity in athletes 733–734
newtons 5
nicotinamide adenine dinucleotide (NAD) 332, 334, 335
nicotinamide adenine dinucleotide phosphate (NADP) 338, 339
nicotine 444–445
  infusion 445
nifedipine 622
night pain 769
night splints 781
nitric oxide 803
  muscle blood flow control 97
  role in inflammation 802–803
  synthesis 97, 803

vasodilatation due to 97
nitric oxide synthase 803
nitrogen
    balance, protein intake and 413
    disposal 414
    negative balance, high altitude 618
nitrogen dioxide 297, 634
Nobel–Robertson model 375, 375
non-steroidal anti-inflammatory
        drugs (NSAIDs) 575, 781, 808
    complications 808
    mechanism of action 803, 808
noradrenaline (norepinephrine) 184,
        185
    age-related response 107
    levels reduced by exercise 696
    overtraining marker 494
    response to endurance exercise
        184, 185
Northern blot 341
nuclear magnetic resonance (NMR),
        muscle 343
nuclei, muscle cells 123–124
nutrient deficiencies, children 513
nutrition
    advice for competition preparation
        654
    central fatigue and 418–419
    children 513–514
    gender differences in requirements
        205–206
    injury prevention 477
    mountaineers 939
    pregnancy 537
    preparation for international
        competition 654–656
    rugby football 915
    strategy 409
    tissue injury and inflammation
        affected 806–807
    women 525–526
    see also diet; foods
nutritional supplements 414–415,
        415–417
    cyclists 869–870, 870
    role on immune system 731, 740

obesity 574–575, 698
    avoidance 756–757
    benefits of exercise 698, 756–757
    injury prevention 574
    training recommendations
        574–575
obturator nerve 792
oedema 622
    see also cerebral oedema;
        pulmonary oedema
oestrogen
    menstrual cycle 719
    replacement therapy 576, 719
    response to exercise 188
    supplementation 514

Ohm's law 22, 88
oligomenorrhoea 361
    see also amenorrhoea
Olympic Games
    1968 (Mexico) 12, 42, 616, 619
    blood doping ban 427
    cross-country skiing 844
    erythropoietin doping ban 430
    Seoul Congress 400
    women participation 517
omeprazole 808
one-leg model 341, 342
'open window' theory 731, 735–740
orienteering 945
orthopaedic conditions 575–577
orthotics, shoe 482
    Achilles tendon injuries 782
    biomechanical goals 482
    injury prevention 482
    leg length discrepancy 469
    malalignment correction 469
    patellofemoral pain syndrome 776
    stress fracture prevention 774
Osgood–Schlatter disease 467, 473
osteitis pubis 793–794
osteoarthritis 468, 575
    after anterior cruciate ligament
        injury 472, 473
    post-traumatic 471
    risk in athletes 751–752
    vitamin E supplements 806
osteopenia 576
osteoporosis 514, 551, 575–576
    effects of exercise training 576
    menstrual disorders causing 718
    postmenopausal 576
    premature 361
    risk after hypoestrogenaemia 514
    spinal cord injuries 579
    training recommendation 576
    treatment 576
ovarian axis see
        hypothalamic–pituitary–ovari
        an (HPO) axis
ovarian follicles 719
overfatigue see overtraining
overhydration 598
overload 147, 710
    musculotendinous junction 803
overpronation 778
overreaching 486, 488, 500
    continuum with training/
        overtraining 501, 501
    see also overtraining
over-the-counter medicines 657
overtraining 4, 656–657, 766
    avoidance 527–528, 742
    child athletes 515
    cold tolerance compromised 294
    continuum with training 501, 501
    definition and terminology
        486–487

diagnosis 656–657
effect on maximum oxygen intake
        309
framework 499–502
immune system impairment
        731–732
incidence 487, 487
infection association 494, 712, 732,
        749–750
monitoring 486–504
mood disturbances 214
need for redefinition 500–501
potential markers 488–499, 489,
        656, 743
    biochemical 491–492
    central fatigue mechanisms 499
    hormonal 492–494, 656
    immunological 494–496, 656
    performance 488–491
    psychological 496–499
preparation for international
        competition 656–657
prevention 501, 657
research 486, 487–488
signs and symptoms 487, 528, 656
swimmers 830
women 527–528
overuse injuries/syndromes
        766–799, 803
    Achilles tendon see Achilles tendon
        overuse injuries
    adductor injuries 792–793
    aetiological mechanism 461,
        803–804
    causes 462, 462
    children/adolescents 462, 466–467
    definition 803
    elderly 468
    epiphyseal 513
    groin pain 791–792
    hamstring injuries 789–791
    incidence 458
    inflammatory response 800, 804
    muscle injuries 788–789
    osteitis pubis 793–794
    patellar tendinitis see patellar
        tendinitis
    patellofemoral pain see
        patellofemoral pain syndrome
        (PFPS)
    plantar fasciitis 785–789
    prevention 579, 766, 807
        rest periods 766–767
    slow progression to prevent 475
    stress fractures see stress fractures
    tennis 463
    triathlons 876, 877
    types 766
    women 466
E-oxidation see fatty acids, oxidation
oxidation–reduction, muscle 334
oxidative burst 733, 737

oxidative enzymes
  adaptation to chronic stimulation 120
  fat metabolism and 131, 132
  glycogen depletion relationship 131
  motoneurones 140
  muscle *see* muscle metabolism
  muscle blood flow and 87–89
  regression of adaptations after training cessation 130
  soccer players 907
  thigh muscle 127
  training effects 122–124, 124, 125, 224
oxidative phosphorylation 137, 153
oxygen
  arteriovenous difference *see* arteriovenous oxygen difference
  consumption
    blood flow relationship 103, 104
    energy costs determination 813
    muscle 103, 260, 303
    'plateau' 301, 302
    splanchnic tissue 103
    swimming 827
    see also oxygen intake
  costs of skiing 851
  costs of ventilation 53–54
  deficit *see* accumulated oxygen deficit (AOD)
  'deficit,' rowers 840
  delivery 93
    oxygen extraction relationship 103–104, 104
  demand
    benefit of exercise 695, 696
    exceeding intake 11
    increased myocardial 653
  desaturation, high altitude 933
  diffusion, high altitude effect 933
  diffusive flux 89, 90–91
  excess post-exercise consumption (EPOC) 574
  exchange capacity 84–91
    blood–muscle 89
    muscle oxidative capacity and 89–90
    training effect 90–91
  haemoglobin affinity at high altitude 934, 934
  kinetics, measurement 282, 283
  maximum consumption *see* maximal oxygen intake ($\dot{V}O_{2max}$)
  myocardial supply/demand 653, 695
  partial pressure 22
    by altitude 932
    arterial 52
    capillary (high altitude) 933, 933

at high altitudes 295, 295, 615–616, 931
  intracellular 96
  radicals 801, 802, 806
  requirements, intermittent exercise 10
  saturation, high altitude and 616, 933, 934
  solubility factor 23, 23
  sources 329
  submaximal cost 47–48, 48, 283
  supply in intermittent exercise 9–10
oxygen dissociation curve 423, 616
  left shift
    by carboxyhaemoglobin 635
    at very high altitude 935
  right shift in altitude acclimatization 618, 935
oxygen intake
  children 509
  heat generation 26
  high altitude effect 12
  intermittent exercise 9
  interval exercise 11
  maximal *see* maximal oxygen intake ($\dot{V}O_{2max}$)
  measurement in swimmers 827
  mountaineers 938
  peak, effect on heat flux 27
  'plateau' 301, 302
  reduction by respiratory muscle unloading 58–59
  rowers 285, 839
  running 11
  skeletal muscle fibre types 85, 85
  skiing 849
  stroke volume relationship 12
  'supramaximal' 311
  swimmers 824, 825
  see also aerobic power
oxygen transport 22–24, 423
  altitude training in women 526–527
  from alveoli to blood 23
  athletic selection 4
  barriers (air to muscle) 23, 23, 24
  benefits of endurance exercise 753
  blood volume role 431–435
  conductance determinants 23, 23–24
  conductance theory 22–24
  driving pressure and 22–23, 24
  effect of training 4
  fatigue development 31
  haemoglobin role 423–431
  maximal 4, 12, 24
  mountaineering 933
  to muscle 682
  performance limitation 55
  rowers 841

rugby football and altitude effect 911
ozone 53, 628–633
  acute inhalation effects 630, 632
  concentrations and effects 629
  effect on maximal oxygen intake 631–632
  endurance performance 629–631, 630
  exercise interactions 628
  at high altitude 623
  interventions 633
  mechanisms of adverse effects 632–633
  pollution 297

pace strategy, perceived effort 387
pace training, women 519, 521
pain
  Achilles tendon 780
  cognitive control strategies 456
  defective recognition and tissue injury 800
  inhibition, dangers 477
  input to perception of effort 379, 380
  knee 775
  night 769
  osteitis pubis 793
  perception 802
  perseverance and psychological aspects 453
  referred, knee 775
  spinal cord injuries 579
  stress fractures 769
  tolerance 217
pain relief
  Achilles tendon injuries 781
  counterproductive effects 800
  mechanisms 803
  patellofemoral pain syndrome 776
pancreas, E cell changes 189
pancreatic enzyme supplements 571
pancreatic hormones 189–190
parallel processing hypothesis 375, 380
paraplegia 578
parasympathetic system 107
paratenon 777
paratenonitis 777–778, 780
  tendinosis with 778, 780, 781–783
  treatment 781–783
Parkinson's disease 584
PARmed-X for Pregnancy 536, 537, 538, 543–545
pars interarticularis, stress fracture 768, 771
patella
  bracing/taping 469, 776
  hypermobile 776
  stabilizing brace 776, 785
  subluxation prevention 480

patella alta 469, 473, 775, 776
patella baja 775, 776
patellar tendinitis 775, 783–785
　aetiology 784
　anatomy and classification
　　783–784
　diagnosis and differential
　　diagnosis 784
　treatment and prevention 785
patellar tendon 783
patellar tracking 774, 775, 776
patellofemoral ligaments 774
patellofemoral pain syndrome (PFPS)
　469, 766, 774–777
　anatomy and aetiology 774–775
　diagnosis/differential diagnosis
　　775
　investigations 776
　treatment/prevention 480,
　　776–777
peak height velocity (PHV) age 397,
　398
perceived effort 33, 374–394
　endurance relationship 385
　intensity inputs 377
　measurement 383–384, 384
　models 375, 375, 380
　physiological inputs 376–380, 387
　　non-specific mediators 379–380
　　peripheral mediators 378–379,
　　　387, 391–392
　　respiratory–metabolic mediators
　　　376–378, 391
　　thresholds 377–378
　practical applications 385–391
　　performance 385–389
　　training 389–391
　psychological inputs 380–384, 388
　　dispositional factors 382–383
　　situtational factors 380–382, 382,
　　　392
　psychophysiological model
　　374–376
　rating see rating of perceived effort
　　(RPE)
perception 374
　of health see health, perceived
performance
　blood volume role 431–435
　body composition and 349–350
　body size consequences 48–50, 49
　cognitive factors 216–217
　deterioration in fatigue 28
　determinants 224, 271, 272, 423,
　　451, 501
　at early age and prediction of
　　success 399
　environmental extremes see specific
　　environmental extremes
　gender differences 523
　genetic determinants see genetic
　　determinants

glucose administration 29
improvement, pulmonary system
　62–64
　respiratory muscle training
　　61–62, 62
jet lag effect 642–644, 643, 644
limitations by pulmonary system
　54–59
mental health model 211–212
overtraining effect 488–491, 490,
　528
ozone exposure affecting 629–631,
　630
peak oxygen deficit and 312
perception of physical effort
　374–394
　applications 385–389
　see also perceived effort
personality and 369–370
pregnancy effects 532, 532–533
psychological aspects 214–215,
　452–453
psychological interventions
　215–216
women and training relationship
　522
see also individual sports
performance-enhancing drugs
　657–658
see also banned substances; doping
perfusion pressure 32
periodization 501, 527
peripheral arterial disease 91, 568
peripheral blood flow, fatigue
　development 34
peripheral limitations of effort 34–35
　see also fatigue, peripheral
peripheral vascular disease 91
　elderly 549
peripheral vascular resistance, in heat
　stroke 604
peritendon 777
personality 217, 366–373
　athletes from different sports
　　369–370
　athletes of different skill levels 370
　athlete vs non-athletes 369
　controversies 366
　definition 366
　iceberg profile 370
　impact on sport 211–212
　implications for practitioners
　　370–371
　input to perception of effort 382
　interactional theory of assessment
　　370
　measurement 366–369
　sports performance and 369–370
　theories 366, 368–369, 370
　traits in endurance athletes 370
Perthes' disease 473
pes cavus-type foot 786

pH
　blood 52, 321, 378
　intracellular, high-intensity
　　exercise 95
　as marker for training intensity
　　389–390
phagocytosis 735, 736, 801
phenotypes 223–224
phenylpropanolamine 442–443
phlebotomy 427
phosphate 21, 166
phosphate-binding agents 572
phosphate compounds, high-energy
　21
phosphocreatine 332, 334
　ATP production in muscle 334
　cycling 861, 863
　intermittent exercise 10–11
　threshold, cycling 863
phosphofructokinase 118
photosynthesis, products 329
phrenic nerve, supramaximal
　stimulation 56
physical activity 3
　minimal and optimal levels 699,
　　700, 747
　see also exercise
Physical Activity Readiness Medical
　Examination for Pregnancy
　536, 537, 538, 543–545
physical fitness see fitness
physicians
　legal aspects of cardiovascular
　　screening 672
　malpractice liability 672
　requirements for wilderness
　　expeditions 664
physiological fatigue see fatigue
physiotherapy, at race finish 611
physique 37–38, 38–40, 346
　genetic influences 232–233
　individual variability 42–43
　see also body size; height
phyto-haemagglutinin, response to
　495, 732, 733
piroxicam 808
pituitary hormones 185–189
placental growth, endurance exercise
　effect 535
placental injury 539
plantar aponeurosis, tear/strain
　785–789
plantar fasciitis 785–789
　aetiology 786
　anatomy 785–786
　diagnosis/differential diagnosis
　　786–787
　investigations 787
　treatment and prevention 787–788
plantaris muscle 147, 777
plasma volume 682
　altitude training in women 527

plasma volume (*continued*)
  decrease 432
    at high altitude 619
    spaceflight 683
  effect on hormone measurements
    191
  increased 432, 682
    at sea-level 620
  response to training, adolescents
    511
  see also blood volume
plasticity
  muscle fibre types 136
  myofibrillar proteins 168
  sensorimotor systems 144
  see also adaptation(s)
Poiseuille's law 94
poliomyelitis, anterior 581–582
polycythaemia, high altitude-
    induced 619
polymerase chain reaction (PCR) 341
polymorphonuclear neutrophils *see*
    neutrophils
polysaccharides, for cyclists 869
polyunsaturated fatty acids (PUFAs)
    807
positron emission tomography (PET)
    343–344
postmenopausal women 468, 576
post-polio syndrome 581–582
post-tetanic potentiation 163
postural hypotension 603
  after exercise 607
  collapse after exercise 594–595
  heat exhaustion and 594
posture
  blood pressure changes in elderly
    549
  hockey players 925
  muscle pump control of blood flow
    97
postviral fatigue syndrome *see*
    chronic fatigue syndrome
potassium
  in fatigue 30, 95
  interstitial 95
  raised levels 550
  regulation 95
  release from muscle 30, 95
  serum levels, elderly 550
potassium spectroscopy 347
power 6, 13
'power strokes' 161, 166
pre-eclampsia 536, 539
pregnancy 531–546
  acid–base balance 532
  aerobic exercise 537
  'anabolic phase' 531
  blood flow and redistribution 535
  carbohydrate metabolism 531
  disorders 536
  duration of exercise 538

effects on performance 532,
    532–533
  effects on response to aerobic
    conditioning 533–534
  fetal response to maternal exercise
    534, 534–535
  gestational diabetes 534, 572–573
  heart and circulation 531–532, 537,
    538
    response to conditioning
      533–534
  heart rate 533, 537, 538
  medical screening 536–537
  nutrition 537
  outcomes 535–536
  physiological effects 531–532
  practical advice 546
  reasons to contact physician 539,
    546
  respiration 532
  response to strenuous exercise 533
  safe limits for conditioning
    536–538
  safety considerations 546
  thermoregulation 532
  training after childbirth 539
  twin 536–537
  unintended due to menstrual
    disorders 718
preload 34, 70, 70
premature labour 536–537, 539
premenstrual syndrome 805
preparticipation screening,
    cardiovascular *see*
    cardiovascular screening
prerace organization 607–608
  collapse reduction 608–609
  mass participation events 660–661
  see also international competition
prerace seminars 608–609
pressure sores, spinal cord injuries
    579
Profile of Mood States (POMS) 212,
    212, 368–369, 370, 371
  identification of 'distress' 497
  overtraining marker 496–497
  rating of perceived effort and
    498–499
progesterone 188
  menstrual cycle 719
  suppression in athletes 718
prolactin 188
pronation 780
  control by shoe orthotics 482
  increased 468, 469, 778
  maximum point 468
  plantar fasciitis 786
proprioceptive training, injury
    prevention 476, 476
prostaglandin E$_1$ analogue 808
prostaglandin E$_2$ 633, 802
prostaglandins 802, 803

prostate cancer 758
prostatitis 792
protective equipment 458, 478,
    478–479
protein 197–207, 203
  catabolism
    cycling 865, 868
    prolonged exercise 203
  as energy source 329, 414
  in fat-free mass 346, 348
  high protein meals, jet lag
    prevention 646
  intake 203–204, 413, 413–414, 414
    cyclists 869, 870, 870
    monitoring in high-risk groups
      203
    recommended 413
  oxidation to energy 414
  requirements 203, 413, 413–414
    women athletes 205
  vegetarian diets 203
proton accumulation 11
  see also hydrogen ions; pH
pseudoephedrine 442–443
psychological aspects 211–221
  benefits of regular exercise
    759–760
  challenges/demands in endurance
    sport 453–454
  chronic pulmonary disease 569
  group (nomothetic) factors 217
  individual (ideographic) factors
    217
  input to perception of effort
    380–384, 388, 392
  mental health model 211–212
  muscular dystrophy 580–581
  pain tolerance 217
  performance 454–455
    characteristics related to
      452–453
    impact on 451–452
    interventions 215–216
    precompetition anxiety 214–215
  'profile of mood states' *see* Profile
    of Mood States (POMS)
  response to endurance training
    212–214
psychological markers, overtraining
    496–499
psychological preparation 451–457
  factors included 452–453
psychological skills training 454–
    455
psychological toughness 8, 21
psychopathology, sport capacity and
    211
psychophysiological model,
    perceived effort 374–376, 375
psychosocial variables
  children 514–515
  input to perception of effort 380

psychotherapy, overtraining
prevention 657
puberty, maximal oxygen intake and
510
pubic rami, stress fracture 794
pulmonary arterial pressure 52–53
high altitude 617, 933
pulmonary blood flow 53
pulmonary blood–gas barrier,
impairment 53
pulmonary diffusing capacity ($\dot{D}$Lco)
53, 59, 682, 683–685, 684
postexercise reduction 682, 684,
684
pulmonary disease see lung disease
pulmonary function see lung function
pulmonary oedema 53, 604
chest X-ray 623
at high altitudes 296, 622
high-permeability type 622
management 622
presentation and risk factors 622
pulmonary vasoconstriction 622
pulse pressure, rowers 840
pygmies, running and energy costs
818
pyruvate 25, 335

quadriceps
fatigue in cycling 34
fibre type distribution 86
strength and injuries 470
strengthening exercises 776
tendonitis 775
wasting 775
quadriceps tendon, pull during
contraction 774
quadriplegia 464, 578, 579
quality-adjusted life expectancy 714,
748
quality of life 714, 748–750, 749
Québec Family Study 233, 234, 238
questionnaires, personality
assessment 367–369

race organizers 661
races (sports)
casualty number prediction
607–608
cool/warm conditions 608
participant screening/qualification
608
planning course 608
plans 453–454
scheduling 608
seminars before 608–609
see also mass participation events
racial aspects see ethnic aspects
racquet sports 945
radiation see ultraviolet radiation
radioactive techniques, muscle
metabolism analysis 341–342

radiography
cardiac hypertrophy 708
neoplasms associated 758
osteitis pubis 794
stress fractures 771–772
rain suits 600
rating of perceived effort (RPE) 374,
376, 377, 378, 392
constant level 386–387
continuous vs interval training 391
disabled persons 565
elderly 559
exercise duration and 389
overtraining marker 498
peripheral arterial disease 568
POMS scale relationship 498–499
pregnancy 538
scale 384, 384
submaximal exercise intensity
390
for training 390, 391, 392, 568
women during sustained distance
training 518
rating scales, personality 367
reactive oxygen species (ROS) 801,
802, 806
see also free radicals
recovery area, for mass participation
events 662
rectal temperature
circadian rhythm 640, 645
collapse 601, 663
heat exhaustion and 593, 594
heatstroke 604
hot environment 289, 290
mass participation events 663
raised 604
emergency management 601,
604
malignant hyperthermia 605
rugby footballers 911
swimmers 266
unconscious patients 603
rectus femoris, injury 788
red blood cells
altitude acclimatization 297, 618,
934
in bronchoalveolar lavage fluid
53
counts 424, 618, 934
erythropoietin role 428
mass 682
testosterone effect 511
volume expansion, high altitude
297
redox reactions 334
'reducers,' input to perception of
effort 382–383
refrigerator facility 610
regattas 836–837
regulatory proteins 164–165
see also tropomyosin; troponin

rehabilitation, chronic pulmonary
disease 570, 750
rehydration, rugby footballers 911
reinjury 470
renal blood flow
elderly 549–550
reduced during exercise 599
renal failure 32, 571–572, 606
NSAIDs causing 808
transient 599
renal function, elderly 549–550
renal vasoconstriction 105, 106
renin–angiotensin–aldosterone
system 190, 550
repetitive activity
Ca^{2+}-release channel 175
cytoskeletal proteins in muscle 178
excitation–contraction coupling
174–176
myofibrillar proteins 165–167
Na^+/K^+ pump changes 174, 175
reproductive changes 718–730
females see menstrual cycle;
menstrual disorders
males 723
resistance training 526
ACSM recommendations 554
adaptations 168
fast-velocity and slow-velocity 526
fat-free mass 555
post-polio syndrome 582
women 526
respiration see breathing; ventilation
respiratory acidosis, compensated
321
respiratory alkalaemia 932
respiratory alkalosis 321, 532
respiratory chain 332, 335, 337
ATP production 334
enzymes 119
function and structure 337
respiratory discomfort, air pollution
628
respiratory exchange ratio (RER) 533
respiratory infections, management
659
respiratory muscles 52
accessory 54
endurance increase 63
exercise stress and maximum
blood flow 60
expiratory 57, 63
fatigue 56–57, 57, 61
reduction by training 63
fibre hypertrophy 62–63
increased activity in exercise 53
loading/unloading effects 58, 63
performance limitation 57–59
prolonged exercise 53, 56
recruitment 57
steal of locomotor muscle
perfusion 57–59, 63

respiratory muscles (*continued*)
   training *see* respiratory muscle
      training (RMT)
   work 56, 63
      cardiovascular consequences
         57–58
respiratory muscle training (RMT)
      60, 61–62, 62
   adaptations due to 62–64
respiratory quotient (RQ) 24, 338,
      813, 830
respiratory rate (f_B), input to
      perception of effort 376
respiratory system 52–67
   adaptations by training 59, 61–64
   alcohol effects 446
   benefits of exercise 750
   endurance training effect 59–61
   failure and performance
      limitations 52, 54–59
   function 52
   improvement of performance
      62–64
   input to perception of effort
      376–378, 391
   respiratory muscle training 61–62
   response to exercise 52–54
respiratory therapists 570
rest periods, importance 766–767
restricted fragment length
      polymorphism (RFLP) 237
retinal haemorrhage 621, 622
retinal oedema 622
rhabdomyolysis 597
rheumatic disorders 779
rheumatoid arthritis 575, 752
right ventricular dysplasia 670, 676
right ventricular hypertrophy 69
risk, sports and sudden death 671
roller-skiing training 854
Rorschach test 367
rowing and rowers 836–843
   ACE gene alleles 235
   aerobic metabolism 839–840
   age, body size and physique 38, 40
   altitude training 841–842
   anaerobic metabolism 840
   biomechanics 838
   blood lactate 840
   blood pressure 840, 841
   boat weights and type 836, 837
   body fat 352–353
   body mass 43
   central venous pressure 840–841,
      841
   cerebral oxygenation 841, 842
   circulation and cardiac output 836,
      840–841
   competitions 836
      duration 837–838
   coxswain 836
   distance and speed improvement

      837
   drag force 838, 838
   energy costs 839
      per unit of body mass 250
   ergometers 275, 275–276, 276
   health problems 836
   immune system changes 732,
      734
   maximal oxygen intake 840
   muscle strength 838–839
   oxygen intake measurement 285
   oxygen transport 841
   regattas 836–837
   sculling 836
   sweep rowing 836
   training 842
      15:15 training method 831
   ventilation 841
   weight categories and gender
      837–838
   work components 246, 246
'rowing strength' 838
rugby football 909–915
   aerobic measures 914
   altitude training 911
   anaerobic threshold 914
   anthropometry 912
   blood lactate 910–911
   body mass 912
   dehydration and body temperature
      911
   demands of specific position 909,
      912
   diet and nutrition 915
   distance covered in game 910
   energy expenditure 911
   environmental factors 911
   field tests 913
   fitness 912–915
   heart rate 914
   historical aspects 909–910
   injuries 911
   lifestyle 915
   low-intensity/high-intensity
      activity 910
   MAOD test 913
   maximal oxygen intake 914, 914
   muscle fibre types 913
   muscle glycogen 911
   muscle strength and endurance
      912–913
   training 915
   women 909–910
   work rate 910–911, 911–912
Rugby League 912
Rugby Union 909, 912, 913
   work rate 910–911
rules
   ineffective and injuries due to 464
   for sport in environmental
      conditions 465
'runner's high' 749, 759

'runner's trots' 662, 758
running and runners 9, 813–823
   association and dissociation
      methods 216, 454
   blood flow to legs 7, 34
   body fat 349, 352
   body size and 39, 40, 42, 43,
      817–819
   cardiac parameters, track *vs*
      treadmill 281
   cortisol levels, perception of effort
      380
   cross-country, rating of perceived
      effort 390
   decreased atmospheric density
      615
   dehydration in triathlon 874
   distance, age, body size and
      physique 39, 40
   economy 247, 402–403, 407
      hill training 403, 407, 407
      lower limb flexibility 249
      maximum oxygen intake *vs* 403,
         405
      performance relationship 524
      speed and 250
      training effects 406–407
   elderly 560
   endurance conditioning 402–408
   energetics 813–823
      bottleneck affecting (equation)
         815, 817
      long-distance running 815–
         817
      middle-distance 819–822
      treadmill 813
   energy costs (C_r) 281, 517, 813–817,
      814
      accleration from start 821
      body mass relationship 250,
         817–818
      ground contact time 285
      increase with distance 817
      interindividual variability 813
      long-distance running 815–817
      track *vs* treadmill 281
   energy expenditure 814, 815
   energy intake 410, 410
   fat mass and performance 349
   fluid ingestion 597
   genetic determinants 227
   gravity effect 614
   heatstroke, management 604
   hill training 403, 407, 407
   hypothermia 599–600
   imagery use 215–216
   injuries 462, 468, 469, 482, 766
   lactate levels and 312
   left ventricle dimensions 76
   limitation by central *vs* peripheral
      factors 34–35
   malalignment injuries 468, 469

marathon *see* marathon runners
maximal aerobic speed 818, 819
maximal metabolic power (E_{max}) 815
maximal oxygen intake 11, 815, 852
    training effect 406, *406*
mechanical power and economy 247
metabolic power (E_r) 815
metabolic rate 409
middle-distance 819–822
    theoretical *vs* best times 821, *821*
mileage link to injury 805
'miserable malalignment syndrome' 469
muscle fibre recruitment patterns 127
oestradiol level prediction by energy balance 724
overuse injuries 766
pace strategy 387
performance and body size 817–819
physiological variable affecting performance 402–404, *404*
pregnancy 537
repeated overload 461
shielding from air resistance 254
shoes 481
speed 250, 815, *816*, 816
    maximal oxygen intake correlation 308
    protection against hypothermia 600
strength training in elderly 559–560
stress fractures 768, 770
stretch–shortening cycle contribution 248, *249*
submaximal oxygen cost 47–48, *48*
sudden deaths 670
technique assessment (video) 770
training errors 462
triathlon 874, 883
velocity (V_{La4}) 403–404
visual impairment and 586
warm-up exercises 474
wind speed/direction effect 253
work and energy expenditure 248
work components 246, *246*
see also marathon runners
ryanodine receptor 597

sacroiliac joint, dysfunction 472, 793
sarcolemma 169, 171–172
sarcomeres, structure 159, *159*–160
sarcoplasmic reticulum 169–170, 172–173
    Ca^{2+}-ATPase 172–173
    characteristics 172–173, *173*
    function 172

repetitive activity effect 175–176
T tubule–Ca^{2+} channel interface 173–174
T tubule coupling failure 176
satisfaction, in athletes 749
scaffold proteins 179–180
scaling and scaling factors 43–50
    allometry applications 44–45
    for body size 43–44, 48–50
    children/adolescents 48, *49*
    $\dot{V}O_{2max}$ 45, 45–47, *46*, *47*
    $\dot{V}O_{2submax}$ 47–48, *48*, *49*
    definition 43
    historical background 44–45
    isometric 44
    non-isometric (allometric) 44, 50
    principles 44–45
scars 472
school athletes, cardiovascular screening 671, 672–673
Schwinn Air-Dyne 577, 578
scientific stretching for sport (3S system) 476
screening *see* medical screening
sculling 836
SDS-PAGE 340–341
sedatives 646–647
Seldinger technique 341
selenium 806–807
self-efficacy, input to perception of effort 383
self-esteem 757, 759
self-presentation theory 380–381
Selye's stress reaction 32
sensation 374
sensorimotor systems 153
    adaptive response 152–153
    overloading 147–149
    plasticity 144
    reducing loading 144, 146, 149, 151
    see also motoneurones; sensory neurones
Sensor-Medics metabolic cart 305
sensory disorders 584–586
sensory neurones 136–157
    dorsal root ganglion 142–144
    morphological/physiological properties 151
    overloading effect 147–149
    reduced loading (spaceflight) effect 151–152
    soma size and enzyme activities 142–144, *143*
septal hypertrophy 710, 712
serotonin (5-hydroxytryptamine) 205
    agonists 499
    branched-chain amino acids effect 655
    elevated 205
    melatonin synthesis from 639
    overtraining marker 499

receptor 499
    role in central fatigue 419
serotoninergic challenge, response 499
serotonin uptake inhibitors 574
sesamoids, stress fractures 771
sex hormone(s) 188, 805
sex hormone-binding globulin, overtraining marker 493
sexual maturation, children 514
shielding, economy of movement and 254
shinty 926
shivering 28–29, 260
shock absorption, by shoes 481
shoe orthotics *see* orthotics
shoes *see* footwear
shoulder, tennis 467, *467*
shoulder pads 479
shuttle run test 913
sickle cell disease 623
Siggard–Andersen nomogram 321
sign language systems 586
sinoatrial node 107
Siri equation 347, 349
SI system of units 5, 6
site visit, preliminary, for international competition 658
skating 847
    classic skiing comparison 847, 849
    shielding from air resistance 254
    work components 246, *246*
skeletal muscle *see* muscle
skeletal muscle-specific creatine kinase *see* creatine kinase
skiing and skiers
    adaptation to training 854
    aerobic metabolism 846
    age, body size and physique 39, *40*
    anaerobic metabolism 847
    blood lactate 847
    body fat 353
    body mass 850, *850*
    body position 849
    classic technique 846, 847, *848*, 849
        skating comparison 847, 849
    cold injury 855
    competitions 844–846
    cross-country 844–857
    distance–velocity relationships 846
    double pole techniques 847, *848*, 849–850
    economy of movement 251
    élite skiers, characteristics 850–852
    energy yield 846–847
    ergometers 276, *277*
    freestyle technique 847, *848*
    heart rate 849
    heat balance 855
    improvement of endurance 844, 845

skiing and skiers (*continued*)
  injuries 463
  lifespan 760, *760, 761*
  maximal oxygen intake 400, 847, 850, 851, 852
  muscle adaptation 852, 854
  muscle fibres 851
  oxygen costs 851
  oxygen intake 849
  performance 846
    prediction 852, 853
  race types 844
  racing course and terrain 844–845, 849
  racing styles 846, 847–850, 854
  roller-skiing training 854
  slow-twitch muscle fibres 13
  speeds in championships 844, *845*
  stretch–shortening cycle 248
  sweating 855
  training 852–855
    amounts 854, *854*
    poling techniques 854, 855
    types and benefits 852, 854
  velocity decrease with distance (males) 846
  viscous work 5–6
  work components 246, *246*
skin
  atrophy 807
  blood flow *see* cutaneous blood flow
  cancer 758
  thermal gradient and heat transfer 27
  water vapour pressure 261
ski-walking 854
sleep
  adequacy 742
  deprivation, jet lag 646
  EEG 646
  loss, effects 642, *643*
  partial deprivation 642
sleep–wake cycle 639, 642, 644
sliding filament theory 159
slow-twitch muscle fibres *see* muscle fibre types
smoking 444–445
  adverse effects 445
  body mass 757
  carboxyhaemoglobin levels 635
  cessation 760
  nicotine effects 444–445
  respiratory diseases 750
smooth muscle, vascular, relaxation 94, 95, 96
soccer 900–930, 908, *909*, 945
  anaerobic threshold 902–903
  backwards/sideways movements 907
  blood lactate 905, 905–906, 906–907

categories of activity 901, *902*
clothing 905
dietary practices 908
distance covered per game 901, *901, 903*
dribbling ball, physiological responses 906, *906*
early selection 399
energy expenditure 903, 906, 907
  training 908, 908, *909*
environmental conditions 904–905
fatigue 903–905
fitness measures 907
goalkeeper 902
goal scoring 904
groin pain 791
heart rate 905, 908
immune system 908–909
low-intensity/high-intensity exercise 902
maximal oxygen intake 902–903, 905, 907
mental fatigue 904
metabolic data 282
metabolic loading 905
oxidative enzymes 907
physiological demands/responses 900–909
  game-related activities 906–907
  match-play 905–906
  roles of individual players 902
  training and habitual activities 907–909, *908*
    intensity 907
    tapering off phase 908
  work-rates
    factors affecting 902–903
    profiles 900–902
social competence, training of children and 515
society, costs of injuries 458
sodium
  addition to drinks 420, 421
  high sodium solutions 606
  imbalance, heat cramps and 593
  renal loss 190
  retention 190
  see also hyponatraemia
sodium cromolyn 571
sodium pump *see* Na⁺/K⁺ pump
softball, area equipment 463–464
soleus muscle 777
somatotype 37–38, *38–40*, 41, 232, 233
Southern blot 341
soybeans 203
spaceflight 144, 146, 149, 151
  plasma volume reduction 683
spasticity, amyotrophic lateral sclerosis 582
speed 247
  stride length and cadence 250–251
spinal cord injury 147, 578–579

spinal fractures 718
spinal motoneurones 149–151
  lack of adaptation 150
splanchnic circulation 103, *106*
  elderly 548
  reduction in exercise 104–105, 106, 107, 112
splenic rupture 623
splints, plantar fasciitis 787
spondylolisthesis 467
spondylolysis 771
spondylosis 467
sports, classification 7
'sports anaemia' 190, 424–425
sports drinks
  carbohydrate 200, 201
  exercise-associated collapse 607
  see also carbohydrate beverages
sports hernia 794–796
sports injury *see* injury, sports
sports psychologists 370–371
sports surfaces
  injury prevention 462–463
  overuse injuries 769, 774, 778, 784
sportswear *see* clothing
sprinting 902, 918
squash, sudden cardiac death 79
3S system 476
stabilization, spinal cord injuries 579
staleness 4, 32, 214
  overtraining marker 497
standard international (SI) units 5, 6
Starling effect 520, 548, 683
state–trait controversy 366, 368–369, 370
statistical methods 44
statistical modelling, maximal oxygen intake 226
stature
  children and adolescents 41, 42
  for specific sports *38–40*
  see also body size; height
'steal effect,' of respiratory muscles 57–59, 63
steroids
  Achilles tendon injuries 779
  anabolic *see* anabolic–androgenic steroids (AAS)
  replacement therapy 719
  see also corticosteroids; hormones
Stevens' power law 374
stiffness, morning 786
stimulants
  adverse effects and injury 477
  banned 439
  caffeine 441
  ephedrine 442–443
  jet lag management 647
  see also amphetamine
stimulus intensity, input to perception of effort 382–383
strength, definition 7–8

strength athletes, left ventricle
    dimensions 76, 77
strength events 7
strength training
    elderly 559–560
    negative effect on flexibility 475
    osteoporosis 576
stress
    exercise, menstrual disorders 723,
        724–725
    musculoskeletal adaptation 475
    reduction by exercise 573
    responses 184
    training, effect on mood 213, 214
stress (force), definition 768
stress fractures 753, 767–774, 794
    aetiology 466, 768–769
    anatomy 769
    at-risk 770–771, 773, 774
    children 513
    definition 767
    diagnosis and examination 466,
        769–770
    differential diagnosis 771
    incidence 767–768
    investigation 771–772
    prevention 773–774
    risk factors 466, 773
    sites 767, 768
    treatment 773
stress hormones 184, 185
    immune system and 735, 740
    see also cortisol
stress hypothesis, menstrual
        disorders 723, 724–725
stretchers 609
stretching
    Achilles tendon injury treatment
        781
    adductor longus injury treatment
        793
    in cool down period 474–475
    dynamic and static 476
    flexibility training 476
    hamstring and calf 776
    pre-exercise, hamstring injury
        prevention 791
stretch–shortening cycle 248–250
    contributions, source 248–249
    flexibility effect 471
    muscle training to prevent injury
        475
    running and jumping 249
    training and flexibility 249–250
stride length, speed and cadence
        250–251
stroke (cerebrovascular) 577–578, 578
    aetiology and risk factors 696
    mortality reduced by exercise 697
    risk reduction by exercise 696–698
stroke volume
    children 510, 511, 513

decrease, exercise in hot
    environment 263
high altitude 617
increase with cardiac hypertrophy
    713
maximal aerobic power definition
    259
maximum 12
pregnancy 531–532, 533, 534
triathlon 873
women 519, 520
substrate availability
    input to perception of effort 379,
        387
    see also carbohydrate(s); fatty acids
succinate dehydrogenase 119, 127,
        129
    dorsal root ganglion 142, 143,
        151–152
    motoneurones and muscle fibres
        148, 148–149
    swimming training interruption
        831
    ventral horn neurones 149
sudden cardiac death 69, 77–80,
        667–681
    cardiomyopathy see hypertrophic
        cardiomyopathy (HCM)
    causes 668, 668–671, 708, 711–712
    disorders predisposing 653
    exercise-related 77–78, 711–712
    myocardial infarction, reduced by
        exercise 694
    non-exercise-related 78
    potential triggers 79–80
    prevalence and scope 78, 668, 671
    race and gender aspects 677–678,
        678
    screening see cardiovascular
        screening
    ventricular hypertrophy and 710
    young athletes 654, 667–681
sudden deaths 667, 671
    erythropoietin use 429
    non-cardiac 670
sudden exercise, sudden death 79, 80
sulphur dioxide 297, 634–635
Super Bowl 915
'supramaximal' effort 311
supraspinal input, motor units
        recruitment 136–137
surface friction 246, 246
surgery, tendon injuries 782,
        790–791, 793
sustained distance training, women
        518
sweat, evaporation 260–261
sweat glands 261
sweating 261
    cold environments 294
    pregnancy 532
    rates 419

skiers 855
threshold temperature for 108
sweat-suits, hyperthermia from 917
swimming and swimmers 824–835
    aerobic metabolism 824, 825
    aerobic power due to workouts
        824
    aerodynamic clothing 253
    age, body size and physique 38,
        39, 40, 42
    anaerobic events 824
    anaerobic metabolism 824, 825
    as 'arm and upper body sport' 825
    benefits in asthma 750
    blood lactate 827, 827–828
        performance profile 828, 829,
            830, 832
    body fat 292–293, 293, 353
    body weight in water and 826
    channel swimmers 266, 600
    cold stress 265–266
    critical swim speed 828–829
    detraining and inactivity 831
    drag forces 253
    economy 824, 884
    endurance testing 826–829
    endurance training 830
        15:15 training method 831
        aerobic exercise 824
        controlled-intensity 830
        effectiveness assessment 833
        fast-speed 831
        glycogen depletion 830
        interval approach 830
        low-speed 830, 831
        patterns for Soviet swimmers
            833, 833
        risks 830–831
        tapering phase 828, 831–832
        whole stroke 830
    energy balance, negative 830–831
    energy costs per unit of body mass
        250
    fat mass 350
    heart rate 826–827, 827
    heat conductance 27
    heat transfer coefficient 265
    hypothermia 600
    long-distance, training 830
    lower extremity amputees 577
    maximal oxygen intake 824, 825,
        826
        land and hydrostatic weight
            comparison 826, 826
    mechanical power and economy
        247
    medals for East Germany 400, 400
    net efficiency 6
    neuromuscular problems 831
    overtraining 487, 497, 830
    oxygen consumption 827
    performance 829–830

swimming and swimmers (*continued*)
  periodization and 527
  pregnancy 537
  psychological response 213, *213*
  tissue insulation in cold water
      292–293, *293*
  triathlon 829, 872–873, *874*, 884
  twin, trained 271, *273*
  work and energy expenditure 248
swimming flumes 277, *277*
sympathetic system 107, 190, 683
sympathoadrenal hormones 184–185
sympathomimetics 442–443, 570, 574
syncope 654
  see also heat exhaustion (syncope)
systemic vascular resistance 94
systolic blood pressure
  canoeists 896
  elderly 549
  'heat exhaustion' and 594
systolic function 70, 75
systolic phase, duration 711

table tennis 945
tachycardia 320, 594
tachypnoea 64, 633
tachypnoeic drift 54
talent, identification and
      development 400
tape, medical 481
task aversion 33, 374
task failure 158, 166–167
T cells 732
  helper to suppressor ratio 656
  mitogen-induced proliferative
      response 732, 738
  overtraining marker 495, 656
  proliferation, overtraining 495, 496
team sports 9, 669
telemetry 281
temazepam 646
temperature, body
  changes during exercise 262, *263*
  circadian rhythm 640, *640*, 644
  core 26, 32
    see also rectal temperature
  effect on motivation 419
  fatigue relationship 32, 111, 419
  gradient during early exercise 260
  heart rate relationship 110
  heatstroke 595
  increases 108, 660
  in infections 660
  input to perception of effort 379,
      380
  low, fatigue 32
  melatonin level changes 640, 647
  muscle, warm-up exercise 474
  oral, avoidance 663
  pregnancy 532
  rectal *see* rectal temperature
  regulation *see* thermoregulation

skin 26
skin blood flow relationship
      107–108, *108*
  steady-state 262
  upper limits 108, *109*
temperature, environmental 259–
      267
  drop with altitude 615
  hypothermia due to 600
  intolerance by elderly 548
  wet bulb globe temperature
      (WBGT) 287
  see also cold environment; hot
      environment
tendinitis 778, 780
  see also patellar tendinitis
tendinosis 778, 780
  paratenonitis with 778, 780,
      781–783
tendon
  benefit of exercise 751–752
  failure 778
  injuries 779, 805
    classification 777–778
  rupture, corticosteroid injections
      809
  strains, elderly athletes 468
  structure 777
  see also Achilles tendon
tennis 945
  early specialization 399
  elderly 468
  overuse injuries 463
  racquet size/stringing and 463
tennis elbow 463, 480
tennis shoulder 467
testosterone
  actions 511
  analogues 443–444
  cortisol ratio 493, 656
  free 492, 493
  levels at puberty 511
  overtraining marker 492, 493
  reduced levels in athletes 723
  response to exercise 188
  as skeletal muscle pump 511
tetraplegia 578
theatre-goer's sign 775
thermal conductivity 27, 43
thermal gradient, skin to air 27
thermal pants 791
thermal sensors 262
thermodilution 341
thermodynamics 21, 88
thermogenesis 7, 26, 108, 260
  shivering 260
thermography 772
thermoregulation 107–108, 259–262,
      596
  body surface area and 43
  children 514
  control 262

endurance exercise influence 110,
      112, 293
  during exercise 262
  exercise in obesity 575
  hot environments 262, 288
  hyperhydration effects 290
  influence on endurance exercise
      110–111
  pregnancy 532
  'set point' 110
  triathlon 872–873
  variations 108
  water immersion 292
thermoregulatory centre 262
Thompson's squeeze test 781
throwing, fat-free mass and
      performance 350
thyroid hormones 187, 719, 723
thyroxine (T$_4$) 187
tibia
  anterior cortical fracture ('dreaded
      black line') 770
  internal rotation 468, 778
  stress fracture 768, 770
tidal volume 53
time zones 639–650
  adjustment and effect of direction
      645
  body temperature 645
  jet lag adverse effects 643–644
  light/dark adjustments 648
  sleeping difficulty after crossing
      642
  see also circadian rhythm; jet lag
tiredness 32
  overtraining marker 499
  see also fatigue
tissue adaptation, mountaineering
      935
tissue injury, exercise-induced
  causes 803–804
  factors influencing 804–807
  nutritional influences 806–807
  prevention and treatment 807–809
  process/reaction 801
  training form and status affecting
      804–805
  see also inflammation
toilet facilities 609, 662
  wheelchair athletes 662
total aerobic running capacity 403
total body mechanical power 246
total body water (TBW) 347
total lung capacity (TLC) 629
Tour de France
  drug use 439
  energy expenditure 655
  erythropoietin and 431
  free fatty acids administration 655
  training 860
tracer techniques 341–342
training 438

ACSM recommendations 554
acute fatigue 501
adaptation *see* adaptation(s)
after childbirth 539
American football 916–917
anaerobic metabolism response
312
Australian Rules football 919
children *see* children
cold stress strategy 293–294
continuous *vs* interval 391
continuum with overtraining 501,
501
contraindications
aneurysms 568–569
diabetics 573
elderly 551
diet *see* diet
diffusive oxygen flux response
90–91
disabled persons *see* disability,
persons with
discontinuation, regression of
adaptations after 130
'distress' signs 487
duration *see* duration of
exercise/training
effect on athletes 405–406
elderly 552–555, *554*
E-endorphin response 189
enzyme adaptation induction
mechanisms 131–133
errors 462, *462*, 766–767
Achilles tendon injuries 778
patellar tendinitis 784
plantar fasciitis 786
tissue injury and inflammation
804–805
see also individual overuse injuries
erythropoietin response 429–430
excitation–contraction coupling
178–179
Gaelic football 919
glucagon response 190
glycolytic enzymes after 127–129
goal 518
growth hormone response
187–188
heart rate recommendation 14
heterogeneity in response 227, *229*,
238
high altitude 12, 296–297, 321–322
high-intensity 180, 231, 232
high resistance 168, 179
hill 403, 407, *407*
hockey 925, 926
imbalance *see* overtraining
injury prevention *see* injury
prevention
insulin response 190
intensity *see* intensity of
exercise/training

interval *see* interval training
lung volumes 59–60
markers, running velocity ($\dot{V}_{La4}$)
403–404
maximal oxygen intake response
14, 227–228, 406, *406*
menarche timing and 399
mitochondrial enzymes increase
90
mood disturbances 213–214
motivation maintenance 453
motor unit changes 147
mountaineering 937–939
muscle adaptation *see* muscle,
adaptation
muscle capillarization 122,
127–129, *128*, *130*
muscle contractile characteristics
130
muscle fibre types 127–129, 147,
168
muscle sensitivity to epinephrine
130
muscle triglycerides 201
for muscular endurance 314
myofibrillar function/composition
changes 167–169
myofibrillary plasticity 168
Na^+/K^+ pump increase 176, 179
need for recovery period after 501
objectives 767
optimal balance 486
optimum programmes 405–406
pace, women 519, 521
perception of physical effort 33,
374–394
applications 389–391
see also perceived effort
periodization 501, 527
phases 767
physiological effects 406–408
pituitary–adrenal activation 186
prerace advice to athletes 608–
609
psychological response 212–214
pulmonary system response 59–61
regional blood flow capacity
response 90–91
regression of adaptation after
discontinuation 130
respiratory muscles response 60
rowers 842
rugby football 915
skiing 852–855
soccer 907–909
sport-specific, for injury
prevention 476–477
stress hormone response 185
stretch–shortening cycle and
249–250
tempo (pace) 518
thyroid hormone response 187

tissue injury and inflammation
804–805
total aerobic running capacity and
403
ventricular performance response
69–70
women *see* women
see also individual sports
training cycle 767
training surfaces, overuse injuries
769, 774, 778, 784
tranquillizers, minor 646
transdiaphragmatic pressure 57
transforming growth factor (TGF) 71
transmural pressure, muscle blood
flow control 96
transport chain 22
transversalis fascia, weakness 794
trauma *see* injury, sports
travel fatigue 639
traveller's diarrhoea 659
treadmill 274
energy costs 813
external/internal locus of control
383
graded exercise test, disabled
persons 565
maximal oxygen intake 12, 304
in wind tunnel 279
triacylglycerol *see* triglycerides
triage 602, 604
mass participation events 663
triathlon and triathletes 872–887
acute effects of sequential exercise
874–875
aerobic power 880–882, *881*, *882*
air resistance 878–879
anaerobic threshold 883
back pain 877
body composition 879–880
body mass 878, 879, *879*
cardiac output 873
characteristics of triathletes
877–885
physical 877–880
physiological 880–885
cycling 857, 858, 873, 874, 885
dehydration 873–874
demands 872–875
economy of movement 875,
884–885
fatigue 874, 875
fractional utilization of $\dot{V}O_{2max}$
882–884
'heavy-weight' 880
height 877–878, *878*
hyponatraemia 874
injury sites 876–877
Ironman 872, 875–876
lactate threshold and performance
525
mixed ability 881

triathlon and triathletes (*continued*)
  muscle fatigue 874
  overuse injuries 876, 877
  performance, training effect 875–876
  running 874, 883
  stroke volume 873
  swimming 829, 872–873, 874, 884
  swimsuits *vs* wetsuits 872–873
  thermoregulation 872–873
  training 875–877
    BRICK 874
    rating of perceived effort 390
  training and performance in women 522
  wetsuit 872–873, 885
tricarboxylic acid cycle *see* citric acid (Krebs) cycle
triceps surae 777, 781
'trigger hypothesis' 510
triglycerides
  content of muscle, cyclists 864
  medium-chain (MCTs) 202
  metabolism/metabolites 28, 312
  reduction by exercise 698–699
  stores 201
trochanteric bursitis 462
tropomyosin 160, 164, 165
  structure and isoforms 164–165
troponin 160, 164
troponin C 164
troponin I 164, 669
troponin T 164
tryptophan
  branched chain amino acid relationship 499
  circadian rhythm adjustment 646
  transport 205
T tubules
  excitation–contraction coupling 170
  Na⁺/K⁺ pump 169, 171–172
    Na^+/K^+ pump 169, 171–172
  sarcoplasmic reticulum Ca^{2+} channel interface 173–174
  sarcoplasmic reticulum coupling failure 176
  terminal cisternae 172
'tube breathing' 322, 620
tumour necrosis factor-Δ (TNF-Δ) 738–739, 801
tuning fork test 769–770
turbulence, high altitude and 615
'turf toe' injury 771
twin studies
  maximal oxygen intake 225–227, 226
  response to training 227–228, 229
  swimmers and training effect 271, 273
tyrosine, circadian rhythm 646

ultra-long distance events

emergency therapy of collapse 602
glycogen depletion and metabolism 313
muscle function 313
nutritional supplements 740
performance 7
plasma volume expansion for 432–433
ultrasound
  Achilles tendon injury 781
  hamstring injuries 790
  patellar tendinitis 785
  plantar fasciitis 787
  sports hernia 795
ultraviolet radiation
  high altitudes and 615, 623
  skin cancer risk 758
unconsciousness
  cerebral oedema 606
  diagnostic steps 602–604
  differential diagnosis 602–603
  management protocols 604–606
underarousal 33
underwater athletes 24, 31
upper motor neurones, degeneration 582
upper respiratory tract infections (URTI) 731–732
  overtraining association 494
  prevention 742
urea serum levels, cycling 865, 868
urine, concentrating ability, elderly 550
US
  cardiovascular screening 672–673
  year 2000 goals for exercise 701
uterine blood flow 107, 535
uterine cancer, risk reduction 758

vaccination, recommended schedule 658
valine, supplements 204
valvular heart disease 676
vascular control models 94–98
  see also muscle blood flow, regulation
vascular resistance 104–105, 105
  increase 104
  reduction 94, 98, 99
vasoconstriction
  ageing effect 107
  cerebral, altitude acclimatization 617
  cutaneous 108–109
  graded responses in exercise 105–107
  during hyperthermic exercise 111–112
  peripheral 104–105
  reflex response to exercise 104, 105–107
    by respiratory muscles 57–58

renal 105, 106
splanchnic *see* splanchnic circulation
  thermoregulatory-induced 110–111
vasodilatation
  cutaneous 108
  factors causing 95–96
  gastrointestinal circulation 105
  impairment, congestive heart failure 91, 92
  intermittent exercise 9
  muscle blood flow and 94, 95, 99, 104
vasodilators 567, 578
vasomotor collapse 594
vasopressin (antidiuretic hormone) 190, 432, 447
vastus lateralis muscle, fibre area in cyclists 863
vastus medialis obliques (VMO) 774, 775, 776
vegan diets 203
vegetarian diets 203, 415
vegetarians 415, 416
vehicular accidents 577
venous return 70, 97
venous sampling, lactate 315
venous valves 97
ventilation ($\dot{V}_E$)
  air pollutants and 53
  anaerobic threshold and 13
  circadian rhythm 640, 641
  high altitude 296, 936, 936
  increase with training 683
  input to perception of effort 376–377
  lactate relationship 60
  mountaineering 932, 932, 938–939
  oxygen costs 53–54
  regulation 54
  rowing 841
  see also breathing
ventilation curve, anaerobic threshold and 318–319
ventilation–perfusion ratio ($\dot{V}:\dot{Q}$) 55
ventilatory drift 54
ventilatory threshold 13, 318, 319
  estimation/measurement 304, 320
  hockey 924
  lactate threshold relationship 54
ventral horn neurones 149–151
ventricles
  dimensions 229, 710
  performance and training effects 69–70
  see also left ventricle
ventricular diastolic filling 548
ventricular fibrillation 306, 696
ventricular hypertrophy 710, 714
  see also cardiac hypertrophy

ventricular performance 69–70
ventricular remodelling 69–70, 77
ventricular wall tension 711
vertebral column
    decreased bone density 752–753
    fractures 576
    hypermobility 467, 467
very low density lipoproteins (VLDL)
        201, 574
veteran élite athletes, injuries 468
violent death 760
visceral blood flow, restriction 32
visual impairment 586
visualizations 215
vitamin B group 656
vitamin C 417, 656, 740
vitamin D, supplements 753
vitamin E 417
    administration 656
    increased requirement, high
        altitude 618
    inflammation regulation 806
    lipid peroxidation reduction 806
vitamins, fat-soluble, deficiency 202
volleyball 464, 945
volume expanders 432, 433
volume loading 432–434
    antidiuretic hormone and 432
    cardiac hypertrophy due to 70
    detection 434–435
volume-regulating hormones
        432–433
    acute supplementation effects
        433
    levels and detection 434–435

walking
    energy costs 282
    fast, elderly 559
    speed, perceived effort 378
    visual impairment and 586
walk/jogging (W/J) programme
        558–559
walk-run programme, after overuse
    injuries 781, 782, 785, 788
warm-up exercises
    elderly athletes 557
    functions and importance 474
    injury prevention 458, 474, 791
water
    excessive intake 662
    in fat-free mass 346, 348
    ingestion, during exercise 200
    loss 190
    for mass participation events
        661–662
    pathogen transmission 658
    purification/sterilization 658
    requirements 419

temperature for triathlons 872–873
thermal conductivity 27, 292
vapour pressure at skin 261
    see also fluid
water immersion 292
    body fat and insulation 292–293,
        293
    heat conductance 292
    heat transfer coefficient 265
    hypothermia risk 261, 266
    survival time by temperature 292
    see also swimming and swimmers
watts 6
weight
    child athletes 514
    energy expenditure importance
        700
    excess, injury risk 468
    gain, maternal 538
    hydrostatic 826
    loss
        critical levels 362
        exercise role in obesity 574, 698
        risk of extreme leanness 362
weightlifting 350, 409
weight training, elderly 560
Weil–Blakesley conchotome 342,
        343
Western blotting 338, 340
wet bulb globe temperature (WBGT)
        287
wetsuit 872, 873, 885
wheelchair athletes
    adapted toilet facilities 662
    ergometers 278, 278
    mass participation events 662
    maximal oxygen intake 34
    training 579
whitewater canoeing 888, 889, 893
wilderness trips 663–664
wind, velocity and skiing 855
wind chill 291–292, 294
wind chill index (WCI) 291
wind resistance
    cycling speeds 279, 280
    at high altitudes 614–615
wind speed/direction 253, 291
wind tunnel 279–284
W/J programme (walk/jog), elderly
        558–559
Wolff–Parkinson–White syndrome
        79, 670
Wolff's law 768
women (athletes) 517–530
    age, body size and physique 40
    altitude training 526–527
    body composition 351
    body fat, by sport type 353
    body mass distribution 41

bone mineral density 355, 357,
        360–361, 415, 551
    endurance sport needs 517–518
    energy intake 202, 205, 410
    exercise and benefits 693
    fat-free mass 354–355, 355
    hockey 921, 922–924
    injuries 465–466
        intrinsic factors predisposing
            465–466
    iron losses 425
    left ventricle size 75–76
    nutritional modification 525–526
    in Olympic Games 517
    overtraining avoidance 527–528
    overuse injuries 466
    performance relationship 522–525
        economy of movement 524
        gender differences and 523
        lactate threshold 524–525
        maximal oxygen intake 522–524
    resistance training 526
    rowers 837–838
    rugby football 909–910
    stress fractures 767, 769
    stroke volume 519, 520
    sudden death 678
    training
        aerobic interval 518–519
        pace 519
        periodization 527
        practices to enhance 525–528
        requirements 518
        sustained distance 518
        techniques 518–519
    training-induced physiological
            adaptations 519–522
        economy of movement 521
        lactate threshold 521–522
        maximal oxygen intake 519–520
    triad of disorders 769, 772, 774
work 5–6
    of breathing 58
    components in different sports
        246, 246
    energy expenditure 248
    energy relationship 6
    against gravity 246, 246
    viscous 5–6
World Health Organization (WHO),
        vaccination 658
'worldloppet' 844, 851
wrestlers 217, 452

young athletes see adolescents;
        children

Z disc 159, 164
zinc oxide powder 663

Printed and bound in the UK by
CPI Antony Rowe, Eastbourne